Diagnostic Ultrasound *for* Sonographers

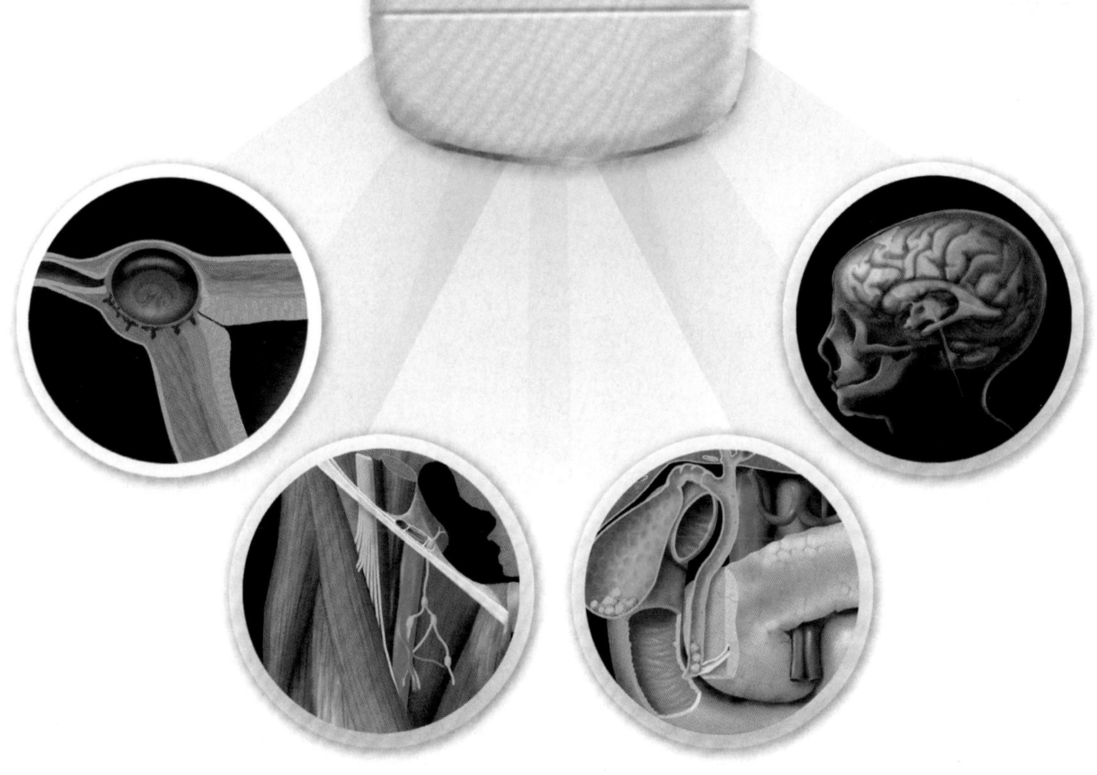

Kamaya | Wong-You-Cheong | Woodward
Kennedy | Sohaey | Yuan | Del Barco | Burke

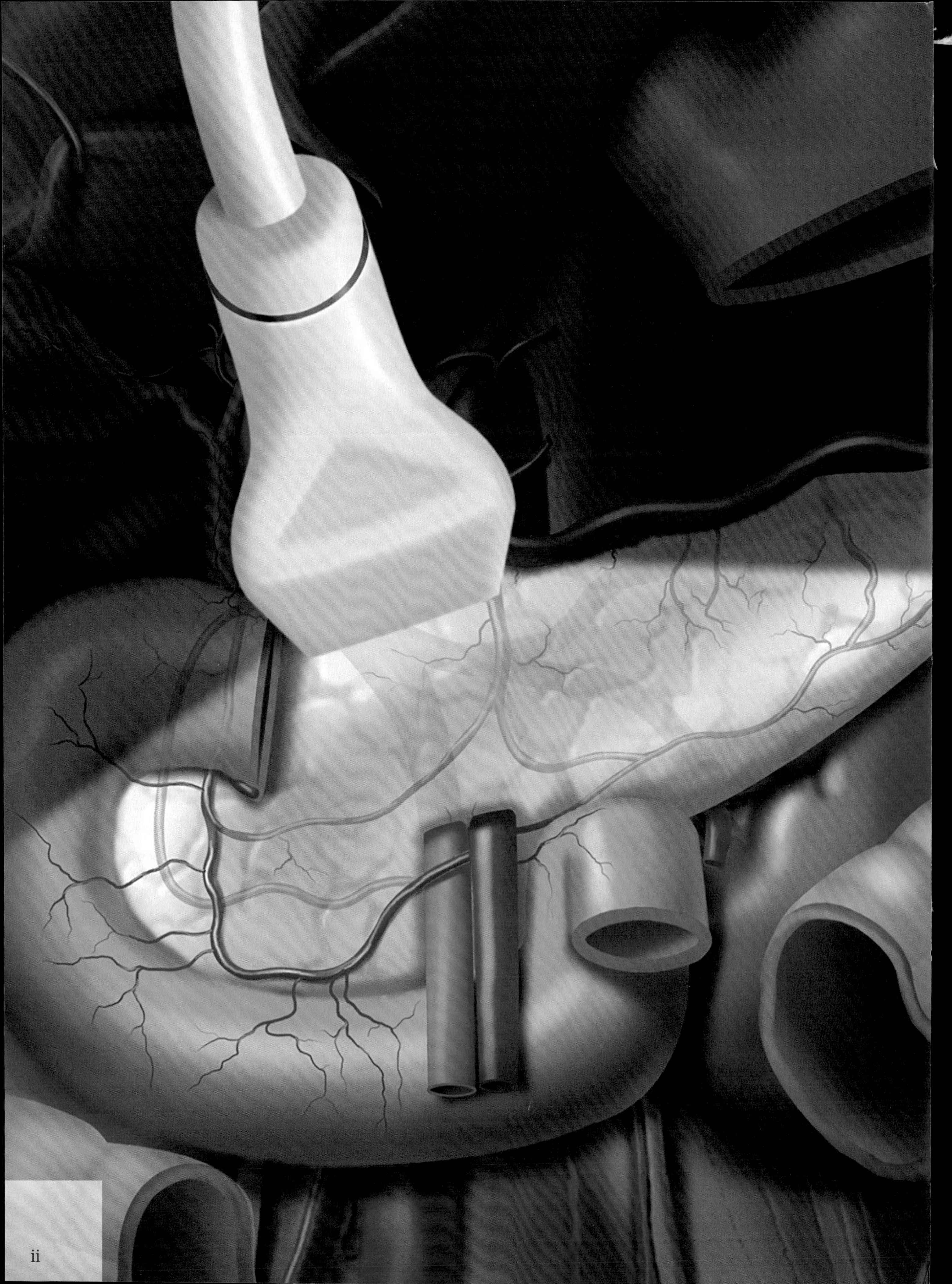

Diagnostic Ultrasound *for* Sonographers

Aya Kamaya, MD, FSRU, FSAR
Associate Professor of Radiology
Director, Stanford Body Imaging Fellowship
Director, Ultrasound
Stanford University School of Medicine
Stanford, California

Jade Wong-You-Cheong, MBChB, MRCP, FRCR
Professor
Department of Diagnostic Radiology and Nuclear Medicine
University of Maryland School of Medicine
Director of Ultrasound
University of Maryland Medical Center
Baltimore, Maryland

Paula J. Woodward, MD
Professor of Radiology
David G. Bragg, MD and Marcia R. Bragg Presidential Endowed Chair in Oncologic Imaging
Adjunct Professor of Obstetrics and Gynecology
University of Utah School of Medicine
Salt Lake City, Utah

Anne M. Kennedy, MD
Professor of Radiology
Adjunct Professor of Obstetrics and Gynecology
Chief Value Officer Radiology
Codirector of Maternal Fetal Diagnostic Center
University of Utah School of Medicine
Salt Lake City, Utah

Roya Sohaey, MD
Professor of Radiology
Affiliate Professor of Obstetrics and Gynecology
Director of Fetal Imaging
Director of Academic Advancement
Oregon Health & Science University
Portland, Oregon

Xin Yuan, MS, RDMS, RVT, RMSK
Ultrasound Quality Coordinator
Stanford Health Care
Radiology/Ultrasound Department
Stanford, California

Oscar R. Del Barco, MS, RDMS, RVT, RT(R)
Department of Diagnostic Radiology
and Nuclear Medicine
Manager, Ultrasound Department
University of Maryland Medical Center
Baltimore, Maryland

Jenny Burke, BS, RDMS
Lead Diagnostic Medical Sonographer
Clinical Instructor for Sonography Students
Oregon Health & Science University
Portland, Oregon

ELSEVIER

1600 John F. Kennedy Blvd.
Ste 1800
Philadelphia, PA 19103-2899

DIAGNOSTIC ULTRASOUND FOR SONOGRAPHERS ISBN: 978-0-323-62516-6

Notices

Practitioners and researchers must always rely on their own experience and knowledge in evaluating and using any information, methods, compounds or experiments described herein. Because of rapid advances in the medical sciences, in particular, independent verification of diagnoses and drug dosages should be made. To the fullest extent of the law, no responsibility is assumed by Elsevier, authors, editors or contributors for any injury and/or damage to persons or property as a matter of products liability, negligence or otherwise, or from any use or operation of any methods, products, instructions, or ideas contained in the material herein.

Library of Congress Control Number: 2018953147

Cover Designer: Tom M. Olson, BA
Printed in Canada by Friesens, Altona, Manitoba, Canada

Last digit is the print number: 9 8 7 6 5 4 3 2 1

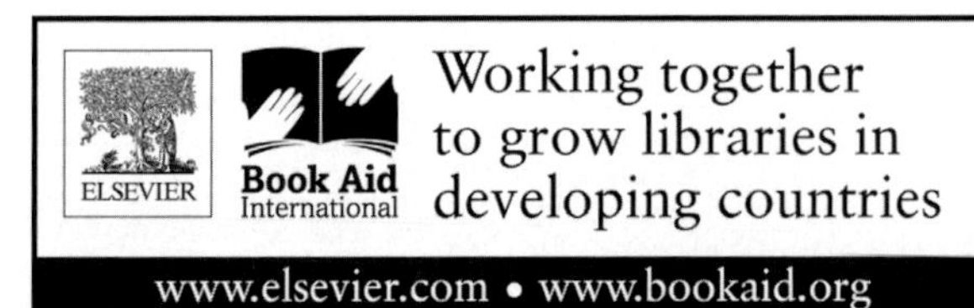

Dedications

To my amazing husband, Yuji, and our kids, Mika (5) and Kenzo (8), whose unconditional love make it all worthwhile; to my parents, Yoko and Hiroshi, who made it possible; to my parents-in-law, Keiko and John, who make it possible now; and to the great sonographers at Stanford, who inspired the creation of this book.

AK

To the many sonographers I have had the privilege and pleasure of working with. Without you, there would be no book.

JWYC

To our sonographers.
Your dedication to patient care and enthusiasm for learning bring us joy every day.
We love your obsession with "book-worthy" images.

PJW & AMK

Dedicated to the OHSU sonographers. You are the warriors that make us look good EVERY DAY. I am grateful.

RS

I would like to thank Dr. Kamaya and my parents for their encouragement and my husband, Jun, and my daughter, Michelle, for their daily support!

XY

To my wife, Roxana, for guiding and supporting me.
To Alexandra and Sergio, for giving me purpose.
To all the radiologists who have mentored me and shaped my career as a sonographer.

ORDB

To my parents, Denny and Judy, for your endless support and love.
And to Michael, whose love makes everything possible. Thank you.

JB

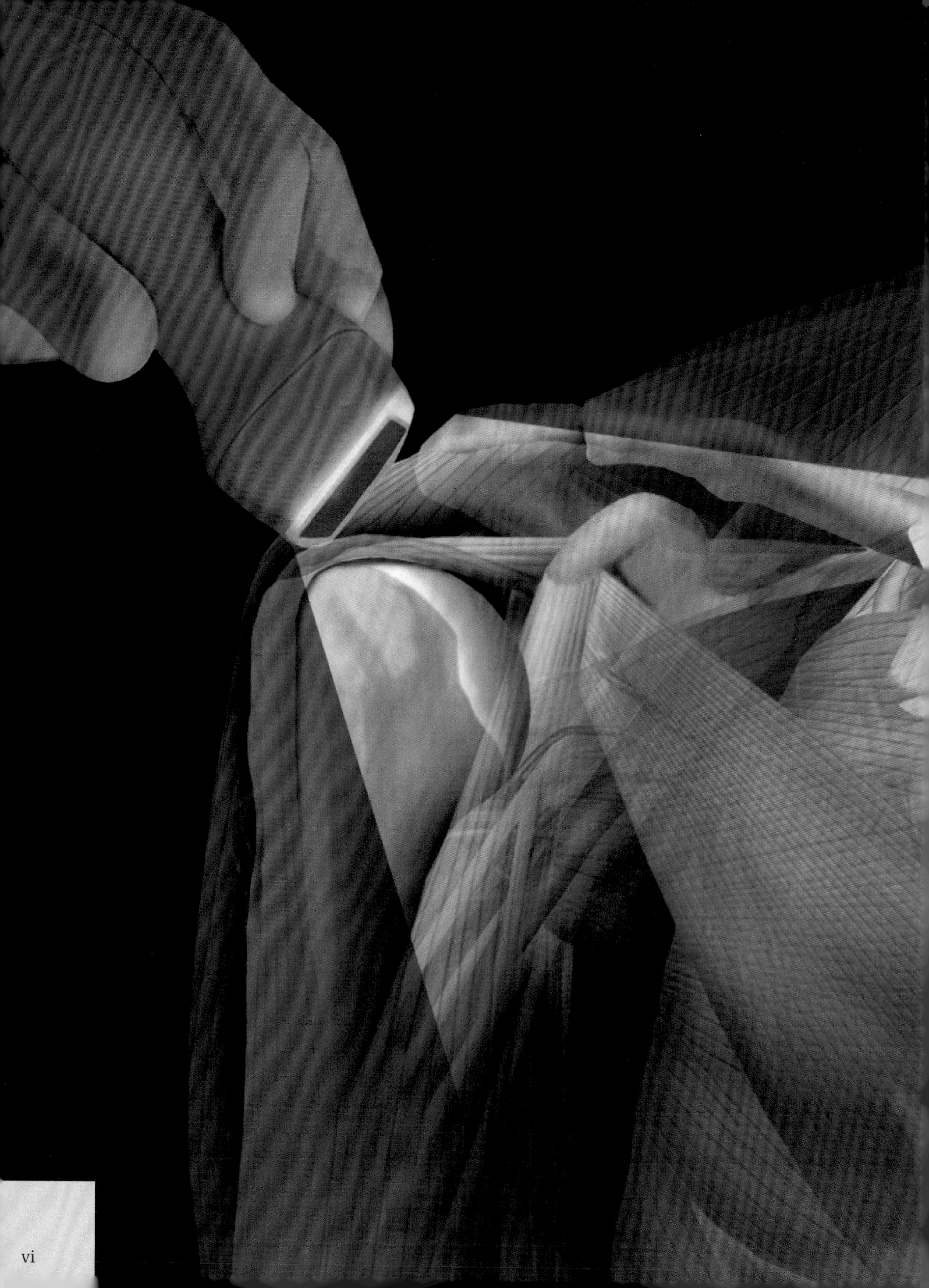

Contributing Authors

Tara Morgan, MD
Assistant Professor of Radiology and Biomedical Imaging
Co-Director, Musculoskeletal Ultrasound
University of California San Francisco
San Francisco, California

Additional Contributors

Jill M. Abrigo, MD, DPBR

Anil T. Ahuja, MD, FRCR

Gregory E. Antonio, MD, DRANZCR, FHKCR

Tanzilah Afzal Barrow, MBChB, BA, MA (Oxon), FRCR

Shweta Bhatt, MD

Constantine Burgan, MD

Janice L. B. Byrne, MD

Amit B. Desai, MD

Richard E. Fan, PhD

Bryan R. Foster, MD

Mary Frates, MD

James F. Griffith, MD, MRCP, FRCR

Simon S. M. Ho, MBBS, FRCR

Stella Sin Yee Ho, RDMS, RVT, PhD

Keegan Hovis, MD

Esther H. Y. Hung, MBChB, FRCR, FHKCR, FHKAM (Radiology)

Sonya Y. Khan, MD

Asef Khwaja, MD

Jane S. Kim, MD

Barton F. Lane, MD

Ryan K. L. Lee, MBChB, FRCR, FHKAM (Radiology)

Yolanda Y. P. Lee, MBChB, FRCR

Eric K. H. Liu, PhD, RDMS

Rachel F. Magennis, MBChB, DMRD, FRCR

Katherine E. Maturen, MD, MS

Adnaan Moin, MD

L. Nayeli Morimoto, MD

Mariam Moshiri, MD, FSAR

Alex W. H. Ng, MBChB, FRCR, FHKCR, FHKAM (Radiology)

Hammed Ninalowo, MD

Karen Y. Oh, MD

Hee Sun Park, MD, PhD

Bhawan K. Paunipagar, MBBS, MD, DNB

Danielle Richman, MD

Nicole Roy, MD

Narendra Shet, MD

Sathi A. Sukumar, MBBS, FRCP (UK), FRCR

Ali M. Tahvildari, MD

Katherine To'o, MD

Fauzia Vandermeer, MD

Ashish P. Wasnik, MD

K. T. Wong, MBChB, FRCR

H. Y. Yuen, MBChB, FRCR

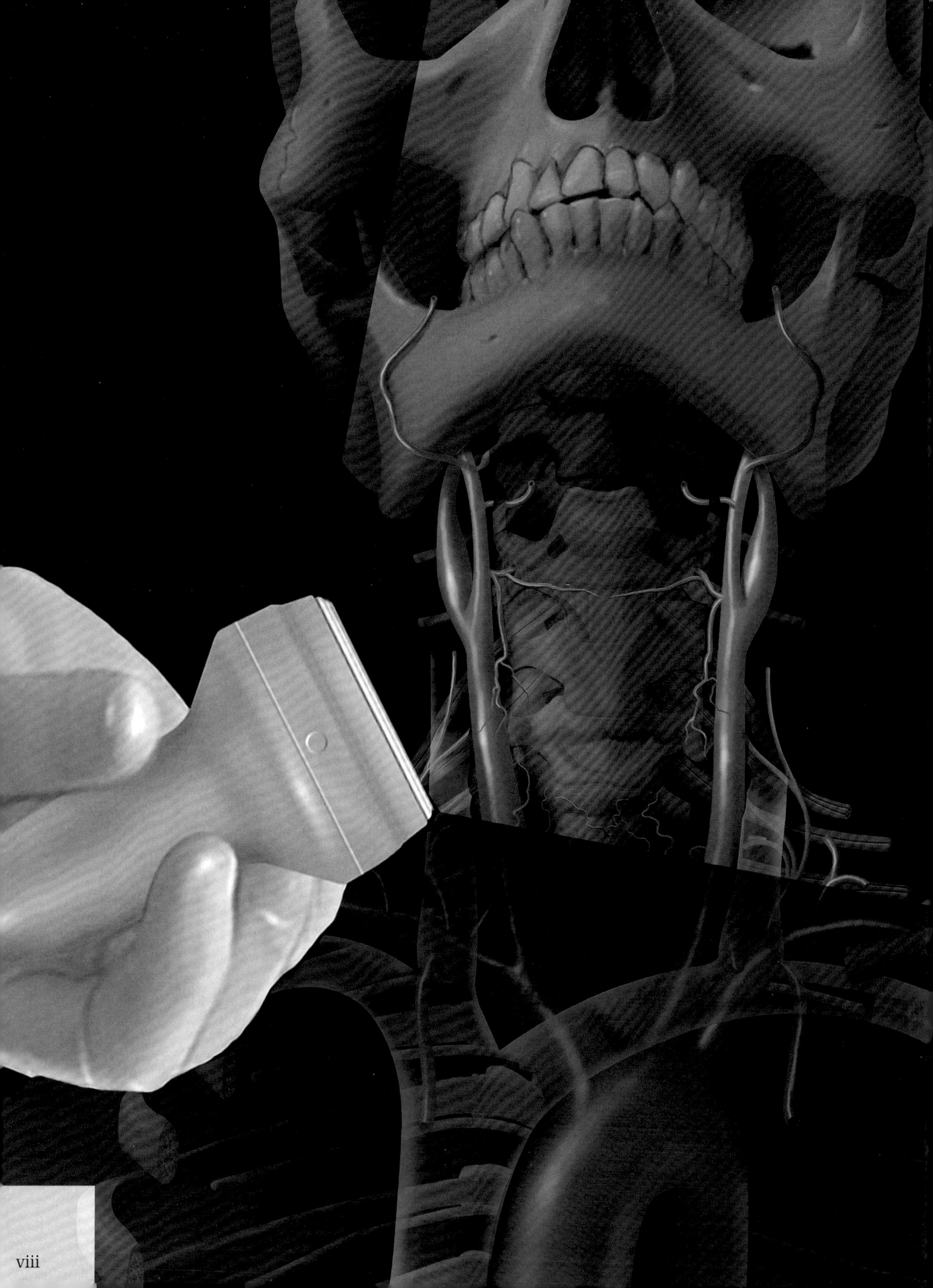

Preface

The sonographers at Stanford constantly impress me with their ability to capture exquisite ultrasound images and cine clips. I attribute this to their thirst for understanding the pathophysiology and diagnosis behind the image. We foster this learning atmosphere with interesting case conferences and monthly didactic lectures that result in an exceptional fund of knowledge. However, our sonographers want to learn more!

This drive for understanding the patient behind the image is, of course, not unique to Stanford; this is a trait common to all great sonographers. Sonographers are different from other technologists, as they are truly instrumental in sonographic diagnosis; they interact with patients, often obtaining a better history than provided by referring clinicians, make observations, and problem solve while obtaining diagnostic images that depict the findings. Great sonographers not only obtain beautiful images, but they also think beyond to what is needed to clinch the diagnosis.

Our sonographers loved our 1st book, *Diagnostic Ultrasound: Abdomen and Pelvis*, which is a 1000+-page, image-rich textbook of abdominal and pelvic ultrasound geared to practicing radiologists, but it is perhaps too detailed and pricy for the typical sonographer. Moreover, it does not cover the full range of what all sonographers do in a typical practice.

It became clear that there is a huge need for a diagnostic ultrasound textbook geared toward sonographers, a book that is focused on disease entities along with dedicated ultrasound scanning tips and tricks, i.e., this book! Our book is intended to be a reference for sonographers but will be useful to radiology residents, abdominal/body/women's imaging fellows, and practicing radiologists alike. We cover the gamut of ultrasound imaging, including abdomen and pelvis, obstetrics, vascular, head and neck, and musculoskeletal sonography.

With input from expert sonographers on special "scanning tips," we have crafted a unique textbook filled with images and key facts on each specific diagnosis. Gorgeous artistic renderings with labeled anatomy as well as thumbnails showing where a transducer should be placed to acquire representative images complement detailed anatomy chapters at the beginning of each section. Within each section, key diagnoses most commonly encountered in practice (as well as a few more unusual diagnoses important to understand) are described with multiple ultrasound examples and detailed annotated descriptions. We hope this book will enhance your practice and that it becomes an essential part of your library.

Aya Kamaya, MD, FSRU, FSAR

Associate Professor of Radiology
Director, Stanford Body Imaging Fellowship
Director, Ultrasound
Stanford University School of Medicine
Stanford, California

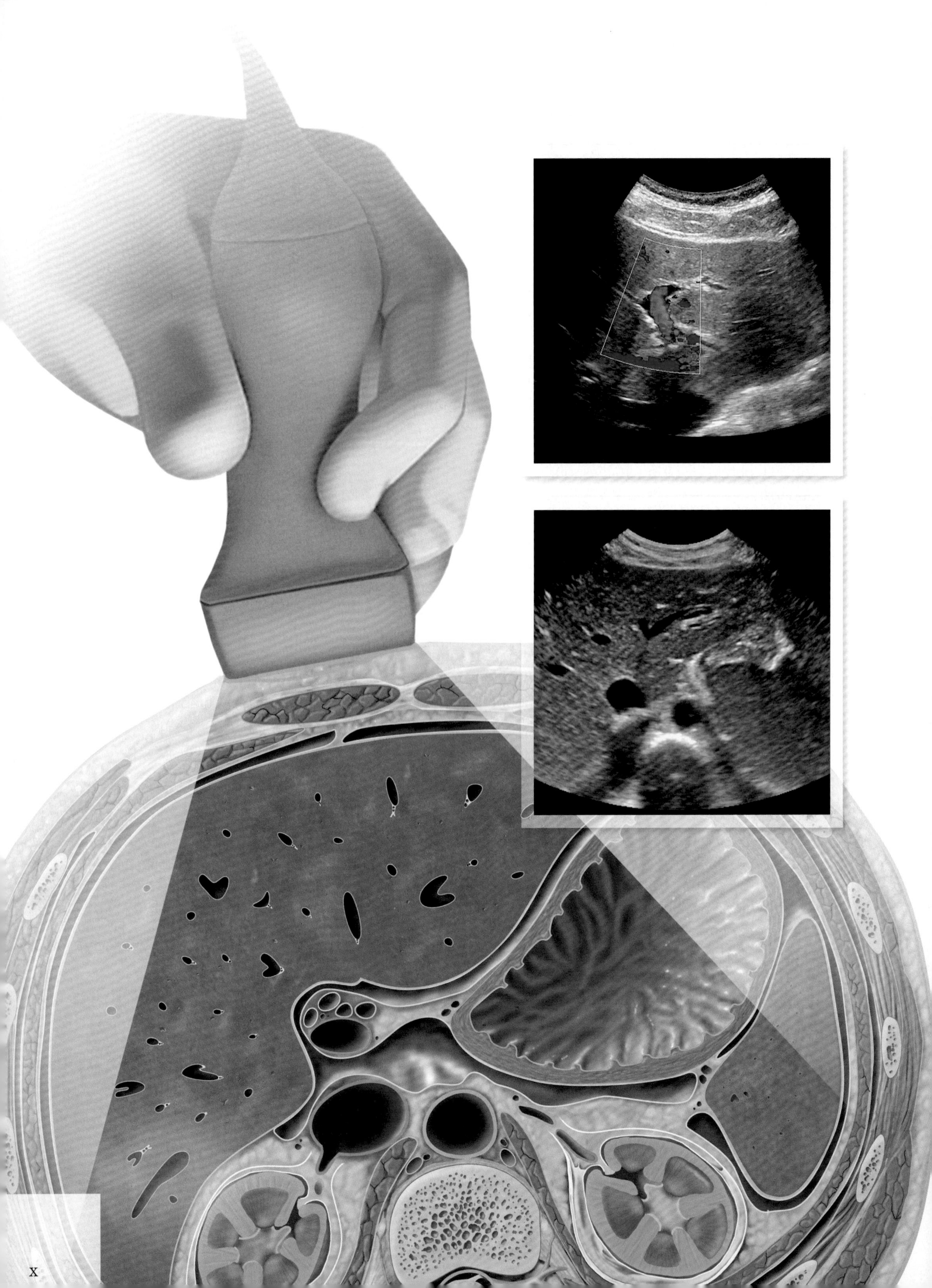

Acknowledgments

Lead Editor

Matt W. Hoecherl, BS

Text Editors

Arthur G. Gelsinger, MA
Rebecca L. Bluth, BA
Nina I. Bennett, BA
Terry W. Ferrell, MS
Megg Morin, BA
Joshua Reynolds, PhD

Image Editors

Jeffrey J. Marmorstone, BS
Lisa A. M. Steadman, BS

Illustrations

Richard Coombs, MS
Lane R. Bennion, MS
Laura C. Wissler, MA

Art Direction and Design

Tom M. Olson, BA
Laura C. Wissler, MA

Production Coordinators

Emily C. Fassett, BA
Angela M. G. Terry, BA
Alexander Eakins, BA

ELSEVIER

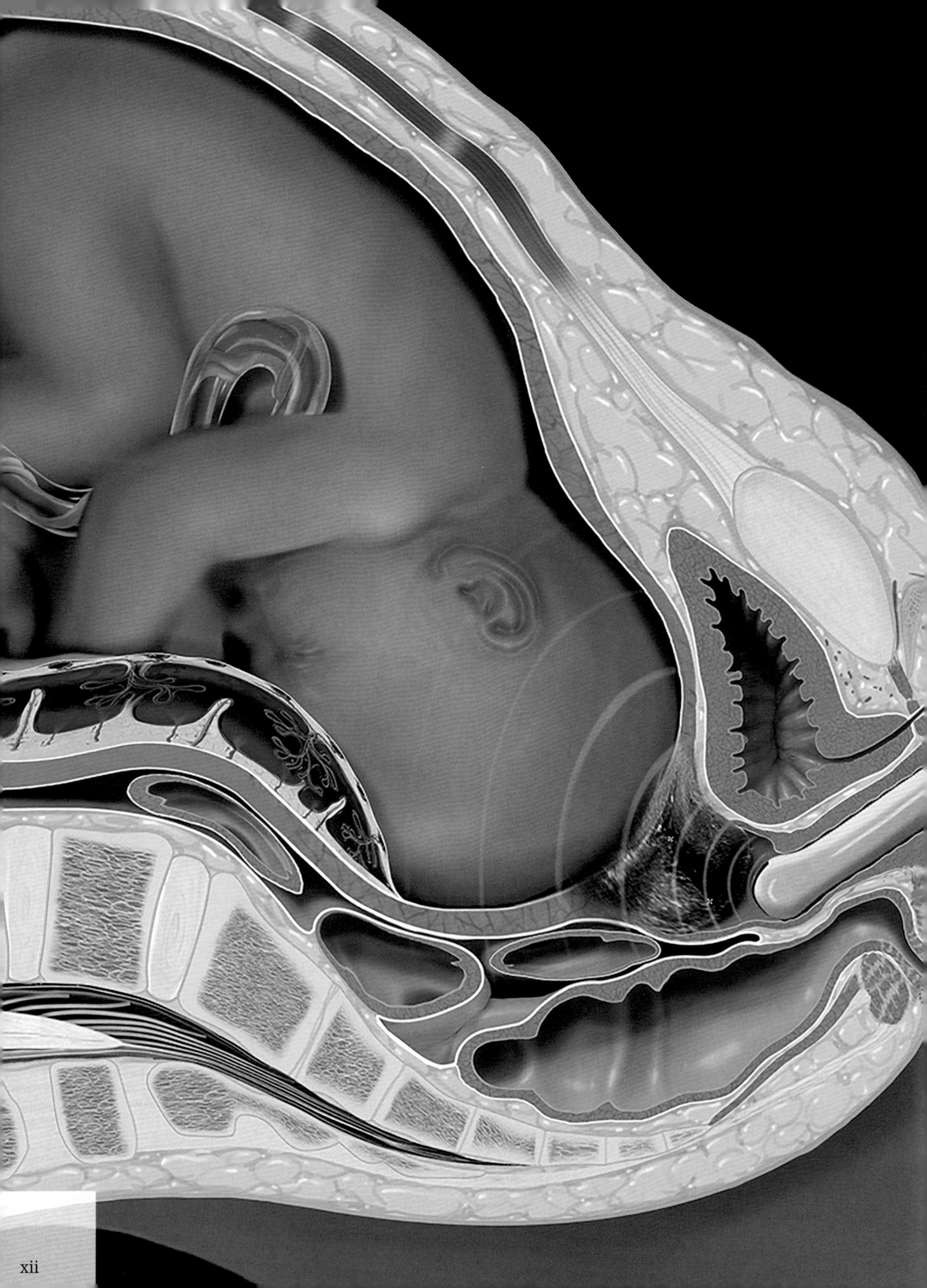

Sections

TABLE OF CONTENTS

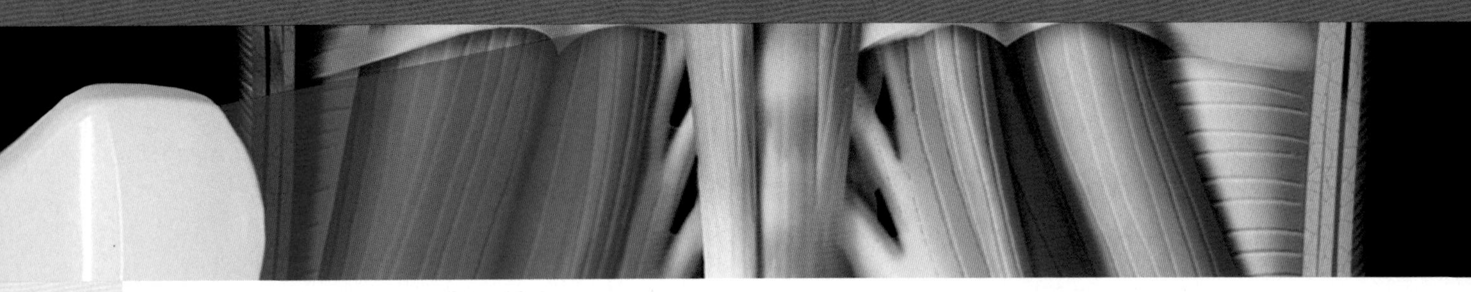

Part I: Abdomen

SECTION 1: LIVER

SECTION 2: BILIARY SYSTEM

TABLE OF CONTENTS

TABLE OF CONTENTS

TABLE OF CONTENTS

TABLE OF CONTENTS

TABLE OF CONTENTS

Part IV: Vascular

SECTION 1: ANATOMY AND APPROACH

SECTION 2: VASCULAR LESIONS

Part V: Musculoskeletal

SECTION 1: ANATOMY AND APPROACH

SECTION 2: MUSCULOSKELETAL LESIONS

TABLE OF CONTENTS

Part VI: Obstetrics

TABLE OF CONTENTS

TABLE OF CONTENTS

Diagnostic Ultrasound *for* Sonographers

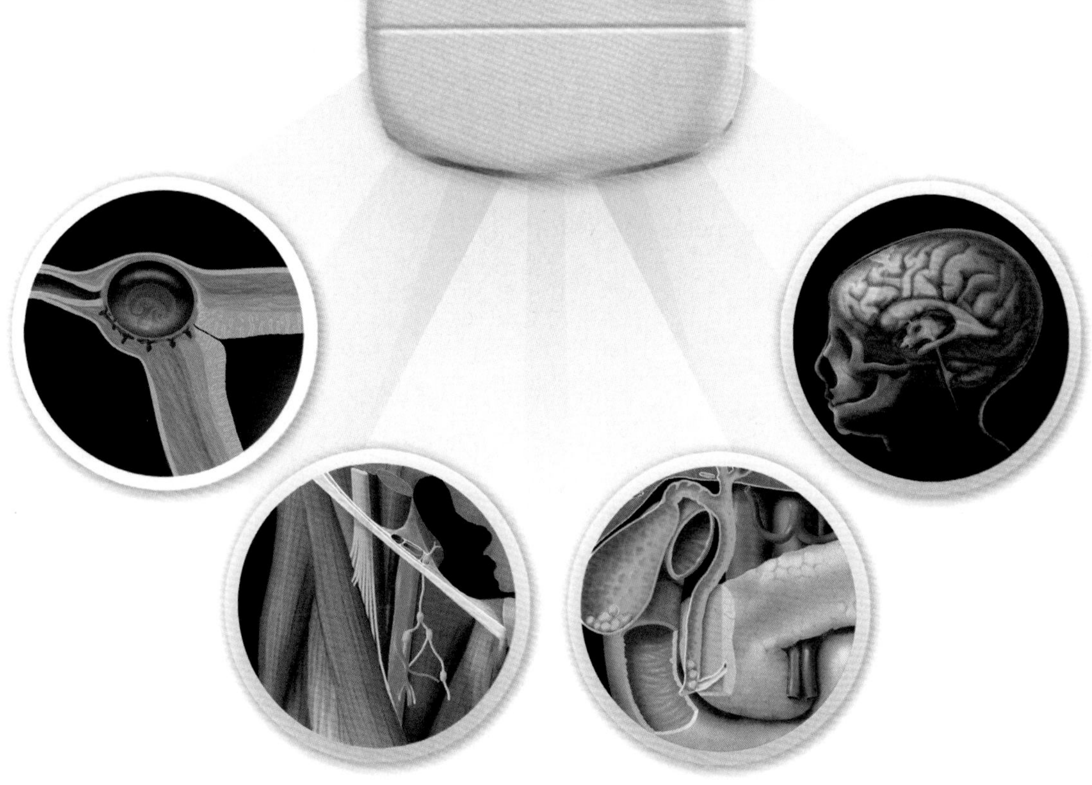

Kamaya | Wong-You-Cheong | Woodward
Kennedy | Sohaey | Yuan | Del Barco | Burke

PART I
SECTION 1
Liver

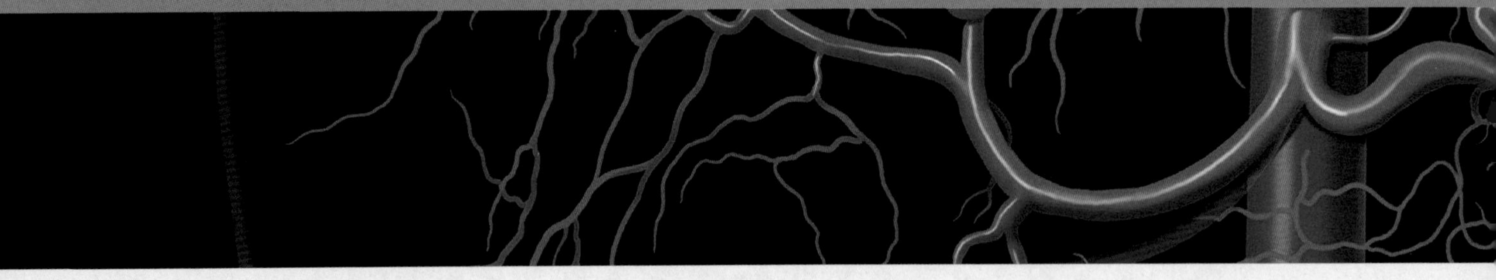

Anatomy and Approach

Diffuse Parenchymal Disease

Cysts and Cyst-Like Lesions

Focal Solid Masses

Vascular Conditions

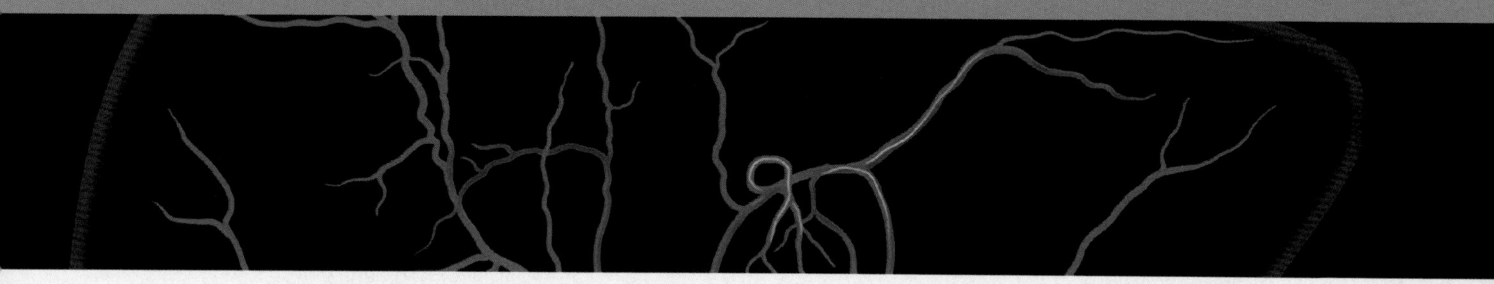

Liver Transplants

GROSS ANATOMY

Overview

- Liver: Largest gland and largest internal organ (average weight: 1,500 g)
  - Functions
    - Processes all nutrients (except fats) absorbed from gastrointestinal (GI) tract; conveyed via portal vein
    - Stores glycogen, secretes bile
  - Relations
    - Anterior and superior surfaces smooth and convex
    - Posterior and inferior surfaces indented by colon, stomach, right kidney, duodenum, inferior vena cava (IVC), and gallbladder
  - Covered by peritoneum except along gallbladder fossa, porta hepatis, and bare area
    - **Bare area**: Nonperitoneal posterior superior surface where liver abuts diaphragm
    - **Porta hepatis**: Portal vein, hepatic artery, and bile duct located within hepatoduodenal ligament
  - **Falciform ligament**
    - Extends from liver to anterior abdominal wall
    - Separates right and left subphrenic peritoneal recesses (between liver and diaphragm)
    - Marks plane separating medial and lateral segments of left hepatic lobe
    - Carries round ligament (ligamentum teres), fibrous remnant of umbilical vein
  - **Ligamentum venosum**
    - Remnant of ductus venosus
    - Separates caudate from left hepatic lobe
- **Vascular anatomy (unique dual afferent blood supply)**
  - **Portal vein**
    - Carries nutrients from gut and hepatotrophic hormones from pancreas to liver along with oxygen
      - Contains 40% more oxygen than systemic venous blood
    - 75-80% of blood supply to liver
  - **Hepatic artery**
    - Supplies 20-25% of blood
    - Liver less dependent than biliary tree on hepatic arterial blood supply
    - Usually arises from celiac artery
    - Variations common, including arteries arising from superior mesenteric artery
  - **Hepatic veins**
    - Usually 3 (right, middle, and left)
    - Many variations and accessory veins
    - Collect blood from liver and return it to IVC
    - Confluence of hepatic veins just below diaphragm and entrance of IVC into right atrium
  - **Portal triad**
    - At all levels of size and subdivision, branches of hepatic artery, portal vein, and bile ducts travel together
    - Blood flows into hepatic sinusoids from interlobular branches of hepatic artery and portal vein → hepatocytes, which detoxify blood and produce bile
      - Blood collects into central veins → hepatic veins
      - Bile collects into ducts → stored in gallbladder and excreted into duodenum
- **Segmental anatomy**
  - 8 hepatic segments
    - Each receives secondary or tertiary branch of hepatic artery and portal vein
    - Each drained by its own bile duct (intrahepatic) and hepatic vein branch
  - Caudate lobe = segment 1
    - Has independent portal triads and hepatic venous drainage to IVC
  - Left lobe
    - Lateral superior = segment 2
    - Lateral inferior = segment 3
    - Medial superior = segment 4a
    - Medial inferior = segment 4b
  - Right lobe
    - Anterior inferior = segment 5
    - Posterior inferior = segment 6
    - Posterior superior = segment 7
    - Anterior superior = segment 8

IMAGING ANATOMY

Internal Contents

- **Capsule**
  - Reflective Glisson capsule making borders of liver well defined
- **Left lobe**
  - Contains segments 2, 3, 4a, and 4b
  - Longitudinal scan
    - Triangular in shape
    - Rounded upper surface
    - Sharp inferior border
  - Transverse scan
    - Wedge-shaped tapering to left
  - Liver parenchyma echoes are midgray with uniform, sponge-like pattern interrupted by vessels
- **Right lobe**
  - Contains segments 5, 6, 7, and 8
  - Liver parenchymal echoes similar to left lobe
  - Sections of right lobe show same basic shape, though right lobe usually larger than left
- **Caudate lobe**
  - Longitudinal scan
    - Almond-shaped structure posterior to left lobe
  - Transverse scan
    - Seen as extension of right lobe
- **Portal veins**
  - Have thicker reflective walls than hepatic veins; portal veins have fibromuscular walls
  - Wall reflectivity also depends on angle of interrogation; portal veins cut at more oblique angle, may have less apparent wall
  - Can be traced back toward porta hepatis
  - Normal portal flow is hepatopetal on color Doppler; absent or reversal of flow may be seen in portal hypertension
  - Normal velocity: 13-55 cm/s
  - Normal diameter: < 13 mm

- Portal waveform has undulating appearance due to variations with cardiac activity and respiration
- Branches run in transverse plane
- Hepatic portal vein anatomy is variable

- **Hepatic veins**
  - Appear as echolucent tubular structures within liver parenchyma with no reflective wall: Large sinusoids with thin or absent wall
  - Branches enlarge and can be traced toward IVC
  - Flow pattern has triphasic waveform
    - Resulting from transmission of right atrial pulsations into veins
      - A wave: Atrial contraction
      - S wave: Systole (tricuspid valve moves toward apex)
      - D wave: Diastole
  - Right hepatic vein
    - Runs in coronal plane between anterior and posterior segments of right hepatic lobe
  - Middle hepatic vein
    - Lies in sagittal or parasagittal plane between right and left hepatic lobe
  - Left hepatic vein
    - Runs between medial and lateral segments of left hepatic lobe
    - Frequently duplicated
  - 1 of 3 major branches of hepatic veins may be absent
    - Absent right hepatic vein: ~ 6%
    - Less commonly middle and left hepatic vein
- **Hepatic artery**
  - Flow pattern has low-resistance characteristics with large amount of continuous forward flow throughout diastole
    - Normal velocity of proper hepatic artery: 40-80 cm/s
    - Resistive index ranges 0.5-0.8, increases after meal
  - Common hepatic artery usually arises from celiac axis
  - Classic configuration: 72%
    - Celiac axis → common hepatic artery → gastroduodenal artery and proper hepatic artery → latter gives rise to right and left hepatic artery
  - Variations from classic configuration
    - Common hepatic artery arising from superior mesenteric artery (replaced hepatic artery): 4%
    - Right hepatic artery arising from superior mesenteric artery (replaced right hepatic artery): 11%
    - Left hepatic artery arising from left gastric artery (replaced left hepatic artery): 10%
- **Bile ducts**
  - Normal peripheral intrahepatic bile ducts too small to be demonstrated
  - Normal right and left hepatic ducts measuring few millimeters usually visible
  - Normal common duct
    - Most visible in its proximal portion just caudal to porta hepatis: < 5 mm
    - Distal common duct should typically measure < 6-7 mm
    - In elderly, generalized loss of tissue elasticity with advancing age leads to increase in bile duct diameter: < 8 mm (somewhat controversial)

ANATOMY IMAGING ISSUES

Imaging Recommendations

- Transducer
  - 2.5- to 6.0-MHz curvilinear or vector transducer generally most suitable
  - Higher frequency linear transducer (i.e., 7-12 MHz) useful for evaluation of liver capsule and superficial portions of liver
- Left lobe
  - Subcostal window with full inspiration generally most suitable
- Right lobe
  - Subcostal window
    - Cranial and rightward angulation useful for visualization of right lobe below dome of hemidiaphragm
    - Can sometimes be obscured by bowel gas
  - Intercostal window
    - Usually gives better resolution for parenchyma without influence from bowel gas
    - Right lobe just below hemidiaphragm may not be visible due to obscuration from lung bases
    - Important to tilt transducer parallel to intercostal space to minimize shadowing from ribs

Imaging Pitfalls

- Because of variations of vascular and biliary branching within liver (common), frequently impossible to designate precise boundaries between hepatic segments on imaging studies

CLINICAL IMPLICATIONS

Clinical Importance

- Liver ultrasound often 1st-line imaging modality in evaluation for elevated liver enzymes
  - Diffuse liver disease, such as hepatic steatosis, cirrhosis, hepatomegaly, hepatitis, and biliary ductal dilatation, well visualized on ultrasound
  - Documentation of patency of portal vein, hepatic vein waveforms, and hepatic arterial velocities helpful in evaluation for etiologies of elevated liver function tests
- Liver metastases common
  - Primary carcinomas of colon, pancreas, and stomach commonly metastasize to liver
    - Portal venous drainage usually results in liver being initial site of metastatic spread from these tumors
  - Metastases from other non-GI primaries (breast, lung, etc.) commonly spread to liver hematogenously
- Primary hepatocellular carcinoma
  - Common worldwide
    - Risk factors include cirrhosis of any etiology and chronic viral hepatitis B in certain populations
    - Chronic hepatitis C with stage 3 fibrosis and nonalcoholic steatohepatitis may also have increased risk of hepatocellular carcinoma
    - Ultrasound commonly used for screening and surveillance in patients at risk for development of hepatocellular carcinoma typically at 6-month intervals

HEPATIC VISCERAL SURFACE

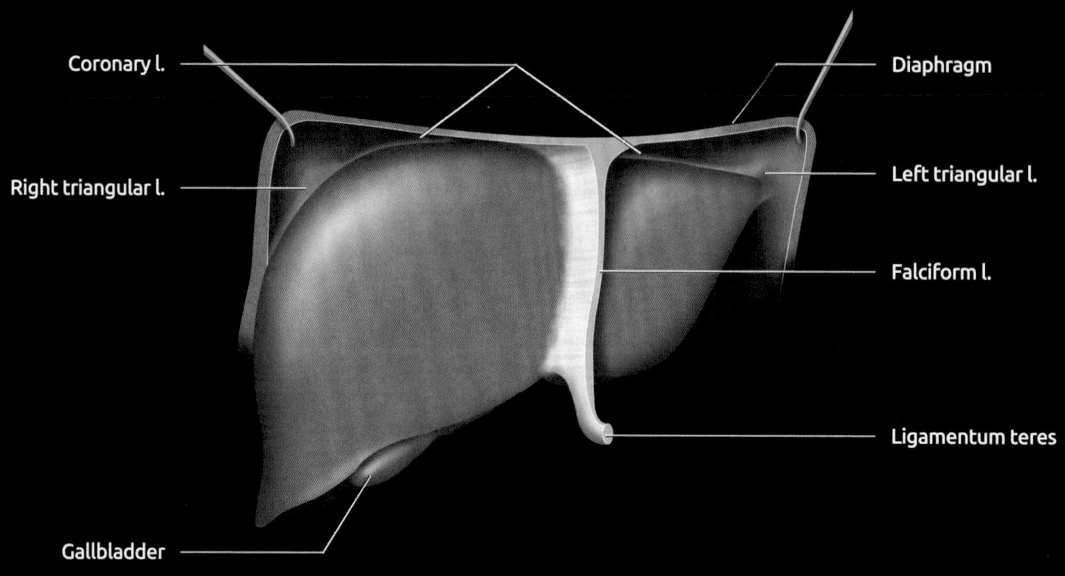

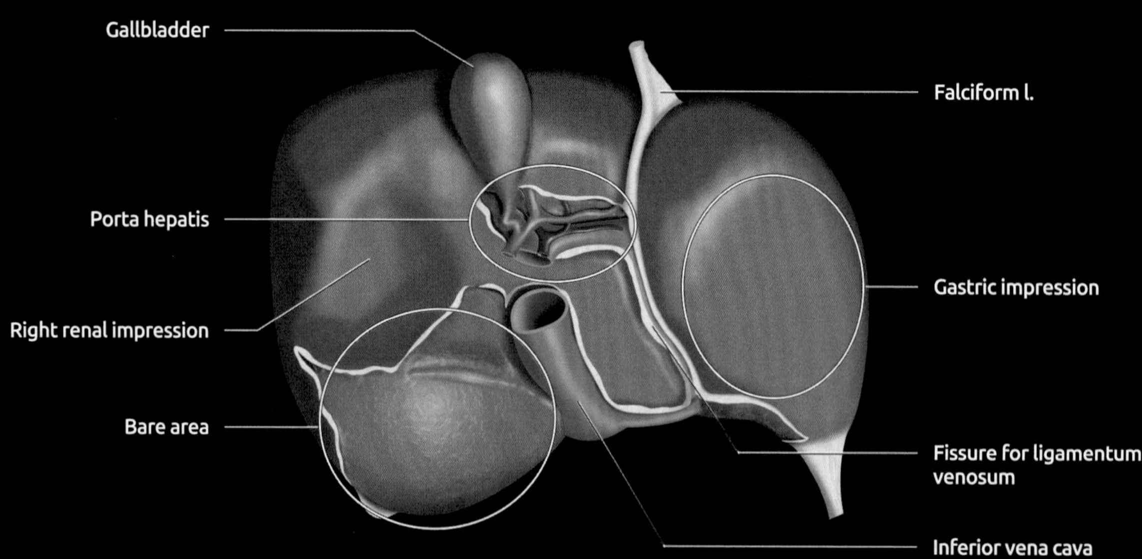

(Top) *The anterior surface of the liver is smooth and molds to the diaphragm and anterior abdominal wall. Generally, only the anterior/inferior edge of the liver is palpable on a physical exam. The liver is covered with peritoneum, except for the gallbladder bed, porta hepatis, and the bare area. Peritoneal reflections form various ligaments that connect the liver to the diaphragm and abdominal wall, including the falciform ligament, the inferior edge that contains the ligamentum teres, and the obliterated remnant of the umbilical vein.* **(Bottom)** *Graphic shows the liver inverted, which is somewhat similar to the surgeon's view of the upwardly retracted liver. The structures in the porta hepatis include the portal vein (blue), hepatic artery (red), and the bile ducts (green). The visceral surface of the liver is indented by adjacent viscera. The bare area is not easily accessible.*

HEPATIC ATTACHMENTS AND RELATIONS

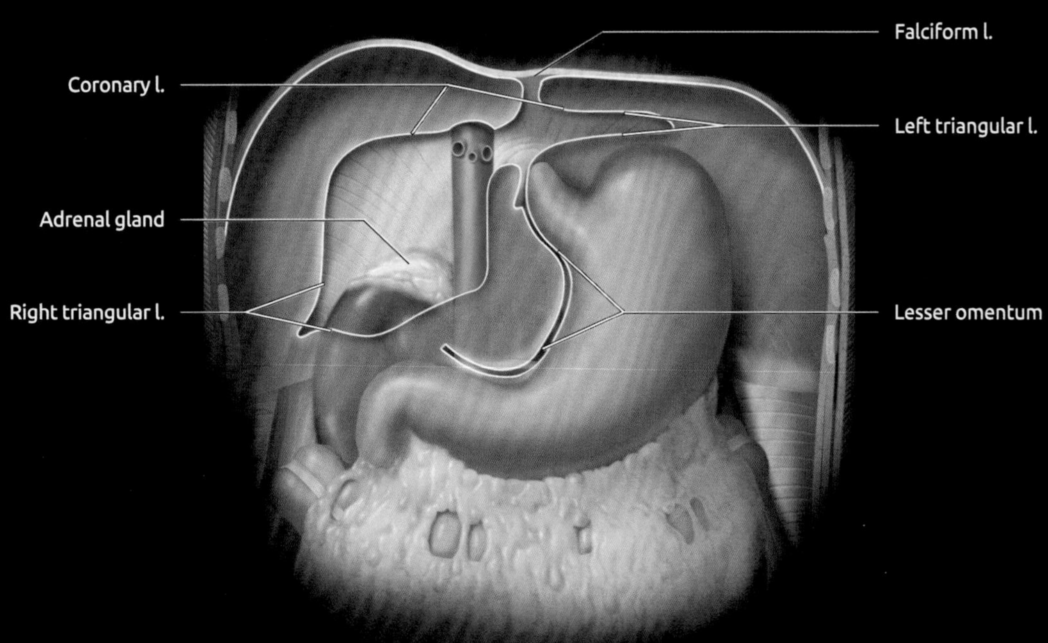

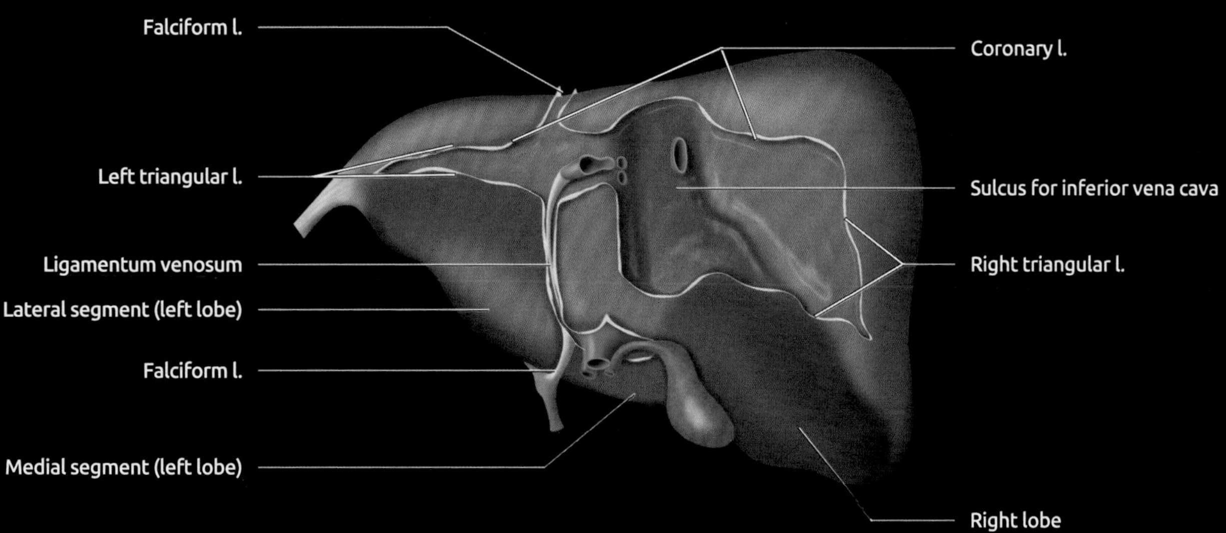

(Top) *The liver is attached to the posterior abdominal wall and diaphragm by the left and right triangular and coronary ligaments. The falciform ligament attaches the liver to the anterior abdominal wall. The bare area is in direct contact with the right adrenal gland, kidney, and inferior vena cava (IVC).* **(Bottom)** *Posterior view of the liver shows the ligamentous attachments. While these may help to fix the liver in position, abdominal pressure alone is sufficient, as evidenced by orthotopic liver transplantation, after which the ligamentous attachments are lost without the liver shifting position. The diaphragmatic peritoneal reflection is the coronary ligament whose lateral extensions are the right and left triangular ligaments. The falciform ligament separates the medial and lateral segments of the left lobe.*

HEPATIC VESSELS AND BILE DUCTS

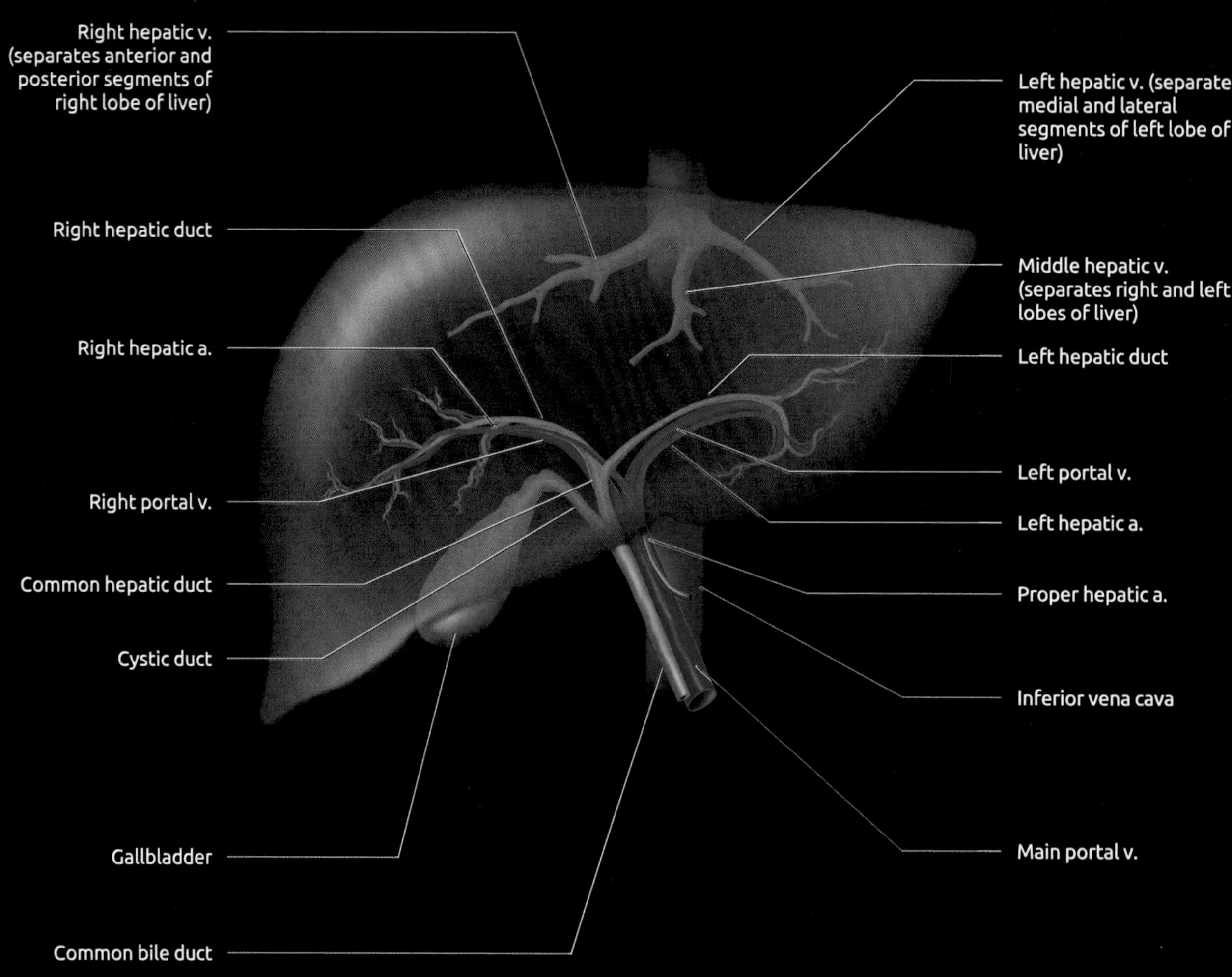

Graphic emphasizes that at every level of branching and subdivision, the portal veins, hepatic arteries, and bile ducts course together, constituting the portal triad. Each segment of the liver is supplied by branches of these vessels. Conversely, hepatic venous branches lie between hepatic segments and interdigitate with the portal triads but never run parallel to them.

HEPATIC ARTERIAL ANATOMY

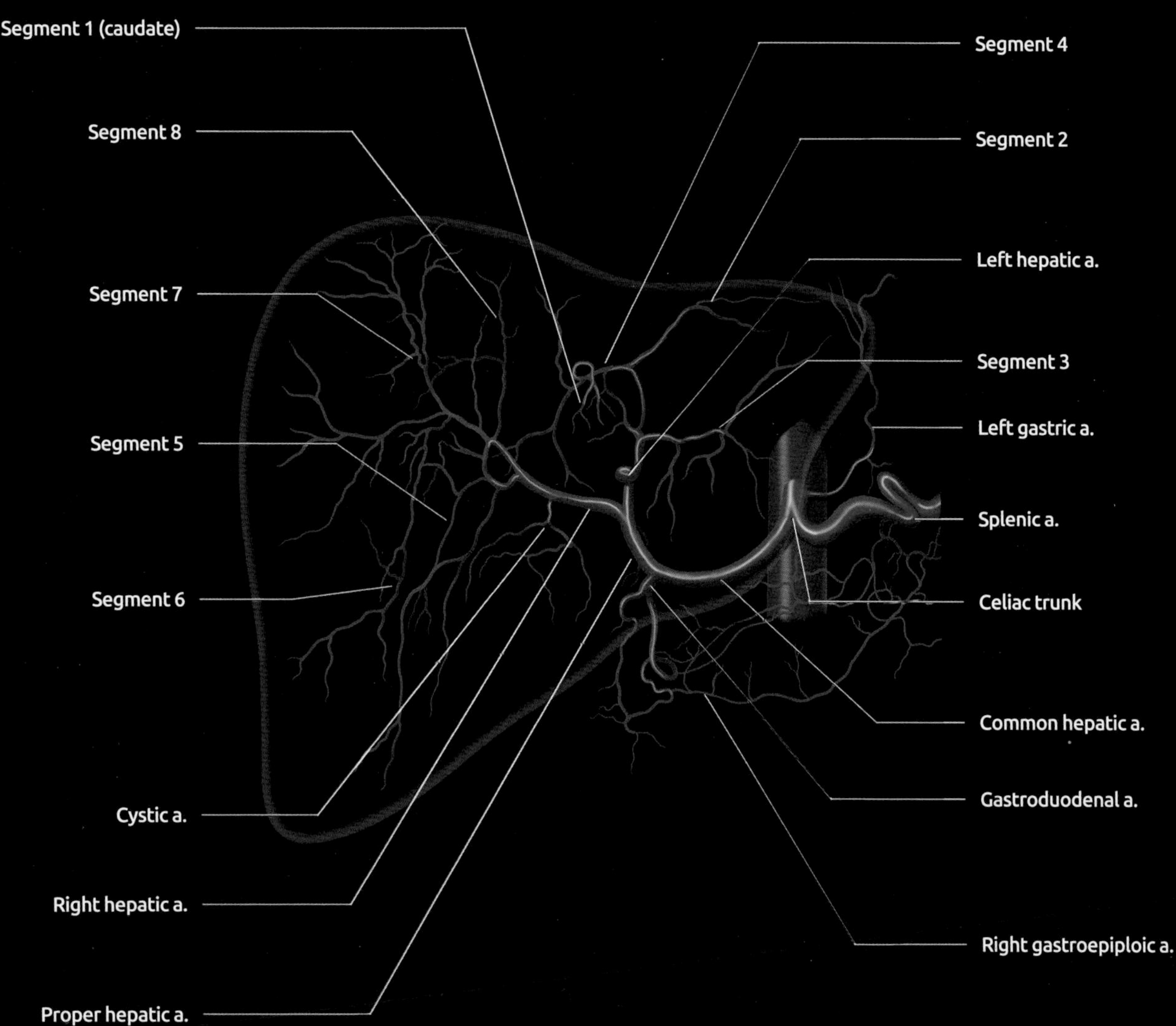

Graphic demonstrates the conventional hepatic arterial supply to the liver. The celiac artery arises at roughly the T12 level before dividing into the common hepatic artery, left gastric artery, and splenic artery. The common hepatic artery gives off the gastroduodenal artery inferiorly and becomes the proper hepatic artery, which then divides into the right and left hepatic arteries at the liver hilum. The left hepatic artery courses superiorly and slightly to the left before giving off branches to segments 2-4. In some instances, the segment 4 artery may arise directly from the proper hepatic artery and is then termed the middle hepatic artery. The right hepatic artery divides into anterior and posterior branches, which take an upward vertical course and horizontal course, respectively. The anterior branch gives off arteries supplying segments 5 and 8, while the posterior branches supplies segments 6 and 7. Segment 1 (caudate) is typically supplied by small branches of either the right or left hepatic arteries (or both).

LEFT LOBE OF LIVER: LEFT HEPATIC VEIN

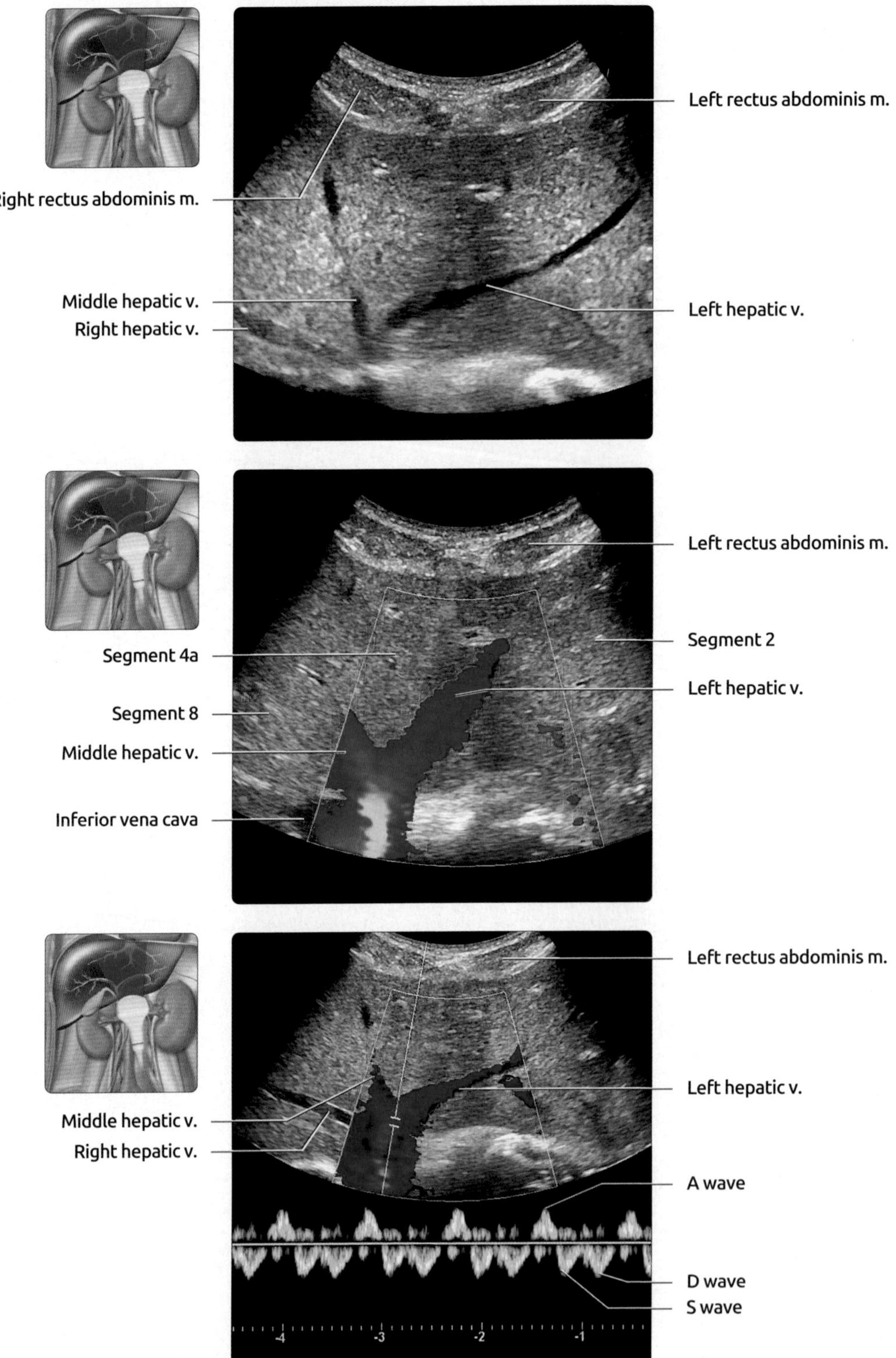

(Top) *Transverse grayscale ultrasound of the liver centered at the left hepatic lobe shows the right, middle, and left hepatic veins as they join into the intrahepatic IVC.* **(Middle)** *Transverse color Doppler ultrasound of the liver, centered at the confluence of the hepatic veins, shows that the flow direction is away from the transducer, directed toward the IVC.* **(Bottom)** *Spectral tracing of the left hepatic vein near the confluence with the IVC shows a characteristic triphasic waveform pattern, which represents reflection of cardiac motion.*

LONGITUDINAL LEFT LOBE OF LIVER

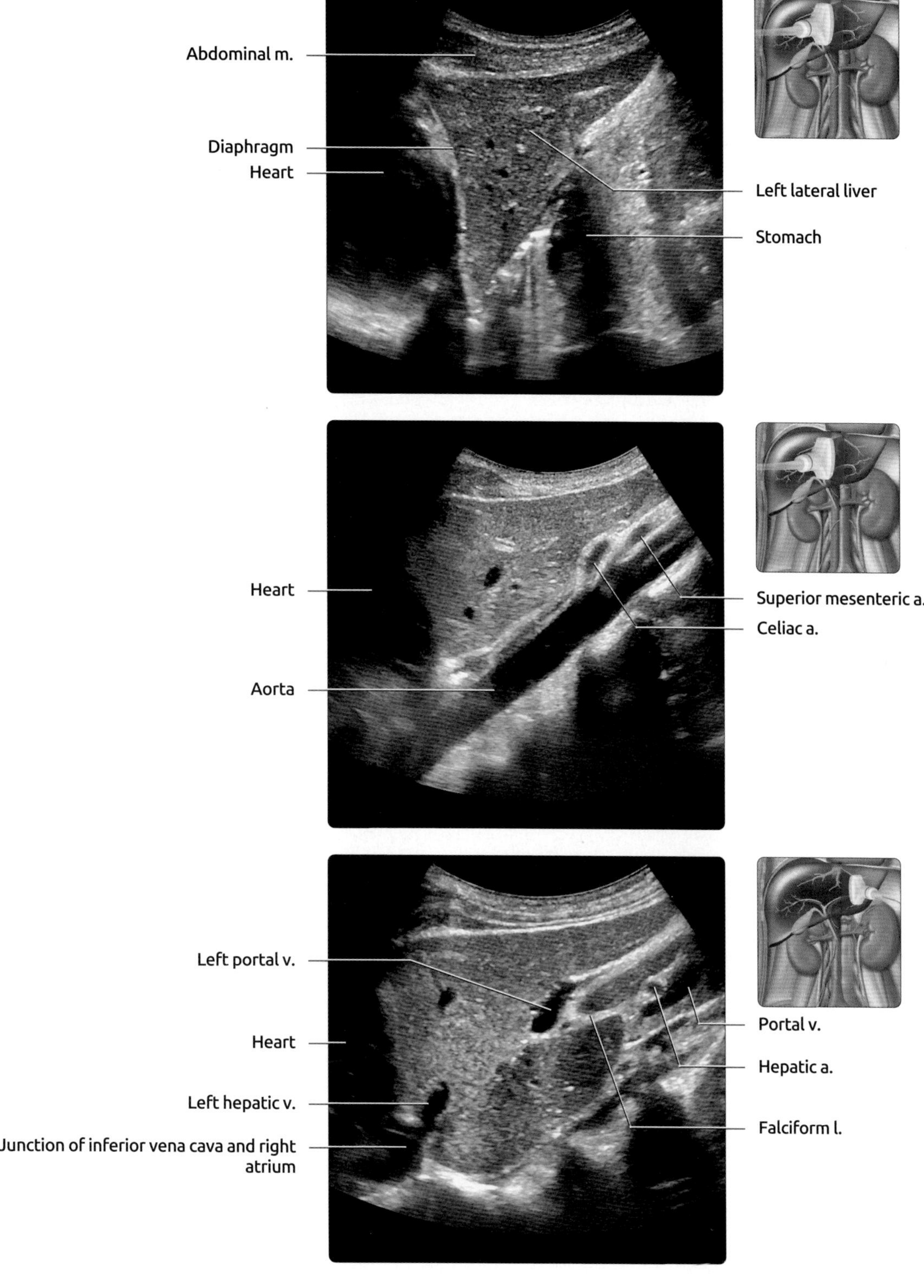

(Top) *Longitudinal grayscale ultrasound of the left lobe of the liver shows a triangular-shaped cross section. The heart is partially visualized above the diaphragm.* **(Middle)** *Longitudinal grayscale ultrasound view of the left lobe of the liver at the level of the aorta shows the aorta posterior to the liver, the celiac artery, and the superior mesenteric artery arising from the aorta.* **(Bottom)** *Longitudinal grayscale ultrasound of the left lobe of the liver shows the left hepatic vein and left portal vein in cross section.*

TRANSVERSE RIGHT LOBE OF LIVER

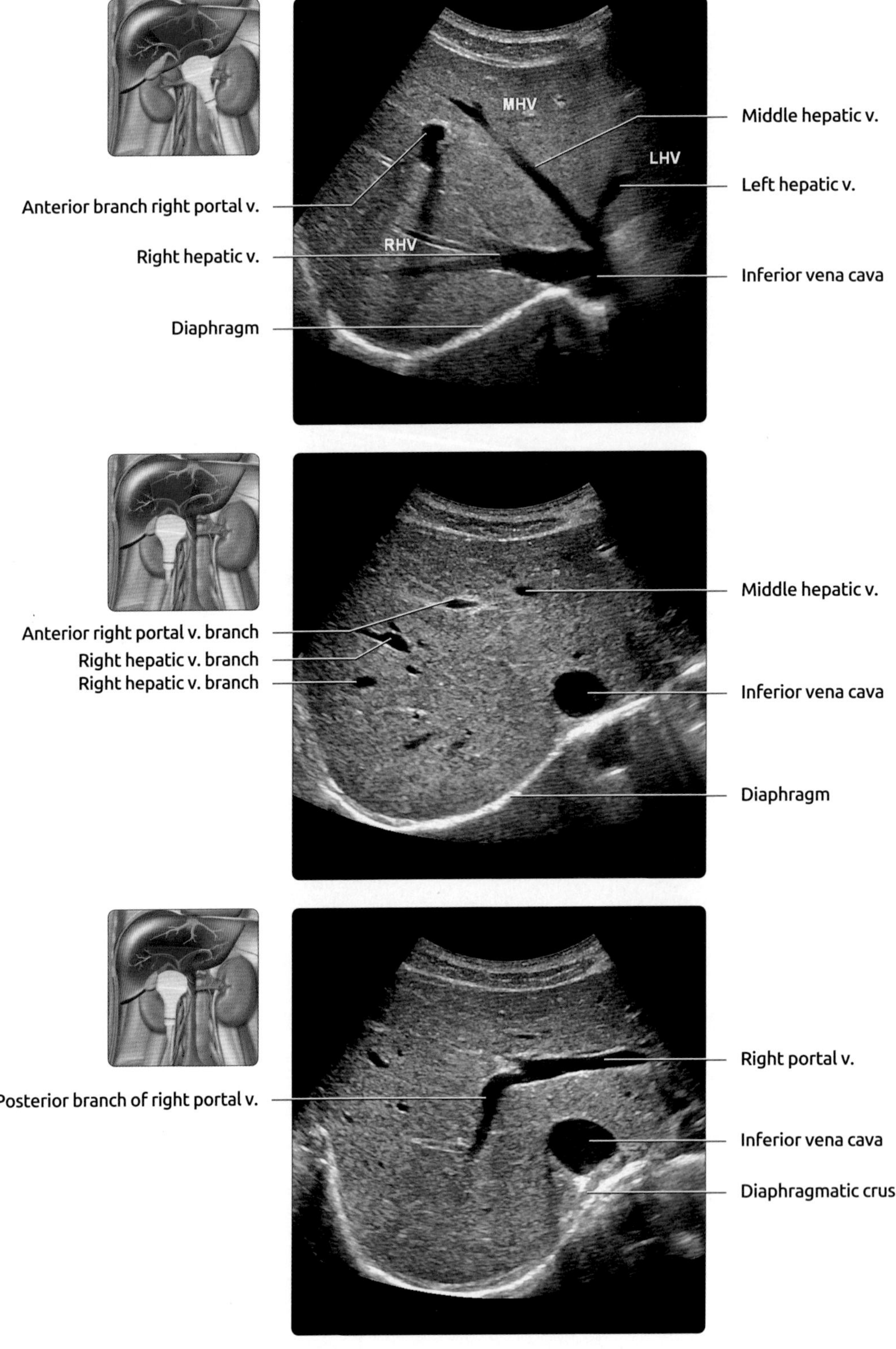

(Top) *Transverse grayscale ultrasound at the level of the hepatic vein confluence shows the right, middle, and left hepatic veins as they join with the IVC posteriorly.* **(Middle)** *Transverse grayscale ultrasound of the liver just below the confluence of the hepatic veins shows the IVC and more peripheral portions of the right and left hepatic veins.* **(Bottom)** *Transverse grayscale ultrasound of the right lobe of the liver, centered at the right portal vein, shows the posterior branch of the right portal vein, which is typically directed away from the transducer.*

RIGHT LOBE OF LIVER: RIGHT HEPATIC VEIN

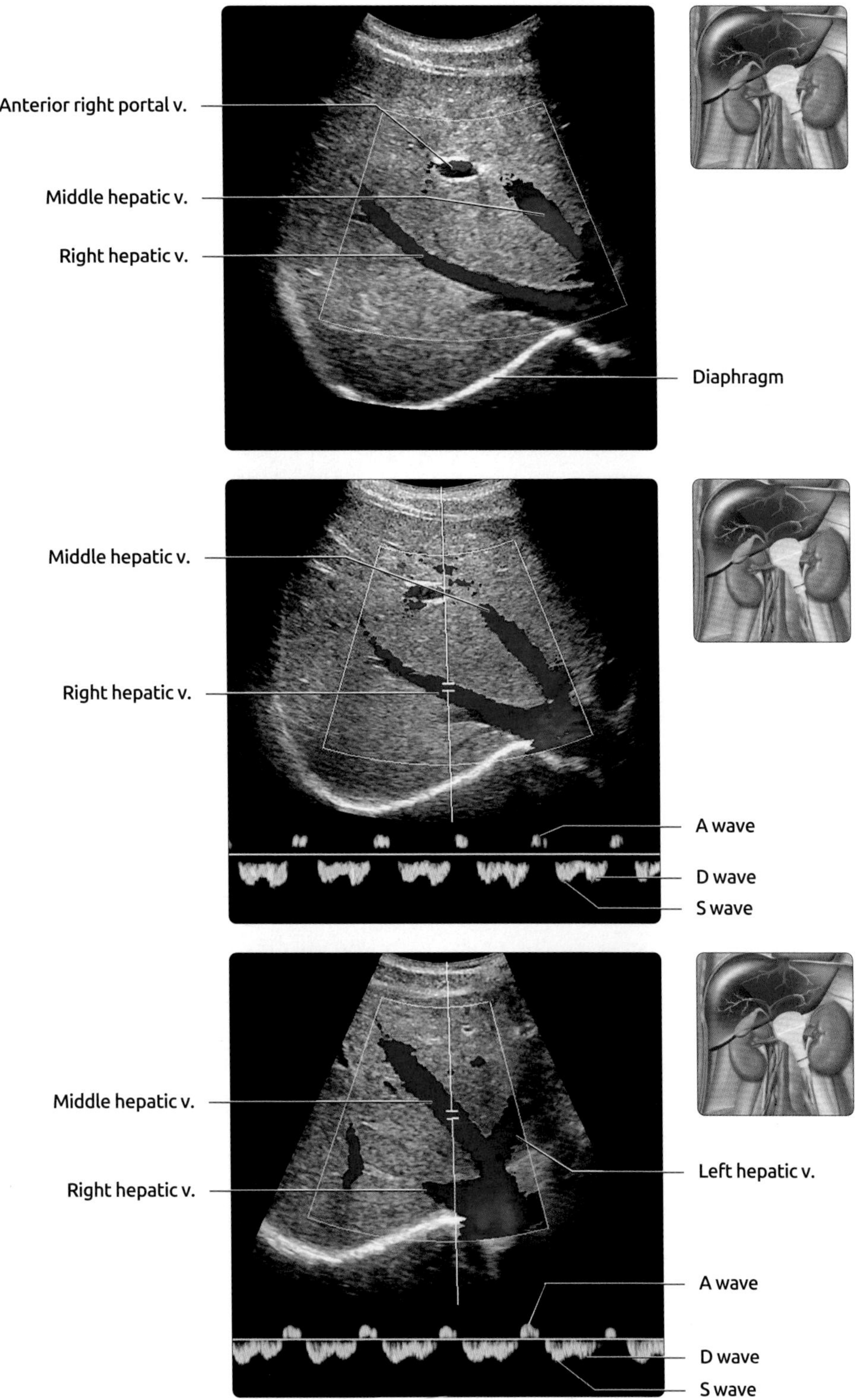

(Top) *Transverse color Doppler ultrasound of the right lobe of the liver shows that the right and middle hepatic veins are directed away from the transducer and flowing toward the IVC.* **(Middle)** *Spectral tracing of the right hepatic vein shows a typical triphasic waveform with A, S, and D waves representing reflection of cardiac motion in the hepatic veins.* **(Bottom)** *Spectral tracing of the middle hepatic vein shows a typical triphasic waveform with A, S, and D waves representing reflection of cardiac motion in the hepatic veins.*

TRANSVERSE LEFT LOBE OF LIVER

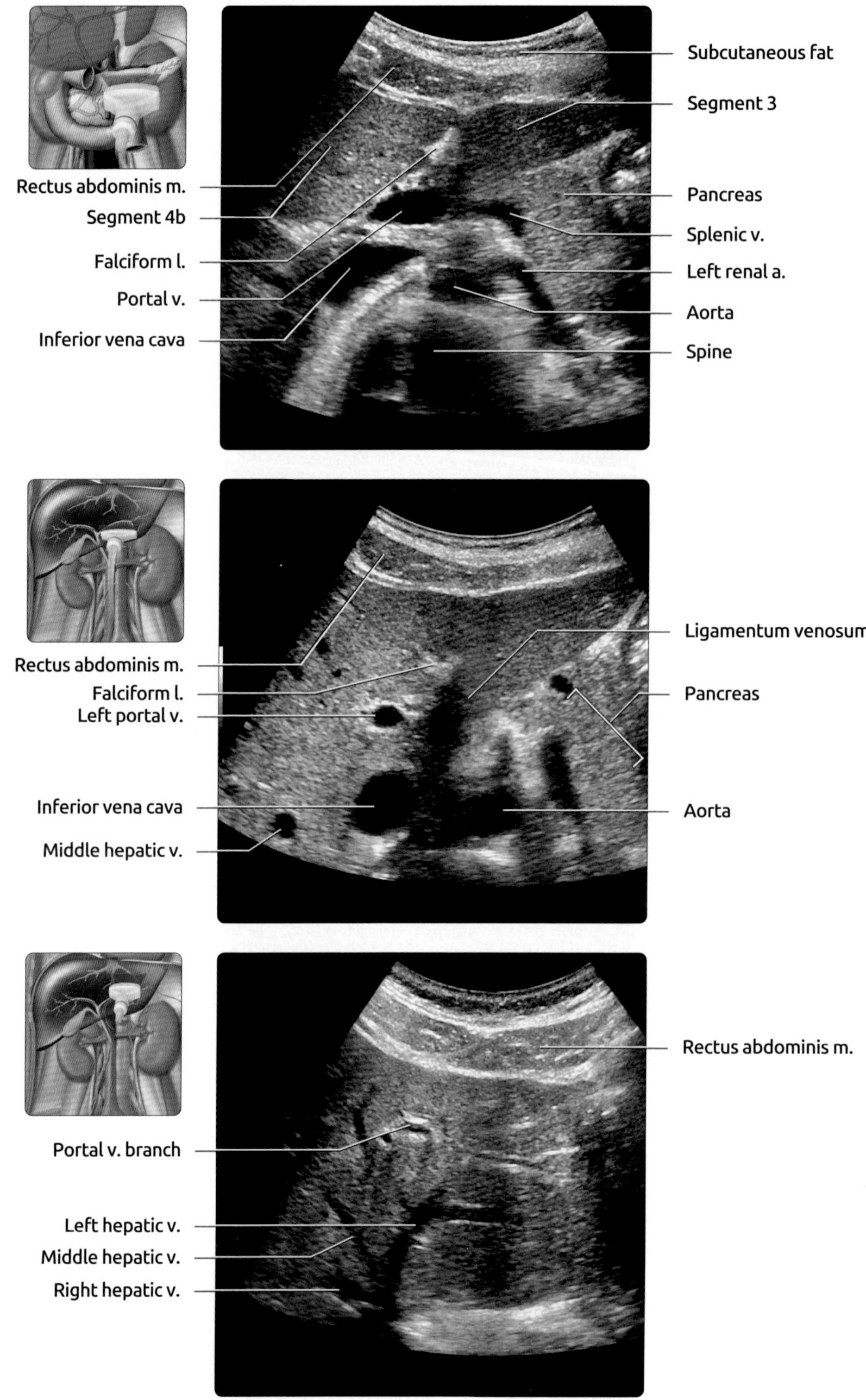

(Top) *Transverse grayscale ultrasound of the left lobe of the liver is shown centered at the level of the falciform ligament and pancreas.* **(Middle)** *Transverse grayscale ultrasound of the left lobe of the liver is shown.* **(Bottom)** *Transverse grayscale ultrasound of the left lobe of the liver is shown centered at the level of the left hepatic vein.*

MAIN PORTAL VEIN

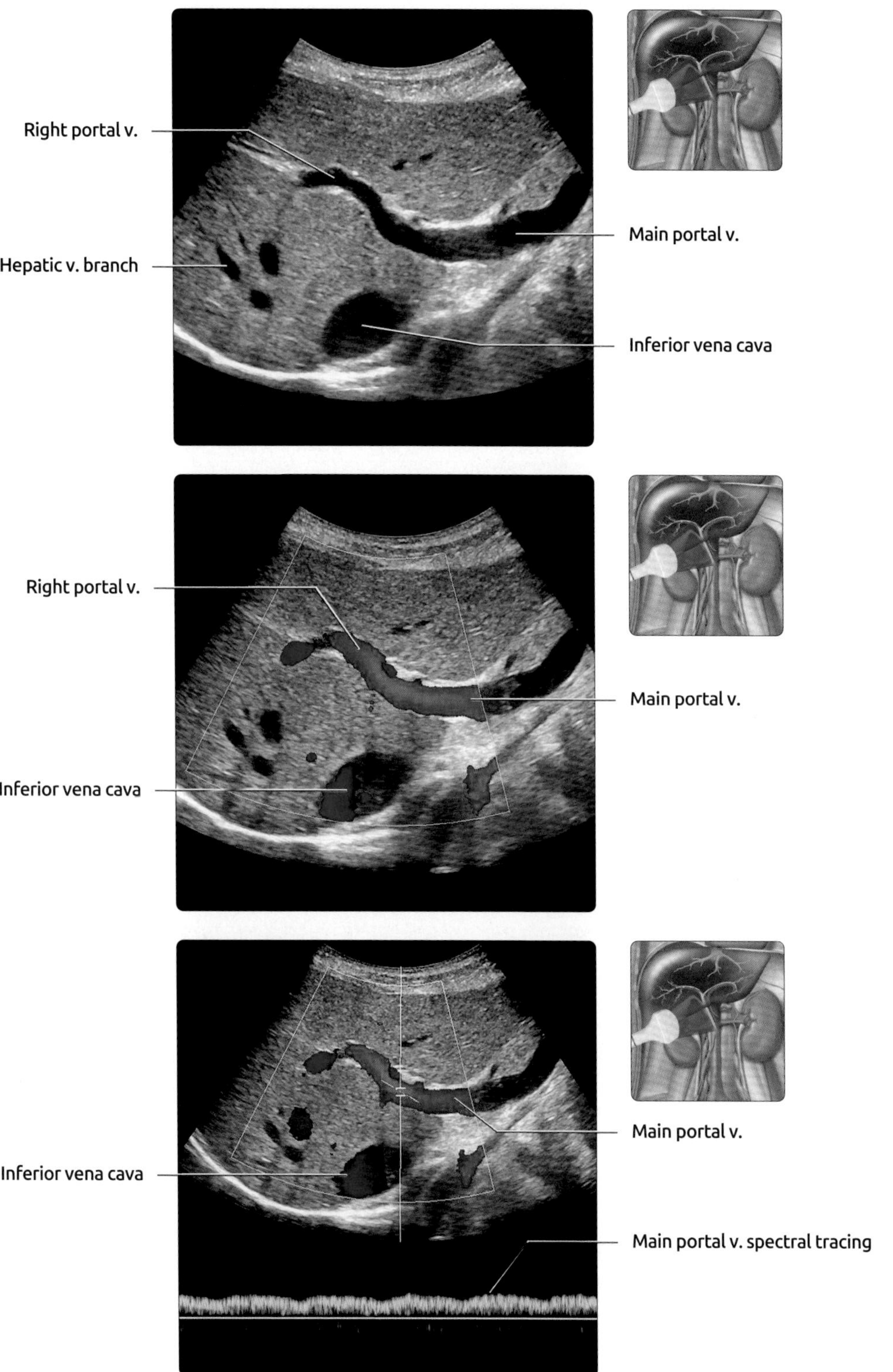

(Top) *Longitudinal oblique grayscale ultrasound is shown centered at the level of the main and right portal veins.* **(Middle)** *Longitudinal oblique color Doppler ultrasound, centered at the level of the main and right portal veins, shows that flow in the portal vein is directed toward the liver (hepatopetal).* **(Bottom)** *Longitudinal oblique spectral Doppler ultrasound of the main portal vein shows that the flow is hepatopetal with gentle undulation reflecting the cardiac and respiratory cycle.*

PORTA HEPATIS

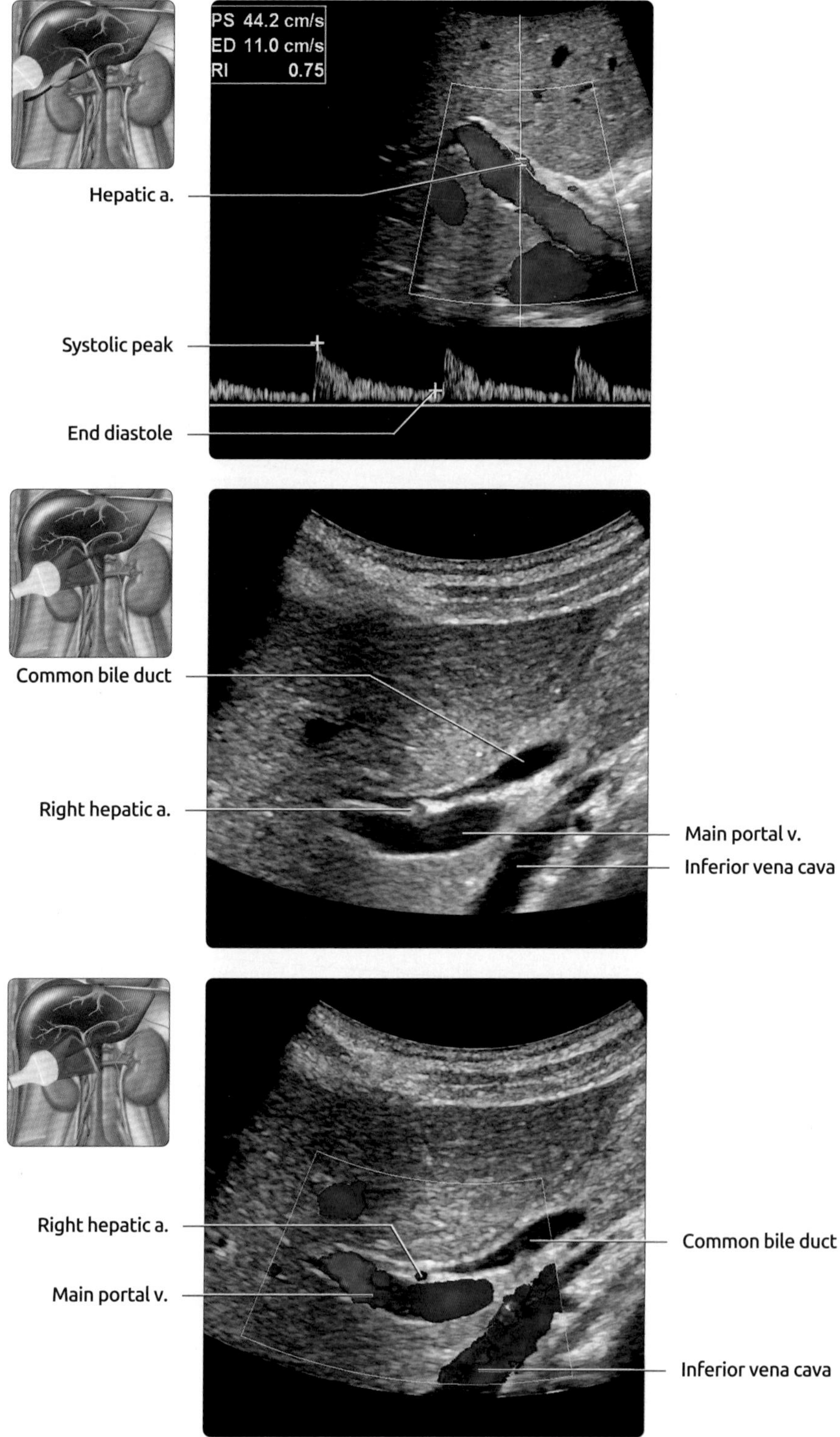

(Top) *Longitudinal oblique spectral tracing of the main hepatic artery shows a typical low-resistance waveform with brisk upstroke and forward diastolic flow. In this case, the hepatic artery velocity is 44 cm/s, which is normal. When measuring velocity, proper angle correction is the key to obtaining accurate velocities.* **(Middle)** *Oblique grayscale ultrasound of the liver, centered at the porta hepatis, shows the common bile duct anterior to the right hepatic artery and portal vein. The IVC is seen posterior to the portal vein.* **(Bottom)** *Oblique color Doppler ultrasound of the liver, centered at the porta hepatis, shows the common bile duct is anterior to the portal vein, and the right hepatic artery is between these 2 structures. This is the typical anatomy in this location, although anatomic variants of the right hepatic artery may occur in which the hepatic artery may be located anterior to the common bile duct.*

LEFT LOBE OF LIVER: LEFT PORTAL VEIN

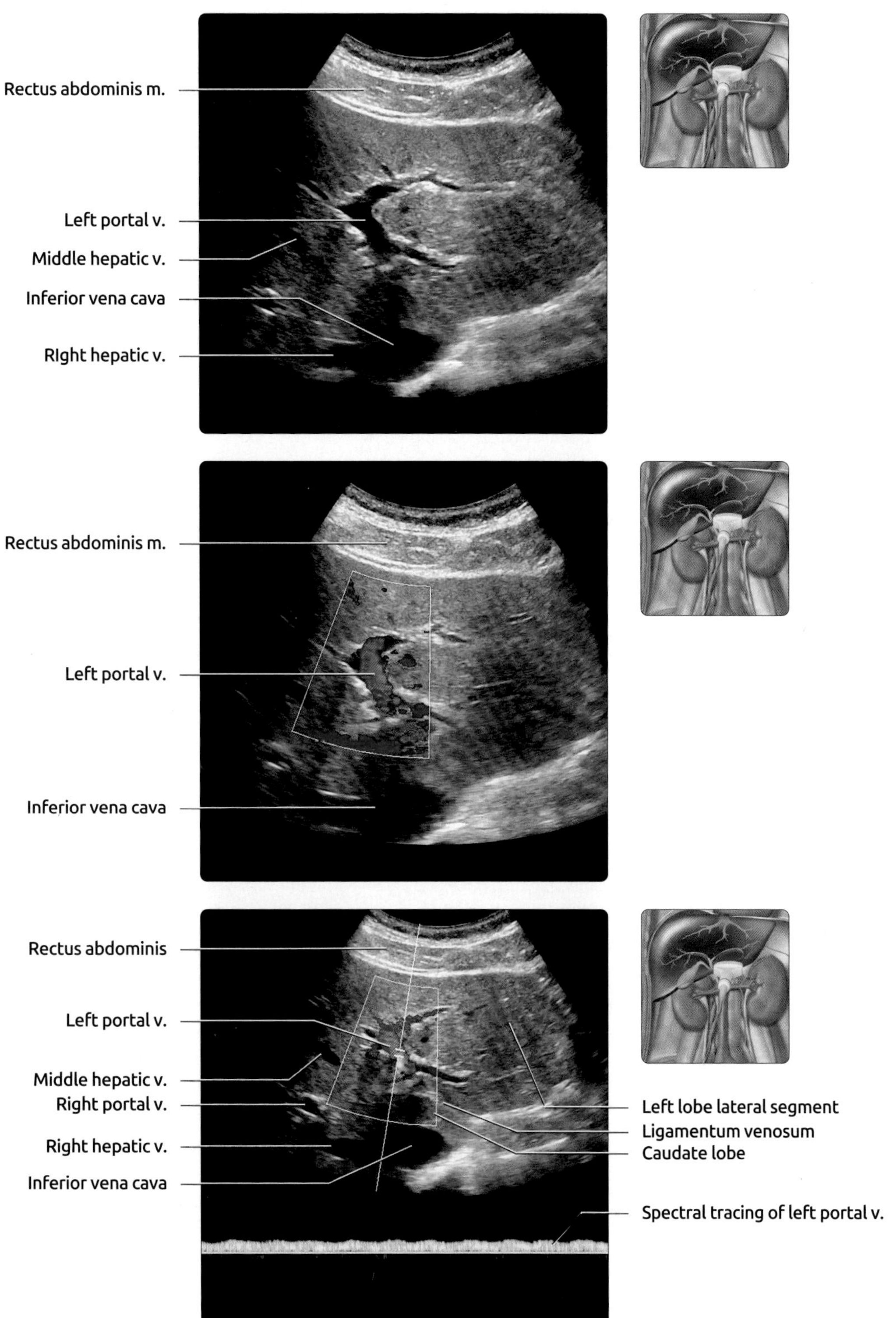

(Top) *Transverse grayscale ultrasound of the left lobe of the liver is shown centered at the left portal vein.* **(Middle)** *Transverse color Doppler ultrasound of the left lobe of the liver is shown centered at the level of the left portal vein. Flow in the left portal vein is directed toward the transducer, indicating that the flow is hepatopetal and therefore normal.* **(Bottom)** *Spectral tracing of the left portal vein on this transverse pulsed Doppler ultrasound shows that the flow is monophasic, directed toward the transducer, with a mildly undulating waveform related to slight transmission of the cardiac cycle, which is a normal appearance for the portal vein.*

LIVER SEGMENTS

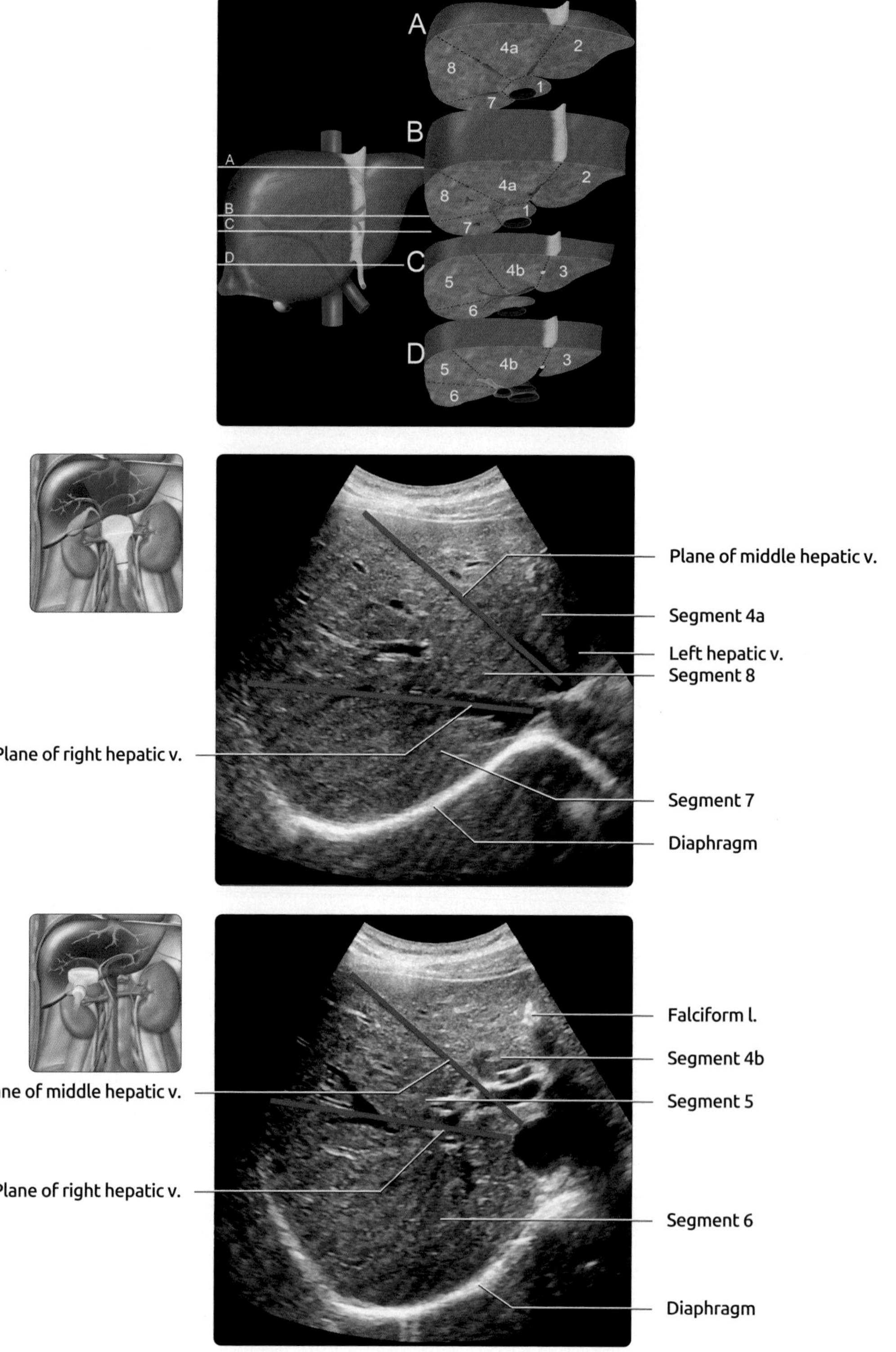

(Top) *Illustration demonstrates the division of the Couinaud segments of the liver at 4 different levels of the liver. The Couinaud segments are defined by the hepatic veins (hepatic vein plane) and the portal veins (portal vein plane).* **(Middle)** *Transverse ultrasound of the right lobe of liver at the level of the confluence of the hepatic veins shows the right hepatic vein separates segment 7 (superior posterior segment of the right lobe of the liver) from segment 8 (superior anterior segment of the right lobe of the liver), and the middle hepatic vein separates segment 8 from segment 4a (superior medial segment of the left lobe of the liver).* **(Bottom)** *Transverse ultrasound of the right lobe of the liver just below the level of the portal vein shows the right hepatic vein, which demarcates the anterior from posterior segments of the right lobe of the liver. The plane of the middle hepatic vein separates the left lobe from the right lobe of the liver. A horizontal plane in line with the main portal vein demarcates the upper from lower liver segments.*

LIVER SEGMENTS

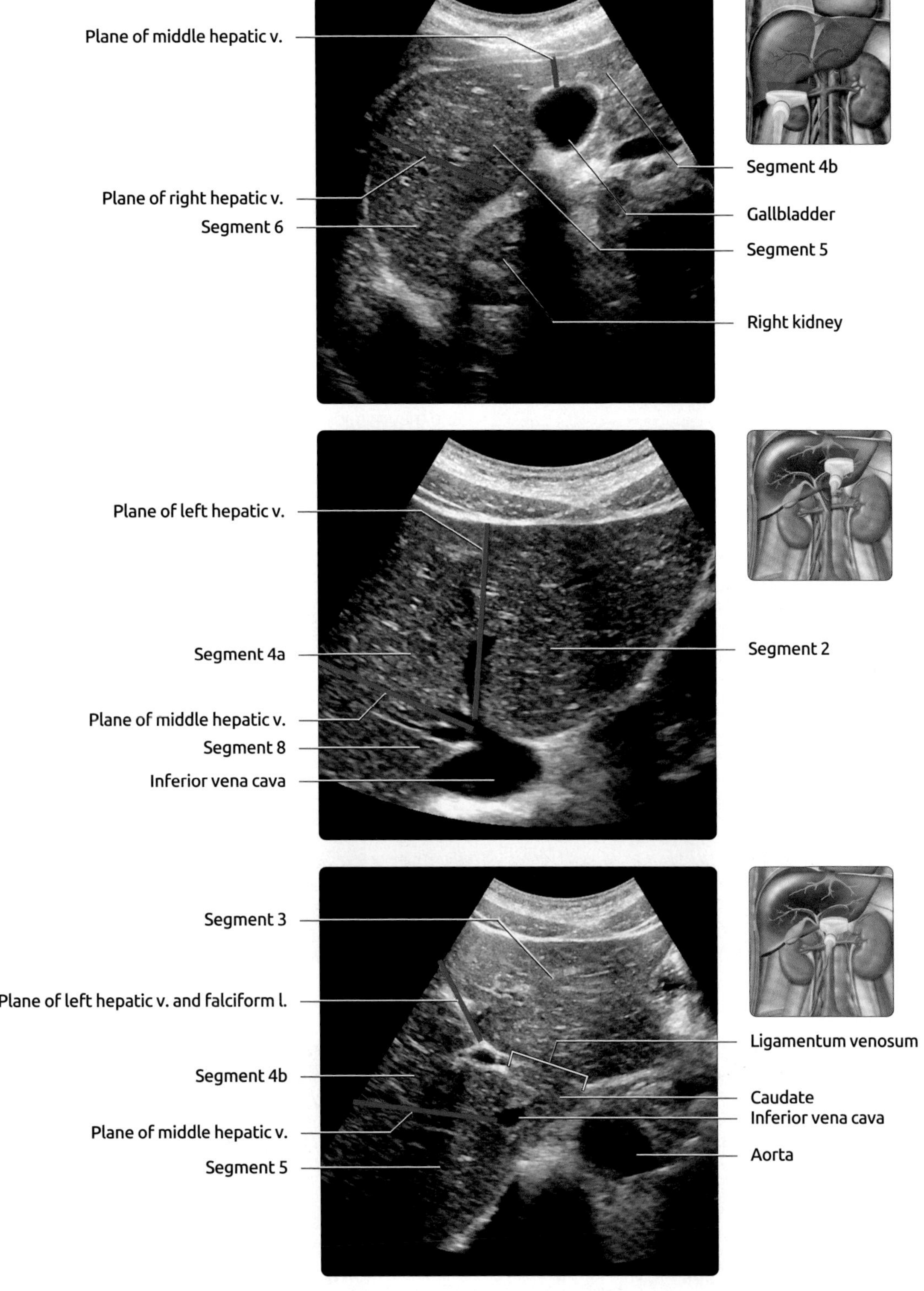

(Top) *Transverse ultrasound of the right lobe of the liver inferiorly at the level of the gallbladder shows the inferior anterior segment of the right lobe of the liver (segment 5) and inferior posterior segment of the right lobe of the liver (segment 6). The demarcation between the 2 segments is created by drawing a plane vertically from the right hepatic vein. A vertically oriented plane at the level of the gallbladder and middle hepatic vein separates the right and left lobe of the liver.* **(Middle)** *Transverse grayscale ultrasound of the left lobe of the liver at the level of the confluence of the hepatic veins and IVC shows the left hepatic vein separates the superior lateral segment of the left lobe of the liver (segment 2) from the superior medial segment of the left lobe of the liver (segment 4a).* **(Bottom)** *Transverse grayscale ultrasound shows the left lobe of the liver at a level just inferior to the left portal vein. The caudate lobe of the liver (segment 1) abuts the ligamentum venosum, IVC, and left portal vein. The falciform ligament separates the inferior lateral segment of the left lobe of the liver (segment 3) from the inferior medial segment of the left lobe of the liver (segment 4b).*

Acute Hepatitis

KEY FACTS

TERMINOLOGY

- Inflammation of liver due to viral infection or toxic agents

IMAGING

- Acute: Enlarged liver
- Chronic: Decrease in liver size
- Grayscale ultrasound
  - Acute hepatitis: Hepatomegaly and diffusely **hypoechoic** parenchyma (variably seen)
  - Steatohepatitis and acute alcoholic hepatitis: Hepatomegaly and diffusely **hyperechoic** liver parenchyma
  - Thickening of gallbladder wall
    - Most pronounced in acute hepatitis A
  - Starry-sky appearance: Portal triads appear markedly echogenic due to periportal edema against background hypoechoic liver (variably seen)
- Pulsed Doppler ultrasound
  - Elevated hepatic arterial velocity

TOP DIFFERENTIAL DIAGNOSES

- Infiltrative hepatocellular carcinoma
- Lymphoma
- Steatosis (fatty liver)

PATHOLOGY

- Viral hepatitis: Caused by 1 of 5 viral agents
  - Hepatitis A (HAV), B (HBV), C (HCV), D (HDV), E (HEV) viruses
- Alcohol abuse
- Autoimmune reactions
- Metabolic disturbances
- Toxic or drug-induced injury

SCANNING TIPS

- Check for tender liver, which may be related to inflammation from acute hepatitis
- Check gain settings, which can affect appearance of liver and may mimic hepatitis or steatosis

(Left) *Transverse transabdominal ultrasound in a patient with acute hepatitis shows diffusely hypoechoic liver parenchyma* ➔ *and hyperechoic portal triad walls* ➔*, creating the starry-sky appearance of acute hepatitis.* **(Right)** *Transverse transabdominal ultrasound in a patient with acute alcoholic hepatitis shows the rounded contour of hepatomegaly* ➔ *with diffusely increased echogenicity* ➔ *throughout the liver, compatible with steatosis.*

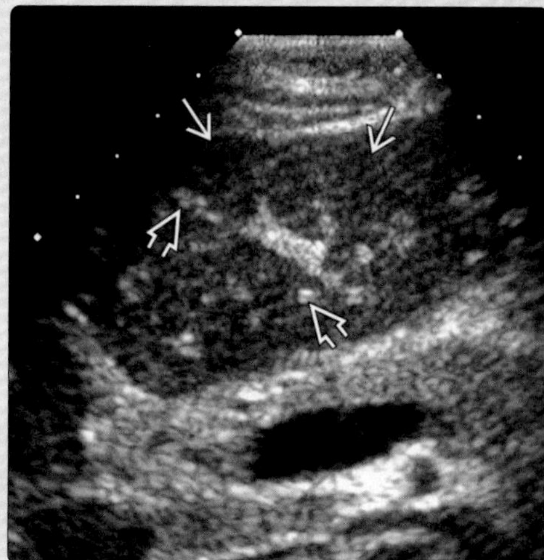

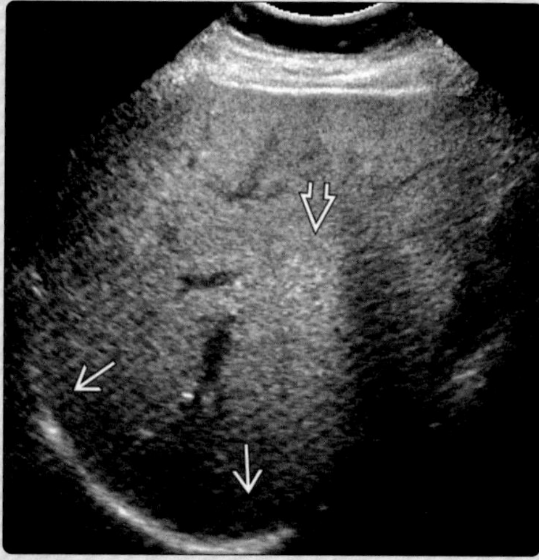

(Left) *Longitudinal oblique transabdominal ultrasound in a patient with acute alcoholic hepatitis shows a markedly enlarged liver with longitudinal extension much greater than the adjacent kidney. Rounded contour* ➔ *is also compatible with hepatomegaly. Of note, the liver is not markedly steatotic.* **(Right)** *Anterior oblique transabdominal US in the same patient demonstrates elevated hepatic artery peak systolic velocity (PSV) of 220 cm/s in acute alcoholic hepatitis. The mean PSV in healthy patients is 66 cm/s.*

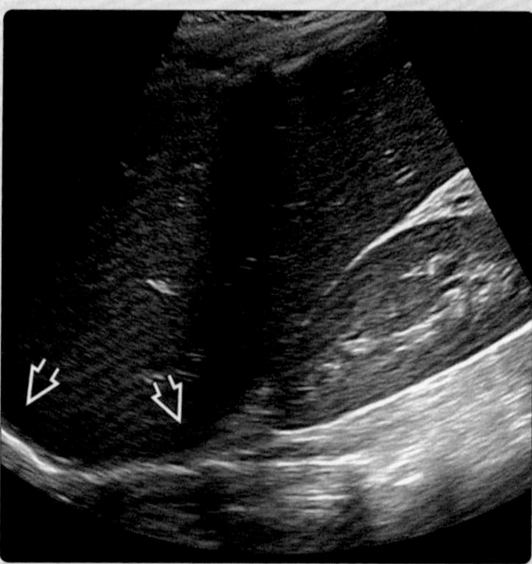

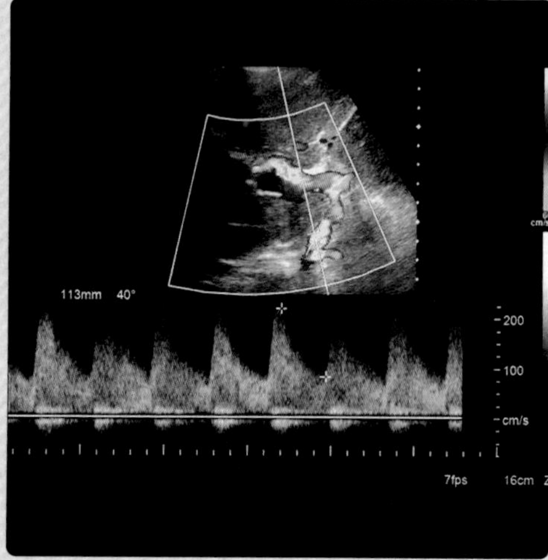

KEY FACTS

TERMINOLOGY

- Common end response of liver to variety of insults, injuries, regeneration, and progressive fibrosis

IMAGING

- Nodular contour, coarse or heterogeneous echotexture ± hypoechoic nodules
- General atrophy with enlargement of caudate/left lobes
- Atrophy of right lobe and medial segment of left lobe
- Coarsened echotexture, increase parenchymal echogenicity
- Regenerating nodules (siderotic)
- Signs of portal hypertension
  - Dilated hepatic and splenic arteries with increased flow
  - Splenomegaly
  - Varices
  - Ascites
- Signs of hypoalbuminemia
  - Edematous, thickened gallbladder wall and bowel wall (especially right colon)
  - Ascites

PATHOLOGY

- Micronodular (Laennec) cirrhosis: Alcohol
- Macronodular (postnecrotic) cirrhosis: Viral
- Nonalcoholic fatty liver disease → nonalcoholic steatohepatitis → fibrosis → cirrhosis
- USA: Alcohol (60-70%), chronic viral hepatitis B or C (10%)

CLINICAL ISSUES

- USA: Hepatitis C (cirrhosis) causes 30-50% of HCC cases
- Japan: Hepatitis C (cirrhosis) causes 70% of HCC cases
- Emerging noninvasive techniques to quantify liver fibrosis
  - US: Transient elastography and shear wave elastography
  - May replace liver biopsy

SCANNING TIPS

- Use linear 9-MHz transducer to evaluate liver capsule for subtle nodularity, which may be early finding in cirrhosis that may otherwise be difficult to visualize

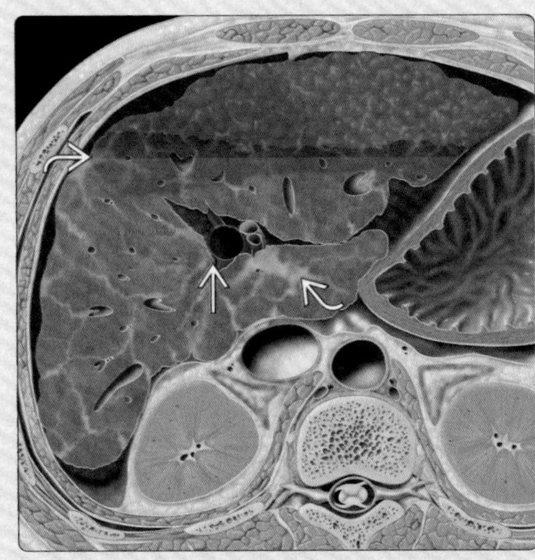

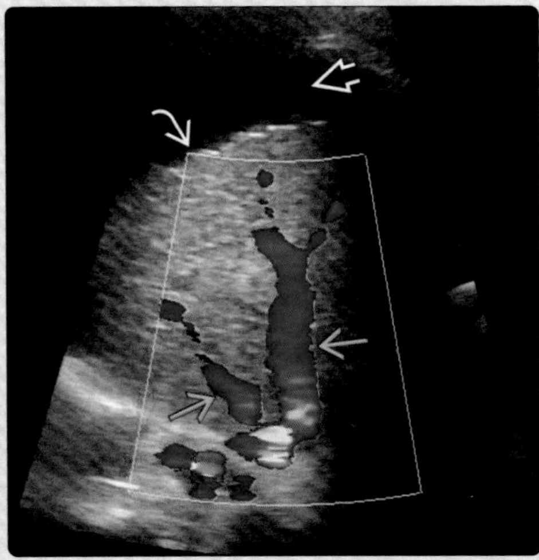

(Left) *Graphic shows a cirrhotic liver with a nodular surface contour and an increase in the caudate:right lobe ratio, measured from the branch point of the right portal vein ➡ to the edges of the caudate and right lobes, respectively. Note the bands of fibrosis ➡ and ascites.* **(Right)** *Transverse color Doppler ultrasound of a cirrhotic liver at the level of the hepatic veins ➡ shows nodular liver capsule ➡ and large-volume ascites ➡.*

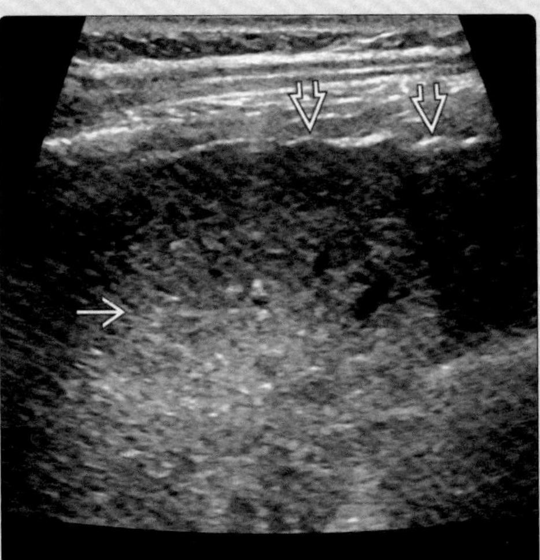

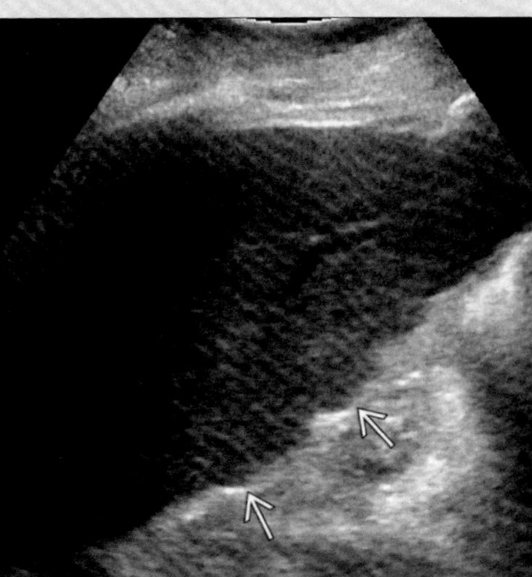

(Left) *Longitudinal high-resolution view of the right liver surface shows a nodular liver capsule ➡ and mildly heterogeneous liver parenchyma ➡ in a patient with liver cirrhosis.* **(Right)** *Longitudinal transabdominal ultrasound shows a nodular liver undersurface ➡ without ascites in a cirrhotic patient. Undersurface nodularity may be an early indicator of cirrhosis.*

Hepatic Steatosis

KEY FACTS

TERMINOLOGY

- Accumulation of triglycerides within hepatocytes

IMAGING

- Diffuse hepatic steatosis
  - Increased echogenicity: Liver more echogenic than kidney
  - Attenuation of US beam results in poor visualization of diaphragm
  - Blurry margins or poorly visualized hepatic and portal veins
- Focal hepatic steatosis
  - Geographic hyperechoic area or multiple confluent hyperechoic lesions
  - No mass effect with vessels running undisplaced through lesion
  - Wedge-shaped/lobar/segmental distribution
- Focal fatty sparing
  - Direct drainage of hepatic blood into systemic circulation
  - Gallbladder bed: Drained by cystic vein
  - Segment 4 or anterior to portal bifurcation: Drained by aberrant gastric vein
  - No mass effect with undisplaced vessel

TOP DIFFERENTIAL DIAGNOSES

- Steatohepatitis
- Fatty cirrhosis
- Hemangioma
- Metastasis or lymphoma

CLINICAL ISSUES

- Nonalcoholic fatty liver disease may progress to nonalcoholic steatohepatitis, which may progress to fibrosis and cirrhosis
- Cirrhosis is major risk factor for hepatocellular carcinoma

SCANNING TIPS

- Ensure overall gain is set correctly; gain set too high can increase apparent echogenicity of liver and mimic steatosis

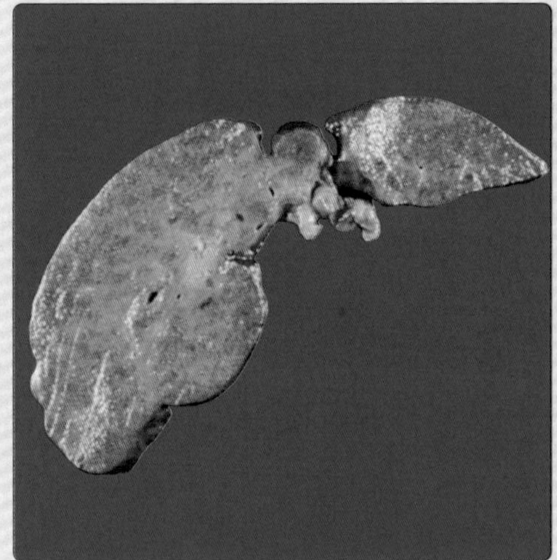

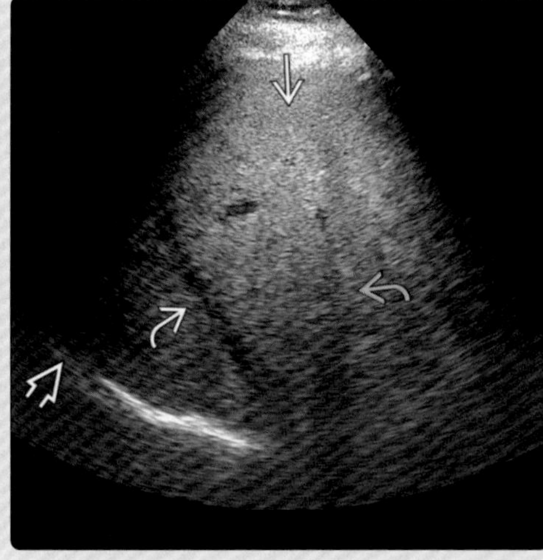

(Left) *Cut section of an explanted liver shows a yellowish, greasy, pale appearance due to steatosis. Steatohepatitis can lead to progressive and irreversible liver failure.* **(Right)** *Transverse abdominal US in a patient with moderate hepatic steatosis shows diffusely increased parenchymal echogenicity ➔ with a poorly delineated right hepatic vein wall ➔ and a hardly visible middle hepatic vein ➔. Part of the diaphragm is not well visualized due to poor acoustic penetration ➔.*

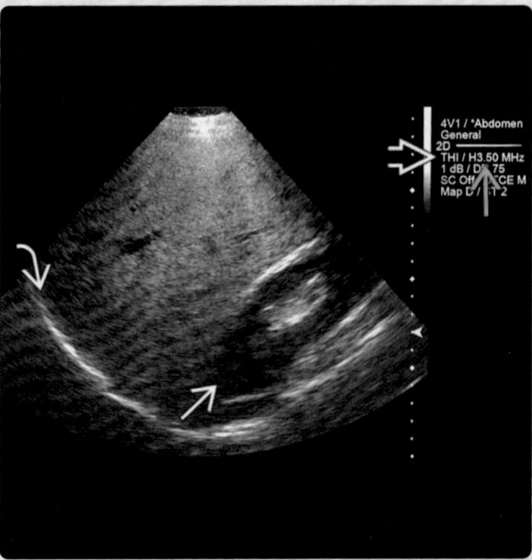

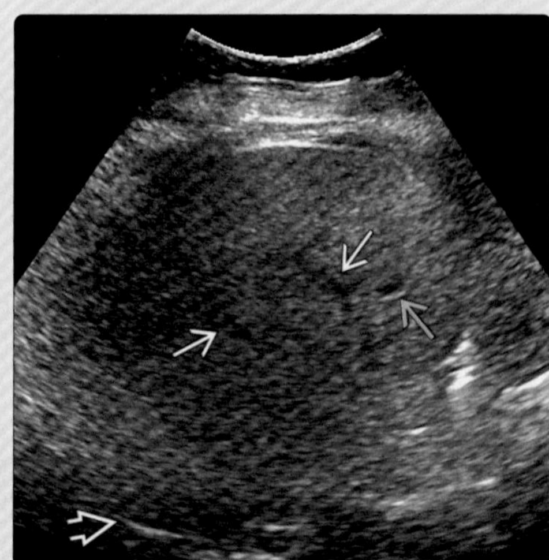

(Left) *Oblique US in a patient with severe steatosis shows diffusely increased liver parenchymal echogenicity in comparison with the right kidney ➔. Lower frequency ➔ vector transducer and harmonic imaging ➔ was applied to optimize penetration, and diaphragm is well visualized ➔.* **(Right)** *Abdominal US shows severe hepatic steatosis with a diffusely echogenic liver, poor visualization of the diaphragm ➔, and decreased visibility of hepatic vein ➔ and portal vein ➔ walls.*

Sinusoidal Obstruction Syndrome (Venoocclusive Disease)

KEY FACTS

TERMINOLOGY

- Hepatic venous outflow obstruction due to occlusion of terminal hepatic venules and sinusoids

IMAGING

- Hepatosplenomegaly, ascites, gallbladder wall thickening
- Narrowing of hepatic veins
- Dilatation of main portal vein
- Appearance or dilatation of paraumbilical vein
- Color Doppler ultrasound
  - Elevated hepatic arterial velocity > 100 cm/s
  - Slow portal venous velocity (< 10 cm/s) or hepatofugal flow

TOP DIFFERENTIAL DIAGNOSES

- Graft-vs.-host disease
- Budd-Chiari syndrome
- Portal vein thrombosis
- Portal hypertension
- Opportunistic infection

PATHOLOGY

- Injury to hepatic venous endothelium
- Progresses to deposition of fibrinogen + factor VIII within venule and sinusoidal walls
- Progressive venular obstruction, centrilobular hemorrhagic necrosis
- Sclerosis of venular wall and intense collagen deposition in sinusoids and venules

CLINICAL ISSUES

- Occurs most frequently following hematopoietic cell transplantation
  - Responsible for 5-15% of deaths in population with VOD
- Signs and symptoms of liver failure with painful hepatomegaly, jaundice, peripheral edema, unexplained weight gain
- Clinical and laboratory features of VOD usually begin within 3 weeks of transplantation

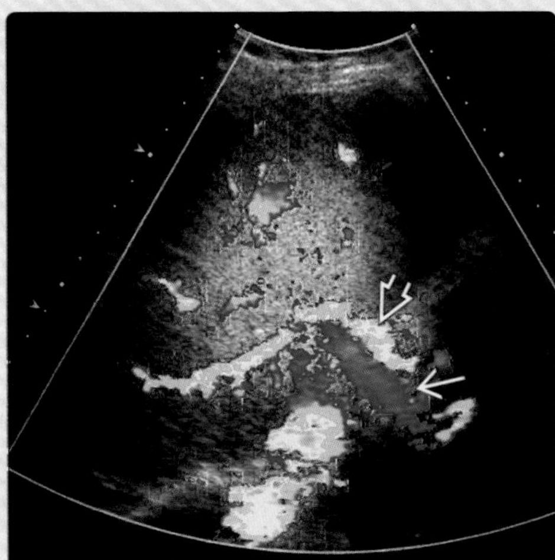

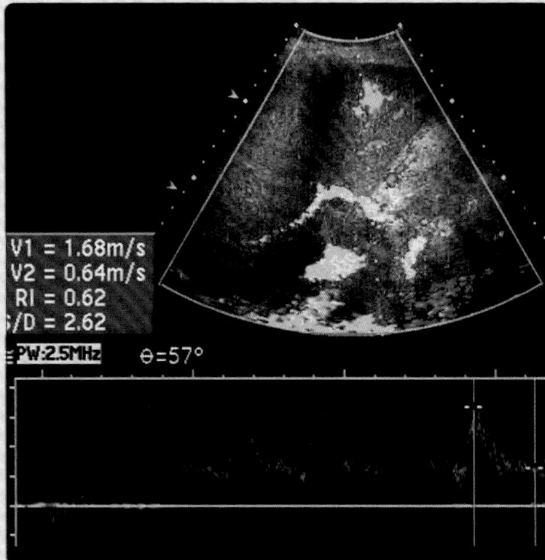

(Left) *Color Doppler US of the liver shows hepatofugal flow in the main portal vein ➡ in a patient with venoocclusive disease (VOD) after bone marrow transplant for AML. Note edematous appearance of the liver and hypertrophied hepatic artery ➡.* **(Right)** *On pulsed Doppler US in the same patient, peak systolic velocity measured at the common hepatic artery is elevated to 168 cm/s, confirming the high-flow state of the hepatic artery related to hepatic arterial buffer response to hepatofugal portal flow.*

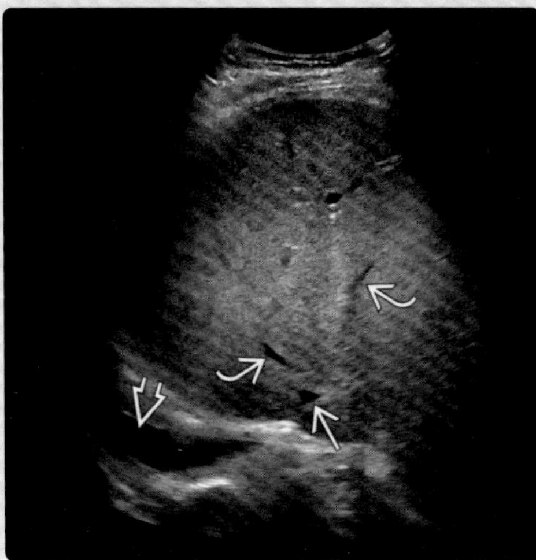

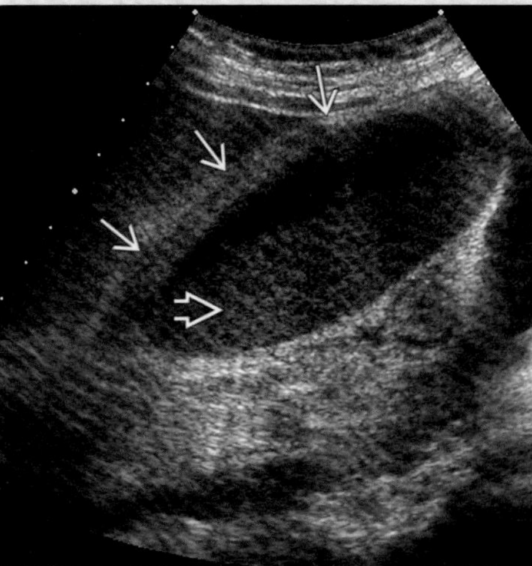

(Left) *Grayscale USshows a markedly edematous and enlarged liver resulting in narrowed hepatic veins ➡ and small-caliber inferior vena cava ➡ in this patient with VOD. A small right pleural effusion ➡ is also evident.* **(Right)** *Grayscale US shows diffuse gallbladder wall thickening ➡ and sludge ➡ in this patient with VOD. Gallbladder wall thickening in isolation is a nonspecific finding. However, in combination with other sonographic findings of VOD, it is supportive of this diagnosis.*

Hepatic Cyst

KEY FACTS

TERMINOLOGY

- Benign, congenital or developmental, fluid-filled space with wall derived from biliary endothelium

IMAGING

- Anechoic lesion with posterior acoustic enhancement, well-defined back wall, and no internal vascularity
- May be unilocular or multilocular with barely perceptible septations
- Ultrasound
  - Often demonstrates septations to better advantage than CT or MR
- Current theory
  - True hepatic cysts arise from hamartomatous tissue
- When > 10 in number, consider fibropolycystic diseases
  - Autosomal dominant polycystic liver disease
  - Autosomal dominant polycystic kidney disease
  - Biliary hamartomas

TOP DIFFERENTIAL DIAGNOSES

- Biliary cystadenoma/cystadenocarcinoma
- Cystic metastases
- Pyogenic abscess
- Echinococcal/hydatid cyst
- Biloma

PATHOLOGY

- Lined by single layer of cuboidal bile duct epithelium
- Surrounding thin rim of fibrous stroma

SCANNING TIPS

- Examine with color or power Doppler to exclude pseudoaneurysm, which can have similar appearance on grayscale imaging
- High-frequency linear transducers with coded harmonic imaging setting can help to demonstrate cystic nature of anterior hepatic cysts

(Left) *Longitudinal oblique grayscale US of the liver shows a cyst ➡ adjacent to the portal vein ⇨. The cyst is anechoic with a well-defined back wall and posterior acoustic enhancement ↪.* **(Right)** *Longitudinal oblique color Doppler US of the same patient shows no internal vascularity in the cyst ➡, confirming the cystic nature of the lesion.*

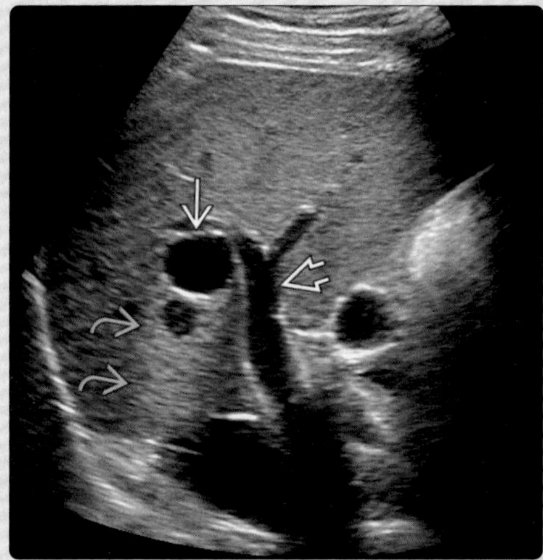

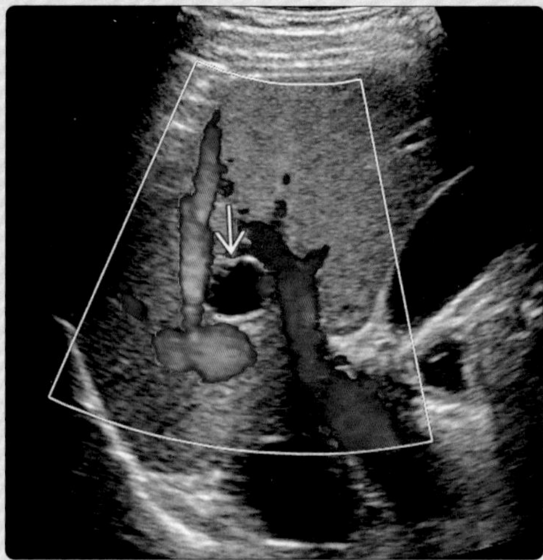

(Left) *Longitudinal color Doppler US of the liver shows a cyst ➡ with an anechoic center, well-defined back wall, and posterior acoustic enhancement ↪.* **(Right)** *Longitudinal oblique grayscale US of the liver shows a bilobed cyst ⇨ with barely perceptible septation ➡ and posterior acoustic enhancement ↪.*

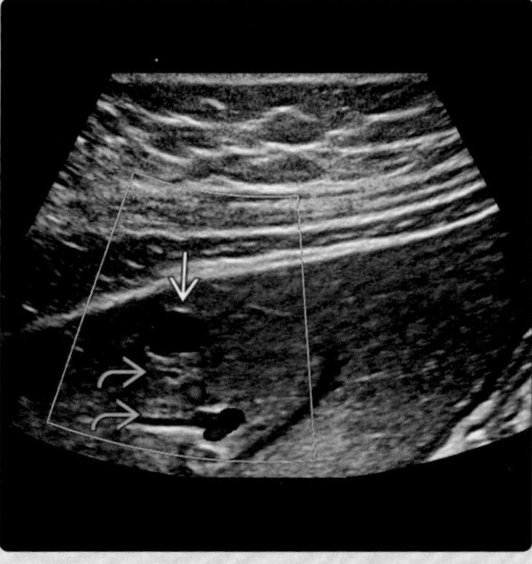

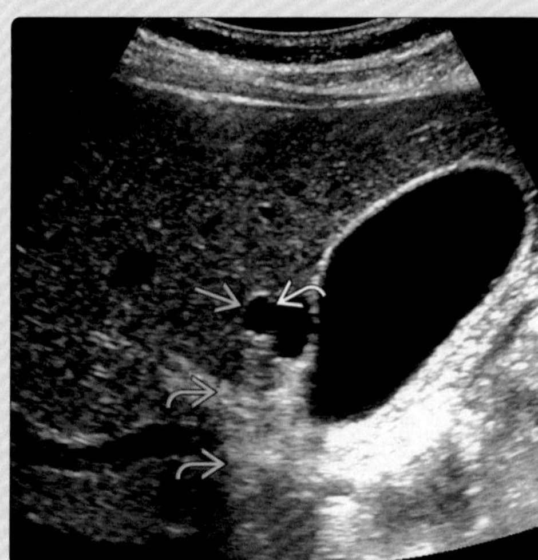

KEY FACTS

TERMINOLOGY

- Benign malformations of biliary tract
- Synonyms: von Meyenburg complex, bile duct hamartoma

IMAGING

- Grayscale ultrasound
  - Numerous small, hypoechoic or hyperechoic foci uniformly distributed throughout liver
    - Leads to inhomogeneous and coarse appearance of liver echotexture
  - Multiple echogenic foci, often with associated comet-tail artifacts
  - Typically smaller lesions appear as echogenic foci whereas larger lesions appear cystic
    - Often extent of echogenic foci on ultrasound is greater than anticipated compared to correlative CT or MR
- Color Doppler ultrasound
  - Twinkling artifact may be seen

TOP DIFFERENTIAL DIAGNOSES

- Multiple simple hepatic cysts
- Multiple small hepatic metastasis
- Hepatic microabscesses
- Autosomal dominant polycystic liver disease
- Caroli disease

CLINICAL ISSUES

- May be misdiagnosed as multiple hepatic metastasis, microabscesses, cirrhosis, lymphoma, leukemia, etc. at initial imaging
- No further evaluation necessary when seen as isolated finding in healthy, nononcologic patient

SCANNING TIPS

- Linear transducers may better demonstrate biliary hamartomas than curved or vector transducers due to higher frequency and greater resolution

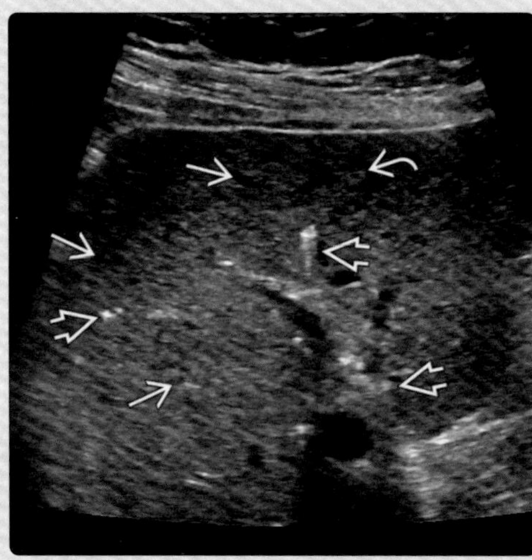

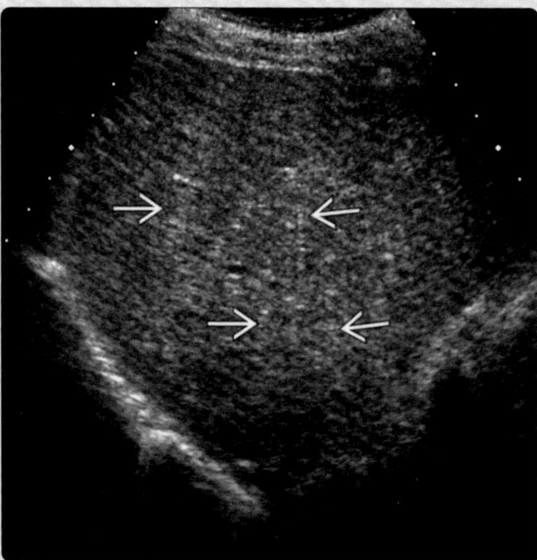

(Left) *Grayscale ultrasound of liver with numerous biliary hamartomas shows diffuse inhomogeneous and coarse parenchymal echotexture with numerous small, hypoechoic ➡ and hyperechoic ➡ foci. Note some echogenic foci have associated comet-tail artifacts ➡.* **(Right)** *Grayscale ultrasound of the liver shows diffuse, coarse, parenchymal echotexture with multiple echogenic foci, some with associated comet-tail artifacts ➡ generated from the biliary hamartomas.*

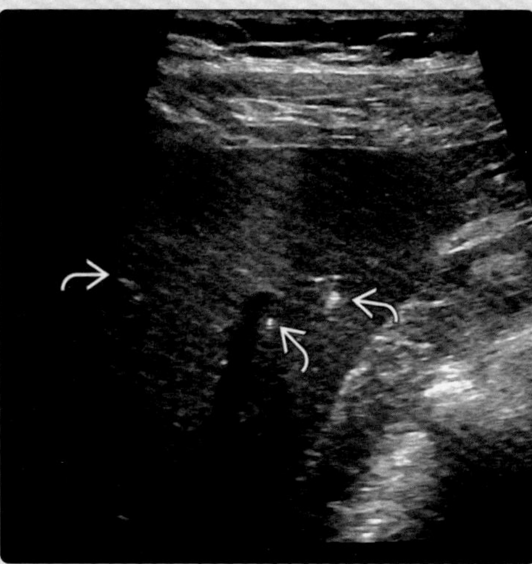

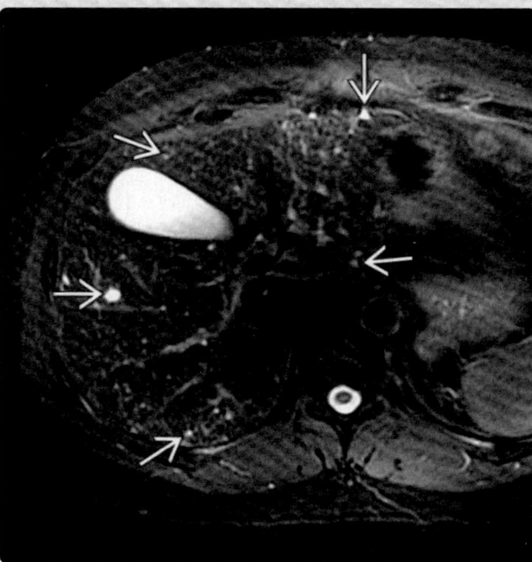

(Left) *Grayscale ultrasound of the liver in a patient with multiple biliary hamartomas as evidenced by multiple tiny echogenic foci, some of which are associated with comet-tail artifacts ➡ is shown.* **(Right)** *Axial T2 FS MR of the liver shows innumerable high signal intensity foci ➡ consistent with biliary hamartomas.*

KEY FACTS

TERMINOLOGY

- Rare premalignant or malignant, unilocular or multilocular cystic tumor arising from biliary epithelium
- Synonyms: Hepatobiliary cystadenoma/carcinoma, biliary cystic tumor, biliary cystic neoplasm, mucinous cystic neoplasm of liver

IMAGING

- Solitary, large, well-defined, multiloculated and multilobulated hepatic cyst
  - Thick, irregular wall and enhancing internal septations
  - May show biliary dilation from mass effect
- Biliary cystadenoma
  - Thin and smooth septa
  - May have fine calcifications and subtle mural nodularity (< 1 cm)
  - Absence of mural nodularity makes cystadenoma more likely
- Biliary cystadenocarcinoma more commonly associated with
  - Thick and irregular septa
  - Mural and septal nodularity (> 1 cm) and papillary projections
  - Coarse calcifications
  - Hemorrhagic internal fluid
- Location
  - Intrahepatic biliary ducts (83%), extrahepatic biliary ducts (13%), gallbladder (0.02%)

TOP DIFFERENTIAL DIAGNOSES

- Simple/complex/complicated hepatic cyst
- Hepatic abscess
- Echinococcal (hydatid) cyst
- Cystic metastases

CLINICAL ISSUES

- Primarily occurs in middle-aged white women

(Left) *Axial graphic shows a biliary cystadenoma ➡ with lobulated contour and multiple, irregular, vascularized septations ⇨.* **(Right)** *Transverse grayscale ultrasound of the liver shows a biliary cystadenoma (with sonographic imaging appearance of a complex cyst) with multiple thickened septations ➡. Most biliary cystadenomas are seen in middle-aged women.*

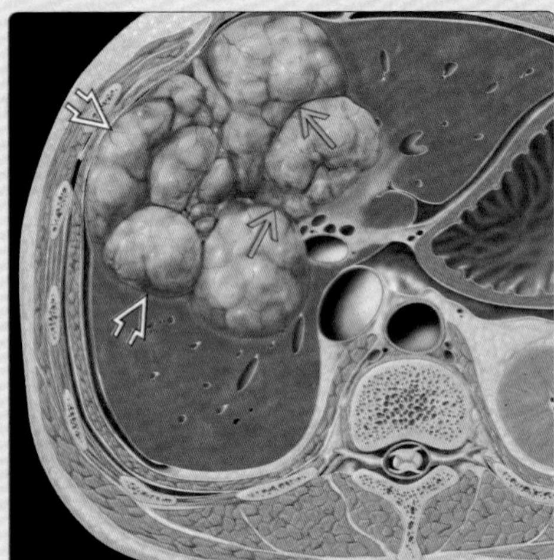

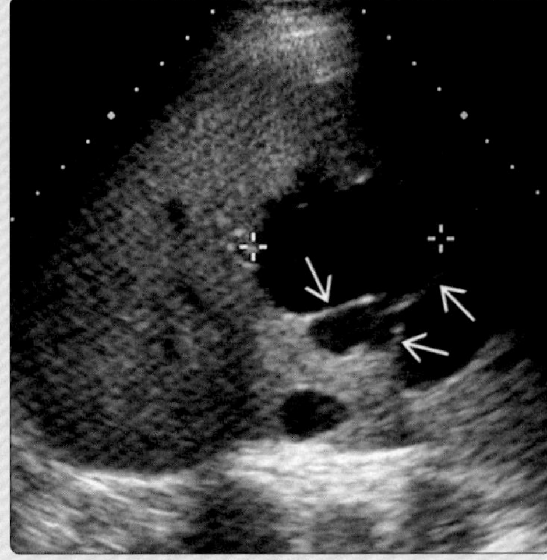

(Left) *Transverse grayscale ultrasound of the liver shows a large, lobulated, multiseptated biliary cystadenoma with thick septations ➡ and layering debris ➡.* **(Right)** *Axial T2-weighted MR with fat saturation of the liver in the same patient shows the large biliary cystadenoma with lobulated contour, multiple thick septations ⇨, and associated mild peripheral biliary ductal dilatation ➡ caused by central mass effect.*

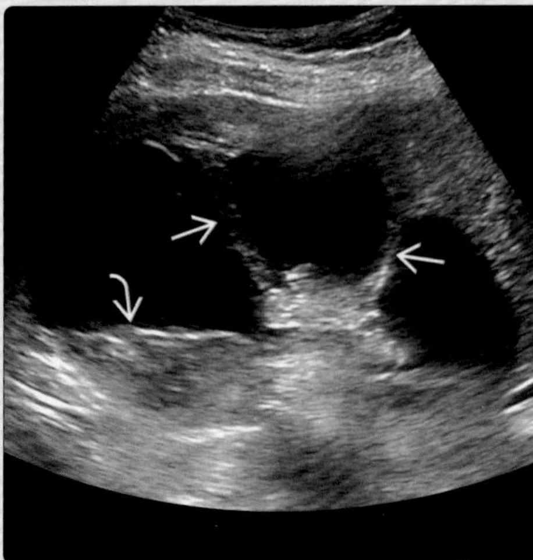

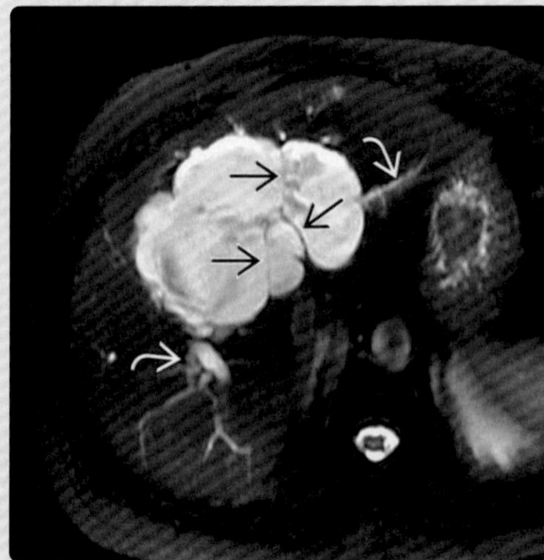

KEY FACTS

TERMINOLOGY

- Encapsulated collection of bile outside biliary tree

IMAGING

- Ultrasound
  - Grayscale ultrasound
    - Focal collection of fluid within liver or close to biliary tree, or in gallbladder fossa in patients with recent cholecystectomy
    - Round or oval in shape, usually unilocular, usually no discernible thin capsule
    - Anechoic fluid content suggests fresh biloma
    - Debris or septa suggest infected biloma
    - May see echogenic foci at periphery related to clips from recent surgery
  - Color Doppler ultrasound
    - No vascularity within lesion
    - For infected biloma, there may be increased vascularity in adjacent tissue
- CECT: Well-defined or slightly irregular cystic lesion without identifiable wall

TOP DIFFERENTIAL DIAGNOSES

- Perihepatic collection/seroma/lymphocele
- Hepatic cyst
- Hepatic abscess
- Intrahepatic hematoma

PATHOLOGY

- Iatrogenic: Laparoscopic cholecystectomy, post liver transplantation, ERCP or other instrumentation of biliary tree, liver biopsy
- Post traumatic: Blunt trauma, motor vehicle accident
- Spontaneous rupture of bile duct

SCANNING TIPS

- Look for low-level echoes within biloma, which can indicate underlying infection

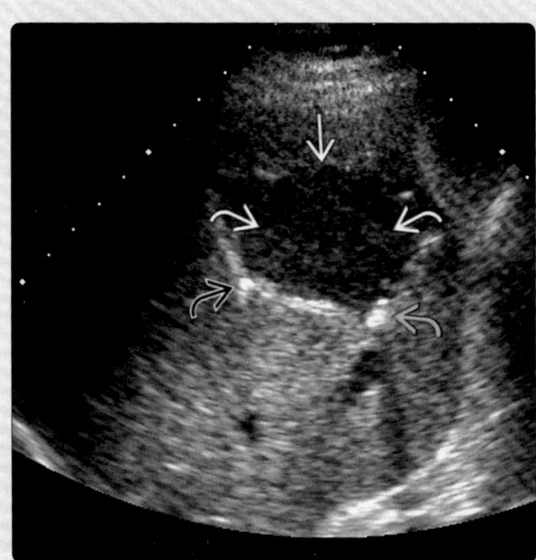

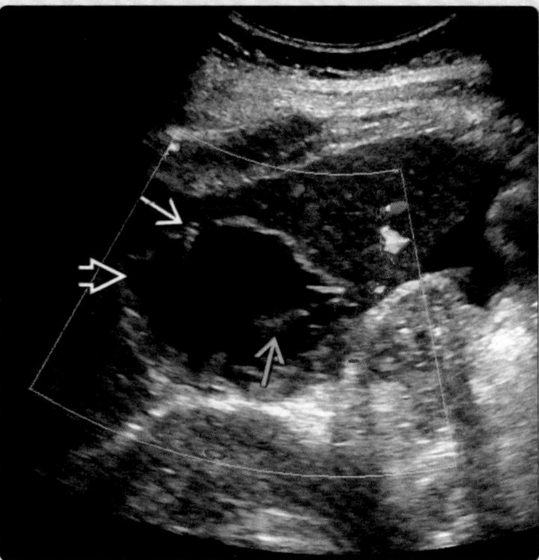

(Left) *Grayscale US shows a biloma ➡ after surgical removal of a liver mass. Low-level internal echoes ➡ suggest infected bile. Peripheral surgical suture with a ring-down artifact ➡ and clip with posterior shadowing ➡ are seen.* **(Right)** *Transverse color Doppler US of the liver shows a biloma ➡ in a resection cavity with peripheral echogenic foci ➡ with posterior ring down, likely related to surgical clip. A small amount of internal debris is seen in the periphery of the biloma ➡.*

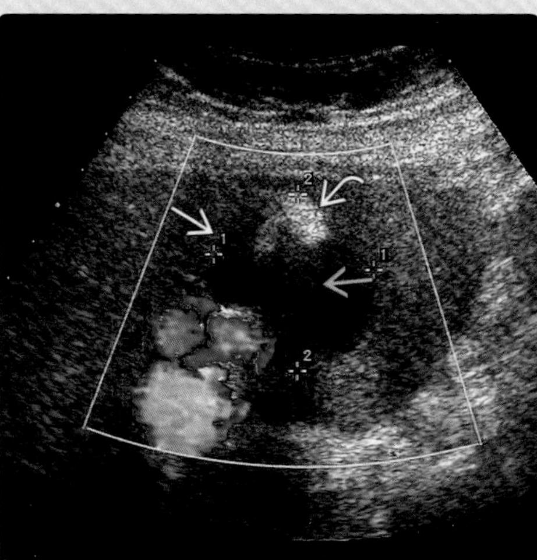

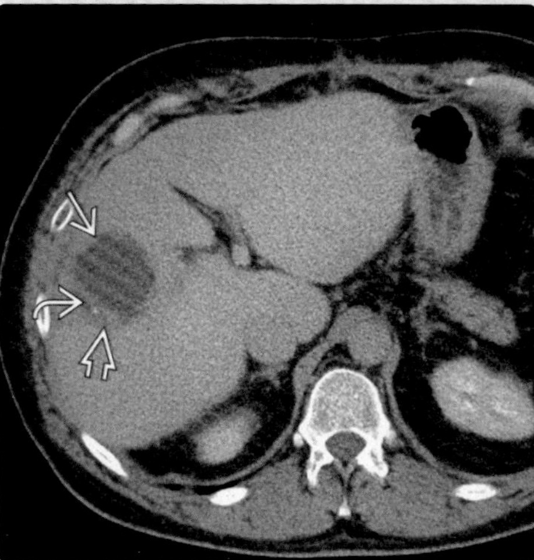

(Left) *Transverse color Doppler US of the liver shows an infected biloma ➡. The lesion is avascular and contains gas ➡ that demonstrates posterior dirty shadowing ➡.* **(Right)** *Delayed-phase CECT shows a round cystic mass without a discernible wall ➡ containing internal debris ➡ and layering debris ➡ in the dependent portion, which suggests infected biloma.*

Pyogenic Hepatic Abscess

KEY FACTS

TERMINOLOGY

- Localized collection of pus in liver due to bacterial infectious process with destruction of hepatic parenchyma and stroma

IMAGING

- Cluster sign: Cluster of small pyogenic abscesses that coalesce into single large cavity
- Early lesions tend to be echogenic and poorly demarcated, evolve into well-demarcated anechoic lesions
- May see central gas or fluid level
- Echogenicity of abscesses
  - Anechoic (50%), hyperechoic (25%), hypoechoic (25%)
- Fluid level or debris, internal septa, and posterior acoustic enhancement

TOP DIFFERENTIAL DIAGNOSES

- Metastasis (post treatment)
- Biliary cystadenocarcinoma
- Amebic abscess
- Hemorrhagic simple cyst
- Hydatid cyst (echinococcal cyst)
- Hepatic infarction in liver transplantation

PATHOLOGY

- Development via 5 major routes: Portal vein, biliary tract, hepatic artery, direct extension, trauma
- Common organisms: *Escherichia coli*, *Klebsiella pneumoniae* (adult), *Staphylococcus aureus* (children)

CLINICAL ISSUES

- Accounts for 88% of all liver abscesses
- Typical presentation: Middle-aged/elderly patient with history of fever, right upper quadrant pain, tender hepatomegaly, leukocytosis

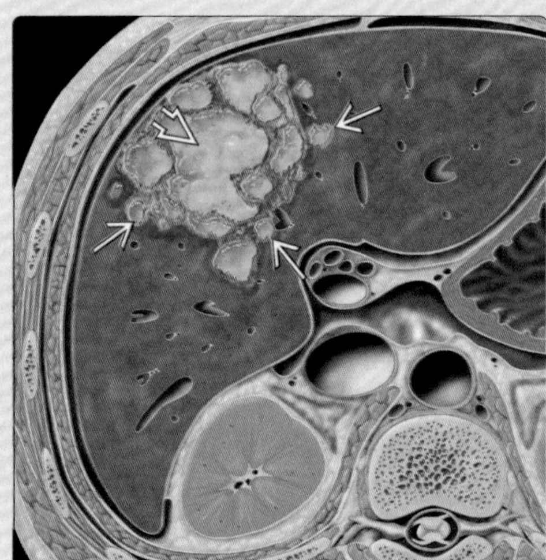
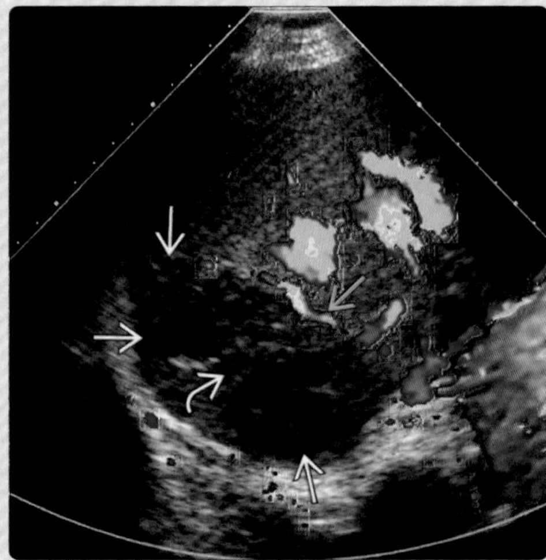

(Left) *Transverse graphic shows a cluster of multiple variably sized pus collections in the right lobe of the liver ➡ coalescing to form a large abscess cavity ➡.* **(Right)** *Oblique transabdominal color Doppler ultrasound shows a cluster of coalescing abscesses ➡ in the right lobe of liver, representing a pyogenic hepatic abscess. The abscess has irregular walls and contains low-level internal echoes ➡. Adjacent hepatic parenchyma is edematous and hypervascular ➡.*

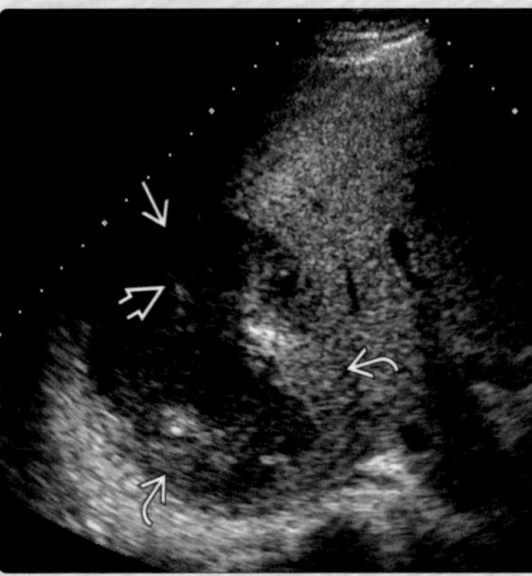
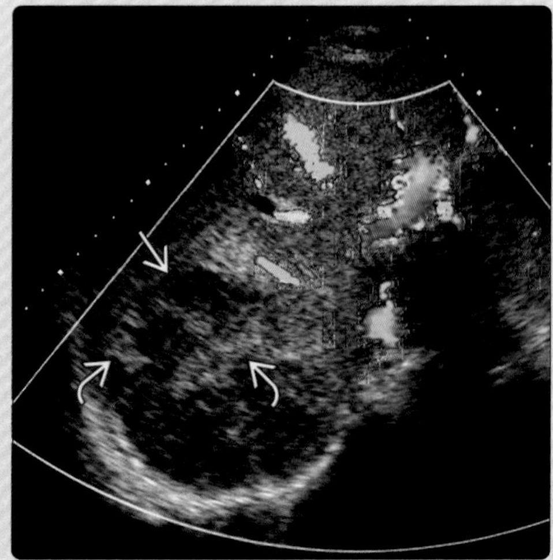

(Left) *Oblique transabdominal grayscale ultrasound shows an irregular-shaped hypoechoic pyogenic abscess ➡ in the right lobe of the liver. Several internal septations ➡ are seen as well as peripheral echogenic components of the abscess ➡.* **(Right)** *Oblique transabdominal color Doppler ultrasound performed in the same patient shows no color flow within the abscess cavity ➡. Note irregular internal echogenic debris ➡ within the abscess cavity.*

Amebic Hepatic Abscess

KEY FACTS

TERMINOLOGY

- Localized pus collection in liver due to *Entamoeba histolytica* with destruction of hepatic parenchyma

IMAGING

- General feature
  - Most often solitary (85%), peripherally located
- Ultrasound
  - Sharply demarcated, round or ovoid mass
  - Hypoechoic with low-level internal echoes
  - May see internal septa or wall nodularity
  - May see posterior acoustic enhancement
- CECT
  - Typically hypoattenuating unilocular lesion
  - Peripheral rim or capsule enhancement
  - May see hypodense halo due to edema

TOP DIFFERENTIAL DIAGNOSES

- Hepatic metastasis (post treatment, cystic, or necrotic)
- Hepatic pyogenic abscess
- Hepatic hydatid cyst
- Biliary cystadenoma/cystadenocarcinoma
- Infarcted liver after transplantation

PATHOLOGY

- Entamoeba histolytica
- Primary source of infection: Human carriers passing amebic cysts into stool

CLINICAL ISSUES

- Right upper quadrant pain, tender hepatomegaly, diarrhea with mucus
- Indirect hemagglutination positive in 90% of cases

SCANNING TIPS

- Rule out pyogenic or fungal abscess, cystic lesions
- Check for history of transplantation, ablation, or chemotherapy for liver tumor or metastasis, which may simulate amebic abscess on imaging

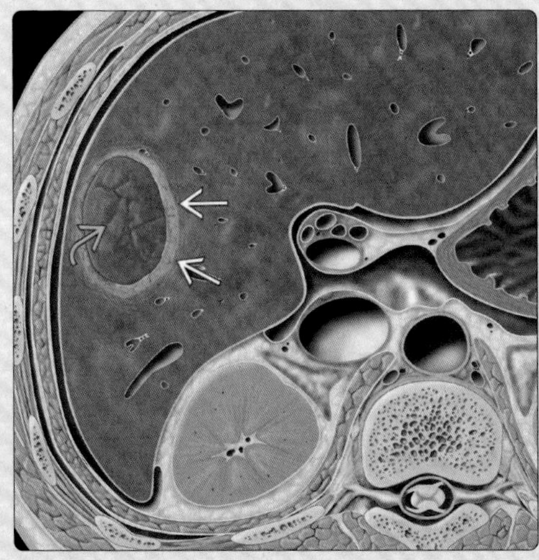

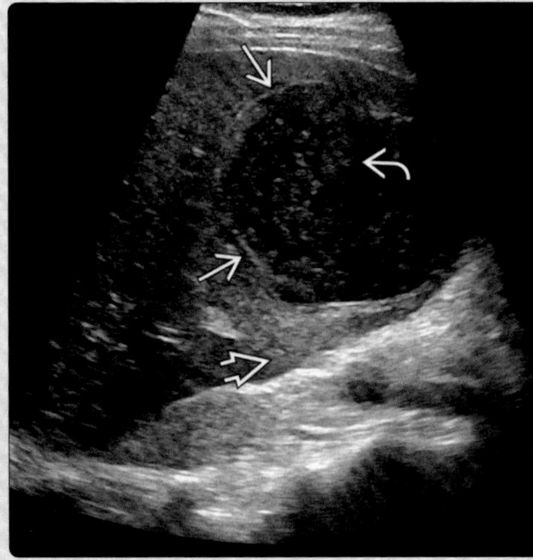

(Left) *Graphic illustration demonstrates a unilocular encapsulated amebic abscess within the liver. Note the surrounding rim of edema and central anchovy paste consistency of contents.* **(Right)** *Sagittal grayscale ultrasound of the liver shows a large, well-demarcated and encapsulated hypoechoic amebic abscess. The contents are heterogeneous due to floating debris. Also note the mild posterior acoustic enhancement.*

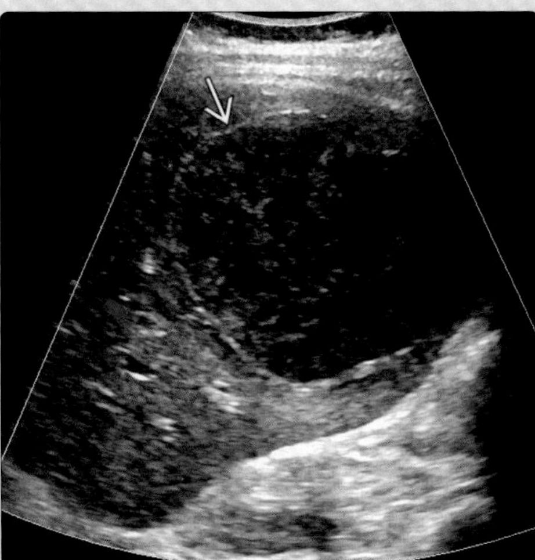

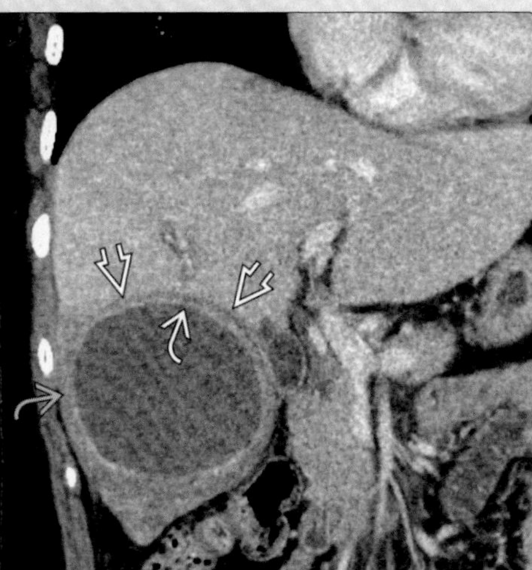

(Left) *Color Doppler ultrasound in the same patient shows no detectable internal vascularity within the lesion.* **(Right)** *Coronal contrast-enhanced CT in the same patient shows a large unilocular amebic abscess in the right lobe of the liver. The abscess is well defined with an enhancing capsule and hypodense halo of edema. Note the abutment with liver capsule.*

Hepatic Hydatid Cyst

KEY FACTS

TERMINOLOGY

- Infection of humans caused by larval stage of *Echinococcus granulosus* or *Echinococcus multilocularis*

IMAGING

- Best diagnostic clue: Membranes ± daughter cysts in complex heterogeneous mass
- *E. granulosus*
  - Anechoic cyst with double echogenic lines separated by hypoechoic layer
  - Honeycomb cyst, multiple septations
  - Water lily sign: Complete detachment of membrane
  - Snowstorm pattern: Anechoic cyst with internal debris and hydatid sand
- *E. multilocularis*
  - Single/multiple echogenic lesions
  - Irregular necrotic lesions with microcalcifications
  - Ill-defined infiltrative solid masses

TOP DIFFERENTIAL DIAGNOSES

- Hemorrhagic or infected cyst
- Complex pyogenic abscess
- "Cystic" metastases
- Biliary cystadenocarcinoma

PATHOLOGY

- Caused by larval stage of *Echinococcus* tapeworm
  - *E. granulosus*
    - Most common form of hydatid disease, unilocular
  - *E. multilocularis*
    - Less common but aggressive

SCANNING TIPS

- Imaging clue: Daughter cysts can float freely within mother cyst
- Altering patient's position may change position of daughter cysts

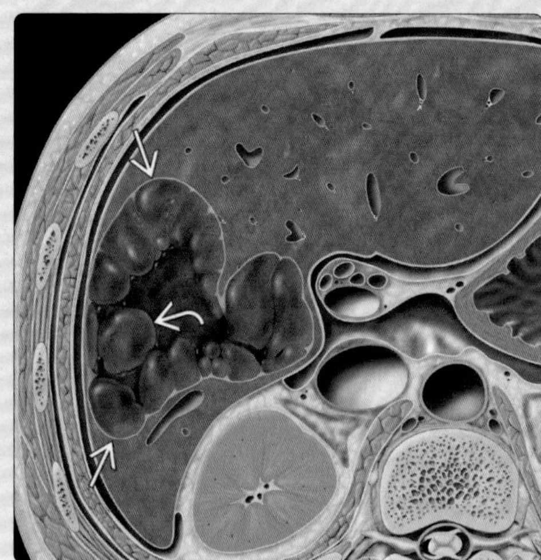

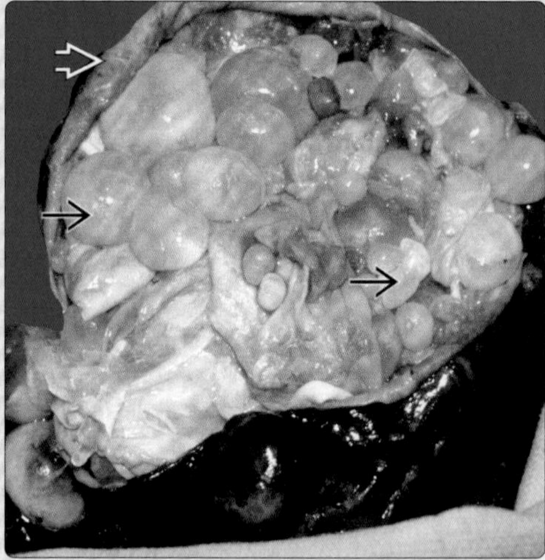

(Left) *Graphic shows an eccentric cystic mass (the pericyst or mother cyst) ➡ with numerous peripheral daughter cysts, or scolices, ➡ within the right lobe of the liver.* **(Right)** *Gross photograph of the liver shows a hydatid cyst containing multiple daughter cysts ➡. The fibrous rim ➡ can be seen surrounding the cyst. (From DP: Spleen.)*

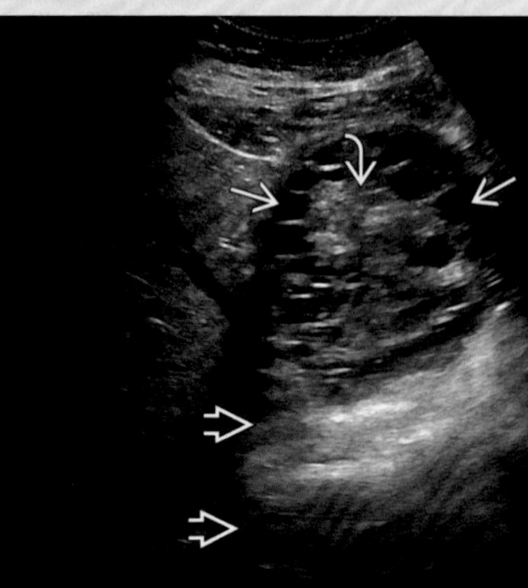

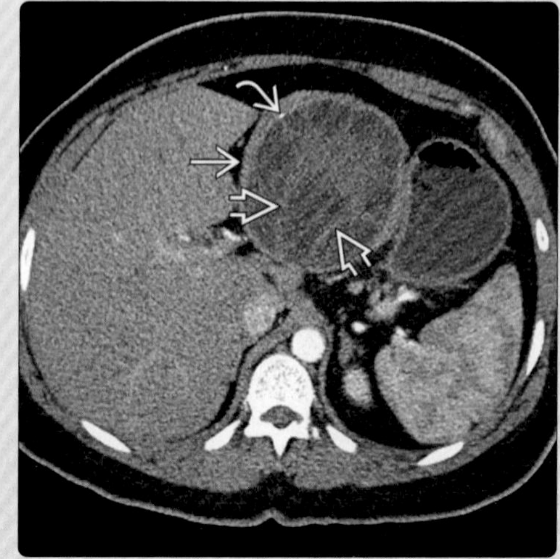

(Left) *Transverse abdominal US shows an echinococcal cyst containing multiple peripheral daughter cysts ➡ and central heterogeneous content ➡ in the left lobe of the liver. Note the posterior acoustic enhancement ➡.* **(Right)** *Axial contrast-enhanced CT performed in the same patient shows a large, multilocular, well-defined cystic mass in the left lobe of the liver ➡. The cystic mass has a thick wall with a tiny focus of calcification ➡ and multiple septations ➡.*

KEY FACTS

TERMINOLOGY

- Typically refers to hepatic *Candida* abscesses in immunocompromised patients

IMAGING

- Multiple small, hypoechoic lesions throughout liver (most common pattern)
- Target sign (hyperechoic center with hypoechoic halo) or bull's-eye configuration
- Wheel within wheel pattern may be present in larger fungal lesions
- Multiple small, hyperechoic foci throughout liver (occurs in later stages)
- Lesions may resolve completely or calcify after successful treatment
- Similar lesions may be found in spleen

TOP DIFFERENTIAL DIAGNOSES

- Simple cysts
- Necrotic metastases
- Hepatic lymphoma
- Sarcoidosis
- Biliary hamartomas

PATHOLOGY

- Fungal infection: Most commonly *Candida albicans* but may also include *Cryptococcus*, histoplasmosis, mucormycosis, *Aspergillus*
    - Occur more commonly in immunocompromised patients (leukemia, lymphoma, AIDS/post transplant)
- Pyogenic infections can appear similarly in patients with GI or biliary tract infection

DIAGNOSTIC CHECKLIST

- Rule out other causes of multiple liver lesions, such as hepatic cysts, hepatic lymphoma, metastases, sarcoidosis
- Liver biopsy with culture often necessary to verify lesions are due to fungal infection

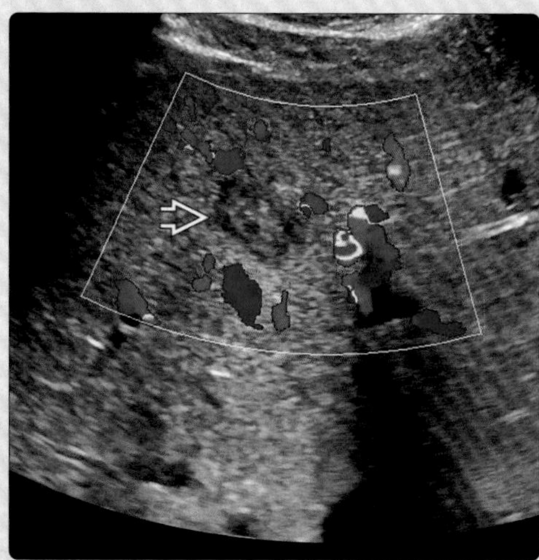

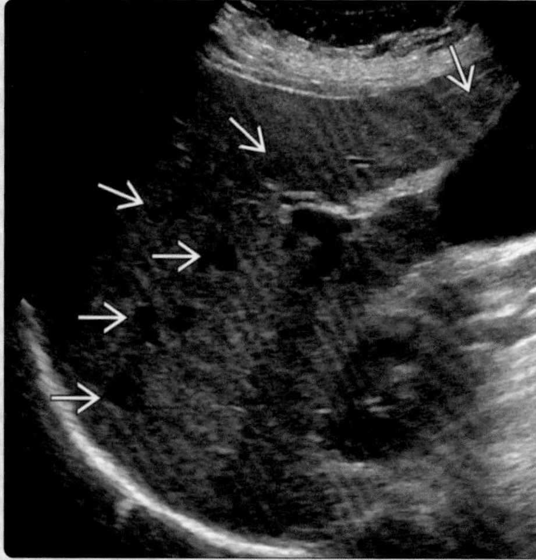

(Left) *Transverse color Doppler ultrasound of a hepatic fungal abscess ➡ shows characteristic wheel within a wheel or target appearance. Notice the fungal abscess is avascular in appearance.* **(Right)** *Longitudinal grayscale ultrasound shows multiple hypoechoic fungal abscesses ➡ throughout the liver in an immunocompromised patient.*

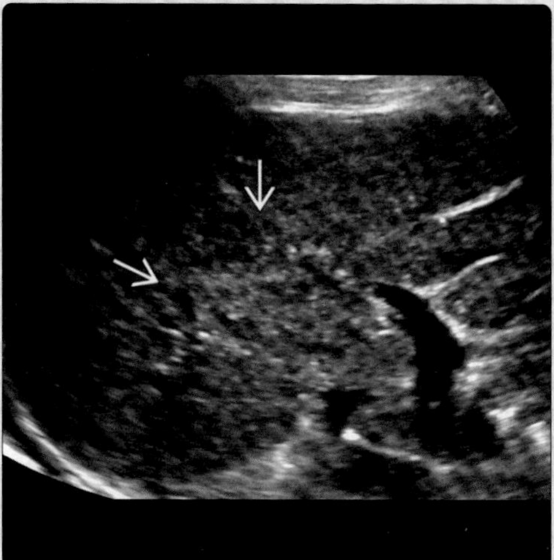

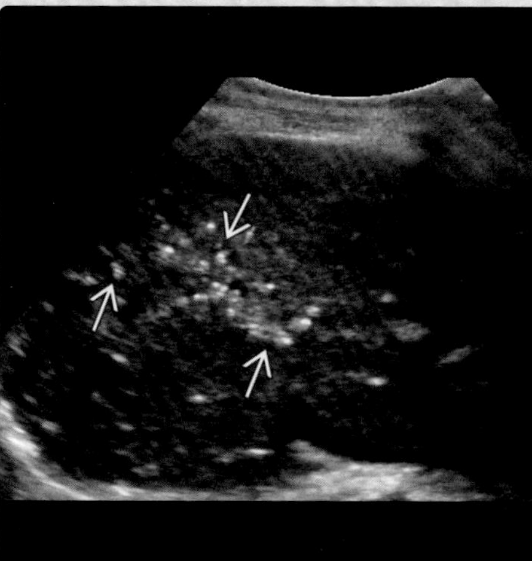

(Left) *Transverse transabdominal ultrasound shows a patchy, heterogeneous echotexture due to diffuse involvement ➡ by Candida microabscesses.* **(Right)** *Longitudinal ultrasound in the same patient 2 years after treatment for disseminated candidiasis shows multiple hyperechoic, punctate parenchymal calcifications ➡ typical of treated Candida microabscesses.*

Peribiliary Cyst

KEY FACTS

TERMINOLOGY

- Cystic dilatation of obstructed periductal glands of bile ducts
- Retention cyst of peribiliary gland

IMAGING

- Well-defined, cystic structures adjacent to portal triads
- Usually multiple; discrete, round/oval/tubular, or confluent configuration
- Variable size, from 2 mm to 2 cm
- Smooth and thin walls without internal echoes
- No enhancement of contents on CECT or MR
- Nonopacification with direct cholangiography or hepatobiliary-phase MR using hepatocyte-specific contrast agent
  - Do not communicate with biliary tree

TOP DIFFERENTIAL DIAGNOSES

- Biliary ductal dilatation
- Caroli disease
- Hepatic autosomal dominant polycystic disease
- Periportal edema/inflammation

PATHOLOGY

- Disturbed portal venous flow, periductal fibrosis, and inflammation → obliteration of neck of peribiliary glands → formation of retention cyst
- Associated with chronic hepatitis, cirrhosis, portal hypertension, portal vein thrombosis, liver transplantation

CLINICAL ISSUES

- Peribiliary cysts are typically asymptomatic; symptoms often related to underlying liver disease
- Obstructive jaundice may occur in end-stage liver cirrhosis or as complication of postliver transplantation

SCANNING TIPS

- Do not confuse peribiliary cysts for biliary ductal dilatation

(Left) *Grayscale ultrasound shows numerous small peribiliary cysts ➡ clustered in a linear configuration located along the portal vein ⇨.* **(Right)** *Color Doppler ultrasound in the same patient confirms the peribiliary cysts ➡ are located adjacent to the portal vein ⇨. Peribiliary cysts should not be confused with biliary ductal dilatation, which would have a more tubular and continuous appearance adjacent to the portal vein.*

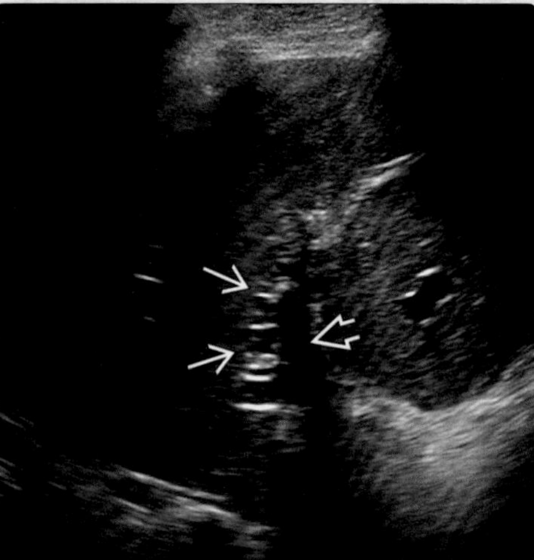

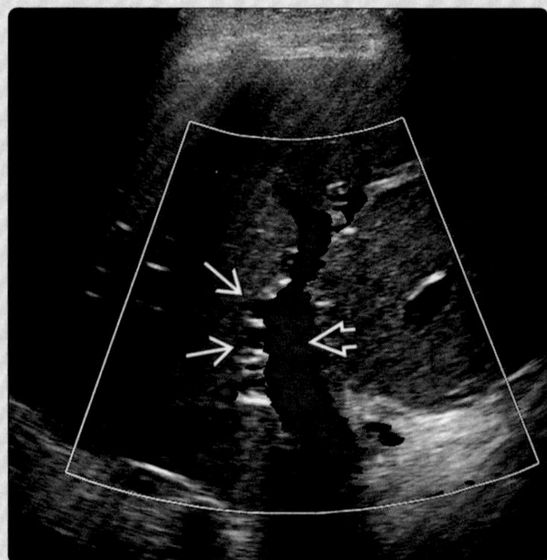

(Left) *Longitudinal grayscale ultrasound shows numerous clustered small peribiliary cysts ➡ coursing along the hepatic hilum.* **(Right)** *Transverse color Doppler ultrasound shows small peribiliary cysts ➡ adjacent to the portal vein ⇨ and a proximal intrahepatic portal vein branch ↗.*

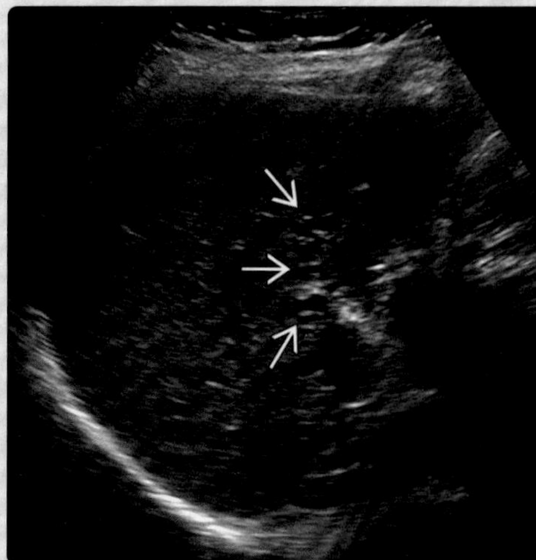

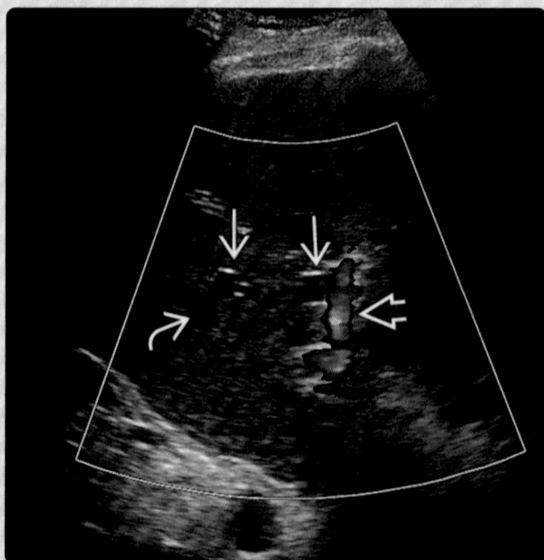

KEY FACTS

TERMINOLOGY

- Benign tumor composed of dilated vascular channels lined by single layer of endothelial cells and supported by thin, fibrous stroma

IMAGING

- Typical hemangioma: Well-defined, uniformly hyperechoic mass
- Internal vascularity often undetectable with color Doppler
- May see posterior acoustic enhancement
- "Typical atypical" hemangioma: Hyperechoic rim with hypoechoic center
- Contrast-enhanced imaging
  - Arterial hyperenhancement: "Flash fill" homogeneous hypervascularity or nodular discontinuous hyperenhancement
  - Centripetal fill-in on later images
  - Enhancement follows blood pool

TOP DIFFERENTIAL DIAGNOSES

- Focal steatosis
- Hepatocellular carcinoma
- Hypervascular metastases
- Focal nodular hyperplasia
- Hepatic adenoma

PATHOLOGY

- Large vascular channels lined by single layer of endothelial cells supported by thin, fibrous septa
- Most common benign tumor of liver

SCANNING TIPS

- Hemangiomas may change in echogenicity at different times of scanning due to rate of blood flow within lesion
- To help improve visualization, try B-color ultrasound or 9-MHz linear transducer for more superficially located lesions

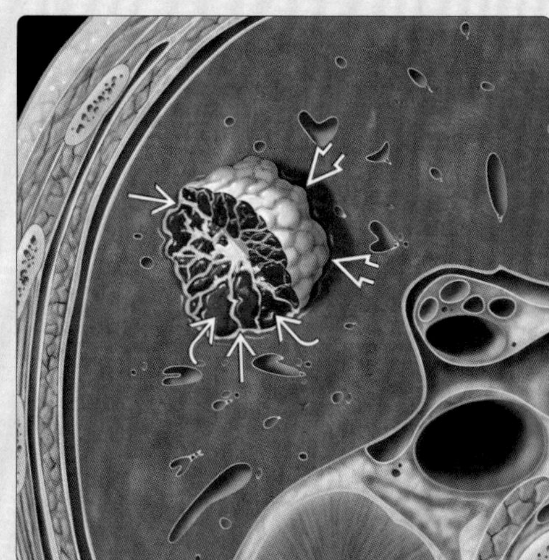

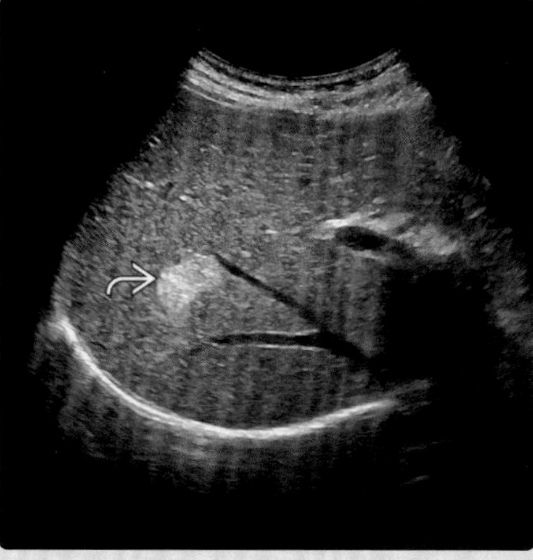

(Left) *Transverse graphic shows a solitary hemangioma, illustrating the lobular contour ➡ and multiple internal fibrous septa ➡, which are separating vascular channels ➡.* **(Right)** *Transverse ultrasound of the right lobe of the liver shows a typical hemangioma ➡, which is homogeneously echogenic with well-defined margins.*

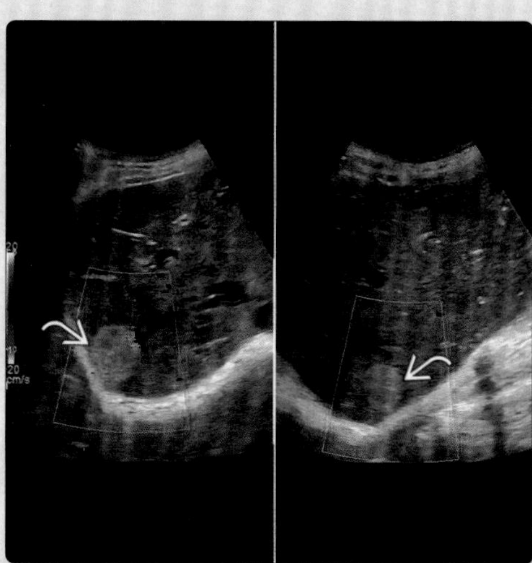

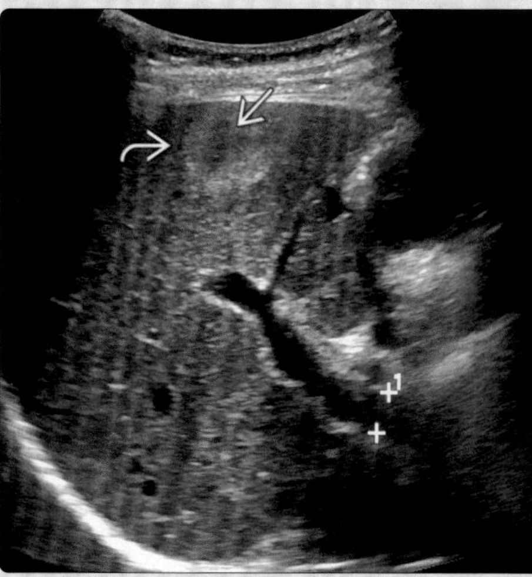

(Left) *Transverse and longitudinal color Doppler ultrasounds show a well-defined, echogenic hemangioma ➡ without detectable internal vascularity.* **(Right)** *Transverse grayscale ultrasound of the liver shows a "typical atypical" hemangioma with a well-defined, echogenic periphery ➡ and hypoechoic center ➡.*

KEY FACTS

TERMINOLOGY

- Focal nodular hyperplasia (FNH)
- Benign tumor of liver caused by hyperplastic response to localized vascular abnormality

IMAGING

- US
  - Usually homogeneous and isoechoic
  - Spoke-wheel pattern on color Doppler US
    - Large central feeding artery with multiple small vessels radiating peripherally
- CEUS/CT/MR
  - Bright, homogeneously enhancing mass in centrifugal direction on arterial phase (CEUS) with delayed enhancement of central scar (CT/MR)
- Gadoxetate-enhanced MR
  - Prolonged enhancement of entire FNH on hepatobiliary phase scan

TOP DIFFERENTIAL DIAGNOSES

- Hepatic adenoma
- Fibrolamellar hepatocellular carcinoma
- Hepatic cavernous hemangioma
- Hypervascular metastasis

PATHOLOGY

- Normal hepatocytes and malformed bile ductules
- Thick-walled arteries in fibrous septa radiating from center to periphery

CLINICAL ISSUES

- Common in young to middle-aged women
- Excellent prognosis

SCANNING TIPS

- Look for radiating vessels that flow in centrifugal direction (away from center) with color Doppler

(Left) *Graphic shows a homogeneous, vascular, nonencapsulated mass ➡ with a central scar and thin, radiating septa dividing the mass into hyperplastic nodules. Note the cluster of small arteries near the central scar.* **(Right)** *Liver wedge resection shows a well-circumscribed nodular lesion with a central stellate scar ⇒, typical of focal nodular hyperplasia. (Courtesy M. Yeh, MD, PhD.)*

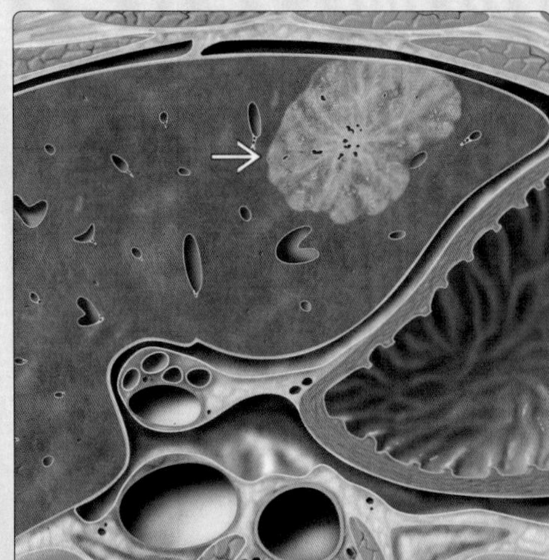

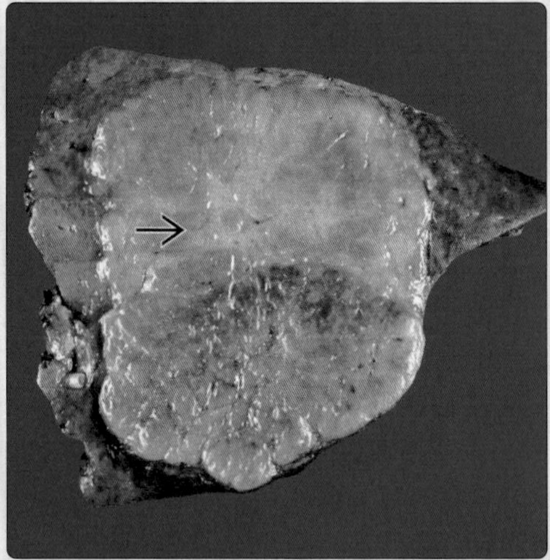

(Left) *Longitudinal transabdominal US shows an isoechoic focal nodular hyperplasia in the caudate lobe of liver ➡. The mass causes contour deformity and mass effect upon the adjacent gallbladder and portal vein ➡. The lesion is difficult to distinguish from the surrounding liver, earning its moniker "stealth lesion."* **(Right)** *Transverse power Doppler US shows centrifugal blood flow away ➡ from the central scar ➡ of a large focal nodular hyperplasia, giving a spoke-wheel vascularity pattern.*

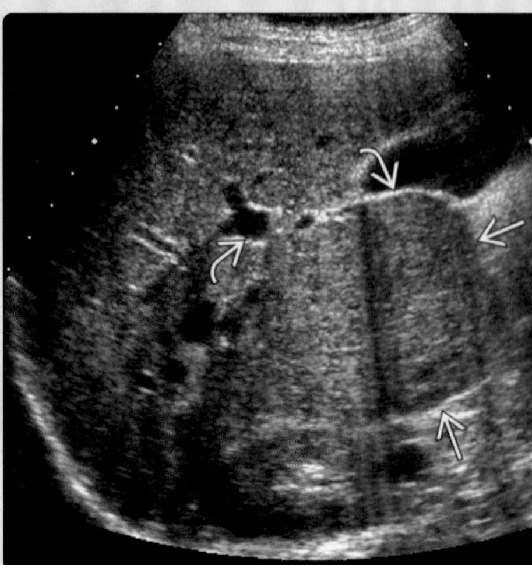

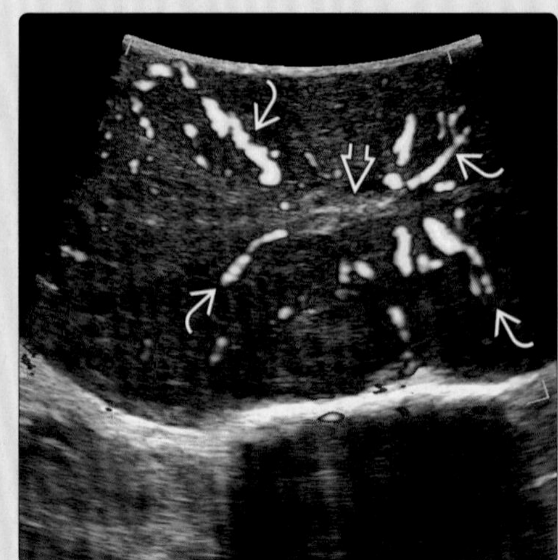

KEY FACTS

TERMINOLOGY

- Hepatocellular adenoma (HCA) or liver cell adenoma
- 2nd most frequent hepatic tumor in young women after focal nodular hyperplasia (FNH)

IMAGING

- Heterogeneous, hypervascular, hypo-/iso-/hyperechoic mass
- Round or mildly lobulated, well-defined borders
- Larger lesions prone to intratumoral hemorrhage or rupture with intraperitoneal hemorrhage

TOP DIFFERENTIAL DIAGNOSES

- Hemangioma
- FNH
- Hepatocellular carcinoma

CLINICAL ISSUES

- Potential complications: ± hemorrhage, malignant degeneration
- More common in younger women on oral contraceptive pill (OCP)
- Definitive diagnosis and subtype with biopsy
- Molecular classification (4 subtypes) helps determine prognosis and management
    - **β-catenin-activated HCA**: 10%
        - Prone to malignant degeneration
    - **Inflammatory (I-HCA)**: 40-50%
        - More common in women on OCP, obese, or metabolic syndrome
        - Greatest risk of hemorrhage (up to 30%)
        - Malignant degeneration: 5-10%
    - **HNF-1α**: 30-35%
        - More common in women on OCP
        - Often asymptomatic, lowest risk of malignant transformation
    - **Unclassified HCA**: 10%

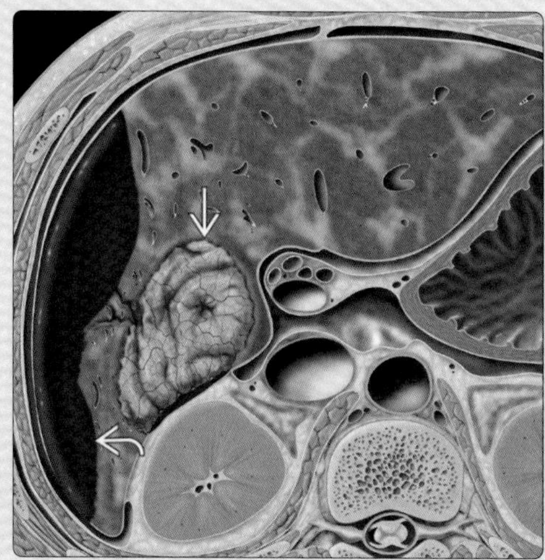

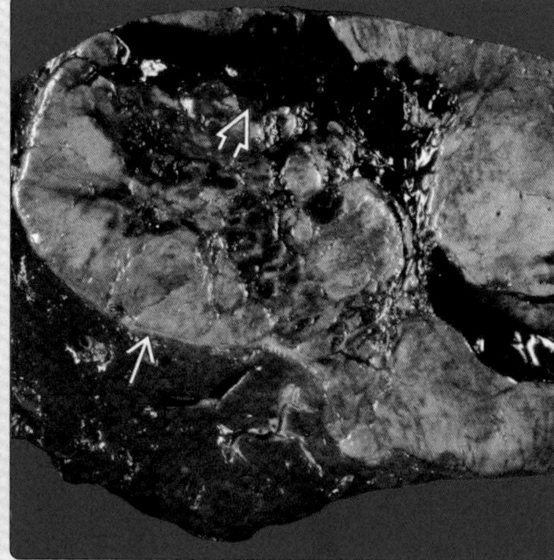

(Left) *Axial graphic shows a hypervascular liver adenoma ➡ in the right lobe and spontaneous subcapsular bleeding ➡, a potential complication of hepatic adenomas.* **(Right)** *Gross photograph of a resected specimen shows a large adenoma ➡ with central areas of rupture and hemorrhage ➡. (Courtesy M. Yeh, MD, PhD.)*

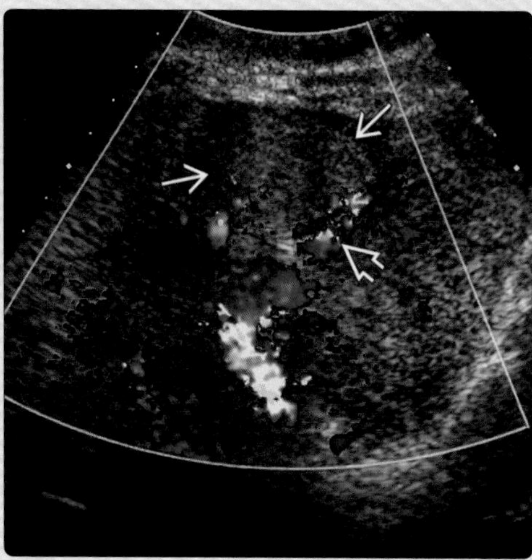

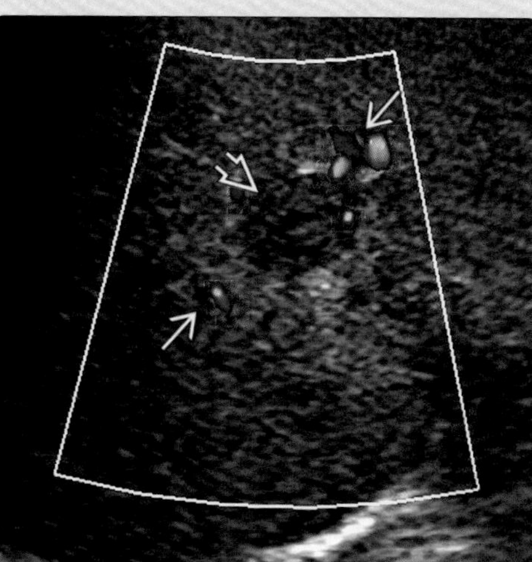

(Left) *Transverse color Doppler ultrasound shows the left lobe of the liver in a patient with a hyperechoic adenoma ➡ with large peripheral vessels ➡.* **(Right)** *Transverse color Doppler ultrasound shows peripheral large vessels ➡ bordering a hypoechoic hepatic adenoma ➡.*

Hepatocellular Carcinoma

KEY FACTS

TERMINOLOGY

- Hepatocellular carcinoma (HCC)
  - Primary malignancy of liver arising from hepatocytes
- Synonyms: Hepatoma, primary liver cancer

IMAGING

- Ultrasound: Primary test for screening/surveillance for HCC
  - Solid, intrahepatic mass may be hypoechoic (most common), hyperechoic, or isoechoic
  - May see hypoechoic halo, mild posterior acoustic enhancement, or internal vascularity on color Doppler
  - Infiltrative tumors often difficult to visualize margins; look for refractive edge shadows, parenchymal distortion, or loss of normal echogenic portal triads, which are helpful secondary findings
  - Portal vein or hepatic vein tumor invasion highly suggestive of HCC
- Contrast-enhanced CT, MR, or CEUS: For characterization
  - Arterial hyperenhancement and portal/delayed washout

CLINICAL ISSUES

- Screening/surveillance ultrasound every 6 months recommended for the following populations in USA
  - Cirrhosis (60-90%) from any cause
  - Noncirrhotic chronic Hepatitis B in certain populations

SCANNING TIPS

- Liver dome lesions are often missed; angle transducer to image above HV to completely visualize liver dome
- RT and LT inferior tip of liver lesions are easily missed; carefully scan through very inferior portions of liver
- Anterior lesions often poorly visualized with curvilinear or vector transducers; diligent use of 9-MHz linear probe helps visualization of superficial portions of liver
- Trying multiple probes, positions, and windows are key to improve detection; some liver lesions may only be seen on left lateral decubitus position (vs. supine) or intercostal approach (vs. subcostal)

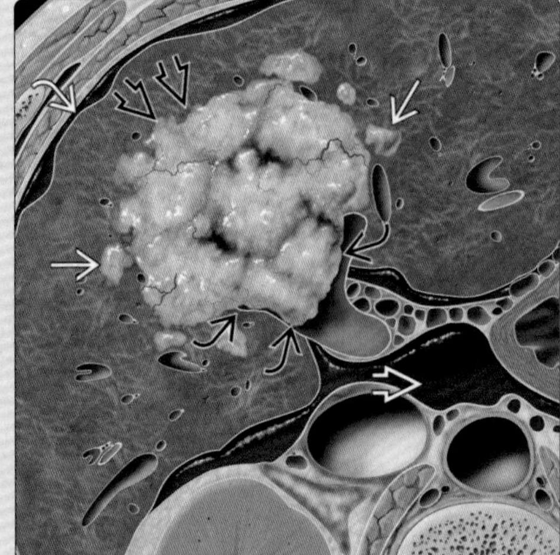

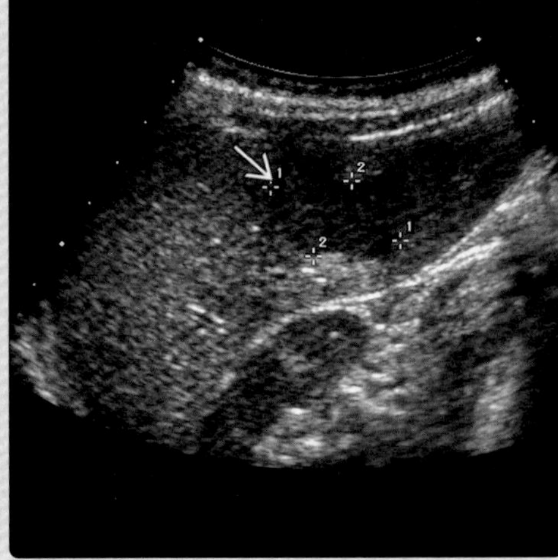

(Left) *Graphic shows a heterogeneous, hypervascular hepatocellular carcinoma (HCC) ➡. Numerous adjacent satellite nodules ➡ and portal vein invasion ➡ are depicted. Underlying liver disease is evident given the nodular liver capsule ➡ and ascites ➡.* **(Right)** *Longitudinal grayscale ultrasound of the liver shows a hypoechoic, solid HCC mass ➡. In the setting of chronic hepatitis, this is suspicious for HCC and should be further characterized with contrast-enhanced multiphasic CT, contrast-enhanced MR, or contrast-enhanced US.*

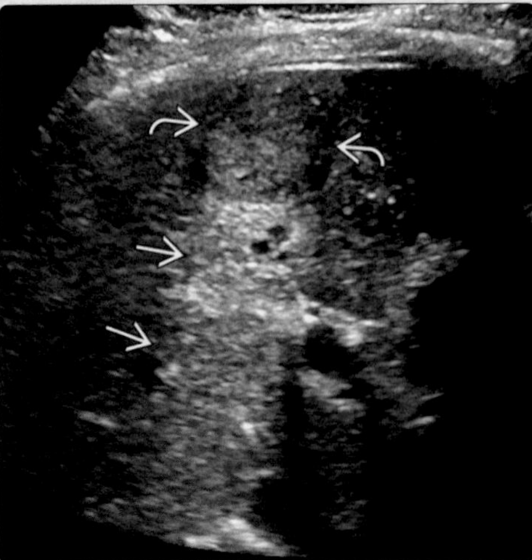

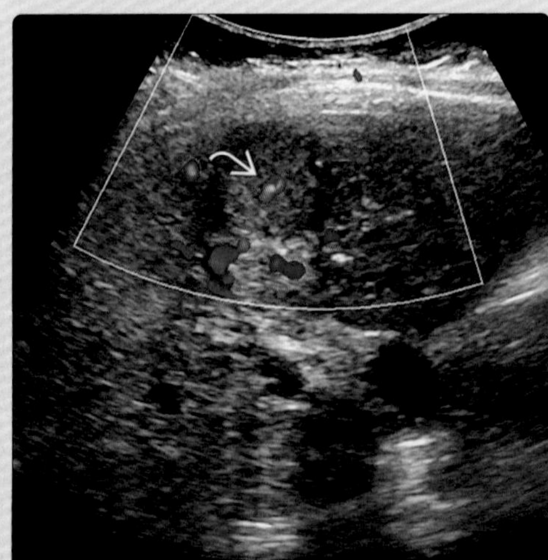

(Left) *Transverse grayscale ultrasound of the liver shows a slightly hyperechoic, solid HCC ➡ with a hypoechoic halo and slight posterior acoustic enhancement ➡, occasionally seen with HCC.* **(Right)** *Color Doppler ultrasound of the same patient shows detectable internal vascularity ➡ in the HCC.*

KEY FACTS

TERMINOLOGY

- Malignant spread of neoplasm to hepatic parenchyma

IMAGING

- Grayscale ultrasound
  - Hypoechoic metastasis: Usually from hypovascular tumors
  - Hyperechoic metastasis: Hypervascular metastasis
  - "Bull's-eye" or "target" metastatic lesions: Solid mass with hypoechoic rim or halo
  - Cystic/necrotic metastases: Mural nodules, thick walls, fluid-fluid levels, internal septa/debris
  - Calcified metastases: Mucinous or ossific primaries
  - Infiltrative/diffuse metastases: Lung or breast primary; may mimic cirrhosis, especially treated breast cancer, which can have pseudocirrhosis appearance
- Color Doppler ultrasound
  - Metastatic lesions follow vascularity of primary tumor
  - Contrast-enhanced ultrasound increases detectability of hepatic metastases

TOP DIFFERENTIAL DIAGNOSES

- Cysts (vs. hypoechoic or cystic metastases)
- Abscesses (vs. hypoechoic metastases)
- Hemangiomas (vs. hyperechoic metastases)
- Multifocal hepatocellular carcinomas or cholangiocarcinomas (vs. "target" lesion)
- Steatosis (vs. hypo-/hyperechoic metastasis)
- Hepatic adenomatosis

CLINICAL ISSUES

- Most common malignant tumor of liver

SCANNING TIPS

- Rule out other other causes of multiple liver lesions, e.g., hepatic cysts, abscesses, or hemangiomas
- Always correlate with clinical history and look for evidence of primary tumor

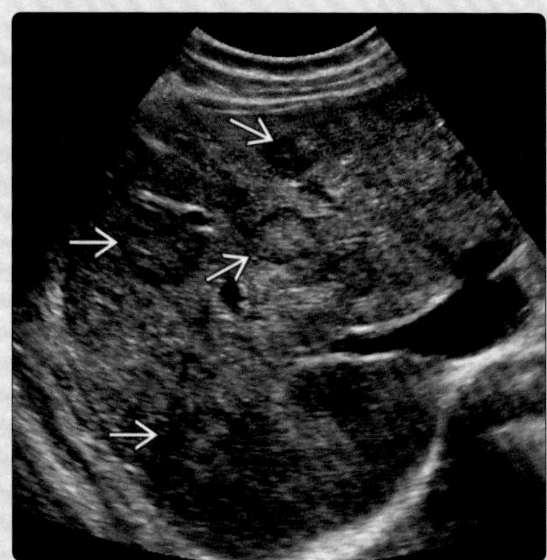

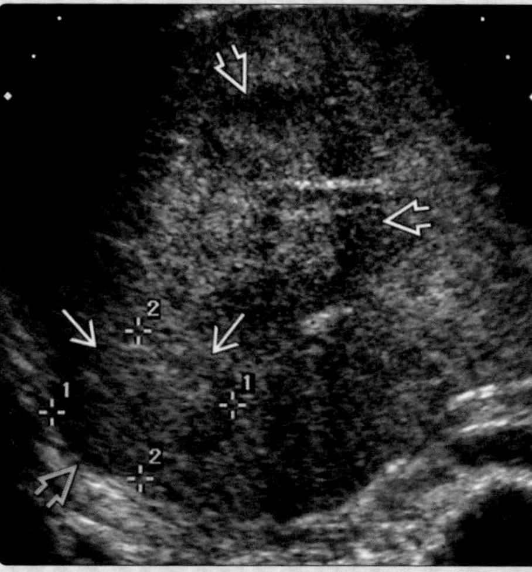

(Left) *Transverse grayscale ultrasound in a patient with breast cancer metastases to the liver shows that the metastases have a classic target appearance ➡ in which rounded lesions are surrounded by a hypoechoic rim.* **(Right)** *Oblique transabdominal ultrasound in a patient with breast cancer shows a minimally hypoechoic, solid metastasis ➡ in the right lobe of the liver, bulging its contour ⇨, as well as other numerous, more subtle, hypoechoic solid masses ➡.*

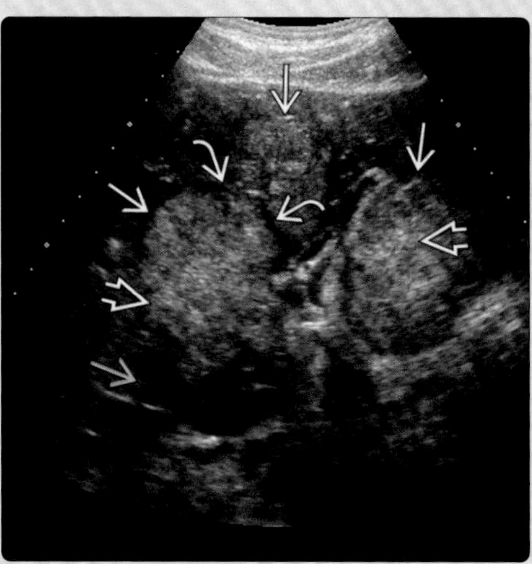

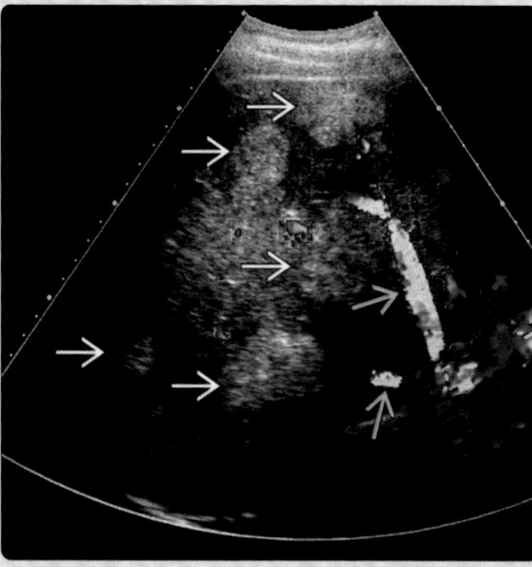

(Left) *Transverse ultrasound in a patient with mucinous colon cancer metastases to the liver demonstrates multiple large, hyperechoic metastases ➡ containing diffuse echogenic foci ➡ related to subtle calcifications. Note posterior acoustic shadowing ⇨ as well as distortion and compression of the right portal vein ➡ by metastases.* **(Right)** *Color Doppler ultrasound of the liver in the same patient with mucinous colon cancer shows multiple hyperechoic metastases ➡ throughout the liver, some of which abut and distort the hepatic veins ⇨.*

Hepatic Lymphoma

KEY FACTS

TERMINOLOGY

- Neoplasm of lymphoid tissues in liver

IMAGING

- Hepatic lymphoma often favors periportal areas due to high content of lymphatic tissue
- Grayscale ultrasound
  - Discrete form: Multiple well-defined, hypoechoic masses
    - Hypoechogenicity due to high cellular density and lack of background stroma
  - Infiltrative form: Innumerable subcentimeter hypoechoic foci, miliary in pattern and periportal in location
    - May be indistinguishable from normal liver
- CECT
  - Solid lesions with poor contrast enhancement
  - Usually homogeneous density and rarely necrotic
  - May have thin rim enhancement
  - Diffuse, infiltrative, low-density areas

TOP DIFFERENTIAL DIAGNOSES

- Metastases
- Multifocal/diffuse hepatocellular carcinoma (HCC)
- Liver abscesses
- Hemangiomas
- Focal fat infiltration/sparing
- Hepatic cysts

CLINICAL ISSUES

- Primary hepatic lymphoma is rare
- Secondary hepatic involvement is more common

SCANNING TIPS

- Hepatic lymphoma often has pseudocystic appearance; lack of specular reflection of backwall is helpful clue that lesions are not cystic and rather solid markedly hypoechoic masses

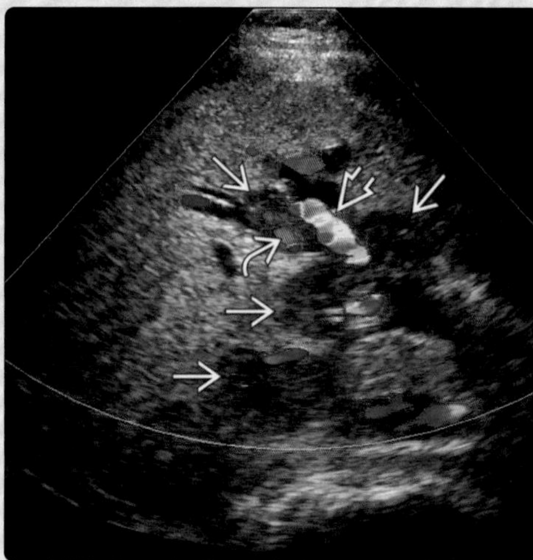

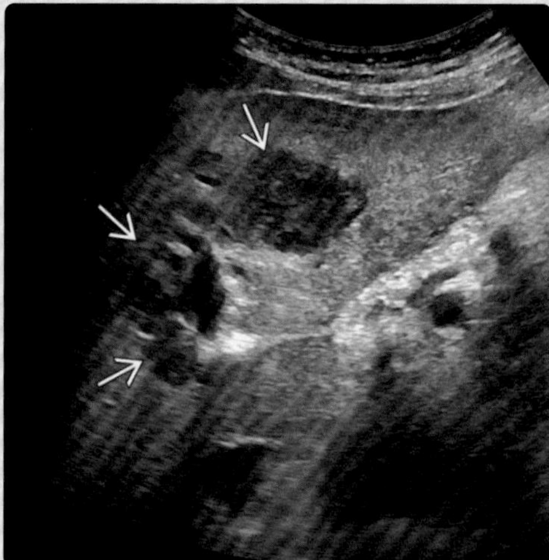

(Left) *Transverse color Doppler ultrasound in a patient with lymphoma involving the liver shows multiple hypoechoic masses ➡ in a periportal distribution (right anterior portal vein) ➡ in the liver. Lesions are predominantly hypovascular with minimal vascularity seen along the periphery ➡.* **(Right)** *Transverse abdominal grayscale ultrasound in a patient with lymphoma shows several hypoechoic masses ➡ in a periportal distribution in the left lobe of the liver.*

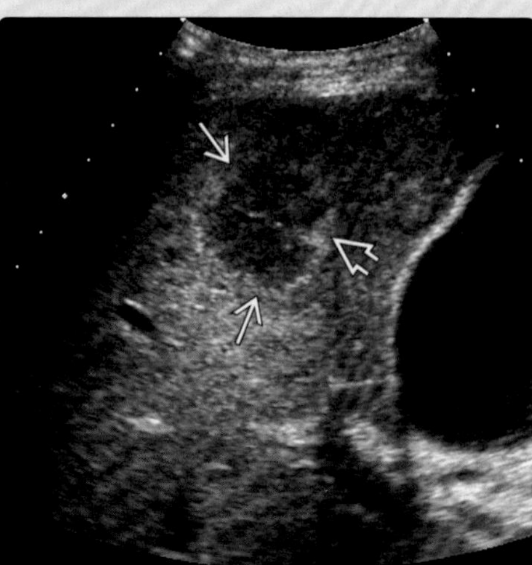

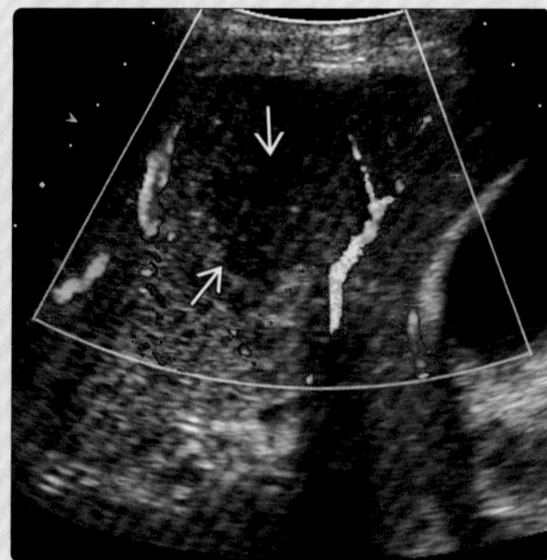

(Left) *Transverse abdominal grayscale ultrasound in the same patient shows a well-defined, hypoechoic mass ➡ with a thin, hyperechoic rim ➡ in segment 5 of the liver.* **(Right)** *Transverse color Doppler ultrasound performed in the same patient shows no detectable vascular flow within the lymphomatous mass ➡.*

KEY FACTS

TERMINOLOGY

- Shunt between main portal vein and hepatic vein created with balloon-expandable covered metallic stent

IMAGING

- Goal of US: Detection of stenosis before shunt occludes or symptoms recur
- Best imaging tool
  - US as primary transjugular intrahepatic portasystemic shunt (TIPS) surveillance tool
  - CTA/MRA indicated if US technically compromised or equivocal
- Doppler US findings of TIPS malfunction
  - Portal vein
    - Hepatofugal flow
    - Peak velocity < 35 cm/s
  - Within shunt
    - Peak velocity < 90 cm/s or > 200 cm/s at any point
    - Temporal change in peak velocity > 50 cm/s

PATHOLOGY

- Stenosis usually secondary to intimal hyperplasia from hepatic venous side
- Hepatic encephalopathy if portal flow bypasses liver

CLINICAL ISSUES

- Most common symptoms/signs of stent malfunction
  - Variceal hemorrhage
  - Signs of worsening portal hypertension with increasing ascites

SCANNING TIPS

- Although typical scanning protocol is to measure velocity at proximal (portal end), mid, and distal (hepatic venous end), look for areas of aliasing and measure flow velocity in these areas to improve sensitivity for stenosis
- Due to high velocities commonly seen in shunts, increase PRF scale to eliminate "artificial" aliasing, which may obscure stenotic areas and direction of flow

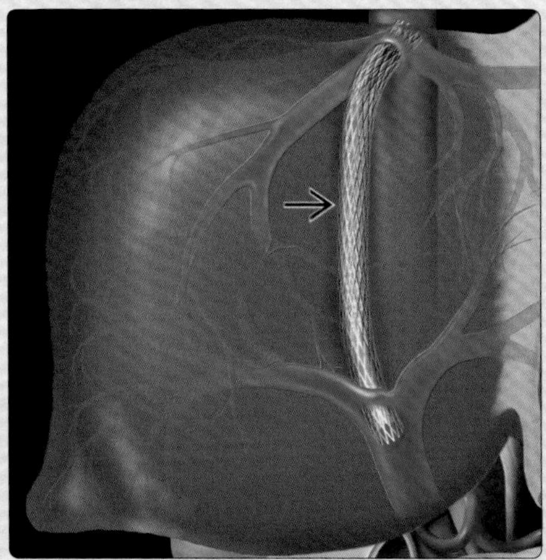

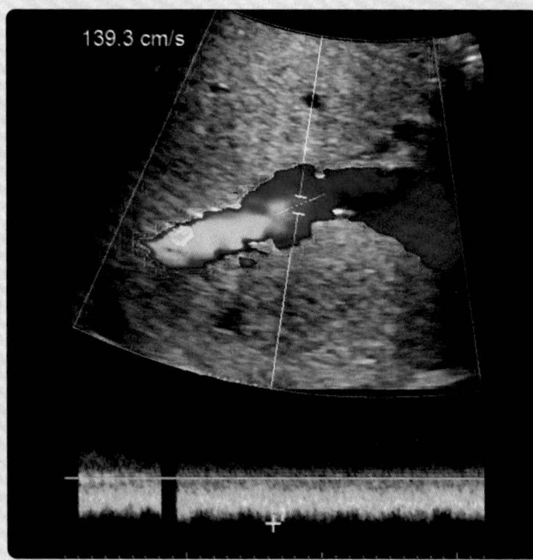

(Left) *Graphic shows transjugular intrahepatic portasystemic shunt (TIPS) shunt creation. The hepatic vein is punctured within 2 cm of the inferior vena cava. A covered stent ➙ is placed between the hepatic venous end and the right portal vein, adjacent to its junction with the main portal vein.* **(Right)** *Spectral Doppler US of a TIPS with interrogation at the proximal (portal venous) portion shows appropriate flow direction and velocity of 139 cm/s.*

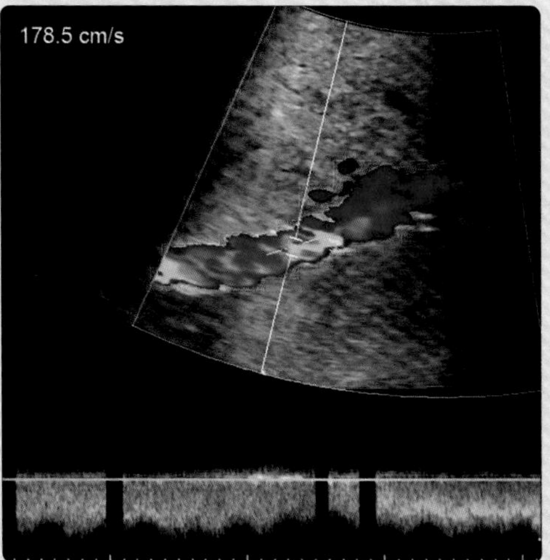

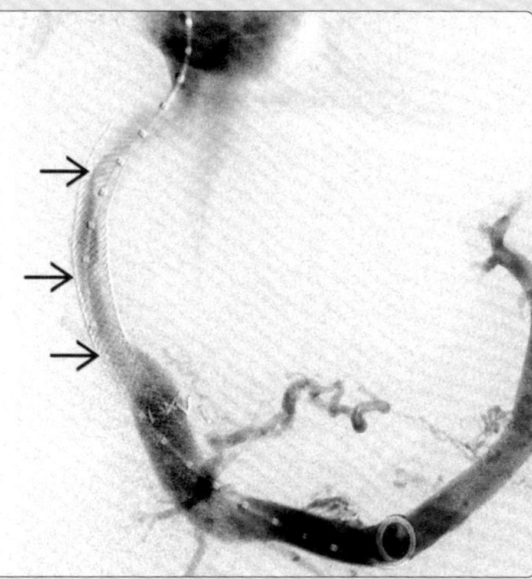

(Left) *Spectral Doppler US in the same patient in the mid TIPS shows slight increase in velocity to 178 cm/s, which is still within normal limits. Angle correction should always be used when evaluating TIPS for accurate velocity measurement.* **(Right)** *Anteroposterior supine portal angiogram in a 66-year-old man with a suspected TIPS stenosis based on Doppler US reveals multiple areas of intimal hyperplasia within the parenchymal portion of the shunt ➙, consistent with stenosis.*

Portal Hypertension

KEY FACTS

TERMINOLOGY

- Portal hypertension: Pressure gradient > 12 mm Hg between main portal vein (PV) and IVC &/or hepatic veins

IMAGING

- Ultrasound for 1st-line evaluation of portal hypertension
  - Best tool for dynamic evaluation of portal venous system
- Large main PV
  - > 16 mm in maximal diameter
- Presence of portosystemic collateral vessels
- May also see slow flow in main PV, to-and-fro or bidirectional PV, or reversal of flow in PVs
- Coronary vein, a.k.a. left gastric vein, can become dilated in portal hypertension
- PVs including main portal, left portal, and anterior and posterior branches of right PV evaluated with both grayscale and color Doppler in longitudinal plane; spectral Doppler waveform analysis also performed on all vessels in longitudinal plane

PATHOLOGY

- Increased portal pressures causes portal blood flow to divert into portosystemic collaterals, eventually resulting in increased resistance and reversal of flow in PVs
- Intrahepatic etiologies most common cause of portal hypertension

CLINICAL ISSUES

- Patients often asymptomatic; clinical manifestations can include splenomegaly, abdominal wall collateral vessels, and thrombocytopenia
- Pathophysiology unclear, but thought to arise from hepatic inflammation with cellular regeneration, resulting in increased pressure in portal venous system

SCANNING TIPS

- PV diameter on deep inspiration higher than on expiration; thus PV diameter measured during deep inspiration may overestimate true diameter

(Left) *Longitudinal grayscale US demonstrates an enlarged main portal vein (calipers) measuring 18 mm.* **(Right)** *Color Doppler US shows a dilated main portal vein.*

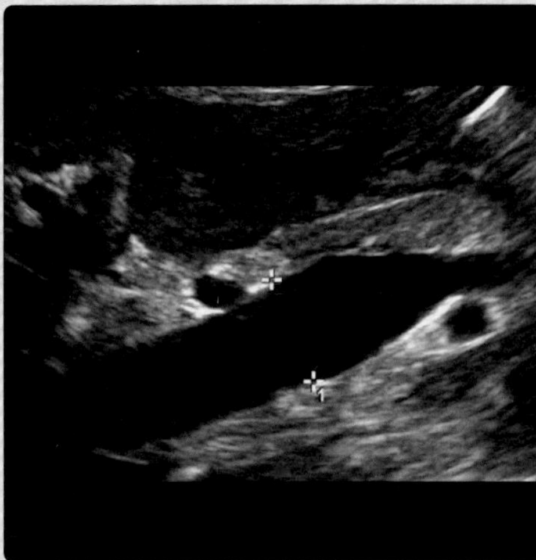

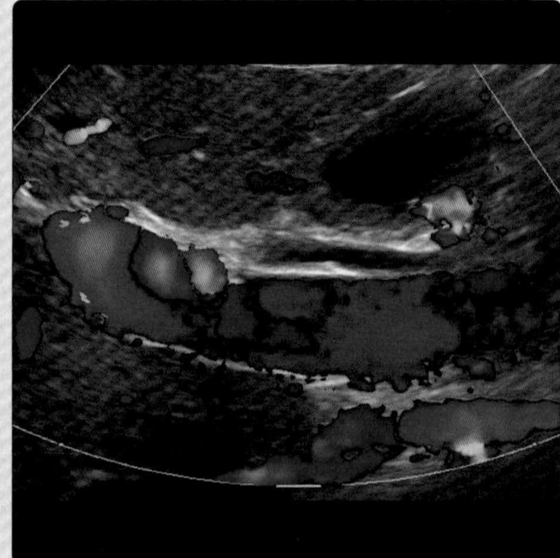

(Left) *Color and spectral Doppler US of a main portal vein demonstrate normal direction of flow with slow flow (velocity 7.9 cm/s).* **(Right)** *Spectral Doppler US of the left portal vein demonstrates to-and-fro flow.*

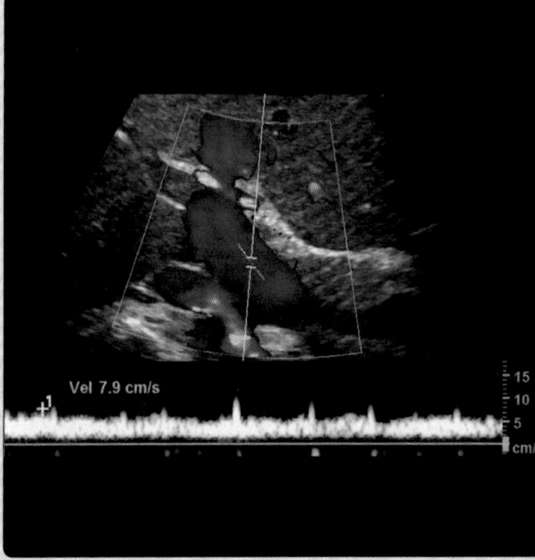

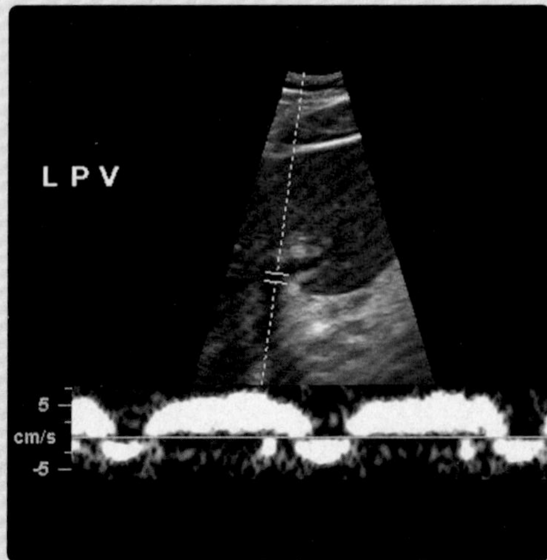

KEY FACTS

TERMINOLOGY

- Definition: Obstruction of PV due to thrombosis

IMAGING

- Absent blood flow within PV on color or spectral Doppler
- Cavernous transformation of PV: Multiple portal venous collaterals develop anterior to thrombosed PV
- May see hypertrophied and high-velocity hepatic artery, which compensates for thrombosed PV

TOP DIFFERENTIAL DIAGNOSES

- Nonocclusive thrombosis
- False-positive PV occlusion
- Tumor in vein (tumor thrombus)
- Splenic vein occlusion
- Dilated bile duct

PATHOLOGY

- Etiology
  - Thrombosis due to flow stasis, hypercoagulability, intraabdominal inflammation
  - Tumor in vein (formerly referred to as tumor thrombus) or direct tumor invasion
- Acute thrombosis
  - Lumen filled with thrombus, diameter may be enlarged
- Chronic thrombosis
  - Thrombosis accompanied by cavernous transformation (collateralization in porta hepatis)

SCANNING TIPS

- Techniques to differentiate very slow flow vs. thrombus: Decrease color box width; place color focus position at or below vessel; decrease scale (PRF); increase color gain; increase color write priority; try B-flow mode; decrease wall filter; push on belly to propel portal venous blood
- Grayscale cine of PV (without moving transducer) may show slow flow not detectable with color Doppler
- Blooming on color Doppler may obscure small thrombus

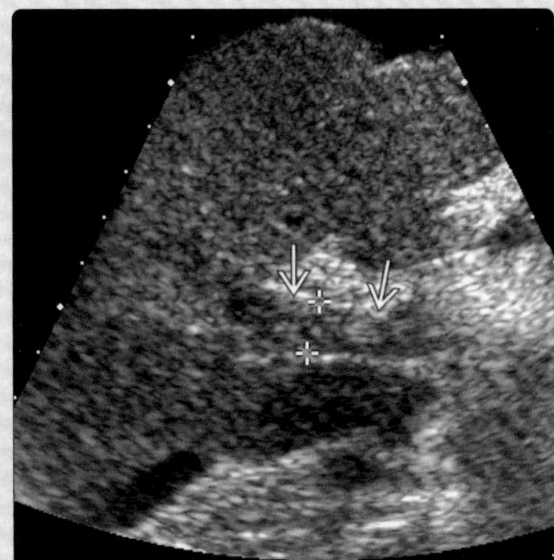

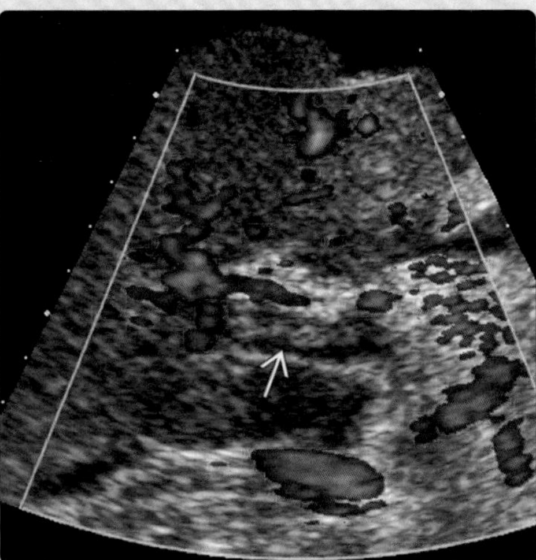

(Left) *Grayscale ultrasound of the liver shows mildly echogenic thrombus ➡ in the main portal vein.* **(Right)** *Power Doppler ultrasound in the same patient confirms absent flow within the thrombosed main portal vein ➡. Note the presence of ascites as well as underlying liver cirrhosis, which is a risk factor for development of portal vein thrombosis.*

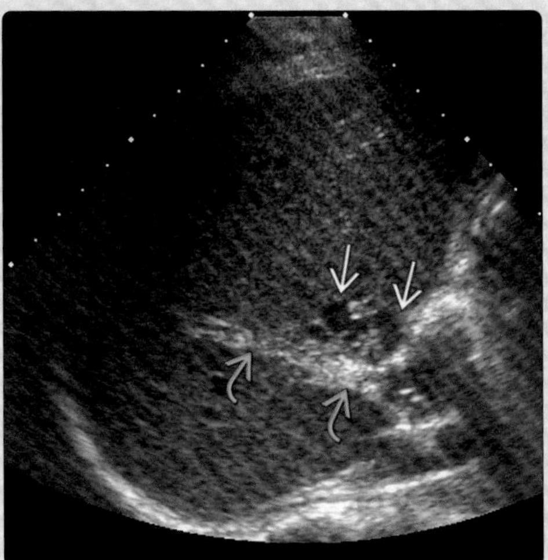

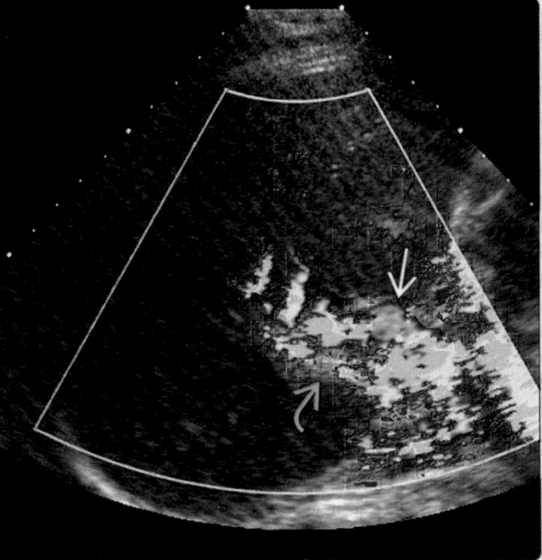

(Left) *Grayscale ultrasound shows an echogenic, chronically thrombosed main portal vein ➡ and adjacent collateralized flow ➡ (cavernous transformation of the portal vein).* **(Right)** *Color Doppler ultrasound in the same patient shows collateralized flow ➡ in the porta hepatis in this patient with chronic portal vein thrombosis ➡. Color Doppler signal is heterogeneous because portal vein collaterals are tortuous, resulting in flow going both toward as well as away from the transducer.*

KEY FACTS

TERMINOLOGY

- Budd-Chiari syndrome: Hepatic venous outflow obstruction
- Global or segmental obstruction of hepatic venous outflow or inferior vena cava (IVC)

IMAGING

- Ultrasound acute phase
  - Absent or restricted flow, possible thrombosis in hepatic veins (HVs)/IVC
  - Intrahepatic collateralization, bicolored HVs: Flow in opposite direction in HV branches with common trunk
  - Reduced velocity, continuous flow in portal vein, possibly hepatofugal flow
- Ultrasound chronic phase
  - Hypertrophy of caudate lobe and unaffected segments, atrophy of involved segments, large regenerative nodules
  - Stenotic or occluded HVs/IVC
  - Intrahepatic &/or extrahepatic collateralization
- CECT: Flip-flop enhancement pattern
  - Early enhancement of caudate lobe and central portion around IVC, decreased peripheral liver enhancement
  - Later decreased enhancement centrally and increased enhancement peripherally

TOP DIFFERENTIAL DIAGNOSES

- Liver cirrhosis
- Portal vein thrombosis
- Acute, severe passive venous congestion

SCANNING TIPS

- Use slow flow settings or B-flow imaging to show lack of flow in thrombosed hepatic veins
- May see bicolored HVs due to intrahepatic collateralization on color Doppler ultrasound
- Thrombosed HVs may be barely discernible or cord-like, requiring extra attention to locate on grayscale

(Left) *Axial graphic of Budd-Chiari syndrome demonstrates ascites, venous collaterals ➡, heterogeneous hepatic parenchyma due to centrilobular necrosis, and hypervascular regenerative nodules ➡. Note the sparing of the caudate lobe with hypertrophy ➡ as well as the thrombosed inferior vena cava (IVC).* **(Right)** *Color Doppler US shows a thrombosed middle hepatic vein ➡. Note tortuous collateral flow around occluded hepatic vein ➡.*

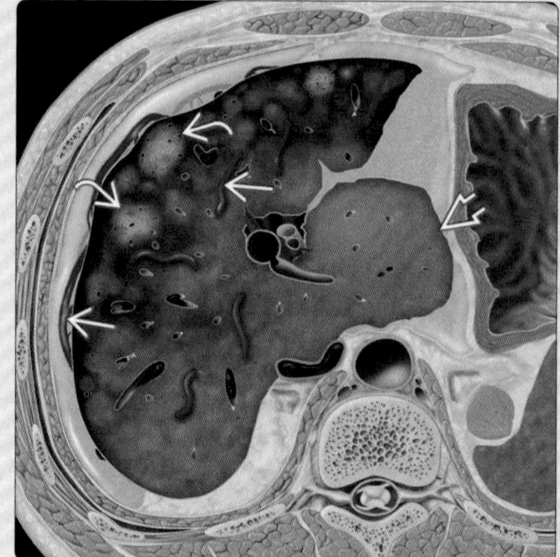

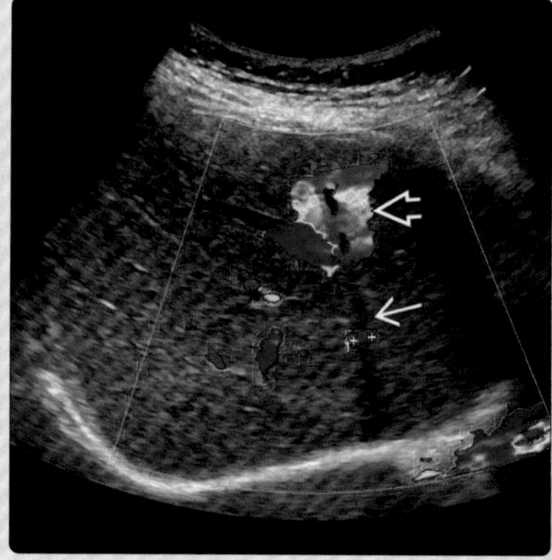

(Left) *Spectral Doppler US in the same patient demonstrates a lack of detectable flow in the middle hepatic vein ➡ on spectral tracing. Only noise ➡ is seen along the baseline of the tracing.* **(Right)** *,Color Doppler US reveals no detectable flow in the right hepatic vein ➡ with tortuous intrahepatic collateral vessels ➡ bypassing the occluded hepatic vein. Middle hepatic vein is bicolored in appearance ➡, and communication with the IVC is not seen.*

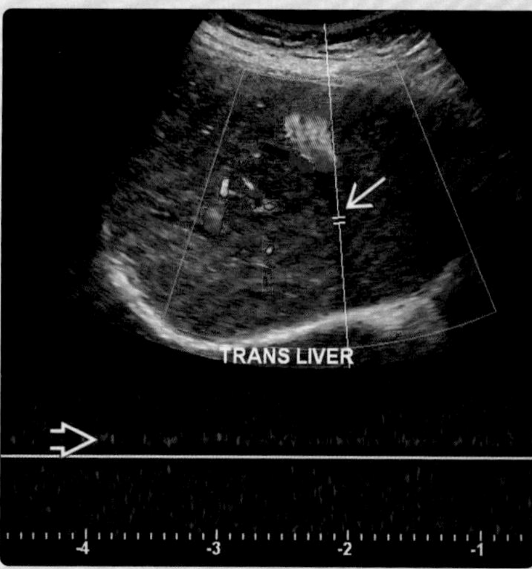

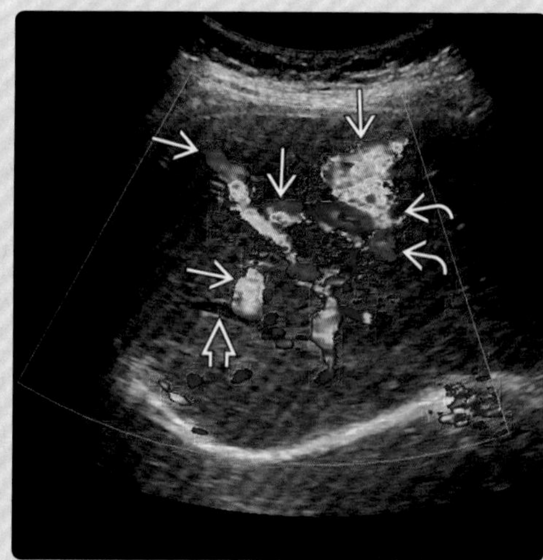

KEY FACTS

TERMINOLOGY

- Gas within portal venous system

IMAGING

- Grayscale ultrasound
  - Highly reflective foci in portal venous system
    - Move along with blood
  - Poorly defined, highly reflective parenchymal foci
    - Scattered small patches to numerous or large areas
- Pulsed Doppler ultrasound
  - High-intensity transient signals (HITS)
    - Strong transient spikes superimposed on portal venous flow pattern
- Color Doppler ultrasound
  - Bright reflectors in portal venous system

TOP DIFFERENTIAL DIAGNOSES

- Biliary tract gas
- Parenchymal abscess
- Biliary calculi/parenchymal calcifications
- Hepatic artery calcification

PATHOLOGY

- Serious conditions
  - Necrotizing enterocolitis, bowel ischemia/infarction
- Benign conditions
  - Bowel distension, intervention-related, benign pneumatosis intestinalis

CLINICAL ISSUES

- Often sign of serious condition; but can sometimes be inconsequential finding

SCANNING TIPS

- To distinguish rouleaux formation in slow-flow veins from gas bubbles, use spectral tracings, which will detect HITs that correspond to gas
- With B-flow imaging, portal venous gas may be more clearly delineated

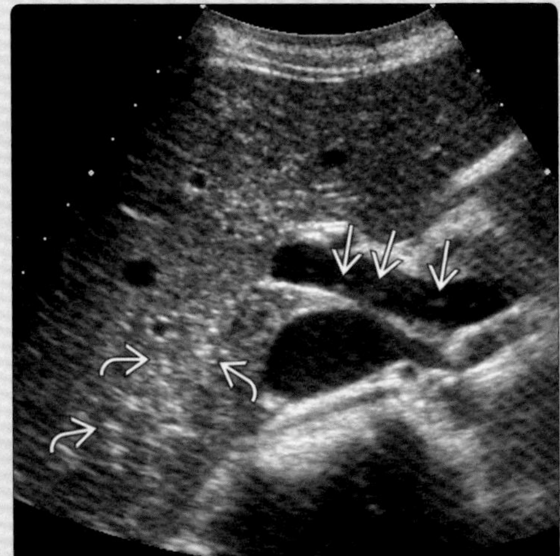

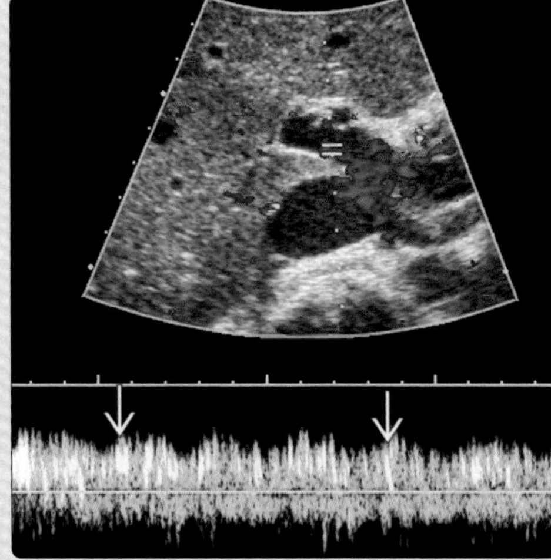

(Left) *Oblique ultrasound of the liver shows several echogenic foci in the portal vein ➡ representing gas bubbles. Brightly echogenic patches ➡ in the liver more peripherally represent parenchymal gas.* **(Right)** *Oblique pulsed Doppler ultrasound in the same patient with portal venous gas shows strong high-intensity transient signals (HITS) ➡ that appear as vertical spikes within the main portal vein interrogation. Spikes are in the same direction as the flow direction of the portal vein.*

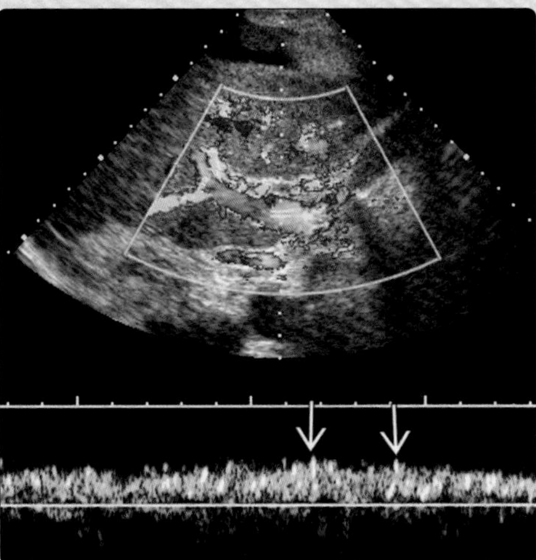

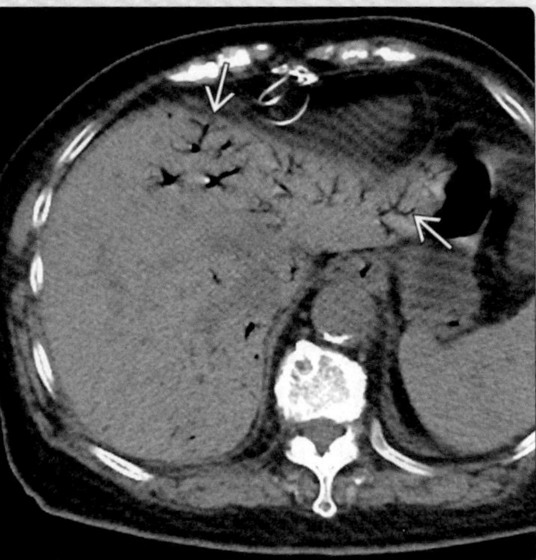

(Left) *Oblique abdominal pulsed Doppler ultrasound in a patient with portal venous gas secondary to small bowel ischemia and pneumatosis shows strong HITS ➡ superimposed upon the main portal vein waveform.* **(Right)** *Axial NECT shows extensive portal venous gas ➡ branching peripherally in the portal veins of the liver. Peripheral predominance of portal venous gas helps distinguish it from biliary gas, which tends to be more centrally located.*

KEY FACTS

IMAGING

- **Hepatic artery stenosis**
  - Elevated peak systolic velocity at anastomosis > 200-250 cm/s
  - Parvus tardus waveforms in intrahepatic arteries
    - Acceleration time > 0.08 s
    - Resistive index < 0.5
- **Hepatic artery thrombosis**
  - No detectable flow in hepatic artery with color or spectral Doppler
  - May see "collateral transformation of hepatic artery"
    - Tortuous collateral arteries in porta hepatis and parvus tardus intrahepatic arterial waveforms

PATHOLOGY

- **Hepatic artery stenosis**
  - Stenosis occurs at anastomosis
  - Usually occurs at > 3 months post transplant
- **Hepatic artery thrombosis**
  - May occur < 15 days or years after transplant
  - Risk factors: Difference in hepatic artery caliber between donor and recipient, prolonged graft ischemia time, ABO blood group incompatibility, CMV infection, acute or chronic rejection, hypercoagulable state, sepsis

CLINICAL ISSUES

- **Hepatic artery stenosis**
  - May be related to injury at time of surgery or disruption of vasa vasorum with ischemia of hepatic artery
- **Hepatic artery thrombosis**
  - Most common immediate vascular complication (2-12%)
  - Complete occlusion of hepatic artery in early transplant period leads to liver failure
    - Up to 75% of patients with hepatic artery thrombosis require retransplantation
  - Biliary ducts in liver transplants supplied only by artery
    - Hepatic artery thrombosis can result in biliary ischemia, bilomas, bile lakes

(Left) *Graphic depicts focal stenosis ➡ of the hepatic artery anastomosis in a liver transplant.* **(Right)** *Spectral Doppler evaluation of the main hepatic artery near the site of anastomosis shows an elevated hepatic artery velocity of 236 cm/s ➡, which is consistent with a stenosis.*

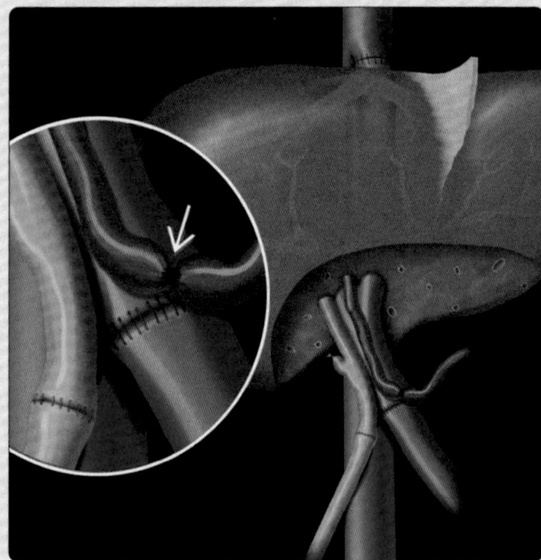

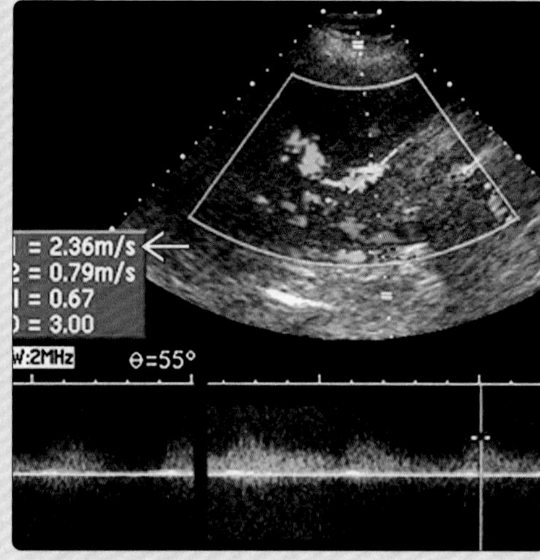

(Left) *Angiographic image in the same patient confirms a focal stenosis ⇨ in the hepatic artery at the level of the anastomosis.* **(Right)** *Volume-rendered CT angiogram of the aorta and celiac artery shows an abrupt termination ➡ of the hepatic artery, consistent with hepatic artery thrombosis in a patient with a liver transplant.*

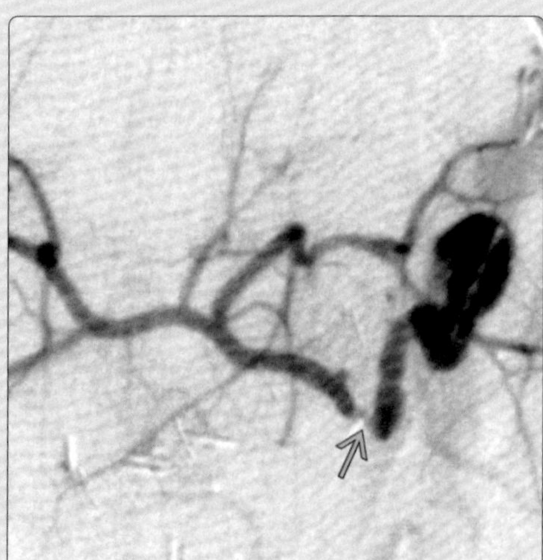

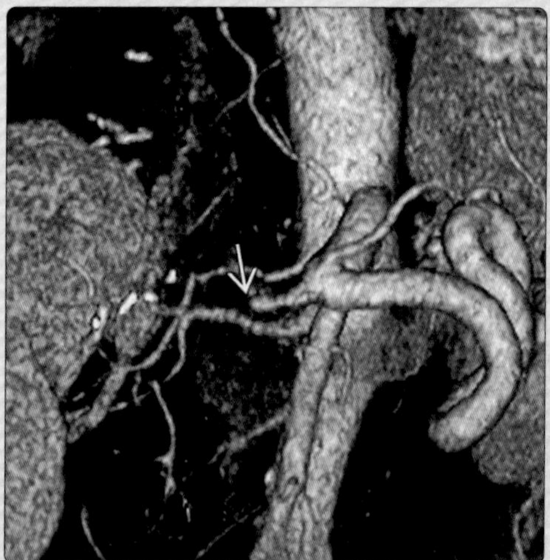

Liver Transplant Portal Vein Stenosis/Thrombosis

KEY FACTS

IMAGING

- **Portal vein stenosis**
  - Elevated portal vein velocity > 125 cm/s at anastomosis
    - Portal vein velocity normally < 60 cm/s
  - Anastomotic:preanastomotic velocity ratio
    - Stenosis: > 3.0
    - Normal: ~ 1.5
- **Portal vein thrombosis**
  - No detectable flow in portal vein
  - May see echogenic thrombus in portal vein, or portal vein may appear markedly hypoechoic or even anechoic
  - May see enlarged hepatic arteries
    - Hepatic arteries compensate for portal vein thrombosis due to hepatic arterial buffer response
  - Bidirectional low-amplitude flow in portal vein may precede portal vein thrombosis

PATHOLOGY

- **Portal vein stenosis**
  - Occurs at site of anastomosis
- **Portal vein thrombosis**
  - Associated with surgical technique
  - Hypercoagulable state

CLINICAL ISSUES

- Portal vein stenosis typically occurs at anastomosis
- Depending on degree of stenosis, may require balloon angioplasty
- Portal vein stenosis and thrombosis are relatively rare, occurring in 1-2.7% of liver transplants

SCANNING TIPS

- In chronic or longstanding portal vein stenosis, may see portal vein aneurysm downstream from anastomosis and helical flow in dilated portion of portal vein

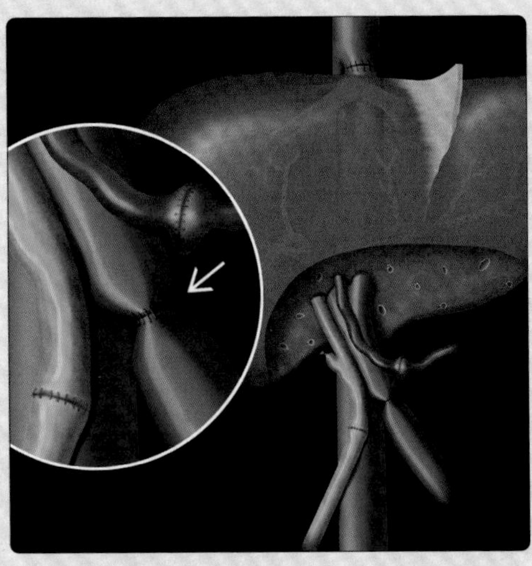

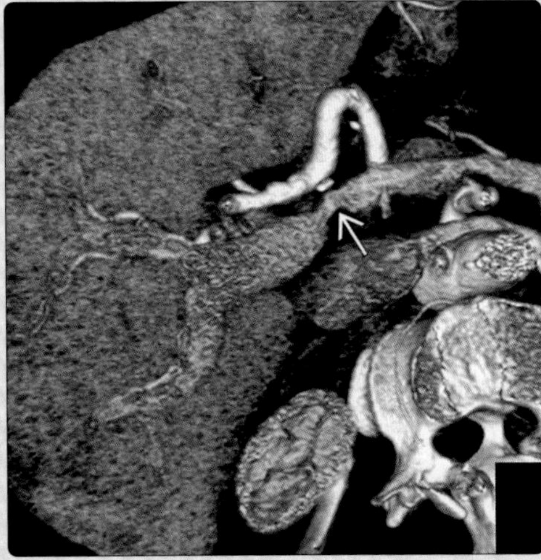

(Left) *Graphic depicts focal stenosis ➡ of the portal vein at the level of the anastomosis in a patient with a liver transplant.* **(Right)** *Volume-rendered CT angiogram in a patient with liver transplant shows a focal caliber change ➡ in the portal vein at the site of anastomosis, consistent with stenosis.*

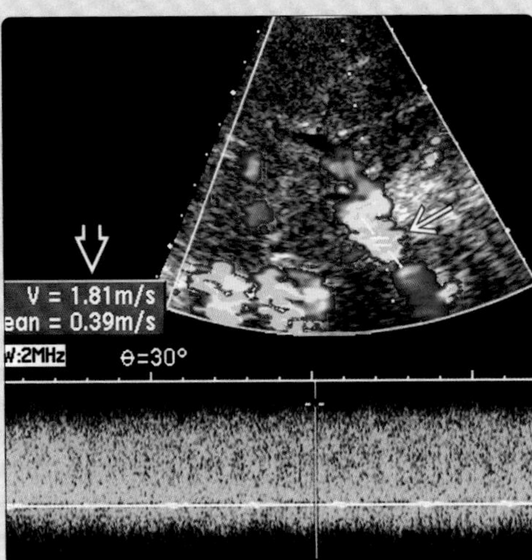

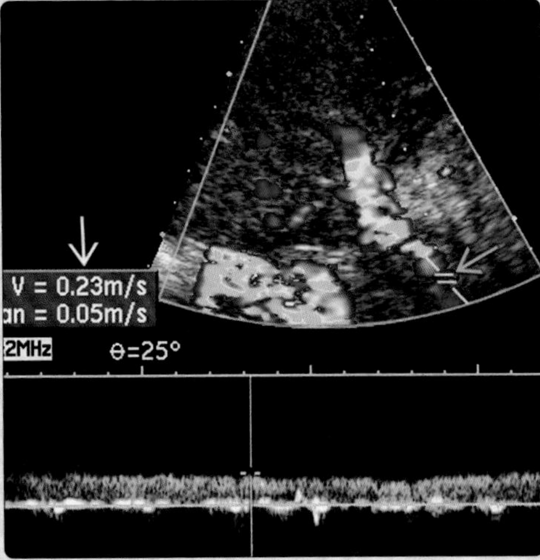

(Left) *Pulsed Doppler evaluation of the main portal vein near the anastomosis shows a focal area of aliasing ➡ as well as corresponding elevated velocities measured to 181 cm/s ➡.* **(Right)** *Pulsed Doppler interrogation in the same patient in the portal vein proximal ➡ to the area of aliasing shows velocity is in a normal range of 23 cm/s ➡. Elevation of velocity at the anastomosis of > 3x the preanastomotic velocity is highly suggestive of stenosis in the portal vein.*

Liver Transplant Hepatic Venous Stenosis/Thrombosis

KEY FACTS

IMAGING

- **Hepatic venous stenosis**
  - Color Doppler
    - May see focal turbulent flow at stenosis and stenotic jet
  - Spectral Doppler
    - Elevated velocity at site of stenosis or < 10 cm/s away from site of stenosis
    - Loss of normal triphasic waveform
      - Most commonly monophasic in appearance
    - May see secondary slow portal vein velocity
  - Angiography
    - Pressure gradient > 5 mm Hg across stenosis
- **Hepatic venous thrombosis**
  - Direct visualization of thrombus in hepatic vein (HV) or lack of detectable flow with color, power, or spectral Doppler

PATHOLOGY

- HV or inferior vena cava (IVC) stenosis results in outflow obstruction of liver
- Immediate posttransplant period: Kinking of vessel
- Delayed presentation: Intimal hyperplasia

CLINICAL ISSUES

- HV stenosis occurs in < 1% of liver transplants, 2-10% of liver transplants when piggyback technique used
- Clinical presentation: Lower extremity edema, Budd-Chiari syndrome, ascites

SCANNING TIPS

- Color Doppler box should always include HV and its IVC confluence because stenoses often occur at the junction
- Obtain HV spectral Doppler tracings within 3 cm of junction with IVC
- If area of aliasing is identified, obtain spectral Doppler with angle correction through the region

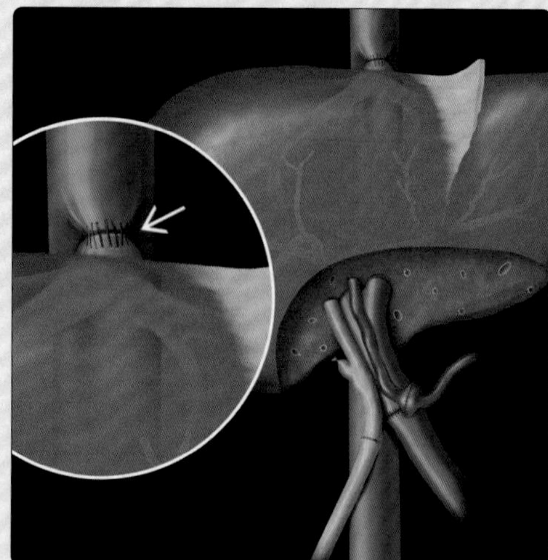

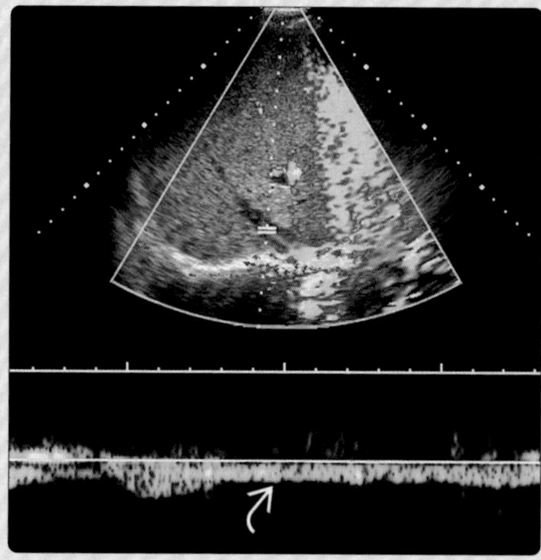

(Left) *Graphic shows stenosis at the piggyback anastomosis ➔ in a liver transplant. In this technique, the donor suprahepatic inferior vena cava (IVC) is anastomosed with the recipient common orifice of all 3 hepatic veins.* **(Right)** *Spectral Doppler US in the right hepatic vein shows monophasic ➔ nonpulsatile waveform. When waveforms that were previously pulsatile become monophasic, a stenosis of the hepatic venous/IVC anastomosis should be suspected and warrants further evaluation.*

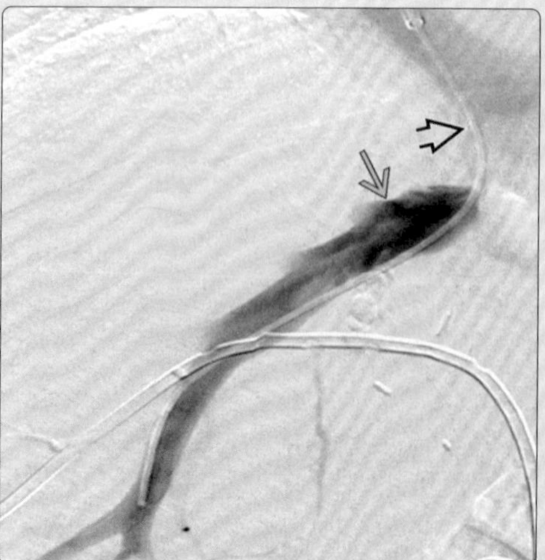

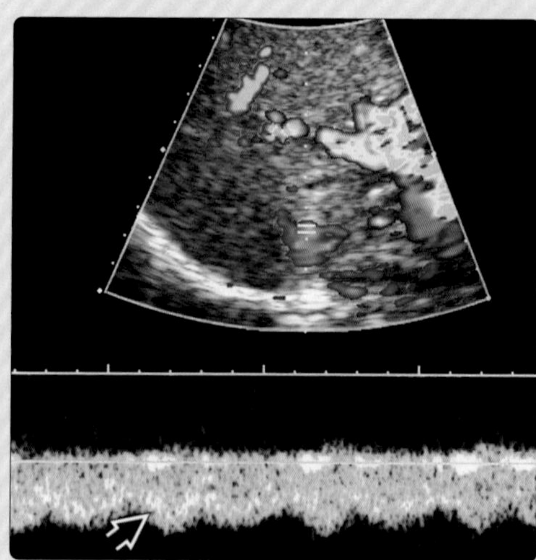

(Left) *Catheter injection of the right hepatic vein in the same patient shows that contrast fills the hepatic vein ➔ but does not reflux readily into the IVC ➔, indicative of stenosis, which was subsequently balloon angioplastied.* **(Right)** *Spectral Doppler US of the right hepatic vein in the same patient after balloon dilation shows increase in pulsatility as well as increased magnitude of flow ➔.*

Liver Transplant Biliary Stricture

KEY FACTS

IMAGING

- Ultrasound
  - Initial imaging modality for evaluation of biliary system
  - Dilated biliary duct proximal to site of anastomosis
  - Focal area of narrowing may be seen in mid common hepatic duct or near hepatic hilum (latter in patients with hepaticojejunostomy)
- Magnetic resonance cholangiopancreatography
  - Heavily T2-weighted image of common hepatic duct shows upstream ductal dilatation and focal narrowing at anastomosis
- Cholangiogram
  - Performed in patients with hepaticojejunostomy in which access to anastomosis difficult with endoscopic retrograde cholangiopancreatography (ERCP)
- ERCP
  - May be diagnostic as well as therapeutic with balloon dilation and plastic stent placement

TOP DIFFERENTIAL DIAGNOSES

- Obstruction from other causes
  - Choledocholithiasis
  - Malignancy
  - Recurrent primary sclerosing cholangitis (PSC) (in patients with prior history of PSC)

PATHOLOGY

- Biliary stricture is most common type of complication after liver transplant, occurring in up to 60%
- In late stricture, > 1 month post transplant, usually related to ischemic injury of bile duct anastomosis

CLINICAL ISSUES

- Early stricture
  - Usually responds well to single endoscopic therapy
- Late stricture
  - Often requires longer treatment regimens

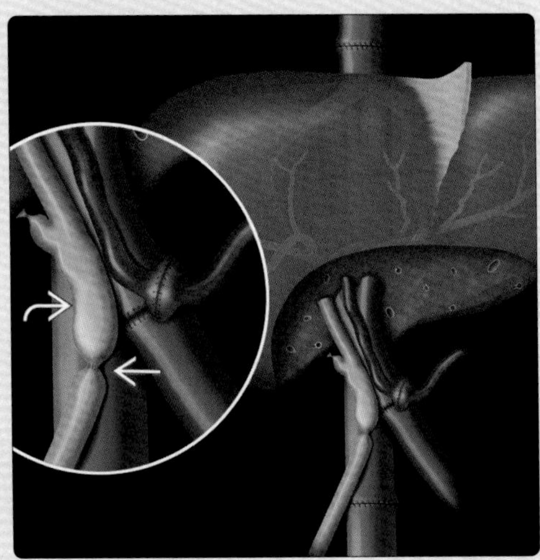

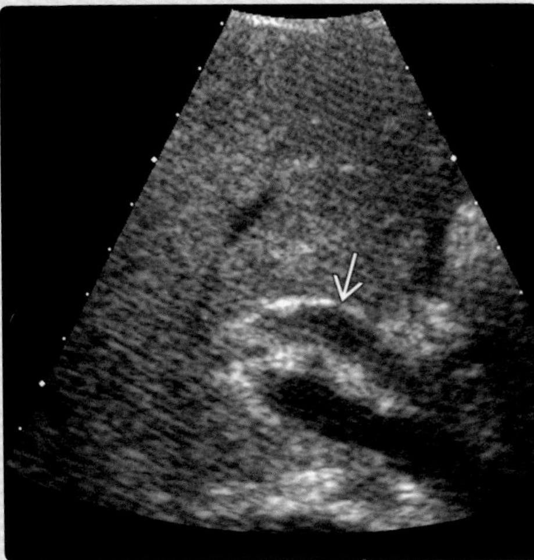

(Left) *Graphic depicts a liver transplant with focal stricture in the common bile duct anastomosis ➡. Notice the mild upstream dilatation ➦, which may be seen with a biliary duct stenosis.* **(Right)** *Transverse grayscale ultrasound of the common bile duct in a patient status post liver transplant shows a moderately dilated common bile duct ➡, which was related to a biliary duct stricture at the anastomosis.*

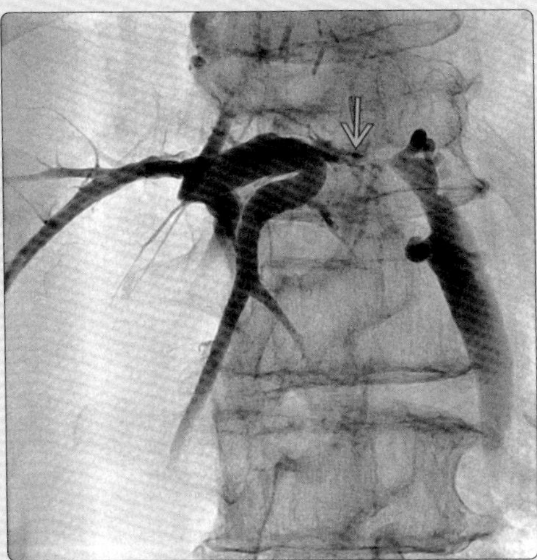

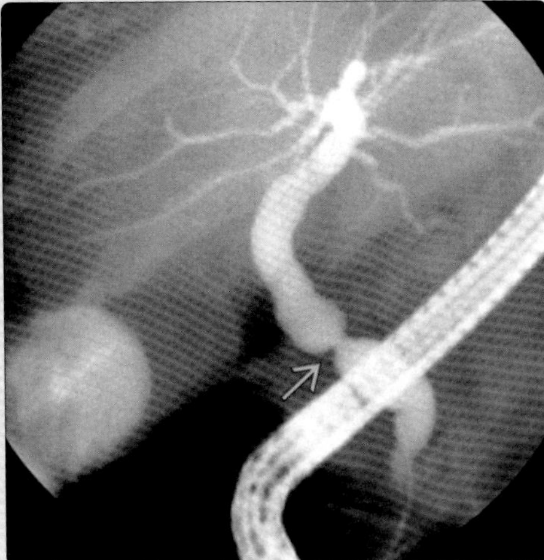

(Left) *Percutaneous transhepatic cholangiogram in a patient with liver transplant and hepaticojejunostomy shows a severe stenosis of the right hepatic duct, at the junction ⇨ of the right and common hepatic duct, near the hepaticojejunostomy site.* **(Right)** *ERCP in a patient after liver transplant shows a focal stenosis ⇨ in the common bile duct at the level of the anastomosis.*

PART I
SECTION 2

Biliary System

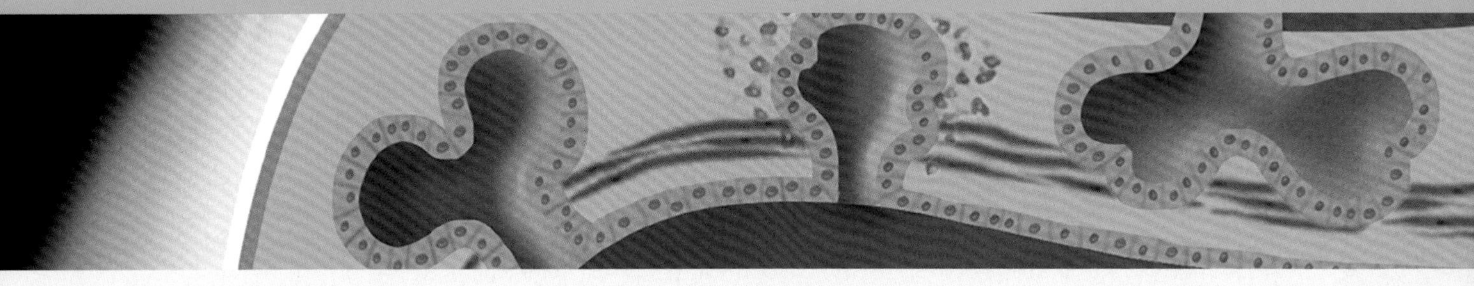

Anatomy and Approach

Gallstones and Mimics

Gallbladder Wall Pathology

Ductal Pathology

TERMINOLOGY

Abbreviations

- Extrahepatic biliary structures
  - Gallbladder (GB)
  - Cystic duct (CD)
  - Right hepatic (RH) and left hepatic (LH) ducts
  - Common hepatic duct (CHD)
  - Common bile duct (CBD)

Definitions

- Proximal/distal biliary tree (follows direction of flow)
  - Proximal refers to portion of biliary tree that is closer in proximity to liver and hepatocytes
  - Distal refers to caudal end closer to ampulla and bowel
- Central/peripheral
  - Central refers to biliary ducts close to porta hepatis
  - Peripheral refers to higher-order branches of intrahepatic biliary tree extending into hepatic parenchyma

IMAGING ANATOMY

Overview

- Biliary ducts carry bile from liver to duodenum
  - Bile is produced continuously by liver, stored and concentrated by GB, and released intermittently by GB contraction in response to presence of fat in duodenum
  - Hepatocytes form bile → bile canaliculi → interlobular biliary ducts → collecting bile ducts → right and left hepatic ducts → CHD → CBD → intestines
- **CBD**
  - Forms in free edge of lesser omentum by **union of CD and CHD**
  - Length of duct: 5-15 cm, depending on point of junction of cystic and CHD
  - Descends posterior and medial to duodenum, lying on dorsal surface of pancreatic head
  - Joins with pancreatic duct to form hepaticopancreatic **ampulla of Vater**
  - Ampulla opens into duodenum through major duodenal (hepaticopancreatic) papilla
  - Distal CBD is thickened into sphincter of Boyden and hepaticopancreatic segment is thickened into sphincter of Oddi
    - Contraction of these sphincters prevents bile from entering duodenum; forces it to collect in GB
    - Relaxation of sphincters in response to parasympathetic stimulation and cholecystokinin (released by duodenum in response to fatty meal)
- Vessels, nerves, and lymphatics
  - **Arteries**
    - Hepatic arteries supply intrahepatic ducts
    - Cystic artery supplies proximal common duct
    - RH artery supplies middle part of common duct
    - Gastroduodenal and pancreaticoduodenal arcade supply distal common duct
    - Cystic artery supplies GB (usually from RH artery; variable)
  - **Veins**
    - From intrahepatic ducts → hepatic veins
    - From common duct → portal vein (in tributaries)
    - From GB directly into liver sinusoids, bypassing portal vein
  - **Nerves**
    - Sensory: Right phrenic nerve
    - Parasympathetic and sympathetic: Celiac ganglion and plexus; contraction of GB and relaxation of biliary sphincters is caused by parasympathetic stimulation, but more important stimulus is from hormone cholecystokinin
  - **Lymphatics**
    - Same course and name as arterial branches
    - Collect at celiac lymph nodes and node of omental foramen
    - Nodes draining GB are prominent in porta hepatis and around pancreatic head
- **Gallbladder**
  - ~ 7-10 cm long, holds up to 50 mL of bile
  - Lies in shallow fossa on visceral surface of liver
  - Vertical plane through GB fossa and middle hepatic vein divides LH and RH lobes
  - May touch and indent duodenum
  - Fundus is covered with peritoneum and relatively mobile; body and neck attached to liver and covered by hepatic capsule
  - Fundus: Wide tip of GB, projects below liver edge (usually)
  - Body: Contacts liver, duodenum, and transverse colon
  - Neck: Narrowed, tapered, and tortuous; joins CD
  - CD: 3-4 cm long, connects GB to CHD; marked by spiral folds of Heister; helps to regulate bile flow to and from GB
- **Normal measurements**
  - CBD/CHD
    - < 6-7 mm in patients without history of biliary disease in most studies
    - Controversy about dilatation related to previous cholecystectomy and old age
  - Intrahepatic ducts
    - Normal diameter of 1st and higher-order branches < 2 mm or < 40% of diameter of adjacent portal vein
    - 1st- (i.e., LH duct and RH duct) and 2nd-order branches are normally visualized
    - Visualization of 3rd and higher-order branches is often abnormal and indicates dilatation

ANATOMY IMAGING ISSUES

Imaging Recommendations

- Patient should fast for at least 4-6 hours prior to US examination to ensure GB is not contracted after meal, ideally fasting for 8-12 hours (overnight)
- Complete assessment includes scanning liver, porta hepatis region, and pancreas in sagittal, transverse, and oblique views
- Subcostal and right intercostal transverse views help align bile ducts and GB along imaging plane for optimal visualization
- Usually structures are better assessed and imaged with patient in full-suspended inspiration and in left lateral oblique position

- Harmonic imaging provides improved contrast between bile ducts and adjacent tissues, leading to improved visualization of bile ducts, luminal content, and wall
- For imaging of gallstone disease, special maneuvers are recommended
  - Move patient from supine to left lateral decubitus position
    - Demonstrates mobility of gallstones
    - Gravitates small gallstones together to appreciate posterior acoustic shadowing
  - Set focal zone at level of posterior acoustic shadowing
    - Maximizes effect of posterior acoustic shadowing to confirm gallstone(s)
- Overall gain is often lowered to remove reverberation artifact from GB; however, do not set gain too low such that true intraluminal echoes are obscured

Imaging Approaches

- Transabdominal US is ideal initial investigation for suspected biliary tree or GB pathology
  - Cystic nature of bile ducts and GB (especially if these are dilated) provides inherently high-contrast resolution
  - Acoustic window provided by liver and modern state-of-the-art US technology provides good spatial resolution
  - Common indications of US for biliary and GB disease include
    - Right upper quadrant/epigastric pain
    - Abnormal liver function test or jaundice
    - Suspected gallstone disease
    - Pancreatitis
  - US plays key role in multimodality evaluation of complex biliary problems
- Supplemented by various imaging modalities, including MR/MRCP and CT

Imaging Pitfalls

- **Common pitfalls in evaluation of GB**
  - Posterior shadowing may arise from GB neck, Heister valves of CD, or adjacent gas-filled bowel loops
    - May mimic cholelithiasis
    - Scan after repositioning patient in prone or left lateral decubitus positions
    - Make sure to increase transducer frequency when evaluating GB after evaluation of liver
  - Food material within gastric antrum/duodenum
    - Mimics GB filled with gallstones or GB containing milk of calcium
    - During real-time scanning, carefully evaluate peristaltic activity of involved bowel with oral administration of water
- **Common pitfalls in evaluation of biliary tree**
  - Redundancy, elongation, or folding of GB neck on itself
    - Mimics dilatation of CHD or proximal CBD
    - Avoided by scanning patient in full-suspended inspiration
    - Careful real-time scanning allows separate visualization of CHD/CBD medial to GB neck
  - Presence of gas-filled bowel loops adjacent to distal extrahepatic bile ducts
    - Obscure distal biliary tree and render detection of choledocholithiasis difficult
    - Scan with patient in decubitus positions or after oral intake of water
  - Gas/particulate material in adjacent duodenum and pancreatic calcification
    - Mimic choledocholithiasis within CBD
  - Presence of gas within biliary tree
    - May mimic choledocholithiasis, differentiated by presence of reverberation artifacts
    - Limits US detection of biliary calculus

Key Concepts

- Direct venous drainage of GB into liver bypasses portal venous system, often results in sparing of adjacent liver from generalized steatosis (fatty liver)
- Nodal metastasis from GB carcinoma to peripancreatic nodes may simulate primary pancreatic tumor
- Sonography: Optimal means of evaluating GB for stones and inflammation (acute cholecystitis); best done in fasting state (distends GB)
- Intrahepatic bile ducts follow branching pattern of portal veins
  - Usually lie immediately anterior to portal vein branch; confluence of hepatic ducts just anterior to bifurcation of right and main portal veins

CLINICAL IMPLICATIONS

Clinical Importance

- In patients with obstructive jaundice, US plays key role
  - Differentiates biliary obstruction from liver parenchymal disease
  - Determines presence, level, and cause of biliary obstruction
- Common variations of biliary arterial and ductal anatomy result in challenges to avoid injury at surgery
  - CD may run in common sheath with bile duct
  - Anomalous RH ducts may be severed at cholecystectomy
- Close apposition of GB to duodenum can result in fistulous connection with chronic cholecystitis and erosion of gallstone into duodenum

Function & Dysfunction

- Obstruction of CBD is common
  - Gallstones in distal bile duct
  - Carcinoma arising in pancreatic head or bile duct
  - Result is jaundice due to back up of bile salts into bloodstream

Embryologic Events

- Abnormal embryological development of fetal ductal plate can lead to spectrum of liver and biliary abnormalities, including
  - Polycystic liver disease
  - Congenital hepatic fibrosis
  - Biliary hamartomas
  - Caroli disease
  - Choledochal cysts

GALLBLADDER IN SITU

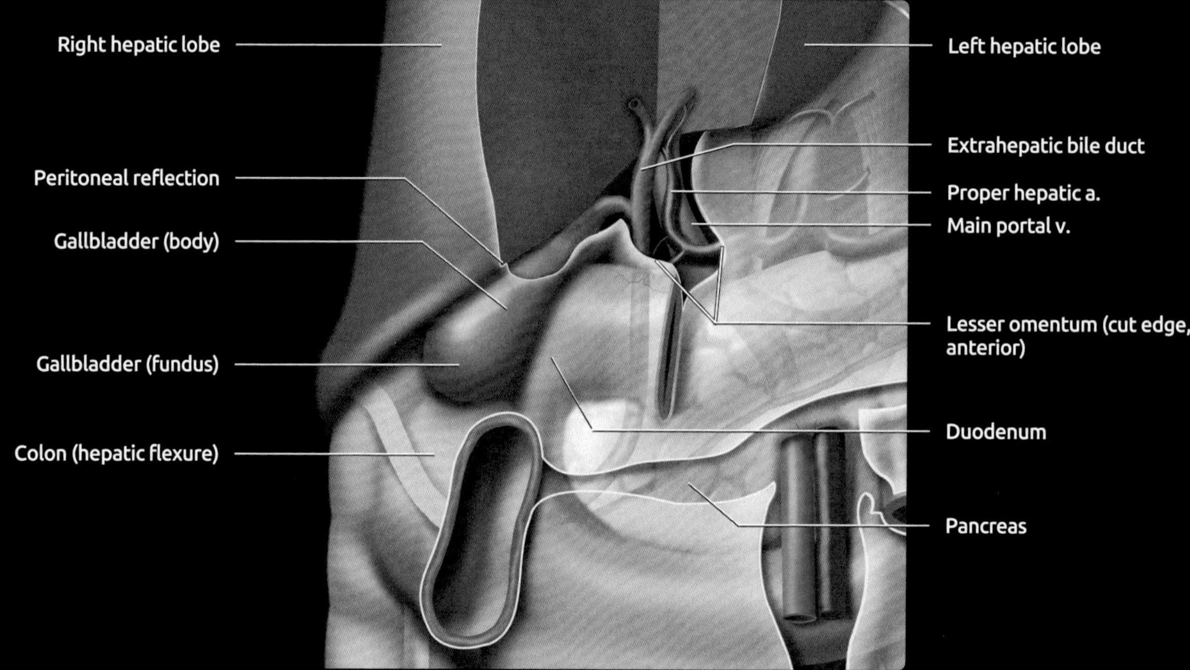

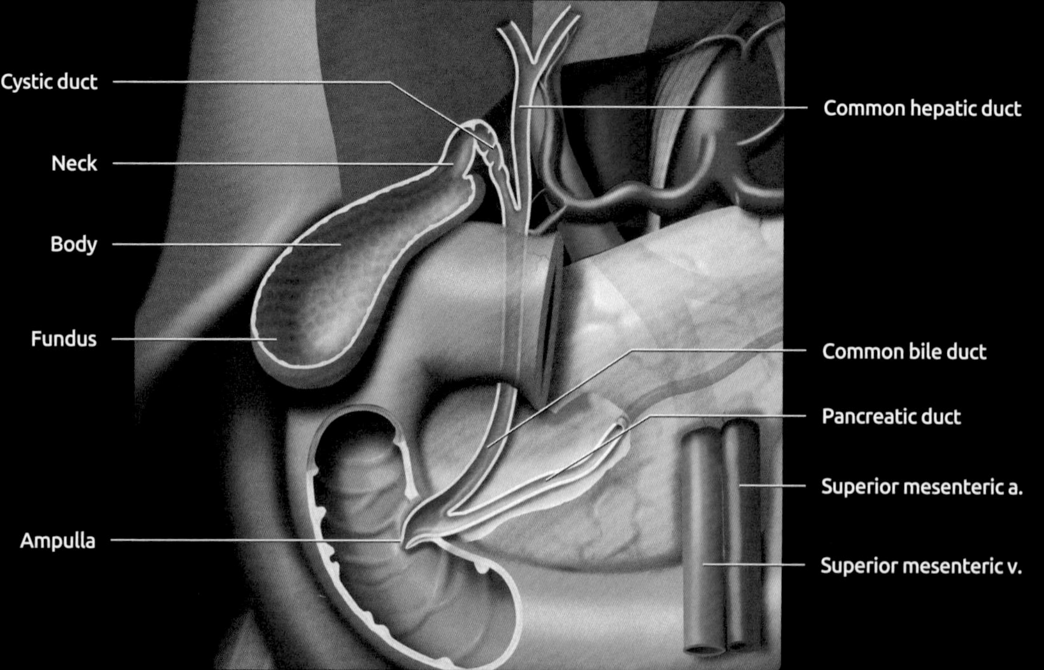

(Top) *Graphic shows that the gallbladder is covered with peritoneum, except where it is attached to the liver. The extrahepatic bile duct, hepatic artery, and portal vein run in the lesser omentum. The fundus of the gallbladder extends beyond the anterior-inferior edge of the liver and can be in contact with the hepatic flexure of the colon. The body (main portion of the gallbladder) is in contact with the duodenum.* **(Bottom)** *The neck of the gallbladder narrows before entering the cystic duct, which is distinguished by its tortuous course and irregular lumen. The duct lumen is irregular due to redundant folds of mucosa, called the spiral folds of Heister, that are believed to regulate the rate of filling and emptying of the gallbladder. The cystic duct joins the hepatic duct to form the common bile duct, which passes behind the duodenum and through the pancreas to enter the duodenum.*

ANATOMIC VARIATIONS OF BILIARY TREE

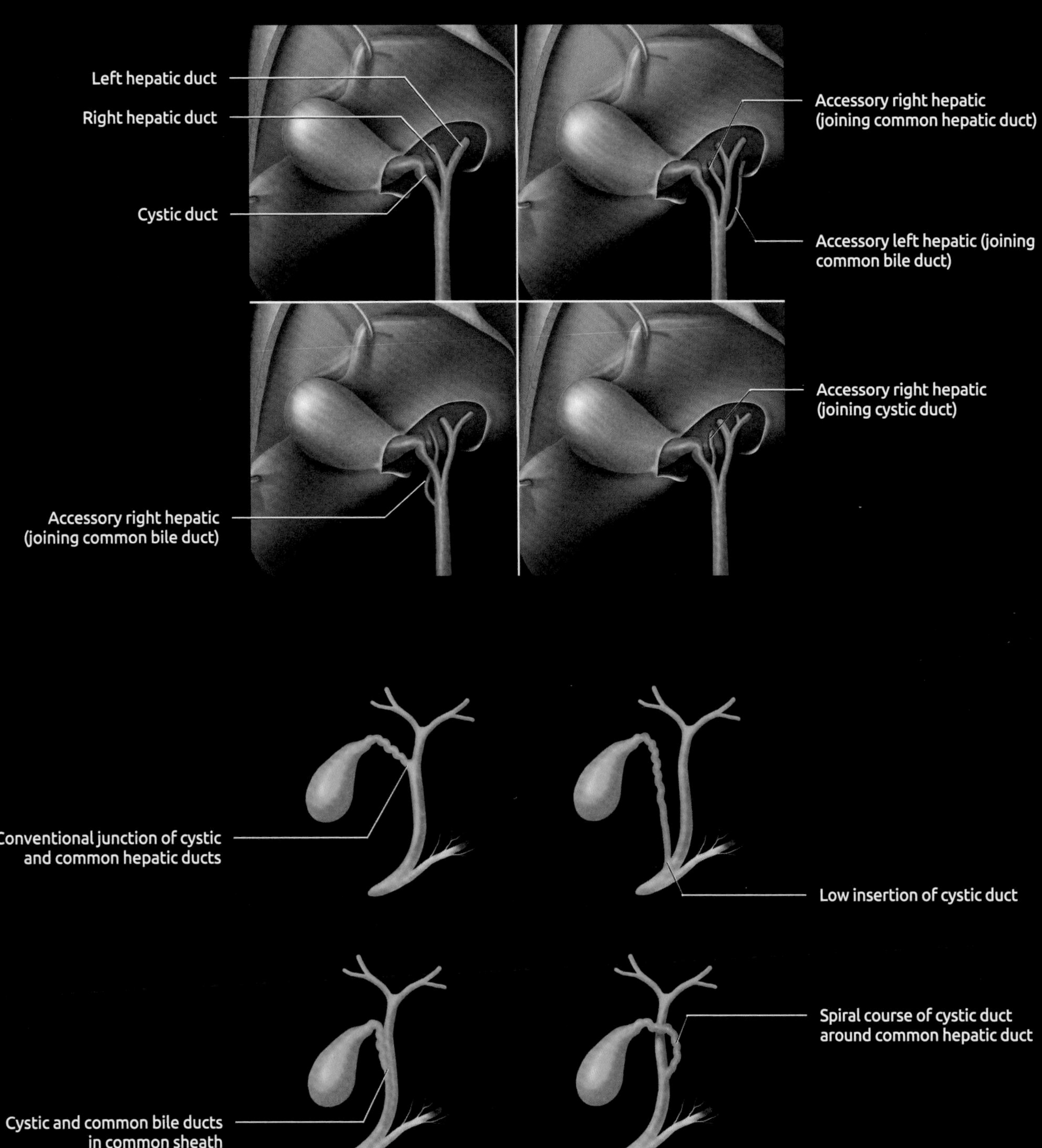

(Top) *Graphic shows the conventional arrangement of the extrahepatic bile ducts, but variations are common (20% of population) and may lead to inadvertent ligation or injury at surgery (such as during cholecystectomy), where the cystic duct is clamped and transected. Most accessory ducts are on the right side and usually enter the common hepatic duct, but they may enter the cystic or common bile duct. Accessory left ducts enter the common bile duct. While referred to as accessory, these ducts are the sole drainage of bile from at least 1 hepatic segment. Ligation or laceration can lead to significant hepatic injury or bile peritonitis.* **(Bottom)** *The course and insertion of the cystic duct are highly variable, leading to difficulty in isolation and ligation at cholecystectomy. The cystic duct may be mistaken for the common hepatic or common bile duct.*

BILIARY TREE

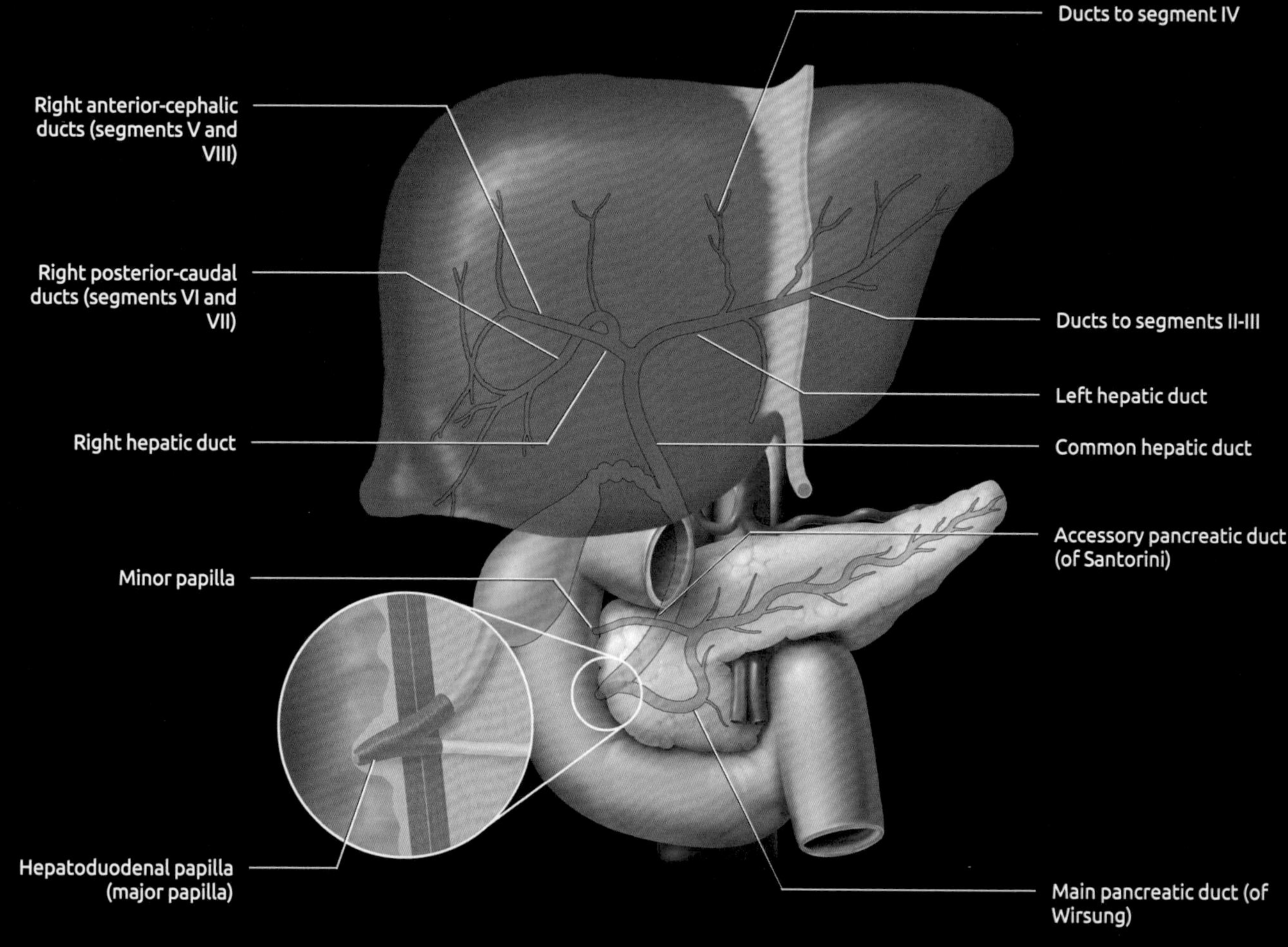

Note the distribution of the larger intrahepatic bile ducts. The common bile duct usually joins with the pancreatic duct in a common channel or ampulla (of Vater) but may enter the major duodenal papilla separately. The distal bile duct has a sphincteric coat of smooth muscle, the choledochal sphincter (of Boyden), which regulates bile emptying into the duodenum. When contracted, this sphincter causes bile to flow retrograde into the gallbladder for storage. The common hepaticopancreatic ampulla may be surrounded by a smooth muscle sphincter (of Oddi).

BILIARY TREE

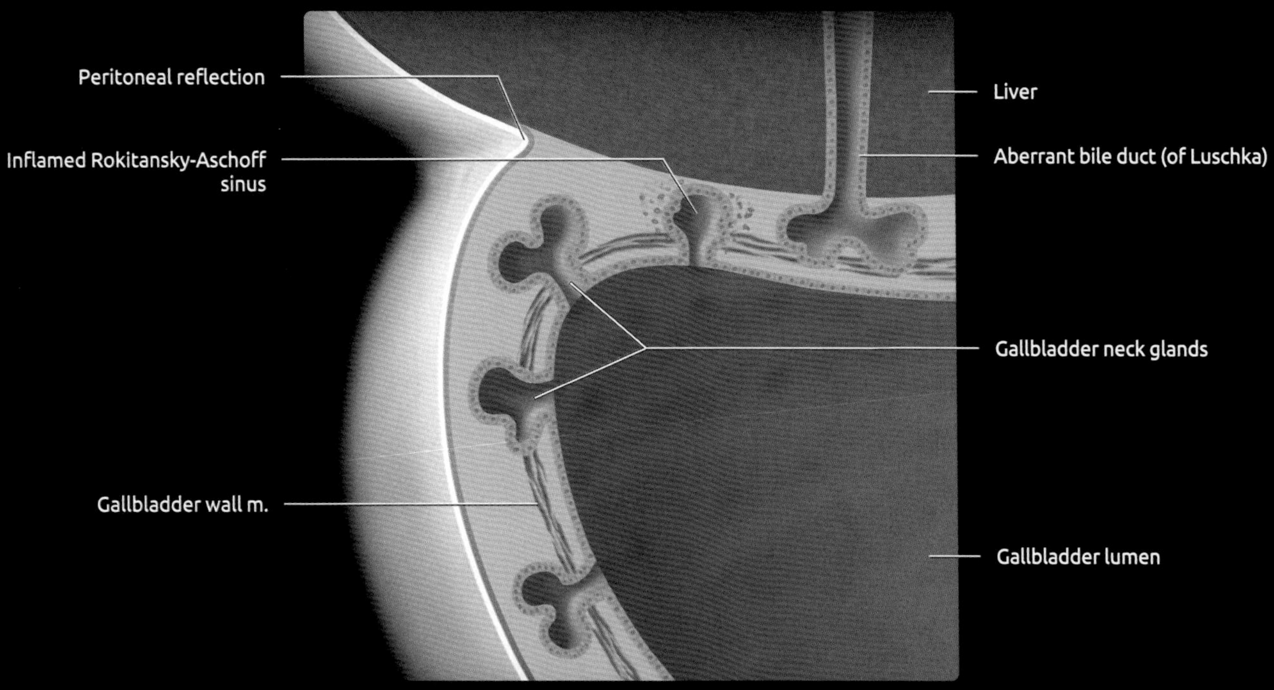

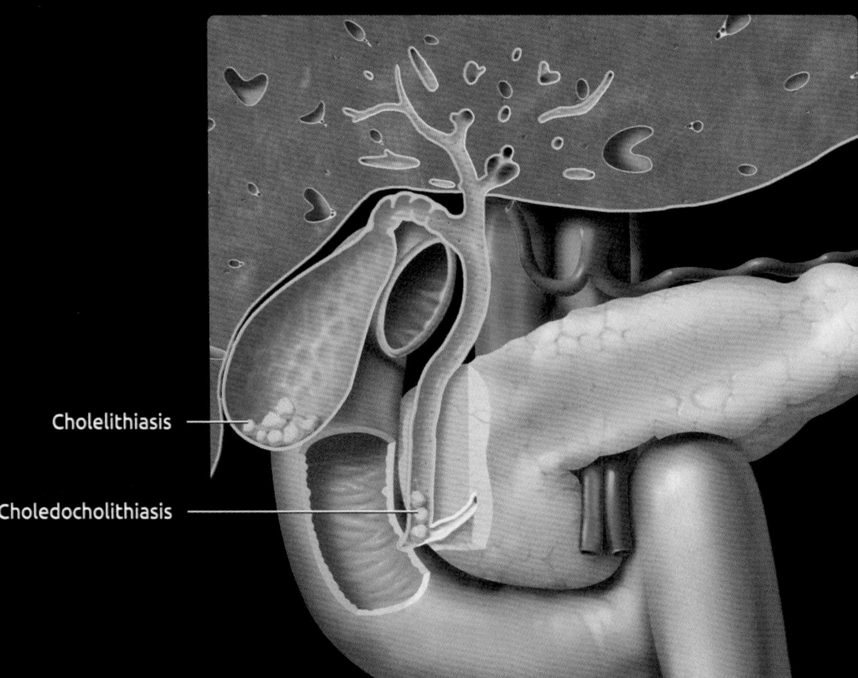

(Top) *The gallbladder body and neck are adherent to the liver and may be bridged by aberrant bile ducts (of Luschka). Mucous glands are found in the gallbladder neck. Rokitansky-Aschoff sinuses are pseudodiverticula that extend into the wall and may collect debris, becoming inflamed.* **(Bottom)** *Graphic demonstrates cholelithiasis (stones in the gallbladder) and choledocholithiasis (stones in the bile ducts). Gallstones are extremely common and may remain asymptomatic. Stones that become impacted, even temporarily, in the gallbladder neck may cause inflammation and distention of the gallbladder, clinically referred to as acute cholecystitis. Stones that pass through the cystic duct often cause biliary colic (spasms of right upper quadrant pain), as they often become trapped within the common bile duct, causing obstruction.*

RIGHT HEPATIC LOBE

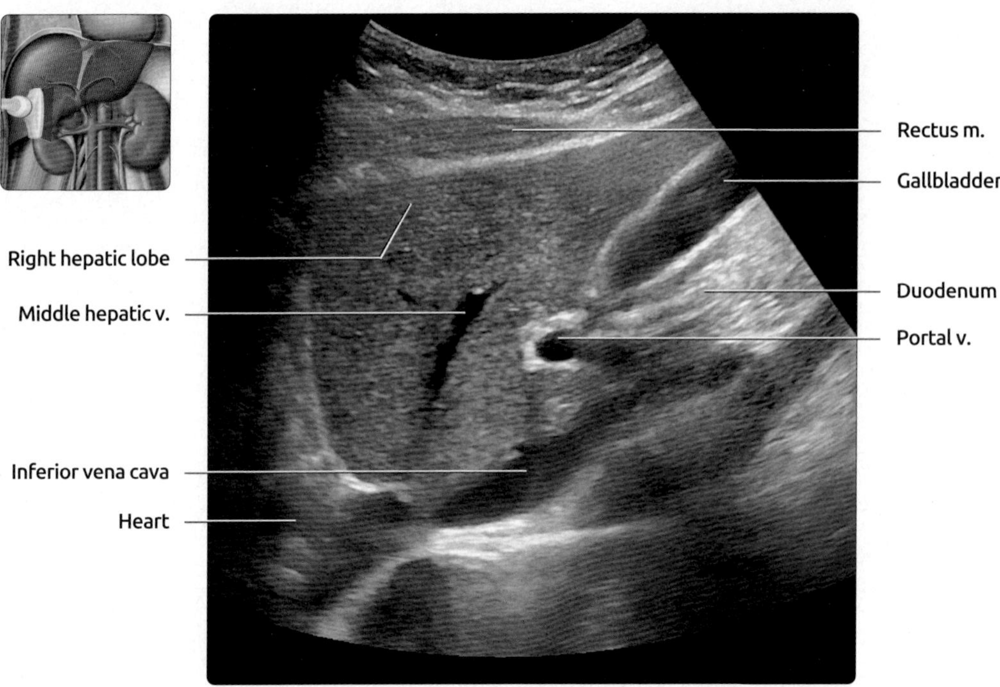

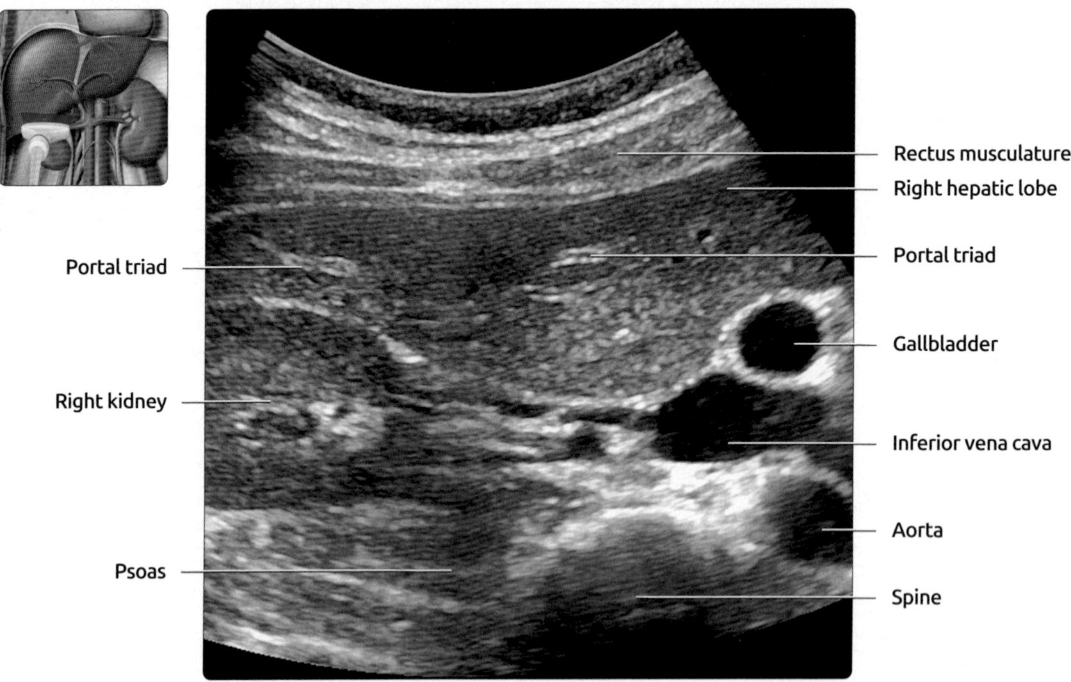

(Top) *Subcostal, longitudinal ultrasound shows the right hepatic lobe and gallbladder with patient in the left lateral decubitus position. Ideally, a patient must fast for at least 4-6 hours to allow for adequate gallbladder distension.* **(Bottom)** *Subcostal, transverse ultrasound of the right hepatic lobe demonstrates its anatomical relationships with major vessels and the right kidney. The intrahepatic bile ducts are localized within the portal triads, which are visible by the prominent echogenic walls of the portal veins in these triads. The portal triad contains the portal vein, bile duct, and hepatic artery. Normally, the intrahepatic bile ducts and hepatic arteries are not readily visible unless they are dilated.*

LEFT HEPATIC LOBE

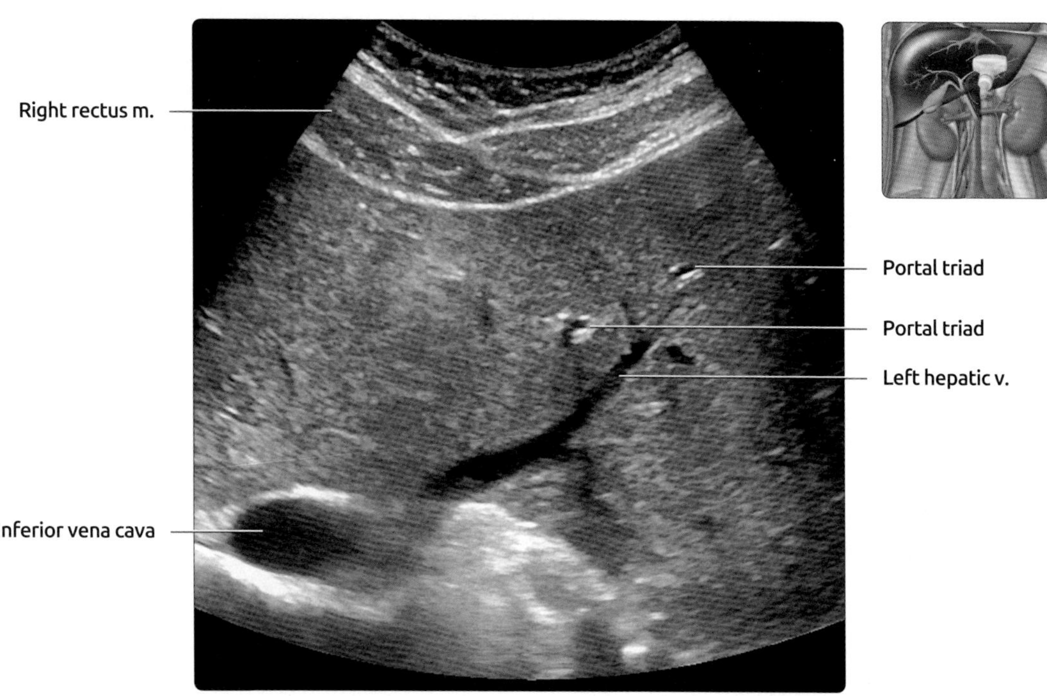

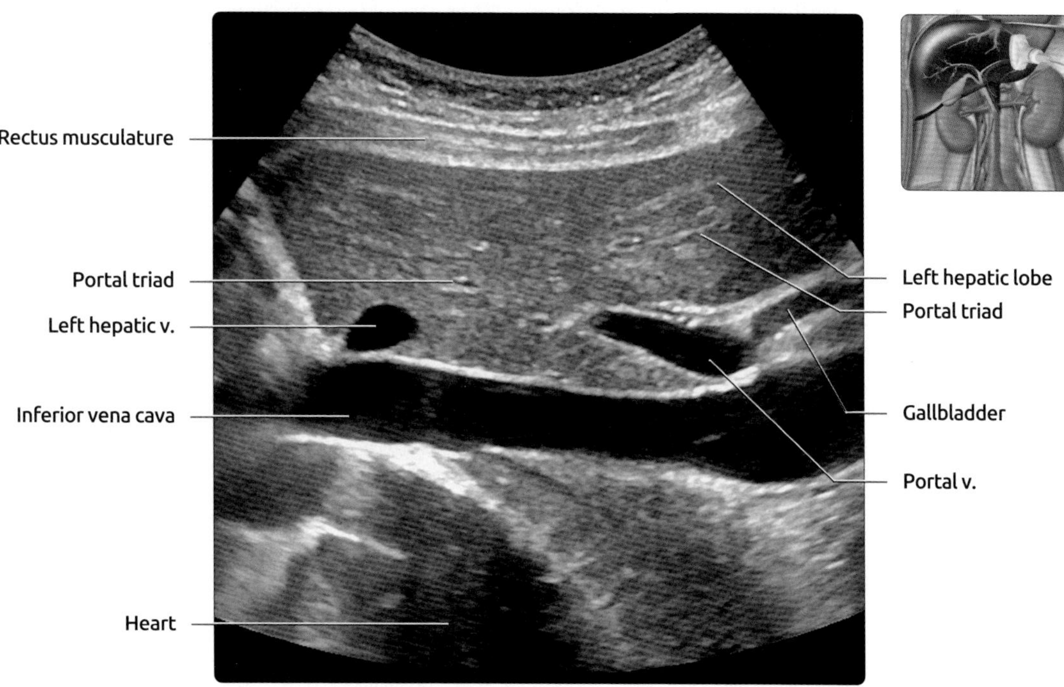

(Top) *Subxiphoid, transverse grayscale ultrasound of the left hepatic lobe shows the left hepatic vein and several portal triads. The portal triads are identified by the prominent echogenic walls of the portal veins. The portal triad contains a portal vein, a bile duct, and a hepatic artery. The hepatic artery and bile duct are not readily visible unless they are dilated.* **(Bottom)** *Longitudinal ultrasound of the left hepatic lobe near the confluence of the left hepatic vein with the inferior vena cava is shown. Portal triads are recognizable by the prominent walls of the portal veins.*

GALLBLADDER

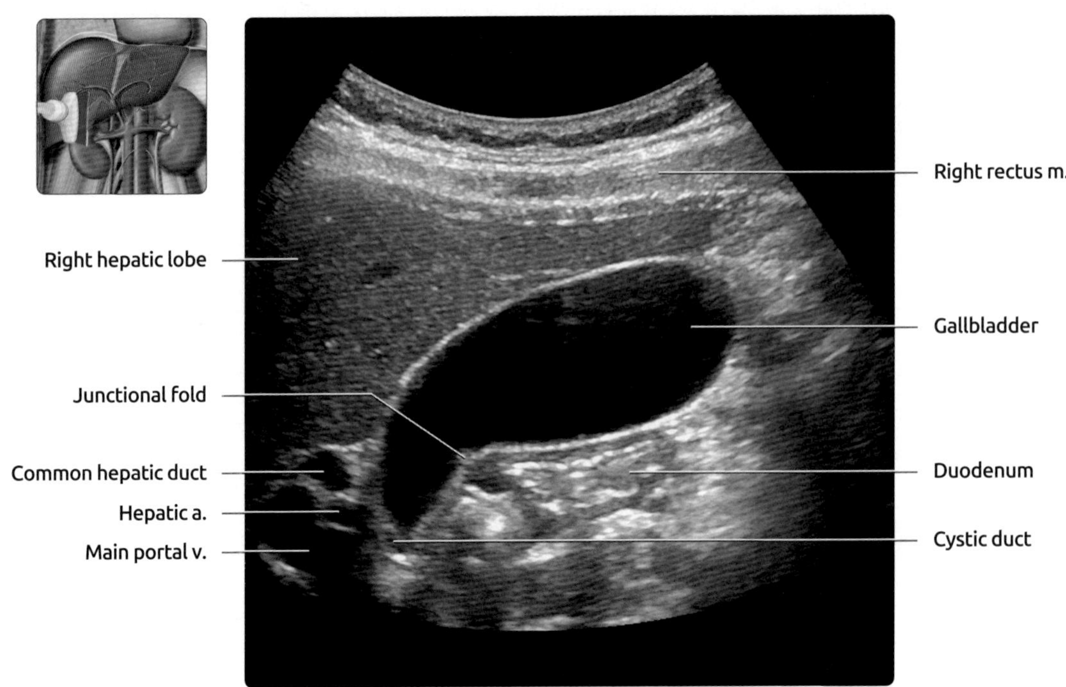

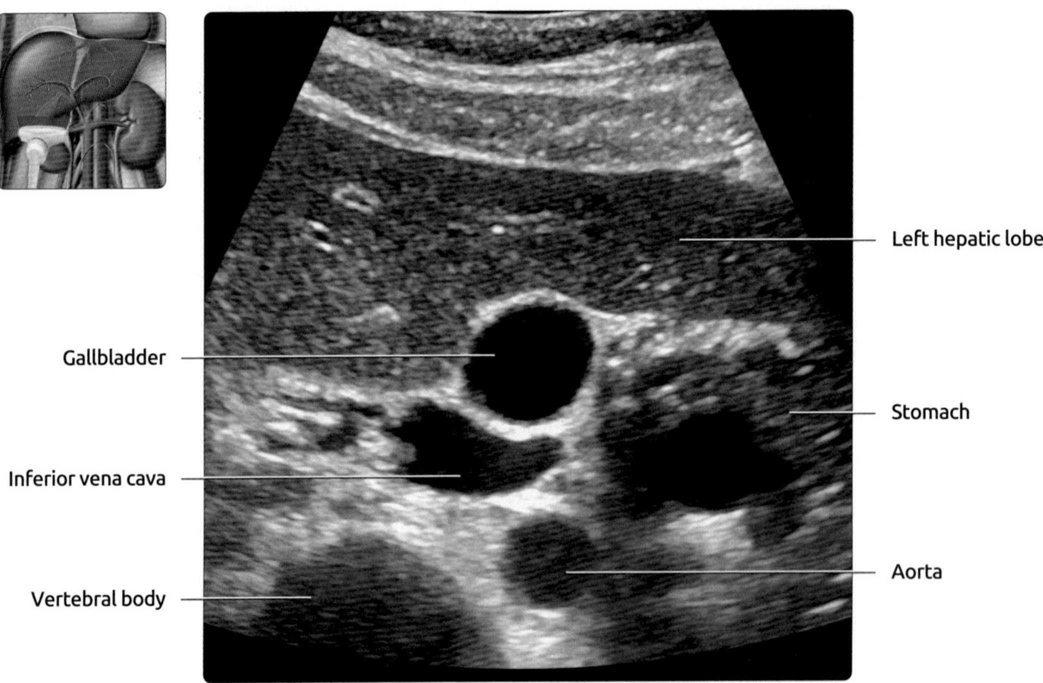

(Top) *Subcostal, longitudinal grayscale ultrasound shows the gallbladder with patient in the left lateral decubitus position. The gallbladder is distended with bile, causing increased transmission of echoes. A patient must fast for at least 4-6 hours to allow for adequate gallbladder distension.* **(Bottom)** *Transverse ultrasound of a distended gallbladder in the left lateral decubitus position is shown. The gallbladder is best evaluated if the patient has fasted at least 4-6 hours, ideally 8-12 hours.*

COMMON BILE DUCT

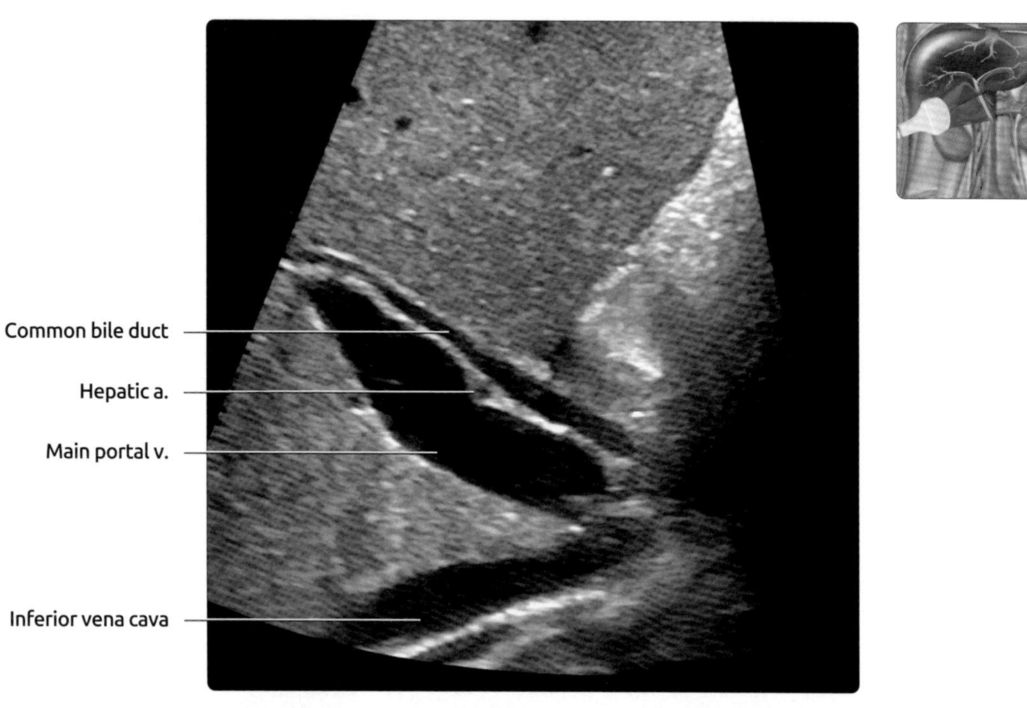

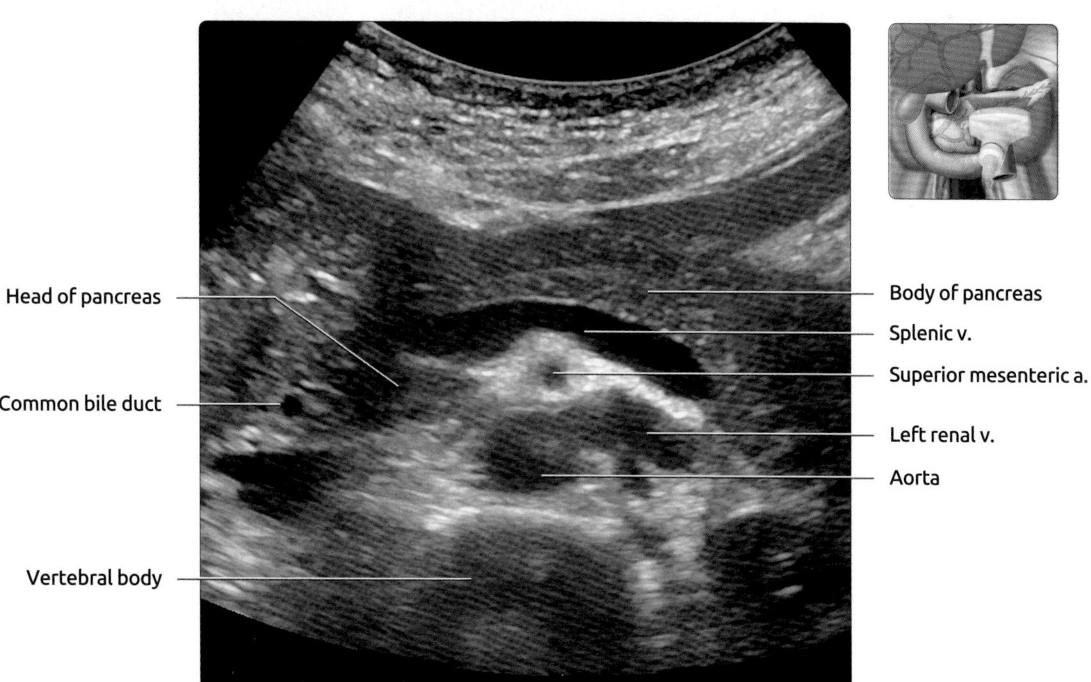

(Top) *Subcostal, longitudinal oblique ultrasound shows the common bile duct and the portal vein in the hepatoduodenal ligament. The common bile duct is normally identified anterior to the portal vein. The distal common bile duct pierces the pancreatic head. Also demonstrated is the hepatic artery, which normally traverses between the portal vein and common bile duct.* **(Bottom)** *Transverse ultrasound at the level of the pancreas demonstrates the distal common bile duct as it pierces the pancreatic head. Overlying bowel gas may obscure this area; positioning the patient upright or in a left lateral decubitus position may help visualization.*

Cholelithiasis

KEY FACTS

IMAGING

- Highly reflective, mobile and gravity-dependent intraluminal structures with posterior clean shadowing
- Variable size; stones < 5 mm may not shadow
- Contracted gallbladder (GB) full of stones may not exhibit mobility and may be mistaken for duodenal bulb
- Wall-echo-shadow (WES) sign: 2 echogenic, curvilinear lines separated by sonolucent line
- Always evaluate for biliary dilatation and signs of cholecystitis, cholangitis, or pancreatitis

TOP DIFFERENTIAL DIAGNOSES

- GB polyp
- GB sludge
- Focal adenomyomatosis
- GB carcinoma

PATHOLOGY

- 80% are cholesterol stones, containing > 50% cholesterol
- 20% are pigmented stones, containing cholesterol and calcium carbonate/bilirubinate

CLINICAL ISSUES

- 10-15% of population; peak: 5th-6th decade, increasing with age; M:F = 1:3
- Right upper quadrant pain/discomfort after fatty meal
- Asymptomatic, incidental finding on imaging
- Complications including acute or chronic cholecystitis, choledocholithiasis, cholangitis, pancreatitis, gallstone ileus, or cancer of GB

SCANNING TIPS

- Patients should fast 6-8 hours
- Optimize parameters to maximize visualization of posterior acoustic shadowing from small stones
- Examine patient in supine and left decubitus/oblique position to demonstrate mobility of gallstone; consider erect or semiprone positions
- Twinkling artifact should not be mistaken for flow

(Left) *Graphic shows multiple small, faceted stones in the gallbladder (GB) ➡ and distal bile duct ➡.* **(Right)** *Left lateral decubitus ultrasound in a patient with acute calculous cholecystitis shows an impacted shadowing stone ➡ in the GB neck. Note acoustic shadowing ➡ and mild GB wall thickening ➡.*

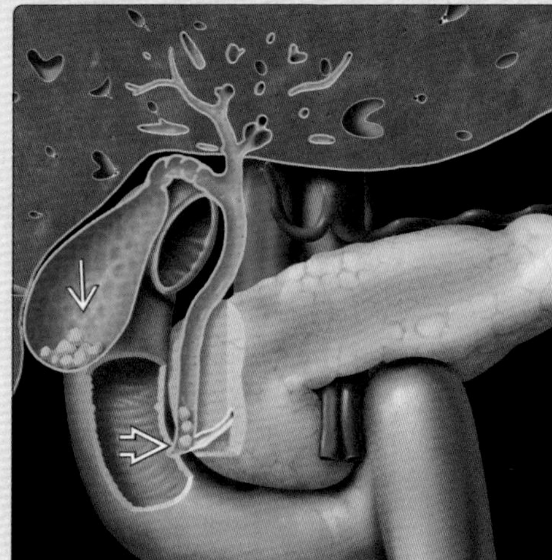

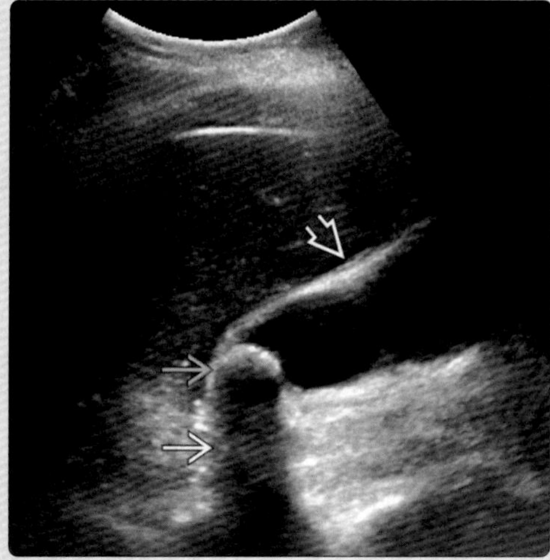

(Left) *Oblique transabdominal ultrasound shows multiple shadowing stones in the GB fundus ➡ with a layer of dependent sludge ➡.* **(Right)** *Transverse ultrasound shows a gallstone filling the GB. Note the wall ➡, echo ➡, and shadow ➡, which together form the WES sign.*

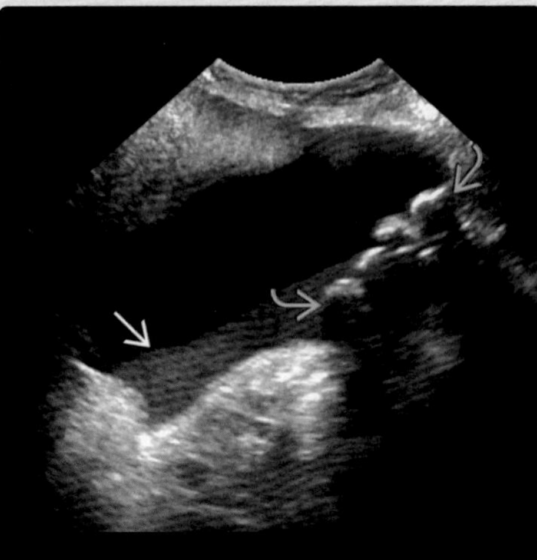

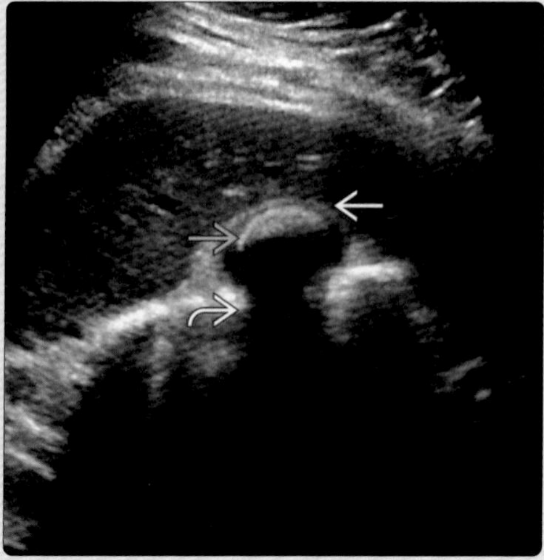

Echogenic Bile

KEY FACTS

IMAGING

- Amorphous, mid-/high-level echoes within gallbladder or bile ducts
- Free floating or mass-like, mobile, settling in dependent position
- Floating punctate echoes may show ring-down artifact
- Occasionally round, low to intermediate echogenicity and mass-like: "Tumefactive" sludge
  - No posterior acoustic shadowing (unlike stones) and no internal color flow (suggesting mass)

TOP DIFFERENTIAL DIAGNOSES

- Cholelithiasis
- Focal adenomyomatosis
- Gallbladder polyp/mass
- Gallbladder pus or blood

PATHOLOGY

- Presence of particulate material in bile
- Larger particles (1-3 mm) are microliths, which may become nidus for gallstones
- Predisposing factors: Prolonged fasting/total parenteral nutrition, pregnancy, rapid weight loss/bariatric surgery, critical illness

CLINICAL ISSUES

- Mostly asymptomatic
- May have clinical symptoms when complications occur
  - Stone formation, biliary colic, acute cholecystitis or pancreatitis

SCANNING TIPS

- Adjust focal zone to gallbladder for optimal resolution
- Distinguish sludge from side lobe artifacts
- Change patient position to demonstrate mobility
- Use color Doppler, but be aware that twinkling artifact may be mistaken for color flow

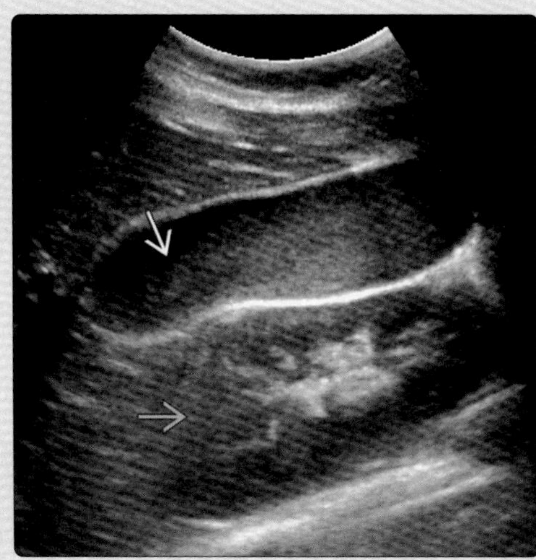

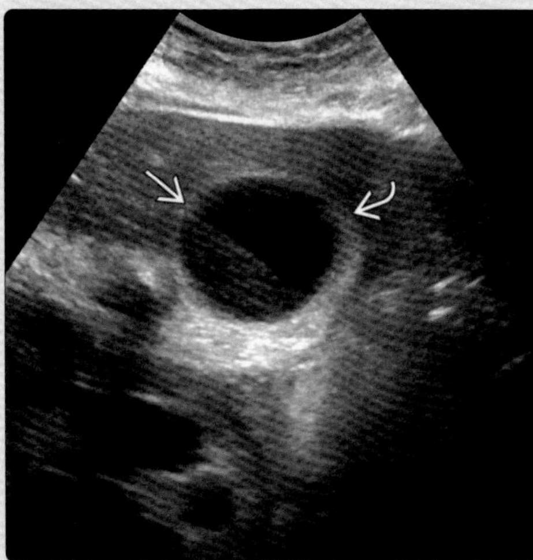

(Left) *Longitudinal ultrasound in a decubitus position shows intraluminal sludge ➡ with a normal wall. The right kidney ⇨ is noted.* **(Right)** *Transverse ultrasound shows a dependent sludge layer in the gallbladder ➡. The gallbladder wall is asymmetrically mildly thickened ➡.*

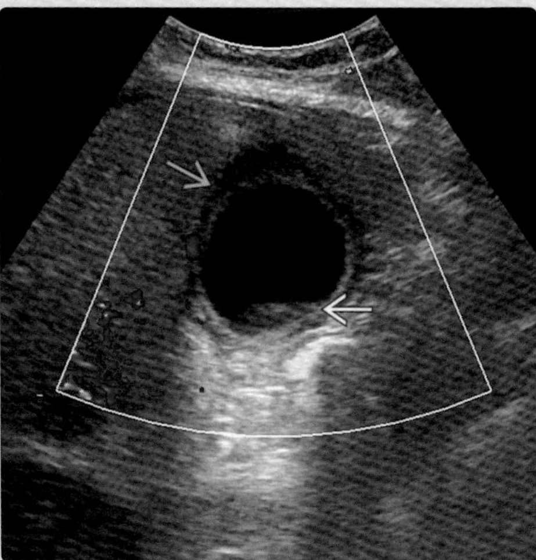

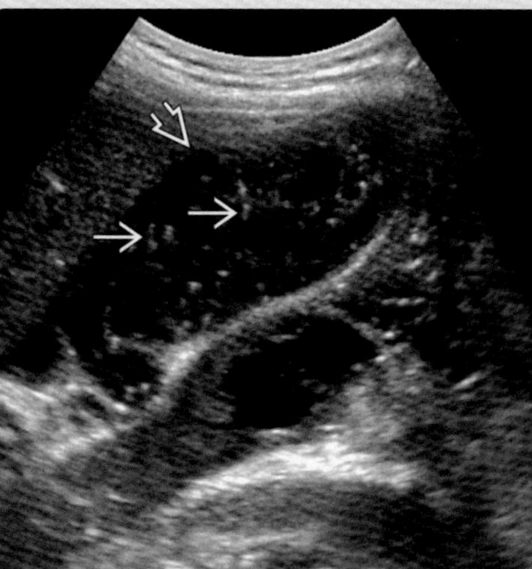

(Left) *Transverse color Doppler ultrasound shows dependent echogenic sludge ➡ with no color flow. The gallbladder wall ⇨ is mildly thickened in this patient with liver disease.* **(Right)** *Longitudinal ultrasound in a decubitus position shows multiple bright intraluminal echoes, which were mobile on real-time imaging. Note the comet-tail artifacts ➡. The gallbladder wall ➡ is normal.*

KEY FACTS

IMAGING

- Single or multiple small, round/ovoid masses attached to gallbladder (GB) wall with no posterior acoustic shadowing
  - Usually sessile but may be pedunculated with well-defined stalk
- Usually 2-10 mm in size, most commonly in middle 1/3 of GB
- Cholesterol polyp: Small with comet-tail artifact
- Avascular or hypovascular on Doppler examination
  - Larger lesions may have slight internal vascularity
- Consider neoplastic GB polyp if size > 10 mm, irregular outline, sessile morphology with abnormal GB wall and invasion of adjacent structures, growth on serial US examinations

TOP DIFFERENTIAL DIAGNOSES

- Hyperplastic cholecystosis/adenomyomatosis
- Nonshadowing cholelithiasis or sludge
- Adenoma
- Carcinoma or metastasis

PATHOLOGY

- Polypoid lesions include cholesterol polyp, adenomyomatosis, and neoplasms such as adenoma, carcinoma, and metastases

CLINICAL ISSUES

- 5% of population have polyps; 50% are cholesterol polyps
- More common in middle age; F > M; incidental finding
  - < 6 mm: No follow-up
  - 7-9 mm: Yearly US follow-up to monitor size
  - > 10 mm: Surgical consult

SCANNING TIPS

- Scan in supine, decubitus (left or right lateral) positions to demonstrate immobility of GB polyp
- Look for color flow in polyp and for any abnormality of adjacent GB wall, which might indicate cancer

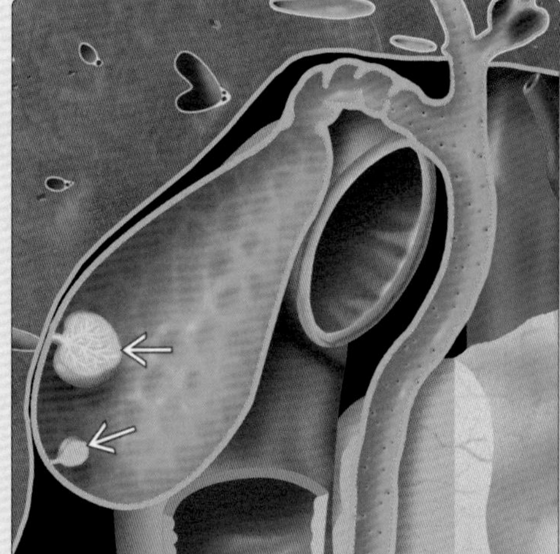

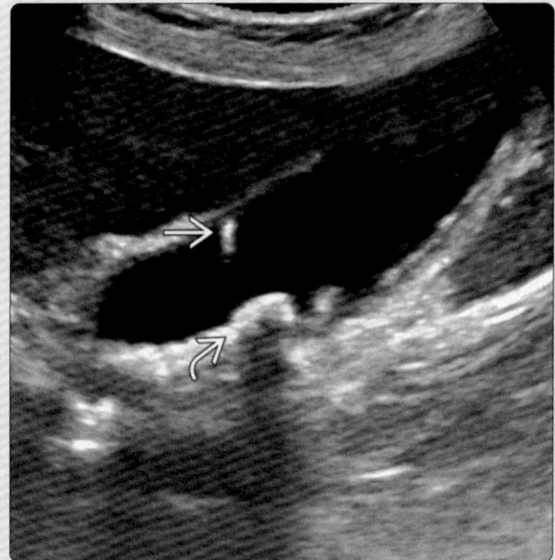

(Left) *Graphic shows well-circumscribed, pedunculated nodules ➡ arising from the gallbladder (GB) wall, compatible with cholesterol polyps. Note the preserved GB wall without invasion to the adjacent liver parenchyma.* **(Right)** *Longitudinal ultrasound shows a cholesterol polyp on the anterior wall of the GB. Note the ring down artifact ➡. There are also dependent stones ↗ with acoustic shadowing.*

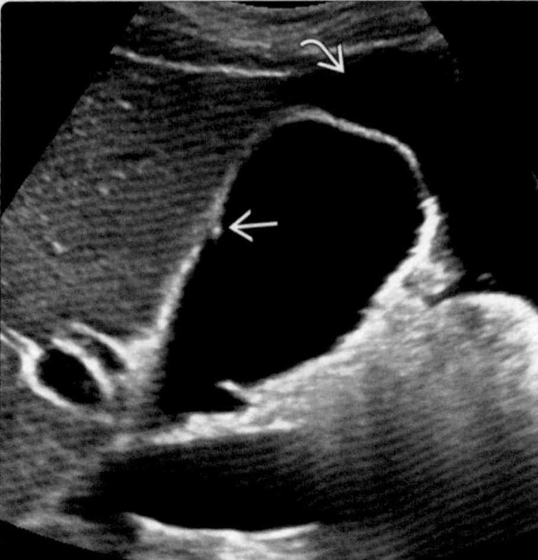

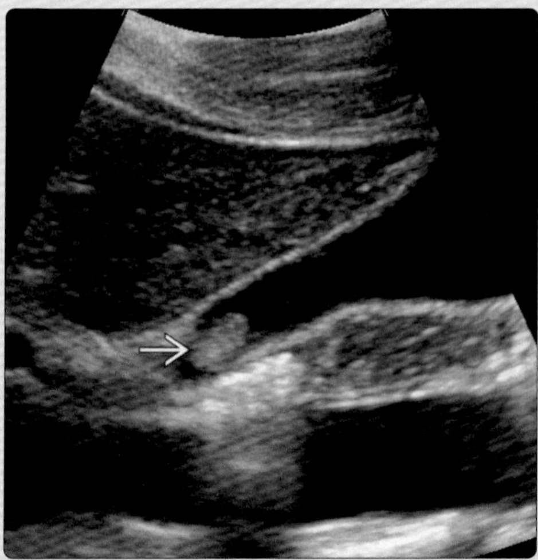

(Left) *Longitudinal oblique ultrasound in the decubitus position shows a cholesterol GB polyp with comet-tail artifact ➡. This was an incidental finding in a patient with chronic liver disease and ascites ↗.* **(Right)** *Longitudinal ultrasound in left lateral decubitus position shows an asymptomatic, fixed polypoid lesion ➡ in the GB neck. Given its size, follow-up is recommended.*

KEY FACTS

TERMINOLOGY

- Acute inflammation of gallbladder (GB) secondary to calculus obstructing cystic duct

IMAGING

- US 1st-line imaging test
- Distended GB (> 5 cm transverse diameter) with rounded/ballooned shape
- Gallstones ± impaction in GB neck or cystic duct
- Diffuse GB wall thickening (> 4-5 mm)
- Hazy delineation of GB wall with echogenic pericholecystic fat ± pericholecystic fluid
- Positive sonographic Murphy sign: Pain and tenderness with transducer pressure directly over GB
- Combination of gallstones, wall thickening, and positive Murphy sign increase specificity
    - Murphy sign may be negative after opioids or when gangrenous
- **Gangrenous cholecystitis**: Asymmetric wall thickening, marked wall irregularities, intraluminal membranes
- **Gallbladder perforation**: Defect in GB wall with pericholecystic abscess or extraluminal stones
- **Emphysematous cholecystitis**: Gas in GB wall/lumen

TOP DIFFERENTIAL DIAGNOSES

- Secondary GB wall thickening or adjacent inflammatory disease

CLINICAL ISSUES

- Typically > 25 years; M:F = 1:3
- Acute right upper quadrant pain, nausea, anorexia, vomiting, local tenderness to palpation
- Increased WBC; mild elevation in liver enzymes

SCANNING TIPS

- Move patient to look for impacted stone in neck/cystic duct, assess Murphy sign and surrounding area

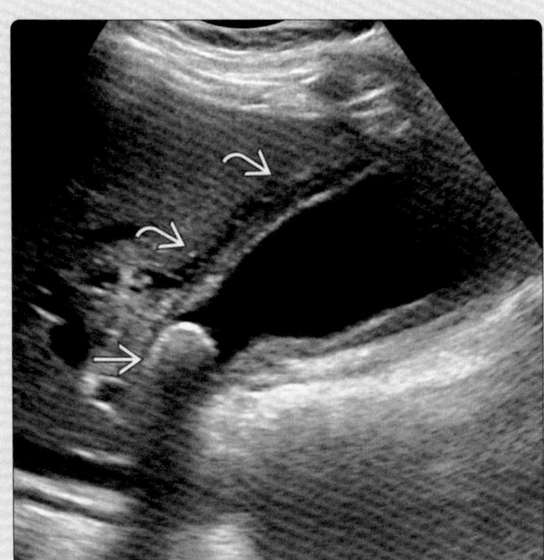

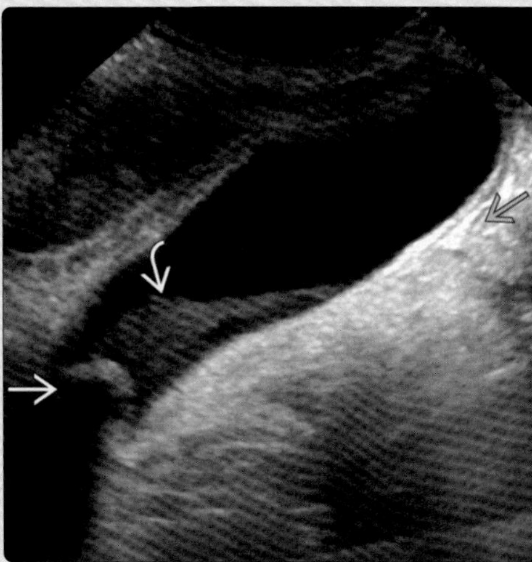

(Left) *Left lateral decubitus ultrasound shows a shadowing stone in the neck of the gallbladder (GB)* ➡. *Note the thick wall with subserosal edema* ➡. *Murphy sign was positive.* **(Right)** *Longitudinal ultrasound in the left lateral decubitus position shows that the GB is distended. There is an impacted stone in the neck* ➡ *with a sludge level* ➡ *and increased echogenicity of the pericholecystic fat* ➡.

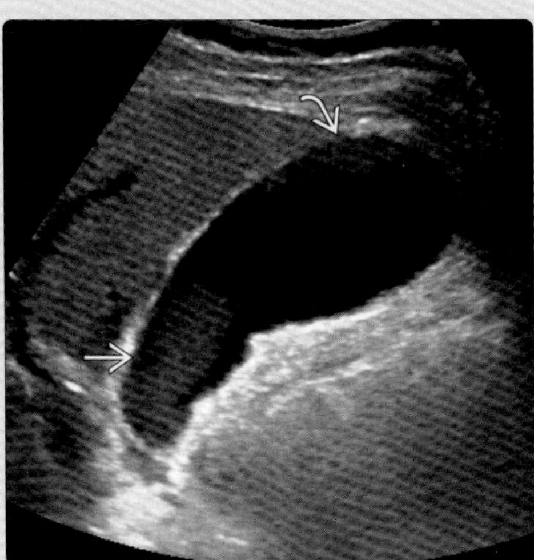

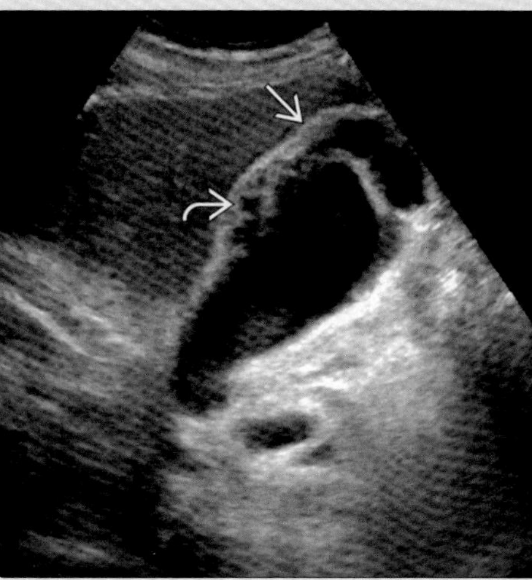

(Left) *Longitudinal ultrasound in the left lateral decubitus position shows a distended GB with a bulging contour* ➡. *Murphy sign was positive. There is sludge* ➡, *but the wall was not thick. Small stones and acute cholecystitis were found at surgery.* **(Right)** *Longitudinal oblique ultrasound shows gangrenous perforated cholecystitis with a shaggy wall* ➡ *and a focal collection at the fundus* ➡. *The lumen is less distended once the wall has perforated.*

Acute Acalculous Cholecystitis

KEY FACTS

TERMINOLOGY

- Acute necroinflammatory disease of gallbladder (GB) secondary to stasis and ischemia, not related to gallstones

IMAGING

- GB wall thickening (> 4 mm) with layered/striated wall
- GB distension
- Positive sonographic Murphy sign, which may not be elicited if patient obtunded, unconscious, or sedated
- US 1st line, HIDA scan for indeterminate US
- 40% develop complications such as gangrene, perforation, and empyema
- CT for complications

TOP DIFFERENTIAL DIAGNOSES

- Acute calculous cholecystitis
- Nonspecific GB wall thickening
- GB mucocele

PATHOLOGY

- Combination of increased bile viscosity and wall Ischemia with secondary infection
- Bile cultures positive in up to 78%
- Pathogenesis multifactorial: Critical illness with sepsis, shock, recent surgery, trauma, or burns

CLINICAL ISSUES

- 0.2-0.4 % of critically ill patients
- Worse prognosis than acute calculous cholecystitis; mortality rate up to 30%
- Acute RUQ pain, fever, sepsis in critically ill patient
- Nonspecific leucocytosis, elevation of liver function tests
- Diagnosis may be challenging in critically ill patient with multiple comorbidities

SCANNING TIPS

- Look for complications such as perforation and abscess

(Left) *Distended gallbladder (GB) with sludge ➡ is shown in a sick patient with a left ventricular assist device. It was not possible to assess the Murphy sign, as the patient was intubated and sedated.* **(Right)** *Longitudinal oblique US of acalculous cholecystitis shows that the GB is distended with sludge and wall thickening ➡. There were no gallstones, but there was a small amount of pericholecystic fluid ➡.*

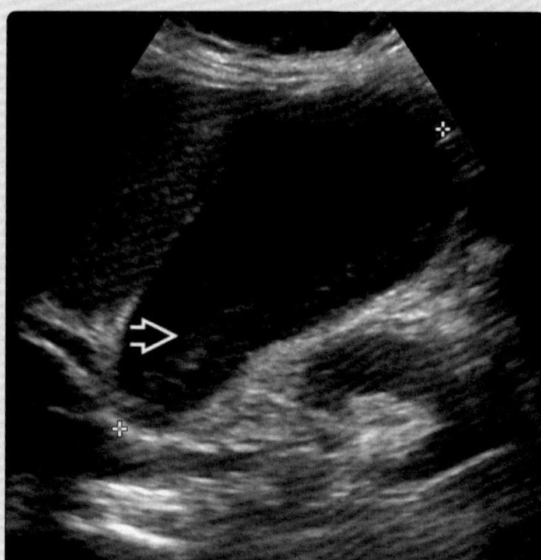

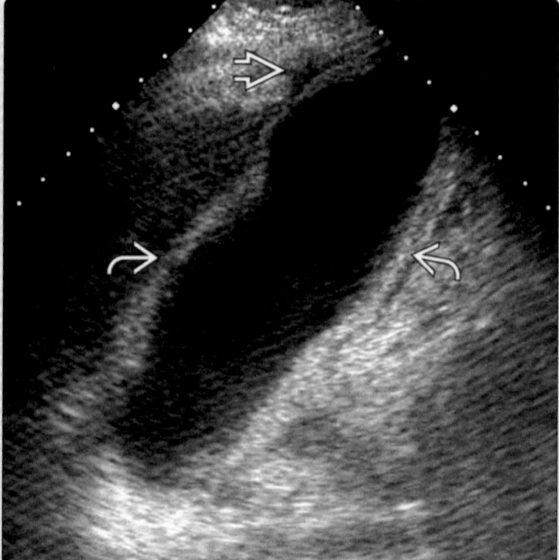

(Left) *Left lateral decubitus US of acalculous cholecystitis shows sludge ➡, wall thickening ➡, and a pericholecystic collection ➡. No gallstones were found.* **(Right)** *Transverse US of perforated acalculous cholecystitis shows an irregularly thickened GB wall ➡ with intramural edema. There is localized pericholecystic fluid ➡ with an abscess that is not shown.*

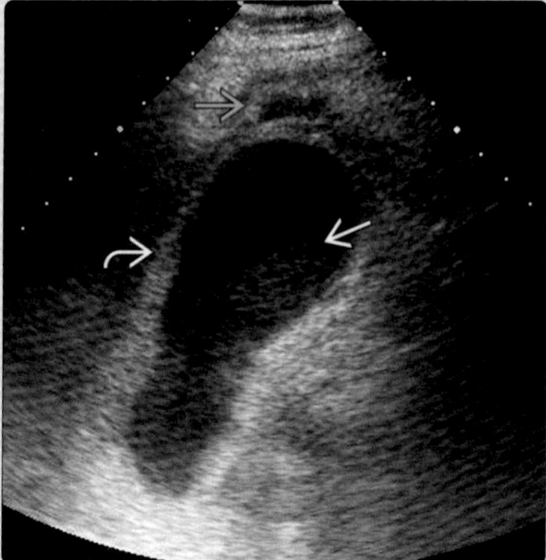

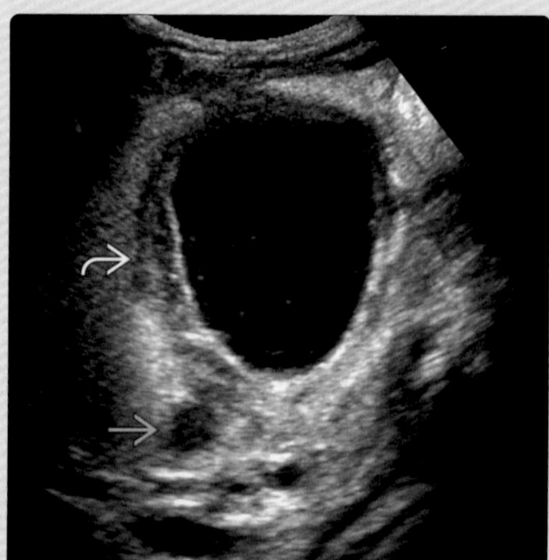

KEY FACTS

TERMINOLOGY

- Chronic inflammation of gallbladder (GB) causing wall thickening and fibrosis

IMAGING

- Presence of gallstones in nearly all cases
- Diffuse symmetric GB wall thickening without hyperemia
- Pericholecystic inflammation usually absent
- Poor GB distension despite fasting
- Localized tenderness usually mild, unlike acute cholecystitis
- US is initial imaging tool
- HIDA scan distinguishes acute from chronic cholecystitis

TOP DIFFERENTIAL DIAGNOSES

- Acute cholecystitis
- Diffuse GB wall thickening from portal hypertension or heart failure
- Adenomyomatosis of GB
- GB carcinoma

PATHOLOGY

- Most common pathology of GB
- 95% associated with gallstone disease
- Intermittent obstruction of cystic duct causes chronic inflammatory infiltration of wall
- Variant: Xanthogranulomatous cholecystitis, mimics carcinoma

CLINICAL ISSUES

- Female > male, middle age, obesity
- Mild intermittent right upper quadrant pain/discomfort after meal or asymptomatic
- Complications include recurrent acute cholecystitis, biliary colic, GB carcinoma, and, rarely, biliary-enteric fistula

SCANNING TIPS

- Look for asymmetric wall thickening, which would suggest malignancy rather than chronic cholecystitis

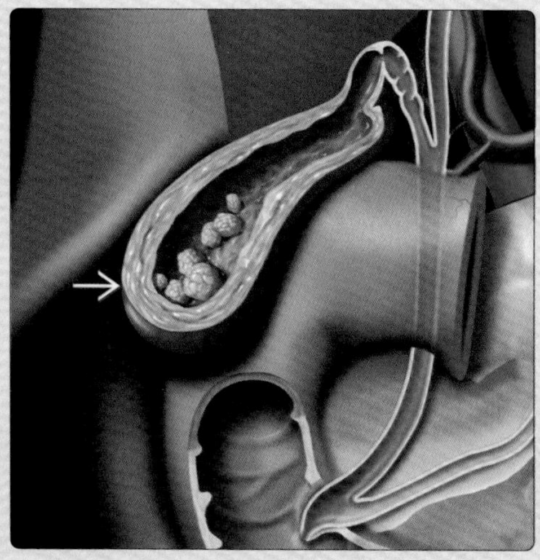

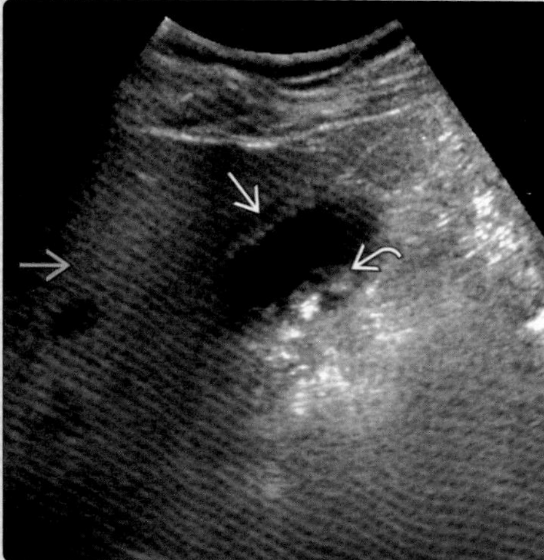

(Left) *Graphic shows multiple gallstones inside a contracted, thick-walled gallbladder ➡, characteristic features of chronic cholecystitis.* **(Right)** *Longitudinal ultrasound of an intubated patient with leucocytosis is shown. The gallbladder is poorly distended despite prolonged fasting. There are stones ➡ and wall thickening ➡. The liver is fatty ➡.*

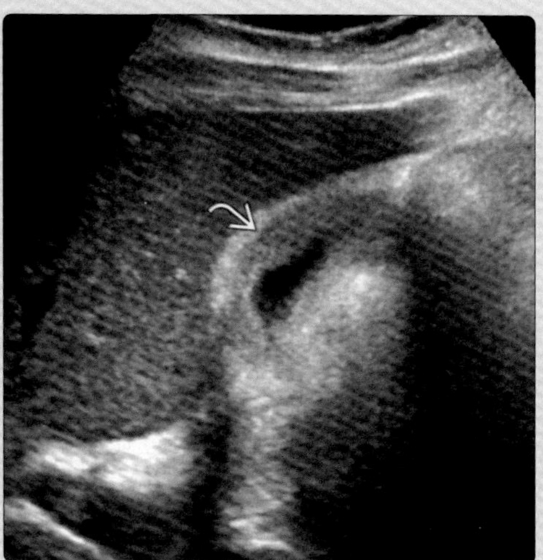

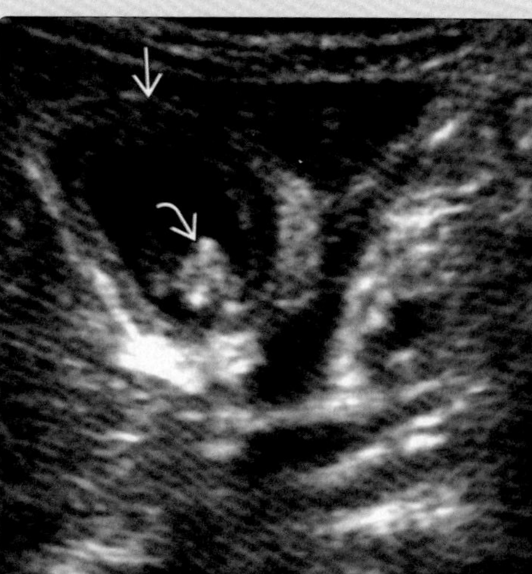

(Left) *Longitudinal ultrasound shows a nondistensible, thick-walled gallbladder ➡ despite prolonged fasting. HIDA scan confirmed chronic cholecystitis.* **(Right)** *Transverse transabdominal ultrasound shows diffuse gallbladder wall thickening ➡ containing an echogenic sludge ball and nonshadowing gallstones ➡.*

Xanthogranulomatous Cholecystitis

KEY FACTS

TERMINOLOGY

- Rare inflammatory process causing focal or diffuse destruction of gallbladder (GB) wall with accumulation of lipid-laden macrophages, fibrous tissue, and acute and chronic inflammatory cells

IMAGING

- Marked GB wall thickening
  - Intramural hypoechoic nodules or bands with continuous mucosa
- Gallstones in 80%
- Absence of hepatic invasion or biliary dilatation when uncomplicated
- Complications in 30%
  - Infiltrative form: GB fossa mass involving adjacent organs and surrounding fat/soft tissue obliterating normal margins, preoperative differentiation from carcinoma nearly impossible
  - Abscesses, fistula

TOP DIFFERENTIAL DIAGNOSES

- GB carcinoma
- Gangrenous cholecystitis
- Hyperplastic cholecystoses

CLINICAL ISSUES

- 1-2% of cholecystectomy specimens
  - Adenocarcinoma seen in up to 10% of resected specimens
- Mean age at presentation: 44-63 years; F > M
- Symptoms of chronic cholecystitis most common, followed by symptoms of acute cholecystitis with leucocytosis
- Less common presentation: Obstructive jaundice, cholangitis, palpable mass
- Treatment: Open cholecystectomy

SCANNING TIPS

- Look for intramural hypoechoic nodules and preservation of mucosal line, which favor this over carcinoma

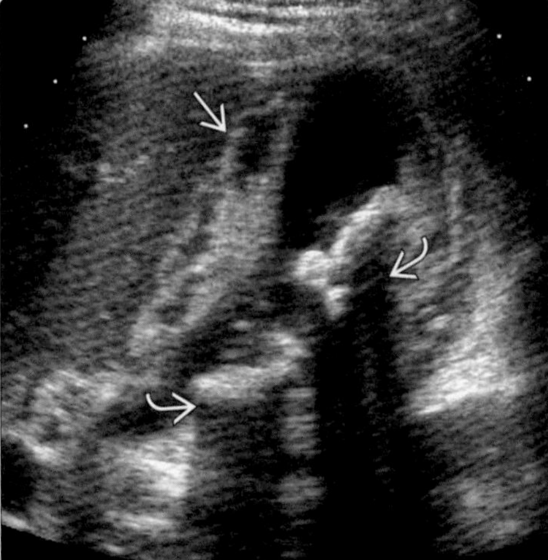

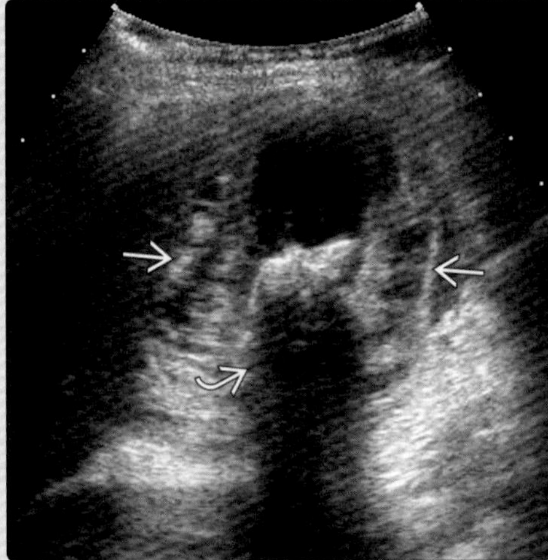

(Left) *Longitudinal ultrasound in an 62-year-old man with right upper quadrant pain and tenderness is shown. There are multiple shadowing stones ➡ and diffuse wall thickening with hypoechoic intramural nodules ➡ compatible with xanthogranulomatous cholecystitis.* **(Right)** *Transverse ultrasound of xanthogranulomatous cholecystitis is shown. The intramural cystic spaces ➡ are not associated with comet-tail artifacts (unlike adenomyomatosis). There are gallstones ➡.*

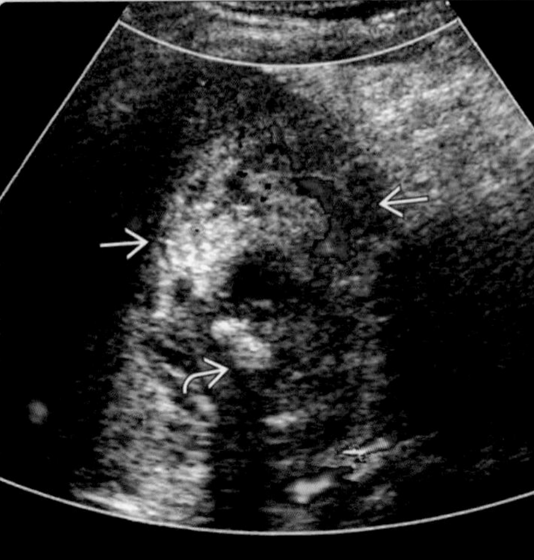

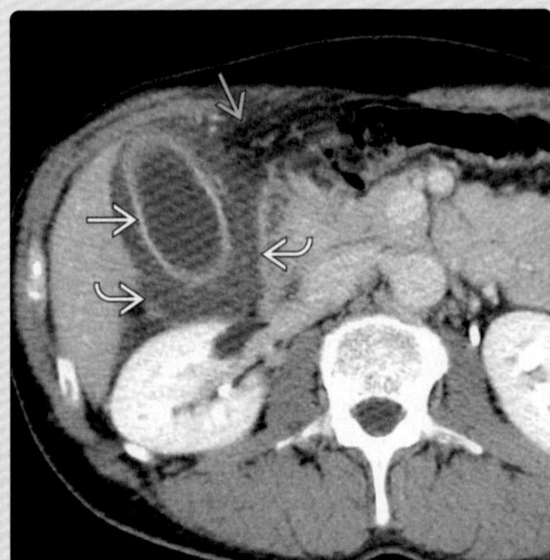

(Left) *Transverse color Doppler ultrasound of xanthogranulomatous cholecystitis is shown. There is color flow in the thickened gallbladder wall ➡ with shadowing stones ➡.* **(Right)** *CT of the same patient from 2 hours prior shows marked wall thickening ➡ and pericholecystic fat stranding ➡. The gallstones were not seen. The CT shows an intact enhancing mucosa ➡.*

KEY FACTS

TERMINOLOGY

- Intramural calcification of gallbladder (GB) wall, uncommon manifestation of chronic cholecystitis

IMAGING

- Variable posterior acoustic shadowing dependent on quantity of calcification
- Complete: Thick, diffuse GB wall calcification
  - Hyperechoic semilunar line in GB fossa
  - Dense posterior acoustic shadowing
- Incomplete: Segmental GB wall calcification
  - Irregular (clumps) hyperechoic foci in GB wall
  - Biconvex curvilinear hyperechogenicity, less shadowing

TOP DIFFERENTIAL DIAGNOSES

- Gallstone-filled GB or large gallstone [wall-echo-shadow (WES) complex]
- Emphysematous cholecystitis
- Hyperplastic cholecystosis

PATHOLOGY

- Associated with gallstones in 95%
- Chronic inflammation/irritation leads to scarring, hyalinization, and dystrophic calcification
- Risk of GB cancer: 0-5% in incomplete type
  - Complete type: No risk, mucosa entirely denuded

CLINICAL ISSUES

- Rare (< 0.1% at autopsy), more common in women (5:1)
- Usually occurs in 6th decade
- Typically asymptomatic; may have biliary-type pain
- Palpable, firm, nontender mass

SCANNING TIPS

- Optimize frequency and focus at level of GB to maximize depiction of calcification and posterior acoustic shadowing
- Look for soft tissue mass, indicating presence of GB carcinoma

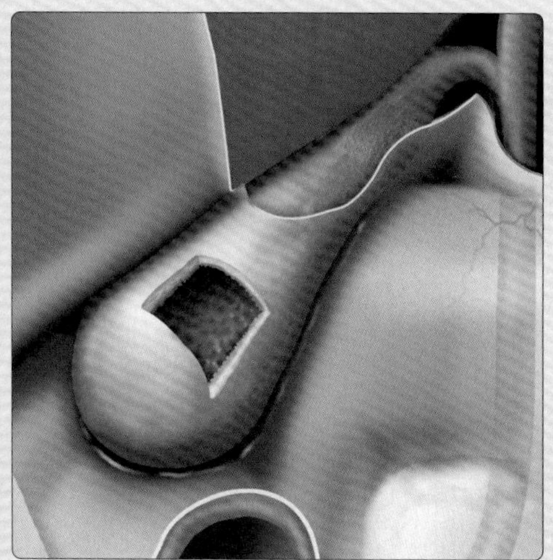

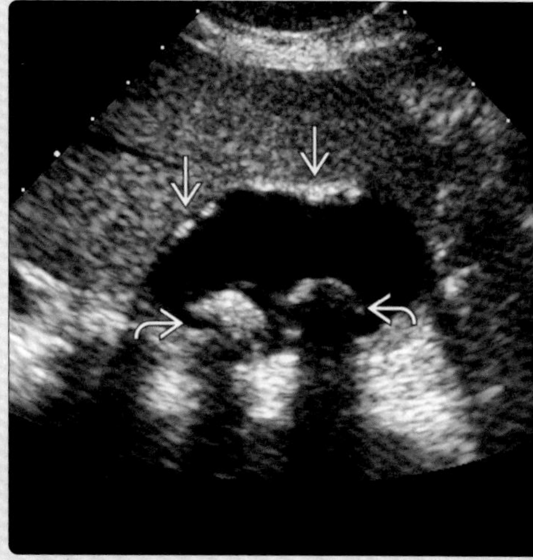

(Left) *Graphic shows diffuse calcifications of the gallbladder walls in a porcelain gallbladder.* **(Right)** *Longitudinal ultrasound of a porcelain gallbladder is shown. There is incomplete anterior wall calcification ➡ with dependent shadowing gallstones ➥.*

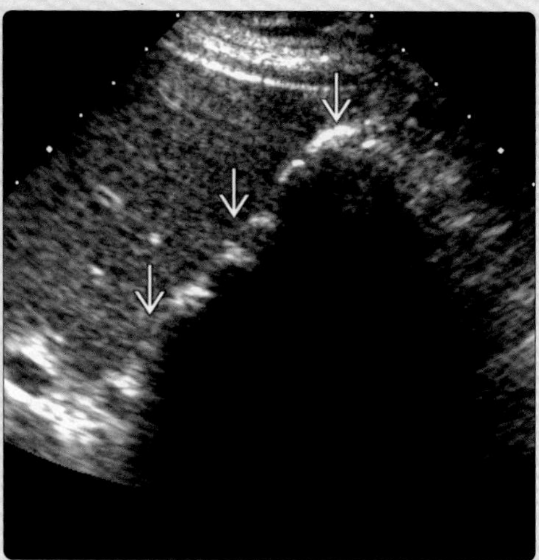

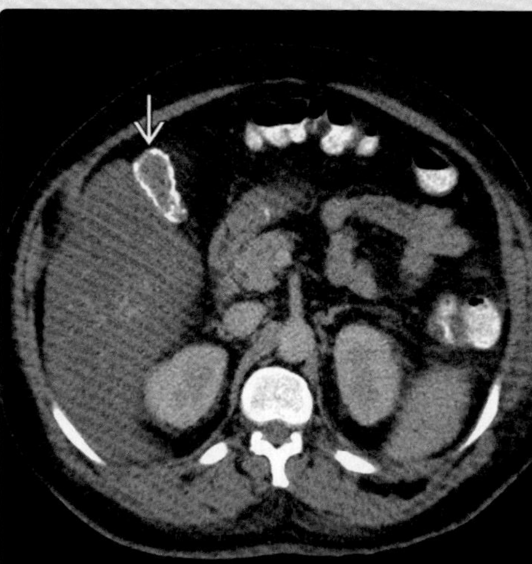

(Left) *Longitudinal ultrasound of a porcelain gallbladder is shown. There is complete anterior wall calcification ➡ with marked acoustic shadowing obscuring the lumen. Note the absence of wall anterior to the calcification, distinguishing this from a gallstone.* **(Right)** *Axial CECT in the same patient shows complete gallbladder wall calcification ➡ and lack of distension.*

Gallbladder Adenomyomatosis

KEY FACTS

IMAGING

- Gallbladder (GB) wall thickening with intramural hyperechoic foci and comet-tail reverberation artifacts
- V-shaped comet-tail artifacts from debris in GB wall cystic spaces
  - Twinkling artifacts from intramural debris on color Doppler examination
- Morphological patterns: Diffuse, segmental, annular, focal
- Annular form: Midbody segmental thickening results in constricting ring around midbody and hourglass shape
- Focal fundal adenomyoma
  - Smooth fundal solitary intraluminal mass, internal cystic spaces, echogenic foci
  - No significant vascularity; ± twinkling artifact

TOP DIFFERENTIAL DIAGNOSES

- GB carcinoma
- Emphysematous cholecystitis
- Chronic cholecystitis
- Adenomatous polyp (fundal form)

PATHOLOGY

- GB wall thickening resulting from epithelial proliferation and muscle hyperplasia leading to formation of intramural diverticula (Rokitansky-Aschoff sinuses) filled with bile, cholesterol crystals, sludge, or calculi
- Gallstones in up to 90%

CLINICAL ISSUES

- 9% prevalence in cholecystectomy specimens
- F > M; mean age: > 50 years
- Most often asymptomatic; or biliary pain/dyspepsia
- No conclusive evidence of increased cancer risk
- No clinical significance in asymptomatic patients when diagnosed correctly and differentiated from carcinoma

SCANNING TIPS

- Use higher frequency transducer for visualization of comet-tail artifacts and cystic spaces; evaluate GB fundus

(Left) *Graphic shows characteristic features of adenomyomatosis. Note the thickened gallbladder wall with multiple intramural cystic spaces ➡.* **(Right)** *Longitudinal ultrasound through the gallbladder shows a focal soft tissue mass at the fundus ➡. There is a comet-tail artifact associated with an echogenic focus ➡ in this patient with fundal adenomyomatosis.*

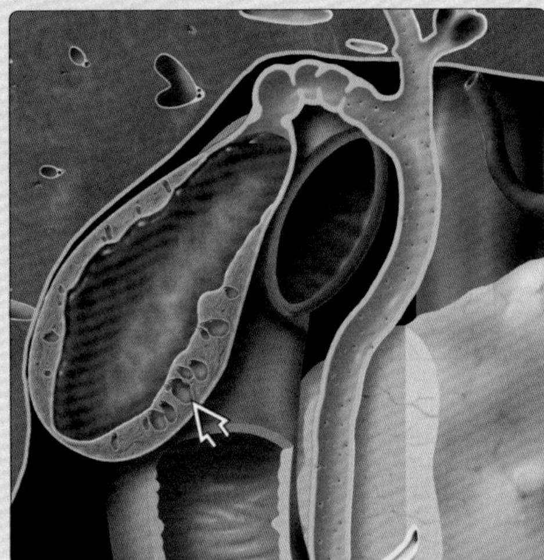

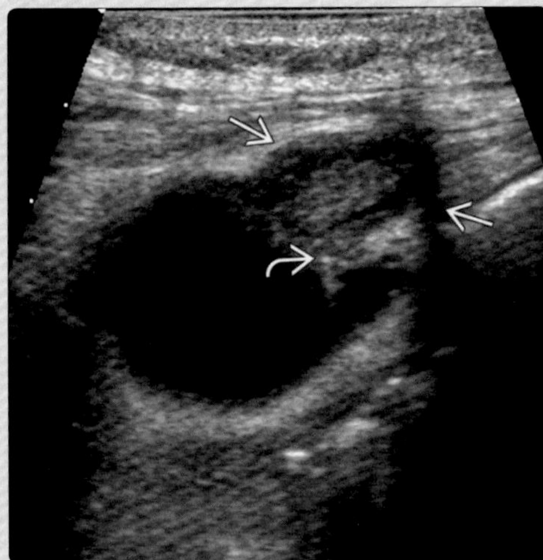

(Left) *Longitudinal ultrasound through segmental gallbladder adenomyomatosis shows proximal wall thickening with comet-tail artifacts ➡. There are stones ➡ in the fundus, where the wall is less thick.* **(Right)** *Transverse oblique ultrasound demonstrates multiple anterior gallbladder wall comet-tail artifacts ➡ emanating from debris in Rokitansky-Aschoff sinuses. The sinuses themselves are not visible. Note reverberation artifact ➡ from adjacent bowel.*

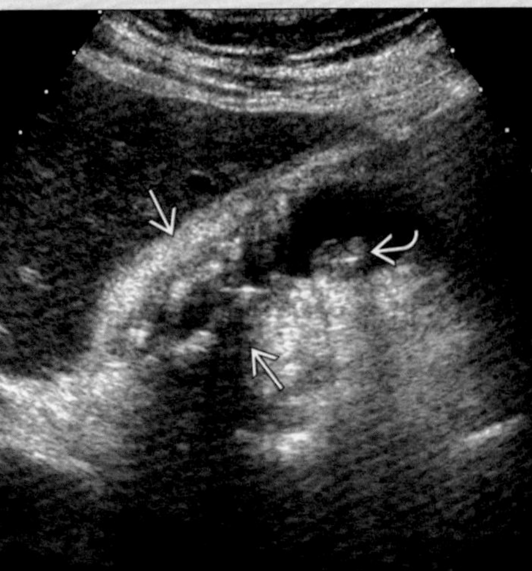

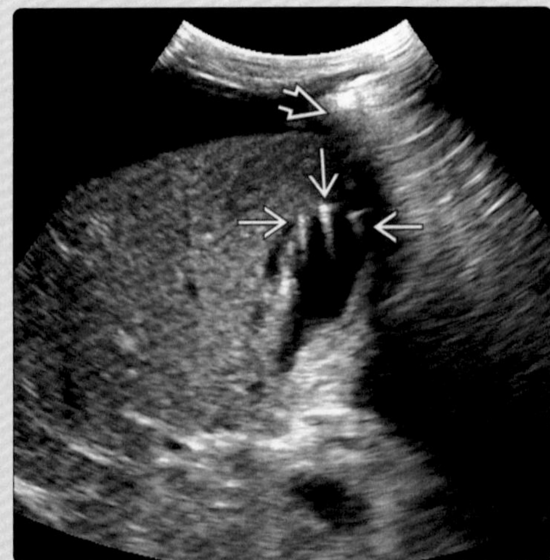

Gallbladder Carcinoma

KEY FACTS

IMAGING

- US for initial detection and characterization, CECT or MR for preoperative assessment and staging
- 3 main morphological types
  - Large soft tissue mass infiltrating gallbladder (GB) fossa/replacing GB, ± invading liver (**most common**)
  - Diffuse or focal GB wall thickening: Asymmetric, irregular, extensive thickening
  - Polypoid intraluminal mass: > 1 cm, thickened base, irregular margins

TOP DIFFERENTIAL DIAGNOSES

- GB polyp
- Chronic or xanthogranulomatous cholecystitis
- Hyperplastic cholecystoses
- Diffuse GB thickening from portal hypertension, heart failure

PATHOLOGY

- Most are adenocarcinoma; mean 5-year survival: 5-10%
- Chronic irritation of GB mucosa by gallstones (GS)
- Malignant degeneration of adenomatous polyps less common
- Spreads by local invasion or hematogenous spread to liver, nodal spread to porta hepatis and paraaortic nodes

CLINICAL ISSUES

- Most common malignancy of biliary tree; prevalence: 3-7%
- F:M = 3:1; mean age: 65 years
- Risk factors: GS, chronic infection and inflammation
- Preoperative diagnosis occurs in < 20% of patients, found at cholecystectomy for stones/cholecystitis
- Right upper quadrant pain, weight loss, anorexia, fever
- Jaundice occurs when tumor invades bile ducts

SCANNING TIPS

- Look for asymmetric mass infiltrating liver

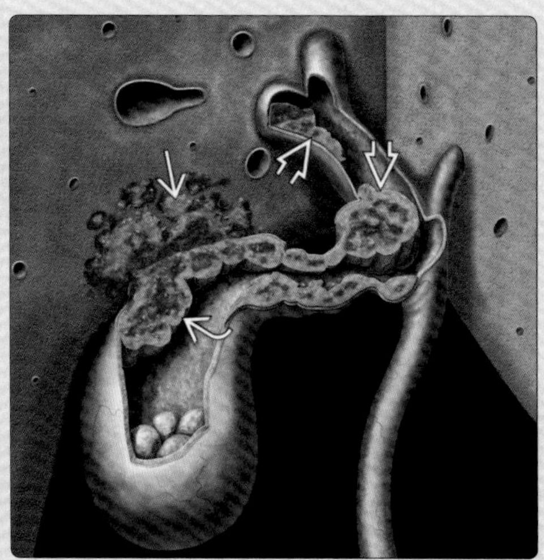

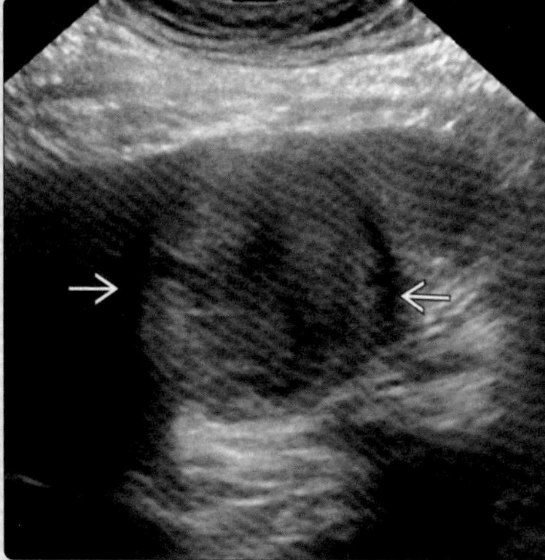

(Left) *Graphic shows pathways of local tumor invasion from carcinoma of gallbladder* ➔*: Direct tumor infiltration to liver parenchyma* ➔ *and retrograde spread along biliary tree* ➔. **(Right)** *Transverse ultrasound shows a distended gallbladder* ➔ *filled with solid tumor proven to be adenocarcinoma. Color Doppler would be useful to confirm that this is a tumor and not sludge.*

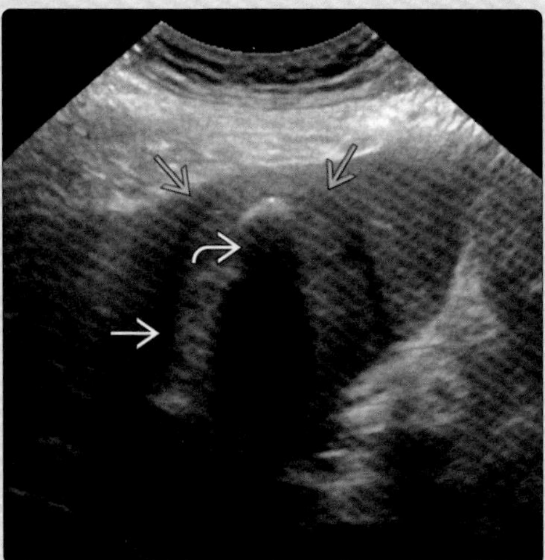

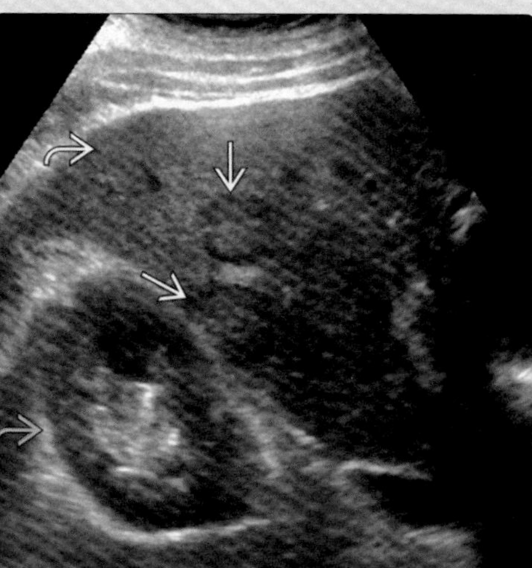

(Left) *Transverse ultrasound of the same patient shows a shadowing gallstone* ➔ *surrounded by tumor* ➔*. The interface* ➔ *between the gallbladder and the liver is indistinct, indicating local invasion.* **(Right)** *Transverse ultrasound of the liver* ➔ *and kidney* ➔ *in the same patient shows liver metastases* ➔*.*

Biliary Ductal Dilatation

KEY FACTS

TERMINOLOGY

- Biliary ductal dilatation, dilated ducts

IMAGING

- Tubular anechoic fluid-filled structures accompanying portal veins in extrahepatic and intrahepatic segments
- Intrahepatic ductal dilatation
  - Dilatation of ductal diameter > 2 mm
- Extrahepatic ductal dilatation
  - Dilatation of common hepatic/bile duct > 6-7 mm or > 40% of diameter of adjacent portal vein

TOP DIFFERENTIAL DIAGNOSES

- Portal vein cavernoma
- Thrombosed portal vein branch
- Venovenous collaterals
- Peribiliary cysts
- Choledochal cyst

PATHOLOGY

- Obstructive causes
  - Intrahepatic: Calculus, recurrent pyogenic cholangitis, sclerosing/AIDS cholangitis, cholangiocarcinoma, etc.
  - Extrahepatic: Calculus, stricture, pancreatic head adenocarcinoma, cholangiocarcinoma, lymph node compression, etc.
- Nonobstructive causes
  - Advanced age
  - Previous cholecystectomy
  - Congenital disease (e.g., choledochal cyst)
  - Hepatic artery stenosis in liver transplant recipients

SCANNING TIPS

- Confirm with color or power Doppler that tubular structure is nonvascular, and follow tubular structure to porta hepatis to confirm communication with common bile duct
- Dilated bile ducts are often tortuous and may demonstrate posterior acoustic enhancement

(Left) *Oblique transabdominal ultrasound through the liver shows moderate dilatation of the common bile duct ➡ and branching intrahepatic ducts ➡ caused by an obstructing pancreatic head tumor (not shown).* **(Right)** *Lack of flow in the dilated tubular structures on this color Doppler ultrasound in the same patient confirms that these are indeed dilated biliary ducts. Color Doppler should be used routinely to confirm biliary ductal dilatation.*

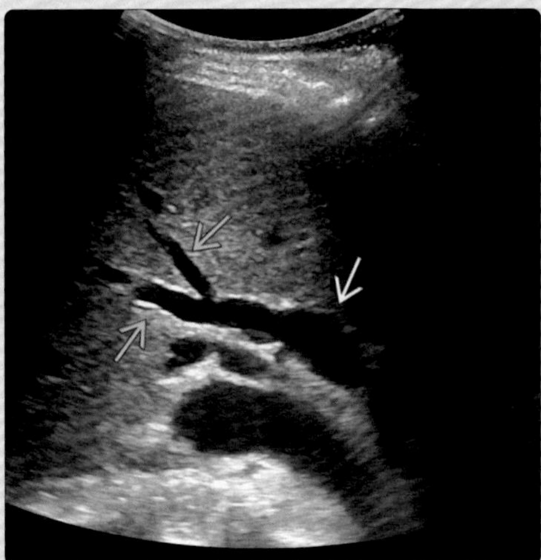

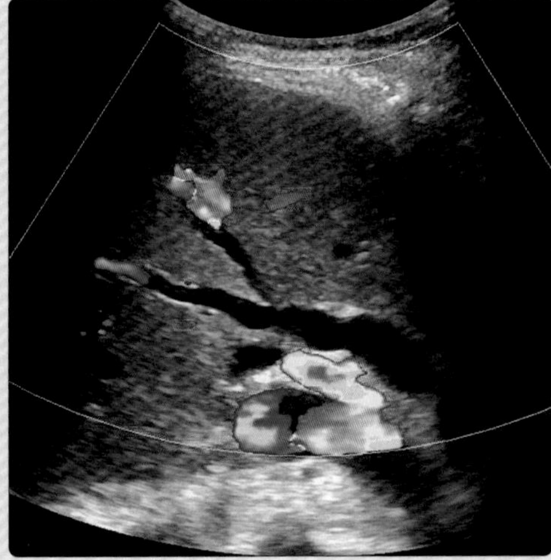

(Left) *Transverse color Doppler ultrasound of the liver shows mild biliary ductal dilatation in the intrahepatic ducts ➡, which measured just over 2 mm in diameter. The cause of mild biliary ductal dilatation was due to an obstructing stone (not shown).* **(Right)** *Transverse color Doppler ultrasound of the liver shows mild biliary ductal dilatation in the intrahepatic ducts ➡ as well as extrahepatic ducts ➡. Patient was found to have both ampullary stenosis as well as cholangitis as the cause of biliary ductal dilatation.*

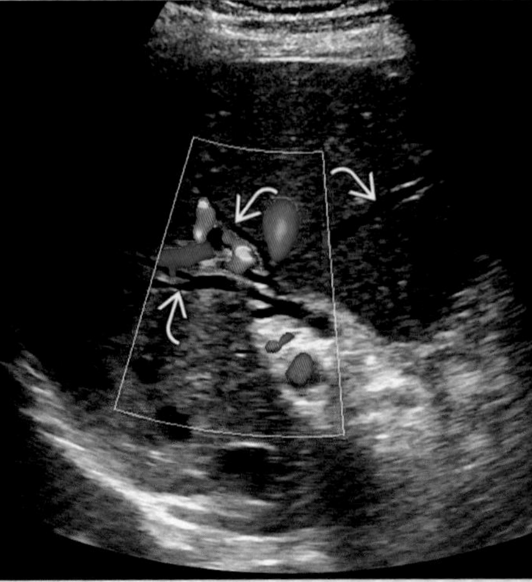

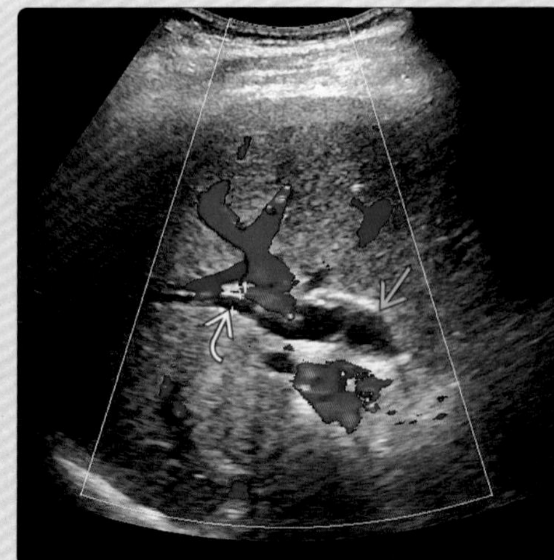

KEY FACTS

TERMINOLOGY

- Spectrum of extrahepatic and intrahepatic bile ducts malformations characterized by fusiform dilatation

IMAGING

- Todani classification
  - Type I: Solitary fusiform or cystic dilatation of common duct
  - Type II: Extrahepatic supraduodenal diverticulum
  - Type III: Choledochocele
  - Type IVa: Both intrahepatic and extrahepatic cysts
  - Type IVb: Multiple extrahepatic cysts without intrahepatic cysts
  - Type V: Single or multiple intrahepatic cysts (Caroli)
- Ultrasound
  - Cystic extrahepatic mass communicating with common hepatic or intrahepatic ducts
  - Intrahepatic ductal dilatation due to simultaneous involvement or secondary to stenosis
  - Abrupt change of caliber at junction of dilated segment to normal ducts

TOP DIFFERENTIAL DIAGNOSES

- Biliary obstruction of various causes
- Pancreatic pseudocyst
- Primary sclerosing cholangitis
- Recurrent pyogenic cholangitis

CLINICAL ISSUES

- Usually diagnosed in childhood (80%)
- Triad: Recurrent right upper quadrant pain, jaundice, palpable mass
- Complications: Biliary calculi, cholangitis, carcinoma
- Surgical excision and enterobiliary reconstruction

SCANNING TIPS

- Caroli disease may appear as unusually shaped cystic structures; look for central dot sign (portal vein within dilated duct) and communication with biliary ducts

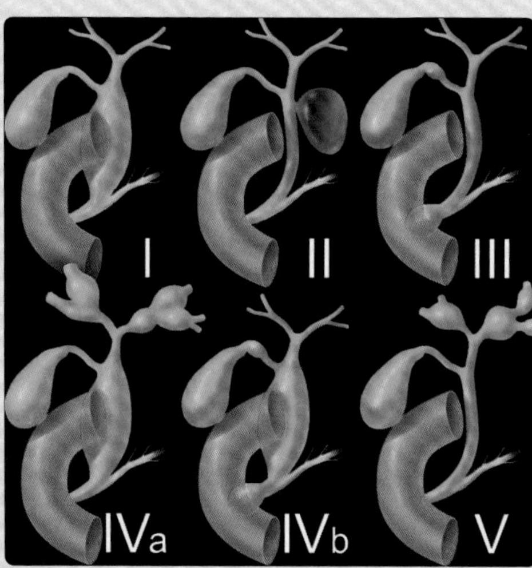

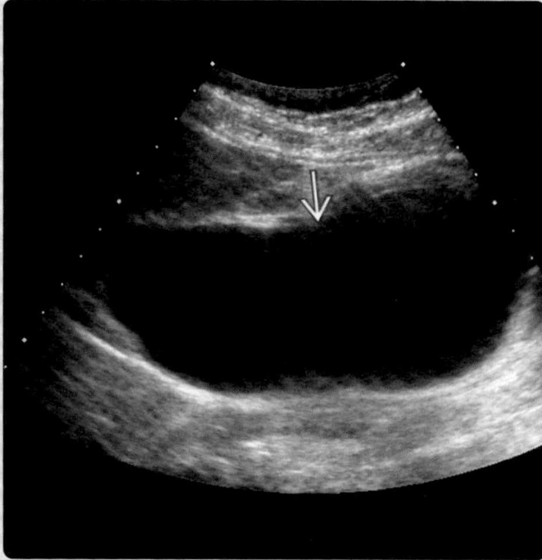

(Left) *Graphic shows Todani classification of choledochal cyst: Type I: Solitary extrahepatic involvement; type II: Diverticulum; type III: Choledochocele; type IVa: Multiple extrahepatic and intrahepatic involvement; type IVb: Multiple extrahepatic involvement without intrahepatic involvement; type V: Caroli disease.* **(Right)** *Longitudinal transabdominal ultrasound shows marked fusiform dilatation of the extrahepatic bile duct ➡ in a patient with type I choledochal cyst.*

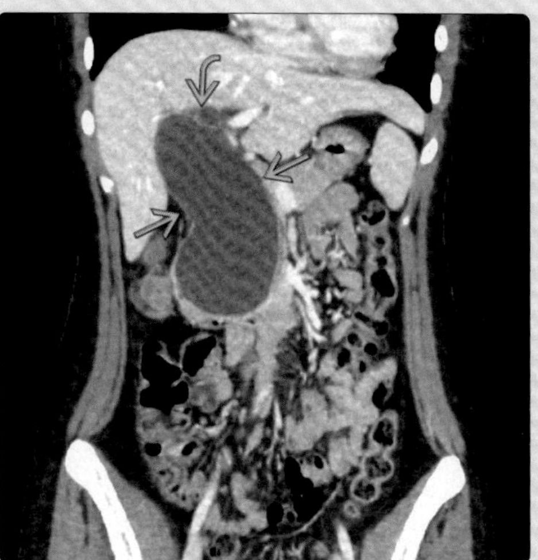

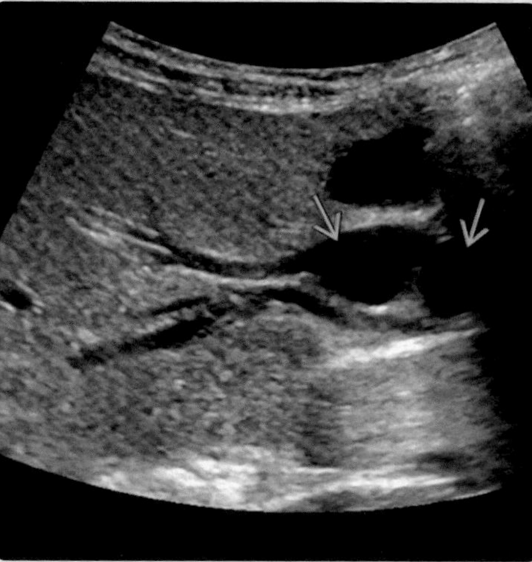

(Left) *Contrast-enhanced coronal CT in the same patient shows marked fusiform dilatation of the common duct ➡ communicating with intrahepatic ducts ➡ consistent with type I choledochal cyst.* **(Right)** *Longitudinal oblique grayscale ultrasound of the porta hepatis shows a multilobulated common duct with 2 distinct lobulations ➡ consistent with type IVb choledochal cyst. (Courtesy S. Bhatt, MBBS.)*

Choledocholithiasis

KEY FACTS

TERMINOLOGY

- Cholangiolithiasis, hepatolithiasis, biliary calculi, common bile duct (CBD) stones

IMAGING

- Most stones are highly echogenic with posterior acoustic shadowing
  - Ultrasound is 1st-line imaging modality
  - Most common in periampullary region/distal CBD
- ERCP: Radiolucent, faceted, or angular filling defects within bile ducts
  - Gold standard is diagnostic and potentially therapeutic
- MRCP: Low-intensity filling defects within increased signal intensity bile ducts

TOP DIFFERENTIAL DIAGNOSES

- Cholangiocarcinoma, ampullary mass
- Ascending cholangitis, recurrent pyogenic cholangitis, or parasitic infection

PATHOLOGY

- Passage of gallstones into biliary ductal system (more common) vs. de novo stone formation within ducts
- Can cause obstruction with subsequent ductal dilation

CLINICAL ISSUES

- Presentation: Right upper quadrant pain, pruritus, jaundice; however, may be asymptomatic
- May present with acute complication: Cholangitis, pancreatitis

SCANNING TIPS

- Most stones will be located in distal CBD; extra effort is required to evaluate entire course of CBD to level of pancreatic head
- Acoustic shadow can be enhanced by using higher frequency transducers or turning off compound imaging
- Gain set too high can obscure posterior acoustic shadowing

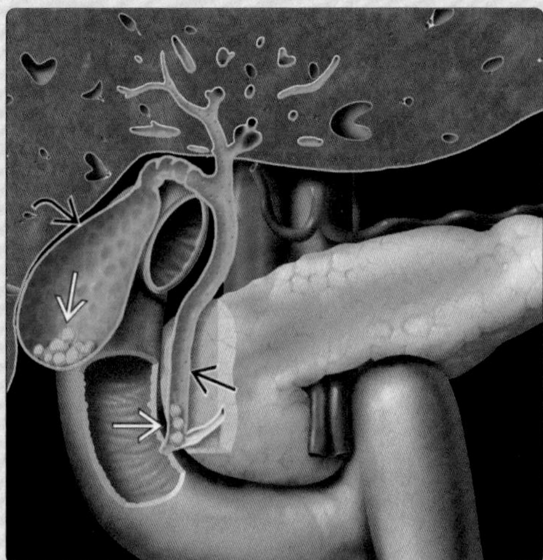

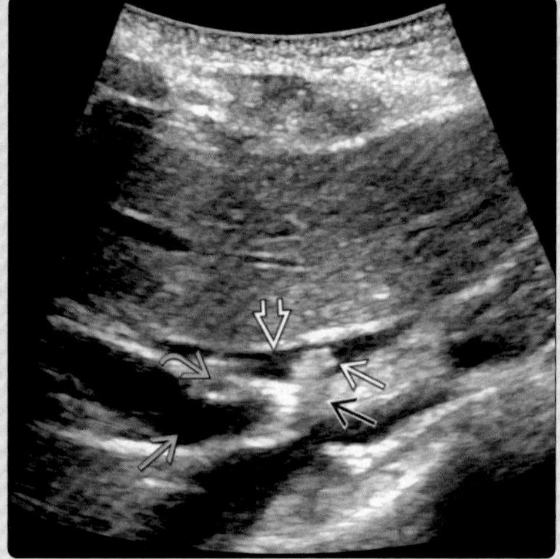

(Left) *Graphic shows multiple nonobstructive stones ➡ in the distal common bile duct (CBD) ➡ and gallbladder ↪.* **(Right)** *An echogenic focus ➡ with posterior shadowing ⇩ that is compatible with a stone is present within the CBD ➡ on this longitudinal US. The CBD is located anterior to the hepatic artery ↪ and the portal vein ➡. The hepatic artery crosses in between the portal vein and CBD.*

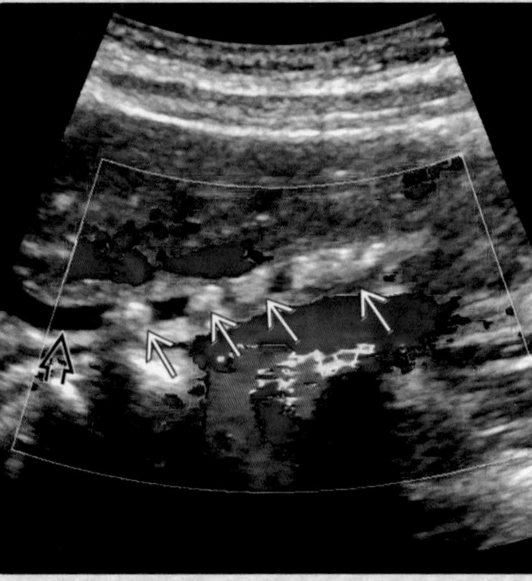

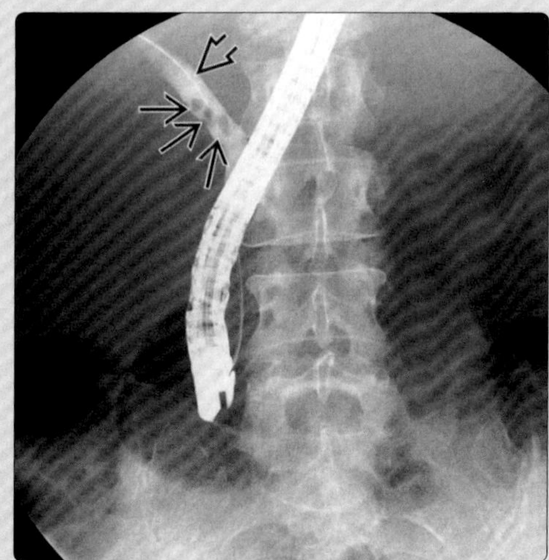

(Left) *More caudally, there are several more stones ➡, which are seen as echogenic shadowing foci within the CBD ⇨ extending to the level of the head of the pancreas. Color Doppler US is helpful to distinguish the biliary ducts from the adjacent vasculature.* **(Right)** *A spot fluoroscopic image from the subsequent endoscopic retrograde cholangiopancreatography procedure demonstrates several filling defects, compatible with stones ➡, within the CBD ⇨.*

Biliary Ductal Gas

KEY FACTS

TERMINOLOGY

- Definition: Gas within biliary tree, including bile ducts or gallbladder
- Synonyms: Pneumobilia, aerobilia

IMAGING

- Bright, echogenic foci in linear/branching configuration following portal triads associated with "dirty" shadowing/ring down artifact
- Most commonly seen within intrahepatic bile ducts, though may also involve extrahepatic bile ducts and gallbladder
- Movement of gas, best demonstrated following change in patient's position

TOP DIFFERENTIAL DIAGNOSES

- Portal venous gas
  - Branching echogenic foci in periphery of liver parenchyma within portal venous radicle
- Intrahepatic ductal stones/sludge
  - Echogenic foci casting dense posterior acoustic shadowing ± dilated duct
- Hepatic arterial calcifications
  - Hyperechoic parallel lines accompanying portal veins
  - More common in chronic dialysis patients

PATHOLOGY

- Etiology
  - Previous biliary intervention, classically papillotomy
  - Cholecystoenteric/choledochoenteric fistula
  - Biliary infection with gas-forming organism
  - Recurrent pyogenic cholangitis

CLINICAL ISSUES

- Majority will resolve spontaneously
- Prognosis depends on underlying etiology

SCANNING TIPS

- Examine patient in supine and oblique positions to demonstrate movement of gas

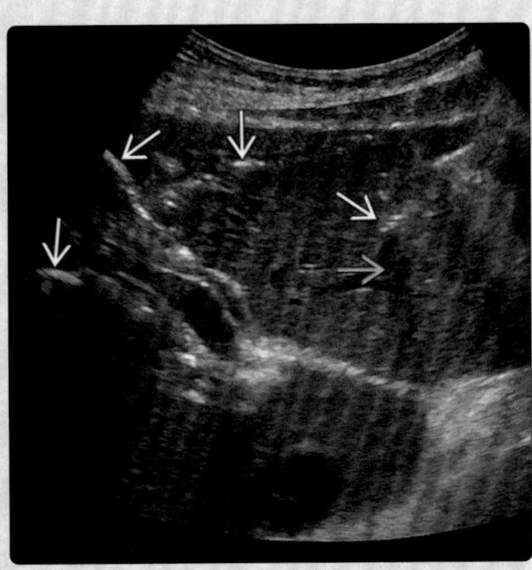

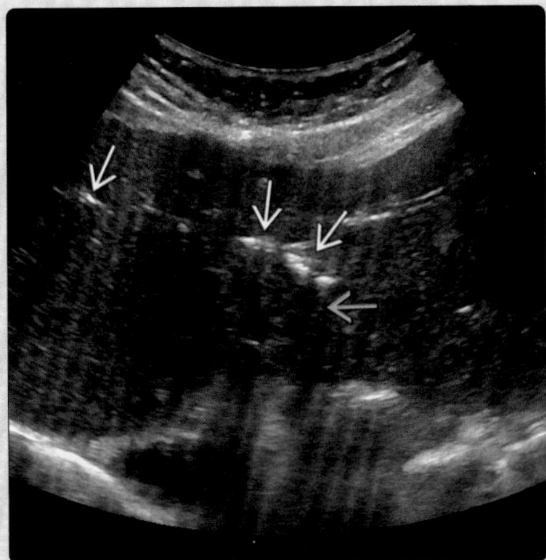

(Left) *Transverse US through the left hepatic lobe demonstrates multiple linear, echogenic areas along the expected course of the biliary tree ➡, some with associated posterior shadowing ⇨, compatible with intrahepatic biliary gas.* **(Right)** *Transverse US through the left hepatic lobe demonstrates linear, echogenic foci ➡ associated with "dirty" posterior shadowing ⇨, compatible with intrahepatic biliary ductal gas.*

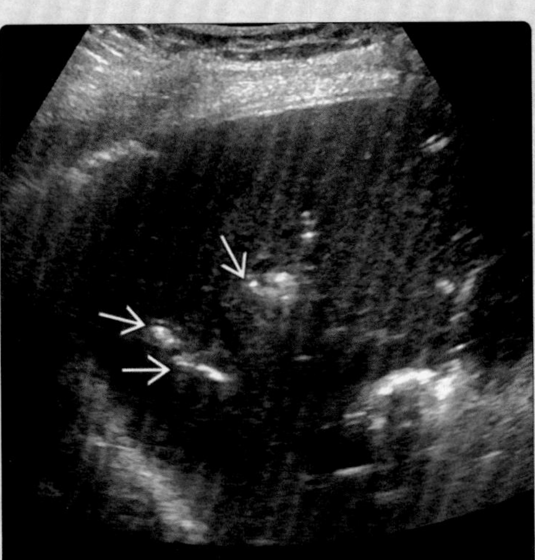

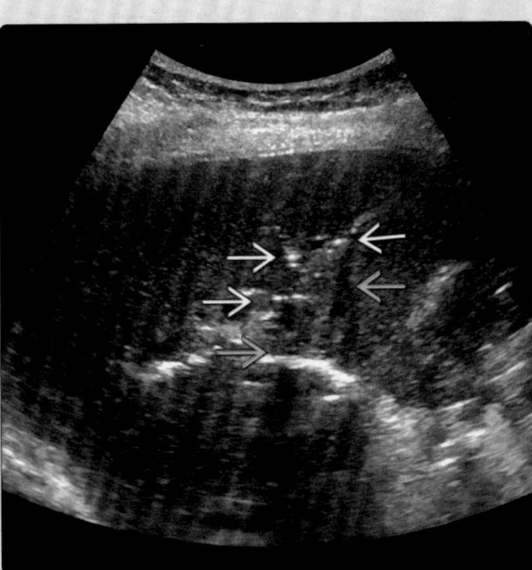

(Left) *Transverse US through the right hepatic lobe demonstrates several echogenic foci ➡ in linear configurations, with "dirty" posterior shadowing, compatible with biliary ductal gas.* **(Right)** *Transverse US through the right hepatic lobe demonstrates several echogenic foci ➡ in linear configurations, with associated "dirty" posterior shadowing ⇨, compatible with biliary ductal gas.*

Cholangiocarcinoma

KEY FACTS

TERMINOLOGY

- Malignancy arising from intrahepatic bile duct (IHBD) or extrahepatic bile duct epithelium

IMAGING

- Best diagnostic clue: Intra- or extrahepatic bile duct mass with upstream bile duct dilatation
- Intrahepatic cholangiocarcinoma
  - Mass with ill-defined margin, heterogeneous echotexture
  - Arise distal to 2nd-order bile ducts
  - Isolated thickening of IHBD or intraductal mass with upstream ductal dilatation
  - May see associated capsular retraction of liver
- Hilar cholangiocarcinoma
  - Nonunion of right and left hepatic ducts due to obstructing mass
  - Primary tumor may not be discernible or appears as small, infiltrative iso-/hyperechoic mass in hilar region
- Extrahepatic cholangiocarcinoma
  - Proportional bile duct dilatation
    - Primary tumor often undetectable due to deep location
  - Ill-defined, solid, heterogeneous mass within or surrounding duct at point of obstruction
  - Polypoidal intraluminal tumor visible as iso-/hyperechoic mass within bile duct

TOP DIFFERENTIAL DIAGNOSES

- Pancreatic head adenocarcinoma
- Choledocholithiasis
- Recurrent pyogenic cholangitis
- Primary sclerosing cholangitis
- Porta hepatis tumor

SCANNING TIPS

- Look for capsular retraction, biliary ductal dilatation, or abrupt cut-off of dilated bile ducts

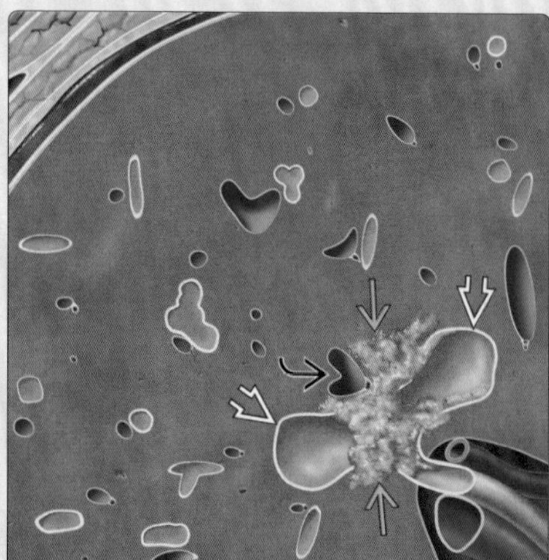

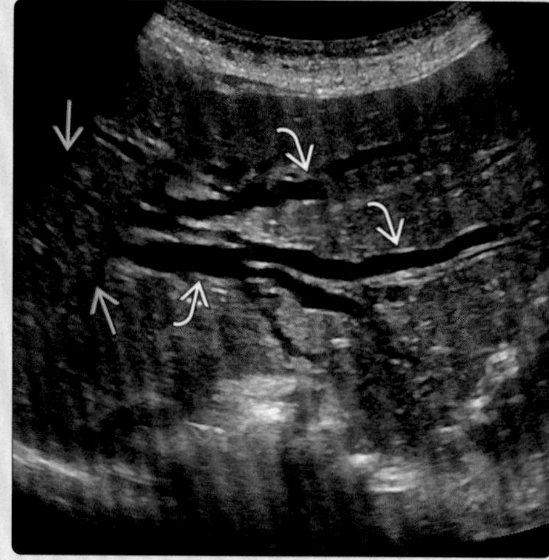

(Left) *Graphic shows an infiltrative mass ➔ at the confluence of the right and left hepatic ducts (Klatskin tumor). The mass invades adjacent liver parenchyma and hepatic veins ➔, a common finding with cholangiocarcinoma. Note upstream dilatation of intrahepatic bile ducts ➔.* **(Right)** *Transverse abdominal grayscale ultrasound shows an ill-defined, isoechoic cholangiocarcinoma ➔ at the hepatic confluence associated with marked left intrahepatic ductal dilatation ➔.*

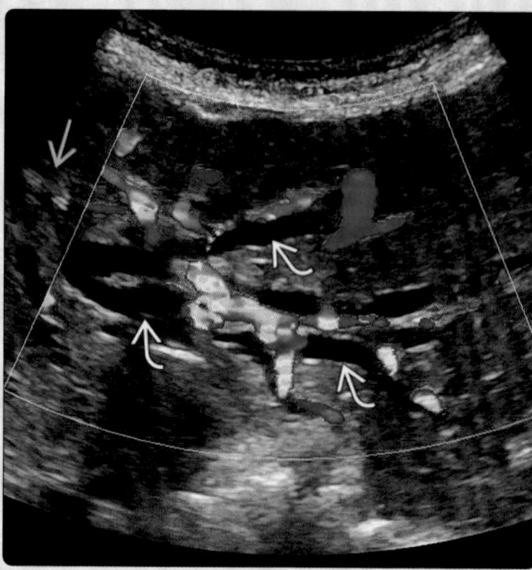

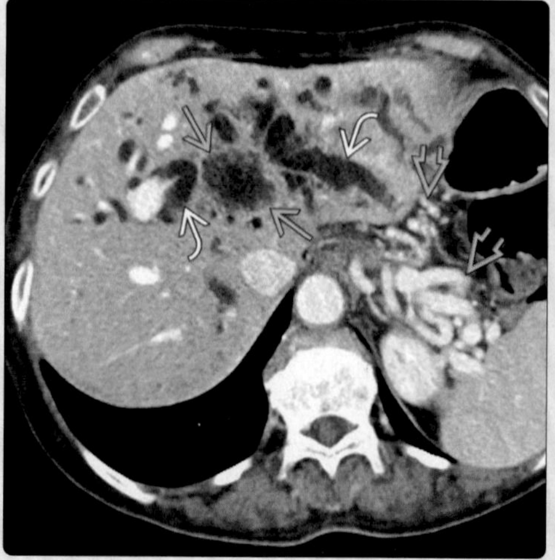

(Left) *Color Doppler ultrasound in the same patient confirms tubular structures are indeed dilated intrahepatic bile ducts ➔ caused by an isoechoic cholangiocarcinoma involving the hepatic confluence ➔.* **(Right)** *Axial CECT shows a hypodense cholangiocarcinoma at the hepatic hilar level invading liver parenchyma ➔ with marked intrahepatic duct dilatation ➔ in right and left lobes. Note gastric/splenic varices ➔ caused by portal vein obliteration (not shown) by the tumor.*

KEY FACTS

TERMINOLOGY

- Inflammation of intra-/extrahepatic bile duct walls due to ductal obstruction and infection

IMAGING

- Dilatation of intra- and extrahepatic bile ducts
  - In cases of early cholangitis or intermittent common bile duct obstruction, bile ducts may not be dilated
- Circumferential thickening of bile duct wall
- Presence of obstructing choledocholithiasis or obstructing tumor
- Periportal hypo-/hyperechogenicity adjacent to dilated intrahepatic ducts
- Presence of purulent bile/sludge
- Multiple small hepatic cholangitic abscesses

TOP DIFFERENTIAL DIAGNOSES

- Cholangiocarcinoma
- Pancreatic ductal carcinoma
- Primary sclerosing cholangitis
- Recurrent pyogenic cholangitis
- Other forms of secondary cholangitis

PATHOLOGY

- Risk factors
  - Choledocholithiasis: Most common
  - Biliary stricture, biliary stent, choledochal surgery, recent biliary manipulation, and sphincter of Oddi dysfunction

CLINICAL ISSUES

- Charcot triad: Right upper quadrant pain, fever, jaundice
- Complications: Cholangitic liver abscesses and septicemia, portal vein thrombosis
- Treatment: Antibiotics and biliary decompression

SCANNING TIPS

- Look for distal obstructing lesion as most cases of cholangitis occur in partially obstructed biliary system

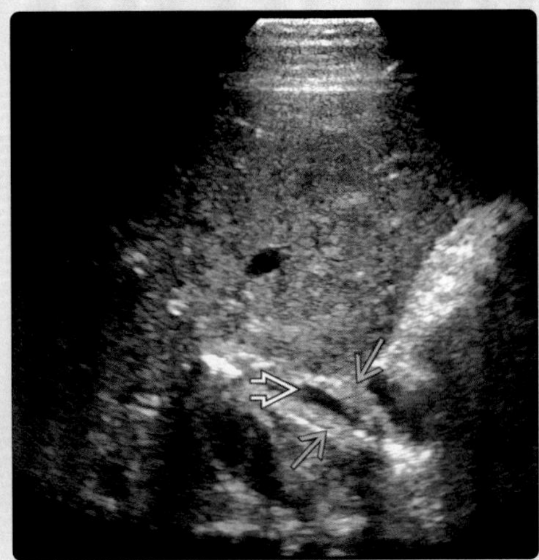

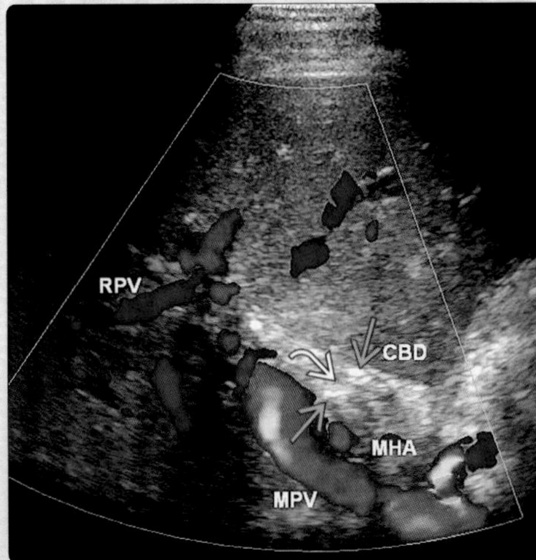

(Left) *Transverse abdominal ultrasound in a patient with ascending cholangitis shows circumferential markedly thickened common bile duct wall (CBD) ➙ with only minimal luminal ➙ distension.* **(Right)** *Transverse color Doppler ultrasound in the same patient with ascending cholangitis shows a lack of detectable vascularity in the thickened CBD ➙. In addition, echogenic debris ➙ within the CBD is evident on this image.*

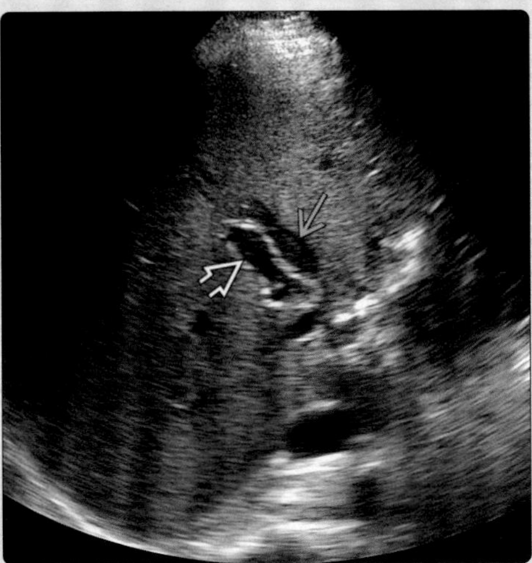

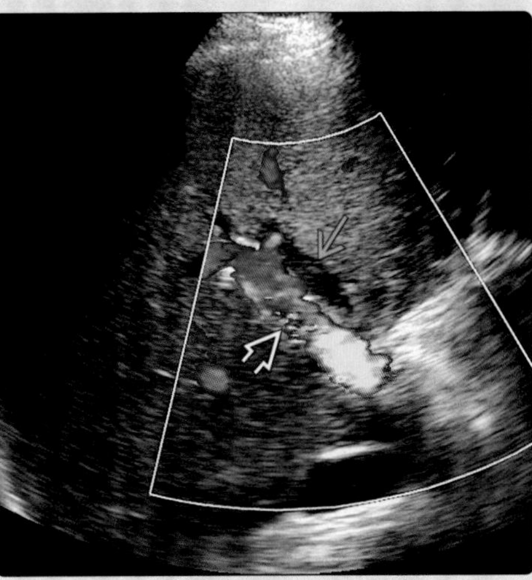

(Left) *Transverse abdominal grayscale ultrasound in a patient with ascending cholangitis shows mildly dilated proximal intrahepatic duct ➙ anterior to right portal vein ➙, consistent with a mild degree of biliary obstruction.* **(Right)** *Transverse abdominal color Doppler ultrasound in the same patient imaged closer to the porta hepatis confirms the tubular structure is a dilated CBD ➙, which lies anterior to the main portal vein ➙.*

Recurrent Pyogenic Cholangitis

KEY FACTS

TERMINOLOGY

- Recurrent episodes of acute pyogenic cholangitis with intra- and extrahepatic biliary pigment stones
- Synonyms: Hepatolithiasis, oriental cholangiohepatitis

IMAGING

- Intra- and extrahepatic biliary ductal dilatations with stones
- Lateral segment of left lobe and posterior segment of right lobe more commonly involved
- Biliary ductal thickening due to repeated inflammation
- Severe atrophy of affected lobe/segment, biliary cirrhosis
- Grayscale ultrasound
  - Presence of echogenic sludge/stones ± posterior acoustic shadowing in intrahepatic and extrahepatic duct
  - Periportal hypo-/hyperechogenicity due to periductal inflammation
  - Ductal rigidity and straightening, rapid tapering of peripheral intrahepatic duct

TOP DIFFERENTIAL DIAGNOSES

- Ascending cholangitis
- Sclerosing cholangitis
- Cholangiocarcinoma
- Intrahepatic stones secondary to biliary stricture
- Caroli disease

CLINICAL ISSUES

- Common symptoms/signs: Recurrent episodes of RUQ pain, fever, and jaundice
- Risk of developing cholangiocarcinoma (5-6%)

SCANNING TIPS

- To better demonstrate posterior acoustic shadowing of intrahepatic stones, consider turning off compounding
- Echogenic sludge may be mistaken for artifact; zooming in or changing windows may help to distinguish real echoes from artifact

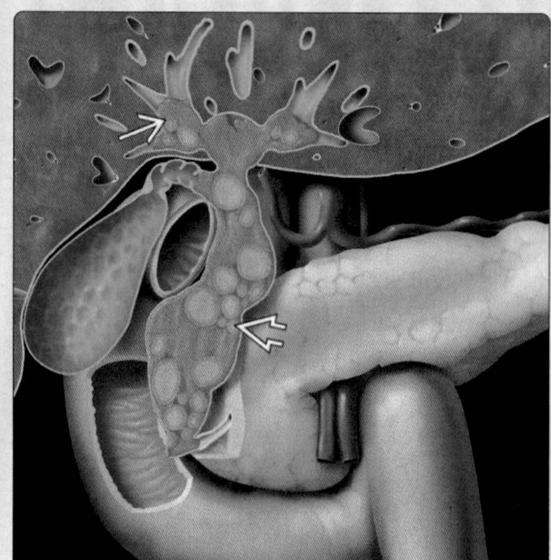

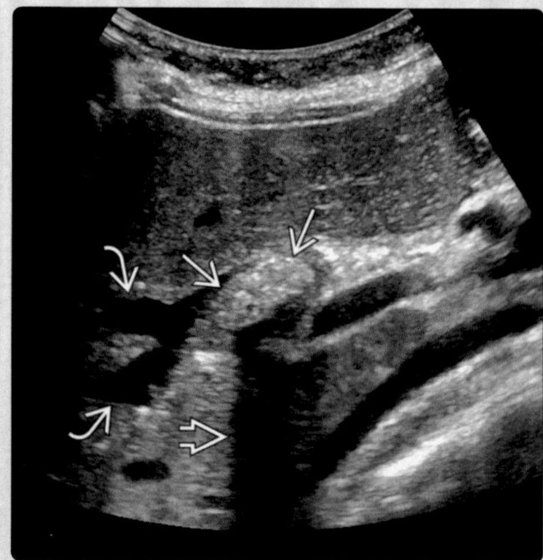

(Left) *Graphic shows recurrent pyogenic cholangitis with marked dilation of intrahepatic* ➡ *and extrahepatic* ⇨ *bile ducts with multiple common bile duct and intrahepatic duct stones. The peripheral intrahepatic duct shows rapid tapering and decreased arborization.* **(Right)** *Grayscale ultrasound shows an ovoid intrahepatic stone* ➡ *with posterior acoustic shadowing* ⇨ *in the right hepatic duct causing upstream intrahepatic bile duct dilatation* ↪.

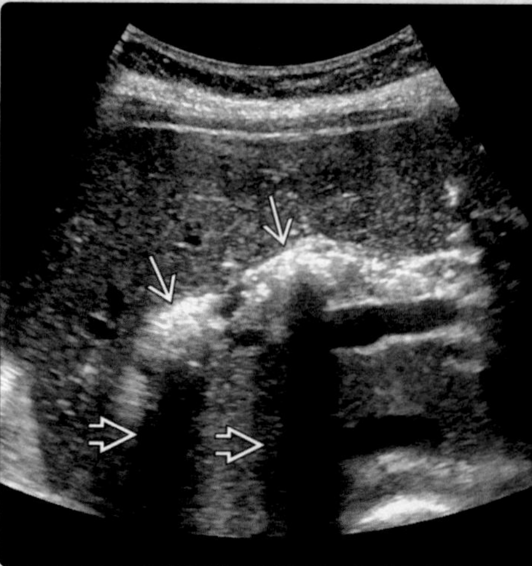

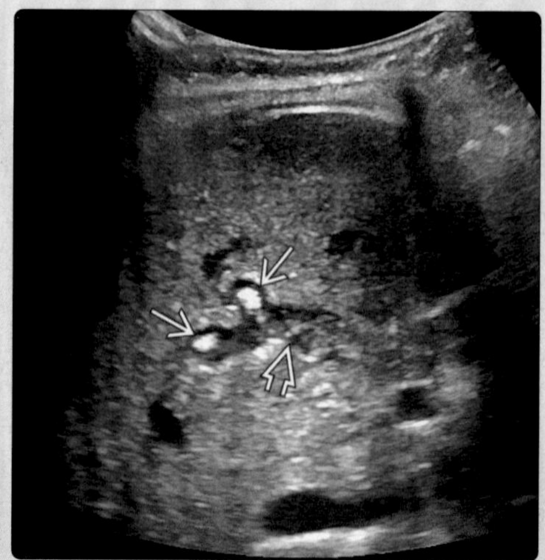

(Left) *Grayscale ultrasound of the liver shows multiple echogenic regions* ➡ *with posterior acoustic shadowing* ⇨ *in the intrahepatic biliary system, consistent with intrahepatic stones in this patient with recurrent pyogenic cholangitis.* **(Right)** *Transverse grayscale ultrasound of the liver shows echogenic stones* ➡ *and sludge* ⇨ *filling moderately dilated intrahepatic ducts.*

HIV-/AIDS-Related Cholangiopathy

KEY FACTS

TERMINOLOGY

- Secondary sclerosing cholangitis usually resulting from opportunistic infection of biliary tract in AIDS patients with CD4 count < 100/mm^3

IMAGING

- Knowledge of HIV/AIDS status is key
- Intra- and extrahepatic bile duct strictures
- Thickened, edematous bile ducts
- Dilated common bile duct from papillary stenosis
- Combination of sclerosing cholangitis and papillary stenosis are unique to AIDS cholangiopathy
- Diffuse gallbladder wall thickening without gallstones
- Ultrasound usually followed by ERCP when tissue can be obtained for culture and therapeutic procedures, such as drainage, can be performed

TOP DIFFERENTIAL DIAGNOSES

- Primary sclerosing cholangitis
- Autoimmune cholangitis
- Ascending cholangitis
- Cholangiocarcinoma

PATHOLOGY

- Chronic inflammation of biliary tract from opportunistic pathogens
- Most common pathogens: Cryptosporidium, CMV
- Favors larger bile ducts

CLINICAL ISSUES

- Epigastric/right upper quadrant, diarrhea
- Fever and jaundice, less common
- Liver function tests may be abnormal
- Decreasing prevalence with improved therapy/prophylaxis of patient with HIV infection

SCANNING TIPS

- Use high-resolution transducer to look for bile duct wall thickening and gallbladder thickening

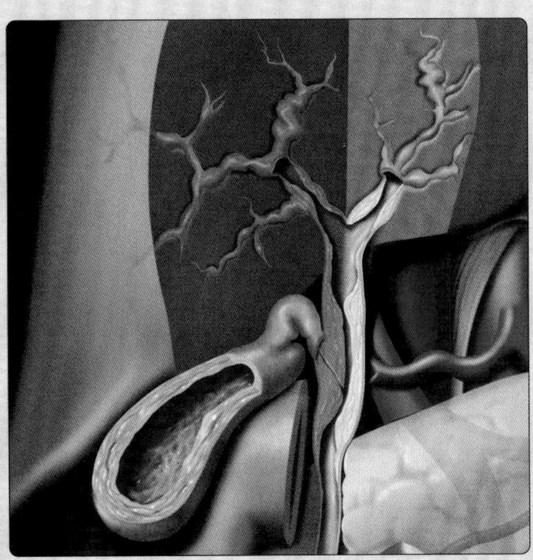

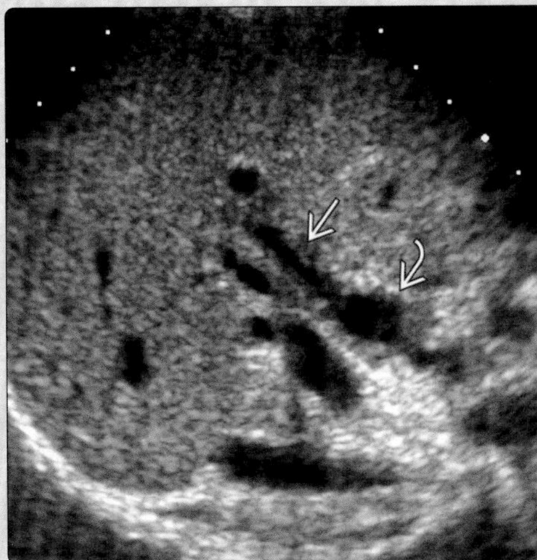

(Left) *Graphic of AIDS-related cholangiopathy shows multiple segments of biliary wall thickening with stenosis involving both the intrahepatic and extrahepatic bile ducts. Also note gallbladder wall thickening.* **(Right)** *Transverse image of the porta hepatis in a patient with HIV/AIDS cholangiopathy is shown. There is bile duct wall thickening and segmental dilatation from a more distal obstruction.*

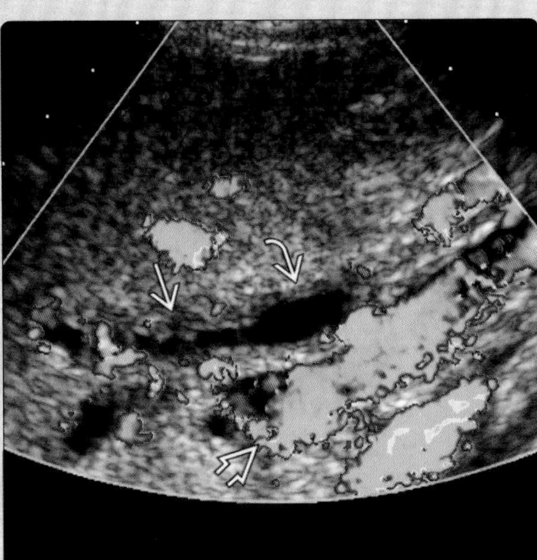

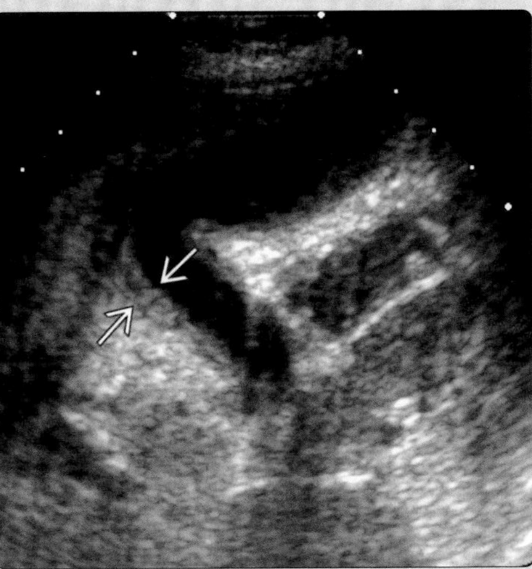

(Left) *Longitudinal color Doppler image of the porta hepatis in a patient with HIV/AIDS cholangiopathy is shown. There is bile duct wall thickening and segmental dilatation from a more distal obstruction. The portal vein is patent.* **(Right)** *Transverse ultrasound of the gallbladder in a patient with HIV/AIDS cholangiopathy is shown. The gallbladder wall is thickened also.*

PART I
SECTION 3
Pancreas

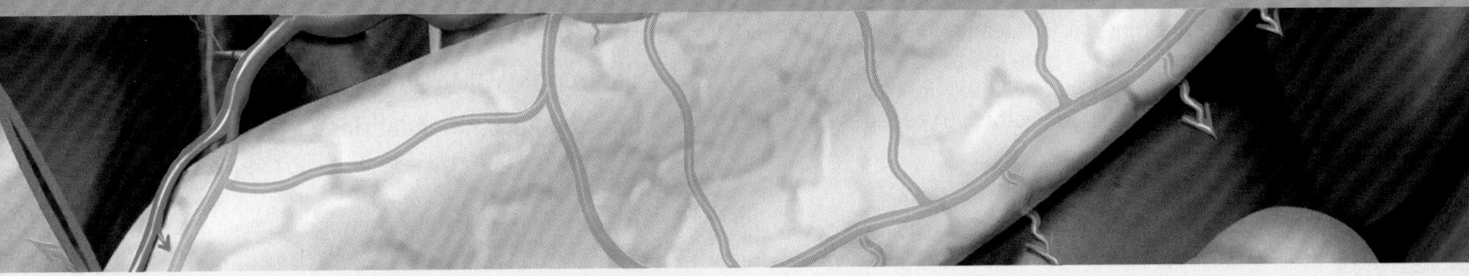

Anatomy and Approach

Pancreatitis

Simple Cysts and Cystic Neoplasms

Solid-Appearing Pancreatic Neoplasms

GROSS ANATOMY

Overview

- Pancreas: Accessory digestive gland lying behind stomach in anterior pararenal space (APS) of retroperitoneum
  - Exocrine function: Pancreatic acinar cells secrete pancreatic juice → pancreatic duct → duodenum
  - Endocrine: Pancreatic islet cells (of Langerhans) secrete insulin, glucagon, and other polypeptides → portal venous system

Divisions

- Head: Thickest part; lies to right of superior mesenteric artery and vein (SMA, SMV)
  - Attached to "C" loop of duodenum (2nd and 3rd parts)
  - Uncinate process: Head extension, posterior to SMV
  - Bile duct lies along posterior surface of head, joins with pancreatic duct (of Wirsung) to form hepatopancreatic ampulla (of Vater)
  - Main pancreatic and bile ducts empty into major papilla in 2nd portion of duodenum
- Neck: Thinnest part; lies anterior to SMA, SMV
  - SMV joins splenic vein behind pancreatic neck to form portal vein
- Body: Main part; lies to left of SMA, SMV
  - Splenic vein lies in groove on posterior surface of body
  - Anterior surface is covered with peritoneum forming back surface of omental bursa (lesser sac)
- Tail: Lies between layers of splenorenal ligament in splenic hilum

Internal Structures

- Pancreatic duct (of Wirsung) runs length of pancreas, turning inferiorly through head to join bile duct
- Accessory pancreatic duct (of Santorini) opens into duodenum at minor duodenal papilla
  - Usually communicates with main pancreatic duct
  - Variations are common, including dominant accessory duct draining most pancreatic juice
- Vessels, nerves, and lymphatics
  - Arteries to head mainly from gastroduodenal artery
    - Pancreaticoduodenal arcade of vessels around head also supplied by SMA branches
  - Arteries to body and tail from splenic artery
  - Veins are tributaries of SMV and splenic vein → portal vein
  - Autonomic nerves from celiac and superior mesenteric plexus
    - Parasympathetic stimulation of pancreatic secretion, but pancreatic juice secretion is mostly under hormonal control (secretin, from duodenum)
  - Lymphatics follow blood vessels
    - Collect in splenic, celiac, superior mesenteric and hepatic nodes

IMAGING ANATOMY

Overview

- Pancreas can be localized on ultrasound by
  - Typical parenchymal architecture: Homogeneously isoechoic/hyperechoic echo pattern when compared with overlying liver
  - Surrounding anatomical landmarks: Body anterior to splenic vein; neck anterior to SMA/SMV
- Variations in reflectivity related to degree of fatty infiltration; uncinate process and posterior pancreatic head are relatively echo poor in 25% of subjects (lack of intraparenchymal fat)

ANATOMY IMAGING ISSUES

Imaging Recommendations

- Use 2- to 5-MHz transducers or up to 9 MHz for smaller patients
- Techniques to combat overlying stomach and bowel gas include
  - Displacement of intervening bowel gas by gentle graded compression with transducer
  - Overnight fasting or fasting > 6-8 hours
  - Noneffervescent fluid can be given orally to fill gastric fundus
    - Scanning delayed for few minutes to allow fluid to settle
    - Patient can lie on left side to allow imaging of body and tail of pancreas
    - Patient can then be turned right to allow gastric fluid to flow to stomach antrum and duodenum, allowing imaging of head and uncinate process
- CT is preferred imaging modality for imaging of pancreas
- MRCP (± secretin) or ERCP useful for defining pancreatic duct

Imaging Pitfalls

- Ultrasound examination of pancreas is often limited by overlying bowel gas

Key Concepts

- Shape, size, and texture of pancreas are quite variable
  - Largest in young adults
  - Atrophy and fatty infiltration with age (> 70), obesity, diabetes, corticosteroids, Cushing disease
  - Pancreatic duct also becomes more prominent with age (normal < 3 mm diameter)
  - Focal bulge or mass effect is abnormal
- Location behind lesser sac
  - Acute pancreatitis often results in lesser sac fluid (may mimic pseudocyst)
- Pancreas lies in APS
  - Inflammation (from pancreatitis) easily spreads to duodenum and descending colon, which are also located in APS
  - Inflammation easily spreads into mesentery and mesocolon; roots of these lie just ventral to pancreas
- Obstruction of pancreatic duct
  - Relatively common result of chronic pancreatitis (fibrosis &/or stone occluding pancreatic duct) or pancreatic ductal carcinoma
- Acute pancreatitis
  - Relatively common result of gallstone (lodged in hepatopancreatic ampulla causing bile to reflux into pancreas) or damage from alcohol abuse

PANCREAS IN SITU

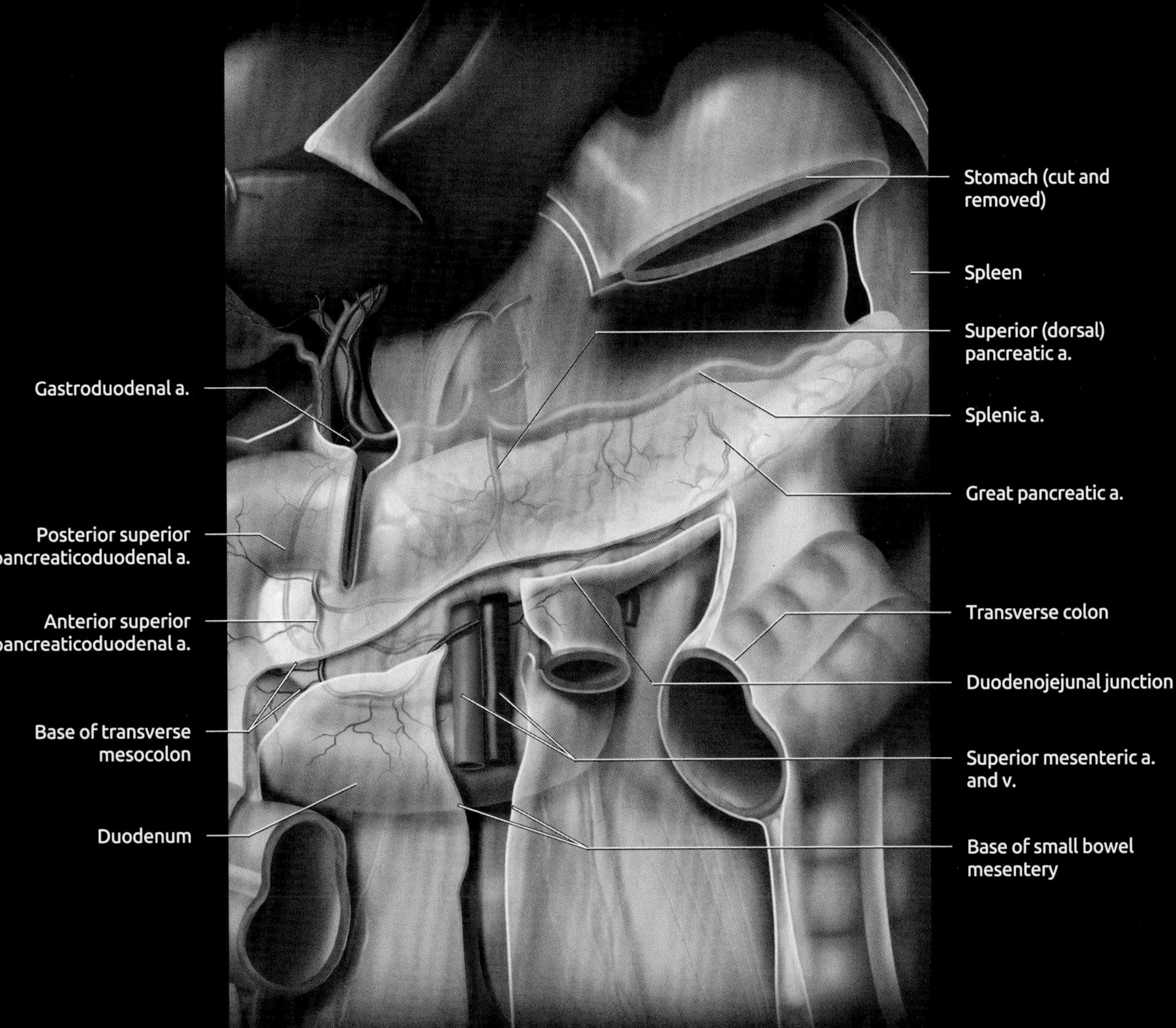

Graphic shows the arterial supply to the body and tail of the pancreas through the terminal branches of the splenic artery, which are variable in number and size. The 2 largest are usually the dorsal (superior) and great pancreatic arteries, which arise from the proximal and distal splenic artery, respectively. The arteries to the pancreatic head and duodenum come from the pancreaticoduodenal arcades that receive flow from the celiac and superior mesenteric arteries. The superior mesenteric vessels pass behind the neck of the pancreas and in front of the 3rd portion of the duodenum. The root of the transverse mesocolon and small bowel mesentery arise from the surface of the pancreas and transmit the blood vessels to the small bowel and transverse colon. The splenic vein runs along the dorsal surface of the pancreas. The splenic vessels and pancreatic tail insert into the splenic hilum.

PANCREAS, TRANSVERSE VIEW

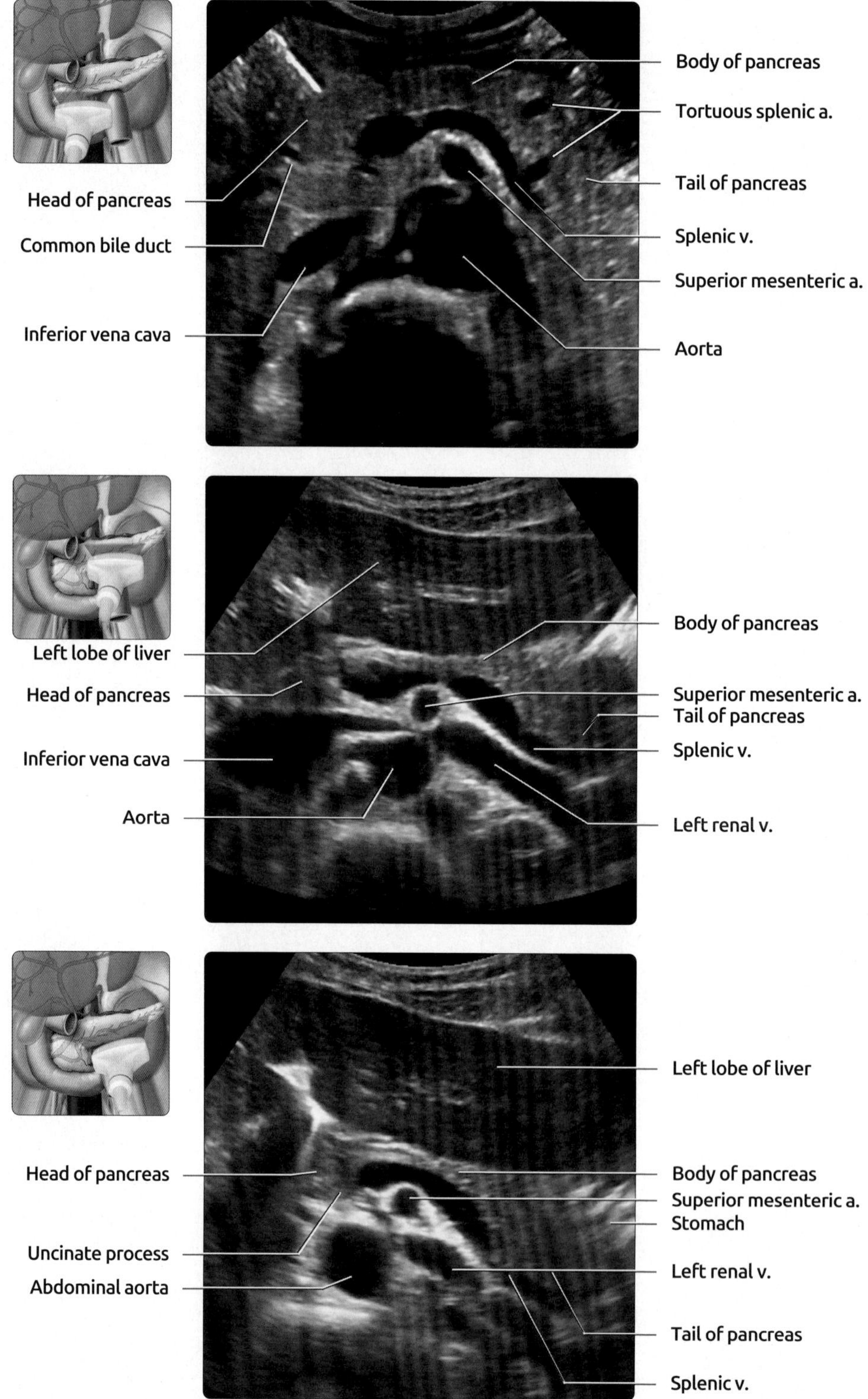

(Top) *Transverse transabdominal grayscale ultrasound at the epigastrium is shown. Anatomically, the pancreatic axis from head to tail is directed superiorly and to the left. This lower transverse section demonstrates the bulk of the pancreatic head.* **(Middle)** *Transverse transabdominal grayscale ultrasound at the epigastrium is shown at a more cephalad angle in the same patient. Note that the pancreatic body and tail have now come into view, but the distal tail is obscured by stomach gas.* **(Bottom)** *Oblique transabdominal grayscale ultrasound at the epigastrium is shown. The transducer is tilted slightly cranially and laterally to the left to follow the pancreatic axis, attempting to imaging the pancreas in its entirety. The splenic vein courses along the posterior pancreas and provides an excellent landmark in locating the pancreas. The superior mesenteric artery is more posteriorly located and has a characteristic dot shape, as it is imaged end on.*

PANCREAS, SAGITTAL VIEW

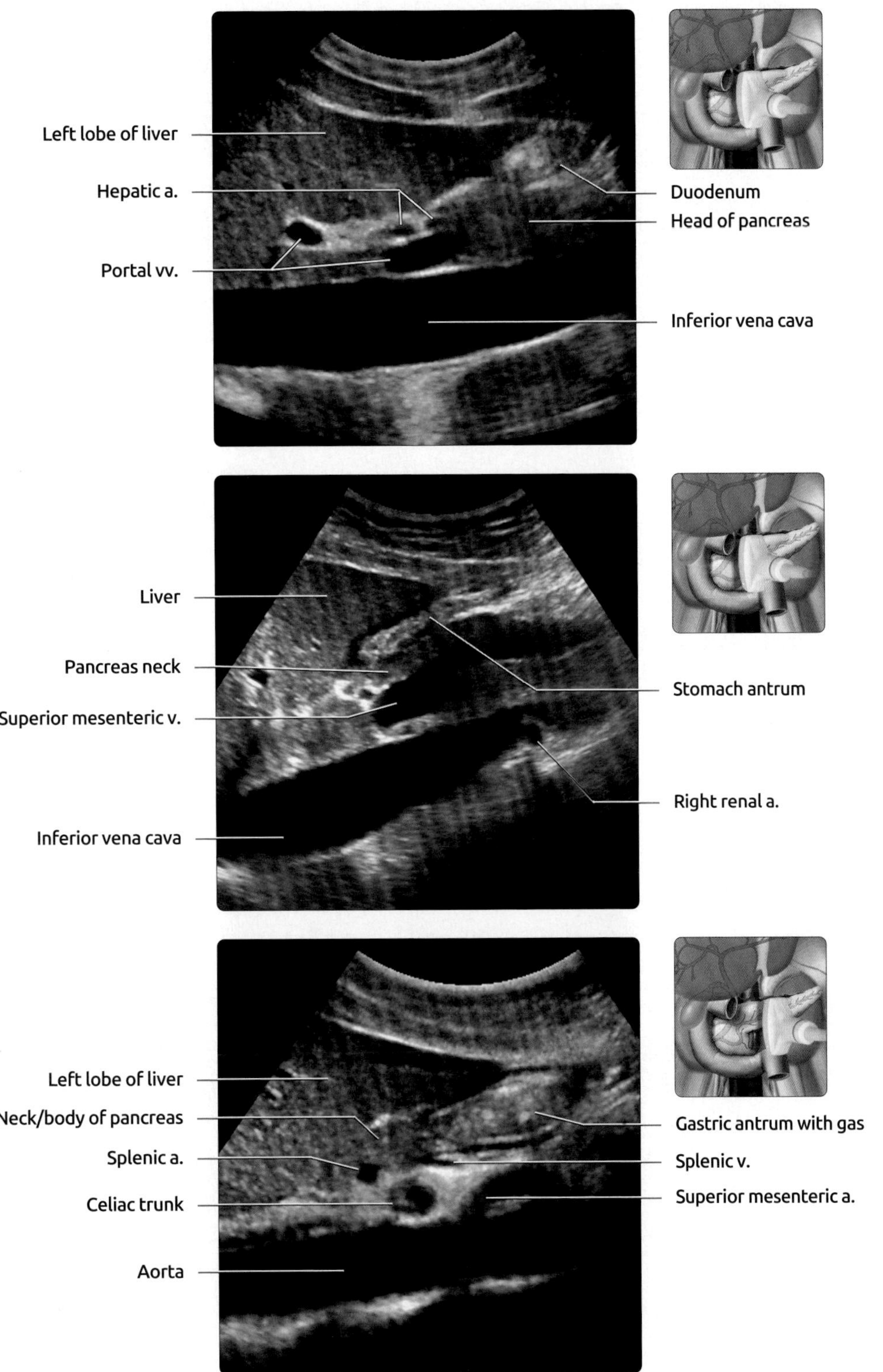

(Top) *Longitudinal transabdominal grayscale ultrasound at the epigastrium, right paramedian region, is shown. Note the relationship of the pancreatic head with the posteriorly located inferior vena cava (IVC).* **(Middle)** *Longitudinal transabdominal grayscale ultrasound at the epigastrium, right paramedian region, is shown continuing medially. Note the superior mesenteric vein coming into view; this is a good landmark for locating the neck of the pancreas on sagittal ultrasound.* **(Bottom)** *Longitudinal transabdominal grayscale ultrasound at the epigastrium, right paramedian region, is shown slightly more medial. The origin of the superior mesenteric artery arising from the abdominal aorta is brought into view. The superior mesenteric artery is also a useful marker for identifying the neck of the pancreas on sagittal ultrasound.*

PANCREATIC ARTERIAL ANATOMY

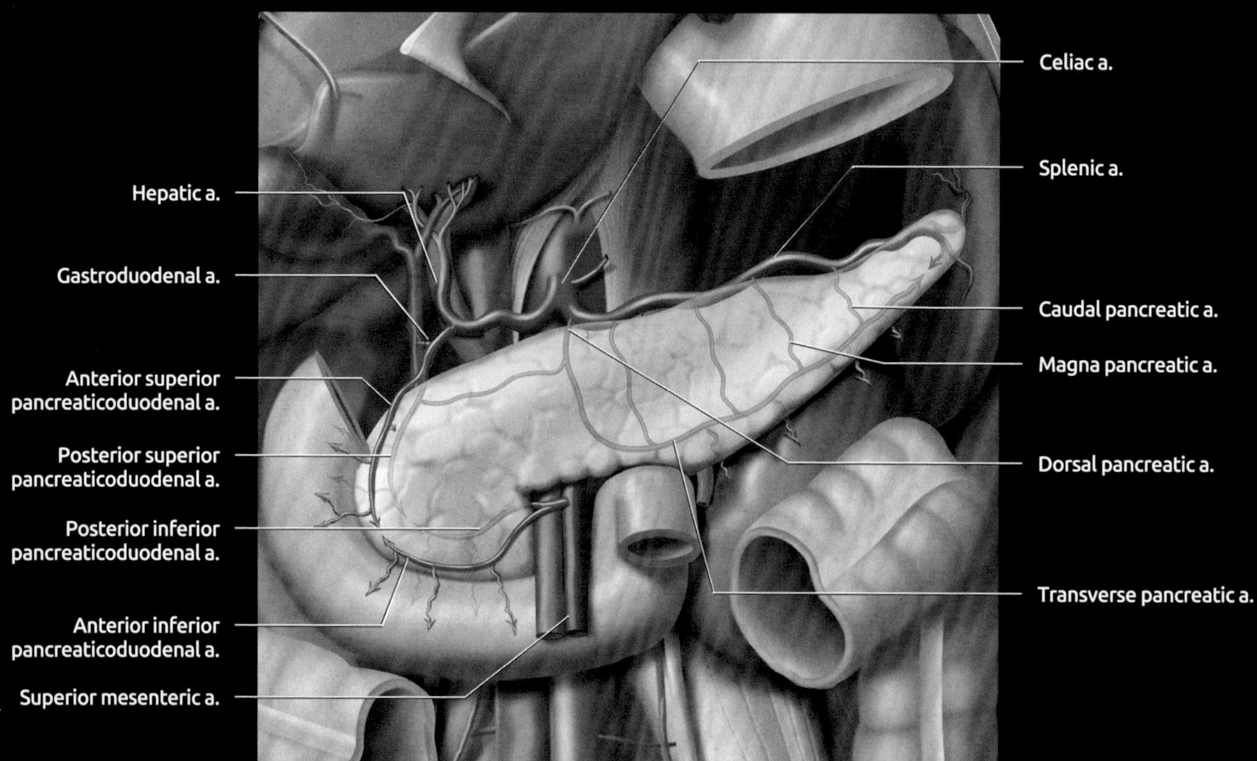

Graphic demonstrates the arterial supply to the pancreas. The pancreatic head is primarily supplied by the anterior and posterior pancreaticoduodenal arcades, including anterior and posterior superior pancreaticoduodenal arteries arising from the gastroduodenal artery and anterior and posterior inferior pancreaticoduodenal arteries arising from the superior mesenteric artery. The blood supply to the body and tail segments is primarily via the splenic artery with the 2 biggest branches, including the dorsal pancreatic artery and the pancreatic great (magna) artery, which arise from proximal and midportions of the splenic artery, respectively.

PANCREAS VASCULATURE, TRANSVERSE VIEW

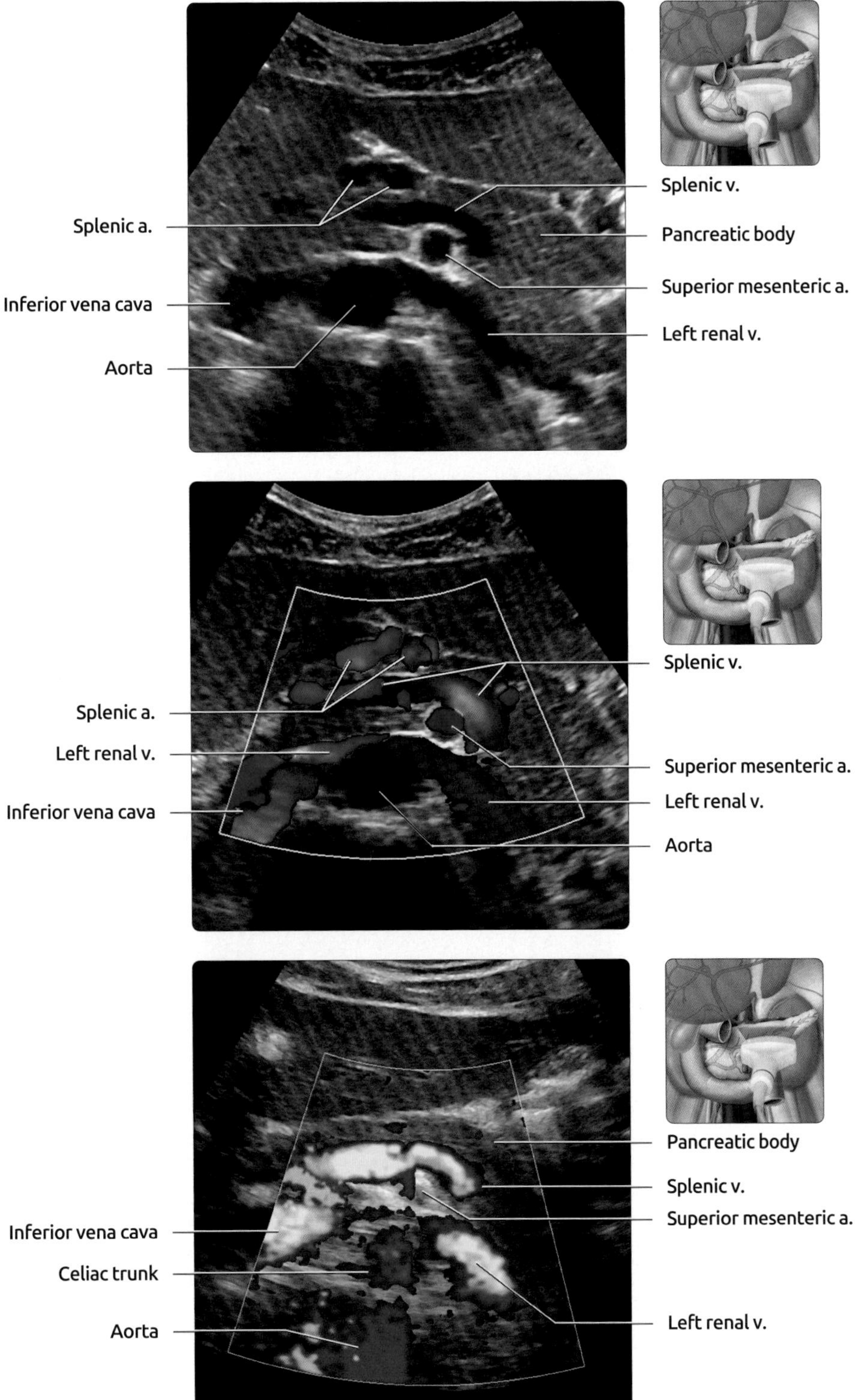

(Top) *Transverse subxiphoid grayscale ultrasound shows the left renal vein coursing posterior to the pancreatic body, superior mesenteric artery, and splenic vein. Two segments of the tortuous splenic artery are visible in cross section anteriorly.* **(Middle)** *Transverse color Doppler ultrasound is shown at the same level. There is a small amount of caudal tilt so that the superior mesenteric artery is blue, away from the transducer, and the IVC is mostly red, toward the transducer. The splenic and left renal veins on the right side of the image are toward the transducer (red), then switch to blue as they travel away from the transducer toward the superior mesenteric vein and IVC, respectively. Note the mixing in the IVC secondary to the left renal vein inflow. The splenic artery is tortuous, and the 2 visible segments appear to flow in opposite directions.* **(Bottom)** *Transverse subxiphoid ultrasound is shown using color power Doppler. This is more sensitive for detecting vascular flow, although there is more flash artifact. Newer machines support directional color power Doppler.*

PANCREAS DUCT, TRANSVERSE VIEW

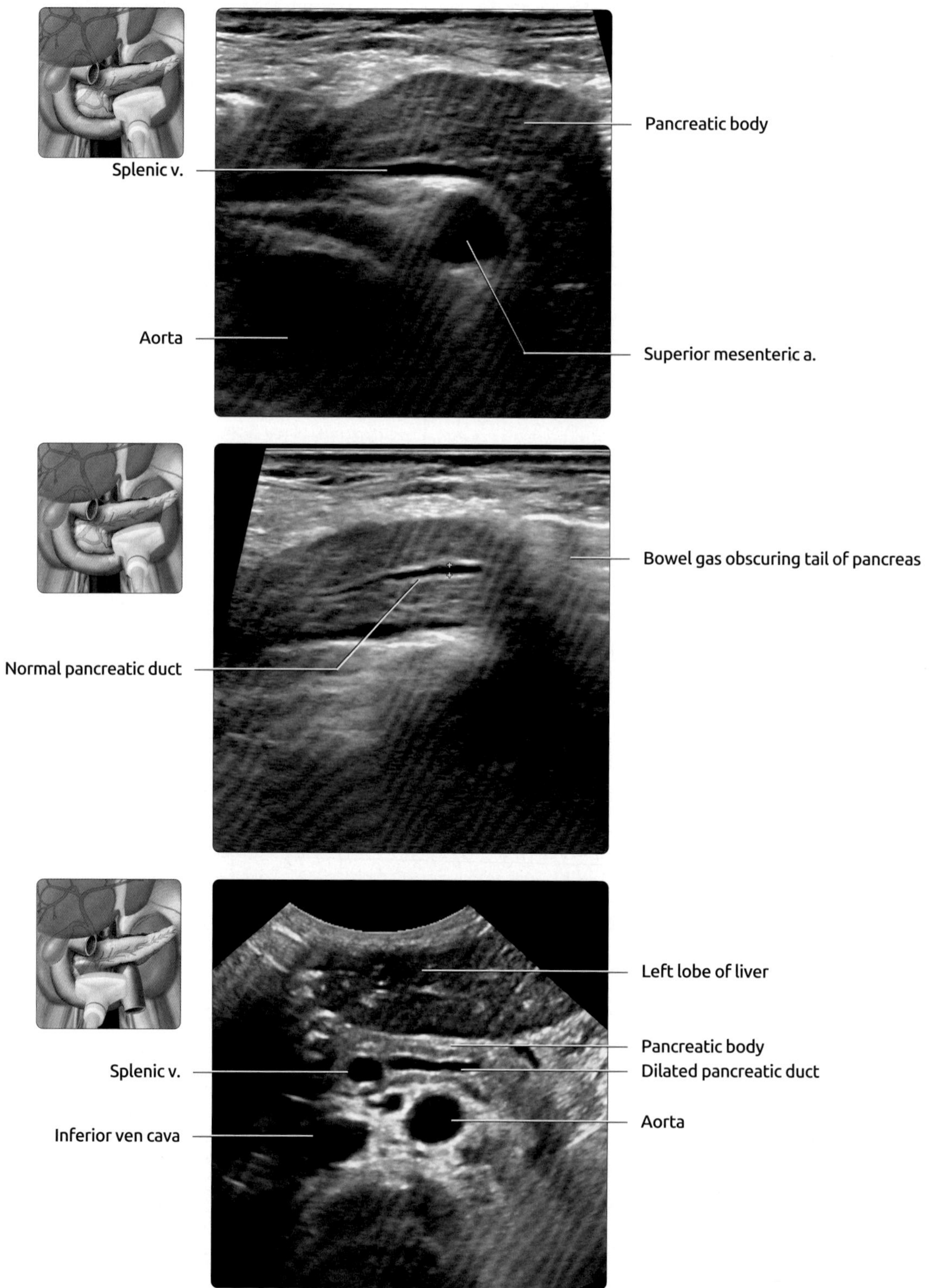

(Top) *Transverse ultrasound of the pancreatic body using a linear 12- to 5-MHz transducer in a thin patient is shown. The texture of the pancreas is finely granular.* **(Middle)** *Transverse ultrasound of the pancreatic body using a linear 12- to 5-MHz transducer in a thin patient is shown. The normal pancreatic duct measures < 3 mm.* **(Bottom)** *Transverse transabdominal ultrasound of the pancreas is shown. There is dilation of the pancreatic duct and atrophy of the parenchyma.*

PANCREATIC DUCT VARIANTS

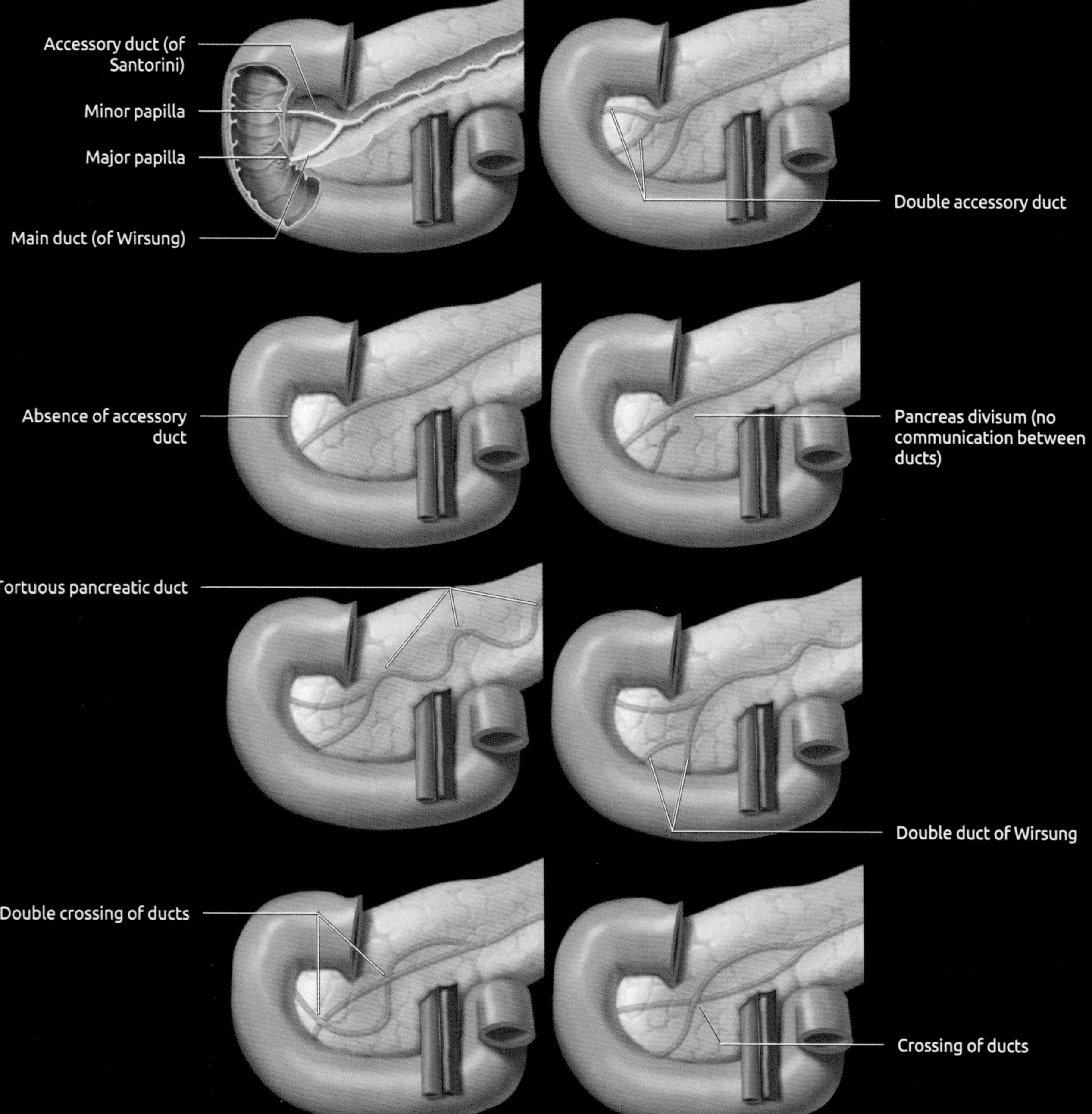

The accessory duct (of Santorini) originates with the dorsal pancreatic anlage, which is the larger bud from the embryologic foregut, composing the pancreatic body and tail. The main duct (of Wirsung) originates with the ventral, smaller, anlage that develops into the pancreatic head and uncinate process. Usually, the main and accessory pancreatic ducts fuse, and the main duct becomes the primary conduit for drainage of secretions into the duodenum. The pancreatic duct courses through the center of the gland and is joined by tributaries that enter it at right angles. In the head, the duct turns caudally and dorsally and runs parallel to the common bile duct before joining it at the ampulla of Vater and entering the major papilla. The accessory duct usually enters the duodenum more proximally through the minor papilla.

ANNULAR PANCREAS

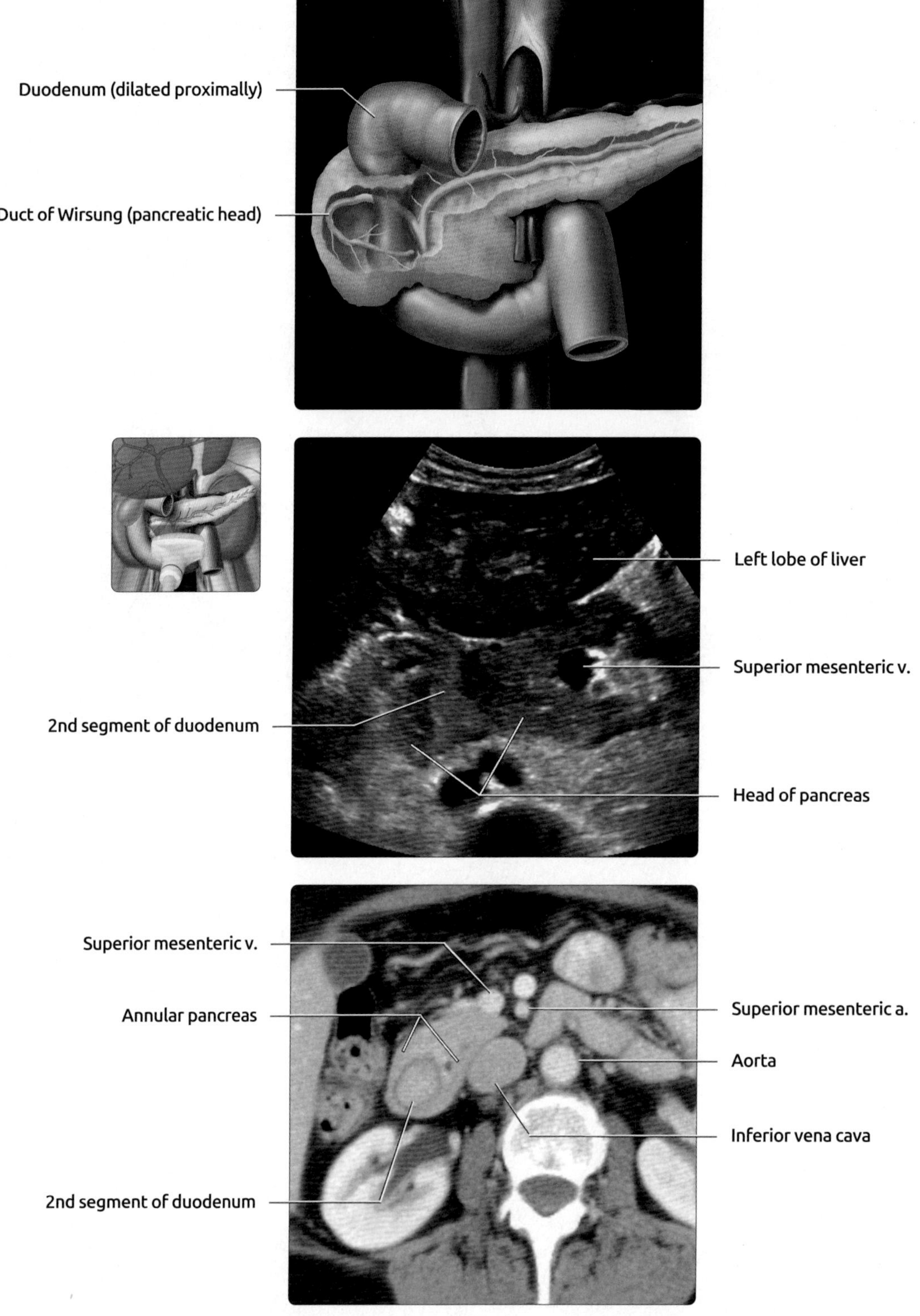

(Top) *Graphic shows the annular pancreas in which there is abnormal rotation and fusion of the ventral and dorsal pancreatic anlage resulting in a circumferential mass of pancreatic tissue that encircles and narrows the duodenum. The duct draining the pancreatic head encircles the 2nd portion of the duodenum. This condition may remain asymptomatic or may result in obstruction of the duodenum, often in neonates.* **(Middle)** *Transverse transabdominal grayscale ultrasound at the midline epigastrium, angled slightly caudally through the liver, shows the descending segment of the duodenum coursing through the pancreatic head in this patient with annular pancreas.* **(Bottom)** *Axial CECT shows the 2nd portion of duodenum completely encircled by pancreatic tissue, consistent with an annular pancreas.*

CT CORRELATION

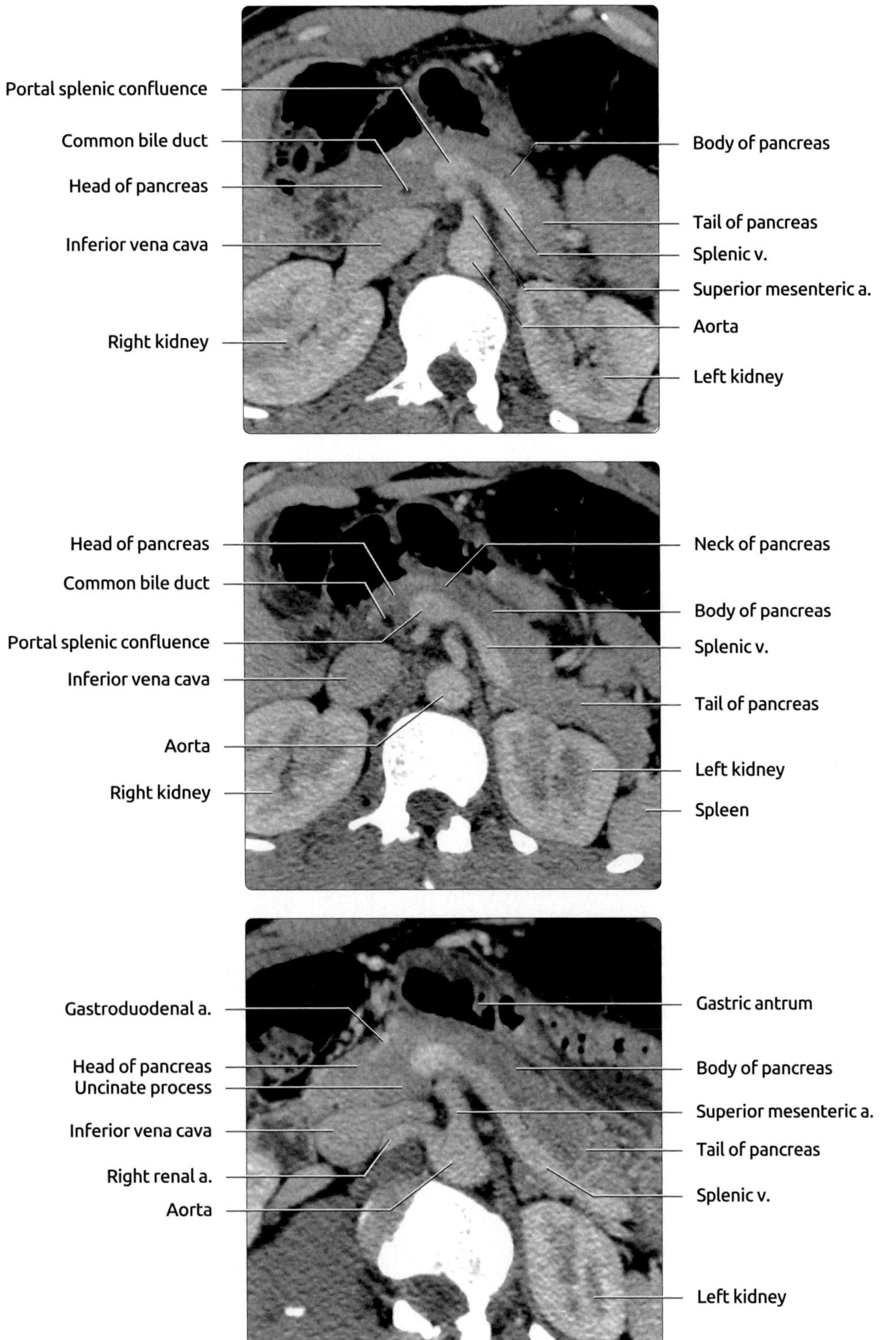

(Top) *Correlative transverse CECT of the pancreas is shown at the level of the origin of the superior mesenteric artery. Note the common bile duct within the pancreatic head before it exits into the duodenum.* **(Middle)** *Correlative transverse CECT of the pancreas shows the course of the pancreatic tail, which goes posteriorly and forms close relations with the left kidney and spleen.* **(Bottom)** *Correlative oblique CECT follows the pancreatic axis and demonstrates its head, body, and tail. The splenic vein courses along the posterior pancreas, following its contour. The anteriorly located stomach may be distended with fluid and used as an acoustic window during ultrasound.*

Acute Pancreatitis

KEY FACTS

TERMINOLOGY

- Acute inflammatory process of pancreas with variable involvement of other local tissues and remote organs
  - Interstitial edematous pancreatitis, necrotizing pancreatitis
  - Acute pancreatic fluid collection ± infection
  - Acute necrotic collection ± infection

IMAGING

- Focal or diffuse enlargement of pancreas
  - In mild pancreatitis, sonographic signs may be subtle or normal
- Blurred pancreatic outline/margin: Pancreatic edema and peripancreatic exudate
- Heterogeneous echotexture due to intrapancreatic necrosis or hemorrhage
- Collections: Anechoic peripancreatic fluid; fluid within pancreatic parenchyma or containing debris
- Presence of gas suggests infection/bowel fistula unless secondary to interventional procedure
- Color Doppler to evaluate for vascular complications: Venous thrombosis, arterial pseudoaneurysms

TOP DIFFERENTIAL DIAGNOSES

- Infiltrating pancreatic carcinoma
- Lymphoma and metastases
- Autoimmune pancreatitis

CLINICAL ISSUES

- Usually young and middle-aged groups, M > F
- Acute-onset epigastric pain, often radiating to back
- Tenderness, fever, nausea, vomiting, ↑ amylase/lipase
- Risk factors: Alcohol, gallstones, metabolic, infection, trauma, drugs, ERCP

SCANNING TIPS

- Ultrasound most useful to rule out cholelithiasis in acute pancreatitis

(Left) *Transverse ultrasound through the pancreas in acute pancreatitis is shown. The pancreas ➔ is hypoechoic but normal in size. The pancreatic duct ➔ is normal. A small amount of peripancreatic fluid ➔ is noted.* **(Right)** *Transverse ultrasound through the pancreas in acute pancreatitis is shown. The pancreas ➔ is enlarged and hypoechoic. Peripancreatic fat planes ➔ are blurred due to inflammation.*

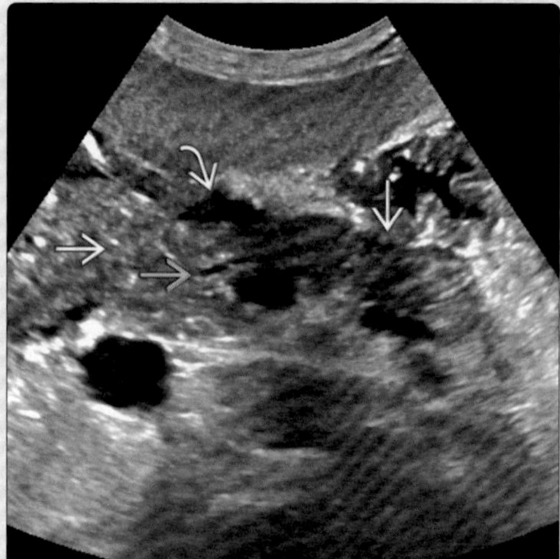

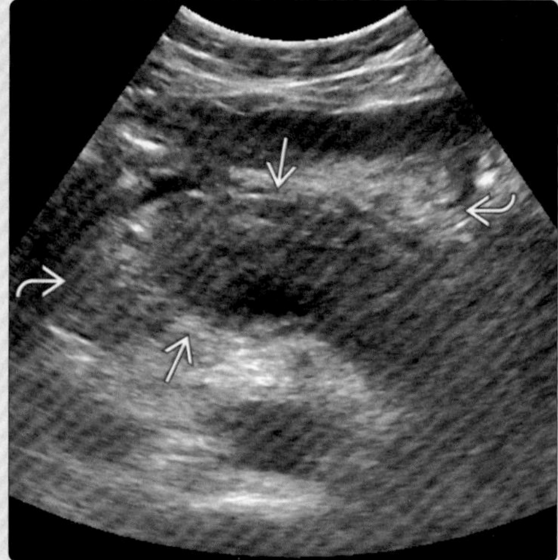

(Left) *Transverse ultrasound through the pancreas in acute necrotizing pancreatitis is shown. The pancreas ➔ is enlarged and heterogeneous with segmental areas of decreased echogenicity ➔ from necrosis. There is peripancreatic fluid ➔.* **(Right)** *Longitudinal ultrasound of the same patient shows a stone ➔ in the common bile duct ➔, the cause of necrotizing pancreatitis.*

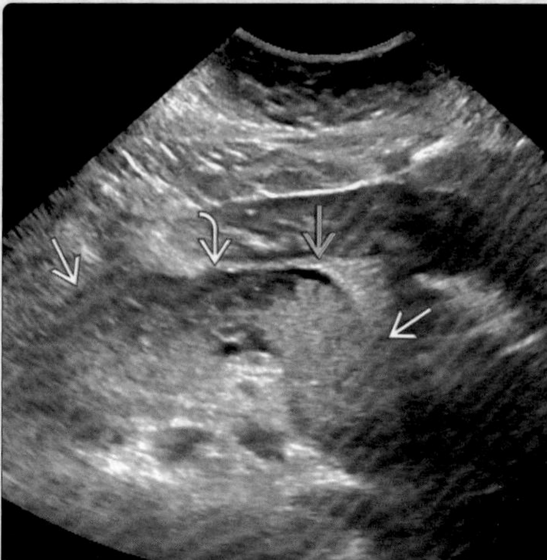

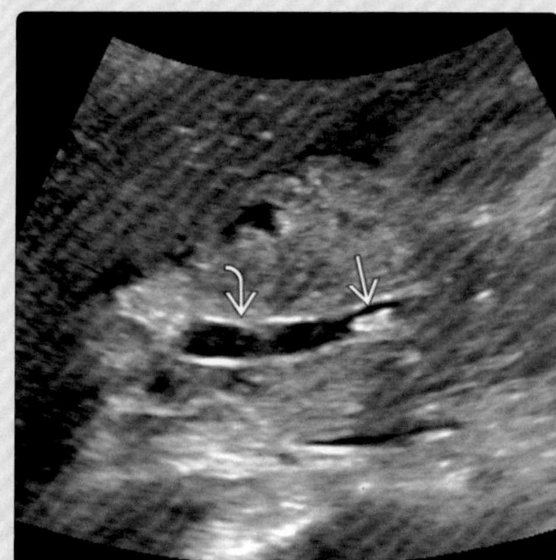

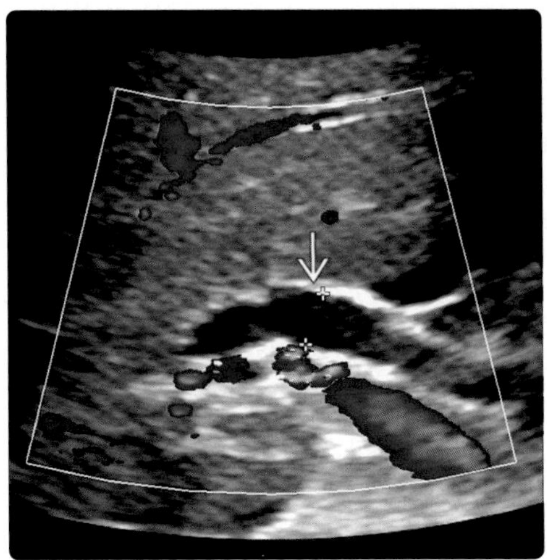

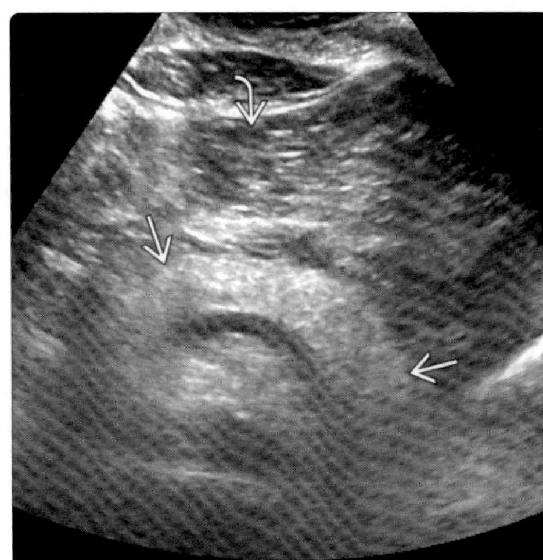

(Left) *Longitudinal oblique color Doppler ultrasound of the same patient with acute gallstone pancreatitis shows a dilated common bile duct ➡ at the porta hepatic. The bile duct should be followed distally to look for a stone.* **(Right)** *Transverse ultrasound of a patient with acute interstitial pancreatitis shows an edematous hyperechoic pancreas ➡. There is a generalized haze through the image secondary to peripancreatic edema ➡.*

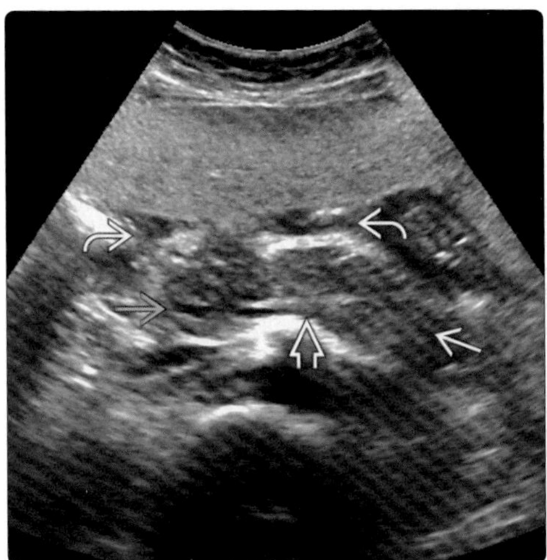

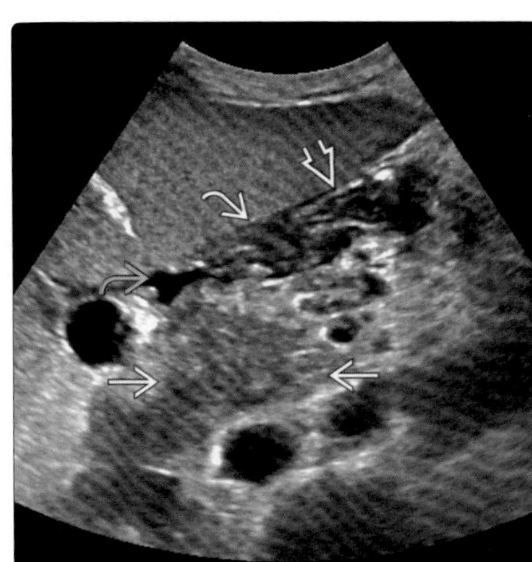

(Left) *Transverse ultrasound shows a mildly enlarged hypoechoic pancreas ➡ with a patent splenic vein ➡ and a normal bile duct ➡. There is edema ➡ anterior to the pancreas.* **(Right)** *Transverse ultrasound shows a swollen pancreatic head ➡ with peripancreatic inflammation ➡ and fluid ➡ adjacent to the gastric antrum ➡.*

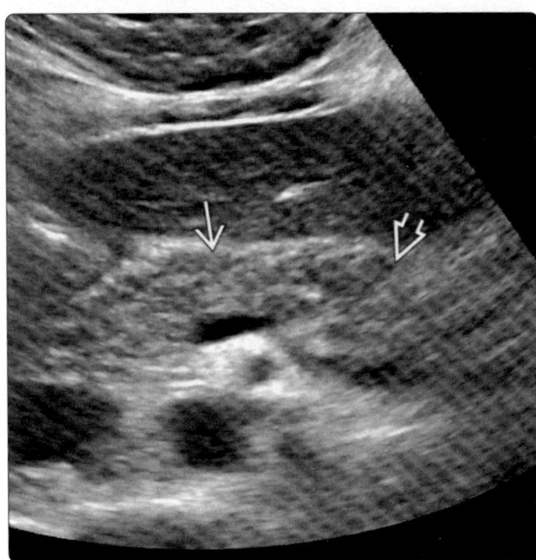

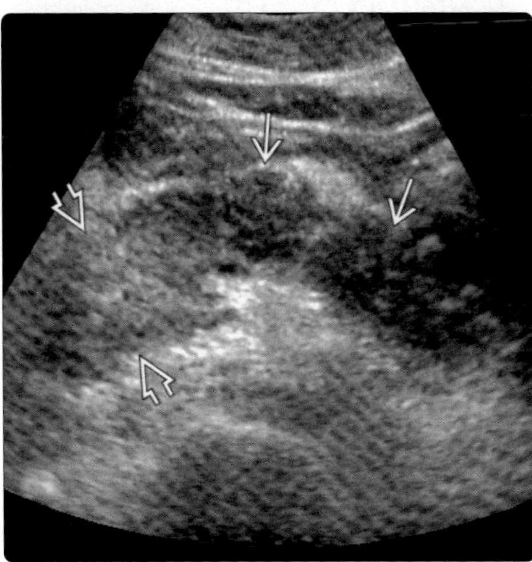

(Left) *Transverse abdominal ultrasound reveals a normal pancreatic head/neck ➡ with focal enlargement, decreased echogenicity, and heterogeneity of the pancreatic body ➡ consistent with focal pancreatitis. There is no associated edema or fluid collection, consistent with mild acute interstitial edematous pancreatitis.* **(Right)** *Transverse ultrasound shows a markedly hypoechoic pancreatic body ➡ suggestive of focal necrosis, relative to the normal echogenicity in the head ➡. This was confirmed with CECT.*

Pancreatic Pseudocyst

KEY FACTS

TERMINOLOGY

- Collection of pancreatic fluid and inflammatory exudate encapsulated by nonepithelial fibrous tissue developing > 4 weeks after acute pancreatic fluid collection

IMAGING

- 2/3 are peripancreatic: Body and tail (85%)
- Uncomplicated pseudocyst: Well-defined, unilocular, peripancreatic cystic mass in setting of prior pancreatitis
  - Smooth-walled, posterior acoustic enhancement
- Complex pseudocysts: Fluid-debris level, internal echoes, or septations (due to hemorrhage/infection); multilocular
- Dilated pancreatic duct and common bile duct
- Wall calcification
- Absence of internal blood flow

TOP DIFFERENTIAL DIAGNOSES

- Mucinous or serous cystic neoplasm
- Intraductal papillary mucinous neoplasm
- Cystic islet cell tumor
- Choledochal cyst

CLINICAL ISSUES

- Associated with acute or chronic pancreatitis; alcoholism, cholelithiasis/choledocholithiasis
- Clinical significance is related to size and complications; however, may be asymptomatic
- Abdominal pain, typically radiating to back; palpable tender mass
- Complications: More common in pseudocysts > 4-5 cm
  - Spontaneous rupture into peritoneal cavity
  - Erosion into adjacent vessel causing pseudoaneurysm or hemorrhage
  - Compression of adjacent bowel or bile duct

SCANNING TIPS

- Turn on color Doppler to look for pseudoaneurysm or active bleeding in pseudocyst

(Left) *Graphic shows a well-circumscribed cystic lesion ➡ in the pancreatic body consistent with a pancreatic pseudocyst. The adjacent pancreatic duct is not compressed or displaced.* **(Right)** *Transverse ultrasound through the left upper quadrant shows a well-circumscribed, unilocular pseudocyst in the pancreatic tail ➡. Posterior acoustic enhancement ➡ is noted. The spleen ➡ provides an acoustic window.*

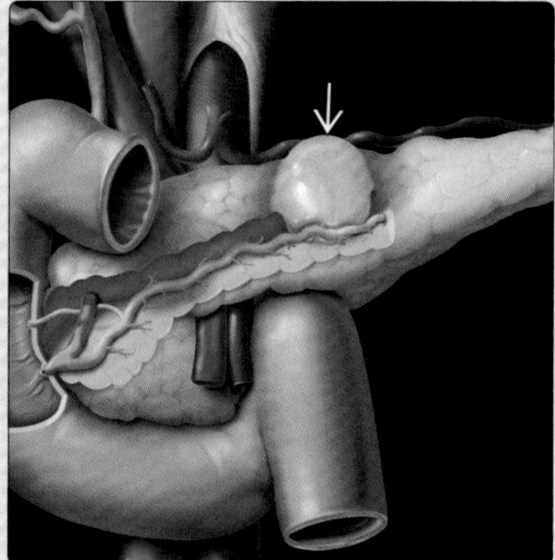

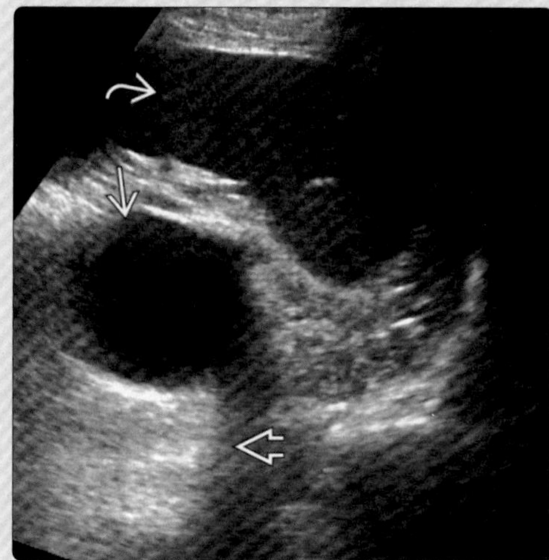

(Left) *Transverse ultrasound through the epigastric region shows a unilocular pseudocyst in the pancreatic body ➡. There is posterior acoustic enhancement ➡. Calcification in the wall ➡ is a sign of chronic pancreatitis.* **(Right)** *Transverse ultrasound of the midbody of the pancreas shows a lobular pseudocyst ➡ in the pancreatic head, separated from the adjacent dilated pancreatic duct ➡ by a thin septation ➡.*

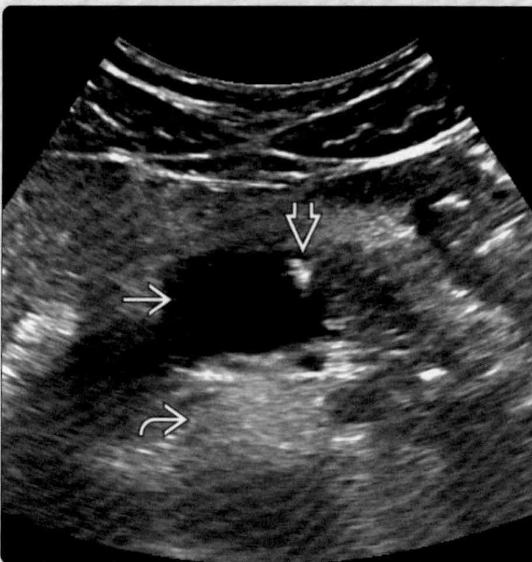

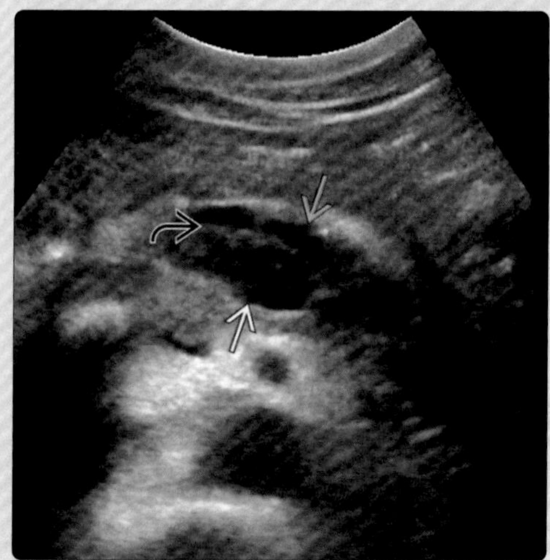

KEY FACTS

TERMINOLOGY

- Progressive, irreversible inflammatory and fibrosing disease

IMAGING

- Dilated main pancreatic duct (MPD) with intraductal calculi is highly specific for chronic pancreatitis
- Gland may be enlarged in early stage of chronic pancreatitis or during acute on chronic episode; focal or diffuse
  - Focal enlargement can mimic adenocarcinoma
- Diffuse fusiform hypoechoic enlargement in autoimmune type > focal or multifocal ± ductal dilation in focal type
- Later: Inflammation and fibrosis causes atrophy
- Calcification/calculi: ~ 90% of calcific pancreatitis caused by alcoholism
- Color Doppler for vascular complications: Portosplenic venous thrombosis (5%); arterial pseudoaneurysm

TOP DIFFERENTIAL DIAGNOSES

- Infiltrating pancreatic carcinoma
- Acute pancreatitis

PATHOLOGY

- Alcohol abuse is most common cause in USA; gallstones not considered risk factor
  - Idiopathic in up to 40%; hyperlipidemia, hyperparathyroidism, hypercalcemia, trauma
  - Cystic fibrosis, hereditary pancreatitis
  - Pancreas divisum or annular pancreas
  - Autoimmune IgG4 related

CLINICAL ISSUES

- Males > females; mean: 5th decade
- Recurrent attacks of epigastric pain, occasionally radiating to back, diarrhea, weight loss, biliary or duodenal obstruction, diabetes

SCANNING TIPS

- Follow pancreatic duct; use higher resolution transducer for the detection of intraductal calculi

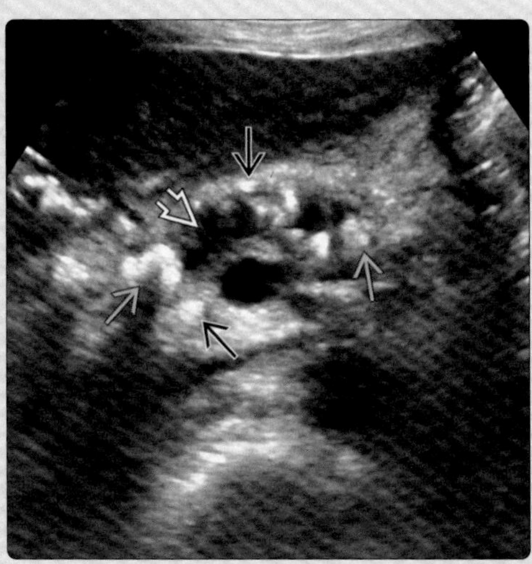

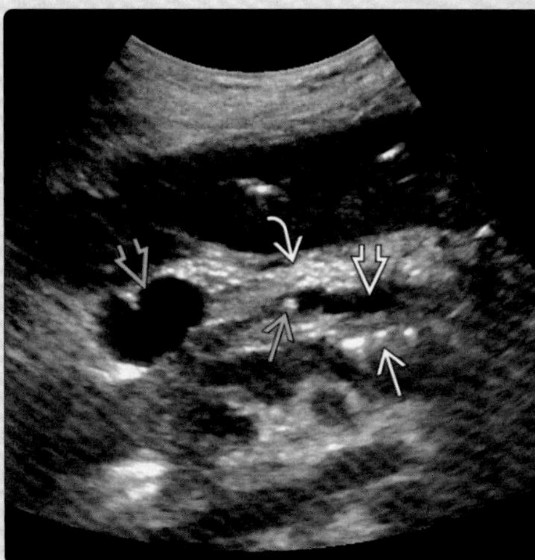

(Left) *Transverse ultrasound demonstrates marked pancreatic ductal dilatation ➡, intraductal stones ➡, and parenchymal calcifications ➡ within the atrophic parenchyma.* **(Right)** *Transverse ultrasound demonstrates a dilated main pancreatic duct ➡ with intraductal calculus ➡ and parenchymal calcifications ➡, consistent with chronic pancreatitis. A bilobed fluid collection in the head ➡ is consistent with a small pseudocyst. The parenchyma ➡ has normal size and echogenicity.*

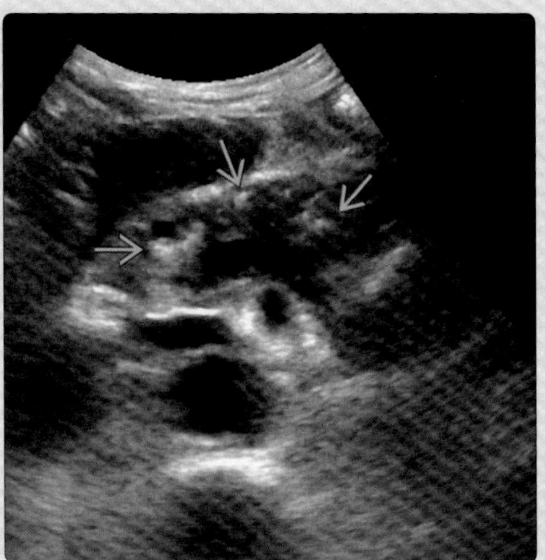

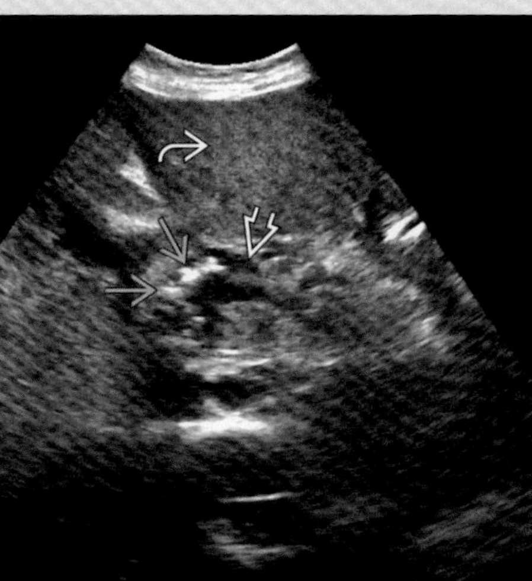

(Left) *Transverse ultrasound shows predominantly parenchymal calcifications ➡ without intraductal calculi. The gland is normal in size in this example.* **(Right)** *Transverse ultrasound demonstrates a dilated pancreatic duct ➡ with intraductal calcifications in the head/neck region ➡. There is a fatty liver ➡.*

Mucinous Cystic Pancreatic Tumor

KEY FACTS

TERMINOLOGY

- Septated cystic neoplasm composed of mucin-producing epithelium and distinctive ovarian-type stroma, ranging in grade from potentially malignant to invasive carcinoma

IMAGING

- Solitary, uni- or multilocular, well-circumscribed cystic lesion in body or tail of pancreas
- Echogenic septations
- Typically < 6 cystic components, which are each > 2 cm in size
- Cyst contents may be anechoic or echogenic with debris representing mucin
- May contain peripheral calcification
- 2 cm to > 10 cm in diameter; mean: 8.7 cm
- No communication with pancreatic duct
- Mural nodularity and solid component suggest malignancy
- Hypovascular on color Doppler (nodules and septations may show flow)

TOP DIFFERENTIAL DIAGNOSES

- Intraductal papillary mucinous neoplasm
- Macrocystic variant of serous cystadenoma
- Solid pseudopapillary tumor
- Pseudocyst
- Cystic pancreatic neuroendocrine tumor

CLINICAL ISSUES

- Seen almost exclusively in middle-aged women; termed "mother lesion"; mean age: 50 years
- 10% of cystic pancreatic tumors
- Often asymptomatic
- May present with epigastric pain, palpable mass, or fullness
- Excellent prognosis without invasive carcinoma
- All tumors in this class are considered surgical lesions

SCANNING TIPS

- Findings on US are nonspecific and further evaluation with CT or MR is necessary

(Left) *Graphic shows a multiseptated, cystic mass ➡ in the tail of the pancreas. Note that the pancreatic duct ➡ is displaced but not obstructed.* **(Right)** *Transverse transabdominal US shows a well-defined, anechoic, cystic lesion ➡ in the body of the pancreas with a few hyperechoic peripheral foci ➡. Note the normal pancreas ➡.*

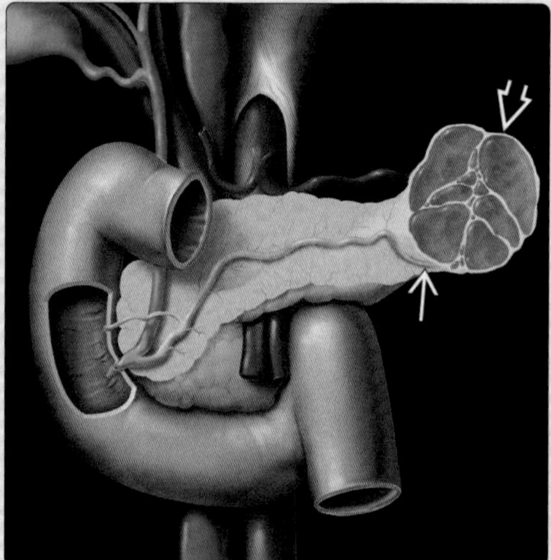

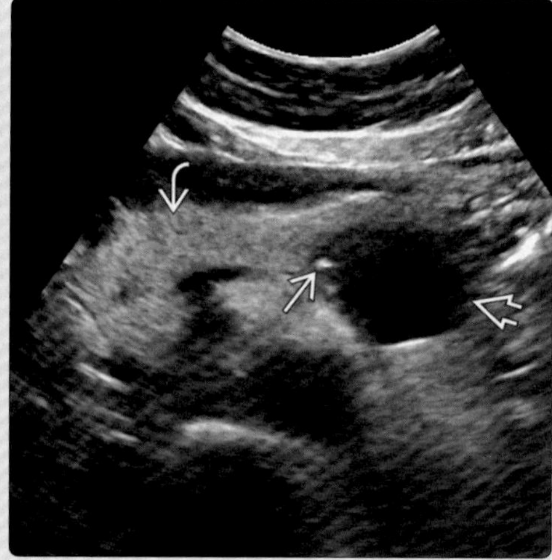

(Left) *Transverse transabdominal US shows a well-defined, complex cystic pancreatic mass (calipers) with thick internal septations ➡.* **(Right)** *Axial CECT of the same lesion shows an encapsulated, complex cystic mass ➡ with internal septations ➡ and peripheral calcification ➡. Note the few, relatively larger cysts and unusual location in the head of the pancreas. Septations are less conspicuous on CT.*

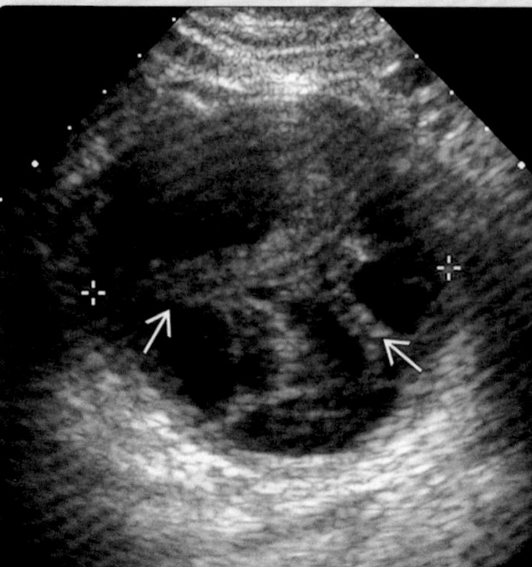

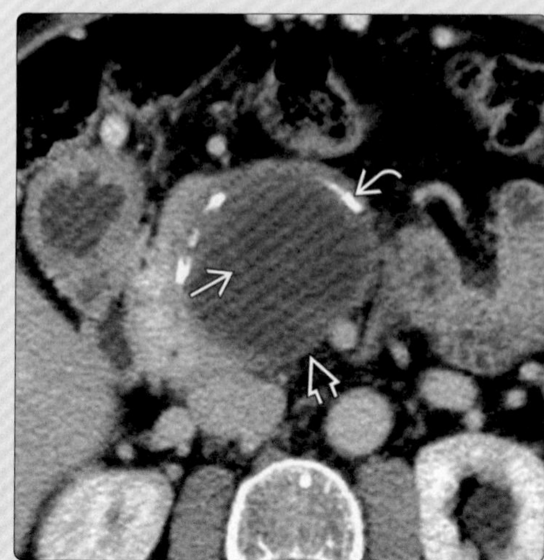

Serous Cystadenoma of Pancreas

KEY FACTS

TERMINOLOGY

- Synonyms: Pancreatic serous cystic neoplasm, microcystic adenoma of pancreas

IMAGING

- Commonly in body and tail; 30% in pancreatic head
- Variable size; mean: 4.9 cm
- Well-demarcated, lobulated, heterogeneous mass with posterior acoustic enhancement
- Microcystic type: "Honeycomb" cystic mass with septa and solid-appearing component
    - Cluster of > 6 cysts; each typically < 1 cm
    - Central echogenic scar (30%); ± calcification
    - Solid, echogenic appearance due to interfaces between microcysts
- Macrocystic type: Unilocular or fewer larger cysts (> 2 cm)
- Pancreatic and common bile duct dilatation not typical
- Increased vascularity within septa

TOP DIFFERENTIAL DIAGNOSES

- Pancreatic pseudocyst
- Mucinous cystadenoma of pancreas
- Intraductal papillary mucinous neoplasm
- Cystic neuroendocrine tumor
- Ductal pancreatic carcinoma

CLINICAL ISSUES

- 20% of all cystic pancreatic lesions; 1% of pancreatic neoplasms
- Middle and elderly age group; mean: 61.5 years, M:F = 1:4
- Typically asymptomatic or vague epigastric pain; may present with nausea, vomiting, weight loss, palpable mass, jaundice

SCANNING TIPS

- Depending on body habitus, consider higher frequency transducers to depict characteristic cluster of small cysts within mass

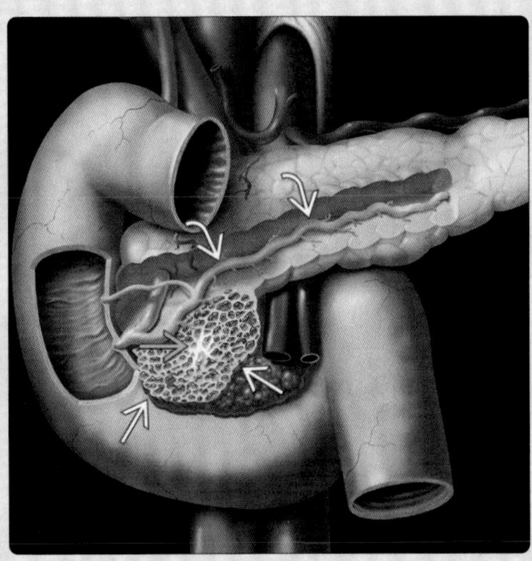

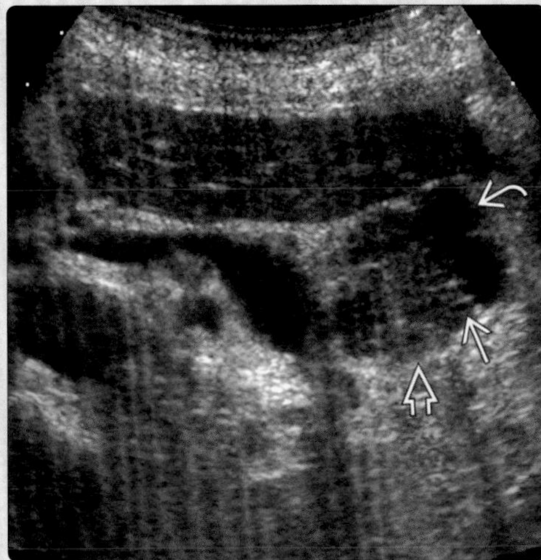

(Left) *Graphic shows a sponge-like or honeycombed mass → in the pancreatic head. Note the presence of innumerable small cysts and a central scar →. The pancreatic duct → is not obstructed.* **(Right)** *Transverse ultrasound shows a well-circumscribed, solid-appearing mass → in the body of the pancreas containing tiny microcysts → and larger peripheral cystic components →. (Courtesy A. Kamaya, MD.)*

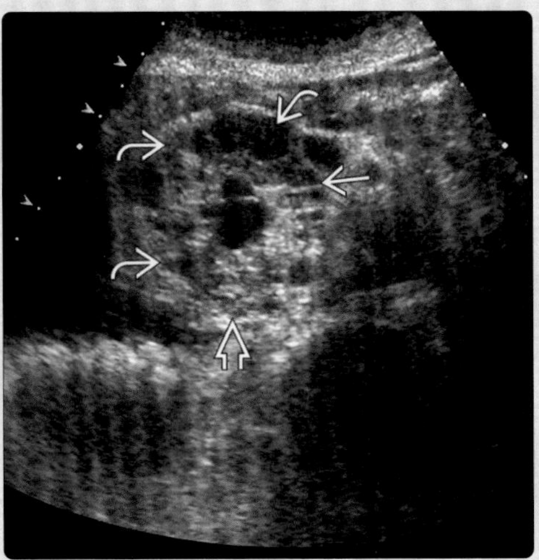

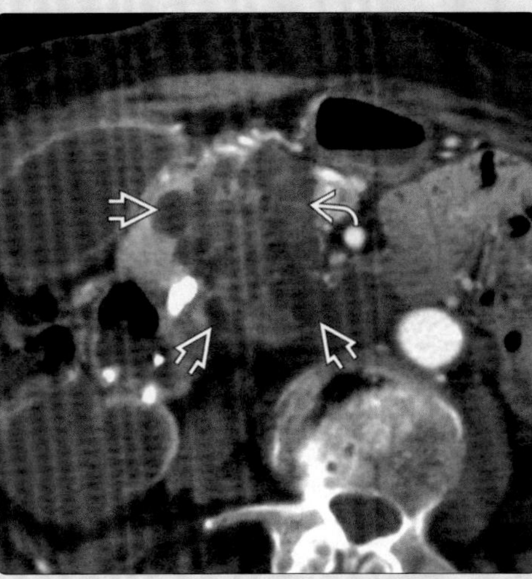

(Left) *Transverse transabdominal ultrasound shows a hyperechoic, solid-appearing mass in the head of the pancreas → with cystic components → of varying sizes and thin intervening septa →.* **(Right)** *Corresponding axial CECT in the same patient demonstrates the mass composed of numerous clustered small cysts → of varying size, separated by thin, enhancing septa →.*

Intraductal Papillary Mucinous Neoplasm (IPMN)

KEY FACTS

TERMINOLOGY

- Cystic neoplasm of pancreas arising from mucin-producing epithelium of main pancreatic duct (MPD) &/or side branch pancreatic ducts (SBD) with variable malignant potential

IMAGING

- US: Not modality of choice: Difficult to evaluate entire pancreas due to bowel gas and limited characterization
- MPD type: Dilated MPD > 5 mm, may contain low-level internal echoes (mucin vs. mural nodule); without obstructive mass
- SBD type: Multicystic, grape-like cluster of anechoic or hypoechoic masses; may see communication with dilated pancreatic duct
- Mixed type: Findings of both types
- Typically in head/uncinate
- May be multiple (21-40%); entire pancreas in up to 20%
- Endoscopic US (EUS): Provides best morphologic evaluation and opportunity for cyst aspiration &/or biopsy

TOP DIFFERENTIAL DIAGNOSES

- Pancreatic pseudocyst
- Chronic pancreatitis
- Mucinous cystic pancreatic neoplasm
- Pancreatic serous cystadenoma
- Pancreatic ductal adenocarcinoma

PATHOLOGY

- Main duct type: Precursor to invasive ductal carcinoma
- Branch duct type: Generally benign, low malignancy risk

CLINICAL ISSUES

- Mean at diagnosis: 68 years; range: 60-80 years; M > F
- Nausea/vomiting, abdominal pain, weight loss, anorexia
- MPD type may result in pancreatitis

SCANNING TIPS

- Look for communication between cystic lesion and pancreatic duct, which may be dilated

(Left) *Graphic demonstrates irregular, dilated main and branch pancreatic ducts within the head and uncinate process of the pancreas, typical of intraductal papillary mucinous neoplasm (IPMN).* **(Right)** *Transabdominal US demonstrates multiple oval and elongated cystic lesions in the pancreatic head/body ➡. Splenic vein ➡ is also noted.*

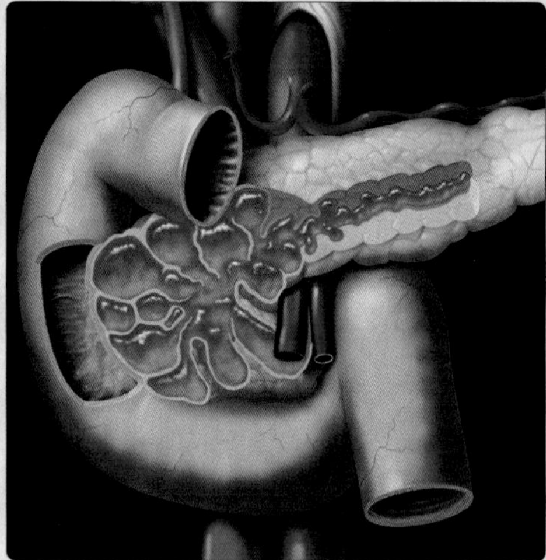

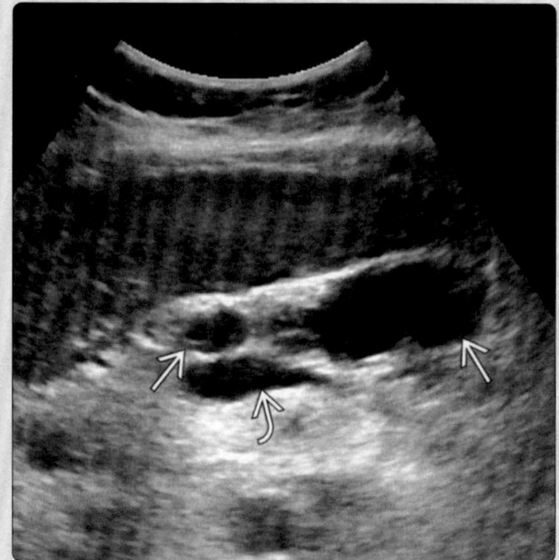

(Left) *Color Doppler transabdominal US demonstrates an anechoic cystic lesion ➡ communicating with a dilated main pancreatic duct ➡.* **(Right)** *Axial T2 MR in the same patient better characterizes the presence of multiple cystic lesions ➡, some of which show communication with the mildly dilated main pancreatic duct ➡.*

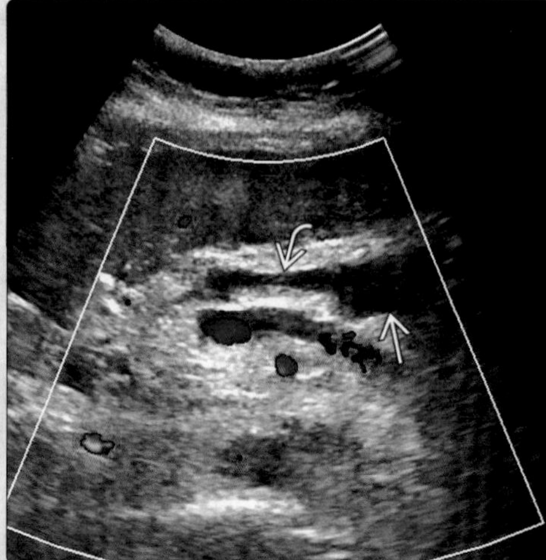

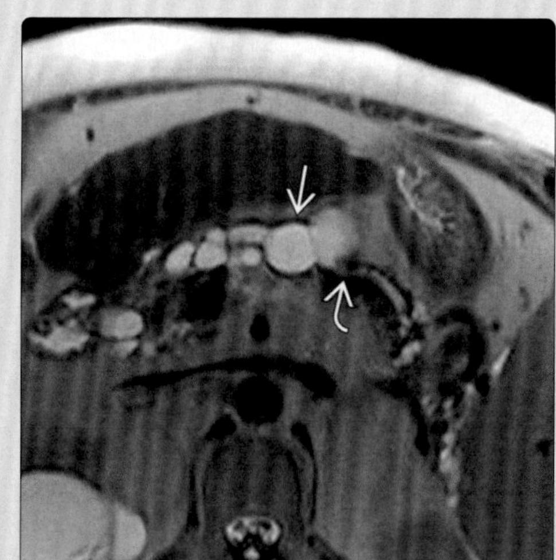

Pancreatic Ductal Carcinoma

KEY FACTS

TERMINOLOGY

- Solid epithelial neoplasm from ductal epithelium of exocrine pancreas

IMAGING

- US often 1st-line imaging to evaluate obstructive jaundice and level of obstruction
  - Not as sensitive as CT or MR for mass or staging
- Hypoechoic, infiltrative mass or isoechoic mass with subtle focal contour deformity
- Variable size
- Pancreatic ductal dilation and bile duct dilation
  - Double duct sign: Dilation of both ducts
- Diffuse glandular tumor involvement can be difficult to differentiate from acute pancreatitis
- Atrophy or pancreatitis proximal to pancreatic ductal obstruction
- Typically hypovascular, but color Doppler may be helpful in assessing vascular encasement or venous obstruction
- Displacement/encasement of adjacent vascular structures, determines resectability (as well as metastases)
- Liver and regional lymph node metastases
- Ascites due to peritoneal metastasis

TOP DIFFERENTIAL DIAGNOSES

- Chronic pancreatitis
- Other primary pancreatic tumors
- Metastases

CLINICAL ISSUES

- Mean at onset: 55 years; peak: 7th decade; M:F = 2:1
- Usually asymptomatic until late in course: Obstructive jaundice, weight loss
- Most commonly presents with distant metastases (~ 65%); least likely to present with tumor confined to pancreas

SCANNING TIPS

- Look carefully at site of transition of dilated bile or pancreatic duct to normal caliber

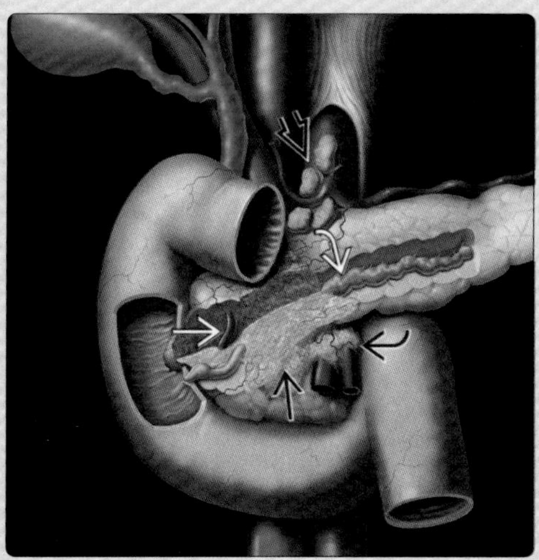

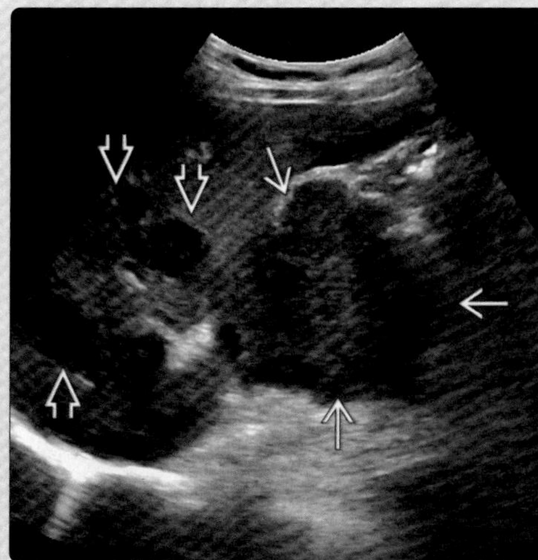

(Left) *Graphic shows an infiltrative mass ⇨ in the pancreatic head partially obstructing the common bile duct ➡ and pancreatic duct ➡. Superior mesenteric vessels are encased ⇨. Celiac nodes ⇨ are present.* **(Right)** *Transverse ultrasound shows a large, lobulated, hypoechoic mass in the pancreatic neck/body ➡. There are multiple liver metastases ➡.*

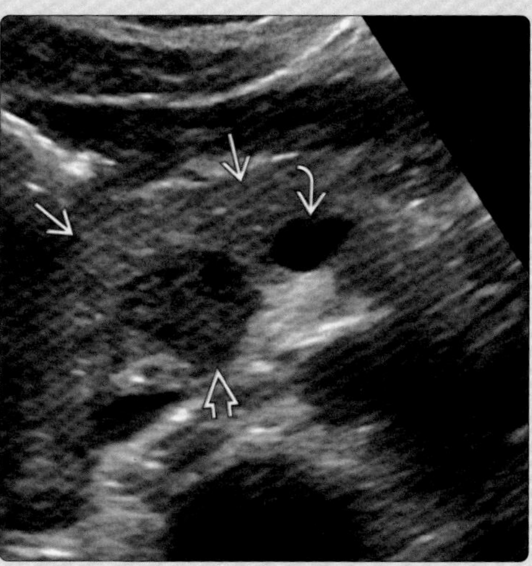

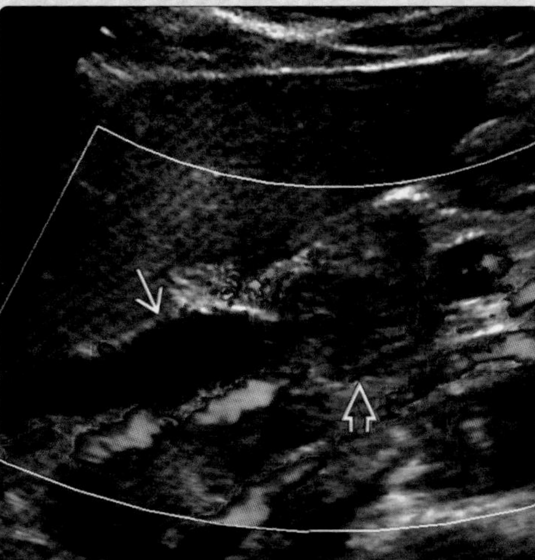

(Left) *Transverse ultrasound shows a rounded hypoechoic mass ➡ in the pancreatic head. The mass is small but conspicuous, as it is less echogenic than a normal pancreas ➡. The superior mesenteric vein ➡ is not involved.* **(Right)** *Longitudinal oblique color Doppler ultrasound shows an ill-defined, solid, hypoechoic mass ➡ in the pancreatic head obstructing the terminal portion of the common bile duct with proximal dilatation ➡.*

Pancreatic Neuroendocrine Tumor

KEY FACTS

TERMINOLOGY

- Historically known as islet cell or carcinoid tumors

IMAGING

- Variable: Range from < 1 cm to > 20 cm; typically 1-5 cm
- Small tumors: Well-defined, round, hypoechoic; can be isoechoic with focal contour deformity
- Larger tumors are well demarcated, lobulated, and more heterogeneous with cystic change/necrosis and calcification
  - Intratumoral calcification suggests malignancy
  - 60-90% have adenopathy and liver metastases at clinical presentation
- Absence of pancreatic ductal dilation
- Color Doppler: Intratumoral flow

TOP DIFFERENTIAL DIAGNOSES

- Mucinous cystic pancreatic neoplasm
- Solid pseudopapillary neoplasm
- Pancreatic ductal carcinoma
- Pancreatic metastases or lymphoma
- Serous cystadenoma of pancreas

CLINICAL ISSUES

- 2-3% of all pancreatic neoplasms; peak: 4th-6th decades; younger in familial cases; most occurring sporadically
- Familial syndromes: Multiple endocrine neoplasia type I; von Hippel-Lindau, neurofibromatosis type 1, tuberous sclerosis
- Functioning tumors: Smaller at time of presentation due to hormonal production of insulin, glucagon, and gastrin
- Nonfunctional tumors (60-80%): Usually asymptomatic but larger size at time of diagnosis; may cause mass effect and abdominal pain from primary or metastases
- Prognosis: Best for insulinomas (most common functional)
- Poor prognostic features: Size > 2-4 cm; cystic change, calcification, necrosis

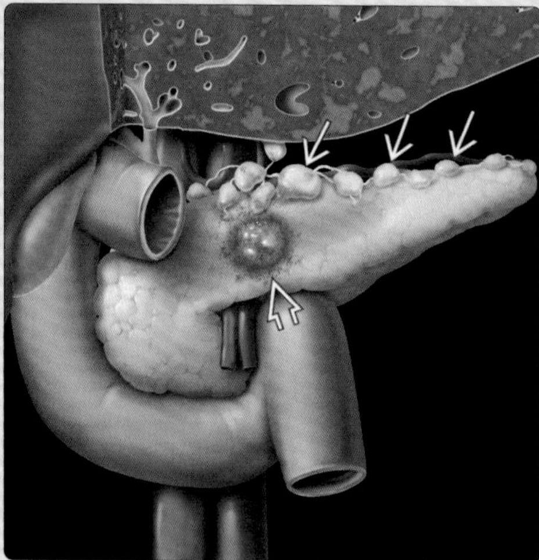

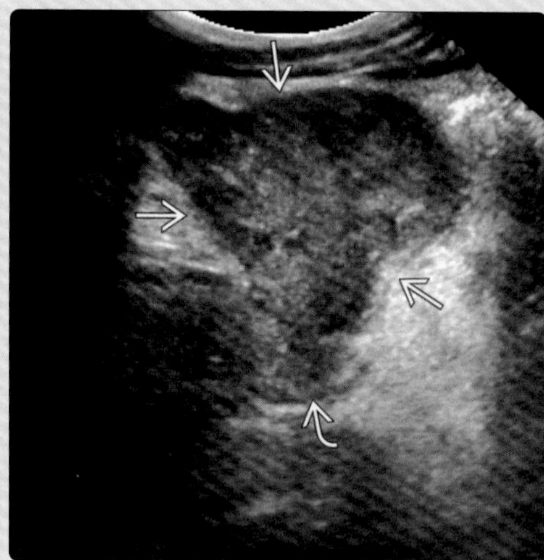

(Left) *Graphic demonstrates a well-circumscribed, round, solid mass ➡ in the pancreatic body with regional metastatic lymphadenopathy ➡.* **(Right)** *Transverse ultrasound through the left upper quadrant shows a large soft tissue mass ➡ arising from the pancreatic tail ➡. This was a nonfunctioning neuroendocrine tumor, proven by biopsy of liver metastases.*

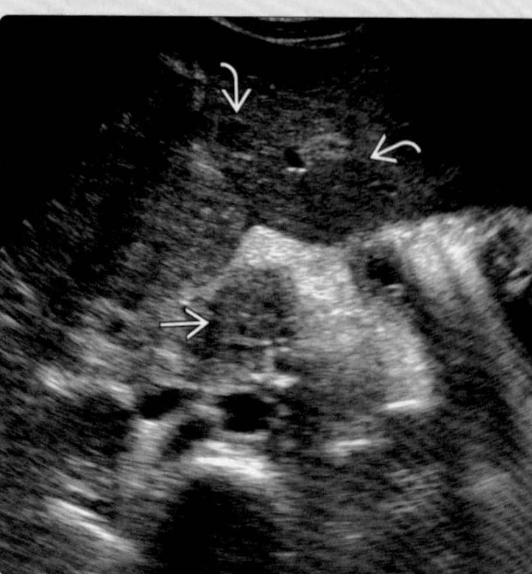

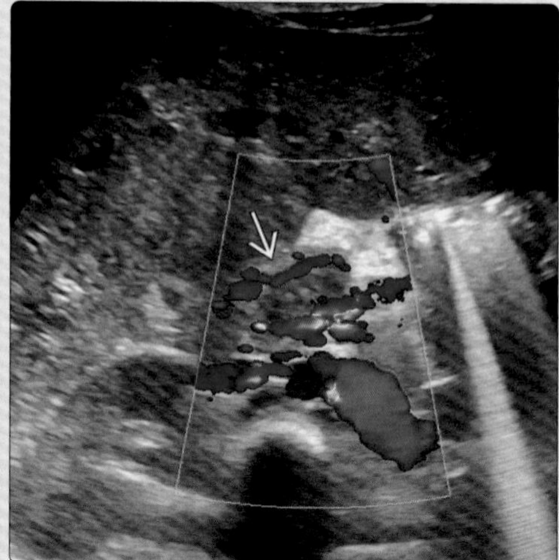

(Left) *Transverse ultrasound through the epigastric region shows a small soft tissue mass ➡ in the pancreatic head in a child who presented with abdominal pain and an enlarged liver. Biopsy of a liver metastasis ➡ revealed the diagnosis of a nonfunctioning neuroendocrine tumor.* **(Right)** *Transverse color Doppler ultrasound of the same patient shows abundant color flow in the pancreatic head nonfunctioning neuroendocrine tumor ➡.*

KEY FACTS

TERMINOLOGY

- Epithelial tumor of exocrine pancreas with low-grade malignant potential and solid and cystic features

IMAGING

- Usually large (average: 10 cm; range: 2.5-20.0 cm)
- Commonly in pancreatic tail
- Lesions < 3 cm with solid, homogeneous appearance
- Larger lesions: Heterogeneous mass with solid and central cystic components (hemorrhage and necrosis), fluid debris level
- May contain dystrophic calcifications
- Color Doppler: Hypovascular, due to areas of necrosis
- Endoscopic ultrasound: More sensitive for small mass; can guide fine-needle aspiration biopsy

TOP DIFFERENTIAL DIAGNOSES

- Mucinous cystic pancreatic tumor
- Pancreatic neuroendocrine tumor
- Pancreatic serous cystadenoma
- Pancreatic ductal carcinoma

PATHOLOGY

- Fibrous, hypervascular capsule with solid and pseudopapillary tissue surrounding hemorrhagic and necrotic center

CLINICAL ISSUES

- Very rare, < 3% of all pancreatic tumors
- Typically in asymptomatic, young, non-Caucasian women
- ~ 90% female; < 35 years of age
- Usually asymptomatic or nonspecific abdominal pain
- May have palpable abdominal mass
- Usually benign but with low malignant potential

SCANNING TIPS

- Look for solid components, which will triage patient to surgery

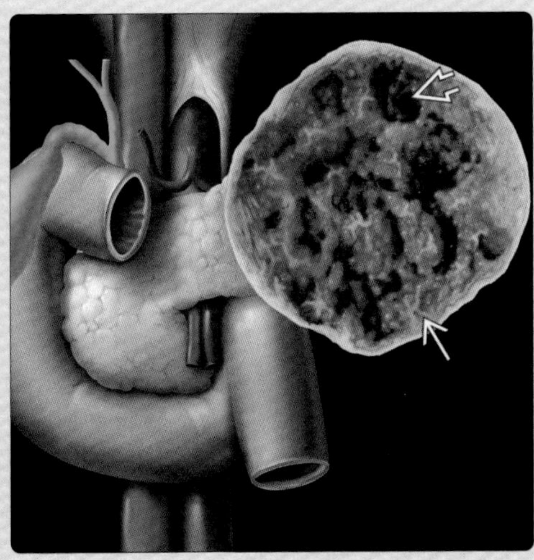

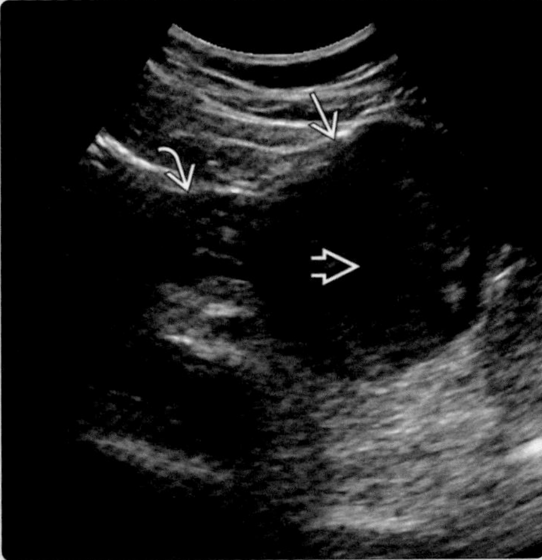

(Left) *Graphic shows a large, encapsulated mass in the pancreatic tail with solid ➡ and cystic or hemorrhagic ⇨ components.* **(Right)** *Transverse ultrasound through the pancreas shows a predominantly solid, lobulated mass ➡ arising from the body of pancreas. The center ⇨ was more cystic. The neck of the pancreas ↪ was normal.*

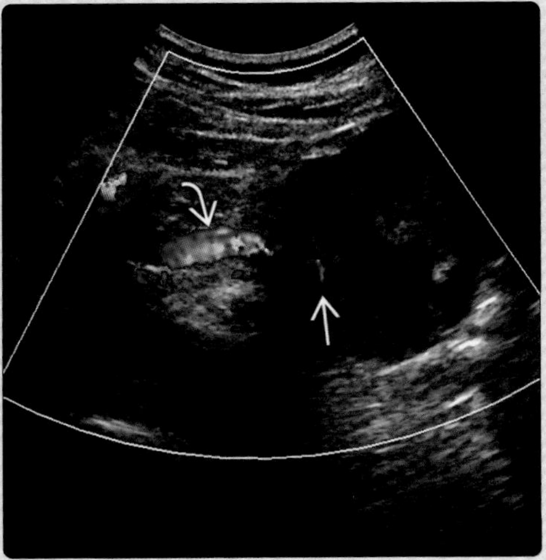

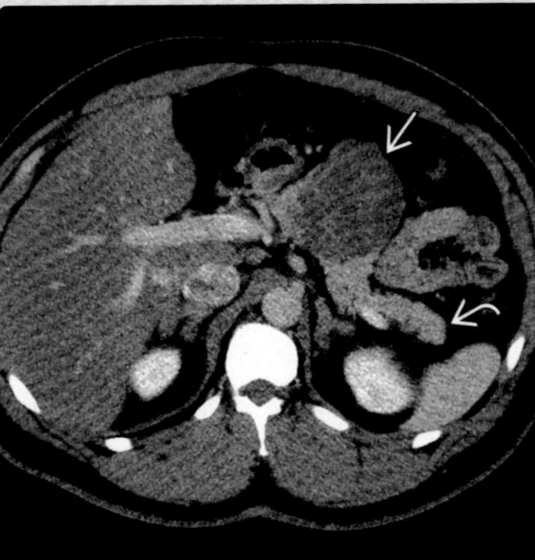

(Left) *Transverse color Doppler ultrasound of the same patient shows color flow ↪ in the solid component of the solid pseudopapillary neoplasm. The splenic vein ➡ was patent.* **(Right)** *Axial CECT of the same patient shows the mixed-density, lobulated, solid pseudopapillary neoplasm ➡ arising exophytically from the body of pancreas. The tail ↪ was normal.*

PART I
SECTION 4
Spleen

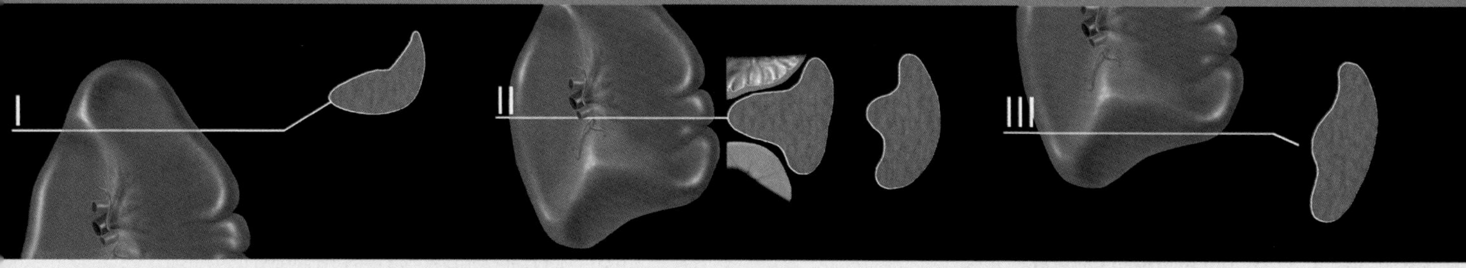

Anatomy and Approach

Splenic Lesions

GROSS ANATOMY

Overview

- Intraperitoneal lymphatic organ located posterior to stomach and intimately associated with retroperitoneum (pancreatic tail and left kidney)
- Surrounded by peritoneum (except at hilum) and suspended by several ligaments
  - **Gastrosplenic ligament**
    - Left anterior margin of lesser sac
    - Connects spleen to greater curvature of stomach
    - Carries short gastrics and left gastroepiploic arteries and venous branches to spleen
  - **Splenorenal ligament**
    - Left posterior margin of lesser sac
    - Connects spleen to left kidney and pancreatic tail
    - Carries splenic artery and vein to splenic hilum
  - Splenocolic ligament: Between spleen and splenic flexure of colon
  - Splenophrenic ligament: Between spleen and inferior surface of diaphragm
- **Normal size is variable**; no universal consensus
  - Generally, normal adult spleen considered 12-cm length x 7-cm width x 4cm thickness
    - Length = longest diameter in longitudinal plane; width = longest transverse (anterior-posterior) diameter; thickness = maximal thickness in transverse plane at hilum
  - Splenic index (product of length, thickness, and width): Normally 120-480 cm^3
- Functions
  - Manufactures lymphocytes, filters blood (removes damaged red blood cells and platelets)
  - Acts as blood reservoir: Can expand or contract in response to changes in blood volume
- Histology
  - Soft organ with fibroelastic capsule and comprised of pulp
    - White pulp: Lymphoid nodules/tissue primarily surrounding vasculature
    - Red pulp: Sinusoidal spaces containing blood
  - Trabeculae: Extensions of capsule into parenchyma; carry arterial and venous branches
  - Splenic cords (plates of cells) lie between sinusoids; red pulp veins drain sinusoids
- **Vasculature**
  - **Splenic artery** arises from celiac axis in > 90%; 8% directly from aorta
    - Often very tortuous
  - **Splenic vein** runs in groove along dorsal surface of pancreatic body and tail
    - Receives inferior mesenteric vein (IMV)
    - Combined splenic vein and IMV join superior mesenteric vein to form portal vein

IMAGING ANATOMY

Overview

- Homogeneous echogenicity
  - Echogenicity: Pancreas > spleen > liver > kidney
  - Radiating pattern of segmental arteries and veins
- **Splenic artery**
  - Low-resistance waveform; tortuosity of vessel results in turbulence and spectral broadening
  - Normal diameter: 4-8 mm; peak systolic velocity (PSV): 25-45 cm/s
- **Splenic vein**
  - Normal diameter: 5-10 mm; PSV: 9-18 cm/s
  - Splenic vein at midline is useful landmark for locating pancreas
    - Pancreas lies anterior to splenic vein
  - Diameter increases between 50-100% from quiet respiration to deep inspiration; increase of < 20% suggests portal hypertension
  - Spectral Doppler waveform typically shows band-like flow profile with minimal respiratory fluctuations

ANATOMY IMAGING ISSUES

Imaging Recommendations

- Patient positioned supine or right decubitus position (left side up) with left arm raised
- Place transducer parallel to ribs in 10th or 11th intercostal space at left midaxillary line, searching for best window
  - Due to rib angle, this results in oblique view, which by convention is called longitudinal or transverse (depending on transducer orientation)
  - Transverse US view of spleen does not correlate directly to axial CT view
- End expiration may be helpful; lung base may obscure spleen in full inspiration
- Spleen poorly accessed from posterior (obscured by left lung base), anterior, or subcostal approach (obscured by stomach and colon)
- Assess splenic vein at hilum and midline for patency and flow direction
- Can use spleen as acoustic window to visualize tail of pancreas

Key Concepts

- Spleen has highly variable size and shape
  - Easily indented and displaced by masses and even loculated fluid collections

EMBRYOLOGY

Practical Implications

- **Accessory spleen** (splenunculus, splenule)
  - Found in 10-30% of population and may be multiple
  - Usually small, near splenic hilum
  - Can enlarge and simulate mass, especially after splenectomy
  - Ectopic intrapancreatic splenule can mimic pancreatic tail mass; should not be > 3 cm from tail tip
- **Wandering spleen**: Spleen may be on long mesentery
  - Found in any abdominopelvic location; risk of torsion
- **Asplenia and polysplenia** (heterotaxy syndromes)
  - Rare congenital conditions of altered left/right orientation of organs
  - Associated with cardiovascular anomalies, intestinal malrotation, etc.
- **Splenosis**: Peritoneal implantation of splenic tissue after traumatic splenic injury, can mimic polysplenia

LIGAMENTS AND VESSELS

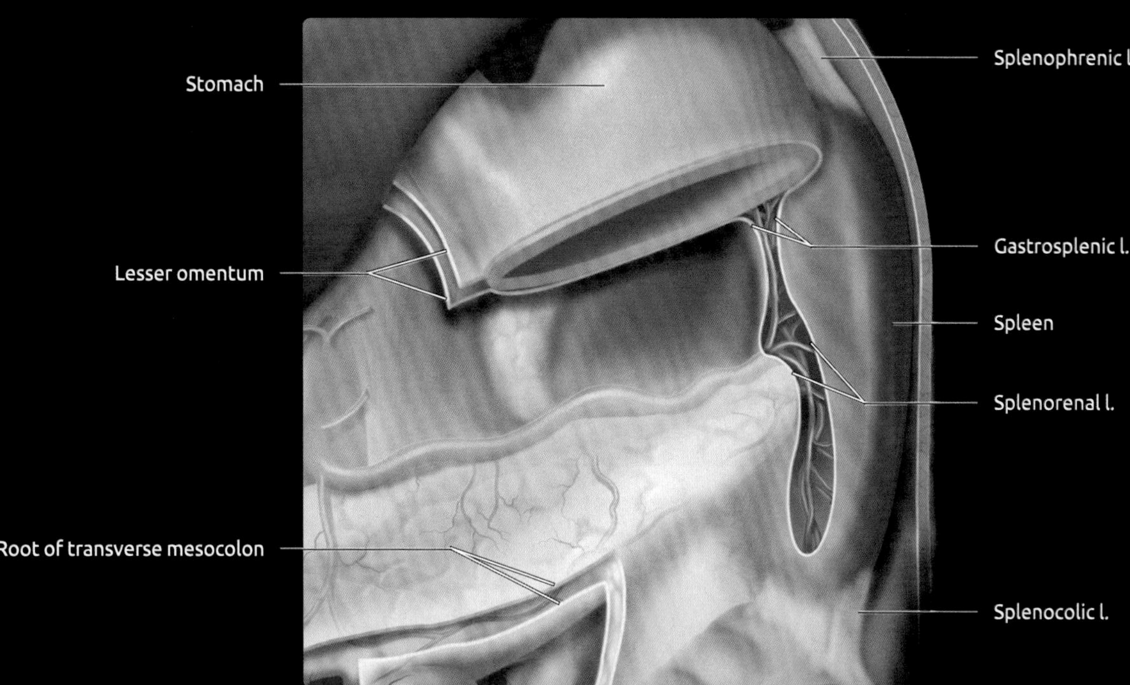

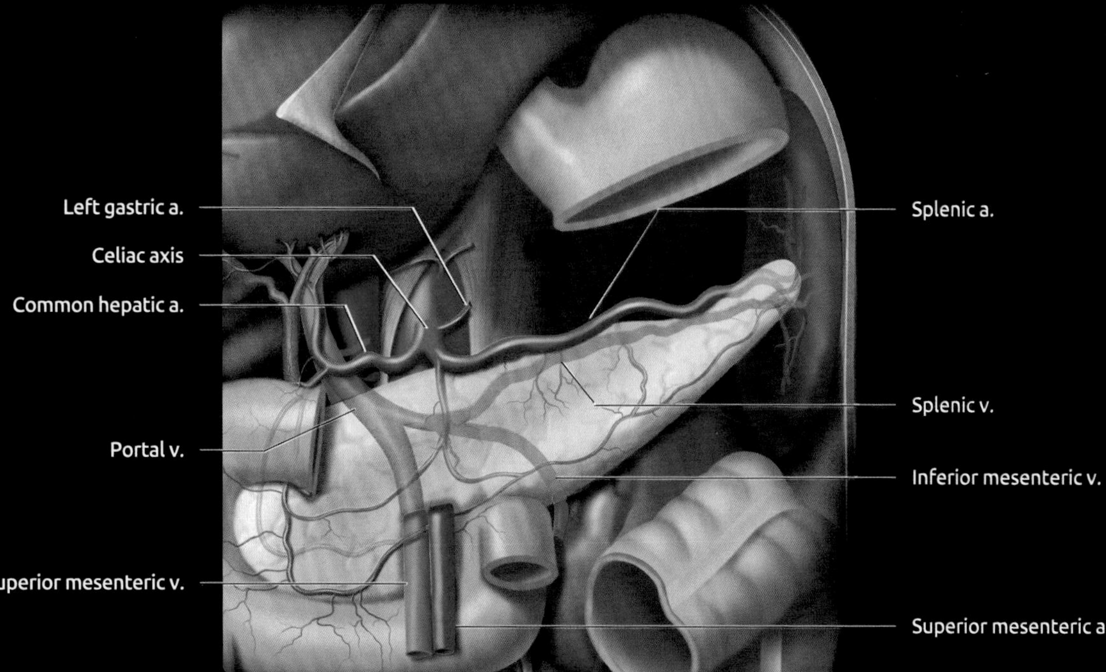

(Top) *Graphic shows the liver is retracted upward and the stomach transected to reveal the pancreas and spleen. The spleen is affixed to surrounding organs by several ligamentous attachments. The gastrosplenic ligament connects the spleen to the greater curve of the stomach and transports the short gastrics and left gastroepiploic vessels. The splenorenal ligament connects the spleen to the left kidney and pancreatic tail and carries the splenic artery and vein into the spleen at the hilum. The splenocolic ligament extends to the splenic flexure of the colon and the splenophrenic ligament to the diaphragm.* **(Bottom)** *Coronal graphic with the mesenteric reflections removed to show the splenic vascular supply. The splenic artery arises from the celiac axis and is often quite tortuous. The splenic vein runs posterior to the body of the pancreas and receives the inferior mesenteric vein. It joins the superior mesenteric vein behind the neck of the pancreas to form the portal vein.*

SPLENIC SHAPE

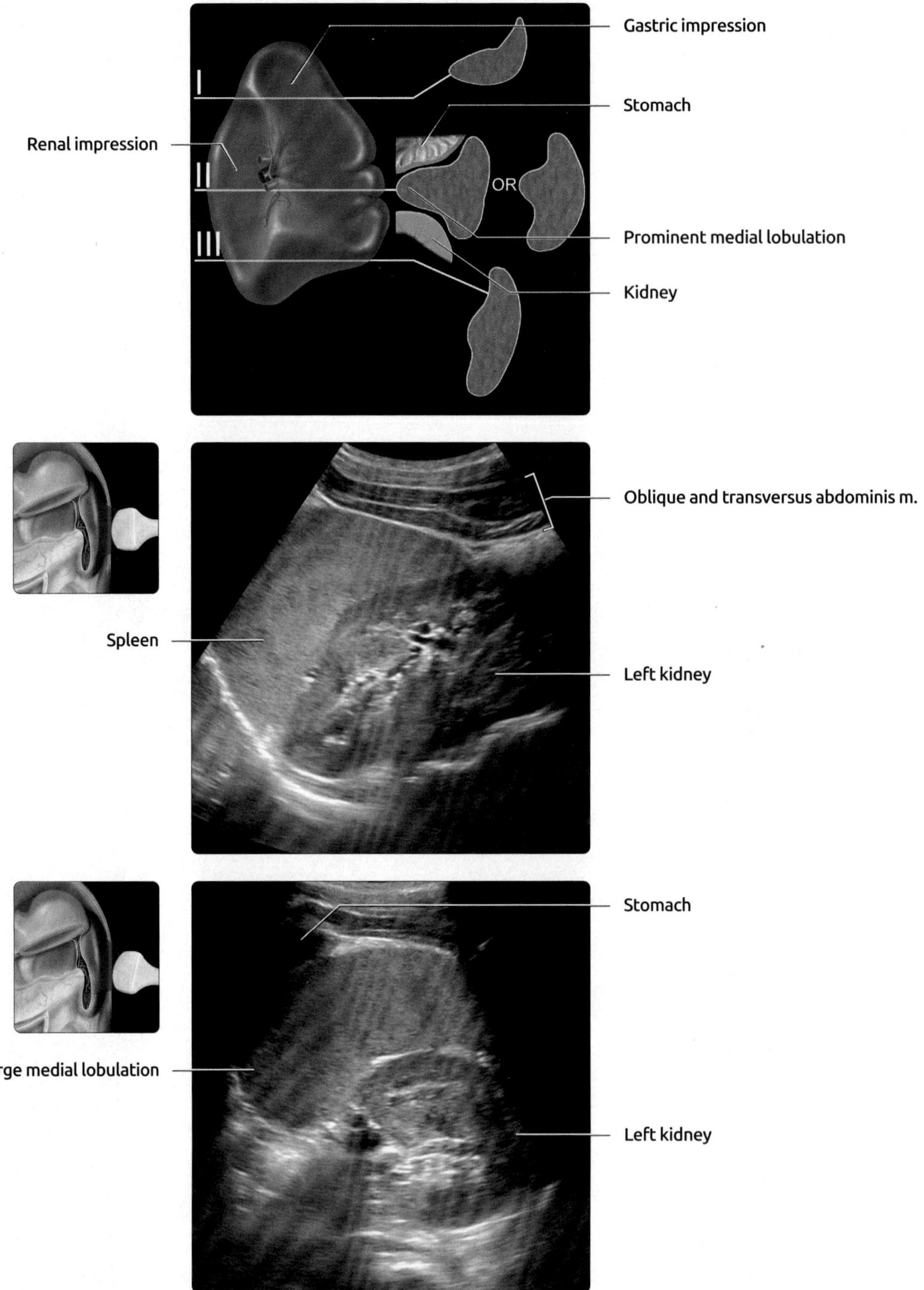

(Top) *Graphic shows the medial surface of the spleen and representative axial sections at 3 levels through the parenchyma. The spleen is of variable shape and size, even within the same individual, varying with states of nutrition and hydration. It is a soft organ that is easily indented by adjacent organs. The medial surface is often quite lobulated as it is interposed between the stomach and the kidney.* **(Middle)** *Longitudinal ultrasound shows the spleen conforming to the shape of the left kidney. In this plane, the spleen appears quite small.* **(Bottom)** *The oblique transverse plane in the same patient shows a large medial lobulation. Volume measurements are more accurate in determining the size of the spleen than any individual measurements, but even that has large individual variability.*

SPLENIC SHAPE

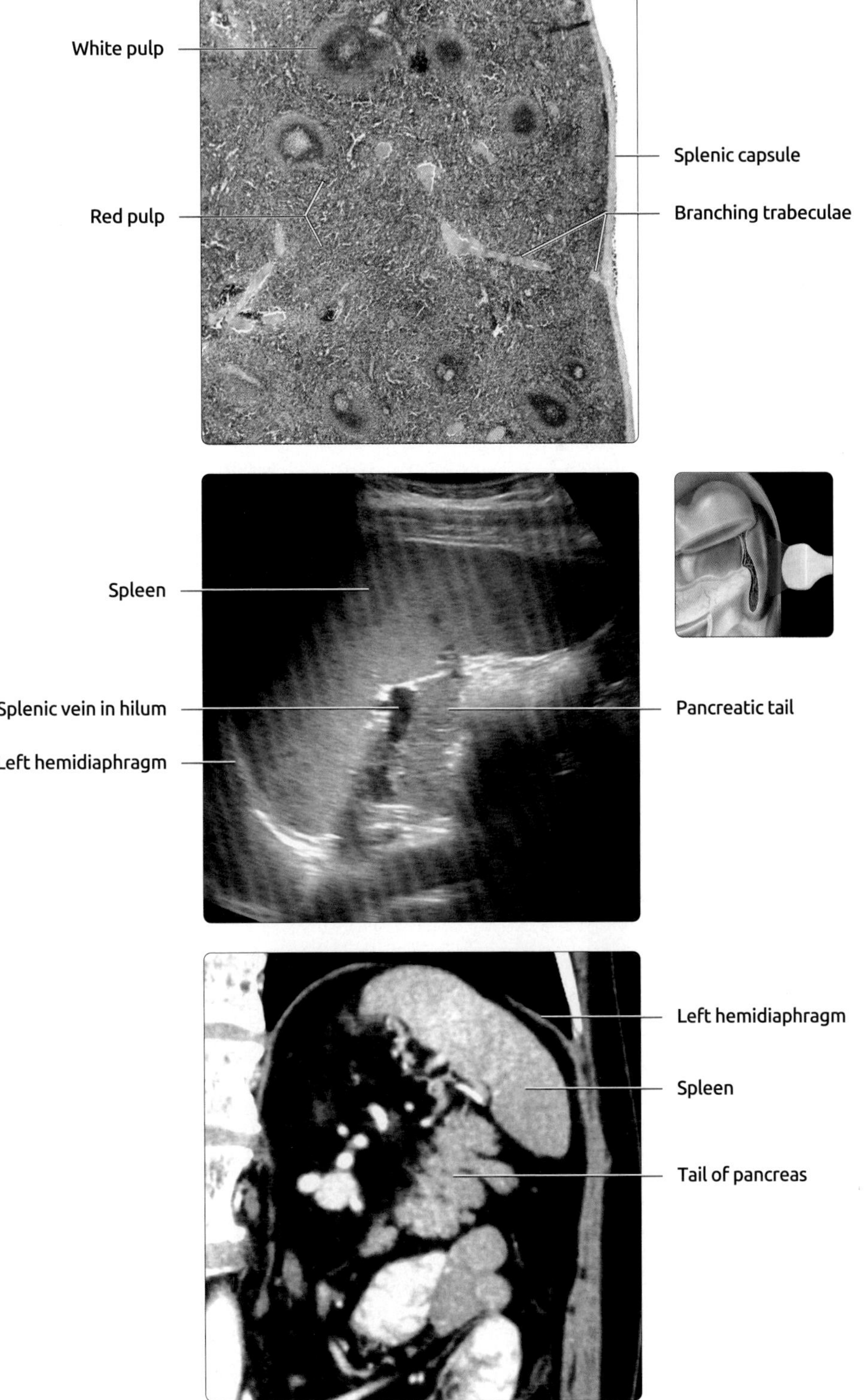

(Top) *Histologic section of a normal spleen viewed at low power shows white pulp and red pulp. A thin splenic capsule with slivers of branching trabeculae is also noted. The red pulp is "spongy" and compressible.* **(Middle)** *This longitudinal view of the spleen through the left flank shows the intimate relationship with the tail of the pancreas. In this case, the spleen was long (13.5 cm), but the splenic index and volume were normal.* **(Bottom)** *Oblique correlative multiplanar reconstruction CT of the spleen is shown. Note the extension of the pancreatic tail toward the splenic hilum. This allows the pancreatic tail to be visualized by ultrasound using the spleen as an acoustic window.*

SPLENIC VESSELS

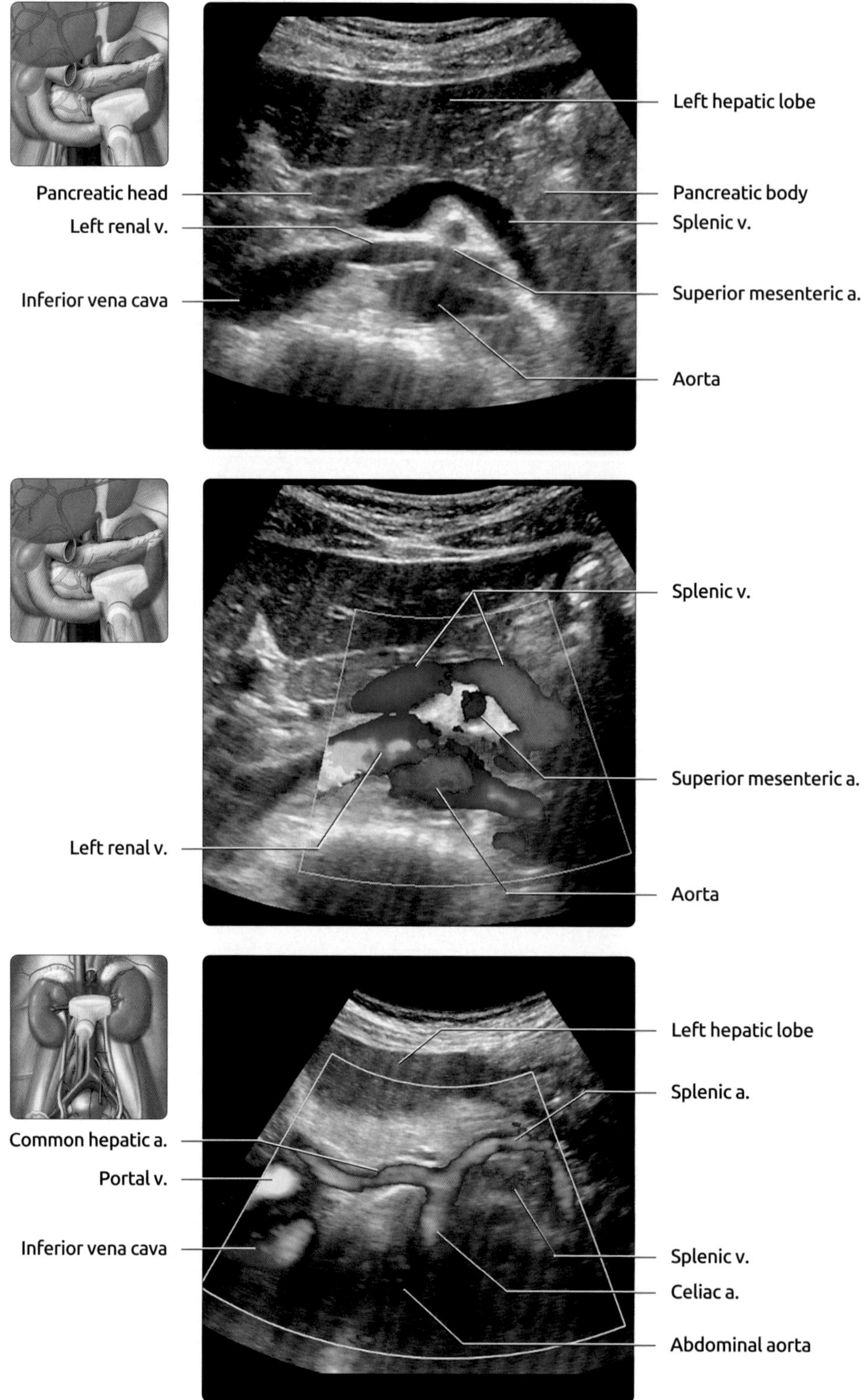

(Top) *Midline transverse anterior grayscale ultrasound of the splenic vein is shown. The splenic vein is located deep to the pancreatic body. Note the left renal vein course between the superior mesenteric artery and aorta.* **(Middle)** *Color Doppler ultrasound of the same area shows the normal direction of flow in the splenic vein toward the liver (hepatopetal). Note the change in color from red to blue, which is due to the position of the transducer, aligned at the midpoint of the vein. Using the information provided by the color bar, the red portion of the splenic vein is blood flowing toward the transducer (away from the spleen), and the blue is blood flowing away from the transducer (toward the the liver).* **(Bottom)** *Power Doppler ultrasound of the upper abdomen at midline shows the origin of the splenic artery from the celiac axis. The celiac artery branches into the splenic artery, common hepatic artery, and left gastric artery (not shown). After its takeoff, the splenic artery typically has a tortuous course. The branching of the celiac axis, as shown in this image, has been referred to as the seagull sign.*

SPLENIC VESSELS

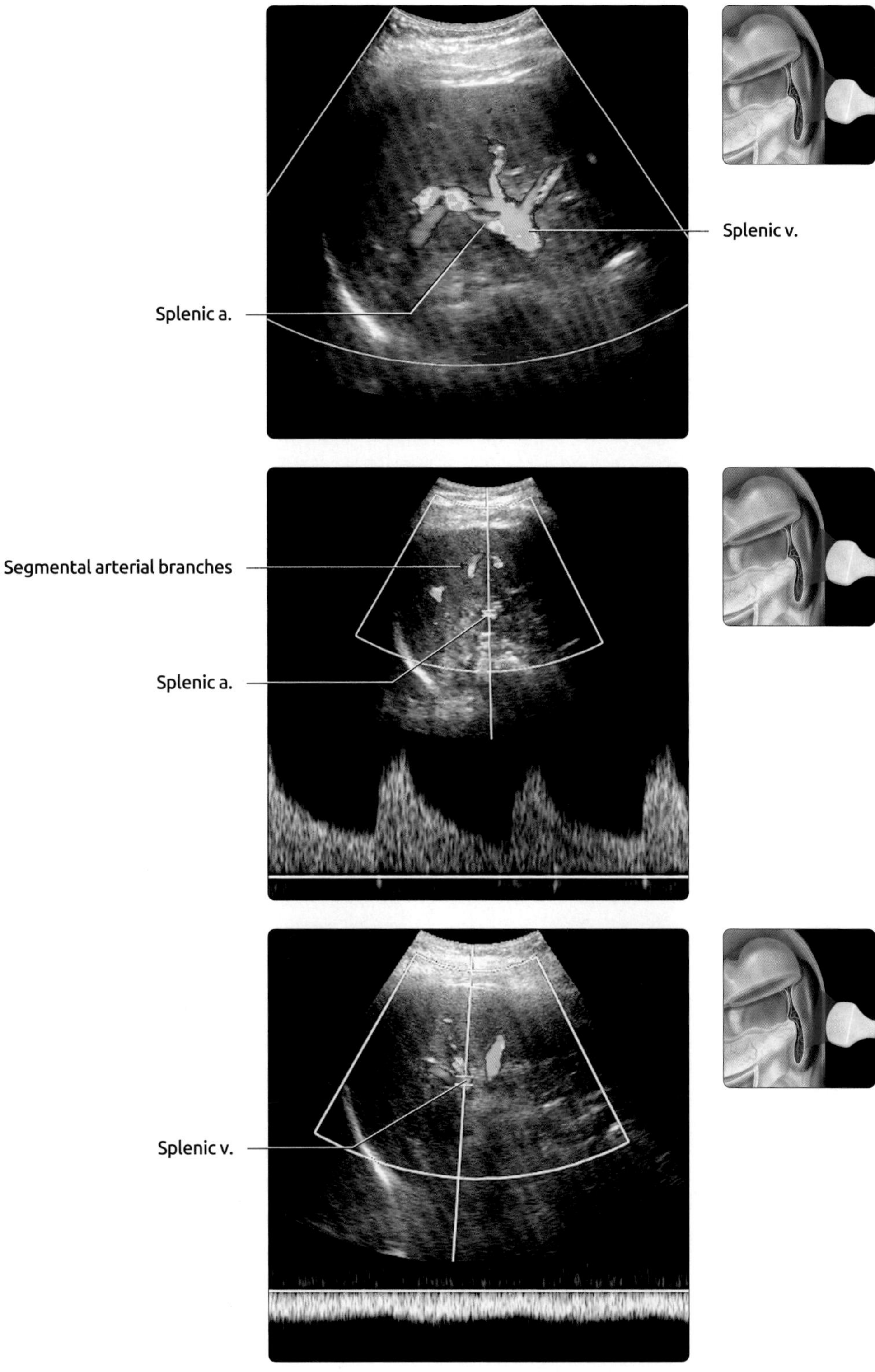

(Top) *Longitudinal oblique color Doppler ultrasound demonstrates the branching of the splenic arteries and veins in the splenic hilum.* **(Middle)** *Spectral Doppler waveform ultrasound of the distal splenic artery at the splenic hilum is shown. Because of a tortuous course, flow in this vessel is typically turbulent. The splenic artery has a low-resistance waveform (ample flow throughout diastole). Normal peak systolic velocity for the splenic artery is 25-45 cm/s.* **(Bottom)** *Spectral Doppler waveform ultrasound of the splenic vein at the hilum shows a typical band-like flow profile with minimal respiratory fluctuations; flow is directed away from the transducer (away from the spleen). Normal peak systolic velocity of the splenic vein is 9-18 cm/s.*

SPLENULE

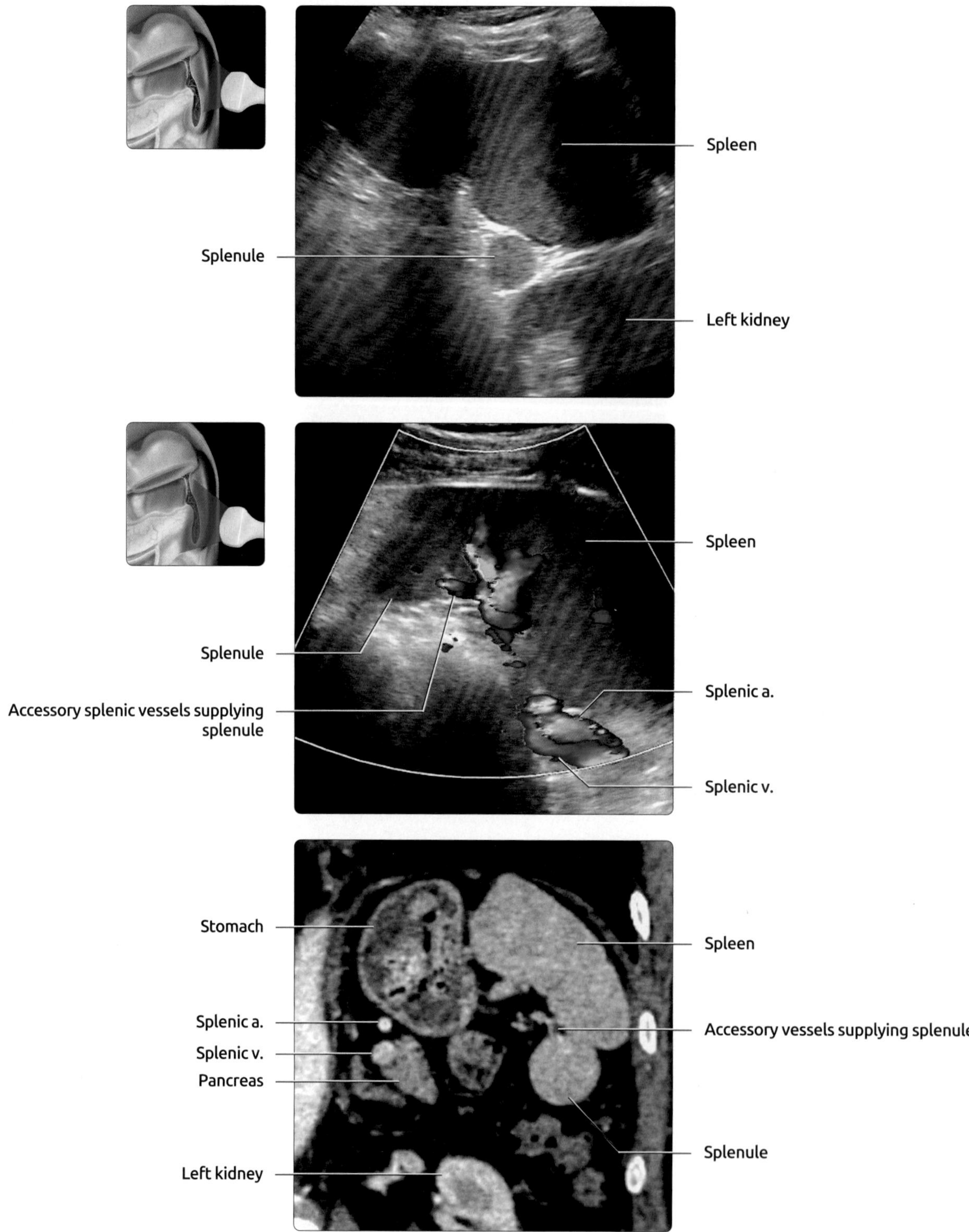

(Top) *Transverse oblique intercostal ultrasound shows a splenule between the spleen and left kidney. Splenules should have the same echogenicity and echotexture as the spleen, though this may depend on the sonographic window.* **(Middle)** *Longitudinal oblique intercostal color Doppler ultrasound shows a splenule adjacent to the spleen tip. The identification of vascular supply from the splenic vessels may also aid in identification of a splenule.* **(Bottom)** *Correlative coronal CECT of the left upper quadrant demonstrates a splenule along the inferior tip of the spleen. Branch vessels from the splenic artery and vein supplying the splenule are visualized.*

SPLENOSIS AND HETEROTAXY

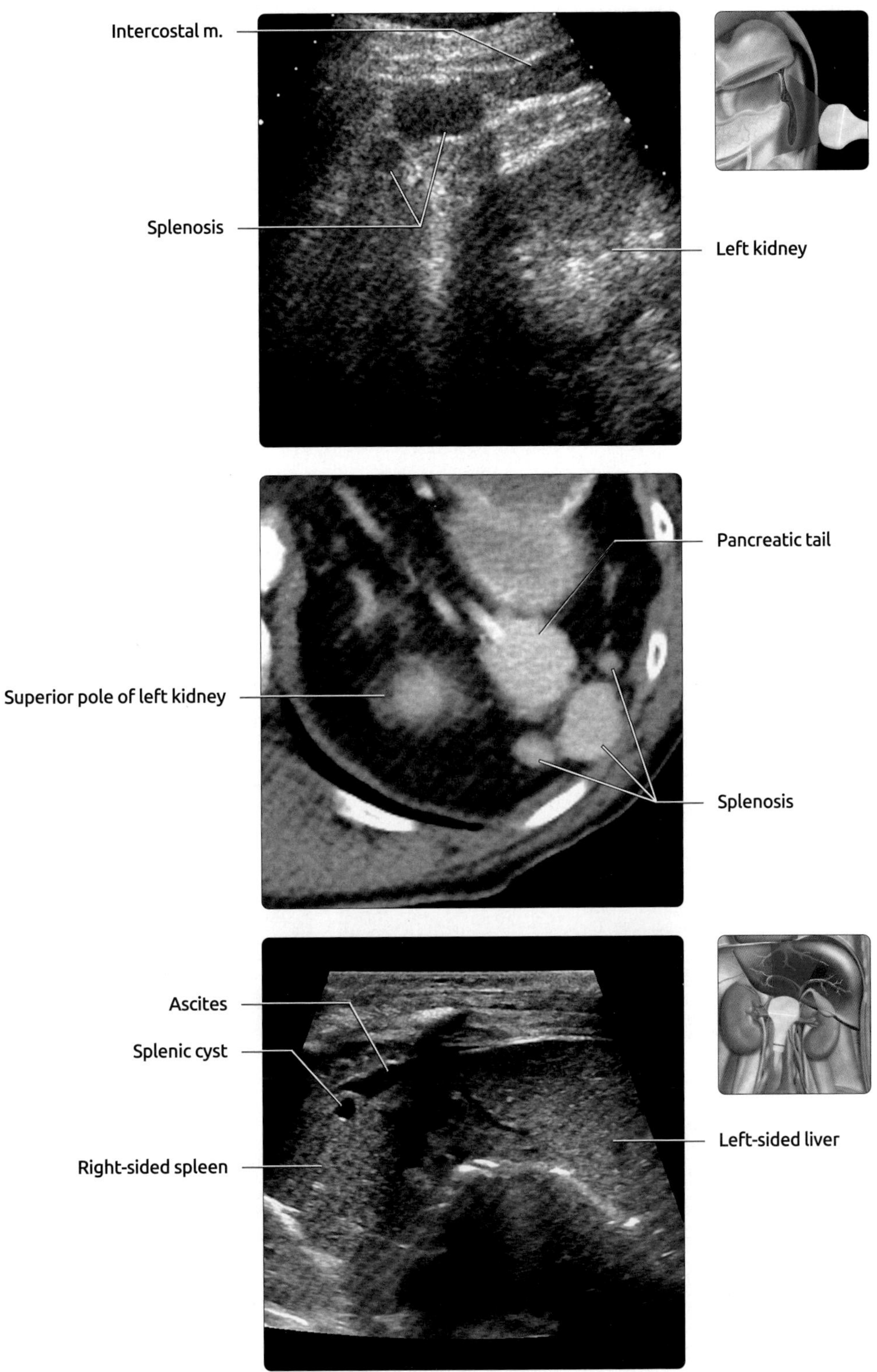

(Top) *Longitudinal oblique intercostal grayscale ultrasound through the left upper quadrant in a patient with prior splenectomy shows rounded, hypoechoic structures adjacent to the upper pole of the left kidney; this represents splenosis.* **(Middle)** *Correlative axial CECT through the left upper quadrant in a patient with prior splenic trauma and splenectomy shows residual splenosis.* **(Bottom)** *Transverse anterior ultrasound in the setting of heterotaxy with polysplenia demonstrates the relationship between the right-sided spleen and the left-sided liver. The classification of heterotaxy syndromes is complex; there is a spectrum ranging from classic asplenia to classic polysplenia. Heterotaxy with polysplenia (i.e., left double sidedness or left isomerism) may present with multiple spleens (resembling splenules) or a single spleen, as in this case.*

Splenomegaly

KEY FACTS

IMAGING

- No universal consensus on splenomegaly (SMG) cut off due to variability in normal adult spleen size
- SMG is diagnosed when length > 13 cm; additional measurements of thickness > 5 cm or width > 8 cm may also be used
- Splenic index (product of length, thickness, and width): Normally 120-480 cm^3; SMG considered index > 500 cm^3
- Color Doppler
  - Portal hypertension: Dilated splenic vein (SV); direction of flow may be reversed; SV thrombus, splenic hilar collaterals, splenorenal shunt, recanalized umbilical vein
- **SMG with normal echogenicity**
  - Infection (mononucleosis, *Salmonella typhi*), congestion (portal hypertension), early sickle cell disease
  - Hereditary spherocytosis, hemolysis, Felty syndrome
  - Wilson disease, polycythemia, myelofibrosis, leukemia
- **SMG with hyperechoic pattern**
  - Leukemia, lymphoma, sarcoidosis, metastasis
  - Infections (malaria, tuberculosis, brucellosis), hematoma
  - Hereditary spherocytosis, polycythemia, myelofibrosis
- **SMG with hypoechoic pattern**
  - Leukemia, lymphoma, sarcoidosis, metastasis
  - Infections (malaria, tuberculosis, brucellosis), hematoma
  - Hereditary spherocytosis, polycythemia, myelofibrosis
- **SMG with mixed echogenic pattern**
  - Abscesses, metastases, infarction, hemorrhage/hematoma in different stages of evolution, primary malignancy (e.g., lymphoma, angiosarcoma)

SCANNING TIPS

- Splenic size correlates with height and can exceed normal size in tall, healthy people
  - If spleen extends below normal left kidney, highly suggestive of SMG
- Spleen thickness should be measured from hilum to outer convex surface of spleen

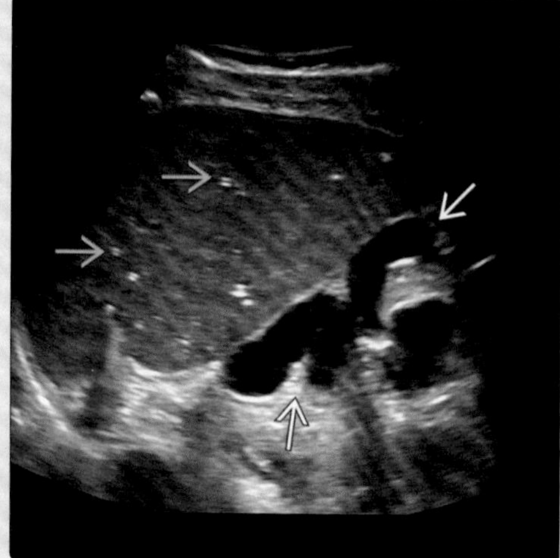

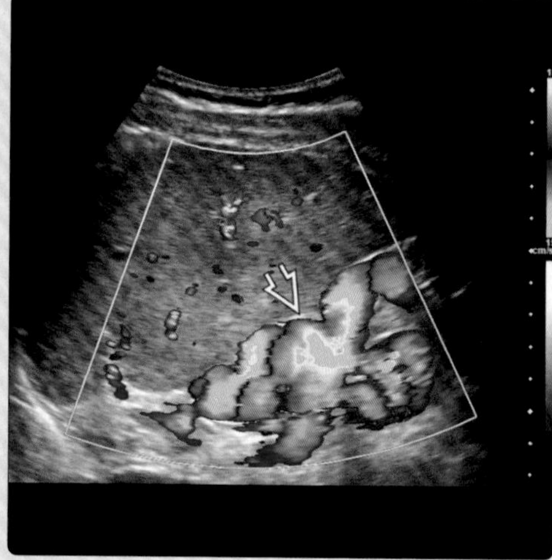

(Left) *US in a 47-year-old man with hepatitis C cirrhosis and splenomegaly (length: 13.5 cm, thickness: 6.5 cm) shows the dilated, tubular anechoic structures at the splenic hilum, consistent with splenic varices ➔. Echogenic foci without posterior acoustic shadowing throughout the spleen represent Gamna-Gandy bodies ➔.* **(Right)** *Color Doppler US in the same patient with portal hypertension confirms dilated splenic hilar varices ➔.*

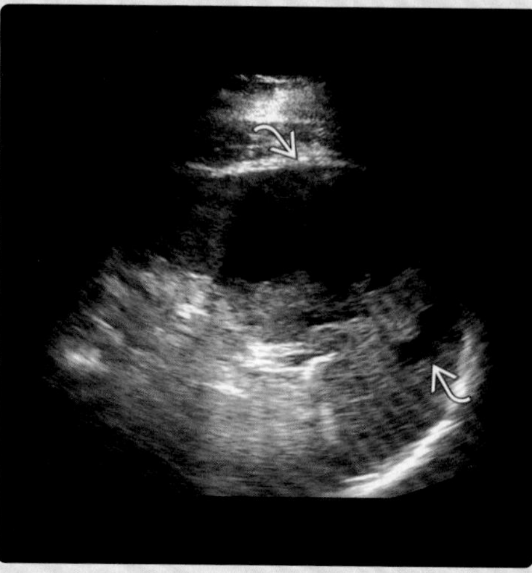

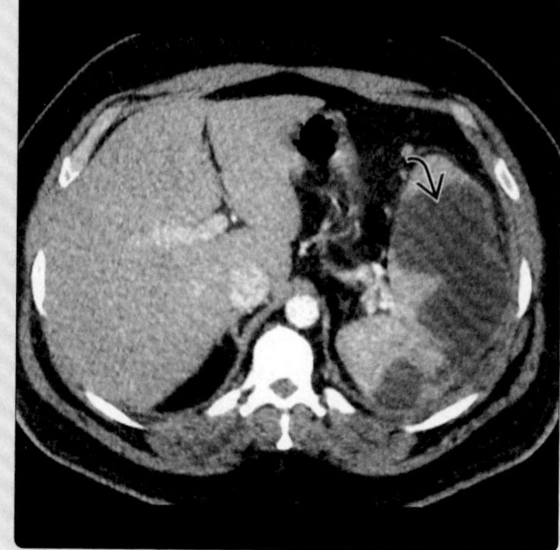

(Left) *US in a 47-year-old man shows splenomegaly (length: 19.5 cm) due to space-occupying hypoechoic masses ➔ without internal vascularity (not pictured). These represented splenic abscesses.* **(Right)** *Axial CECT in the same patient demonstrates large, lobulated, hypodense splenic lesions ➔ resulting in splenomegaly. Pus was revealed on percutaneous drain placement, consistent with splenic abscess.*

KEY FACTS

IMAGING

- Can be classified as primary (congenital) vs. secondary (acquired) **or** true (epithelial lined) vs. false (no epithelial lining)
  - Secondary more common than primary (80% vs. 20%)
  - Hydatid cyst is example of acquired true cyst
- Classically, anechoic to hypoechoic, avascular, sharply defined, spherical lesion with posterior acoustic enhancement
  - Variable presence of internal debris/septation, wall calcification depending on type and etiology

TOP DIFFERENTIAL DIAGNOSES

- Inflammatory or infection
  - Pyogenic, fungal, or granulomatous abscess
- Neoplastic
  - Benign (hemangioma, lymphangioma) or malignant (cystic metastasis, lymphoma)
- Vascular
  - Hematoma, infarction, peliosis, intrasplenic pseudoaneurysm
- Intrasplenic pancreatic pseudocyst

DIAGNOSTIC CHECKLIST

- Rule out infectious, vascular, and neoplastic cystic lesions
- Consider if congenital or acquired cyst
  - Congenital (epidermoid): Typically larger, anechoic, with thin wall; ± calcification or debris (less common)
  - Acquired: Most commonly posttraumatic; usually smaller, often anechoic, but may have debris; thicker wall ± calcification
- Often impossible to distinguish primary vs. secondary (or true vs. false) cysts by imaging

SCANNING TIPS

- Patient is best scanned in supine or right lateral decubitus position following deep inspiration with US transducer angling between ribs

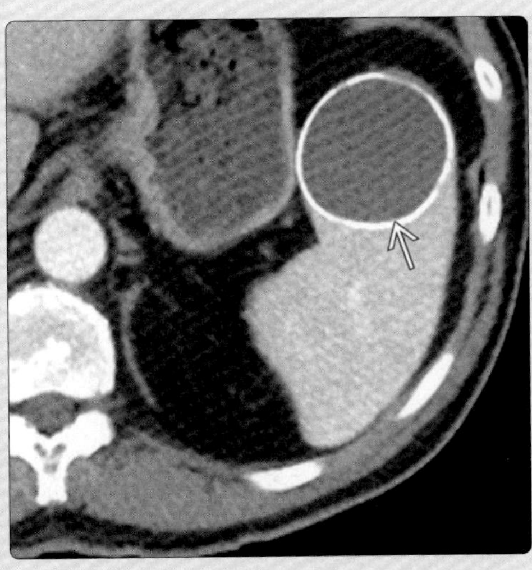

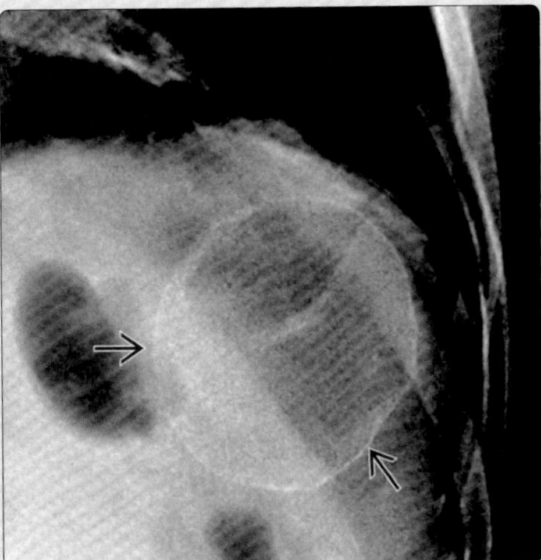

(Left) *Axial CECT of the left upper quadrant shows a large, rim-calcified, posttraumatic pseudocyst in the anterior spleen ➡.* **(Right)** *Zoomed in view of the left subdiaphragmatic space on frontal chest radiograph in the same patient shows the cyst delineated by thin-rim calcification ⇨.*

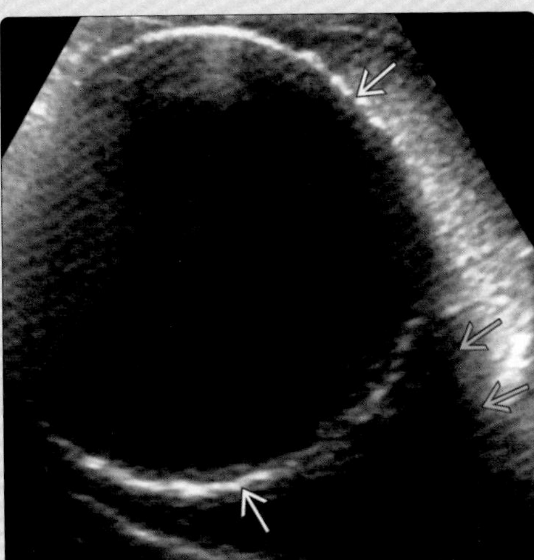

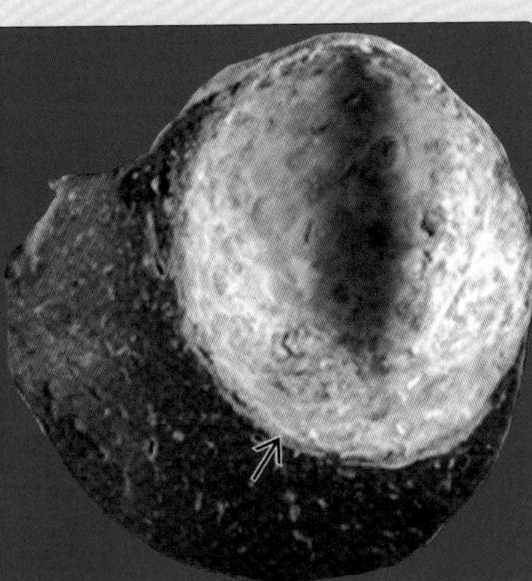

(Left) *Grayscale US shows an anechoic splenic pseudocyst with curvilinear rim calcification ➡, which causes posterior acoustic shadowing ⇨.* **(Right)** *Gross pathology of an acquired pseudocyst in the spleen shows a calcified, fibrous wall ⇨.*

KEY FACTS

IMAGING

- **Benign tumors**
  - Hemangioma: #1 benign splenic tumor; typically small, echogenic, incidental, asymptomatic
  - Hamartoma: Typically echogenic, homogeneous
  - Lymphangioma: Typically hypoechoic, loculated, avascular; younger age
  - Littoral cell angioma: Rare; variable appearance, splenomegaly
- **Malignant tumors**
  - Lymphoma (Hodgkin disease, non-Hodgkin lymphoma, primary splenic, AIDS-related), leukemia, myeloproliferative disorders
    - Classic: Diffuse SMG; if focal: Hypoechoic, indistinct margins
    - 3 macroscopic patterns: Diffuse/infiltrative, miliary/nodular, focal hypoechoic
  - Metastasis (breast, lung, ovary, stomach, melanoma)
    - Cystic, solid, or mixed; can be targetoid lesions
  - Primary splenic malignancies very rare (angiosarcoma most common of these)

TOP DIFFERENTIAL DIAGNOSES

- Splenic infarct
- Splenic infection/abscess
- Splenic cyst
- Splenic hematoma
- Hepatosplenic sarcoidosis

SCANNING TIPS

- Color Doppler vascularity may be helpful if present (to conclude not cyst), but absent color flow does not entirely exclude benign or malignant tumor
- Isolated splenic metastases and primary splenic malignancies are rare; most splenic metastases are seen in setting of widespread metastatic disease, including liver

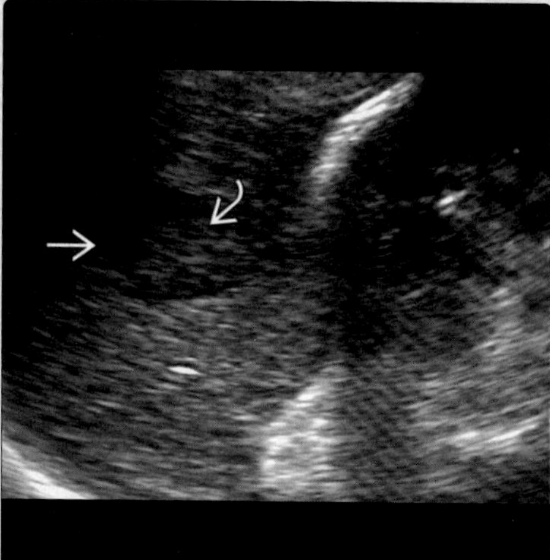

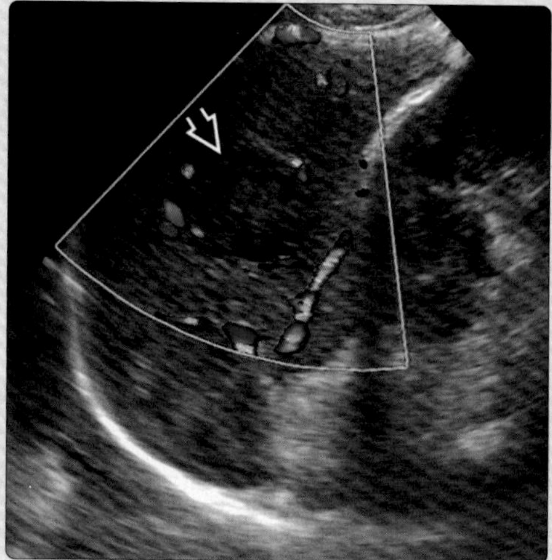

(Left) *Grayscale ultrasound of the spleen in a patient with hepatitis C (HCV) and previously treated hepatocellular carcinoma (HCC) shows a solitary solid mass in the spleen with central hyperechogenicity* ➡ *and peripheral hypoechogenicity* ➡ *(target-like pattern).* **(Right)** *Color Doppler evaluation of the lesion demonstrates a small amount of flow within the lesion* ➡, *confirming its solid (not cystic) nature.*

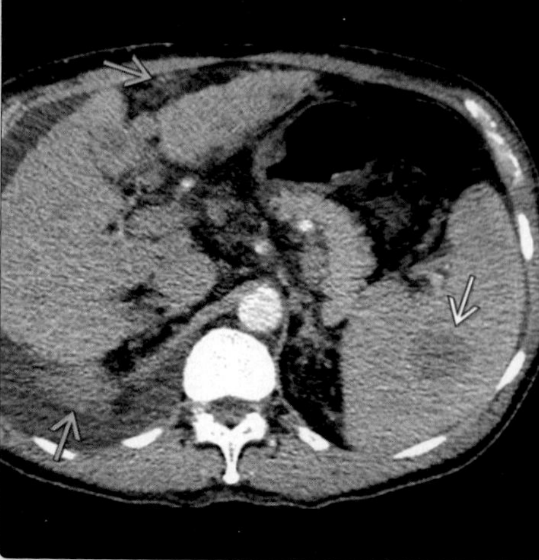

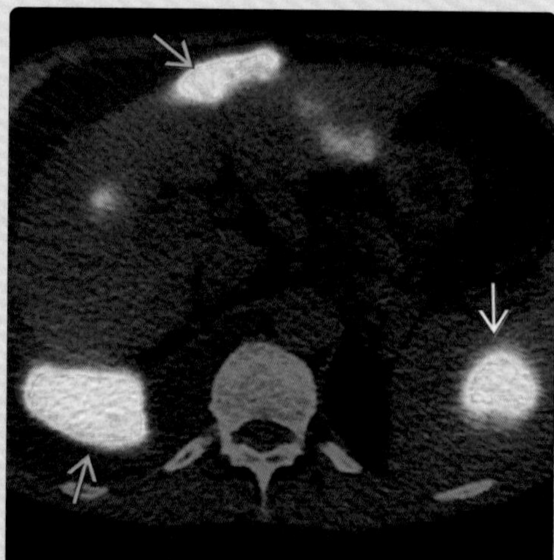

(Left) *Corresponding axial CECT shows the solitary solid hypoattenuating splenic lesion* ➡. *Also note the presence of peritoneal soft tissue implants along the surface of the liver* ➡. **(Right)** *F-18 FDG PET/CT fusion image in the same patient shows intense metabolic activity of the splenic lesion* ➡, *peritoneal implants* ➡, *and sites of hepatic involvement. Histology revealed large B-cell lymphoma. Note that HCC metastasis to the spleen is rare; HCV infection has been linked to B-cell lymphomas.*

KEY FACTS

IMAGING

- Variable sonographic appearance of acute splenic infarction
  - Classic
    - Hypoechoic, peripheral, wedge-shaped, and avascular
  - Nonclassic
    - Rounded or peripheral band morphology
    - Global infarction
    - Isoechoic to hyperechoic
  - **Bright band sign**
    - Parallel, thin specular reflectors perpendicular to US beam within hypoechoic parenchymal lesions
    - Thought to represent preserved fibrous trabeculae within infarcted tissue
- Chronic infarction
  - Atrophic, scarred spleen ± calcification
- Associated findings
  - Splenomegaly, splenic vein occlusion (with large perisplenic varices), splenic artery thrombosis

TOP DIFFERENTIAL DIAGNOSES

- Splenic laceration
- Splenic hematoma
- Splenic mass
- Splenic metastases
- Splenic lymphoma

DIAGNOSTIC CHECKLIST

- Color and power Doppler are critical components of US evaluation of splenic infarct
- Grayscale appearance can be variable depending on morphology, evolution of infarct
- Clinical history is very helpful
  - Multitude of underlying disorders can predispose to splenic infarction

SCANNING TIPS

- Use of slow-flow settings in color or power Doppler helpful to confirm avascular or hypovascular nature of infarct

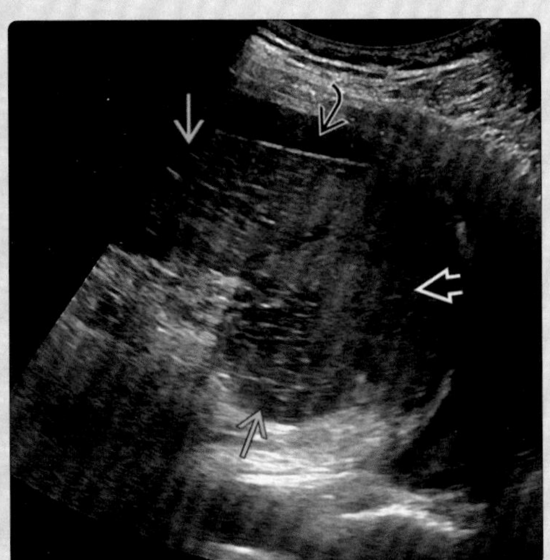

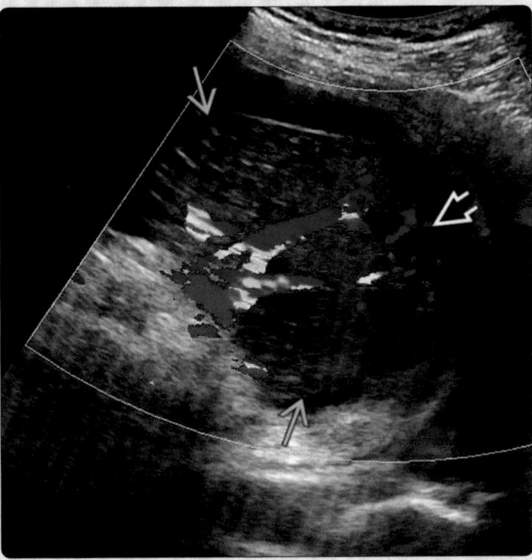

(Left) *Transverse US of the spleen demonstrates inhomogeneity of the splenic echotexture with geographic areas of hypoechogenicity ➞ containing parallel echogenic bands; these regions represent infarct. Compare this to normal parenchyma ➡. Note also the presence of perisplenic fluid ➙.* **(Right)** *Corresponding color Doppler US shows absent vascularity in the infarcted parenchyma ➞ and normal vascularity within the uninvolved parenchyma ➡.*

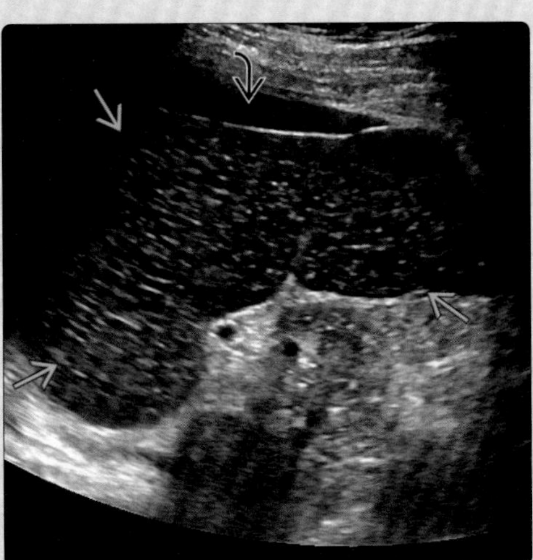

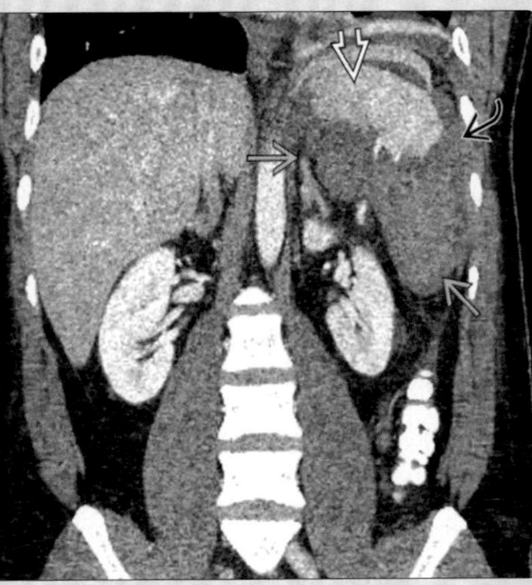

(Left) *Longitudinal splenic US is shown in the same patient. In this plane of view, the extent of the infarct can be appreciated. The infarcted tissue ➞ is hypoechoic with numerous thin, parallel echogenic bands (the bright band sign). Note again the free fluid ➙.* **(Right)** *Corresponding coronal CECT clearly shows areas of nonenhancement ➞ within the inferior 2/3 of the enlarged spleen (splenomegaly). Normal tissue shows enhancement ➡. Fluid ➙ surrounding the spleen indicates rupture.*

PART I
SECTION 5

Urinary Tract

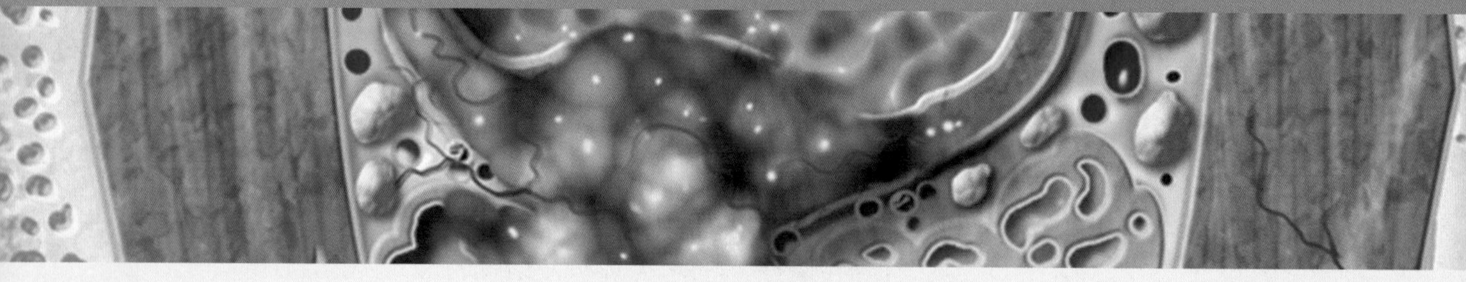

Anatomy and Approach

Normal Variants and Pseudolesions

Calculi and Calcinosis

Cysts and Cystic Disorders

Urinary Tract Infection

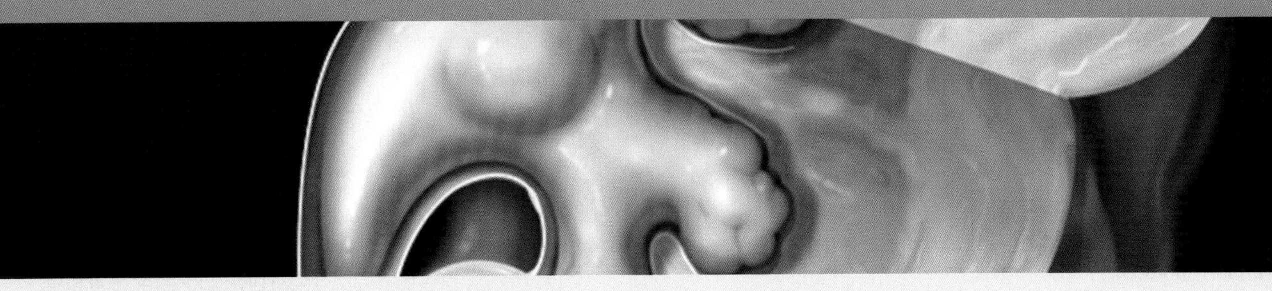

Solid Renal Neoplasms

Vascular Conditions

Bladder

GROSS ANATOMY

Overview

- Kidneys are paired, bean-shaped, retroperitoneal organs
  - Function
    - Removal of excess water, salts, and wastes of protein metabolism from blood
    - Regulation of water and electrolyte balance
    - Secretion of hormones that control blood pressure, bone and blood production

Anatomic Relationships

- Located in retroperitoneum, within perirenal space, surrounded by renal fascia (of Gerota)
- Each adult kidney is ~ 9-14 cm in length, 5 cm in width, 3 cm in thickness
- Both kidneys lie on quadratus lumborum muscles, lateral to psoas muscles, between T12-L3

Internal Structures

- Kidneys are hollow centrally with renal sinus occupied by fat, renal pelvis, calyces, vessels, and nerves
- Renal hilum: Concavity where artery enters and vein and ureter leave renal sinus
- Renal pelvis: Funnel-shaped expansion of upper end of ureter
  - Receives major calyces (infundibula) (2 or 3), each of which receives minor calyces (2-4)
- Renal papilla: Pointed apex of renal pyramid of collecting tubules that excrete urine
  - Each papilla indents a minor calyx
  - 7-10 papilla per kidney
- Renal cortex: Outer part, contains renal corpuscles (glomeruli, vessels), proximal portions of collecting tubules and loop of Henle
- Renal medulla: Inner part, contains renal pyramids, distal parts of collecting tubules, and loops of Henle
- Vessels, nerves, and lymphatics
  - Artery
    - Usually 1 for each kidney
    - Arise from aorta at about L1-L2 vertebral level
  - Vein
    - Usually 1 for each kidney
    - Lies in front of renal artery and renal pelvis
  - Nerves
    - Autonomic from renal and aorticorenal ganglia and plexus
  - Lymphatics
    - To lumbar (aortic and caval) nodes

IMAGING ANATOMY

Overview

- Ultrasound is 1st-line modality for acute or chronic disease, flank pain, and suspected complications of acute pyelonephritis

Internal Contents

- **Renal capsule**
  - Normal kidneys are well-defined due to presence of renal capsule and are less reflective than surrounding fat
- **Renal cortex**
  - Renal cortex has reflectivity that is less than adjacent liver or spleen
  - If renal cortex brighter than normal liver (hyperechoic), high suspicion of renal parenchymal disease
- **Medullary pyramids**
  - Medullary pyramids are less reflective than renal cortex
- **Corticomedullary differentiation**
  - Margin between cortex and pyramids is usually well-defined in normal kidneys
  - Margin between cortex and pyramids may be lost in presence of generalized parenchymal inflammation or edema
- **Renal sinus**
  - Echogenic due to the fat that surrounds blood vessels and collecting systems
  - Outline of renal sinus is variable, smooth to irregular
  - Renal sinus fat may increase in obesity, steroid use, and sinus lipomatosis
  - Renal sinus fat may decrease in cachectic patients and neonates
  - If sinus echoes are indistinct in noncachectic patient, tumor infiltration or edema should be considered
- **Collecting system (renal pelvis and calyces)**
  - Not usually visible in dehydrated patient
    - AP diameter of renal pelvis in adults should be < 10 mm
  - May be seen as physiological "splitting" of renal sinus echoes in patients with a full bladder undergoing diuresis
  - Possible obstruction can be excluded by performing postmicturition images of collecting system and looking for ureteral jets in the bladder with color Doppler
  - Physiological "splitting" of renal sinus echoes is common in pregnancy
    - Causes of dilatation of pelvicalyceal system include mechanical obstruction by enlarging uterus, hormonal factors, increased blood flow, and parenchymal hypertrophy
    - Seen in up to 75% of right kidneys at 20 weeks into pregnancy, less common on left side, thought to be due to cushioning of ureter from gravid uterus by sigmoid colon
    - Changes usually resolve within 48 hours after delivery
- **Renal arteries**
  - Normal caliber 5-8 mm
  - 2/3 of kidneys are supplied by single renal artery arising from aorta
  - 1/3 of kidneys are supplied by 2 or more renal arteries arising from aorta
    - Main renal artery may be duplicated
    - Accessory renal arteries may arise from aorta superior or inferior to main renal artery
    - Accessory renal arteries enter kidney in hilum or at poles
    - Extrahilar accessory renal arteries may arise from ipsilateral renal artery, ipsilateral iliac artery, aorta, or retroperitoneal arteries
  - Spectral Doppler
    - Open systolic window, rapid systolic upstroke occasionally followed by secondary slower rise to peak systole with subsequent diastolic delay but persistent forward flow in diastole

- Continuous diastolic flow is present due to low resistance in renal vascular bed
- Low-resistance flow pattern is also present in intrarenal branches
- Normal peak systolic velocity (PSV) 75-125 cm/s, not more than 180 cm/s
  - > 200 cm/s is abnormal
- Resistive index (RI) is (peak systolic velocity - end diastolic velocity)/peak systolic velocity; normal < 0.7
- Pulsatility index (PI) is (peak systolic velocity - end diastole velocity)/mean velocity, normal < 1.8

- **Renal veins**
  - Normal caliber 4-9 mm
  - Formed from tributaries that coalesce at renal hilum
  - Right renal vein is relatively short and drains directly into IVC
  - Left renal vein receives left adrenal vein from above and left gonadal vein from below
  - Left renal vein crosses midline between aorta and superior mesenteric artery
  - Spectral Doppler
    - Normal PSV 18-33 cm/s
    - Spectral Doppler in right renal vein mirrors pulsatility in IVC
    - Spectral Doppler in left renal vein may show only slight variability of velocities consequent upon cardiac and respiratory activity

Size

- Bipolar length is found by rotating transducer around its vertical axis such that the longest craniocaudal length can be identified
- Normal size between 10-15 cm
- Volume measurements
  - May be more accurate but is time consuming
  - 3D ellipsoidal formula can be used for volume estimation
    - Length x AP diameter x transverse diameter x 0.5
  - Consistency and changes in volume over time more important

ANATOMY IMAGING ISSUES

Imaging Recommendations

- Right kidney
  - Liver used as acoustic window
  - Transducer placed in subcostal or intercostal position
  - Varying degree of respiration is useful
  - Raising patient's right side and scanning laterally/posterolaterally may be useful
- Left kidney
  - More difficult to visualize due to bowel gas from small bowel and splenic flexure
  - Usually easier to search for left kidney using posterolateral approach with left side raised
  - Full right lateral decubitus with pillow under right flank and left arm extended above head may be useful in difficult cases
    - Spleen can be used as acoustic window for imaging upper pole of left kidney
- Posterior approach for both kidneys
  - Useful for interventional procedures such as renal biopsy, nephrostomy
  - Use bolster or pillow under the patient's abdomen to decrease lordosis
  - Image quality may be impaired by thick paraspinal muscles and ribs shadowing
- Renal arteries
  - Origins best seen from midline anterior approach
  - Right renal artery can usually be followed from origin to kidney
  - Left renal artery often requires posterolateral coronal transducer scanning position for visualization
- Renal veins
  - Best seen on transverse scan from anterior approach
  - May also be seen on coronal scan from posterolateral coronal
- Use highest frequency transducer appropriate for patient body habitus: 2-9 MHz curvilinear or 8-12 MHz linear
- Compound and harmonic techniques to decrease artifacts
- Color Doppler for global renal perfusion, presence of flow in lesions, segmental hypoperfusion in acute pyelonephritis/infarcts and bladder jets
- Spectral Doppler: Renal artery stenosis, arteriovenous fistula

Key Concepts

- Accessory renal vessels
  - Accurate diagnosis necessary when planning surgery (e.g., resection, transplantation)
  - Due to limitations of ultrasound, CT arteriography, magnetic resonance angiography, or digital subtraction angiography are more sensitive and accurate
- Normal variants may mimic disease
  - Dromedary hump and hypertrophied column of Bertin may be mistaken for renal tumors
- Congenital anomalies very common
  - Leading cause of renal failure in children
  - Early diagnosis important

EMBRYOLOGY

Embryologic Events

- Congenital structural anomalies include abnormal renal number, position, structure, and vessels
  - Abnormal number: Absence of 1 or both kidneys; supernumerary kidney
  - Abnormal position: Pelvic kidney, crossed-fused renal ectopia, malrotation, ptosis
  - Abnormal structure
    - Duplication: Results from lack of fusion and commonly produces an enlarged kidney with 2 separate hila and pelvicalyceal systems, these may join or continue as 2 ureters
      - Ureters may be completely separate until they join the bladder or join proximal to the bladder
      - "Duplex kidney": Bifid renal pelvis with single ureter
    - Hypertrophied column of Bertin (lobar dysmorphism; fetal lobulation; hilar lip)
    - Pelviureteric junction obstruction
  - Often accompanied by anomalies of other systems

RENAL FASCIA AND PERIRENAL SPACE

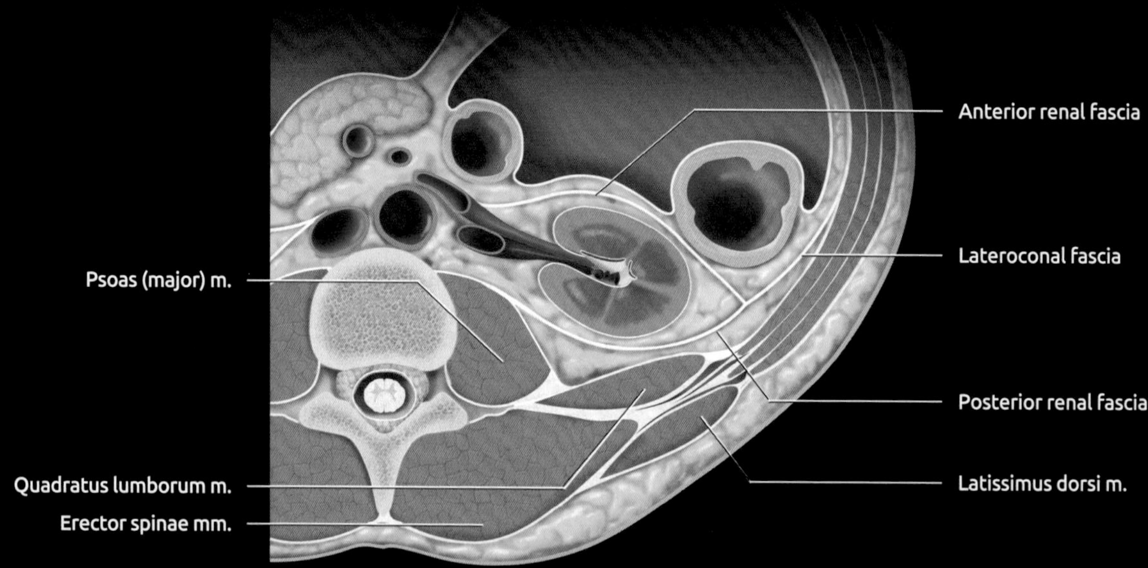

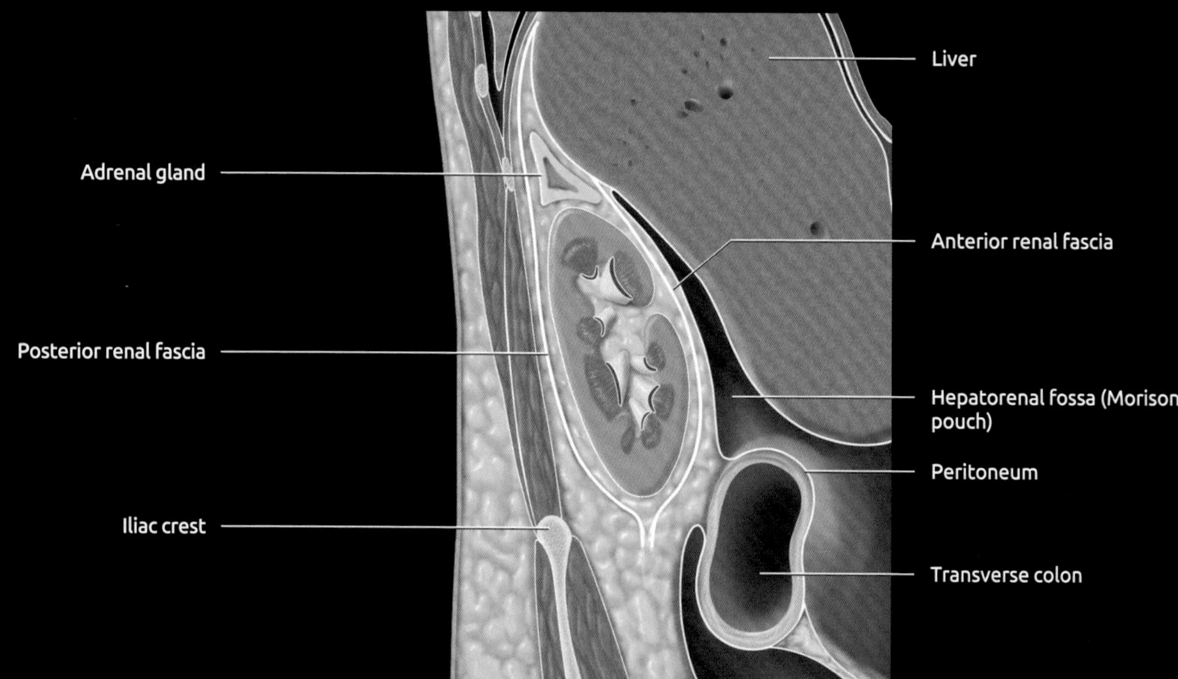

(Top) *The anterior and posterior layers of the renal fascia envelop the kidneys and adrenals along with the perirenal fat. Medial to the kidneys, the course of the renal fascia is variable (and controversial). The posterior layer usually fuses with the psoas or quadratus lumborum fascia. The perirenal spaces do not communicate across the abdominal midline. However, the renal and lateroconal fasciae are laminated structures that may be distended with fluid collections to form interfascial planes that do communicate across the midline and also inferiorly to the extraperitoneal pelvis.* **(Bottom)** *Sagittal section through the right kidney shows the renal fascia enveloping the kidney and adrenal gland. Inferiorly, the anterior and posterior renal fasciae come close together at about the level of the iliac crest. Note the adjacent peritoneal recesses.*

KIDNEYS IN SITU

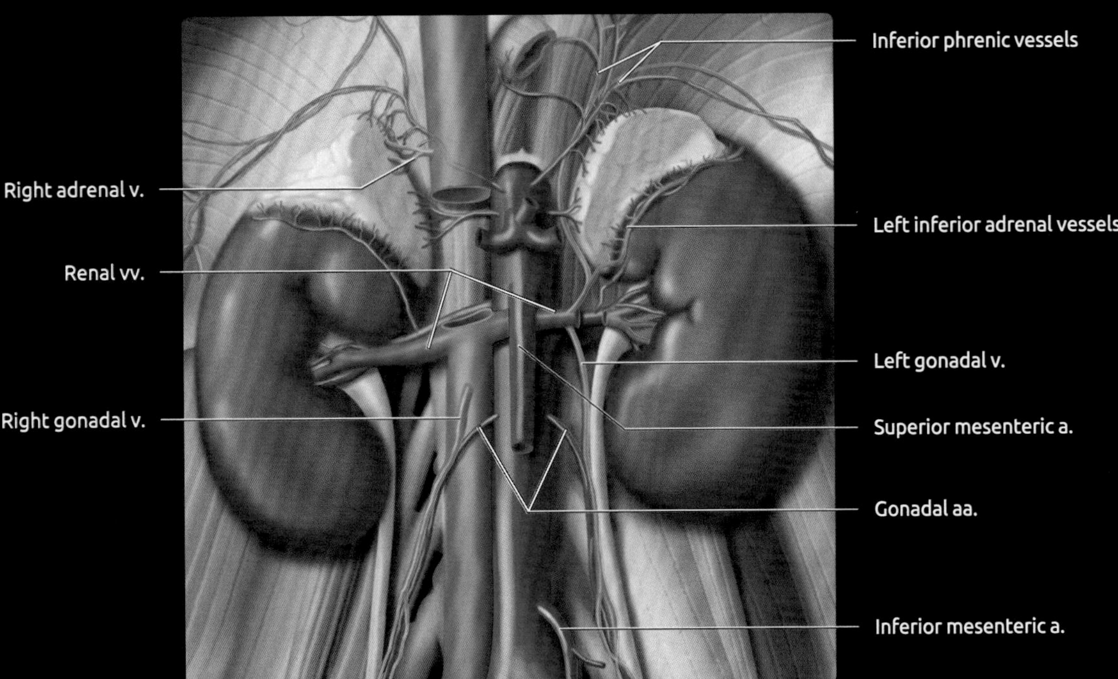

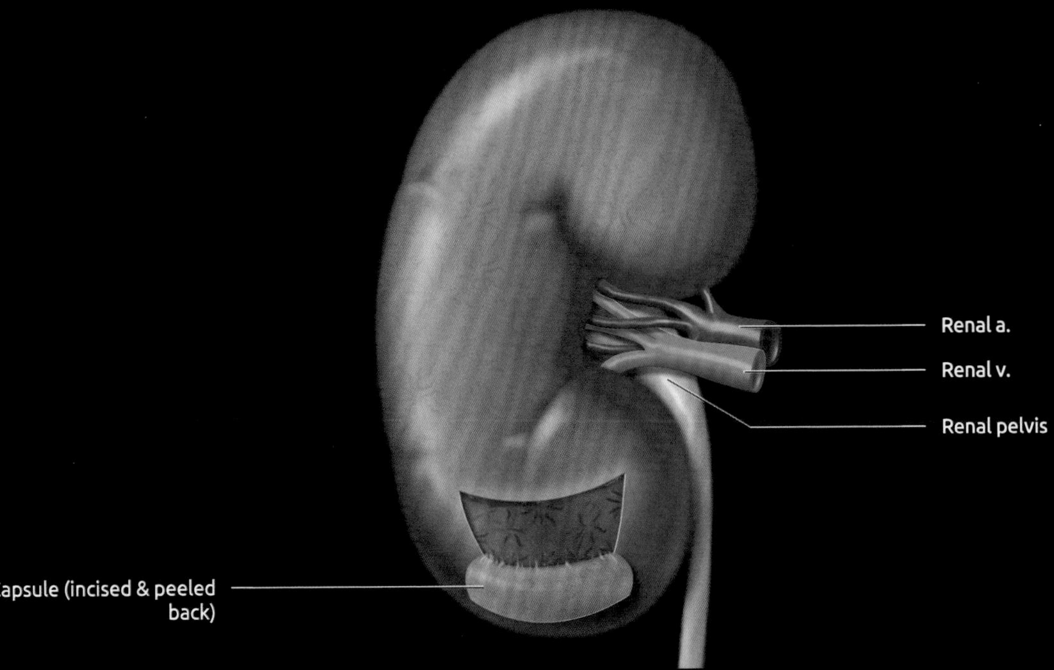

(Top) *The kidneys are retroperitoneal organs that lie lateral to the psoas, on the quadratus lumborum muscles. The oblique course of the psoas muscles results in the lower pole of the kidney lying lateral to the upper pole. The right kidney usually lies 1-2 cm lower than the left, due to inferior displacement by the liver. The adrenal glands lie above and medial to the kidneys, separated by a layer of fat and connective tissue. The peritoneum covers much of the anterior surface of the kidneys. The right kidney abuts the liver and the hepatic flexure of the colon and duodenum, while the left kidney is in close contact with the pancreas (tail), spleen, and splenic flexure.* **(Bottom)** *The fibrous capsule is stripped off with difficulty. Subcapsular hematomas do not spread far along the surface of the kidney, but compress the renal parenchyma, unlike most perirenal collections.*

RENAL ARTERY

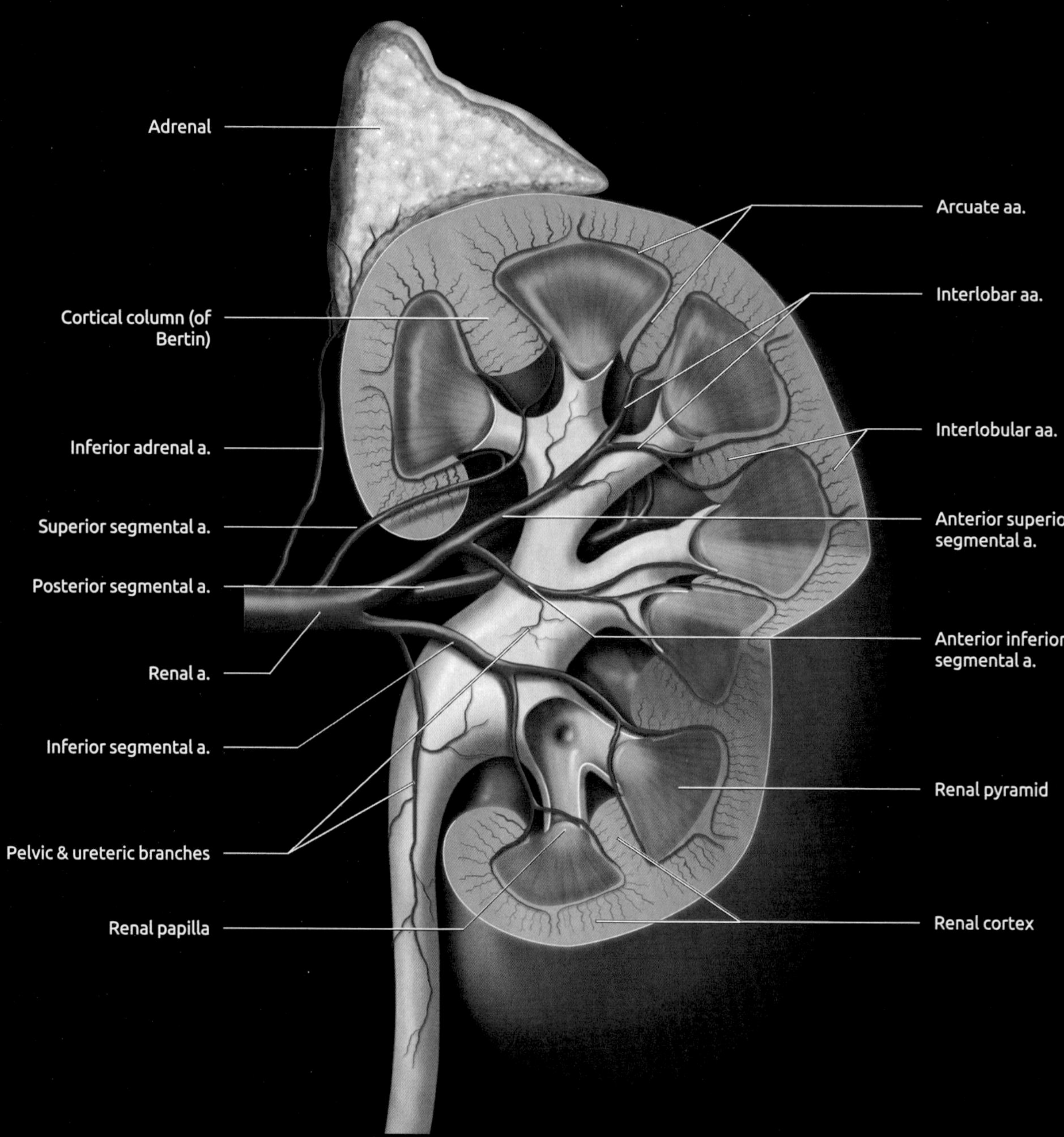

The kidney is usually supplied by a single renal artery, the 1st branch of which is the inferior adrenal artery. It then divides into 5 segmental arteries, only 1 of which (the posterior segmental artery) passes dorsal to the renal pelvis. The segmental arteries divide into the interlobar arteries that lie in the renal sinus fat. Each interlobar artery branches into 4-6 arcuate arteries that follow the convex outer margin of each renal pyramid. The arcuate arteries give rise to the interlobular arteries that lie within the renal cortex, including the cortical columns (of Bertin) that invaginate between the renal pyramids. The interlobular arteries supply the afferent arterioles to the glomeruli. The arterial supply to the kidney is vulnerable, as there are no effective anastomoses between the segmental branches, each of which supplies a wedge-shaped segment of parenchyma.

RIGHT KIDNEY

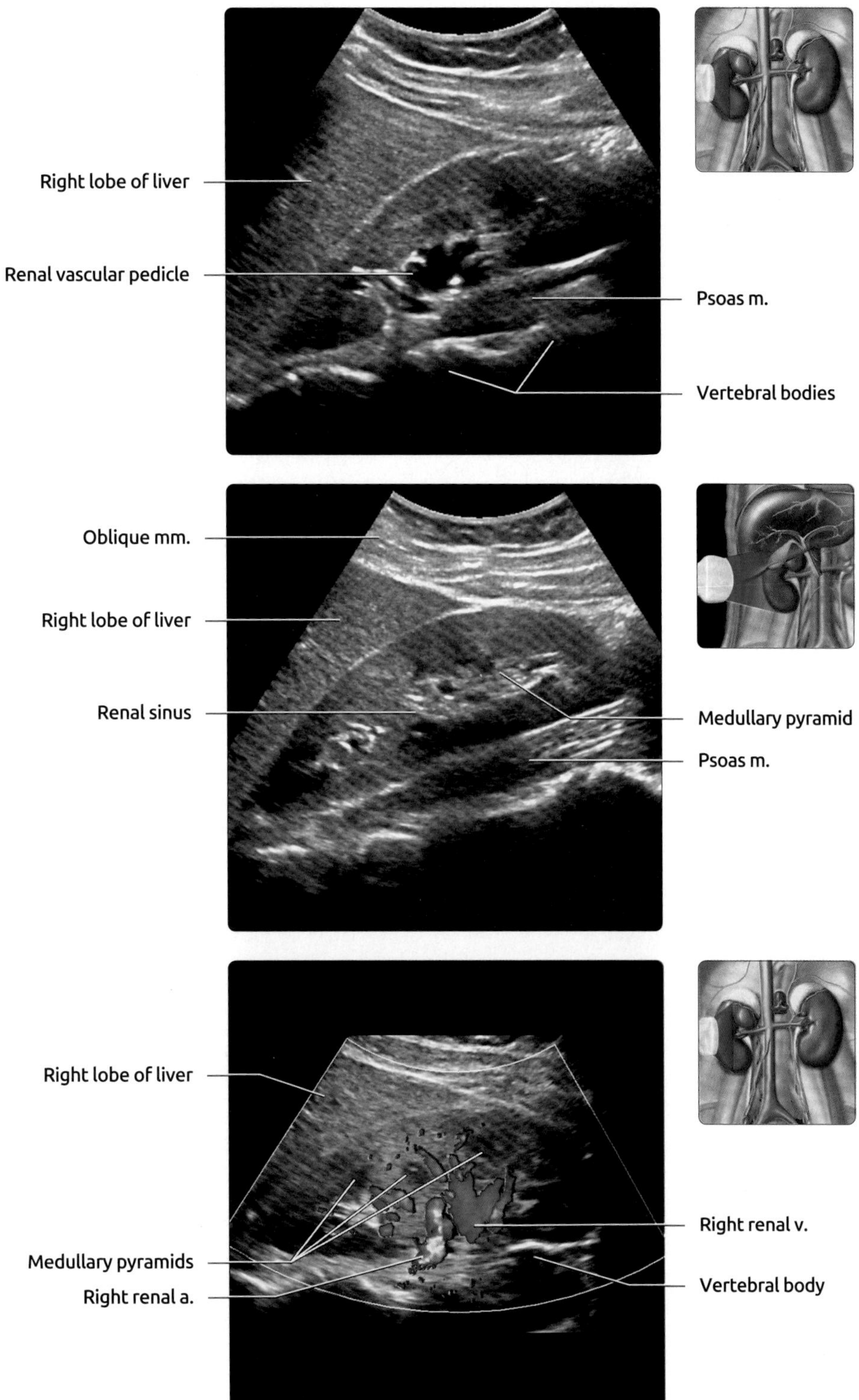

(Top) *Longitudinal oblique grayscale ultrasound shows the right kidney using the liver as an acoustic window with the probe angled medially toward the renal hilum and vascular pedicle.* **(Middle)** *Longitudinal grayscale ultrasound shows the right kidney using the liver as an acoustic window. This approach usually provides excellent visualization of the right kidney and is useful for measuring bipolar renal length.* **(Bottom)** *Longitudinal color Doppler ultrasound of the right kidney obtained through the renal sinus shows the renal artery and vein.*

RIGHT KIDNEY

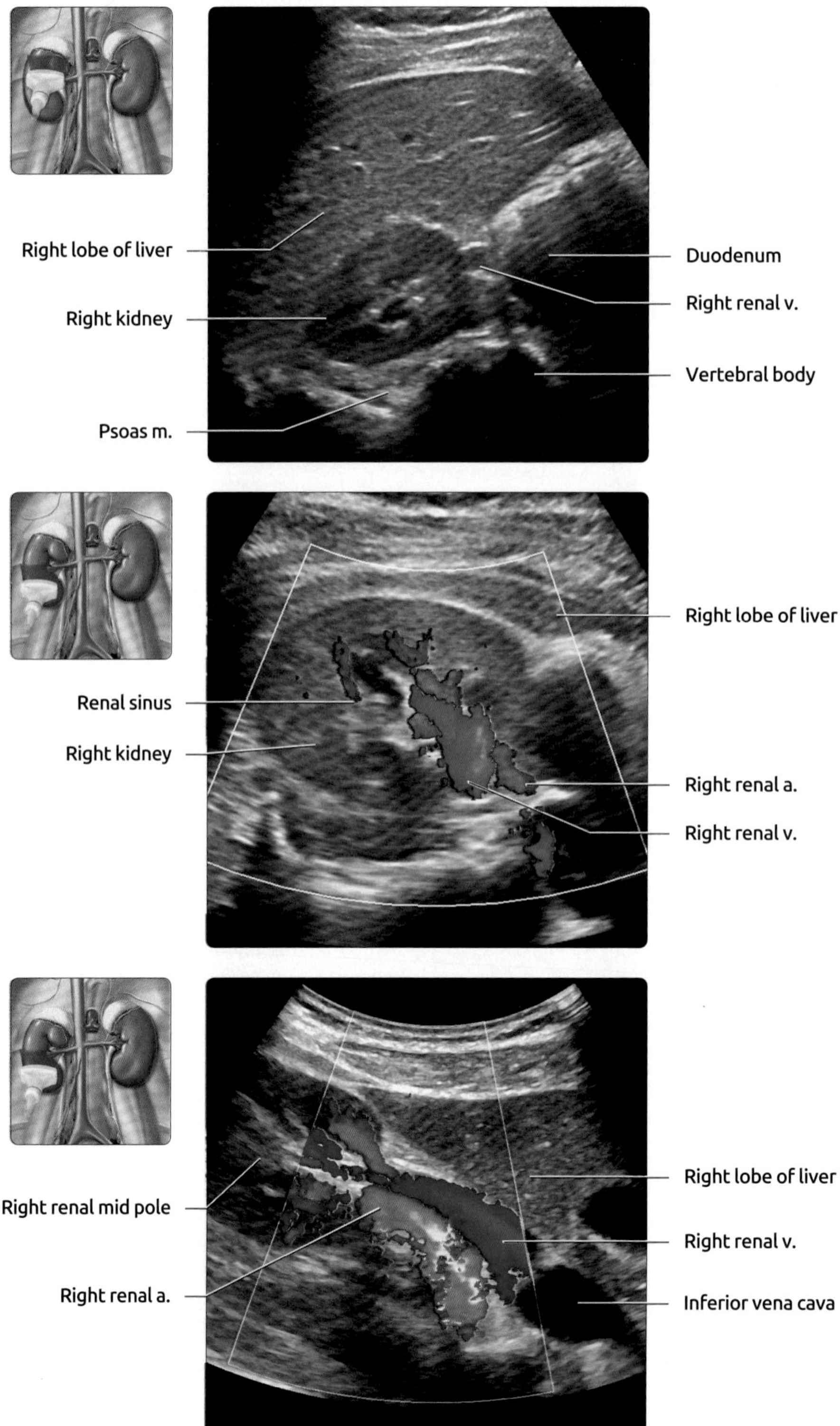

(Top) *Transverse grayscale ultrasound of the upper pole of the right kidney is shown. The liver is used as an acoustic window.* **(Middle)** *Transverse color Doppler ultrasound of the mid right kidney at the hilum shows renal vein and artery.* **(Bottom)** *Transverse color Doppler ultrasound of the right renal vascular pedicle. Note that the renal vein lies anterior to the right renal artery. The renal artery normally measures 5-8 mm in caliber.*

LEFT KIDNEY

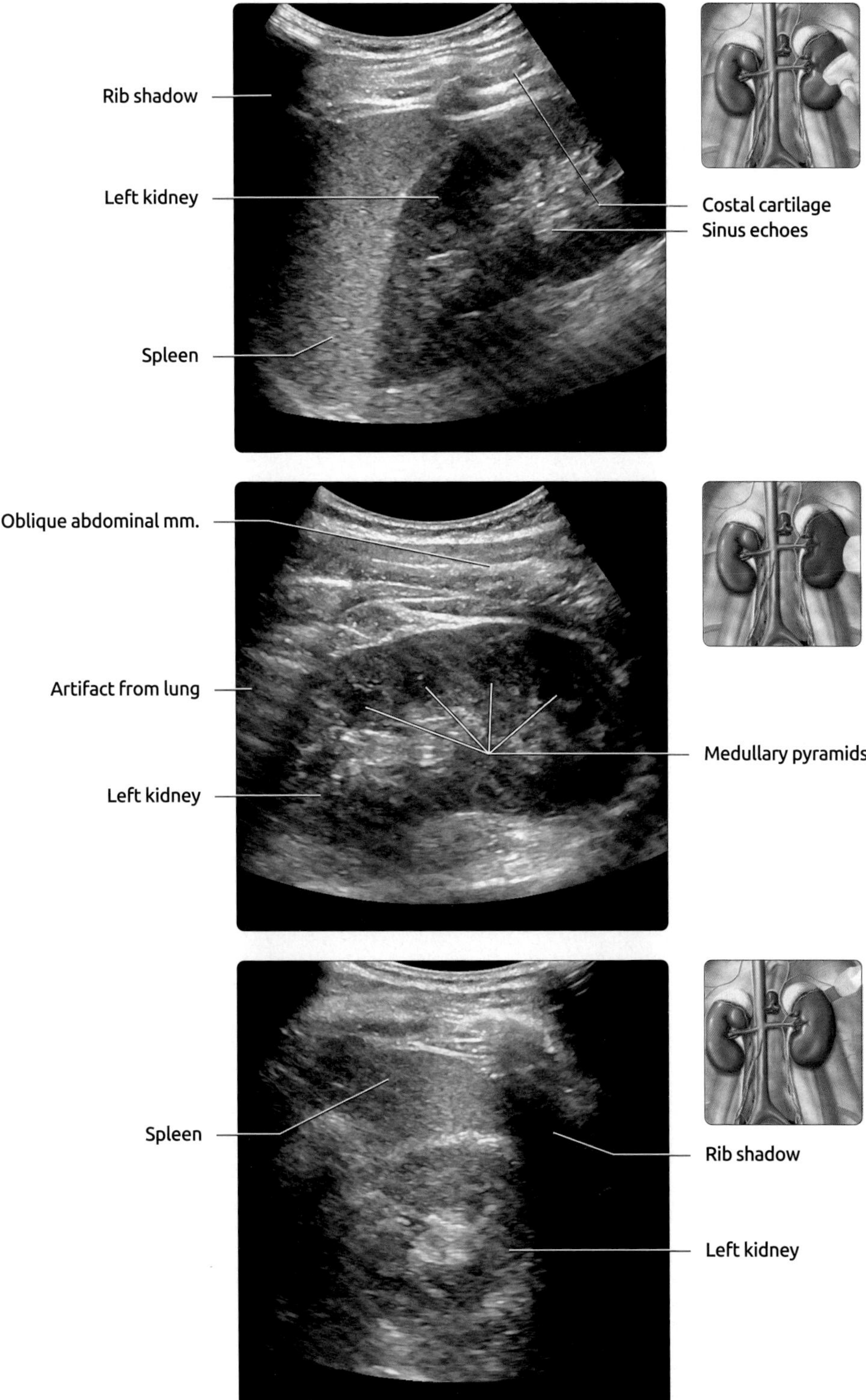

(Top) *Longitudinal grayscale ultrasound shows the upper pole of the left kidney using the anterolateral approach. Note that the spleen may occasionally be used as an acoustic window for the left kidney.* **(Middle)** *Longitudinal grayscale ultrasound shows the left kidney using the anterolateral approach and angling posteriorly. The lung base causes reverberation artifact, which partially obscures the upper pole.* **(Bottom)** *Transverse grayscale ultrasound shows the mid pole of the left kidney using the posterolateral approach.*

LEFT KIDNEY

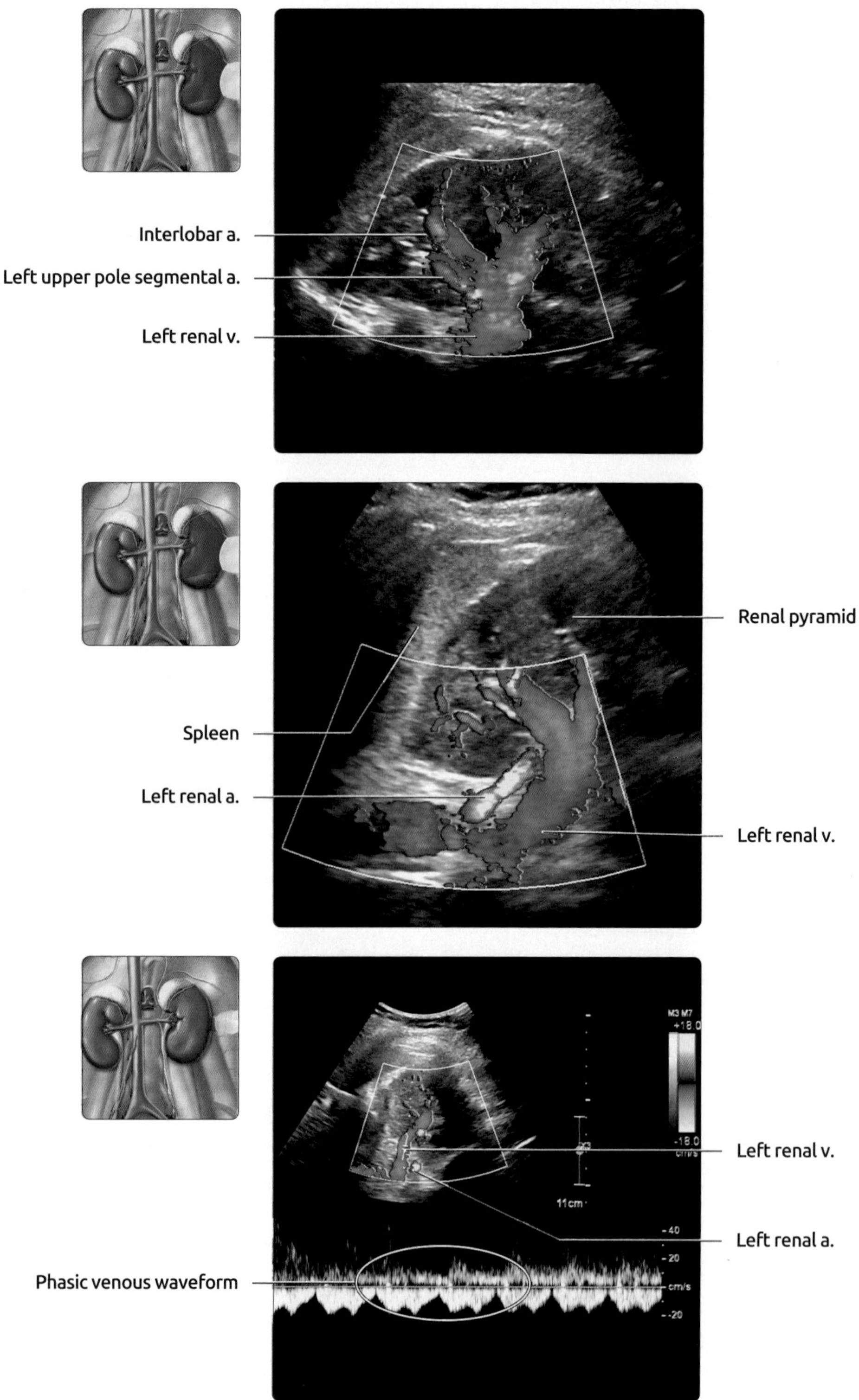

(Top) *Longitudinal color Doppler ultrasound of the left kidney using a posterolateral approach shows the left renal vein. Color Doppler is useful to differentiate a prominent renal vein from hydronephrosis.* **(Middle)** *Color Doppler ultrasound of the left renal artery and vein, using a posterolateral decubitus approach is shown. The origin of the left renal artery was not seen using this approach.* **(Bottom)** *Pulsed Doppler waveform of the left renal vein is shown using a lateral approach. There is variability in venous velocity consequent upon cardiac and respiratory activity. The renal vein normally measures 4-9 mm in caliber with a PSV of 18-33 cm/s.*

RENAL VESSELS

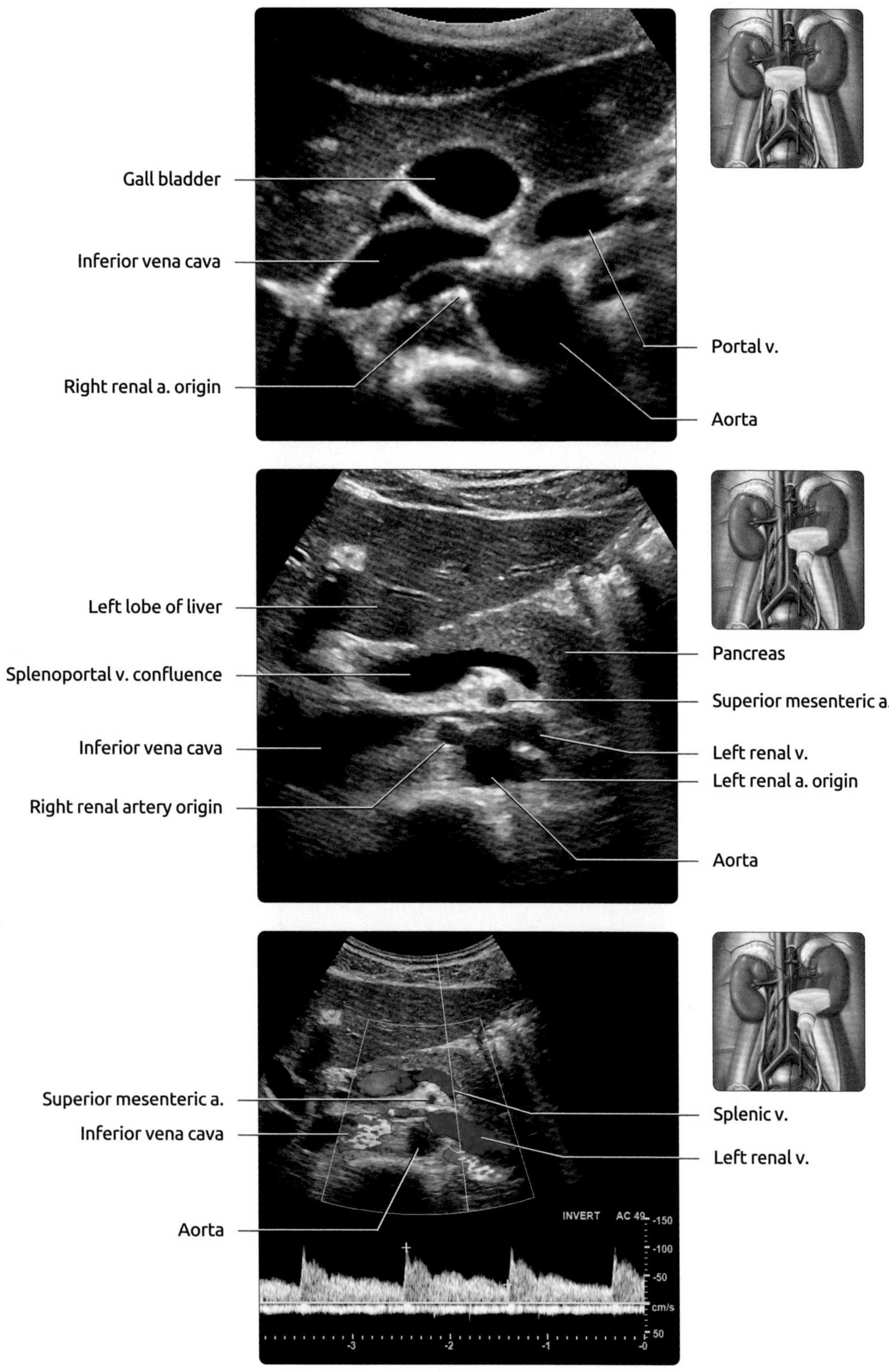

(Top) *Transverse ultrasound of the right renal artery origin is demonstrated using an anterior approach. This approach allows measurement of the PSV in screening for renal artery stenosis. The normal PSV in the artery ranges from 60-140 cm/s with a normal resistive index < 0.7 and pulsatility index < 1.8.* **(Middle)** *Transverse ultrasound of the aorta and renal artery origins using an anterior approach is shown. This approach is ideal for evaluation of renal artery origins but may be limited by bowel gas and body habitus.* **(Bottom)** *Spectral Doppler waveform of the left renal artery is shown using an anterior approach. The normal PSV in the artery ranges from 60-140 cm/s with a normal resistive index < 0.7 and pulsatility index < 1.8. There is variability in venous velocity consequent upon cardiac and respiratory activity. The renal vein normally measures 4-9 mm in caliber with a PSV of 18-33 cm/s.*

RENAL ARTERY VARIANTS

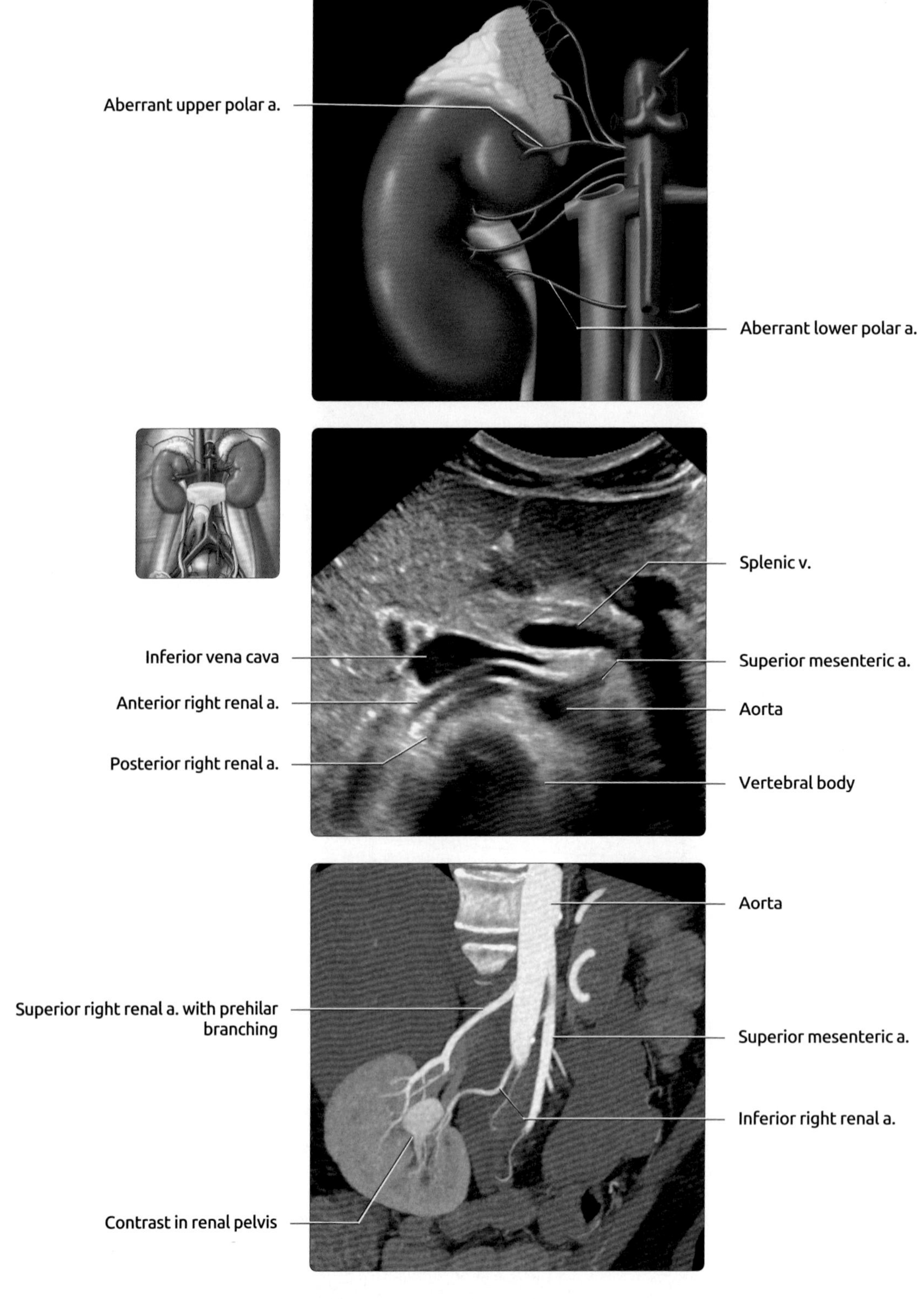

(Top) *Graphic depicts supernumerary renal arteries arising directly from the aorta. Some of these enter the kidney at locations other than the renal hilum, close to the renal poles. These "polar" or "extrahilar" arteries may be ligated or transected unintentionally during renal or other surgeries. These are sometimes referred to as "accessory" renal arteries, but each is an end artery and the sole arterial supply to a substantial portion of the renal parenchyma.* **(Middle)** *Transverse ultrasound shows 2 right renal arteries running posterior to the inferior vena cava.* **(Bottom)** *Combined arterial/excretory phase CT in a potential renal donor shows 2 right renal arteries. Their origins are relatively far apart, which is a factor limiting the sensitivity of ultrasound for multiple renal arteries.*

RENAL VEIN VARIANTS

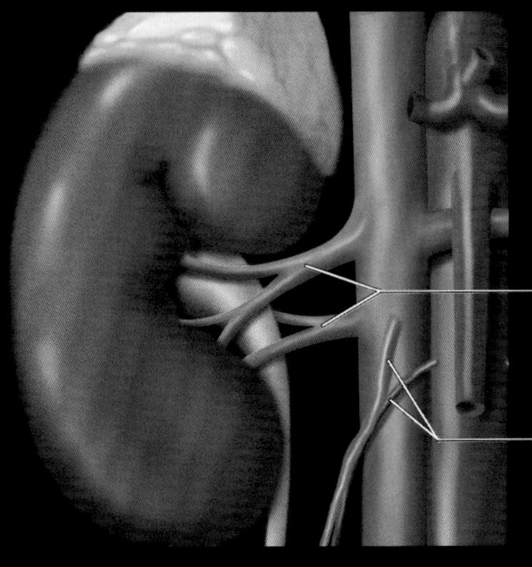

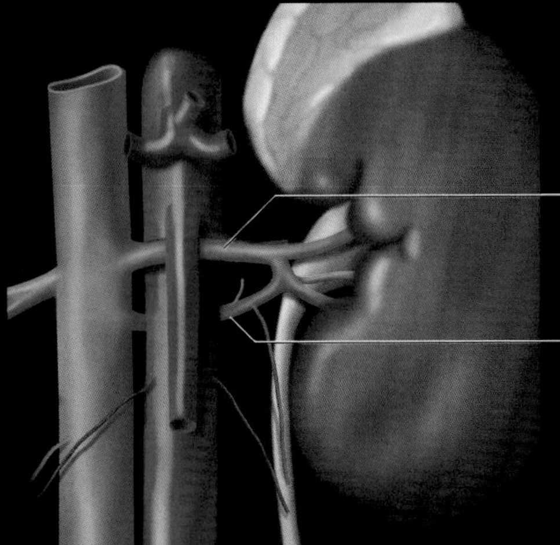

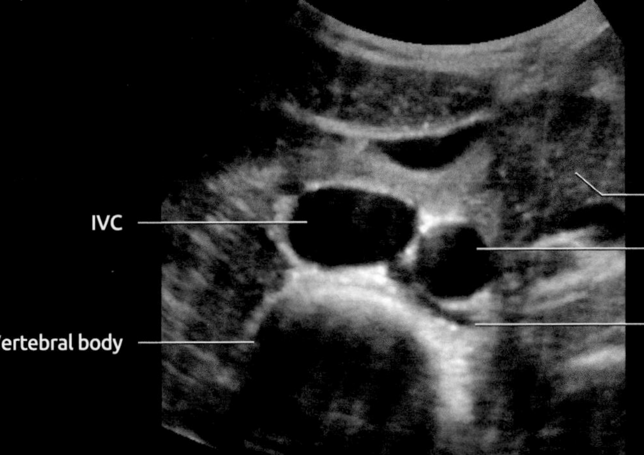

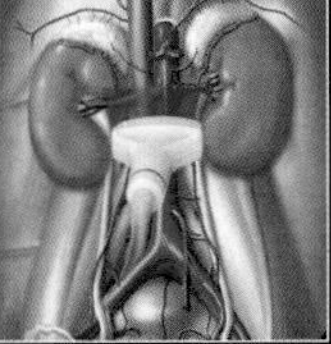

(Top) *Persistence of the collar of veins on the right results in supernumerary right renal veins that encircle the renal pelvis.* **(Middle)** *Anomalies of the renal veins are less common than those of the arteries but are encountered in clinical practice and may have important implications. All anomalies are variations of the embryologic development and persistence of portions of the paired longitudinal channels, the subcardinal and supracardinal veins, which form a ladder-like collar around the aorta. Normally, only the anterior components persist, becoming the renal veins, which course anterior to the aorta. Persistence of the whole collar results in a circumaortic renal vein, which is depicted in this graphic. This anomaly is more common than an isolated retroaortic renal vein.* **(Bottom)** *Transverse oblique ultrasound shows an incidental retroaortic left renal vein.*

GROSS ANATOMY

Ureters

- Muscular tubes (25-30 cm long) that carry urine from kidneys to bladder
- **Course**
  - In abdomen, **retroperitoneal location**
    - Proximal ureters lie in perirenal space
    - Mid ureters lie over psoas muscles slightly medial to tips of L2-L5 transverse process
  - In pelvis, lie anterior to sacroiliac joints crossing common iliac artery bifurcation near pelvic brim
    - **Lie anterior to internal iliac vessels** and course along pelvic sidewall
    - At level of ischial spines, ureters curve anteromedially to enter bladder at level of seminal vesicles (men) or cervix (women)
  - **Ureterovesical junction (UVJ)**: Ureters pass obliquely through muscular wall of bladder for ~ 2 cm
    - Creates valve effect with bladder distension, preventing vesicoureteral reflux (VUR)
- **3 points of physiological narrowing**
  - Ureteropelvic junction
  - Pelvic brim (crossing over common iliac artery)
  - UVJ
- **Vessels, nerves, and lymphatics**
  - Arterial branches are numerous and variable, arising from aorta and renal, gonadal, internal iliac, vesicle, and rectal arteries
  - Venous branches and lymphatics follow arteries with similar names
  - Innervation
    - Autonomic from adjacent sympathetic and parasympathetic plexuses
      - Responsible for ureteral peristalsis
    - Also carry pain (stretch) receptors
      - Stone in abdominal ureter perceived as back and flank pain
      - Stone in pelvic ureter may project to scrotum or labia
  - Lymphatics to external and internal iliac nodes (pelvic ureter), aortocaval nodes (abdomen)

Bladder

- Hollow, distensible viscus with strong, muscular wall and normal adult capacity of 300-600 mL of urine
- Lies in **extraperitoneal** (retroperitoneal) pelvis
- **Peritoneum covers dome** of bladder
  - Reflections of peritoneum form deep recesses in pelvic peritoneal cavity
  - **Rectovesical pouch** (between rectum and bladder) is most dependent recess in men (and in women following hysterectomy)
  - **Vesicouterine pouch** (between bladder and uterus) and **rectouterine pouch of Douglas** (between rectum and uterus)
    - Rectouterine pouch most dependent in women
- Bladder is surrounded by extraperitoneal fat and loose connective tissue
  - **Perivesical space** (contains bladder and urachus)
  - **Prevesical or retropubic space (of Retzius)** between bladder and symphysis pubis
    - Communicates superiorly with infrarenal retroperitoneal compartment
    - Communicates posteriorly with presacral space
  - Spaces can expand to contain large amounts of fluid (as in extraperitoneal rupture of bladder and hemorrhage from pelvic fractures)
- Bladder wall composed mostly of **detrusor muscle**
  - **Trigone** of bladder: Triangular structure at base of bladder with apices marked by 2 ureteral orifices and internal urethral orifice
- **Vessels, nerves, and lymphatics**
  - Arteries from internal iliac
    - Superior vesicle arteries and other branches of internal iliac arteries in both sexes
  - Venous drainage
    - Men: Vesicle and prostatic venous plexuses → internal iliac and internal vertebral veins
    - Women: Vesicle and uterovaginal plexuses → internal iliac vein
  - Autonomic innervation
    - Parasympathetic from pelvic splanchnic and inferior hypogastric nerves (causes contraction of detrusor muscle and relaxation of internal urethral sphincter to permit emptying of bladder)
    - Sensory fibers follow parasympathetic nerves

IMAGING ANATOMY

Overview

- Normal ureters are small in caliber (2-8 mm) and are difficult to appreciate on ultrasound
- Fluid-distended urinary bladder is anechoic with posterior acoustic enhancement
- Urinary bladder changes in shape and position depending on intraluminal volume of urine
  - In its nondistended state, urinary bladder is retropubic in location, lying anterior to uterus in females and rectum in males
  - In markedly distended state, urinary bladder may occupy abdominopelvic area
  - Urinary bladder wall changes in thickness depending on state of distension of urinary bladder and is normally 3-5 mm in thickness

ANATOMY IMAGING ISSUES

Imaging Recommendations

- Transducer: Curvilinear 2-5 MHz
- **Ureters**
  - Ureters are normally not seen on ultrasound unless they are dilated; when dilated, overlying bowel gas may still limit ureteral evaluation in transabdominal approach
    - Proximal dilated ureters may be well seen using kidney as window in coronal oblique plane
    - Middle portion of dilated ureter may be identified in pediatric patients or thin adults using transabdominal approach
    - Dilated terminal ureter/UVJ are seen best along posterolateral aspect of urinary bladder on transverse view

- Can also be evaluated by endovaginal sonography in women
  - Ureteral caliber may slightly increase as result of overfilled urinary bladder
    - Distended bladder may cause ureteral and pelvicalyceal dilation, and rescanning post void is beneficial to exclude obstruction
  - Color Doppler
    - Assess ureteral jets; presence of jets helps exclude complete ureteral obstruction
    - Look for **twinkling artifact** from obstructing stone
- **Bladder**
  - Recommend fluid intake prior to examination to ensure optimal distension of urinary bladder
    - In fully distended state, urinary bladder is easily visualized using transabdominal approach
  - Examine patient in supine position with transabdominal suprapubic approach
    - Perform scanning in sagittal and transverse planes
    - Patient may be placed in decubitus position to determine mobility and differentiated intravesical masses from debris or stones
    - With poor distention, caudal transducer angulation is needed to visualize urinary bladder in its retropubic location
  - Nature of cystic structure in pelvis may be ascertained by asking patient to void or by inserting Foley catheter
  - Transvaginal ultrasound may be used in women for evaluation of suspect bladder neck lesions, UVJ stone, or ureterocele
  - Advantages of ultrasound
    - Radiation-free, real-time assessment with high spatial resolution of bladder and bladder wall
    - Real-time assessment of intraluminal masses in bladder for mobility and vascularity
    - Real-time imaging guidance for bladder intervention, e.g., placement of percutaneous suprapubic catheters
    - Real-time assessment of ureteral jets using color Doppler imaging; particularly useful in pregnant patients with dilated collecting system

Imaging Pitfalls

- **Reverberation artifacts** are commonly encountered behind anterior wall of urinary bladder
  - Appear as regularly spaced lines at increasing depth as result of repeated reflection of ultrasound signals between highly reflective interfaces close to transducer
  - May be reduced or avoided by changing scanning angle or by moving transducer or using spacer
- Underdistended bladder may give false impression of wall thickening and limits intraluminal assessment
  - Have patient drink water and rescan with better distention
- Large midline ovarian or pelvic cystic mass may simulate bladder on transabdominal ultrasound
  - Attention to normal bladder shape, rescanning after voiding to confirm empty bladder, or transvaginal imaging is helpful to differentiate

CLINICAL IMPLICATIONS

Clinical Importance

- Ureters are at high risk of inadvertent injury during abdominal or gynecological surgery due to close proximity to uterine (in uterosacral ligament) and gonadal arteries (at pelvic brim)
- **Ectopic ureter**
  - Usually (80%) associated with complete ureteral duplication; more common in females
  - In complete duplication, upper moiety inserts ectopically inferiorly and distally to lower moiety (**Weigert-Meyer rule**) and can be associated with ureterocele
    - Ureterocele may cause obstruction of upper pole moiety; also distorts UVJ of normally inserting lower pole moiety causing predisposition to VUR
  - Ectopic ureteral insertion in females can occur in urethra or vagina, leading to urinary incontinence
- **Ureterocele**
  - Cystic dilation of intramural portion of ureter bulging into bladder
    - Orthotopic: Normal insertion of single ureter
    - Ectopic: Inserts below trigone, mostly in duplicated system
- **Ureteral duplication**
  - Bifid ureter drains duplex kidney, but ureters unite before entering bladder
- **Urachal anomalies**
  - Patent fetal urachus forms conduit between umbilicus and bladder
  - Urachus is normally obliterated to form median umbilical ligament
  - May persist as cyst, diverticulum, or, rarely, fistula
  - Risk of infection or carcinoma (adenocarcinoma)
- **Bladder diverticula** are common
  - Congenital: Hutch diverticulum (near UVJ)
  - Acquired (usually due to chronic bladder outlet obstruction), associated with trabeculated bladder wall
  - Can lead to infection, stones, tumor
- **Trauma**
  - **Extraperitoneal bladder rupture**
    - Urine and blood distend prevesical space (Retzius)
    - Urine often tracks posteriorly into presacral space, superiorly into retroperitoneal abdomen
    - High association with pelvic fractures
  - **Intraperitoneal bladder rupture**
    - Urine flows up paracolic gutters into peritoneal recesses and surrounds bowel
    - Bladder ruptures along dome, which is in contact with intraperitoneal space
    - Usually caused by blunt trauma to overdistended bladder

URETERS AND URINARY BLADDER IN SITU

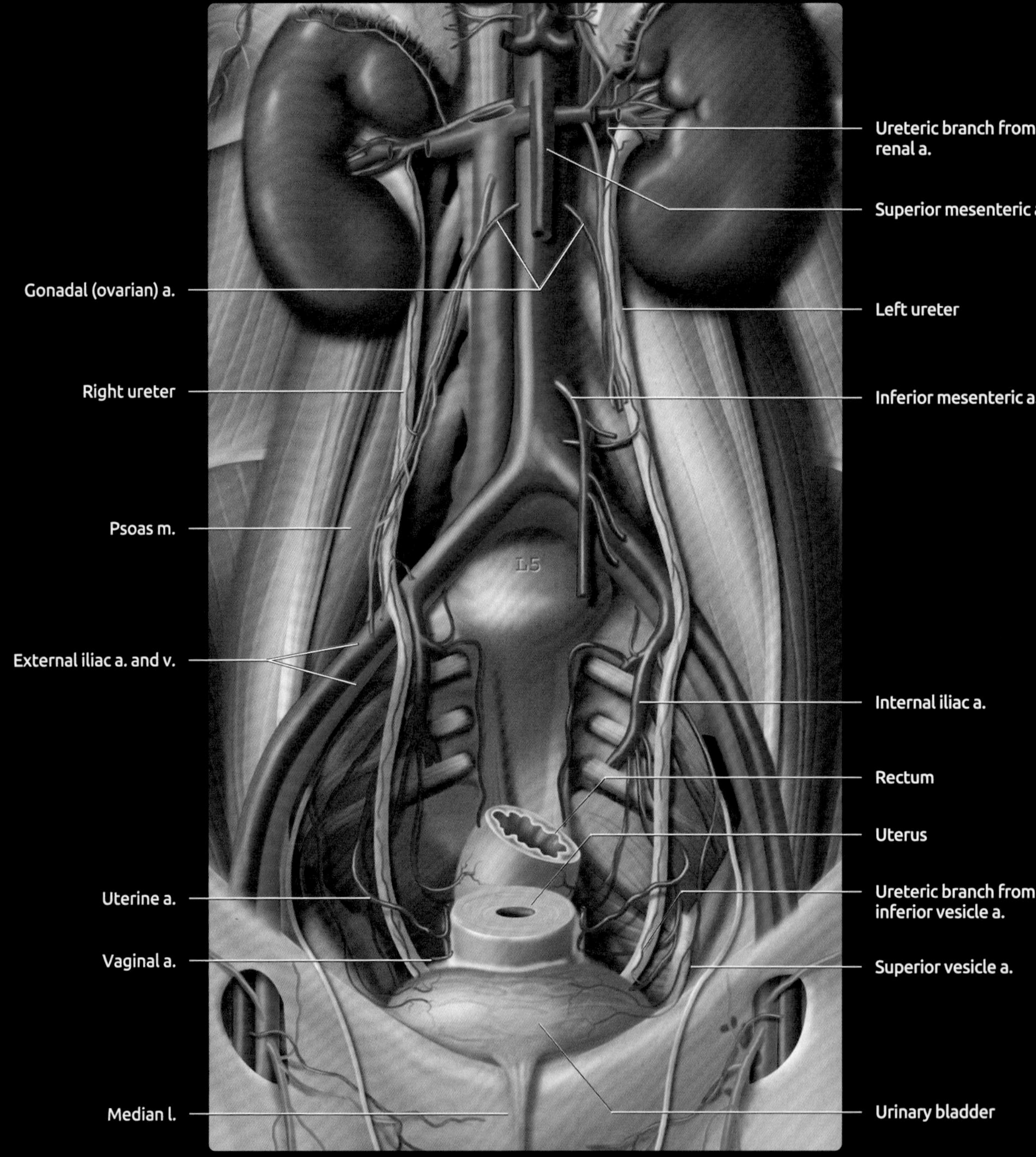

The ureters receive numerous and highly variable arterial branches from the aorta and the renal, gonadal, and internal iliac arteries. These vessels are short and can be easily ruptured by retraction of the ureter during surgical procedures. The arterial supply to the bladder is also quite variable. Both genders receive supply from the superior vesicle arteries and from various branches of the internal iliac arteries. Branches to the prostate and seminal vesicles (men) also send branches to the inferior bladder wall. In women, branches to the vagina send arteries to the base of the bladder. Note how the ureters deviate anteriorly as they cross the external (or common) iliac vessels and pelvic brim. This may constitute a point of relative narrowing where the passage of ureteral calculi (stones) may be impeded. In the abdomen, the ureters course along the psoas muscles.

URINARY BLADDER IN SITU, MALE

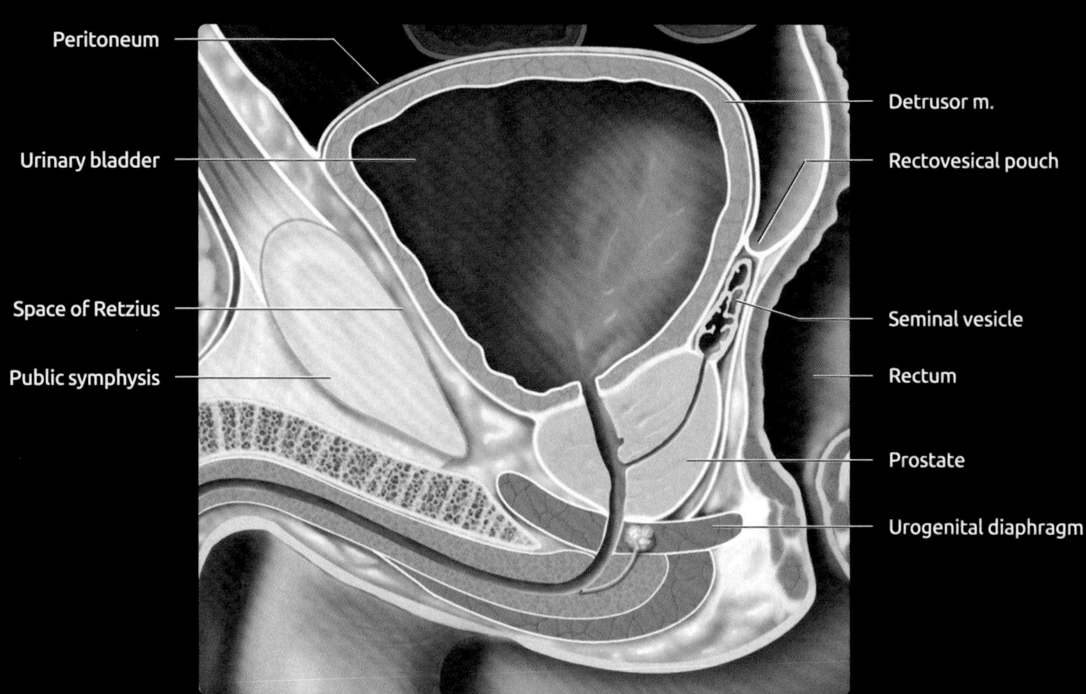

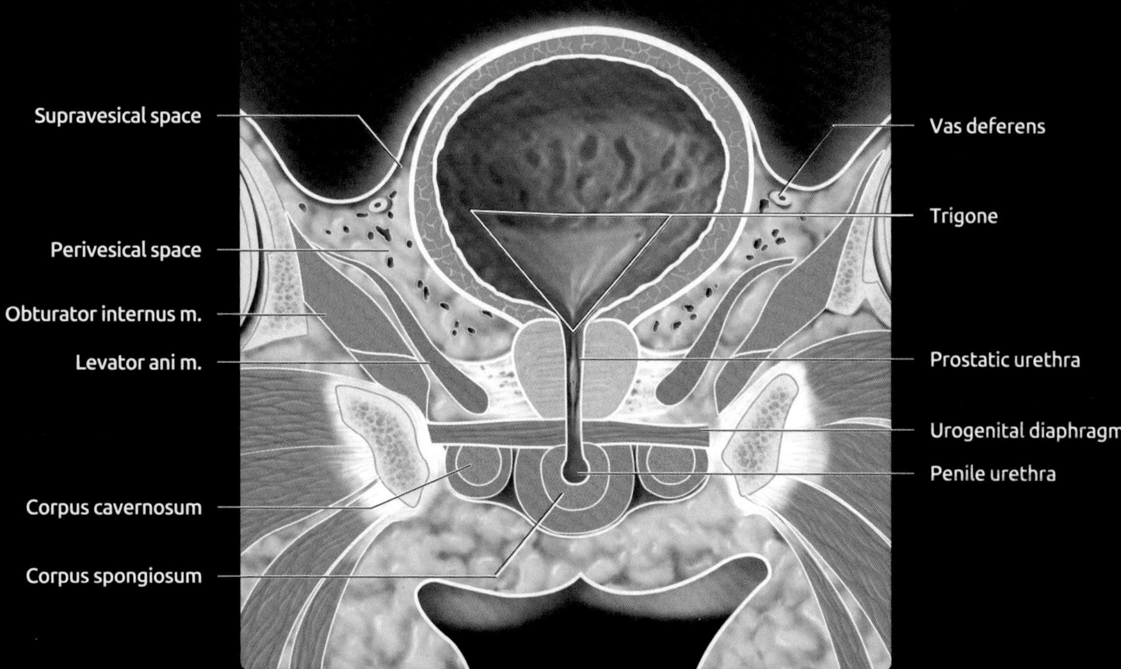

(Top) *Graphic of a sagittal section of the male bladder shows that it rests on the prostate, which separates it from the muscular pelvic floor. The bladder wall is muscular, strong, and very distensible. In males, the urinary bladder is directly anterior to the rectum, and the rectovesical pouch is the deepest point in the pelvis.* **(Bottom)** *A coronal section of the male bladder shows the anatomic relationships of the bladder with its surrounding structures. The trigone is a triangle formed by the ureteral orifices and urethral outlet. The ureters enter the bladder through an oblique anteromedial course that helps to prevent urinary reflux into the ureters.*

URINARY BLADDER IN SITU, FEMALE

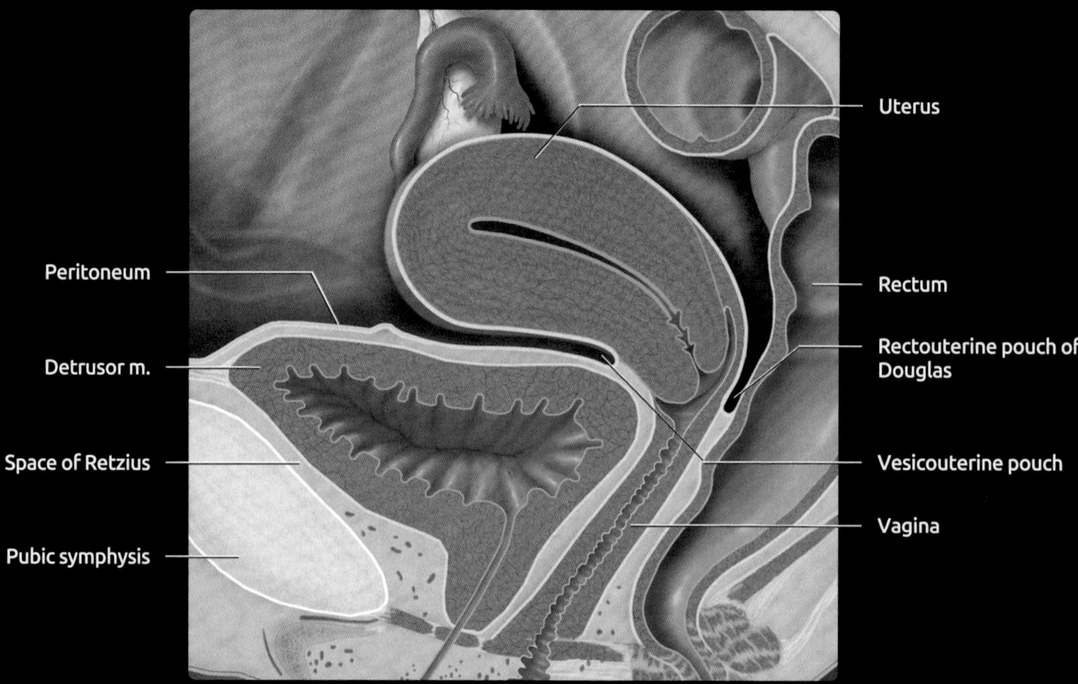

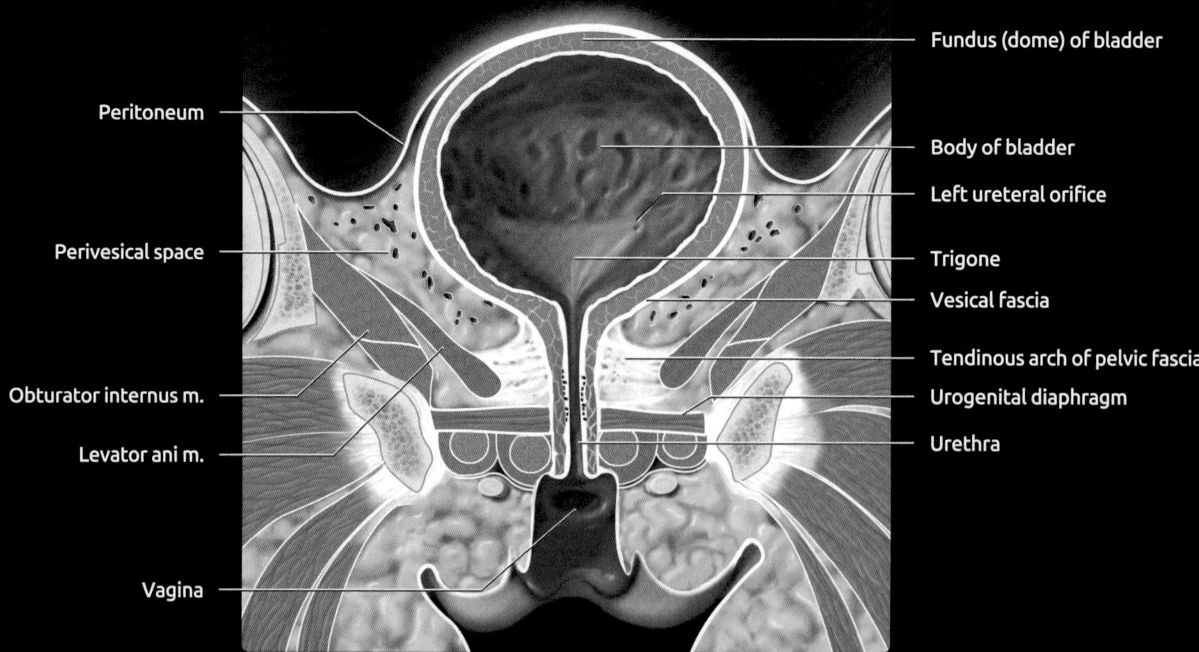

(Top) *Sagittal graphic shows a nondistended bladder in a female patient. When decompressed, the bladder wall can appear quite thick and can erroneously be interpreted as abnormal. The dome of the bladder is covered with peritoneum. The bladder is surrounded by a layer of loose fat and connective tissue (the prevesical space of Retzius and perivesical spaces) that communicate superiorly with the retroperitoneum. Note the vagina/uterus in the female pelvis, which intervenes between the urinary bladder and rectum.* **(Bottom)** *A frontal (coronal) section of the female bladder shows that it rests almost directly on the muscular floor of the pelvis. The dome of the bladder is covered with peritoneum. The trigone is the distinct triangular base of the bladder whose apices are formed by the ureteral and urethral orifices.*

URETERS

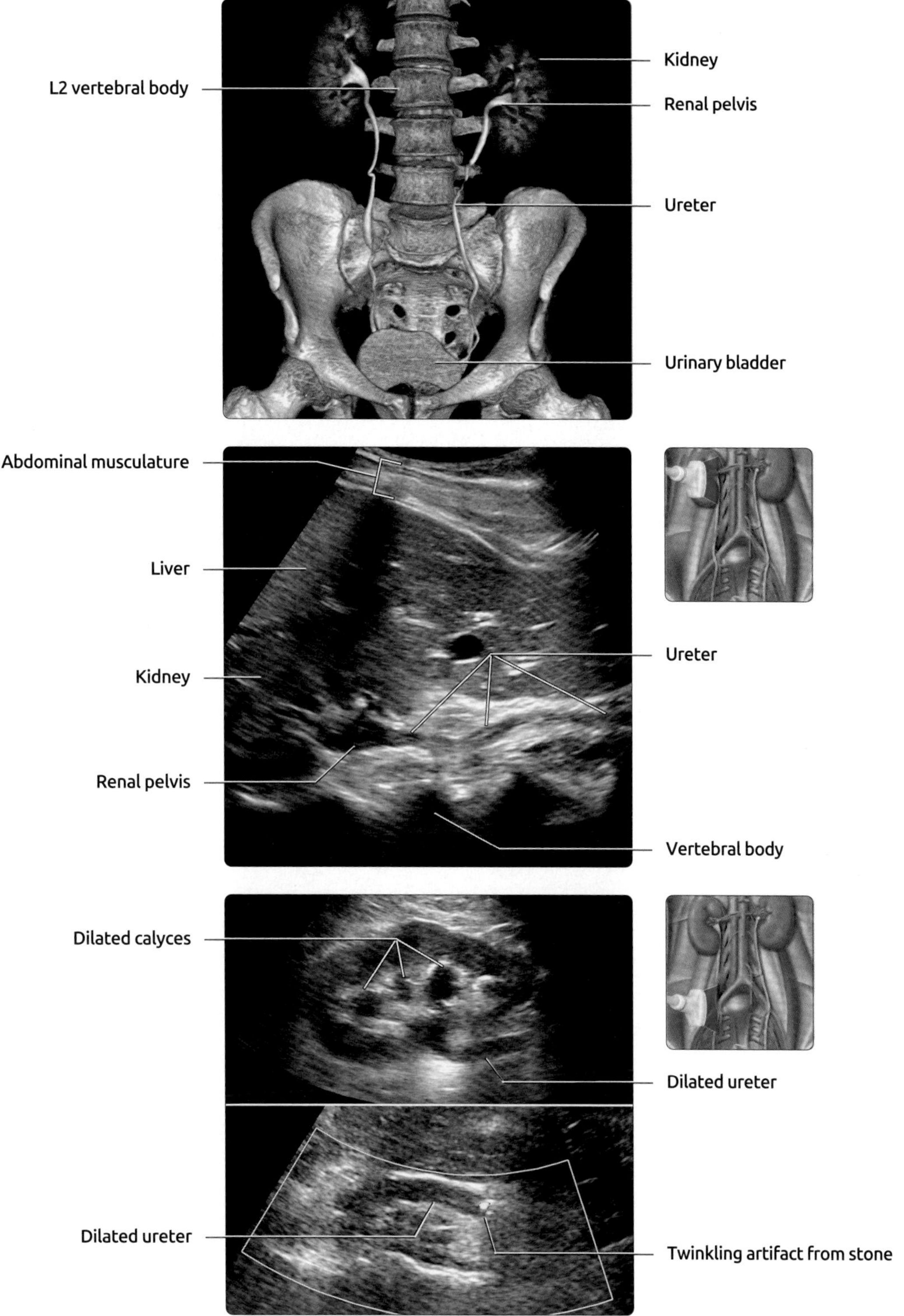

(Top) *Volume-rendered 3D reformatted image from a CT urogram shows the normal course of the ureters overlying the L3-L5 transverse process.* **(Middle)** *The ureter is identified in this very thin teenage girl by scanning through the right flank and using the liver as an acoustic window. Even in thin patients, the ureter is usually not seen secondary to overlying bowel gas.* **(Bottom)** *This composite image shows an obstructing midureteral stone just above the pelvic rim. The pelvic rim, along with the ureteropelvic and ureterovesical junctions, are areas of narrowing and are the most likely locations for a stone to lodge. Even if you can't seen the entire ureter, specifically target these areas on your scan when evaluating for an obstructing stone.*

URETERS

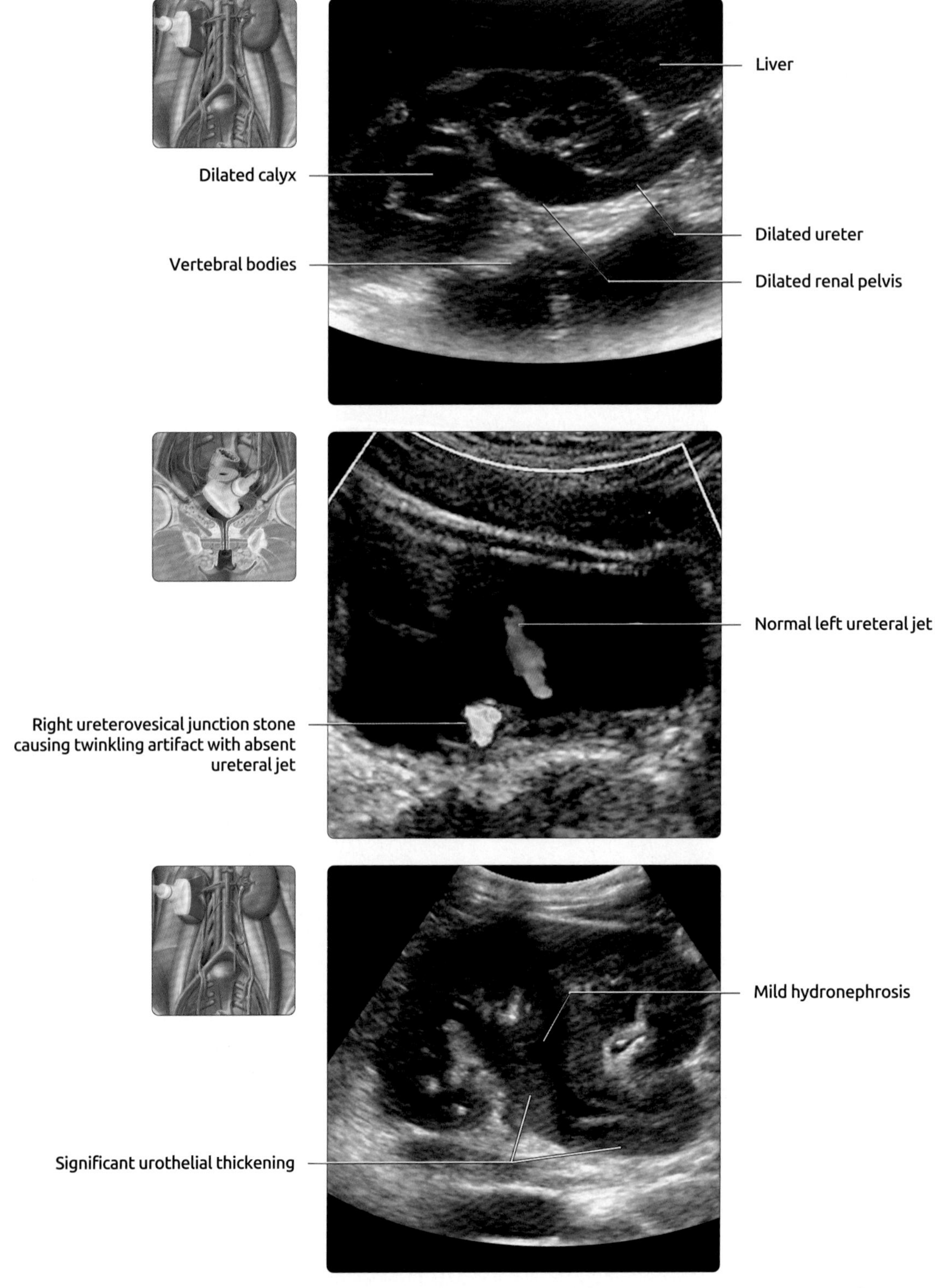

(Top) *Longitudinal transabdominal grayscale ultrasound of the right kidney shows a dilated pelvicalyceal system and proximal ureter. The ureter is normally not visible on ultrasound unless it is dilated, as seen here.* **(Middle)** *Oblique color Doppler ultrasound of the suprapubic region in the same patient shows a calculus at the right ureterovesical junction causing twinkling artifact with an absent ureteral jet. A normal left ureteric jet is seen.* **(Bottom)** *Longitudinal transabdominal ultrasound of the left kidney shows significant urothelial thickening of the pelvicalyceal system and proximal ureter in this patient with known extramedullary hematopoiesis.*

BLADDER

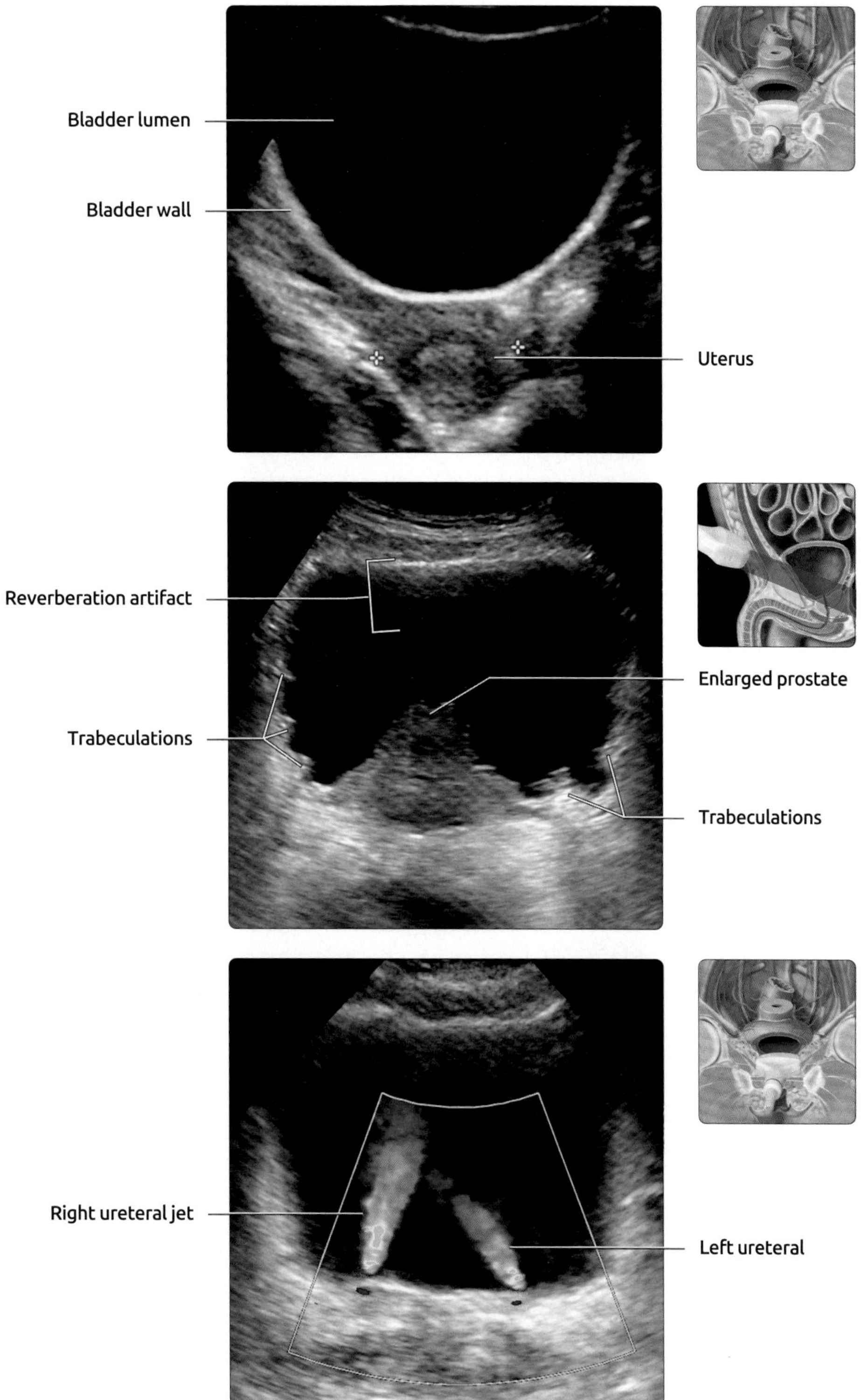

(Top) *Transverse transabdominal grayscale ultrasound shows a distended bladder with a smooth wall. The transducer must be angled caudally to image the urinary bladder, especially when it is not well distended and assumes a retropubic location.* **(Middle)** *Transverse ultrasound of the bladder shows wall thickening and trabeculations in this patient with benign prostatic hypertrophy and chronic bladder outlet obstruction. Note the reverberation artifact, which compromises evaluation of the anterior bladder wall.* **(Bottom)** *Transverse color Doppler ultrasound at the level of the ureteral orifices shows bilateral, symmetric, ureteral jets. Always evaluate for the presence of ureteral jets when evaluating for obstruction.*

URINARY BLADDER

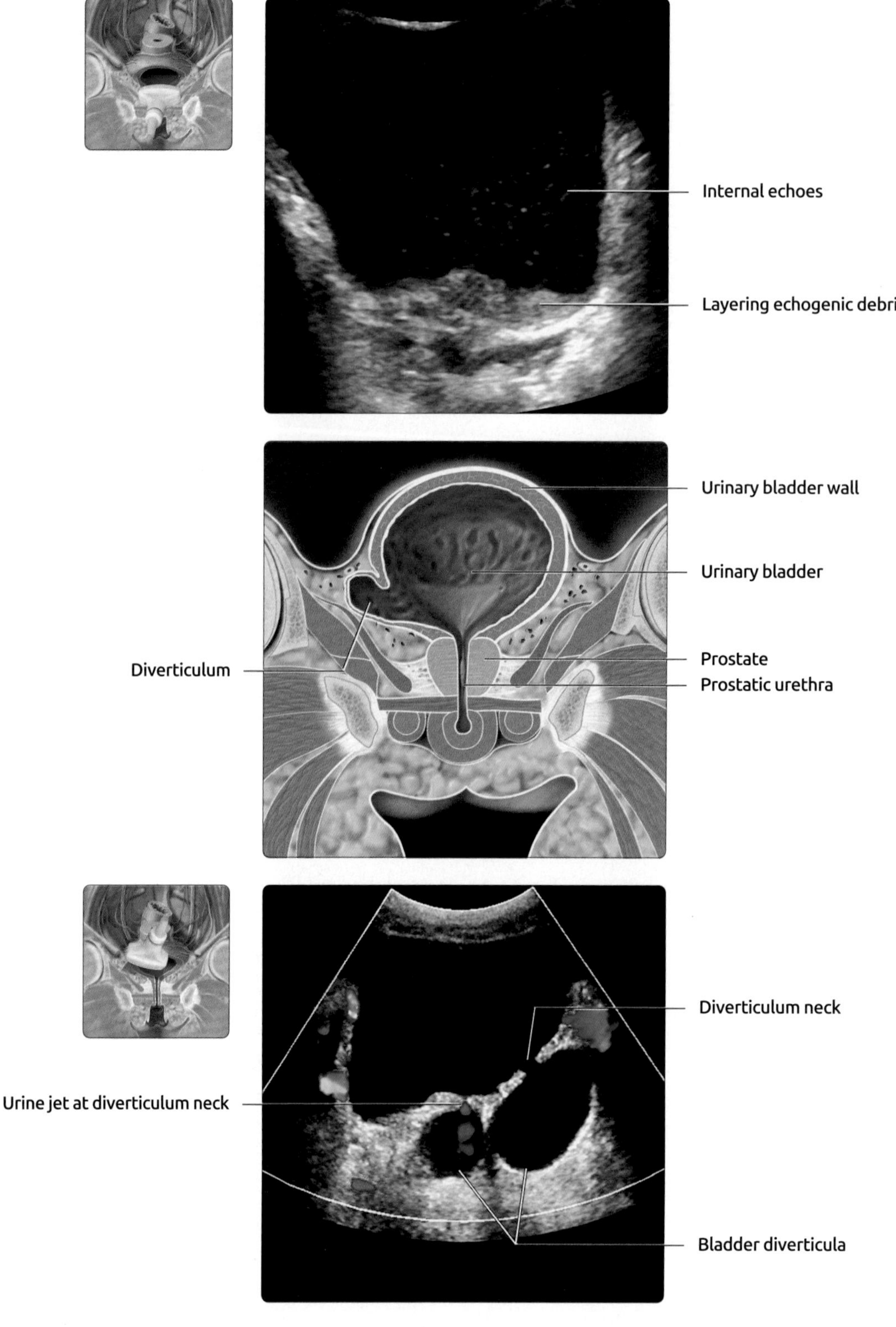

(Top) *Transverse transabdominal ultrasound of the bladder shows floating internal echoes with layering echogenic debris in this patient with cystitis. This could be confused with wall thickening, and the patient should be put in a decubitus position to document debris movement.* **(Middle)** *Graphic shows a diverticulum arising from the lateral urinary bladder wall with herniation of the mucosa and submucosa through the muscular wall.* **(Bottom)** *Transverse oblique transabdominal color Doppler ultrasound through the bladder shows 2 well-distended bladder diverticula along the left posterolateral bladder. A urine jet is identified in one of the diverticular necks.*

WEIGERT-MEYER RULE

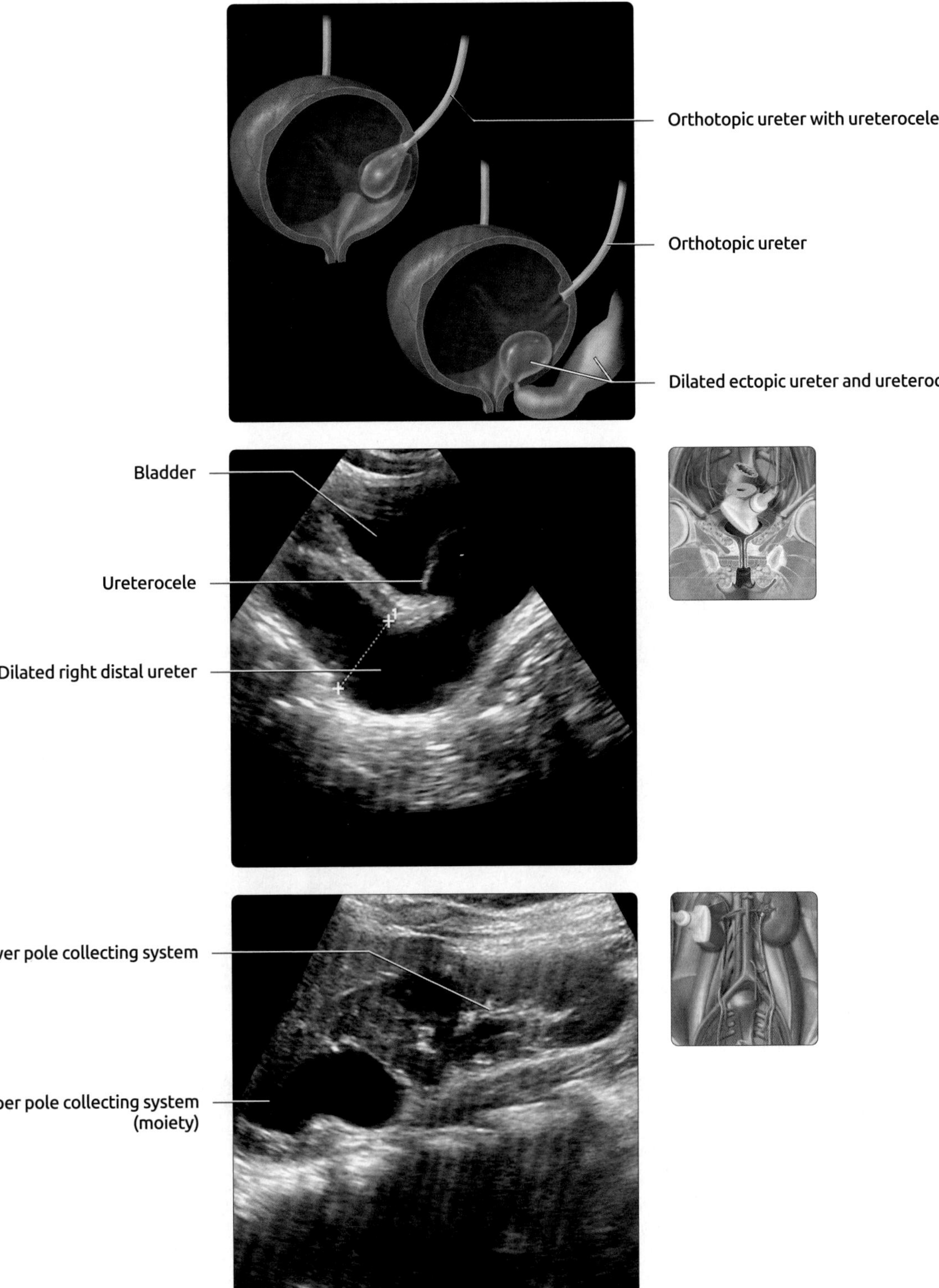

(Top) *Graphic illustrates an orthotopic ureterocele in a single ureter system (left, upper) and an ectopic ureterocele in a duplicated ureter system (right, lower). Note the hydroureter accompanying the ectopic ureterocele. The ectopic ureterocele inserts inferior and medial to the normally inserting ureter (Weigert-Meyer rule).* **(Middle)** *Longitudinal oblique transabdominal grayscale ultrasound at the suprapubic region shows a dilated ureter seen terminating in a ureterocele; the patient had complete duplication of the collecting system.* **(Bottom)** *Longitudinal transabdominal grayscale ultrasound through the right kidney in the same patient shows a dilated, obstructed upper pole moiety with a decompressed inferior moiety. The lower pole moiety is at risk for reflux and may also be dilated.*

KEY FACTS

TERMINOLOGY

- Hypertrophic band of normal cortical tissue that separates pyramids of renal medulla

IMAGING

- Band of tissue isoechoic to cortex and continuous with renal cortex, extending between renal pyramids
  - Echogenicity may be increased because of anisotropy
- At junction of upper and middle 1/3 of kidney
- Left side > right side
- Unilateral > bilateral (18% of cases)
- Measures < 3 cm
- Indents renal sinus laterally
- Normal external renal contour
- No vascular distortion with preserved arcuate arteries surrounding pyramids

TOP DIFFERENTIAL DIAGNOSES

- Renal tumor
- Renal scarring with pseudotumor
- Renal duplication
- Dromedary hump

PATHOLOGY

- Embryology: Incomplete resorption of polar parenchyma of subkidneys that fuse to form normal kidney

CLINICAL ISSUES

- Normal variant, asymptomatic
- Found on imaging
- Most likely to simulate mass on sonography

SCANNING TIPS

- Optimize ultrasound by focusing on lesion and placing it in center of field of view
- Use color Doppler to differentiate from tumor

(Left) *Graphic shows a column of Bertin ➡, which is an extension of renal cortical tissue between the pyramids.* **(Right)** *Longitudinal ultrasound of the right kidney demonstrates a hypertrophied column of Bertin ➡ indenting the sinus fat in the midkidney. Note its isoechogenicity relative to the cortex and the smooth external contour ➡.*

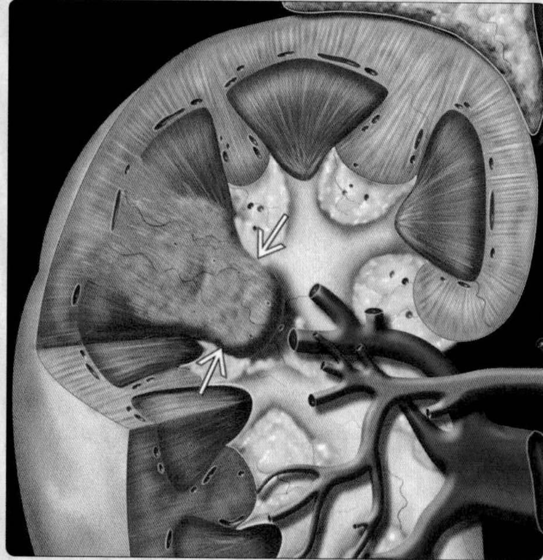

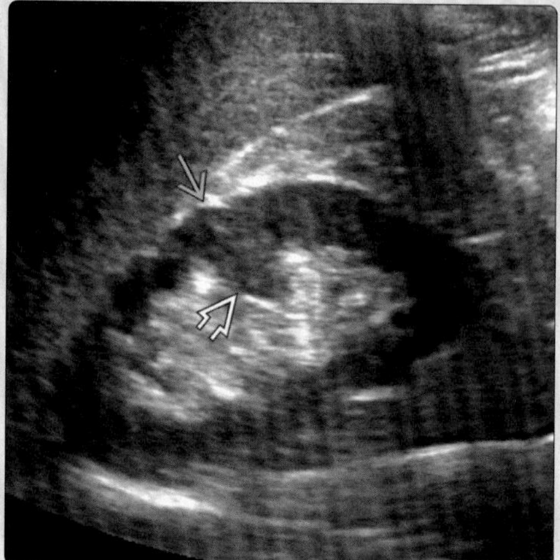

(Left) *Longitudinal ultrasound of the right kidney demonstrates a hypertrophied column of Bertin ➡, which is isoechoic to and contiguous with renal cortex ➡.* **(Right)** *Longitudinal color Doppler ultrasound of the same kidney shows no color flow in the column of Bertin ➡.*

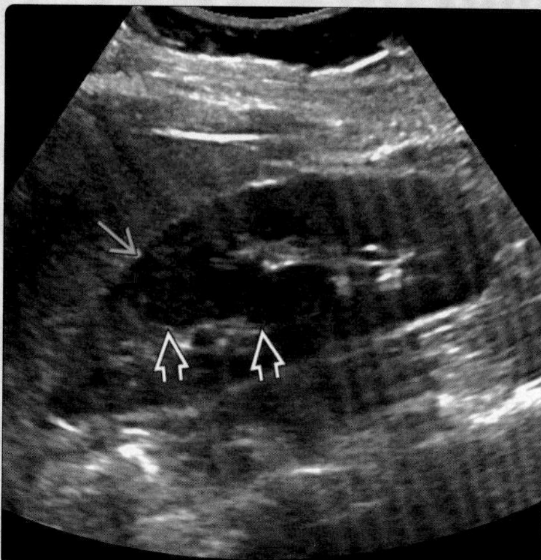

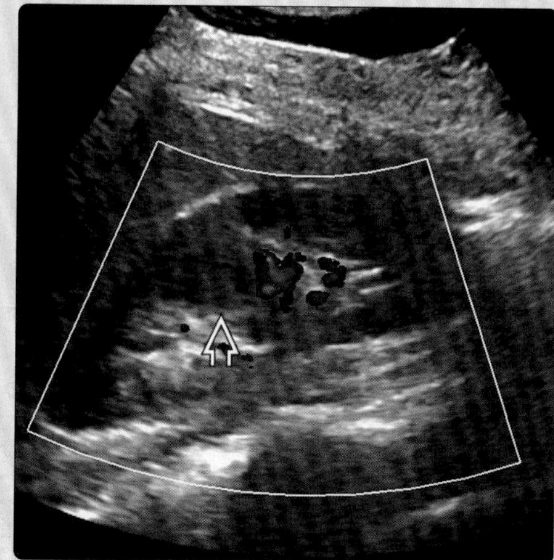

KEY FACTS

TERMINOLOGY

- Definition
  - Defect or line representing incomplete embryologic fusion of 2 primary renal lobes: Upper and lower poles of kidney
- Synonyms
  - Junctional parenchymal defect
  - Interrenuncular septum

IMAGING

- Characteristic location at anterosuperior aspect of kidney, upper to middle 1/3 of kidney
- Wedge-shaped hyperechoic defect or echogenic line
- Variable size of defect
- No associated loss of parenchyma
- More commonly seen on right
- Overlays column of Bertin

TOP DIFFERENTIAL DIAGNOSES

- Scar
- Fetal lobulation
- Angiomyolipoma

PATHOLOGY

- Layer of connective tissue trapped from fusion of 2 metanephric elements in formation of kidney
- Deep diagonal groove extending from anterior surface of upper pole of kidney into hilum

CLINICAL ISSUES

- Normal variant
- No clinical sequelae

SCANNING TIPS

- Absence of parenchymal loss useful to differentiate it from cortical scar
- Increased echogenicity on ultrasound; no disturbance of vessels

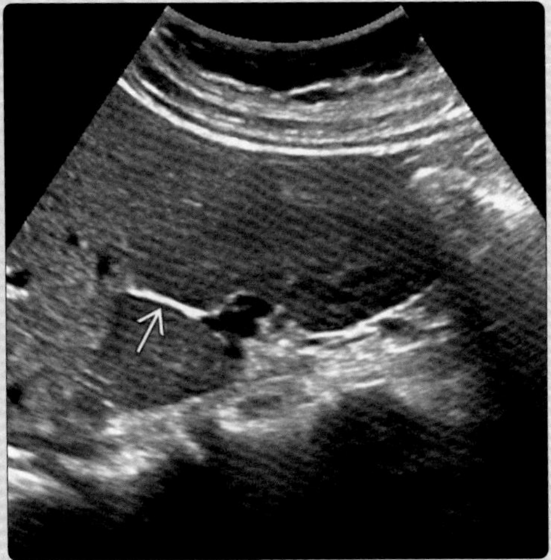

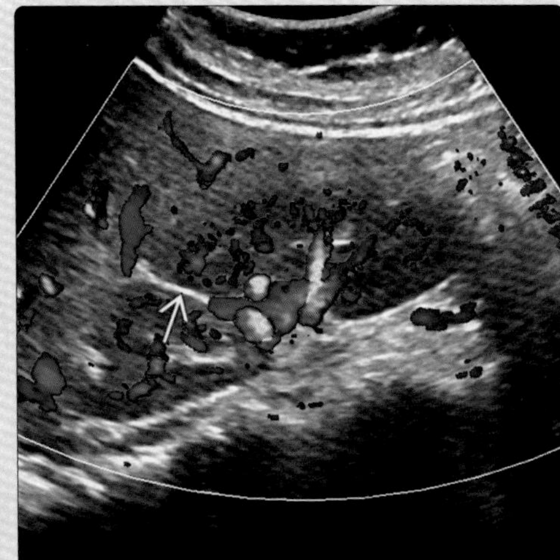

(Left) *Longitudinal ultrasound of the right kidney demonstrates a renal junctional line ➡ as a thin echogenic line communicating with the renal sinus.* **(Right)** *Longitudinal color Doppler ultrasound of the same patient shows no vascular distortion secondary to the junctional line ➡.*

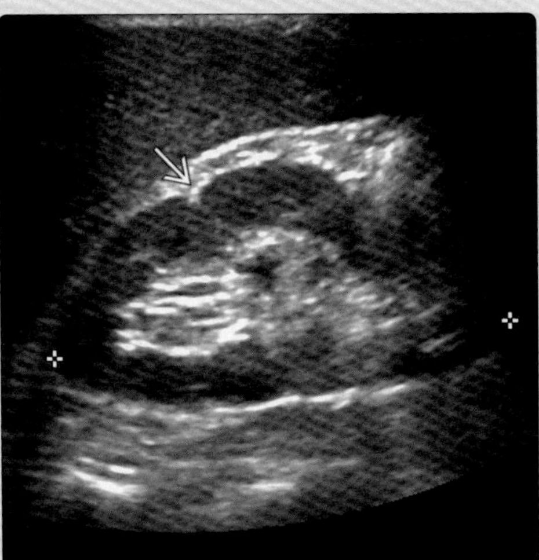

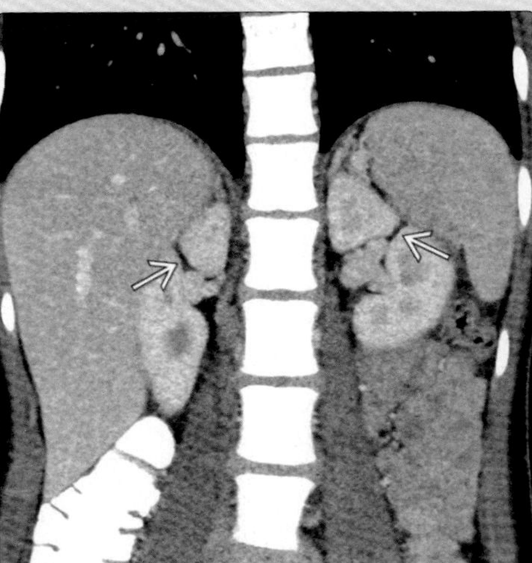

(Left) *Longitudinal ultrasound of the right kidney demonstrates a junctional parenchymal defect ➡ as a small triangular echogenic focus between the upper and middle 1/3 of the kidney.* **(Right)** *Coronal contrast-enhanced CT of the kidneys shows bilateral renal junction lines ➡ as complete clefts extending into the renal sinus.*

Renal Ectopia

KEY FACTS

TERMINOLOGY

- Aberrant location of kidney
- Separated into multiple categories, of which simple renal ectopia (RE) and crossed-fused ectopia (CFE) are most common

IMAGING

- Absence of kidney in expected renal fossa
- RE can range in location from pelvic (most common) to thoracic (rare)
    - Kidney is located ipsilateral to its ureteral insertion
- CFE: Ectopic kidney is malrotated; usually fusion of upper pole of ectopic kidney to lower pole of normally positioned kidney
    - Kidney located contralateral to its ureteral insertion
    - Left kidney more commonly ectopic than right
- CECT and CEMR with urography can better delineate ureteral course and presence of crossing vessels

TOP DIFFERENTIAL DIAGNOSES

- Renal transplant (iatrogenic ectopia)
- Horseshoe kidney
- Ptotic kidney
- Acquired renal displacement

PATHOLOGY

- Arrested migration during embryologic development

CLINICAL ISSUES

- CFE is 2nd most common fusion abnormality
- Associated with anomalies in genitourinary tract in ~ 1/2 of cases and other organ systems in up to 1/3
- Commonly asymptomatic, incidental finding
- ~ 50% have complications related to vesicoureteral reflux, hydronephrosis, stones, and infection

SCANNING TIPS

- When renal fossa is empty, look for ectopic kidney

(Left) *Graphic shows inferior crossed-fused renal ectopia. The left kidney ➡ is fused to the lower pole of the right kidney. Note that the left ureter ➡ crosses midline and inserts in its normal location.* **(Right)** *Grayscale ultrasound demonstrates crossed-fused ectopia on the right side of the abdomen. The right ➡ kidney is in a normal location. The left ➡ kidney has migrated to fuse. Note the anterior orientation of the renal pelvis ➡.*

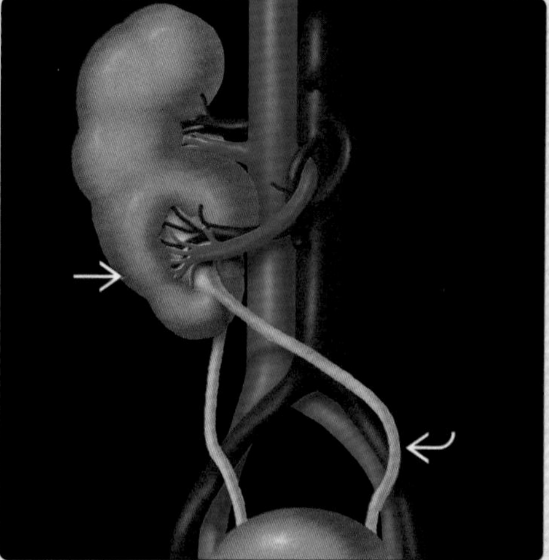

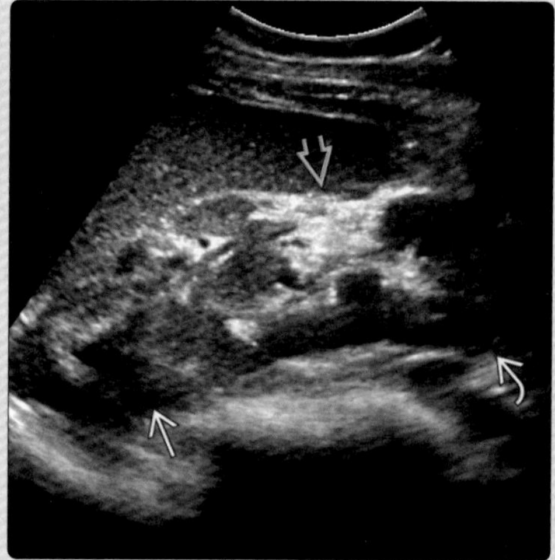

(Left) *Grayscale ultrasound demonstrates ectopic location of the left kidney ➡, which is situated within the pelvis.* **(Right)** *Color Doppler ultrasound demonstrates crossed-fused ectopia ➡ in the left lower quadrant/midline. The kidneys run anterior to the aorta ➡ and vena cava ➡.*

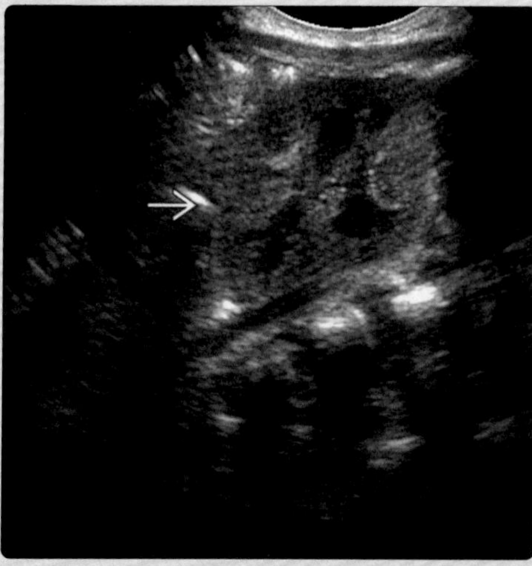

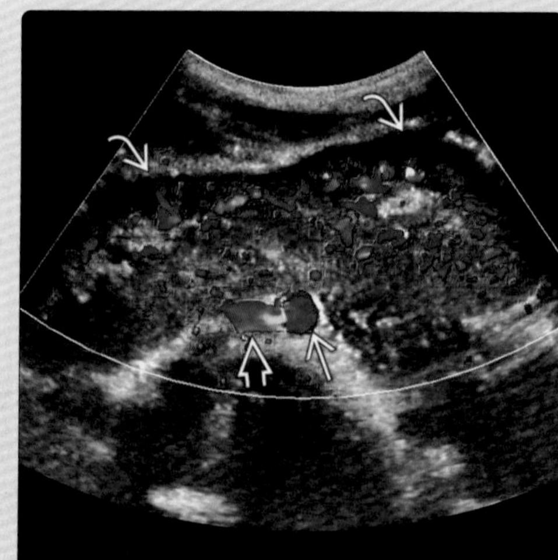

Horseshoe Kidney

KEY FACTS

TERMINOLOGY

- Congenital anomaly in which kidneys are fused at their lower poles in midline

IMAGING

- Kidneys on opposite sides with lower poles fused in midline
  - Note that in crossed-fused ectopia, both kidneys are located on one side
- Presence of isthmus is defining feature; isthmus may be fibrous or functioning renal tissue
  - Isthmus crosses midline anterior to spine and aorta but posterior to inferior mesenteric artery
- Arterial supply and venous drainage may be complex

TOP DIFFERENTIAL DIAGNOSES

- Crossed-fused ectopia
- Paraaortic lymphadenopathy/retroperitoneal mass

PATHOLOGY

- Fusion of kidney precursors in early gestation when still located in pelvis, preventing appropriate ascent

CLINICAL ISSUES

- 1 in 500 children; M:F = 2:1
- 30% asymptomatic
- Up to 2/3 have associated abnormalities (most commonly genitourinary)
- Complications include uretero-pelvic junction obstruction, infection, nephrolithiasis
- Increased risk of malignancy such as Wilms tumor, urothelial carcinoma, and carcinoid

SCANNING TIPS

- Suspect when lower renal poles disappear medially
- Look for isthmus in midline anterior to aorta and posterior to inferior mesenteric artery
- Use compression to displace bowel

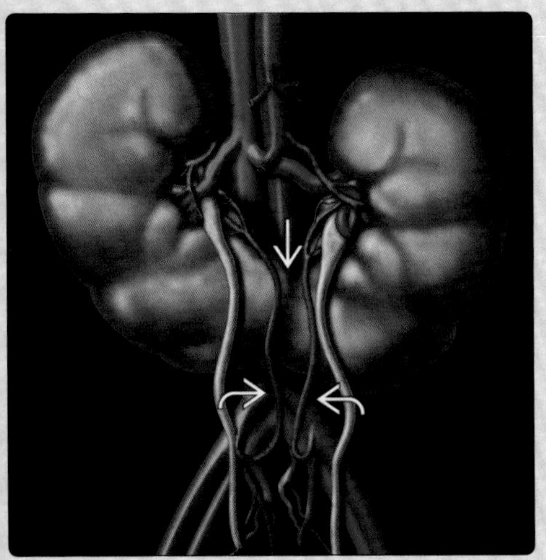

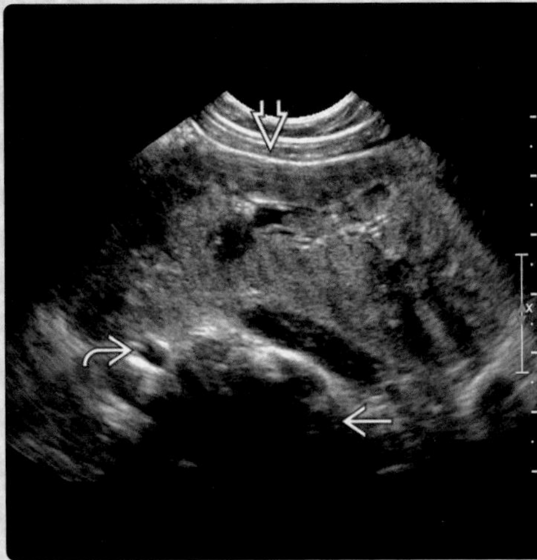

(Left) *Graphic shows a horseshoe kidney with the isthmus ➡ anterior to the aorta and inferior vena cava. Note the additional renal arteries arising from the common iliac arteries ➡.* **(Right)** *Transverse midline ultrasound shows a horseshoe kidney in an infant. The isthmus ➡ of the horseshoe kidney lies anterior to the spine ➡ and vena cava ➡. The isthmus is composed of functioning renal tissue.*

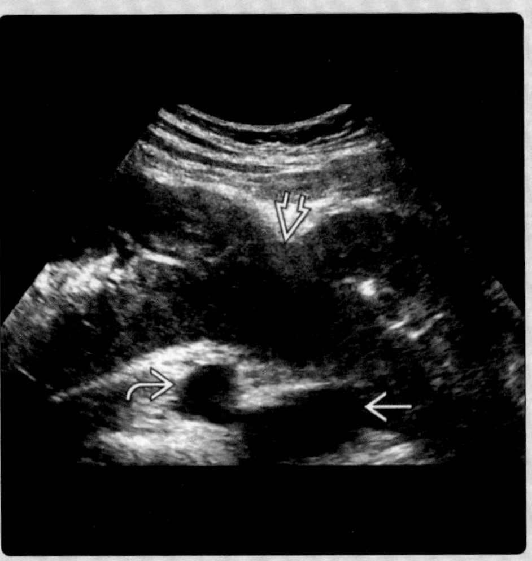

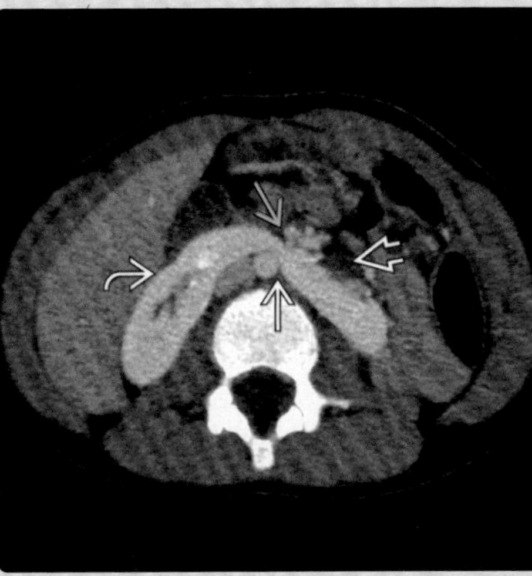

(Left) *Transverse ultrasound in the midline shows a horseshoe kidney. The isthmus ➡ of the horseshoe kidney lies anterior to the aorta ➡ and inferior vena cava ➡. The isthmus is composed of functioning renal tissue.* **(Right)** *Axial CECT in the same patient demonstrates horseshoe kidney ➡ draped over the aorta ➡ in the lower abdomen. The inferior mesenteric artery ➡ prevents ascent of the kidney in utero. The renal pelvis ➡ is malrotated.*

Ureteral Duplication

KEY FACTS

TERMINOLOGY

- Presence of 2 separate pelvicalyceal collecting systems draining 1 kidney, which may join above bladder (partial), drain into bladder separately (complete), or beyond bladder

IMAGING

- Asymmetric renal enlargement, 20% are bilateral
- 2 central echogenic renal sinuses with intervening bridging renal parenchyma
- 2 distinct renal pelves or 2 exiting ureters in single kidney
- Weigert-Meyer rule: Upper moiety ureter inserts inferior and medial to lower moiety ureter
  - Upper pole tends to obstruct
  - Lower pole tends to have vesicoureteral reflux
- Look for ureterocele (cystic structure) in bladder

TOP DIFFERENTIAL DIAGNOSES

- Column of Bertin
- Segmental multicystic dysplastic kidney
- Hydrosalpinx (dilated ureter in pelvis)

PATHOLOGY

- Abnormal bifurcation of ureteral bud
- Increased incidence of ureteropelvic obstruction; genital anomalies found in 50% of affected females

CLINICAL ISSUES

- Symptoms include infection from reflux/stasis, hematuria, abdominal/flank pain from obstruction or calculi
- Ectopic insertion in females: Incontinence due to insertion below bladder sphincter
- Ectopic insertion in males: Prostatitis, epididymitis

SCANNING TIPS

- Color Doppler can be useful to distinguish collecting system from vessel in renal pelvis
- Ureteral jets can be helpful to identify vesicoureteral junction of both upper and lower moieties

(Left) *Graphic shows a left duplex kidney. Upper moiety is hydronephrotic ➡ with hydroureter draining into a ureterocele ➡. Note the upper moiety ureter inserts inferior and medial to lower moiety ureter ➡.* **(Right)** *Longitudinal US demonstrates 2 renal pelves ➡, separated by intervening bridging renal tissue.*

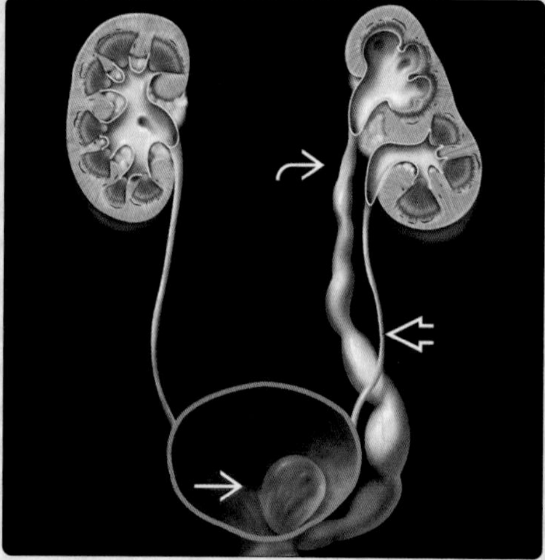

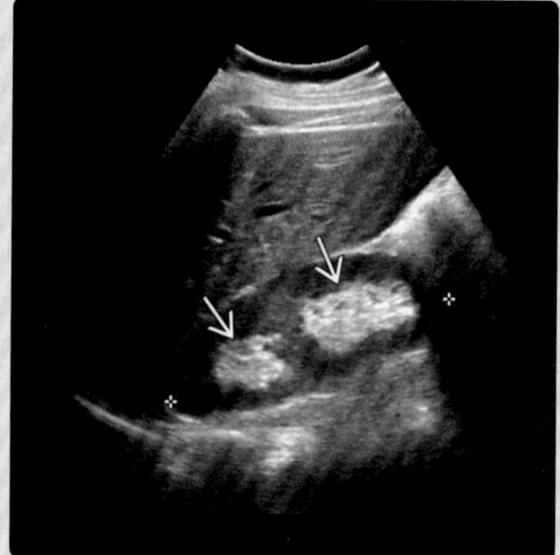

(Left) *Longitudinal US demonstrates a round anechoic structure in the upper pole ➡, reflecting a dilated upper moiety of a duplex kidney. The lower pole ➡ was normal.* **(Right)** *Longitudinal US demonstrates a dividing prominent band of renal tissue ➡ with dilatation of the lower moiety ➡, secondary to reflux.*

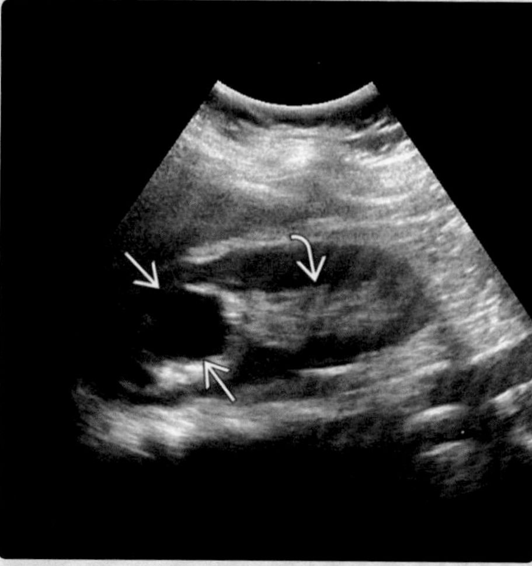

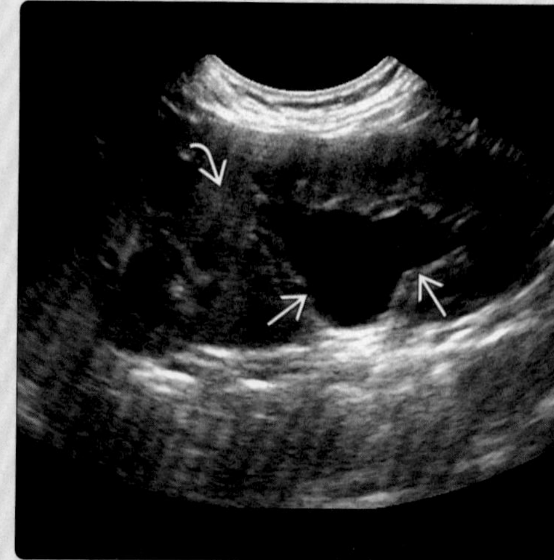

Ureteral Ectopia

KEY FACTS

TERMINOLOGY

- Strict definition: Ureter not inserting into bladder trigone
- Common usage: Ureter terminating outside bladder

IMAGING

- 70-80% have complete ureteral duplication, 5-17% bilateral
- Intravesicular insertion
  - Weigert-Meyer rule: Upper moiety ureter inserts inferior and medial to lower moiety ureter, upper renal moiety obstructs
  - Lower moiety tends to have vesicoureteral reflux
  - Ureterocele may be present if ectopic vesicular insertion
- Extravesicular insertion
  - Dilated ureter extends beyond bladder
  - Males: Prostatic urethra most common insertion site
  - Females: Vestibule or urethra most commonly
- Transrectal/transvaginal US may delineate site of insertion

TOP DIFFERENTIAL DIAGNOSES

- Bladder diverticulum, urachal cyst, or diverticulum
- Hydrosalpinx
- Seminal vesicle, müllerian, ejaculatory duct, utricular cysts

PATHOLOGY

- Failure of separation of ureteral bud from wolffian duct results in caudal ectopia

CLINICAL ISSUES

- M:F = 1:6; predominantly duplicated systems in females (80%) vs. single systems in males
- Recurrent or chronic urinary tract infections, dribbling urinary incontinence in females, chronic or recurrent epididymitis in males

SCANNING TIPS

- Trace dilated ureter to its termination below bladder
- Ureteral jet can be used to identify ectopic intravesicular insertion

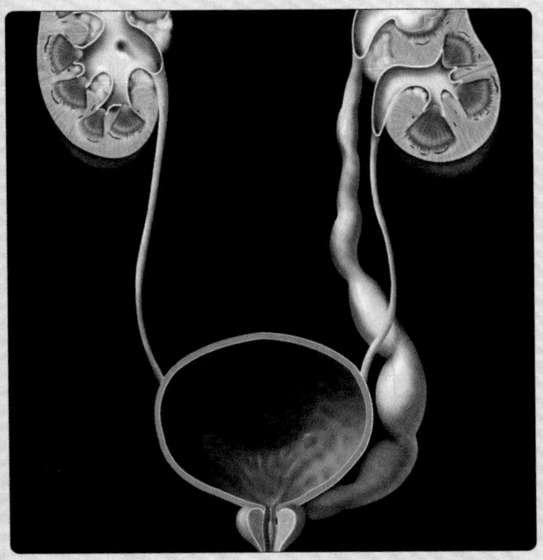

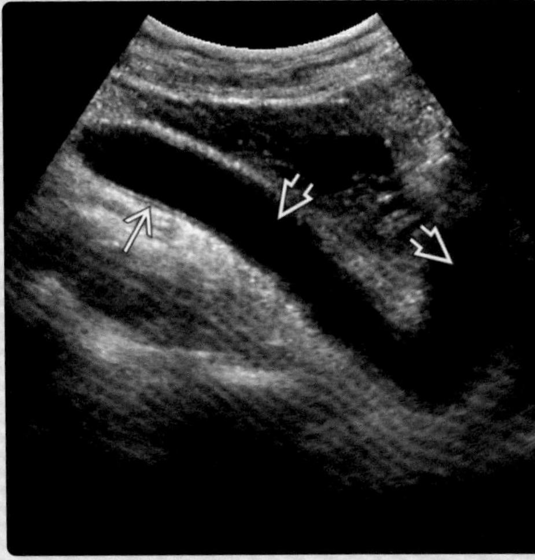

(Left) *Graphic shows a dilated upper moiety ureter of a left duplex kidney with extravesicular ectopic insertion into the prostatic urethra.* **(Right)** *Longitudinal oblique ultrasound of the left pelvis shows a dilated tortuous ureter ➔, which did not insert into the trigone of the bladder. There is mild urothelial thickening ➔.*

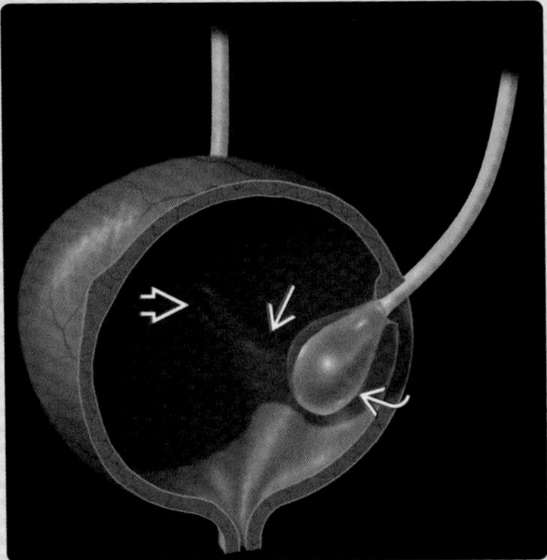

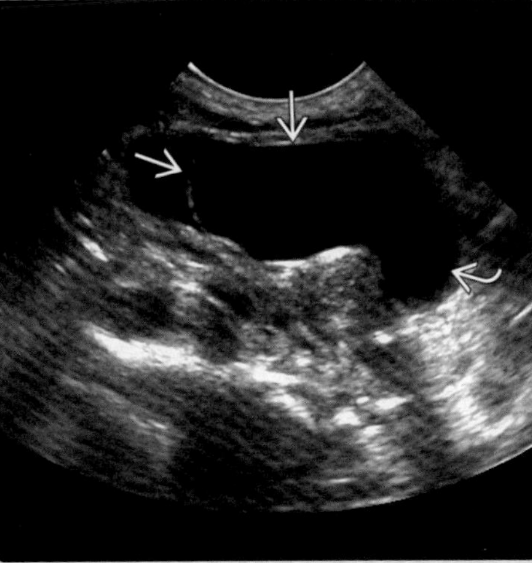

(Left) *Graphic shows intravesicular insertion of a ureter from a duplex left kidney with an associated ureterocele ➔. The interureteric ridge ➔ runs between the ureteral orifices. The right ureteral insertion ➔ was normal.* **(Right)** *Transverse ultrasound of the bladder shows a dilated left ureter ➔ from a duplex left kidney that is terminating as a large ureterocele ➔.*

Ureteropelvic Junction Obstruction

KEY FACTS

TERMINOLOGY

- Also known as pelviureteric junction obstruction
- Obstruction of urine flow at level of UPJ
- Congenital or acquired

IMAGING

- Marked hydronephrosis to level of UPJ without dilatation of ureter
- Renal pelvis disproportionately larger than calyces
- Color Doppler may detect crossing vessel
- Ultrasound is 1st-line modality
- CTA or MRA for vascular evaluation prior to surgery
- Nuclear renal scan to determine relative renal function and confirm obstructive hydronephrosis

TOP DIFFERENTIAL DIAGNOSES

- Multicystic dysplastic kidney
- Hydronephrosis of other etiology
- Extrarenal pelvis
- Pararenal cyst

PATHOLOGY

- Intrinsic causes: Abnormal peristalsis at UPJ, stone, clot, tumor, stenosis, scarring
- Extrinsic causes: Crossing vessels near UPJ
- Associated with renal ectopia and fusion anomalies
- Higher incidence in multicystic dysplastic and duplicated kidneys

CLINICAL ISSUES

- M > F, twice as common on left, 10-30% bilateral
- Most common cause of antenatal and neonatal hydronephrosis, diagnosed by prenatal screening
- Symptoms include: Intermittent abdominal or flank pain, nausea, vomiting, failure to thrive, hematuria, renovascular hypertension (rare)

SCANNING TIPS

- Use color Doppler for bladder jets and crossing vessels

(Left) *Graphic shows a markedly dilated renal pelvis ➡ and calyces ➡ in a ureteropelvic junction obstruction. The ureter ➡ is not dilated.* **(Right)** *Longitudinal ultrasound of the left kidney demonstrates marked dilatation of the renal pelvis ➡ as well as the renal calyces ➡. Note the severe cortical thinning ➡.*

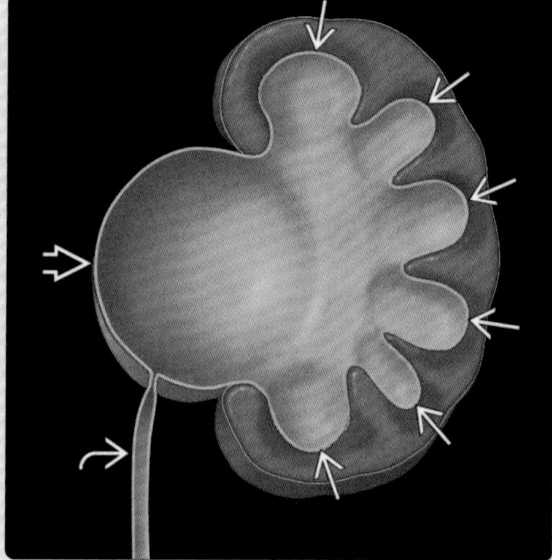

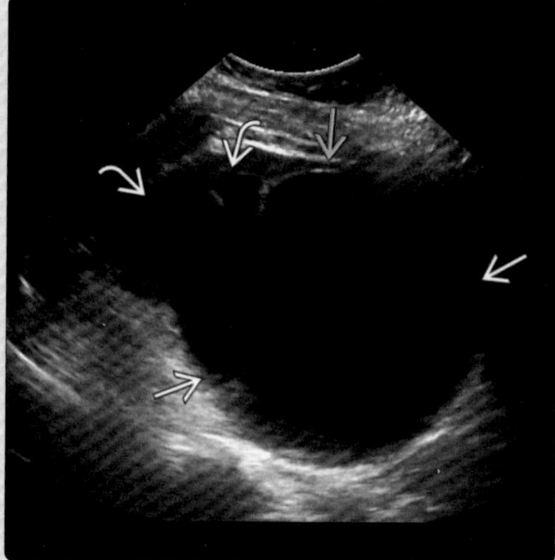

(Left) *Longitudinal ultrasound of the left kidney demonstrates moderate dilatation of the renal pelvis ➡ and the calyces ➡.* **(Right)** *Coronal CT angiogram of a woman with right-sided ureteropelvic junction obstruction is shown. The renal pelvis ➡ is dilated to a greater degree than the calyces ➡. Crossing arteries are seen superior and inferior to the renal pelvis ➡.*

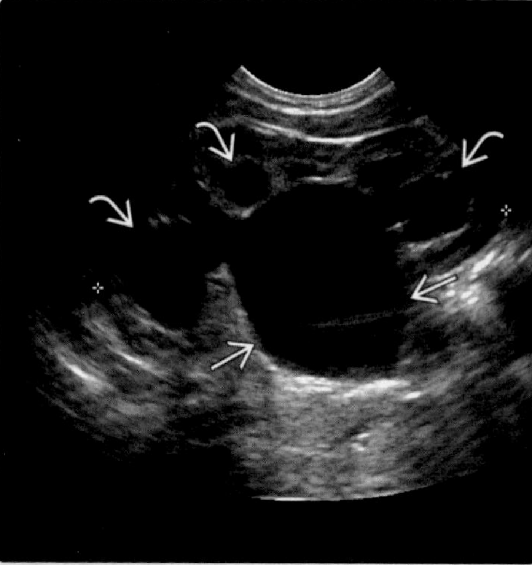

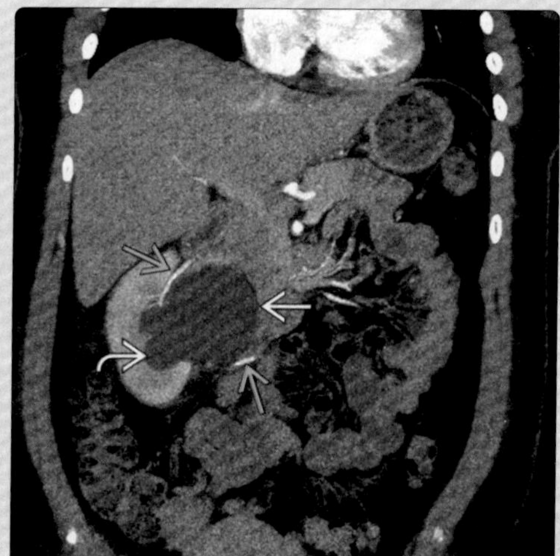

KEY FACTS

TERMINOLOGY

- Urinary tract stone, urinary calculous disease, nephrolithiasis, ureterolithiasis, vesicolithiasis
- Macroscopic concretions of crystals in urinary system, sometimes mixed with proteins

IMAGING

- US has 96% sensitivity, nearly 100% specificity for renal stones > 5 mm
- US is valuable for follow-up imaging, particularly in patients with renal colic & known renal stones or patients not improving on treatment for known stone
- Virtually all stones are visible (including those radiolucent on KUB) on CT except pure matrix stones & protease inhibitor stones (e.g., indinavir, treatment of HIV)
- NECT is preferred imaging modality to confirm stone in adult patients with acute flank pain

TOP DIFFERENTIAL DIAGNOSES

- Milk of calcium in small cyst
- Arterial calcifications
- Nephrocalcinosis
- Emphysematous pyelonephritis

CLINICAL ISSUES

- Size, number, location, evidence of obstruction or infection, & relevant anatomic findings (aberrant vasculature, distorted pelvicalyceal architecture, infundibular orientation) are all imaging findings that impact treatment

SCANNING TIPS

- US protocol: Drink 16-32 oz water prior to examination to fill bladder
- Always include bladder with special attention to UVJ
- Twinkling artifact on color Doppler is useful to identify otherwise occult stone; more sensitive than acoustic shadowing but higher false-positive rate

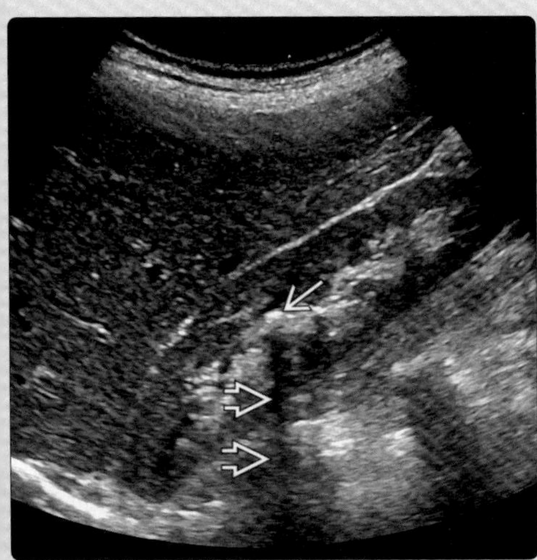

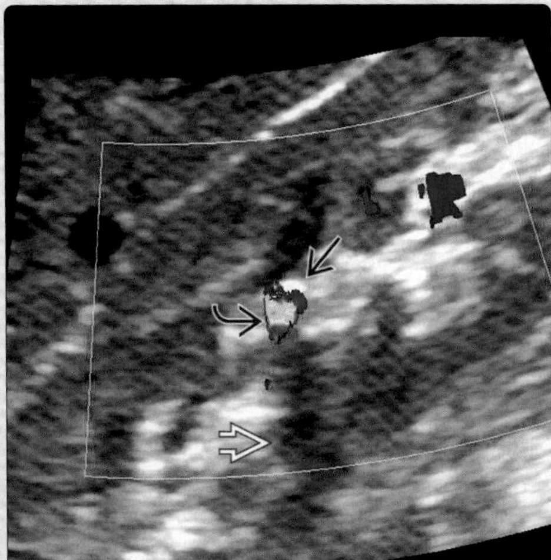

(Left) *Longitudinal US of the right kidney shows an echogenic stone ➡ within the mid right kidney. Posterior acoustic shadowing ➡ helps differentiate this stone from the surrounding sinus fat.* **(Right)** *Zoomed-in longitudinal color Doppler US of the right kidney in the same patient shows the echogenic stone ➡ with twinkling artifact ➡ and posterior acoustic shadowing ➡.*

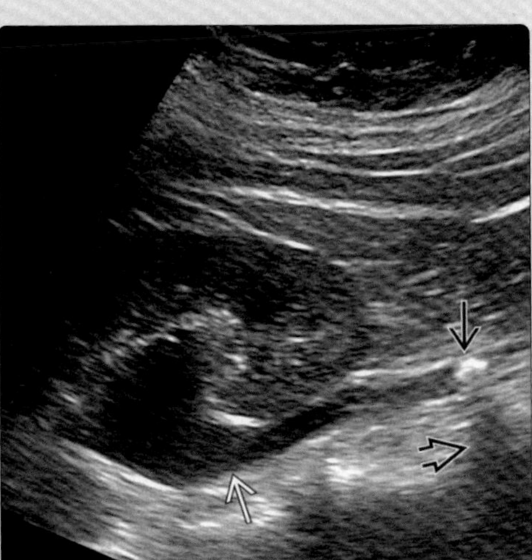

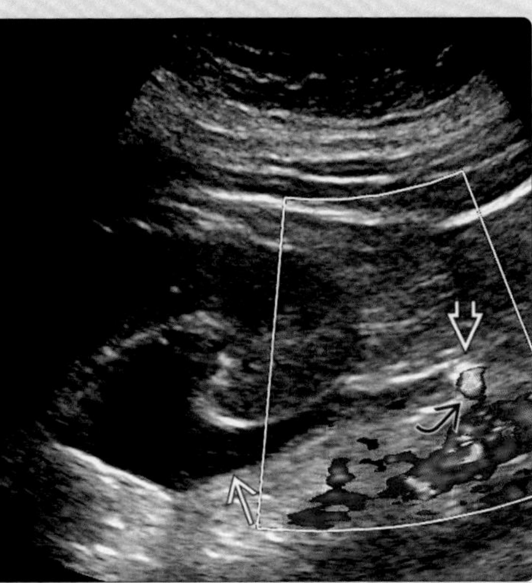

(Left) *Longitudinal US of the inferior pole of the left kidney shows an obstructing proximal ureteral calculus ➡ with posterior acoustic shadowing ➡ and hydroureteronephrosis ➡.* **(Right)** *Longitudinal color Doppler US of the inferior pole of the left kidney in the same patient now shows twinkling artifact ➡ posterior to the proximal ureteral calculus ➡ causing hydroureteronephrosis ➡.*

Nephrocalcinosis

KEY FACTS

TERMINOLOGY

- Medullary nephrocalcinosis (NC), cortical NC
- Calcification of renal parenchyma

IMAGING

- Medullary NC: Generalized increased echogenicity of renal pyramids with reversal of normal corticomedullary differentiation ± shadowing
- Cortical NC: Increased cortical echogenicity ± acoustic shadowing
- Noncontrast CT is best imaging modality in adults
  - Exception: CT intravenous pyelogram may be best for medullary sponge kidney given high sensitivity for stones and collecting tubule dilation
- US is 1st diagnostic imaging option in infants and children with suspected NC

TOP DIFFERENTIAL DIAGNOSES

- Renal calculus
- Emphysematous pyelonephritis
- Other causes of hyperechoic medulla: Metabolic and protein deposition disorders, autosomal recessive polycystic kidney disease

PATHOLOGY

- Most common causes of medullary NC are hyperparathyroidism, renal tubular acidosis type 1 (distal), and medullary sponge kidney
- Most common causes of cortical NC are acute cortical necrosis, chronic glomerulonephritis, and oxalosis
- Medullary and cortical NC are rare and seen in oxalosis

SCANNING TIPS

- NC is often associated with renal calculi
- Look for subtle renal calculi with both color Doppler (twinkling artifact) and confirmation with grayscale (posterior acoustic shadowing)
  - Increase PRF to 60-80 cm/s to distinguish twinkling artifact from aliasing artifact

(Left) *Graphic shows diffuse calcification → in renal the pyramids, representing medullary nephrocalcinosis.* **(Right)** *Longitudinal US of the left kidney shows echogenic pyramids with reversal of the normal corticomedullary differentiation. Note the medullary ring → of hyperechoic rim outlining the pyramid. Posterior acoustic shadowing → helps identify a stone →.*

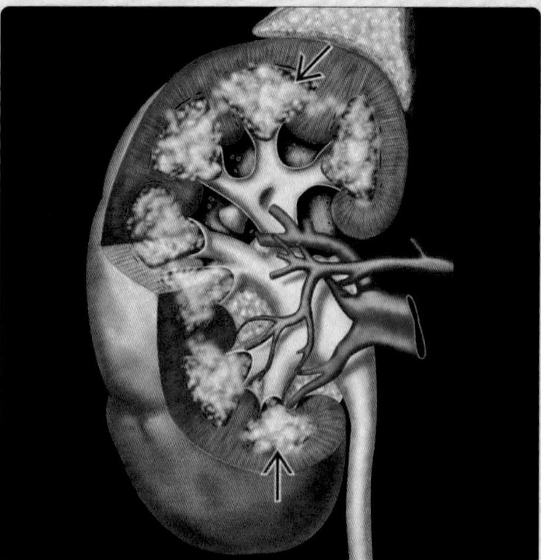

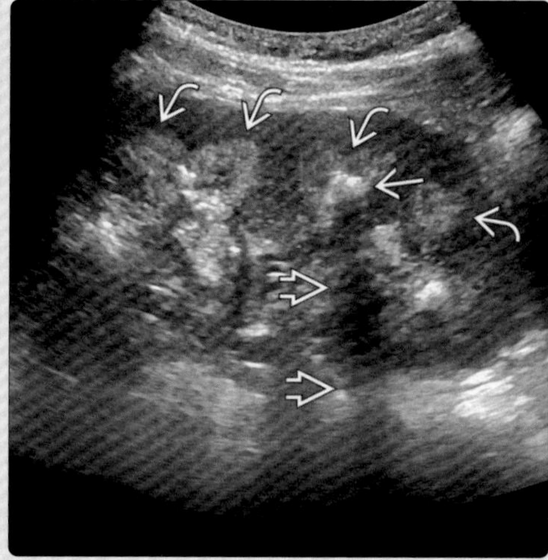

(Left) *Longitudinal US of the right kidney shows hyperechoic pyramids → with reversal of the normal corticomedullary differentiation. Mild fullness of the right renal collecting system → is present.* **(Right)** *Longitudinal color Doppler US of the right kidney in the same patient confirms the hypoechoic spaces represent caliectasis →.*

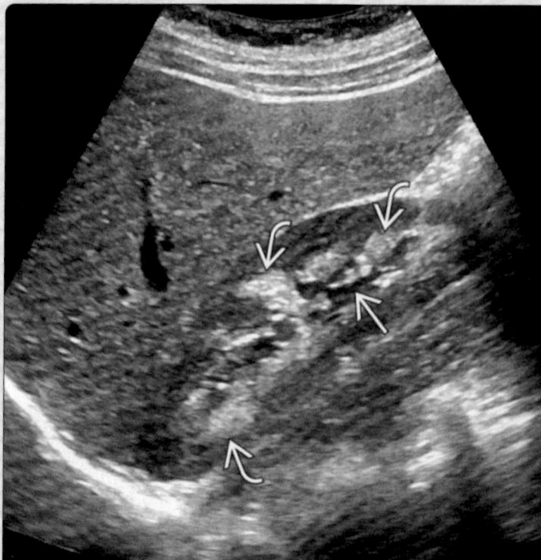

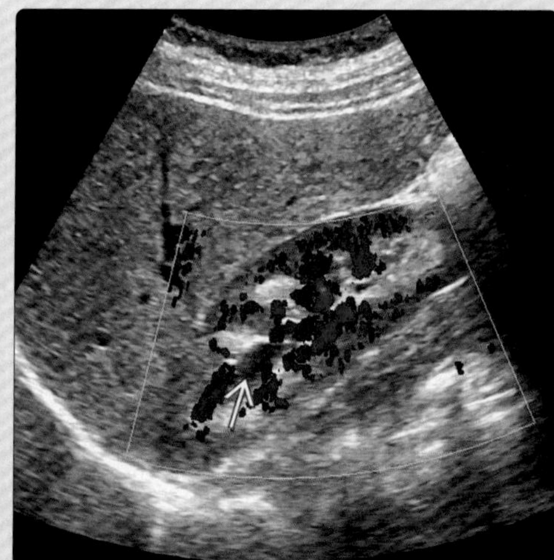

Hydronephrosis

KEY FACTS

TERMINOLOGY

- Dilation of renal collecting (pelvicalyceal) system ± ureteral dilation from intrinsic or extrinsic cause
- Renal collecting system dilation, pelvicalyceal dilatation, pelvocaliectasis

IMAGING

- Dilated intercommunicating fluid-filled anechoic channels (renal calyces and pelvis) in kidney
- Severity of hydronephrosis depends on degree and duration of obstruction
- Presence of internal echoes within dilated collecting system may represent underlying infection/pyonephrosis
- Acute hydronephrosis: RI > 0.70 or RI 0.08-0.10 higher than normal contralateral side in unilateral obstruction

TOP DIFFERENTIAL DIAGNOSES

- Parapelvic cyst
  - Parenchymal cysts that extend into renal pelvis
- Peripelvic cyst
  - Ovoid lymphocysts in pelvic hilum, usually multiple
- Extrarenal pelvis
- Prominent renal vasculature

SCANNING TIPS

- Evaluate with color Doppler to exclude prominent renal vessels in hilum that could mimic hydronephrosis
- Look for debris in collecting system, which could indicate pyonephrosis, urologic emergency
- Evaluate kidneys after voiding, as mild hydronephrosis may be transient with full bladder
- Look for bladder jets, which may help delineate complete from partial obstruction
- Look at ureterovesical junction (UVJ) with color Doppler for subtle twinkling artifact, which may indicate distal ureteral or UVJ stone as etiology of hydronephrosis

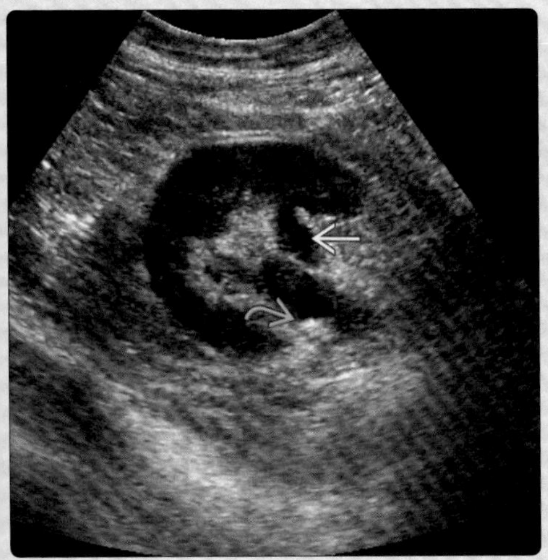

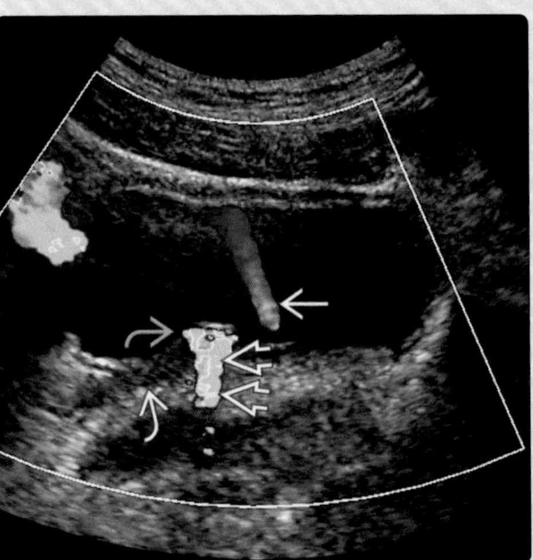

(Left) *Axial transabdominal renal ultrasound shows an echogenic stone in the renal pelvis with mild hydronephrosis.* **(Right)** *Transverse transabdominal color Doppler ultrasound of the urinary bladder shows an obstructing stone at right ureterovesical junction. Twinkling artifact is seen distal to the stone, which can be useful to identify stones in the urinary system. The ureter proximal to the obstructing stone is moderately dilated. A normal left ureteral jet is seen on the contralateral side.*

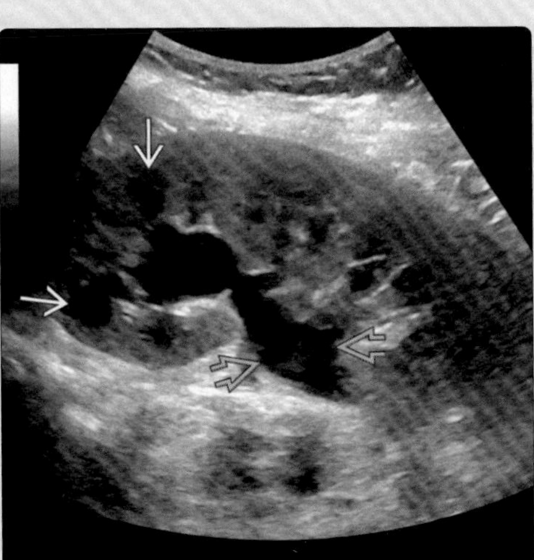

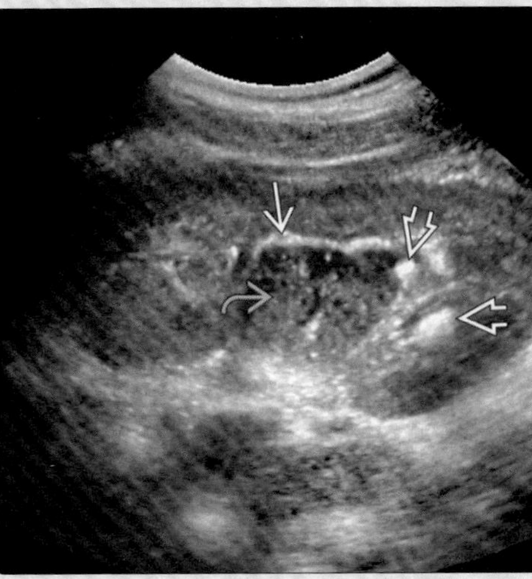

(Left) *Longitudinal transabdominal ultrasound of the right kidney shows moderate hydronephrosis as evidenced by the presence of caliectasis as well as pelviectasis.* **(Right)** *Longitudinal transabdominal ultrasound shows a moderately dilated renal pelvis with echogenic debris, which raises concern for pyonephrosis in the proper clinical setting of superimposed infection. Additional finding of a few echogenic intracalyceal stones may be nidus for infection.*

KEY FACTS

TERMINOLOGY

- Benign, fluid-filled, nonneoplastic renal lesion

IMAGING

- Ultrasound is ideal for characterizing simple or complex renal cysts in nonobese patients
- Unilocular, thin-walled, round/oval renal lesion
- Anechoic: No internal echoes, septations, or solid components; distinct posterior wall
- Increased sound transmission gives rise to characteristic posterior acoustic enhancement
- Variable size
- Location: Intraparenchymal, exophytic, parapelvic

TOP DIFFERENTIAL DIAGNOSES

- Complex renal cyst
- Peripelvic cysts
- Prominent pyramids
- Cystic disease of dialysis
- Perinephric collections
- Pyelogenic cyst/pyelocalyceal diverticulum
- Multilocular cystic nephroma

CLINICAL ISSUES

- In 20-30% of middle-aged adults and 50% > 50 years of age
- Most common renal lesion, usually detected incidentally
- No further imaging or monitoring of cyst is warranted
- May present with pain from bleeding/rupture/infection or mass effect when large
- Multiple renal cysts may indicate syndrome, such as autosomal dominant polycystic kidney disease

SCANNING TIPS

- Distinguish simple renal cysts from complex cystic renal lesions; look for solid nodules and septa
- Optimize ultrasound by adjusting frequency and focal zone; use harmonics and turn off compounding for optimal detection of posterior enhancement

(Left) *Transverse ultrasound shows a typical simple cortical cyst ➡ with complete lack of internal echoes, imperceptible walls, and posterior acoustic enhancement ➡. The gallbladder ➡ was normal.* **(Right)** *Longitudinal ultrasound shows a large parapelvic renal cyst ➡ in addition to multiple smaller cortical cysts ➡. Large cysts may produce distension, pain, or spontaneous hemorrhage.*

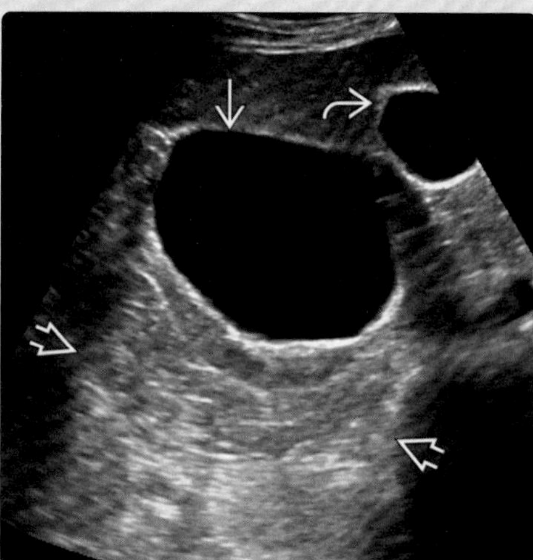

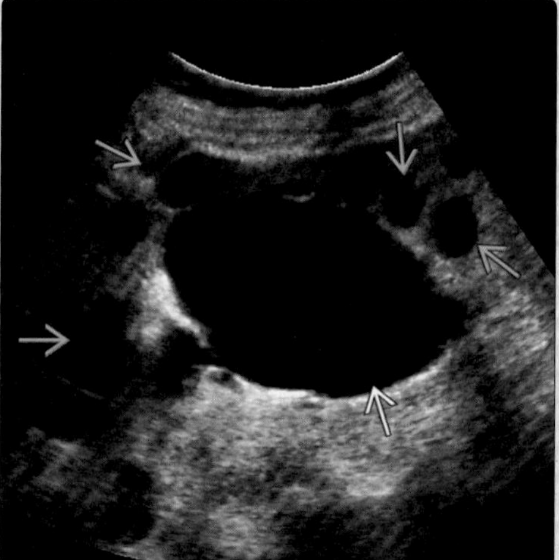

(Left) *Longitudinal color Doppler ultrasound of a simple lower pole renal cyst ➡. Color Doppler should be used to confirm that an anechoic lesion is not vascular.* **(Right)** *Longitudinal ultrasound shows a small renal cyst ➡. Acoustic enhancement ➡ is well seen despite the small size of the cyst.*

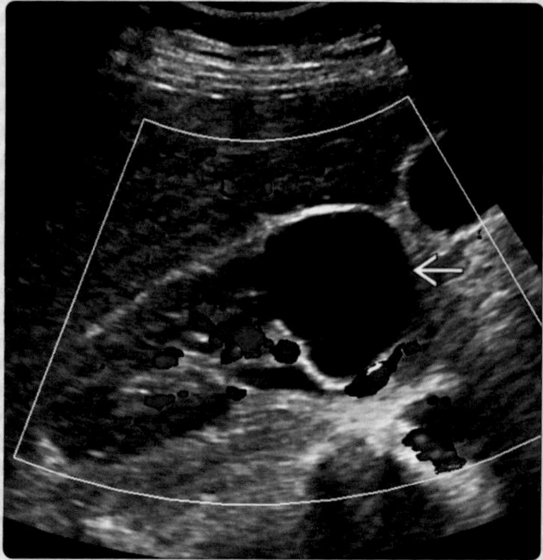

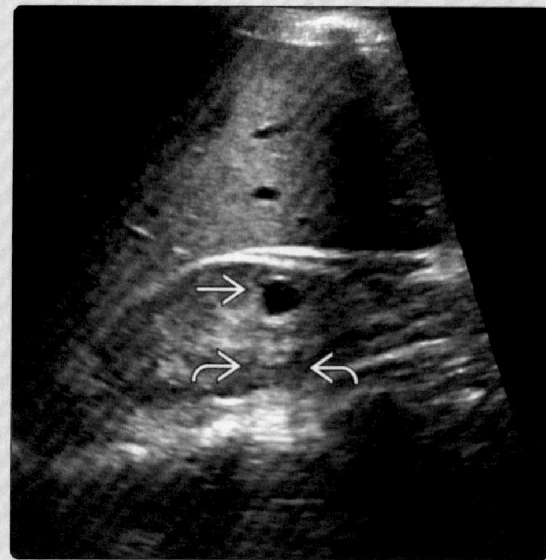

KEY FACTS

TERMINOLOGY

- Benign, fluid-filled nonneoplastic renal lesion not meeting criteria of simple renal cyst, Bosniak classes II, IIF, and III

IMAGING

- Round, oval, or irregular-shaped anechoic lesion
- Hemorrhagic cyst: Variable → echogenic fluid, retracting clot, debris level or septations
- Proteinaceous cyst: Low-level echoes with bright reflectors or even layers of echoes
- Infected cyst: Thick wall with scattered internal echoes ± debris-fluid level
- Calcified cyst: Wall or septal calcification ± shadowing
- Neoplastic features: Solid mural or septal nodules, irregular wall, or irregular septal thickening with color flow
- Complex cysts should be evaluated with CEUS, CECT, or CEMR for decision of surgical intervention
- Contrast uptake on CEUS suspicious for malignancy (other than a few bubbles in thin, smooth septa or wall)
    - Increased sensitivity for detecting malignancy
- Depending on body habitus and number of cysts, US can fully characterize renal cysts/monitor complex renal cysts

TOP DIFFERENTIAL DIAGNOSES

- Renal cell carcinoma (cystic)
- Multilocular cystic nephroma
- Localized cystic disease
- Renal abscess
- Renal metastasis/lymphoma

CLINICAL ISSUES

- 20-30% of middle-aged adults; > 50% of patients > 50 years
- Complications: Hydronephrosis, hemorrhage, infection, cyst rupture

SCANNING TIPS

- Optimize color Doppler settings to detect flow in septa and nodules

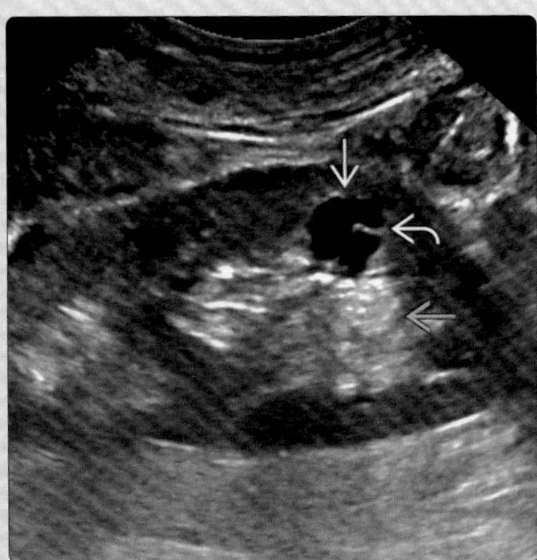

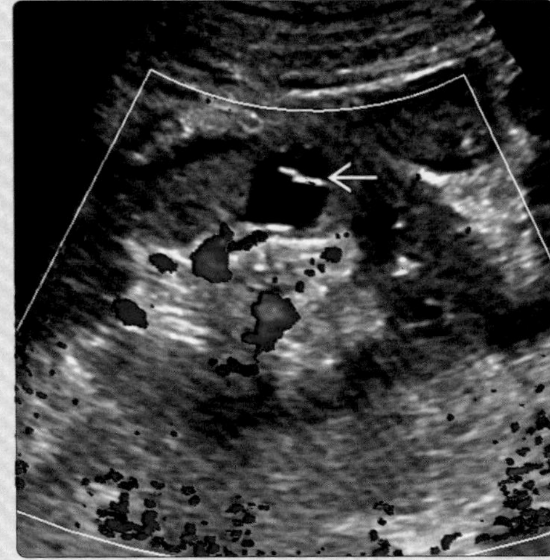

(Left) *Longitudinal US of the right kidney shows a lower pole cyst ➡ with a thin, smooth septation ➡. Posterior acoustic enhancement is present ➡.* **(Right)** *Color Doppler US shows no flow in the septum ➡ of this minimally complex cyst.*

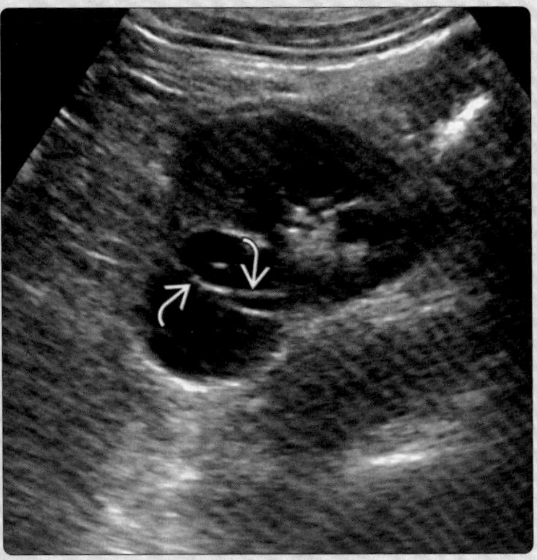

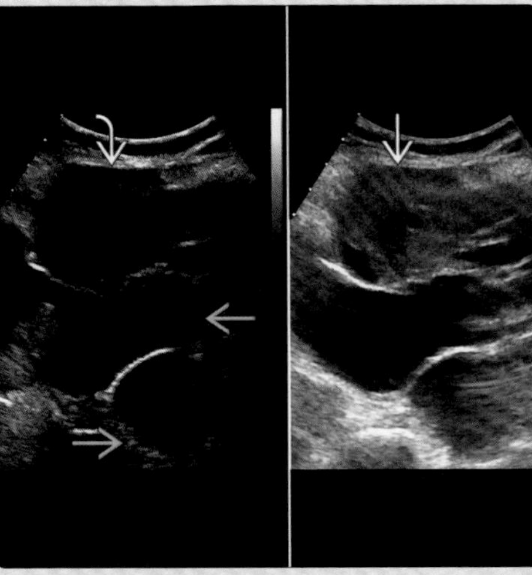

(Left) *Transverse US shows a cystic lesion with multiple thin internal septations ➡, which did not have flow on color Doppler. There are no internal nodules, wall, or septal thickening; this corresponds to a Bosniak II lesion.* **(Right)** *Split-screen contrast-enhanced US of a patient with autosomal dominant polycystic kidney disease shows that 1 cyst has internal echoes ➡. After injecting contrast, there was no internal flow ➡, confirming that this was an intracystic hemorrhage. The other cysts ➡ were simple.*

Cystic Disease of Dialysis

KEY FACTS

TERMINOLOGY

- Presence of 3 or more renal cysts per kidney in patients with chronic kidney disease (CKD) who do not have hereditary cystic disease
- Occurs predominantly in patients on long-term dialysis (peritoneal or hemodialysis)
- In up to 13% of patients with CKD prior to dialysis

IMAGING

- Ultrasound: Study of choice for establishing diagnosis in patients on dialysis
- Multiple bilateral small cysts in normal-sized or atrophic, echogenic kidneys
  - Cysts are usually simple; may be complicated by hemorrhage, leading to internal fluid, solid avascular debris and septa
  - Malignant transformation of cysts typically manifests as papillary growth within the cyst
- Cysts scattered in both renal cortex and medulla
- Kidneys may be enlarged due to cysts
- CEUS, CT, or MR are required to fully evaluate complex cysts and distinguish from renal cell carcinoma

TOP DIFFERENTIAL DIAGNOSES

- Multiple simple cysts
- Adult polycystic kidney disease
- von Hippel-Lindau disease
- Tuberous sclerosis
- Medullary cystic disease

CLINICAL ISSUES

- Most patients are asymptomatic
- Hematuria, flank pain, fever if complications such as hemorrhage or infection occur
- Renal cell carcinoma occurs in up to 7% of patients

SCANNING TIPS

- Look for solid components

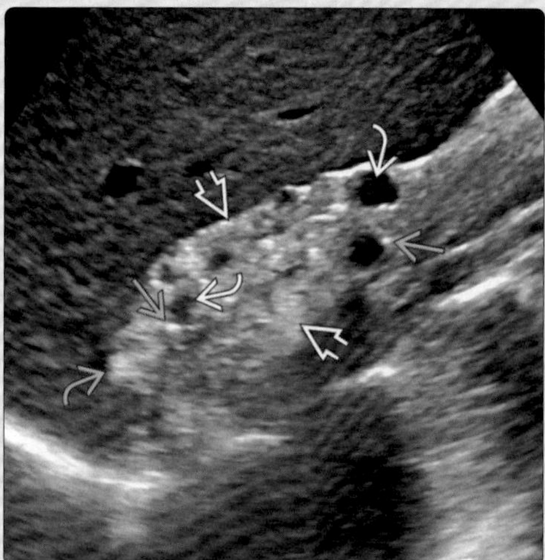
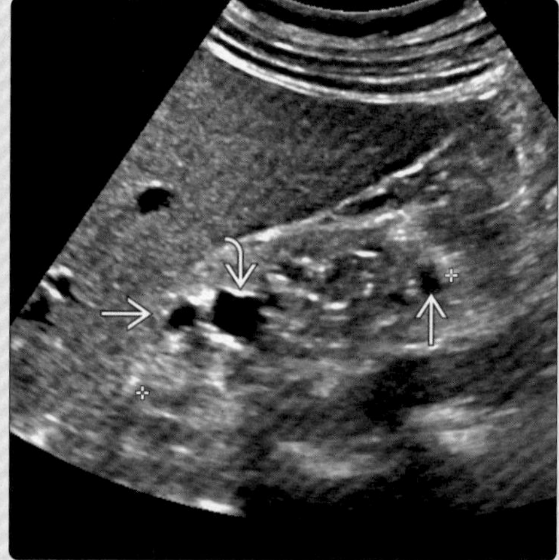

(Left) *US shows a markedly echogenic kidney ➡ with multiple small cortical and medullary cysts ➡. Many of these contain peripheral calcifications ➡, more common in ACKD than in age-related simple renal cysts. One of these is entirely calcified ➡.* **(Right)** *Longitudinal US of the right kidney shows a small (7.9 cm) right kidney with cortical ➡ and medullary ➡ cysts in a patient with chronic kidney disease, not yet on dialysis. The kidney is hyperechoic.*

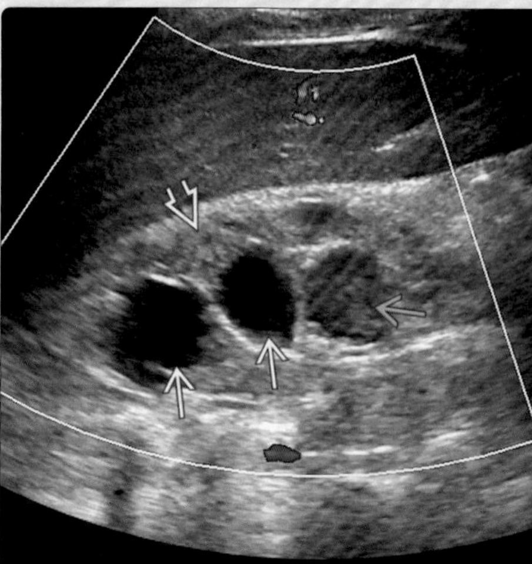
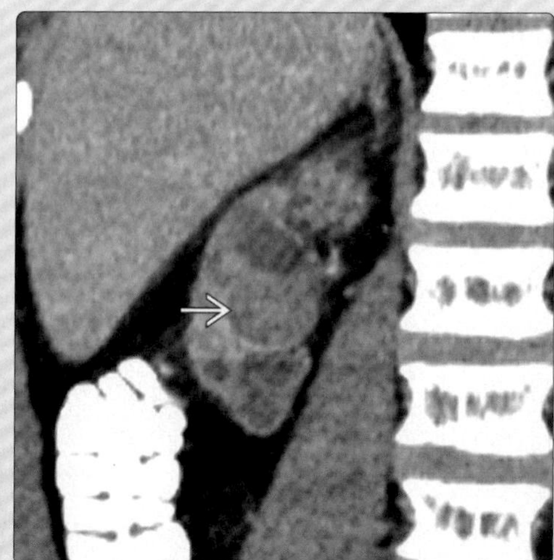

(Left) *Longitudinal color Doppler US shows multiple cysts ➡ within an echogenic right kidney ➡. There is cortical atrophy. The inferior cyst has internal echoes ➡ and lack of color flow, consistent with a hemorrhagic cyst, common in patients with cystic kidney disease of dialysis.* **(Right)** *Coronal CT in the same patient shows the corresponding hyperdense ➡ cyst in the mid to lower pole. There was no evidence of enhancement on this multiphase CT scan, which is consistent with a hemorrhagic cyst.*

Multilocular Cystic Nephroma

KEY FACTS

TERMINOLOGY

- Rare, nonhereditary, benign cystic renal neoplasm containing epithelial and stromal components
- a.k.a. cystic nephroma, multilocular cystic renal tumor, cystic hamartoma

IMAGING

- Multiloculated cystic renal mass; characteristic herniation into renal pelvis/ureter or, rarely, into renal vein/IVC
- Hyperechoic thick fibrous capsule, encapsulating tumor
- Numerous anechoic cysts with hyperechoic septa
- Occasionally more solid appearing due to numerous tiny cysts causing acoustic interfaces
- Fine vessels may be seen within septa on color Doppler
- Contrast uptake within septa and wall on contrast-enhanced US, CT, or MR
- Entire lesion: Few cm to > 30 cm (average: 10 cm)
- May be indistinguishable from cystic renal carcinoma

TOP DIFFERENTIAL DIAGNOSES

- Cystic renal cell carcinoma
- Mixed epithelial and stromal tumor
- Complex renal cyst
- Multicystic dysplastic kidney

CLINICAL ISSUES

- Bimodal age and sex distribution
  - 2-4 years old, M > F; 40-60 years old, F > > M
- Present with hematuria, abdominal/flank pain, palpable mass, or incidental imaging finding
- Complications: Obstructive uropathy, infection, hemorrhage
- Cured with complete surgical excision

SCANNING TIPS

- Lack of solid nodules and presence of enclosing capsule favor multilocular cystic nephroma over cystic renal carcinoma, but pathologic confirmation is required

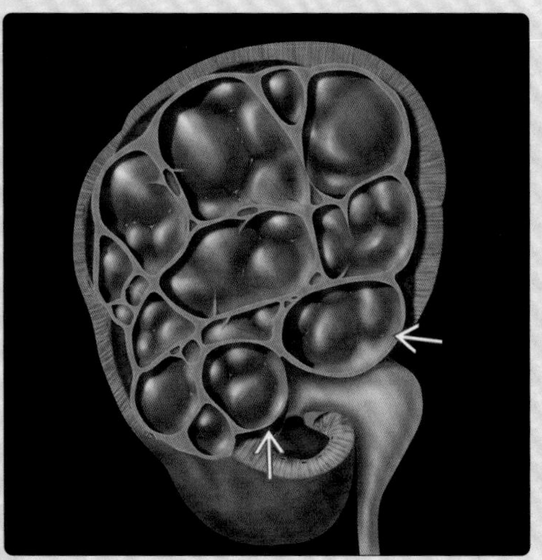

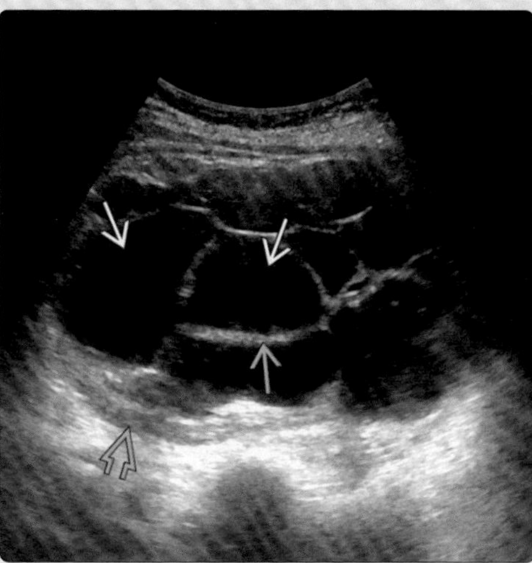

(Left) *Graphic shows multiple noncommunicating cysts separated by thick septa. The multiloculated cystic mass herniates into the renal hilum ➡ but shows no communication with collecting system.* **(Right)** *Longitudinal ultrasound of the left kidney reveals multiple large, anechoic cysts ➡ separated by thick septa ⇨, consistent with a large multilocular cystic nephroma (MLCN). Compressed renal parenchyma is visible at the medial aspect of the kidney ⇨.*

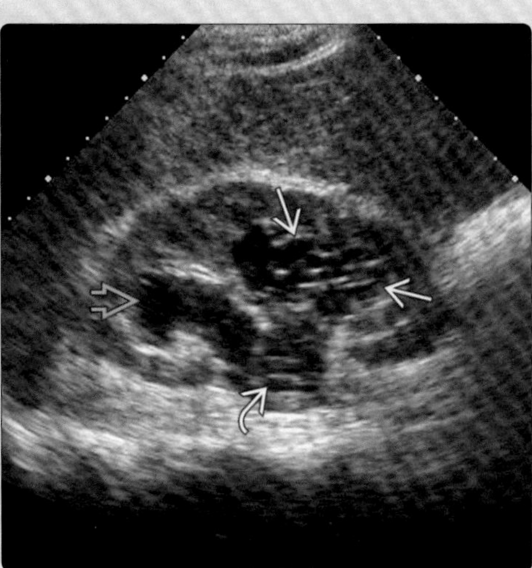

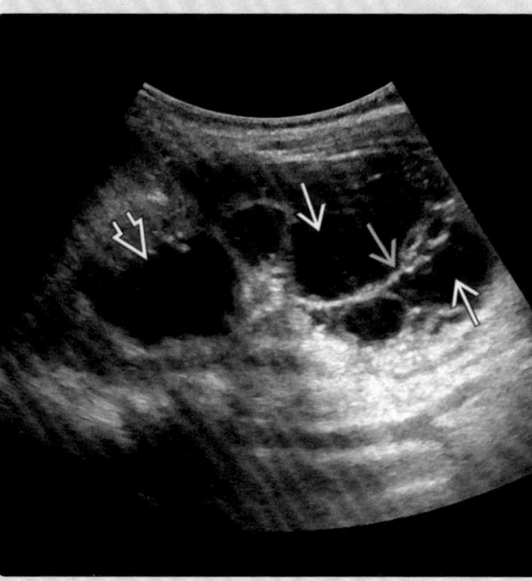

(Left) *Longitudinal view shows a right kidney MLCN. There are numerous small, anechoic cystic locules ➡ in the lower pole, separated by echogenic septa, herniating into the renal hilum ↪, with associated obstruction of the renal pelvis leading to upper pole calyectasis ⇨.* **(Right)** *Longitudinal ultrasound view of the left kidney reveals multiple large, anechoic cysts in the lower pole ➡ separated by thick septa ⇨, consistent with MLCN. The upper pole cystic structure ➡ represents calyceal dilatation secondary to mass effect from the MLCN.*

Acute Pyelonephritis

KEY FACTS

IMAGING

- Findings of acute pyelonephritis (AP) are almost always asymmetric
- Renal enlargement with loss of corticomedullary differentiation
- Geographic areas of altered echogenicity
- Urothelial thickening
- In general, ultrasound is much more sensitive for causes (obstruction) and complications (abscess) of AP than for AP itself, which is clinical diagnosis
- Many kidneys with pyelonephritis will be sonographically normal
- Foci of gas in parenchyma (rare) could indicate emphysematous pyelonephritis; treat as urologic emergency
- Microabscesses or areas of necrosis can emerge after 1-2 weeks of infection

PATHOLOGY

- Most common organism: *Escherichia coli*
- Route of spread of infection: Ascending (85%) > hematogenous (15%)
- Risk factors include obstruction, ureteric reflux, diabetes, pregnancy, lower UTI

SCANNING TIPS

- Pyelonephritis usually asymmetric; sonographic changes may be subtle in acute setting
- Focused US evaluation for ureteral stones if AP is suspected, including transvaginal images for distal ureter stones, because presence of stones would alter management
- Higher frequency linear transducers, especially in thin patients, may help identify subtle areas of involvement
- Best acoustic windows are often through liver or spleen but evaluation with different acoustic windows important for full evaluation

(Left) *Transverse US of the kidney exhibits a geographic area of increased echogenicity in the anterior interpolar region ➔ in an area of focal pyelonephritis.* **(Right)** *Longitudinal US of the kidney illustrates diffuse loss of corticomedullary differentiation, crescentic perinephric fluid ➔, and urothelial thickening ➔ in a patient with acute pyelonephritis.*

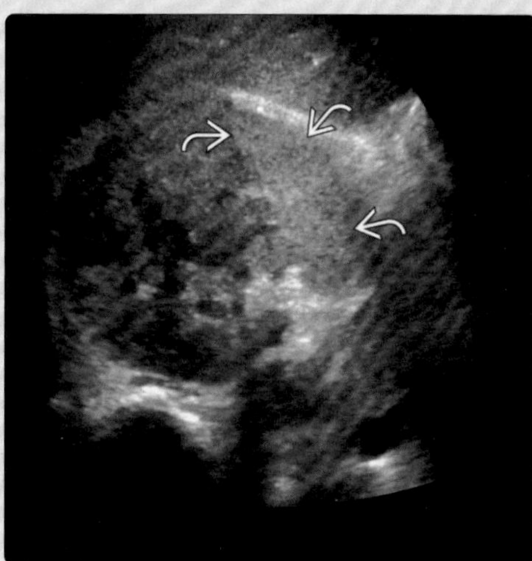

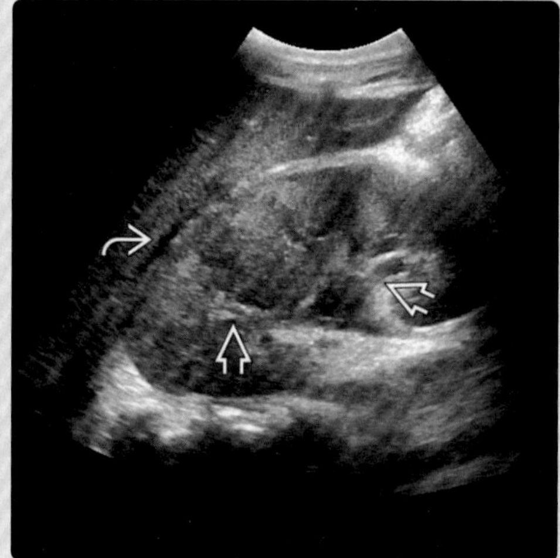

(Left) *Longitudinal US of the kidney illustrates a focal, wedge-shaped area of increased echogenicity ➔ in a patient with pyelonephritis.* **(Right)** *Longitudinal color Doppler US of the same kidney shows a focal area of diminished color flow ➔ corresponding to the hyperechoic wedge in an area of infection.*

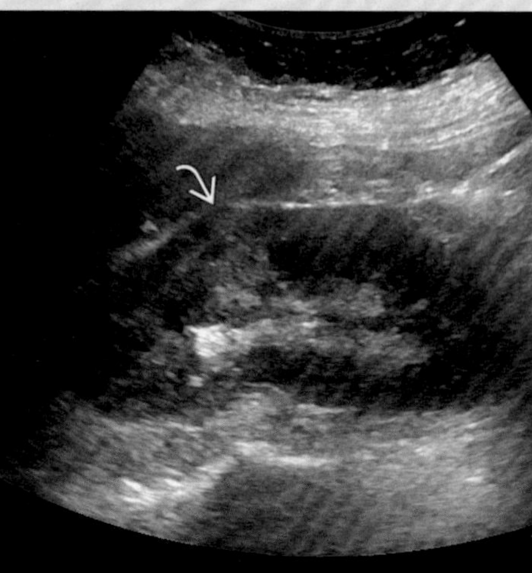

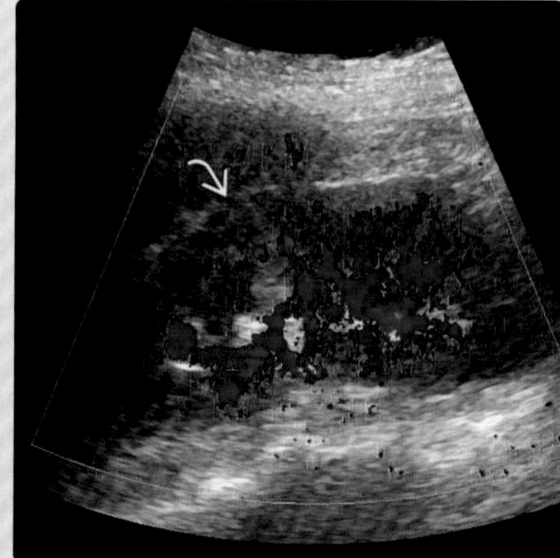

KEY FACTS

TERMINOLOGY

- Purulent &/or necrotic intraparenchymal or perinephric collection arising from unresolved pyelonephritis

IMAGING

- Complex cystic mass, may be sharply marginated or more permeative
- Rim may be hypervascular, or vessels may course to edge of lesion and stop
- Findings of pyelonephritis (renal enlargement, lack of corticomedullary differentiation, and urothelial thickening) may be present
- Internal echogenic foci with "comet tail" may represent gas-forming organisms within abscess

PATHOLOGY

- Ascending urinary tract infections (80%)
  - Corticomedullary abscess by *Escherichia coli* or *Proteus* species
- Hematogenous spread (20%)
  - Cortical abscess by *Staphylococcus aureus*

CLINICAL ISSUES

- Abscess emerges after 10-14 days of untreated or undertreated urinary tract infection, not on 1st day of symptoms
- Antibiotic therapy, usually IV ± percutaneous drainage
- Surgical drainage or nephrectomy are rarely needed

SCANNING TIPS

- Many abscesses appear mass-like and may mimic neoplasms; careful evaluation with color Doppler may show minimal internal vascularity
- Look for surrounding echogenic fat, which indicates associated inflammatory changes
- Because findings can be subtle, change scanning windows and alter phase of respiration while scanning to help attain best image

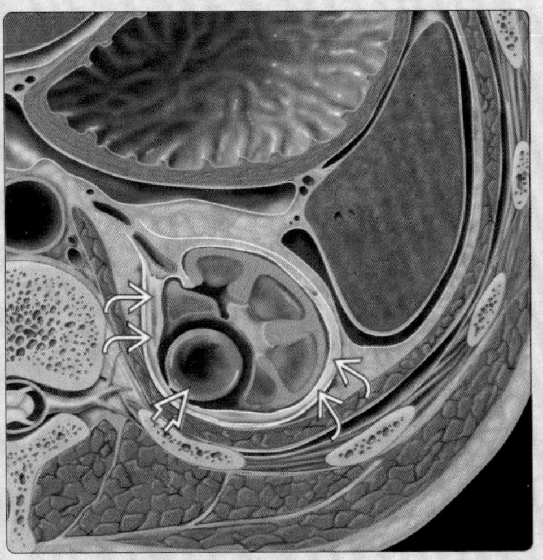

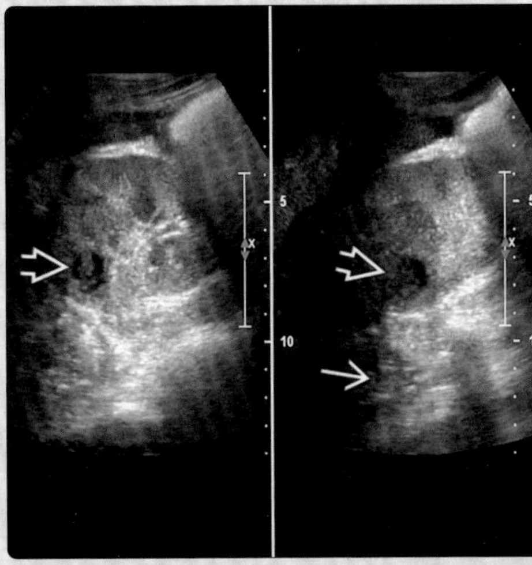

(Left) *Graphic shows a pus-filled cavity within the renal parenchyma* ➡ *and purulent material in the perinephric space* ➡. **(Right)** *Transverse and longitudinal images of the kidney show a well-circumscribed, hypoechoic mass in the posterior kidney* ➡. *Note the posterior acoustic enhancement* ➡.

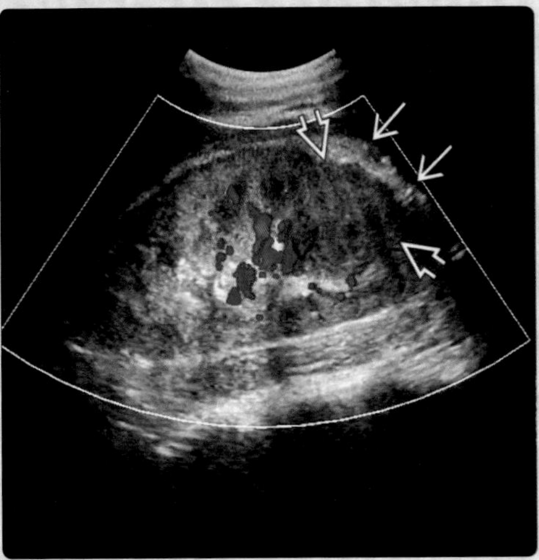

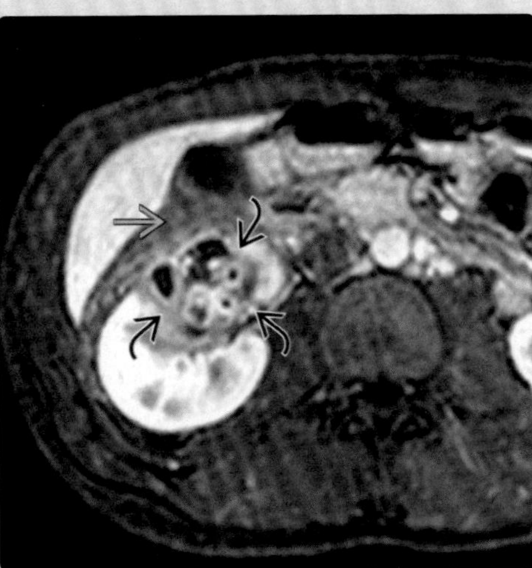

(Left) *Color Doppler US shows lack of vascularity within a lower pole hypoechoic mass (abscess collection)* ➡. *Note the echogenic surrounding fat, indicative of perinephric inflammation* ➡. **(Right)** *T1 C+ FS MR in the same patient shows an irregular lower pole mass containing multiple rim-enhancing locules* ➡. *Because of the resemblance to cystic renal neoplasm, biopsy was performed and abscess was confirmed. However, note the inflammatory change in the anterior pararenal space* ➡, *favoring infection.*

Emphysematous Pyelonephritis

KEY FACTS

TERMINOLOGY

- Gas-forming upper UTI involving renal parenchyma &/or perinephric space

IMAGING

- Highly echogenic areas within renal sinus and parenchyma with "dirty" shadowing
- Ring-down artifacts: Air bubbles trapped in fluid
- Perinephric fluid collections may be seen
- Type I (33%): Parenchymal replacement by gas, ± crescent of subcapsular or perinephric gas
- Type II (66%): Renal or perirenal fluid abscesses with bubbly gas pattern ± gas within renal pelvis
- Evaluation for psoas abscess and spinal osteomyelitis essential
- CT may help further delineate location and extent of renal and perirenal gas

TOP DIFFERENTIAL DIAGNOSES

- Emphysematous pyelitis
    - Gas limited to renal collecting system and pelvis, not parenchyma
    - Less clinically serious than emphysematous pyelonephritis, unless obstructed

PATHOLOGY

- *Escherichia coli* (68%), *Klebsiella pneumoniae* (9%)
- *Proteus mirabilis, Pseudomonas, Enterobacter, Candida, Ilostridia* species

CLINICAL ISSUES

- Extremely ill at presentation: Fever, flank pain, hyperglycemia, acidosis, dehydration, and electrolyte imbalance

SCANNING TIPS

- Gas in perinephric space or perinephric collections may obscure kidney

(Left) *Ill-defined, hyperechoic material in the posterior renal cortex causes posterior acoustic shadowing. However, the shadowing is much less dense, or obscuring, than would be expected for something like a calcification of this size.* **(Right)** *As on the transverse image, gas in the central left kidney is highly echogenic with posterior "dirty" shadowing. The renal sinus is obscured, and it is hard to differentiate emphysematous pyelonephritis from emphysematous pyelitis.*

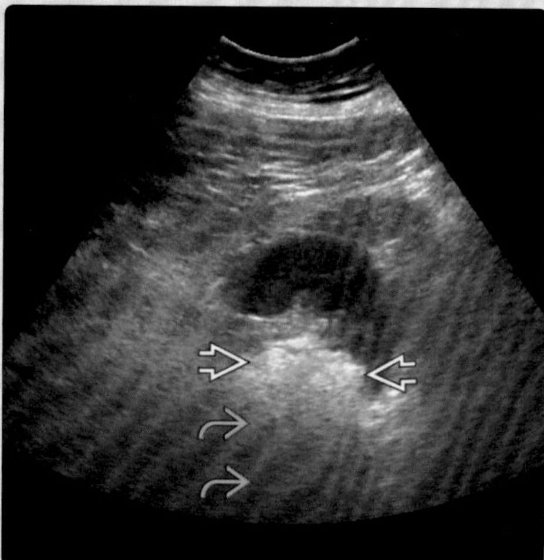

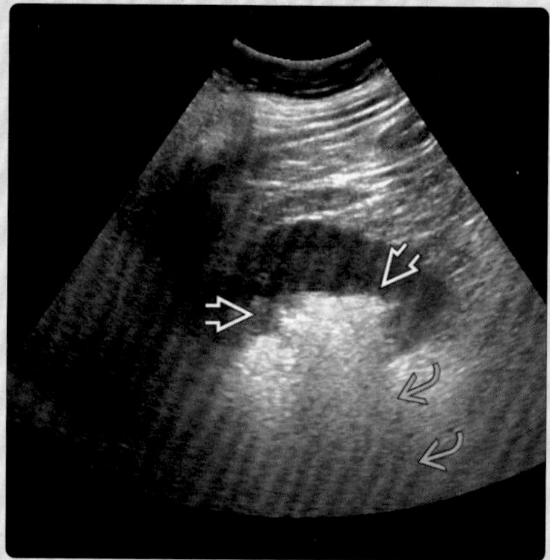

(Left) *NECT in the same patient shows gas in the renal parenchyma and pelvis. The adjacent posterior renal fascia is thickened by edema and inflammation, but there is no perinephric collection.* **(Right)** *Sagittal reconstruction CT shows a lobulated area of intraparenchymal gas with sparing of the renal sinus fat.*

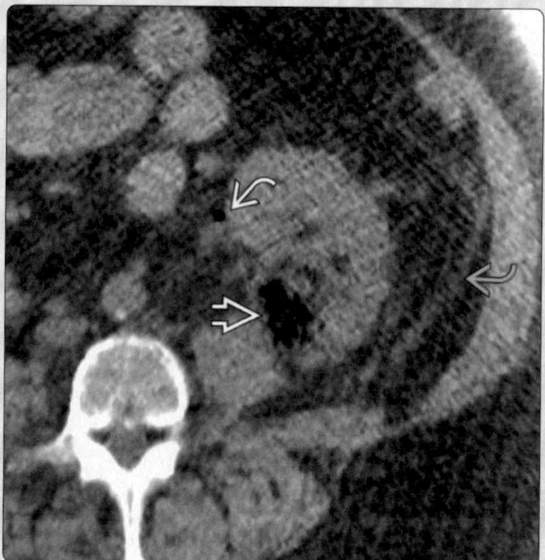

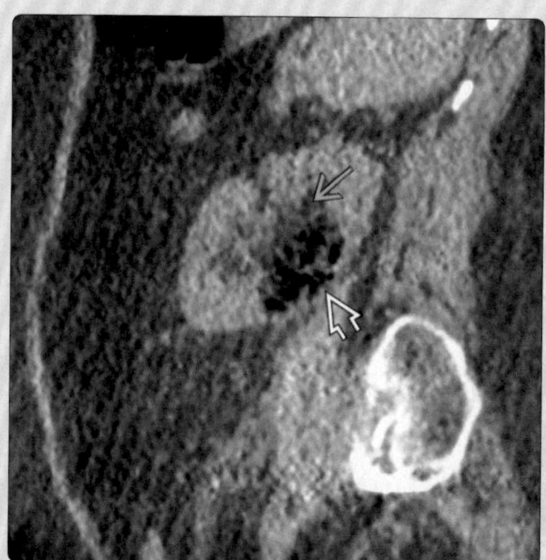

KEY FACTS

TERMINOLOGY

- Obstructed renal collecting system containing pus or infected urine

IMAGING

- Presence of mobile debris and layering of low-amplitude echoes within dilated collecting system on US

TOP DIFFERENTIAL DIAGNOSES

- Sterile hydronephrosis
- Complex renal cyst
- Urothelial carcinoma

PATHOLOGY

- Stagnant urine becomes infected, filled with white blood cells, bacteria, debris, and pus
- Chronic > acute ureteral obstruction

CLINICAL ISSUES

- Urologic emergency: Delay in diagnosis and treatment leads to irreversible renal parenchymal damage and renal failure
  - Progress to bacteremia or septic shock and can lead to 25-50% mortality
- Symptoms include fever, chills, flank pain
- Most common organism: *Escherichia Coli*
- Treatment: Percutaneous nephrostomy
- Diabetes is risk factor for worse clinical outcomes

SCANNING TIPS

- Coronal plane best demonstrates collecting system, renal contour, renal cortex, medulla, and renal vessels
- To obtain good coronal view, place probe between iliac crest and lower costal margin; start with midaxillary window then try posterior axillary line where rib spaces are wider
- Graded probe pressure may help move bowel gas away

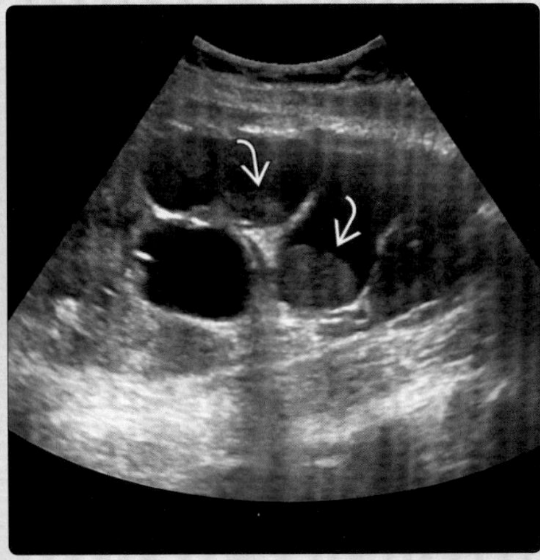

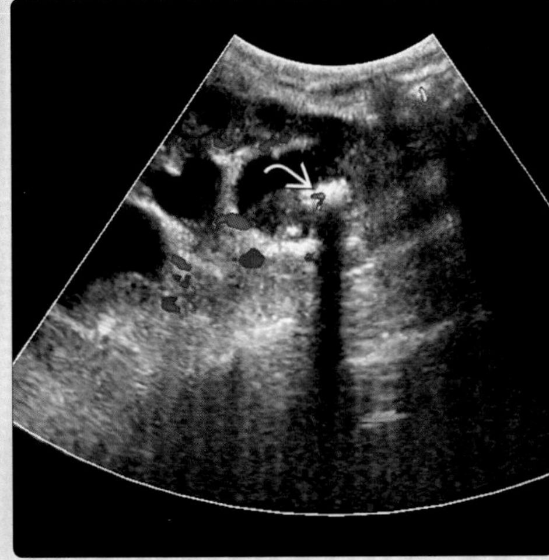

(Left) *Debris layers dependently in a mass-like fashion ➔ in this case of pyonephrosis in an adult patient with multiple sclerosis on grayscale US imaging.* **(Right)** *Note the twinkling artifact on the surface of the stone ➔ in this high-PRF Doppler US.*

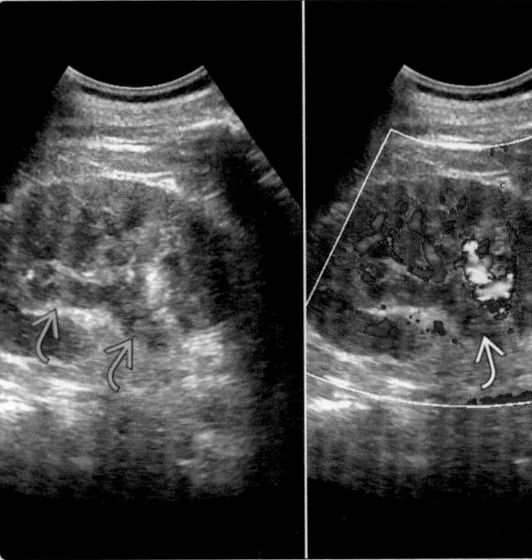

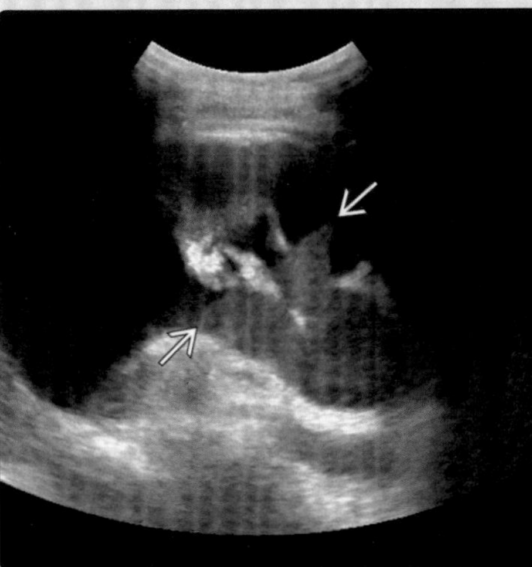

(Left) *Longitudinal grayscale and color Doppler US images show abnormal echogenic material within a mildly dilated collecting system ➔. Note absence of internal vascularity ➔, helping to distinguish this from tumor in the renal pelvis.* **(Right)** *Transverse US of the kidney with the patient in the left lateral decubitus position shows a distinct pus-urine level ➔ in the dilated system in this patient with prostate cancer and pyonephrosis.*

KEY FACTS

TERMINOLOGY

- Chronic renal inflammation usually associated with longstanding urinary calculus obstruction (75%)
- Renal parenchyma is gradually replaced by lipid-laden macrophages
- Diffuse (> 80%) and focal (< 20%) forms
- 3 stages of xanthogranulomatous pyelonephritis: Intrarenal → perirenal → perinephric ± retroperitoneal involvement

IMAGING

- Diffusely enlarged kidney with hypoechoic round masses replacing normal parenchyma on US
- "Staghorn" calculus with renal enlargement and perirenal fibrofatty proliferation
- Perinephric extension ± adjacent organs or structures may include sinus tracts or abscesses
- Multiple focal, low-attenuating renal masses with rim enhancement on CT
- Ultrasound ideal at initial investigation; CT good for assessing excretory function and retroperitoneal involvement

PATHOLOGY

- Lipid-laden, "foamy" macrophages, diffuse infiltration of plasma cells and histiocytes

CLINICAL ISSUES

- Flank pain, fever, palpable mass, and weight loss
- Rare complications: Hepatic dysfunction, extrarenal extension, fistulas
- Long-term chronic process with good prognosis if treated and rare mortality
- Antibiotic treatment is sometimes effective
- Severe disease or perinephric extension usually requires nephrectomy

(Left) *Graphic shows lower pole xanthogranulomatous pyelonephritis (XGP) with a longstanding ureteropelvic obstruction by a large staghorn stone ➔, causing replacement of parenchyma by collections of foamy macrophages ➔.* **(Right)** *Transverse color Doppler US shows a dilated collecting system ➔ with internal debris and an obstructing stone ➔ at the ureteropelvic junction. The parenchyma is replaced by cystic spaces containing debris ➔. Note the lack of vascularity in the expected region of renal parenchyma.*

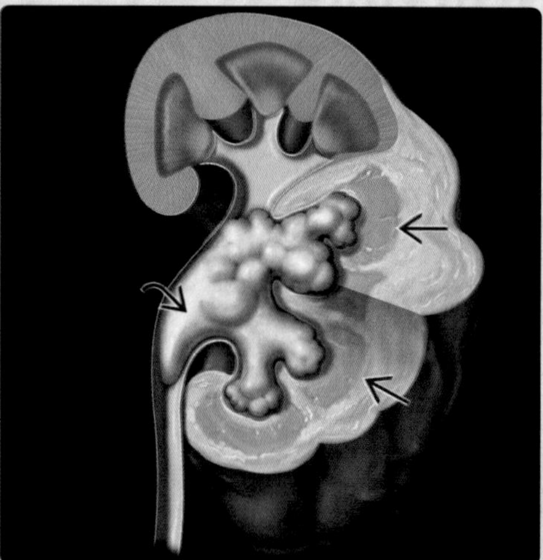

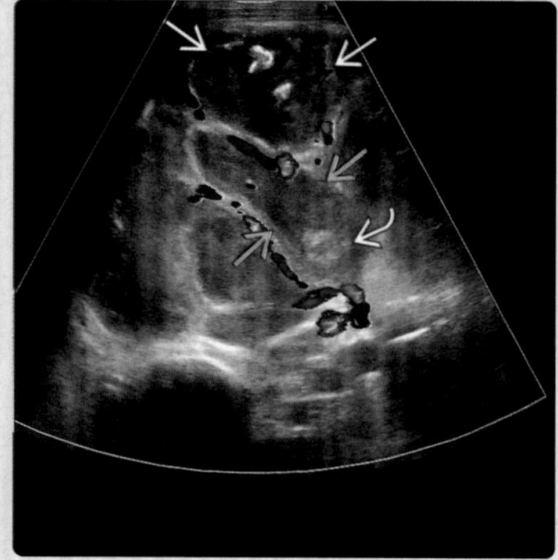

(Left) *Dual US in a patient with XGP shows cystic intraparenchymal spaces ➔ peripheral to calculi (calipers) in the central renal pelvis. Color Doppler US shows twinkling artifact ➔ with stones.* **(Right)** *Axial CECT shows a large central calculus ➔, near-complete replacement of parenchyma by cystic collections ➔, and formation of an abscess and sinus tract ➔ necessitating into adjacent abdominal wall. Proliferation of perinephric fat ➔ in this otherwise cachectic patient is a response to chronic inflammation.*

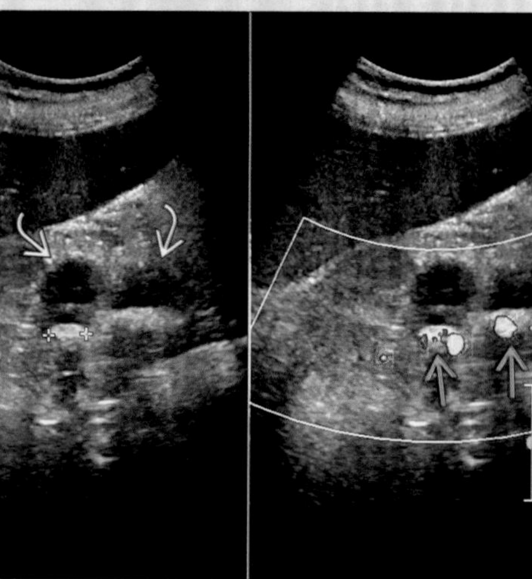

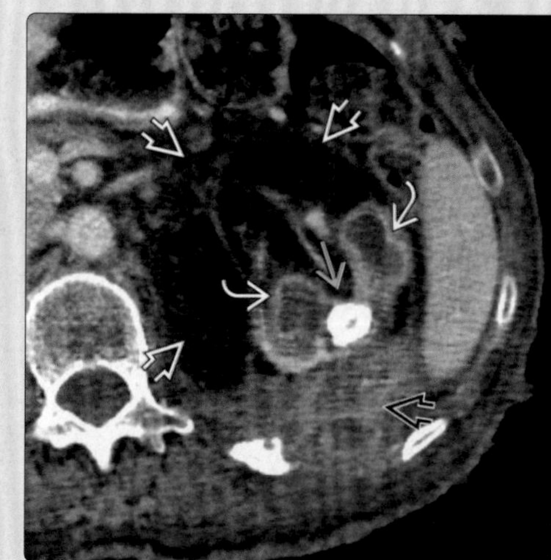

KEY FACTS

TERMINOLOGY

- Urinary tract infection by mycobacterium tuberculosis via hematogenous spread from primary focus, usually lungs

IMAGING

- Depends on stage of disease; may range from caliectasis, abscess, cavities, calcifications, and strictures in urinary tract
- Early stage: Normal kidney or small focal cortical lesions with poorly defined border ± calcification
- Progressive stage: Papillary destruction with echogenic masses near calyces
- Mural thickening ± ureteric and bladder involvement, associated stricture → hydronephrosis
- Small, fibrotic, thick-walled bladder
- Small, shrunken kidney, "paper-thin" cortex, and dystrophic calcification in collecting system
- CECT with CT urogram (CTU) is useful in diagnosing and assessing severity
- Heavily calcified caseous mass surrounded by thin parenchymal shell → "putty kidney"
- Hydrocalyces or "phantom calyx" (nonopacification of calyx due to infiltration and obliteration) proximal to infundibular stricture
- Late stages: Small, poor-functioning, scarred kidneys with dystrophic calcification
- CT (CTU) has replaced IVP for diagnosis and to rule out complications (strictures, abscess) and extrarenal manifestation
- Ultrasound useful in assessing complications (renal abscess, hydronephrosis)

TOP DIFFERENTIAL DIAGNOSES

- Papillary necrosis
- Pyonephrosis
- Xanthogranulomatous pyelonephritis
- Cystitis

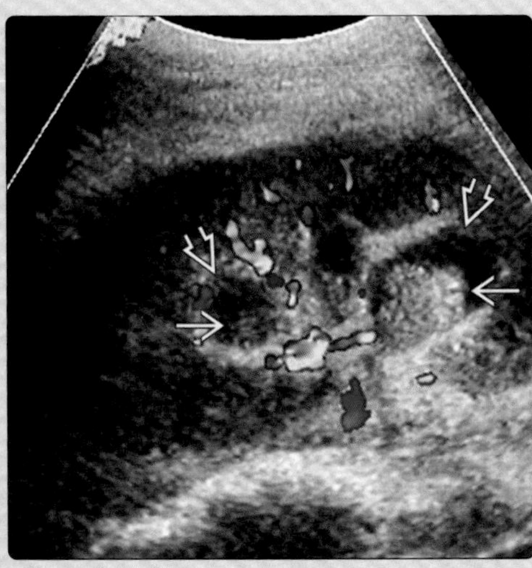

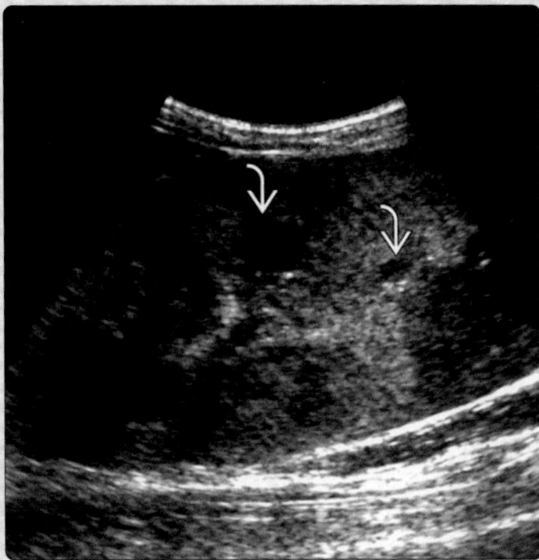

(Left) *Longitudinal transabdominal Color Doppler ultrasound shows renal tuberculosis (TB) with mild hydronephrosis ➡ and avascular internal echogenic debris ➡. (Courtesy A. Pandya, MD.)* **(Right)** *Longitudinal transabdominal ultrasound shows renal TB with distorted renal parenchyma. There are small, irregular, hypoechoic lesions ➡, which represent cavities connecting to the collecting system.*

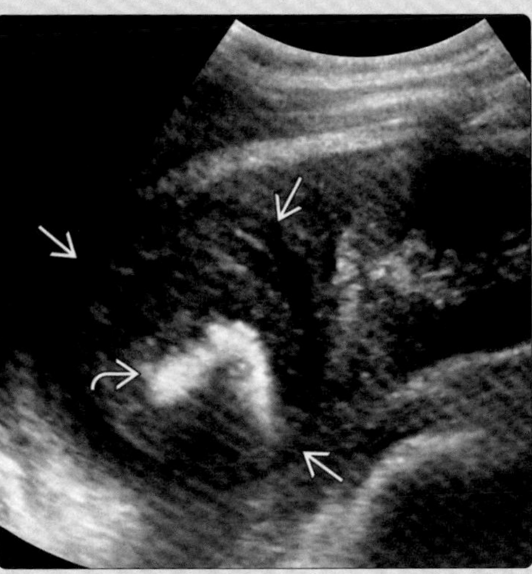

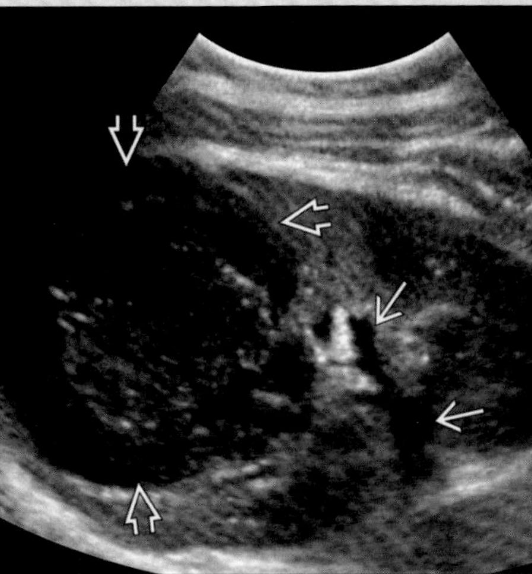

(Left) *Longitudinal transabdominal ultrasound shows renal TB with a large cavity in the upper renal pole ➡ containing gas ➡ consistent with abscess. (Courtesy A. Pandya, MD.)* **(Right)** *Longitudinal transabdominal ultrasound shows a large cavity with internal debris ➡ in the upper renal pole. Note the mild hydronephrosis ➡. (Courtesy A. Pandya, MD.)*

Renal Cell Carcinoma

KEY FACTS

IMAGING

- Variable appearance: Solid, cystic, or complex
- Solid: Homogeneous or heterogeneous, hypervascular soft tissue components and areas of necrosis, calcifications
- Cystic variant: Unilocular or multilocular, fluid-debris levels (hemorrhage and necrosis), thick and irregular wall or septations, nodules
- Use Doppler for detection of internal vascularity
- RCC may be initially detected by US, but CECT and MR are primary tools for characterization and staging
- US may be useful in characterizing complex cystic lesions, indeterminate or equivocal on CECT or MR
- Contrast-enhanced US: Option for detection of perfusion analogous to enhancement on CT/MR

TOP DIFFERENTIAL DIAGNOSES

- Renal angiomyolipoma
- Transitional cell carcinoma (urothelial carcinoma)
- Renal oncocytoma
- Renal metastases and lymphoma
- Column of Bertin

PATHOLOGY

- Most common primary renal malignancy; most sporadic but can be hereditary (~ 4%)
- Risk factors: Smoking, obesity, long-term dialysis
- Variants: Clear cell, papillary, medullary RCC

CLINICAL ISSUES

- 50-70 years of age
- M:F = 2:1; slightly higher in African Americans
- Gross hematuria (60%), flank pain (40%), palpable flank mass (30-40%); classic triad (< 10%)
- Fever, anorexia, weight loss, malaise, nausea, vomiting
- Most tumors now detected incidentally and are smaller

SCANNING TIPS

- Look for unequivocal blood flow in renal lesions, particularly in components of complex cystic lesions

(Left) *Graphic shows a lobulated, solid, upper pole renal cell carcinoma ➡. The renal vein ➡ is expanded with tumor thrombus, which extends into the inferior vena cava ➡. A 2nd tumor nodule is seen ➡.* **(Right)** *Longitudinal ultrasound in a patient with renal cell carcinoma shows a solid, slightly hyperechoic mass within the calipers. There is an incomplete hypoechoic rim ➡. Note posterior acoustic enhancement ➡; however, there was internal flow on color Doppler.*

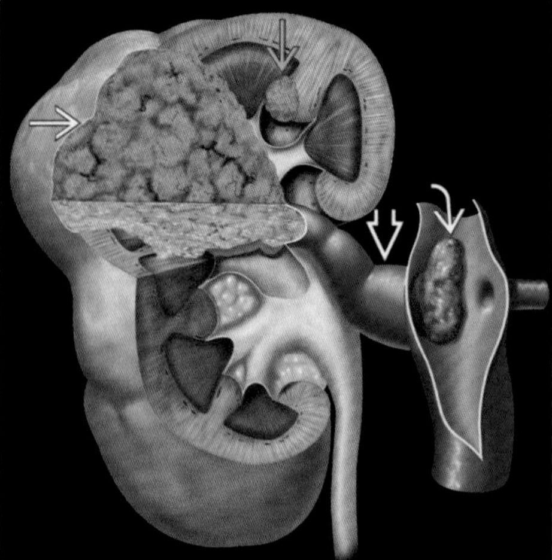

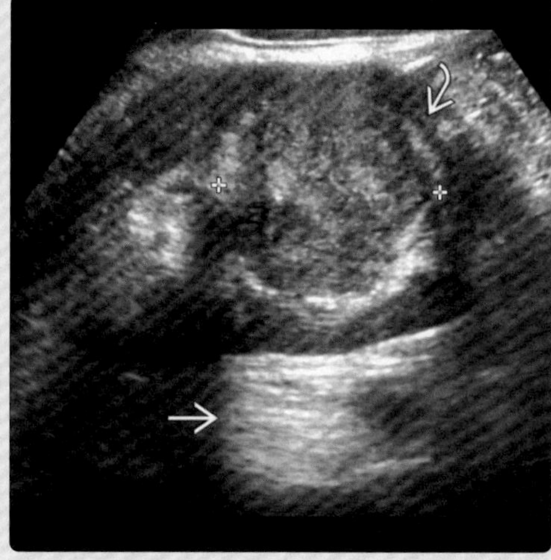

(Left) *Longitudinal ultrasound shows an exophytic, homogeneous, hypoechoic chromophobe variant renal cell carcinoma ➡ with infiltration and distortion of the renal sinus fat ➡.* **(Right)** *Transverse ultrasound of the same patient shows a solid, hypoechoic, exophytic chromophobe variant renal cell carcinoma ➡ with peripheral ➡ and internal color flow ➡.*

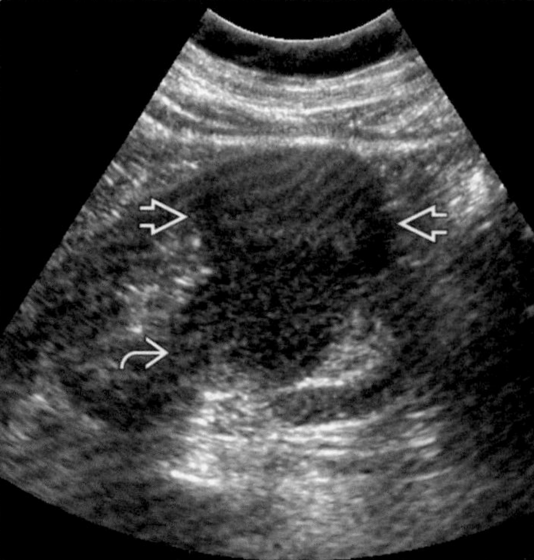

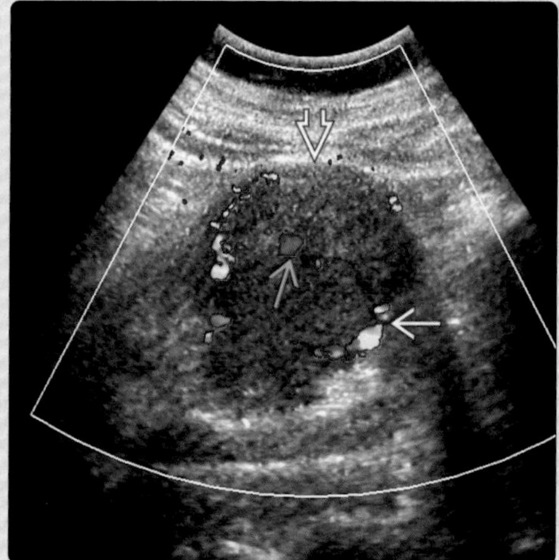

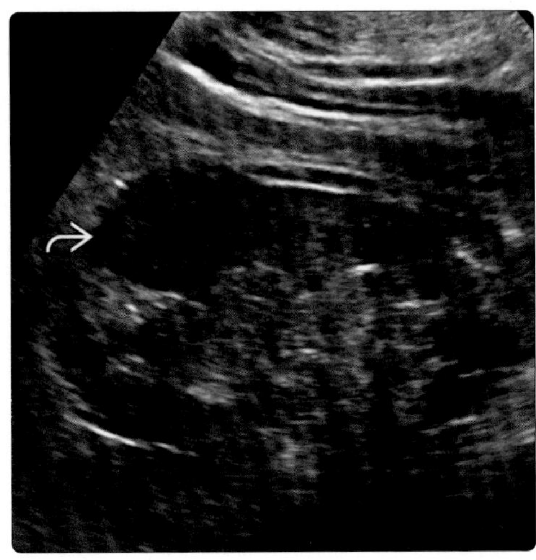

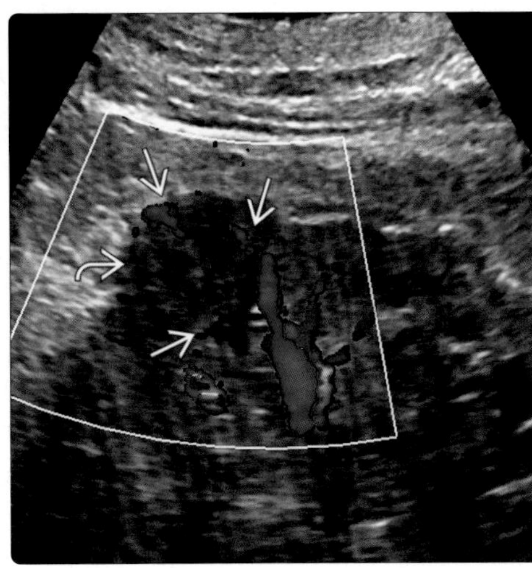

(Left) *Longitudinal ultrasound of the kidney in a patient with chronic kidney disease shows a partially exophytic hypoechoic mass that was a clear cell renal carcinoma.* **(Right)** *Longitudinal color Doppler ultrasound of the same patient with chronic kidney disease shows color flow in the partially exophytic hypoechoic mass.*

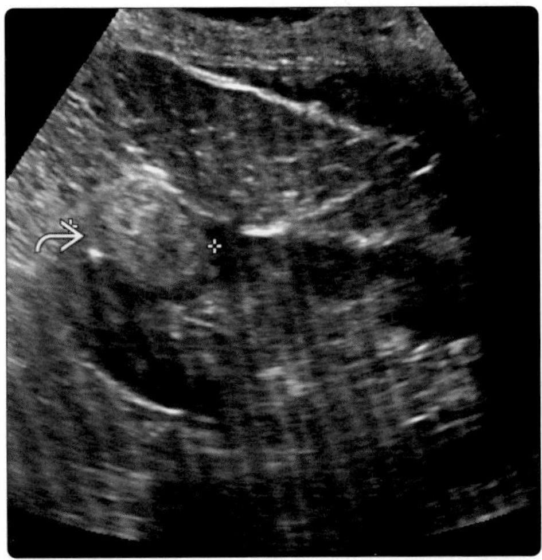

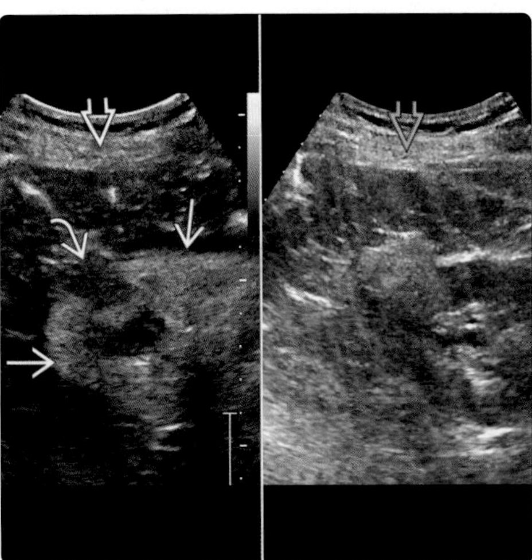

(Left) *Longitudinal ultrasound of the kidney in a patient with chronic kidney disease shows a partially exophytic hyperechoic mass.* **(Right)** *Longitudinal contrast-enhanced ultrasound of the same patient. The split screen shows the contrast image on the left with the simultaneous gray scale image on the right. There is enhancement within the mass, although to a lesser degree than normal kidney.*

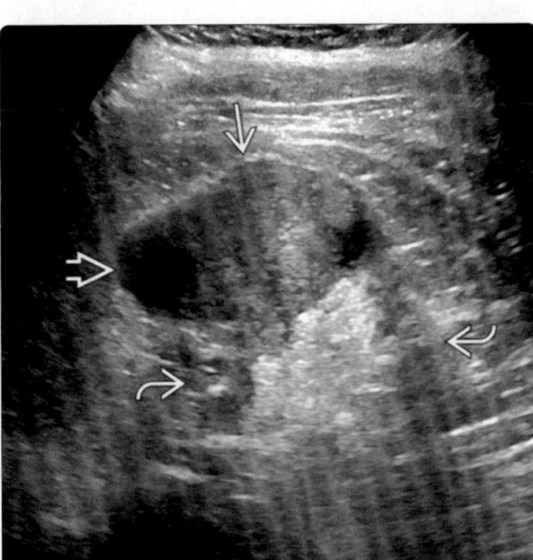

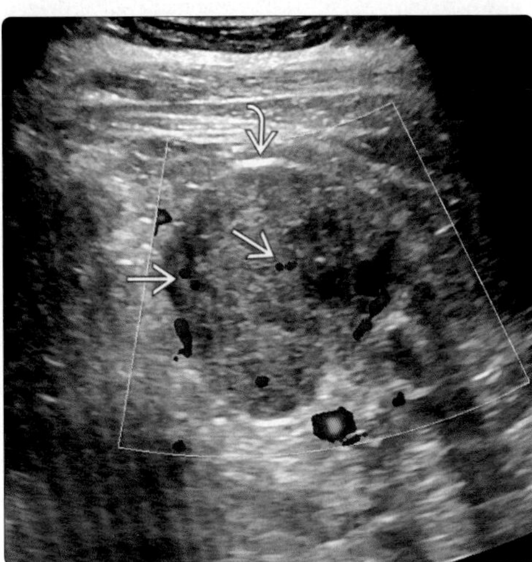

(Left) *Longitudinal ultrasound of the kidney in a patient with chronic kidney disease shows a hypoechoic mass with a cystic component arising from the kidney, which was atrophic.* **(Right)** *Transverse power Doppler ultrasound of the same patient shows color flow in the solid components of the mass. This was a papillary renal carcinoma.*

Renal Metastases

KEY FACTS

IMAGING

- Usually small and round, may be wedge-shaped
- Usually cortical; rarely disrupting renal contour or capsule
  - Large, exophytic metastases may be encountered
- Hypoechoic, hyperechoic, or sonographically occult
- Occasionally infiltrative
- Perinephric infiltration from tumor extension or hemorrhage may be seen (melanoma)
- Mostly avascular or hypovascular using low-flow Doppler settings
- Melanoma (and other hypervascular primary tumors) metastasis can be hypervascular, simulating renal carcinoma

TOP DIFFERENTIAL DIAGNOSES

- Primary renal malignancy
- Renal angiomyolipoma
- Renal cysts (complex)
- Renal lymphoma or leukemia
- Renal infection
- Renal infarction

CLINICAL ISSUES

- May have hematuria or microhematuria (12-31%)
- Most are clinically occult and found on imaging or at autopsy
- Most common malignant renal tumor at autopsy (7-13% of autopsies); 20% of patients dying of disseminated malignancy
- Most patients have metastatic tumor at other locations
- Lung cancer most common primary site followed by breast, gastric cancer, melanoma, and lymphoma
- Prognosis very poor

SCANNING TIPS

- Metastases may be subtle on ultrasound; use color Doppler at low-flow settings
- Presence of disseminated malignancy suggests metastases as cause of abnormal renal ultrasound

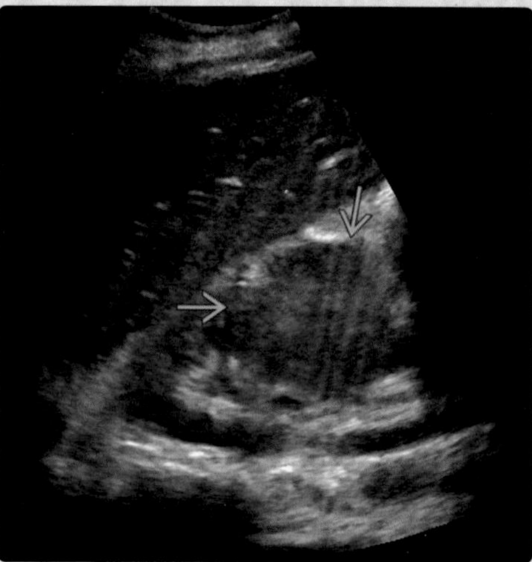

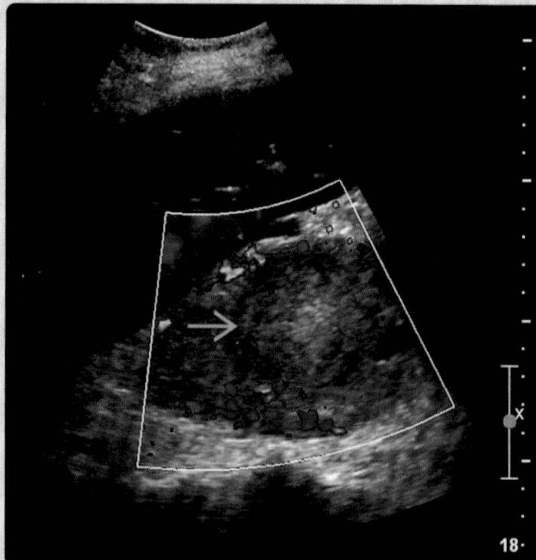

(Left) *Longitudinal ultrasound of the right kidney shows a midpole solid, homogeneous, slightly hyperechoic mass ⇒ representing metastatic melanoma. This cannot be distinguished from renal cell carcinoma.* **(Right)** *Corresponding color Doppler ultrasound shows no significant color flow within the mass ⇒. While the grayscale features are indistinguishable from renal cell carcinoma, metastases are typically hypovascular compared to renal cell carcinoma.*

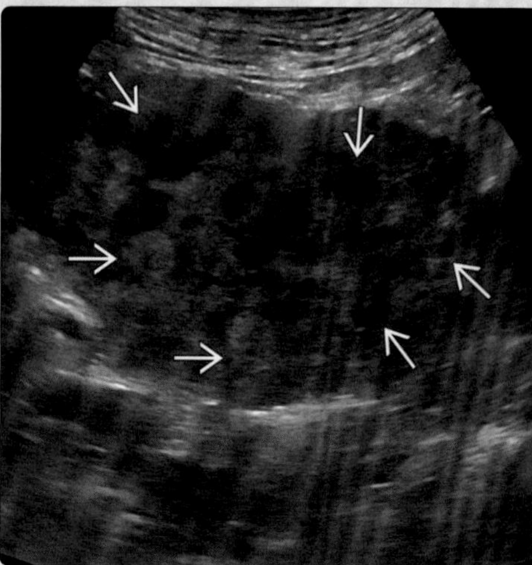

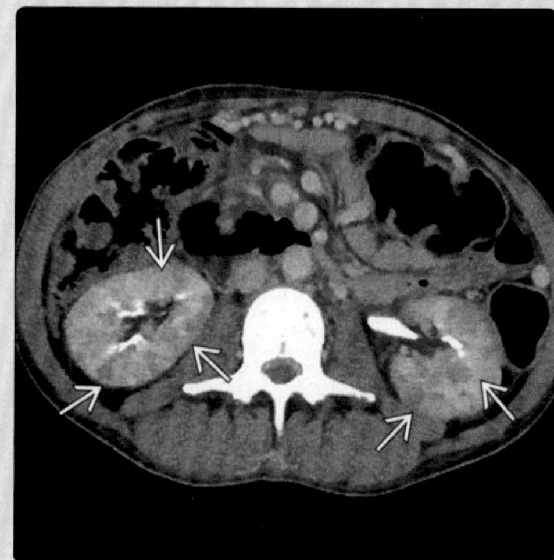

(Left) *Longitudinal ultrasound of the left kidney in a patient with a metastatic neuroendocrine tumor is shown. The kidney is abnormal with small hypoechoic and hyperechoic masses ➡.* **(Right)** *Axial CECT of the same patient shows numerous bilateral, small renal metastases ➡. These have indistinct borders but are much easier to identify on CT than ultrasound.*

Renal Angiomyolipoma

KEY FACTS

IMAGING

- Discrete renal mass with varying amounts of dysmorphic blood vessels, smooth muscle, and mature adipose tissue
- Variable size, can be very large
- Single or multiple
- Classic angiomyolipoma (AML): Lipid-rich echogenic mass with posterior acoustic shadowing
- Fat-poor subtype ("AML with minimal fat"): Usually hyperechoic but fat not detected by CT or MR
- Color Doppler: Absent from fatty component, may be present in soft tissue/vascular components

TOP DIFFERENTIAL DIAGNOSES

- Renal cell carcinoma
- Wilms tumor
- Renal oncocytoma
- Deep cortical scar with fat
- Cortical milk of calcium cyst

CLINICAL ISSUES

- Most common benign solid renal neoplasm
- 80% sporadic; prevalence: 0.2%; 4th-6th decades; usually unilateral and solitary; F:M = 3:1
- 20% associated with tuberous sclerosis complex; mean age: younger; 55-75% of these patients will have AML by 3rd decade; any subtype of AML, multiple and bilateral
- Tend to grow faster when > 4 cm
- Size > 3-4 cm or aneurysm size > 5 mm → bleeding
- Majority detected as incidental finding on imaging and asymptomatic, during screening of tuberous sclerosis
- Can present with spontaneous renal hemorrhage, which may obscure mass

SCANNING TIPS

- Echogenic masses detected by US should be further evaluated with CT or MR to confirm presence of fat

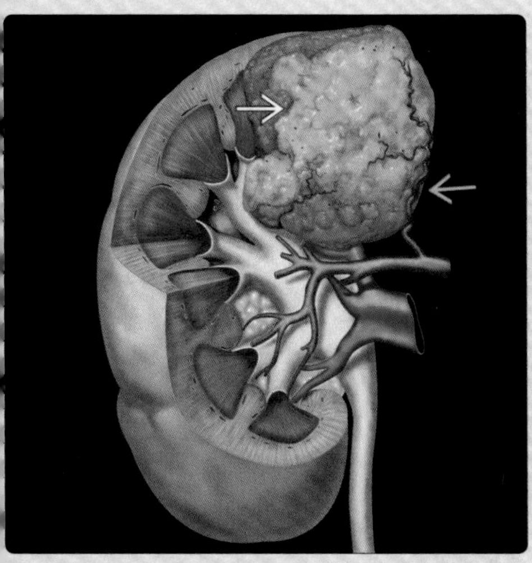

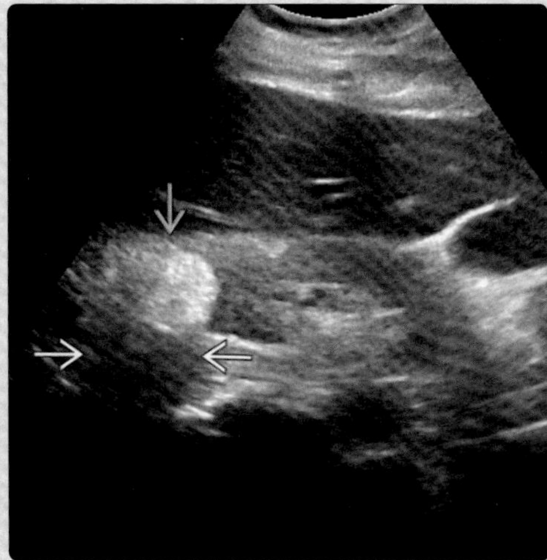

(Left) *Graphic shows a vascular renal mass containing predominantly adipose ➡ components. Note the tortuous feeding artery ➡ arising from the main renal artery.* **(Right)** *Longitudinal oblique US shows an echogenic angiomyolipoma (AML) ➡ in the upper pole of the kidney. Note the posterior acoustic shadowing ➡.*

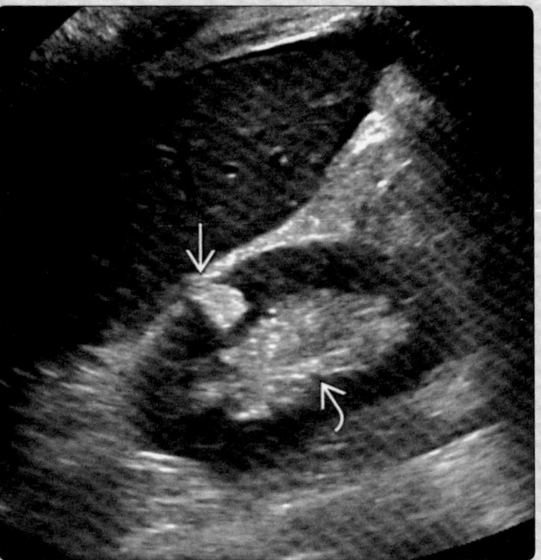

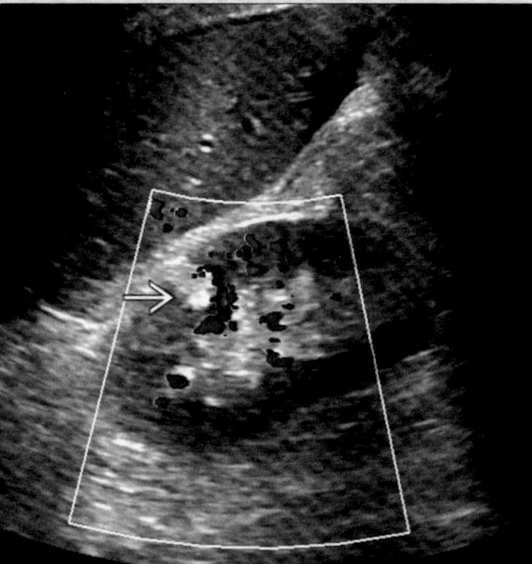

(Left) *Longitudinal US shows an echogenic AML ➡ in the anterior renal cortex of the right kidney. The echogenicity of the AML is similar to the renal sinus fat ➡.* **(Right)** *Longitudinal color Doppler US shows no detectable color flow in the AML ➡. Color flow is not expected in homogeneous lipid-rich AML.*

KEY FACTS

TERMINOLOGY

- a.k.a. transitional cell carcinoma

IMAGING

- Hypoechoic infiltrative tumor in renal pelvis or ureter
- Wall thickening or intraluminal soft tissue mass
- Papillary or sessile mass
- Secondary hydronephrosis and calyceal dilatation
- Advanced tumor: Diffusely infiltrating renal mass, invading sinus fat but with preservation of renal contour
- Hypovascular on color Doppler
- Contrast-enhanced US may be option in patients unable to have enhanced CT or MR but limited for staging

TOP DIFFERENTIAL DIAGNOSES

- Renal cell carcinoma
- Lymphoma
- Blood clot or hemonephrosis
- Other causes of obstruction or urothelial thickening

PATHOLOGY

- 10% of all renal tumors: Renal pelvis: 8%; ureter: 2%
- Multifocality with synchronous and metachronous tumors; most common in bladder
- Highest recurrence rate of any cancer
- Risk factors include: Tobacco use, chemical carcinogens, recurrent urinary infections and stones

CLINICAL ISSUES

- Gross or microscopic hematuria (70-80%), flank pain (20-40%), lumbar mass (10-20%)
- Peak incidence: 70-80 years (M:F = 3:1)

SCANNING TIPS

- Look for upper tract lesions in setting of bladder cancer
- Use color Doppler to differentiate tumor from clot/debris
- Follow dilated collecting system to point of transition and look for pathology there

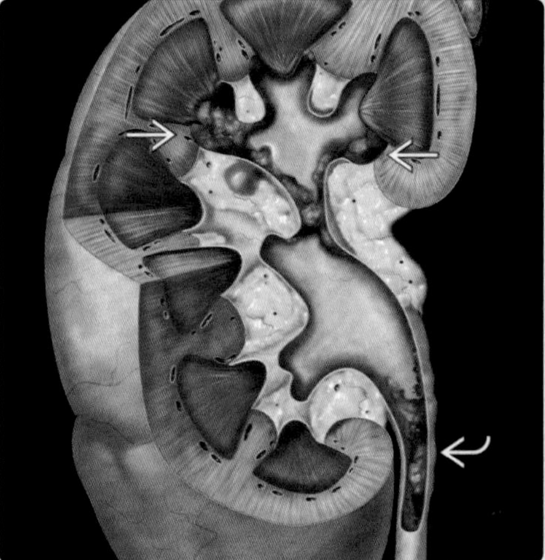

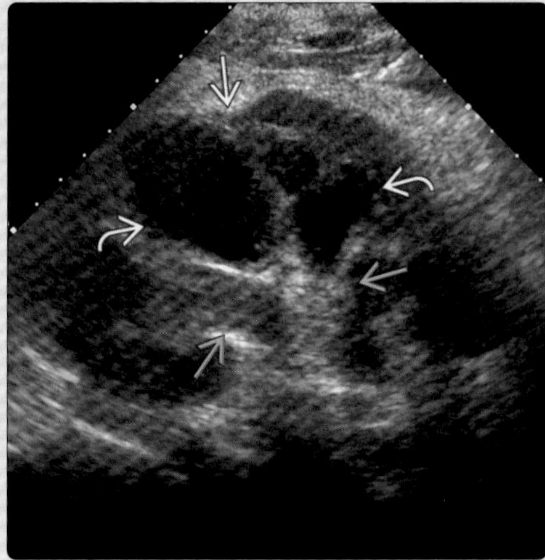

(Left) *Graphic shows a multifocal urothelial carcinoma involving the upper pole calyces ➡ and the proximal ureter ⮩. Hydronephrosis ± dilated calyces are commonly associated with upper tract urothelial carcinoma.* **(Right)** *Longitudinal ultrasound of the left kidney shows dilated calyces ⮫ and cortical loss ➡ secondary to a poorly defined hyperechoic mass in the renal pelvis ⇨. The patient had liver metastases from this upper tract urothelial cancer.*

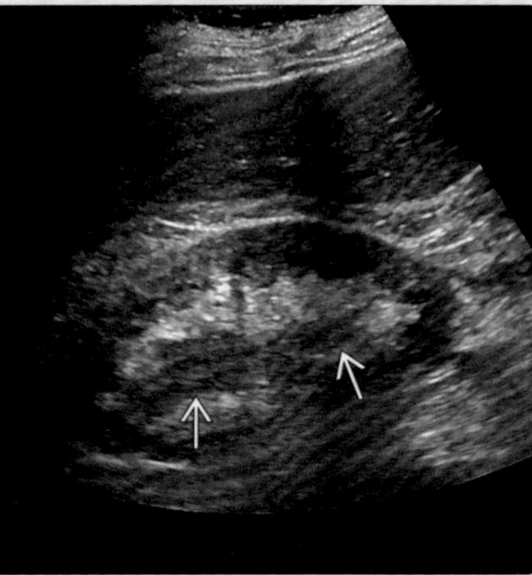

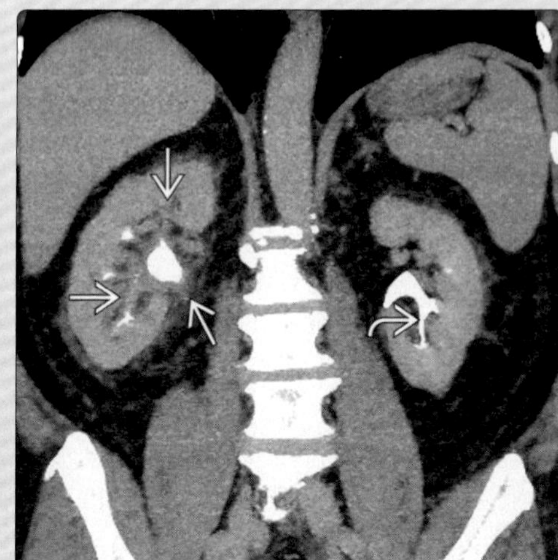

(Left) *Longitudinal ultrasound of the right kidney in a patient with hematuria is shown. There is tumor, isoechoic to the renal cortex, in the renal sinus ➡. Smaller tumors may be occult on ultrasound.* **(Right)** *Delayed phase of a contrast-enhanced CT urogram in the same patient shows diffuse, irregular wall thickening of the renal pelvis ➡ extending into the calyces. The contralateral renal pelvis ⮫ was normal.*

KEY FACTS

IMAGING

- Multiple hypoenhancing/hypoechoic masses; may see posterior acoustic enhancement from "pseudocystic" nature
- Direct extension from retroperitoneal adenopathy, associated hydronephrosis
- Solitary hypoenhancing/hypoechoic mass
- Bilateral renal enlargement
- Perinephric disease
- Vascular invasion rare
- Multisystem involvement, such as liver, lung, CNS, bone marrow, and gastrointestinal tract

TOP DIFFERENTIAL DIAGNOSES

- Renal cell carcinoma
- Transitional cell carcinoma
- Metastases

PATHOLOGY

- Primary: Involvement of kidneys only
- Secondary: Dissemination of extrarenal lymphoma by hematogenous spread (90%) or direct extension via retroperitoneal lymphatic channels
- Usually non-Hodgkin lymphoma, typically B-cell or Burkitt type; involvement by Hodgkin disease very rare

CLINICAL ISSUES

- Any age (middle aged to elderly more common)
- Symptoms related to extent of lymphoma, diffuse tumor may cause functional renal impairment
- Other complications: Renal or perinephric hemorrhage, renal obstruction, renovascular hypertension

SCANNING TIPS

- Look for extrarenal nodal and other organ disease
- Optimize color sensitivity to detect flow in markedly hypoechoic masses

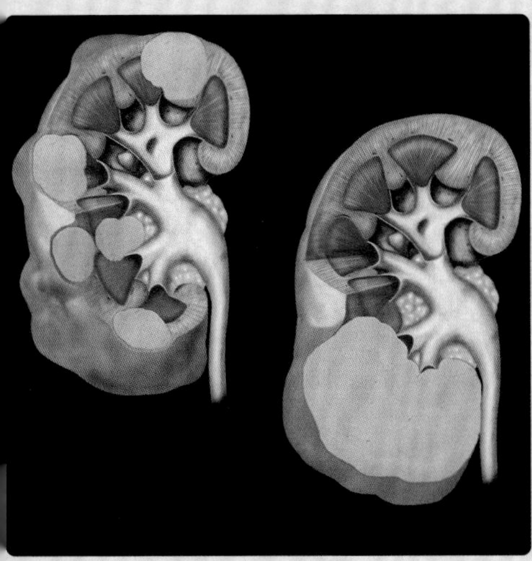

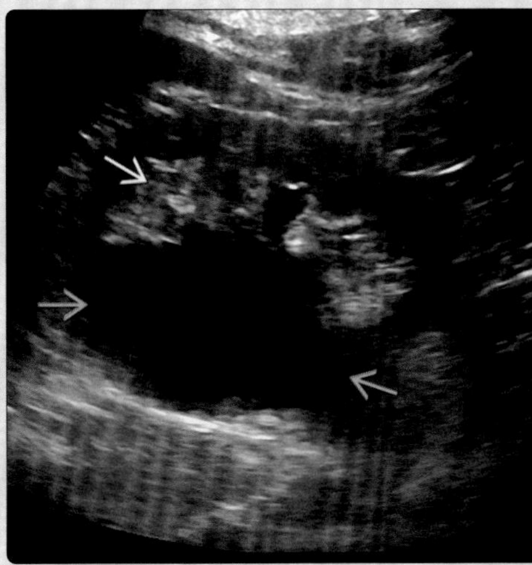

(Left) *Graphic shows different manifestations of renal lymphoma. Multiple masses are depicted in variable locations in renal parenchyma (left), whereas a solitary mass replaces a lobar segment (right).* **(Right)** *US shows a markedly hypoechoic mass ⇒ medial to the left kidney. The mass infiltrates the sinus fat ➡. It could be misinterpreted as being cystic, but there are internal echoes. Color Doppler should be used to find internal vascularity.*

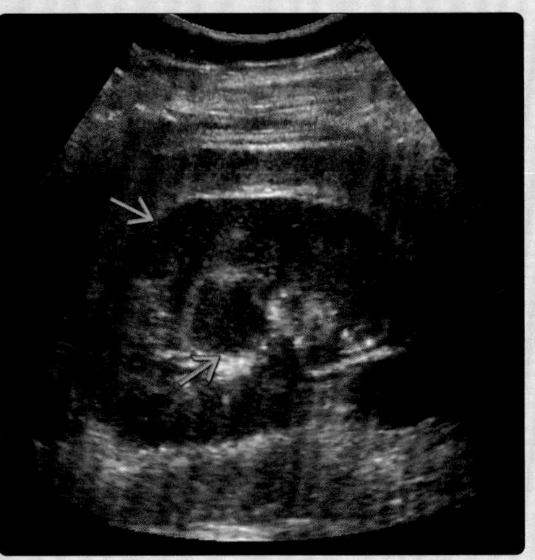

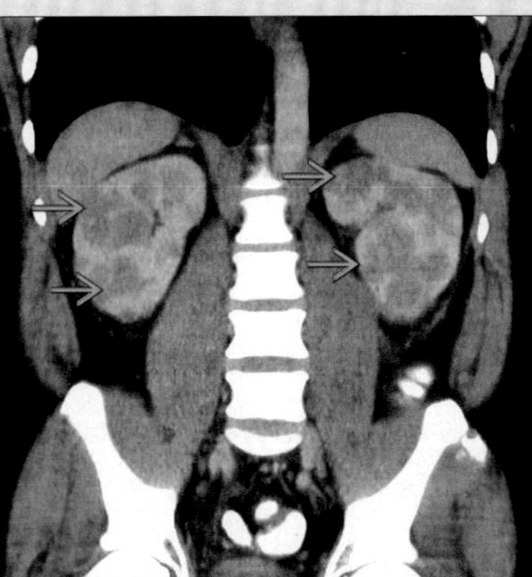

(Left) *Longitudinal US shows an enlarged right kidney with loss of normal morphology. There are multiple ill-defined, solid, hypoechoic masses ⇒ secondary to Burkitt lymphoma.* **(Right)** *Portal-phase CECT in the coronal plane of the same patient with Burkitt lymphoma shows multiple hypodense deposits of lymphoma in both kidneys ⇒. The masses are distributed in the cortex and medulla.*

Renal Artery Stenosis

KEY FACTS

TERMINOLOGY

- Hemodynamically significant narrowing of renal artery (RA)

IMAGING

- Poststenotic "jet" and turbulent flow on color Doppler
  - Peak systolic velocity in and immediately distal to stenosis ≥ 180-200 cm/s
- Diminished downstream systolic peaks
  - Abnormally low peak systolic velocity in arcuate arteries with diminished resistive indices
  - Tardus et parvus waveform shape
    - Low resistive index < 0.5 due to dampened systolic peaks and normal diastolic flow
    - Acceleration time (time to peak systole) > 0.07 s
    - Acceleration index < 3 m/s^2

PATHOLOGY

- Atherosclerosis: Ostium or proximal 2 cm of RA
- Fibromuscular dysplasia: Mid or distal main RA
- Aortic dissection or aneurysm (RA compression)
- Thromboembolism
- Other vasculitides
- Retroperitoneal fibrosis
- Trauma with RA dissection

SCANNING TIPS

- Scanning in decubitus or oblique position in coronal plane through posterior axillary line will allow improved Doppler evaluation of segmental arteries
- Evaluation of RA ostium can be best achieved via epigastric window; use superior mesenteric artery or renal vein as landmarks; if this window is obscured by bowel gas, left lateral decubitus position with probe in sagittal orientation from below ribs may be used
- Right RA can be seen arising from aorta via longitudinal transhepatic view; by angling probe, both RAs can be seen arising from aorta in this view, creating "banana peel" view, which demonstrates both RA origins in 1 image

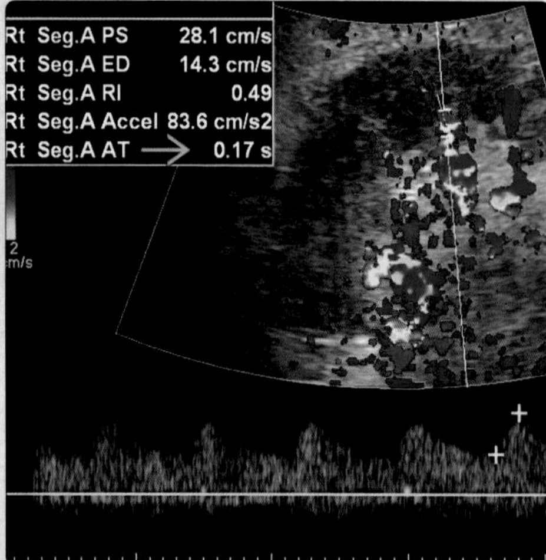

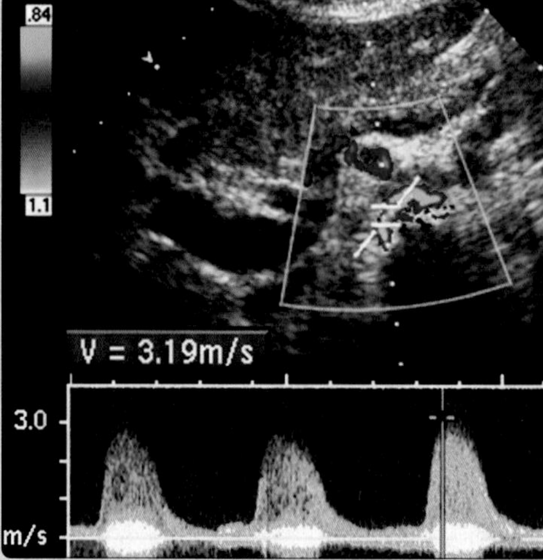

(Left) *Renal artery stenosis and tardus et parvus waveform due to aortic dissection are shown. Note the prolonged acceleration time ➙.* **(Right)** *Spectral Doppler ultrasound shows a peak systolic velocity of 319 cm/s at the location of aliasing, consistent with high-grade stenosis. The renal:aortic ratio was 4.0.*

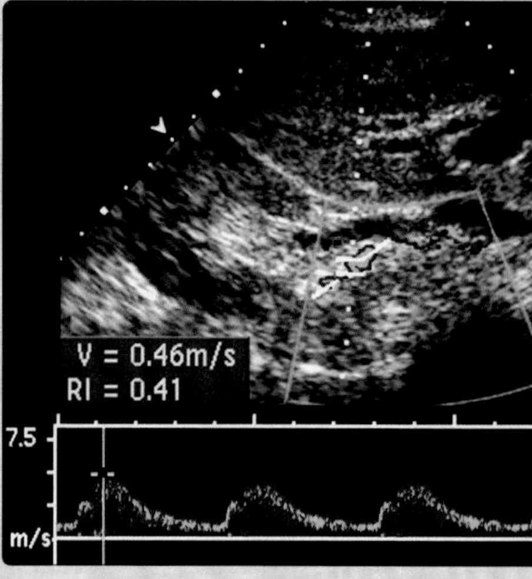

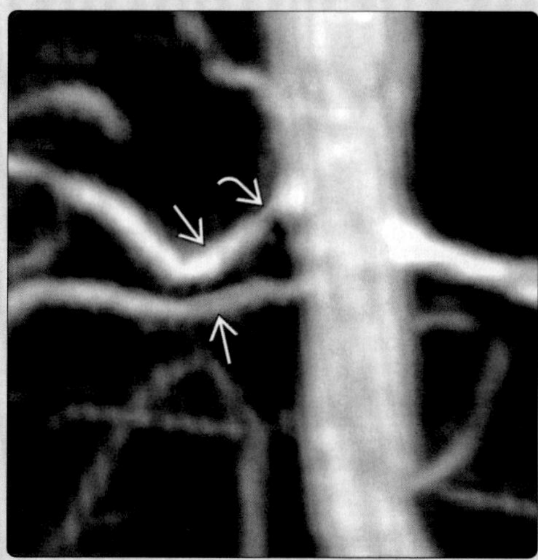

(Left) *Transverse spectral Doppler ultrasound in the same patient illustrates diminished systolic peaks and resistive indices < 0.5 distal to the right renal artery stenosis.* **(Right)** *Oblique maximum intensity projection from MRA shows duplicated right renal arteries ➡ with the more superior exhibiting a significant stenosis ➘. It is easy to envision why renal artery duplication is often missed with ultrasound and complicates assessment of intrarenal flow dynamics.*

KEY FACTS

TERMINOLOGY

- Clot formation in renal vein

IMAGING

- Unilateral > bilateral
- Kidney enlarged acutely in 75% cases
- Renal vein dilated acutely
- Possible inferior vena cava (IVC) thrombus extension
- **Altered renal artery spectral waveforms**
  - ↑ systolic pulsatility (narrow, sharp systolic peaks)
  - Persistent retrograde diastolic flow

PATHOLOGY

- Nephrotic syndrome: Most common cause of renal vein thrombosis in adults
- Hypovolemia/renal hypoperfusion: Most common cause of renal vein thrombosis in children
- Risk in neonates is associated with fetal distress, perinatal asphyxia, diabetic mothers, and volume contraction

CLINICAL ISSUES

- Outcome depends on cause, time to diagnosis, duration of occlusion, recanalization, collateralization
- Prognosis overall good; frequent spontaneous recovery
- Anticoagulation: Heparin then Coumadin or low-molecular-weight heparin for maintenance
- Thrombolysis/surgical thrombectomy: Heroic measure for life-threatening situations
- Suprarenal caval filter (IVC thrombus)

SCANNING TIPS

- Renal vein can be scanned from flank or epigastric window; flank window is more frequently used because it is less affected by body habitus and has fewer surrounding vessels
- Do not mistake splenic vein for left renal vein (when using epigastric window)
  - Splenic vein **anterior** to superior mesenteric artery
  - Left renal vein **posterior** to superior mesenteric artery

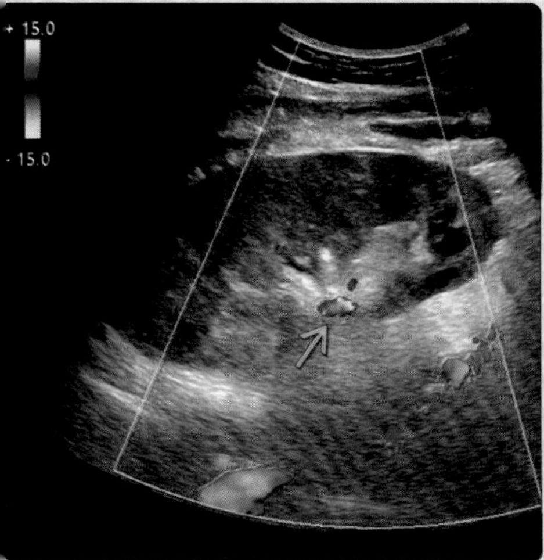

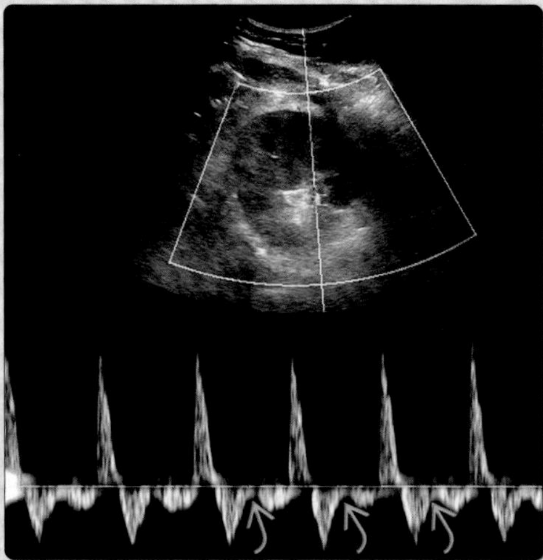

(Left) *Longitudinal color Doppler ultrasound of a renal transplant on postoperative day 1 reveals no detectable parenchymal vascularity. The only area of detectable vascularity is an arterial signal at the hilum ➡.* **(Right)** *Spectral Doppler in the same patient reveals pandiastolic reversal of flow ➡ in the main renal artery, which occurred secondary to acute renal vein thrombosis. Renal vein patency could not be restored in this patient, and the patient required explantation on day 3.*

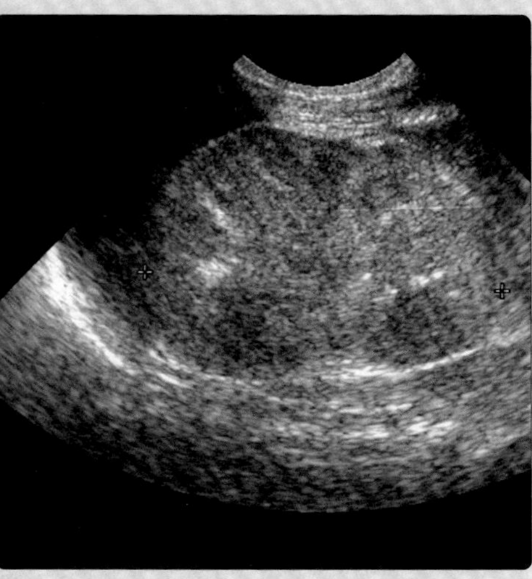

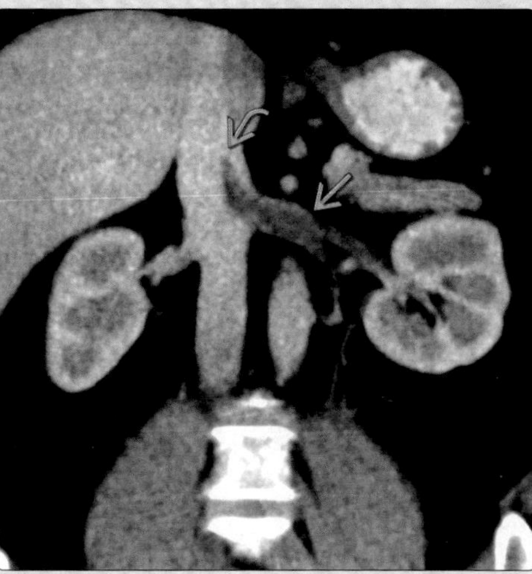

(Left) *Longitudinal ultrasound of the left kidney in a premature infant shows an edematous and nearly featureless kidney caused by acute renal vein thrombosis.* **(Right)** *Coronal reformatted CT in a patient with nephrotic syndrome shows diffuse left renal vein thrombosis ➡ with extension into the inferior vena cava ➡. This patient later suffered a small pulmonary embolism.*

Renal Infarct

KEY FACTS

TERMINOLOGY

- Global or focal renal hypoperfusion → tissue ischemia and eventually, parenchymal loss

IMAGING

- ± alteration in grayscale appearance with ↓ corticomedullary differentiation
- Focally diminished or absent Doppler flow
- May involve all or part of 1 kidney
- Insults to accessory renal arteries tend to cause polar infarcts
- Wedge-shaped, corresponding to vascular territory in kidney
- May be hypoechoic or hyperechoic, depending on timing
- When focal, tends to be wedge-shaped and extend all the way from hilum to capsule
- Focal or global loss of parenchymal flow

PATHOLOGY

- Arterial disease: Trauma, atherosclerosis, vasculitis, dissection
- Embolism: Endocarditis, arrhythmias with clot
- Thrombosis: Trauma or hypercoagulability
- Iatrogenic: Small polar arteries may be sacrificed in AAA repair or transplant harvest

SCANNING TIPS

- Scanning in lateral decubitus or oblique position in coronal scan plane through posterior axillary line results in shorter Doppler distance and improved color Doppler sensitivity
- Make sure to scan kidneys in horizontal presentation such that both upper pole and lower poles are located at similar depth from transducer; this will ensure entire kidney is interrogated equally with color Doppler

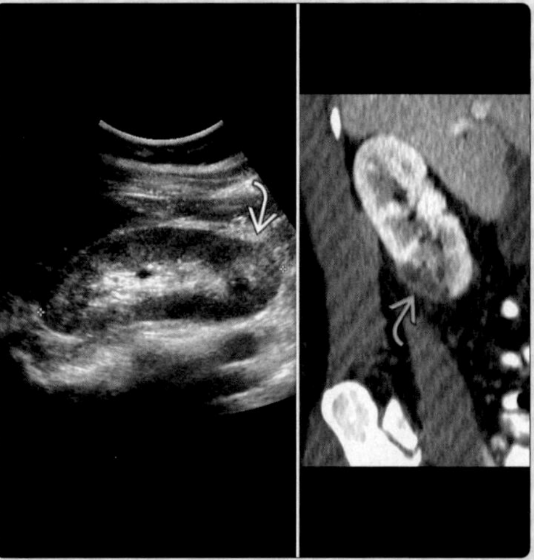

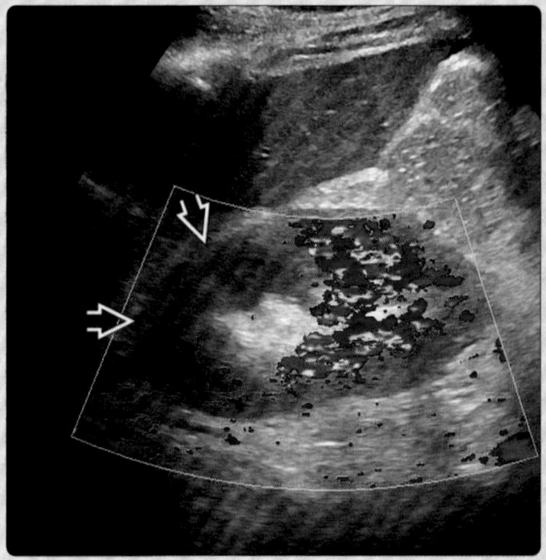

(Left) *US shows a subtle, wedge-shaped, hyperechoic infarct ➡ in the lower pole of the right kidney in a patient with dilated cardiomyopathy. Correlative CECT demonstrates the corresponding enhancement defect ➡. Note the preserved capsular enhancement, a.k.a. the cortical rim sign, due to patent capsular arteries that perfuse the capsule.* **(Right)** *Absent color Doppler flow ➡ is shown in the upper pole of a patient with segmental renal infarct.*

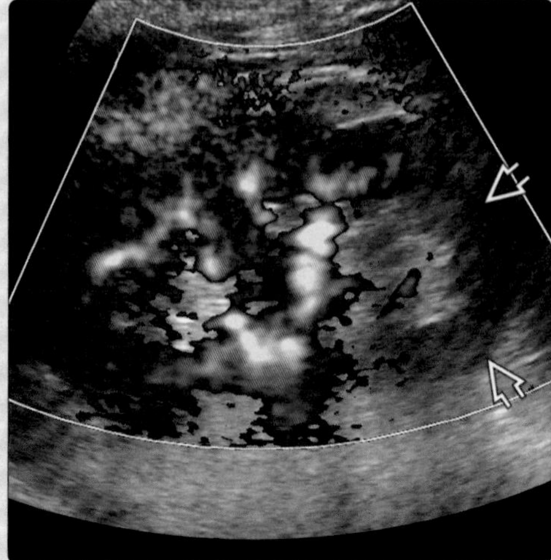

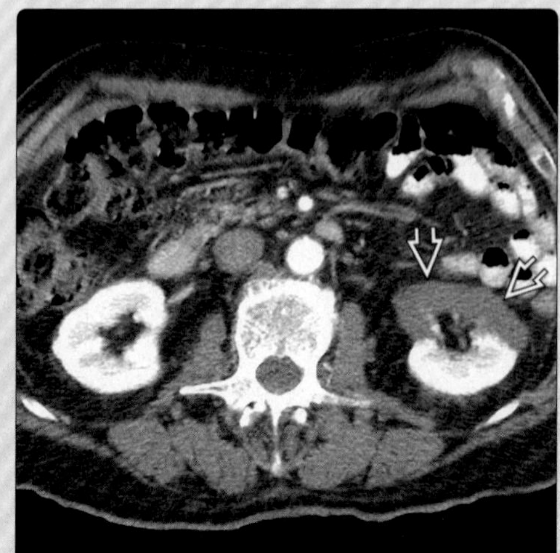

(Left) *Absent power Doppler flow ➡ is shown in the lower pole of a patient with renal infarct from atrial fibrillation. Power Doppler is most sensitive for slow flow and should be used as a confirmatory test when infarct is suspected.* **(Right)** *CECT in the same patient shows absent perfusion ➡ in the anterior cortex of the kidney.*

KEY FACTS

TERMINOLOGY

- Hemorrhagic collection in perinephric spaces: Subcapsular, perirenal, anterior and posterior pararenal

IMAGING

- Avascular solid or cystic masses in 1 or more perinephric spaces
- Echogenicity of blood changes over time
- Sonographic features vary over time
  - Acute: Highly echogenic perinephric mass
  - Subacute: Partial liquefaction, echogenic debris, retractile clot with thick septa
  - Chronic: May be almost anechoic

TOP DIFFERENTIAL DIAGNOSES

- Lymphoma infiltration
- Cystic lymphangioma
- Perinephric abscess

PATHOLOGY

- Causes include trauma, renal biopsy, renal cyst or tumor rupture, anticoagulation, aneurysm rupture

CLINICAL ISSUES

- Hematoma without underlying significant pathology usually resolves spontaneously
- Flank pain, often severe, palpable mass, shock
- Subcapsular hematoma may cause hypertension due to renin-angiotensin-aldosterone cascade (Page kidney)

SCANNING TIPS

- Look for underlying malignancy, which can often be cause of spontaneous perinephric hematoma
- Use power Doppler to show perinephric hematoma is avascular and to distinguish from adjacent renal cortex
- Perinephric fat in diabetic patients (often hypoechoic) may mimic perinephric hematoma; compare with contralateral side to demonstrate bilaterality

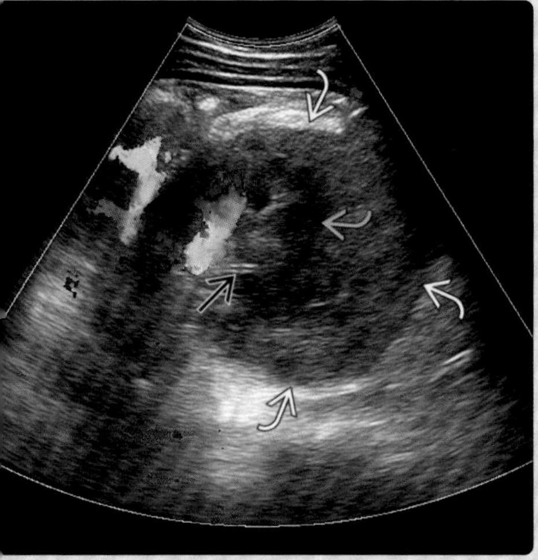

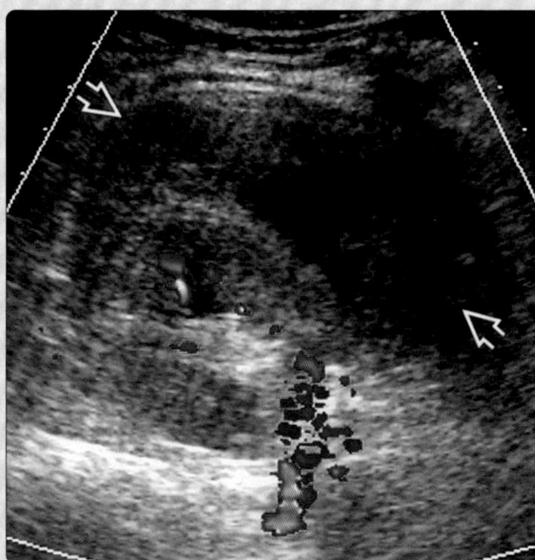

(Left) *Transverse color Doppler US of a 6 year old after stent placement ➡ shows a grossly enlarged renal contour ➡ due to large echogenic perinephric hematoma. The relatively hypoechoic kidney is seen in the center of the mass ➡, demonstrating how hyperechoic acute blood can obscure normal structures.* **(Right)** *Transverse color Doppler US shows a large, spontaneous perinephric hematoma with mixed echogenicity ➡. Note occult RCC must be considered in spontaneous hemorrhage.*

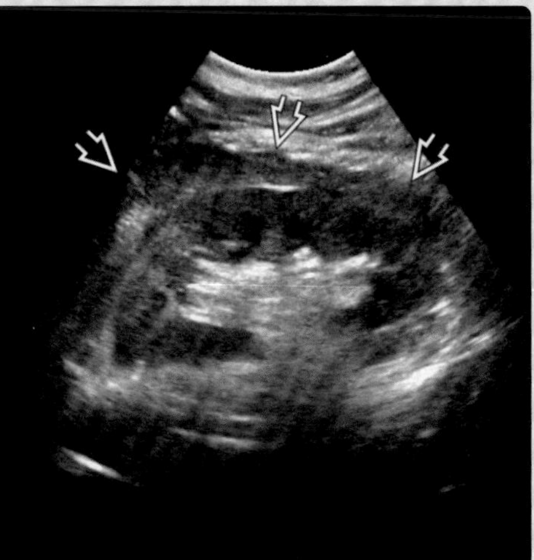

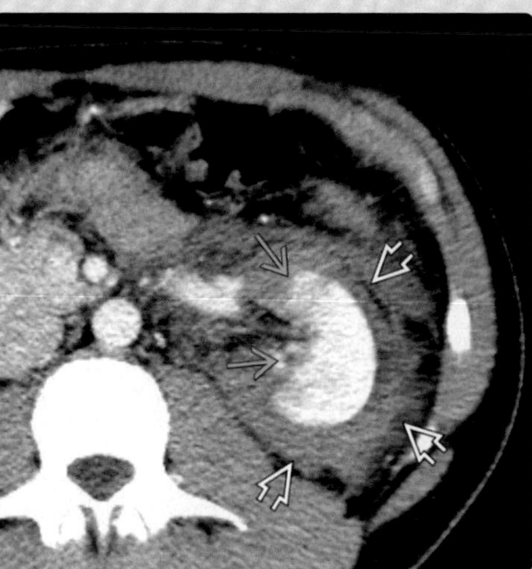

(Left) *Longitudinal US in a young man with left flank pain after collision during a soccer game illustrates a thick, irregular soft tissue rind ➡ of blood surrounding the left kidney.* **(Right)** *CT confirms an extensive perinephric hematoma ➡ in the same patient, with associated renal lacerations ➡.*

Bladder Carcinoma

KEY FACTS

TERMINOLOGY

- Malignant tumor of bladder [95% transitional cell (urothelial) carcinoma]

IMAGING

- Focal bladder wall thickening with intraluminal extension as mass
- Grayscale US: Immobile polypoidal or broad-based mass along bladder wall, may present as focal wall thickening
  - May see associated calcification
- Color Doppler US shows increased vascularity in large tumors; power Doppler more sensitive in detection of vascularity in small tumors
  - Useful for bladder tumor screening in patients with schistosomiasis, tumor within diverticulum
- ± enlarged (> 10 mm) metastatic lymph nodes

TOP DIFFERENTIAL DIAGNOSES

- Benign prostatic hypertrophy
- Bladder debris &/or blood clot
- Extrinsic tumor/mass
- Bladder inflammation

PATHOLOGY

- Superficial (70-80%) and are usually papillary (70%)

CLINICAL ISSUES

- Painless hematuria
- If tumor near UVJ, may cause hydronephrosis

SCANNING TIPS

- Check kidneys, ureters for synchronous and metachronous tumors
- Optimize color and power Doppler frequency and scale to demonstrate subtle vascularity
- Roll patient or ask patient to cough to demonstrate if bladder lesion is attached to wall
- Layering debris or blood clot often present and may obscure delineation of tumor

(Left) *Graphic shows an irregular bladder tumor ⇨ infiltrating beyond the muscular layer of the bladder wall and invading the right seminal vesicle ⇨. There is a hematogenous metastasis to the right pubic symphysis ⇨.* **(Right)** *Transverse and longitudinal transabdominal US of the bladder shows a broad-based, immobile, polypoidal mass (bladder transitional cell cancer) ➡.*

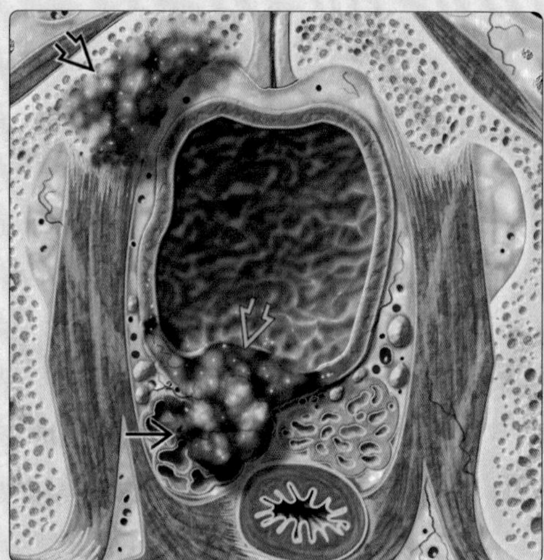

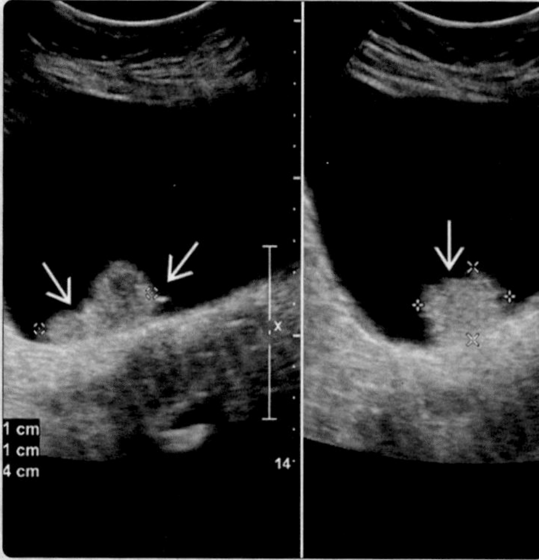

(Left) *Transverse transabdominal color Doppler US of the bladder shows a solid intraluminal mass ➡ with internal vascularity ➡, consistent with bladder carcinoma.* **(Right)** *Axial CT urography of the pelvis in the same patient confirms the lobulated mass ⇨ arises from the left posterolateral bladder wall. Margins are well delineated as a filling defect in the contrast-opacified bladder. The left ureter ⇨ is noted.*

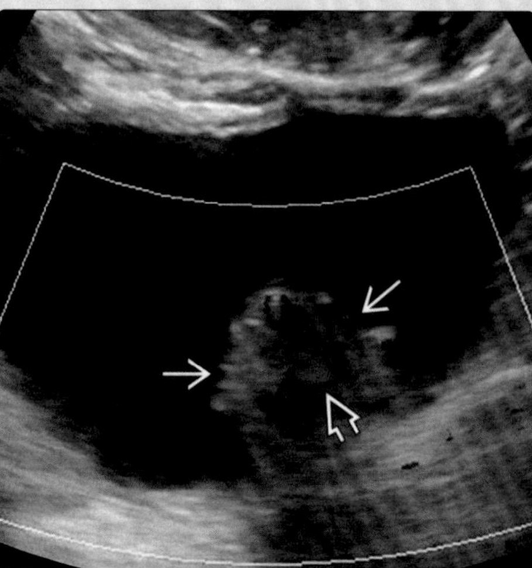

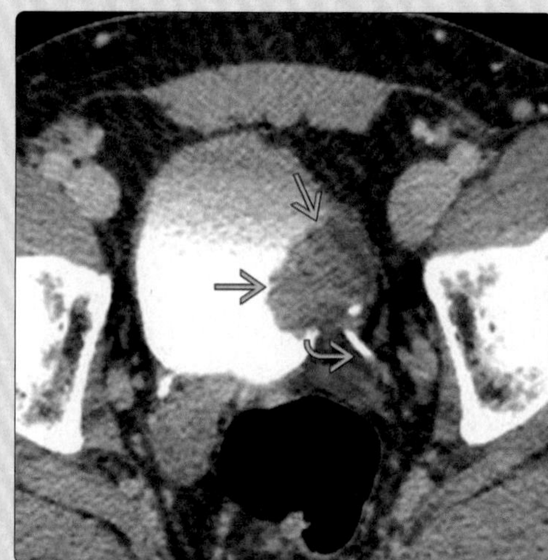

KEY FACTS

TERMINOLOGY

- Cystic, balloon-like dilatation of intramural portion of distal ureter bulging into bladder
- **Orthotopic ureterocele (less common)**: Normal insertion at trigone and otherwise normal ureter
- **Ectopic ureterocele (more common)**: Inserts below trigone
- Duplicated collecting system in 80%

IMAGING

- Ectopic: 50% in bladder and 50% in posterior urethra; 10% bilateral
- Thin-walled, cystic intravesical mass continuous with distal ureter
- Changes in size with degree of ureteral dilation
- Dilated ureter in ectopic lower moiety, changes in size with degree of ureteral dilation
- Obtain images when bladder is reasonably full

PATHOLOGY

- Single system ectopic ureteroceles: Associated with cardiac and genital anomalies
- Complete duplicated system: Commonly upper moiety ureter associated with ureterocele

SCANNING TIPS

- Look for ureterocele in reasonably full bladder if duplex renal system detected
  - Ureteroceles can be missed if bladder is empty and ureterocele is collapsed
- Look for ureteroceles at ureterovesical junction, which should always be included in bladder protocol
- Ureteroceles are highly dynamic and will "inflate" and "deflate" during peristaltic activity of ureter; adequate scanning time is required to visualize "inflation" stage of ureterocele

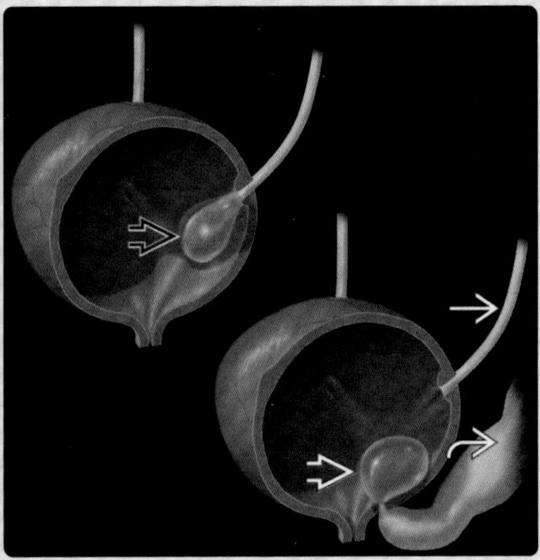

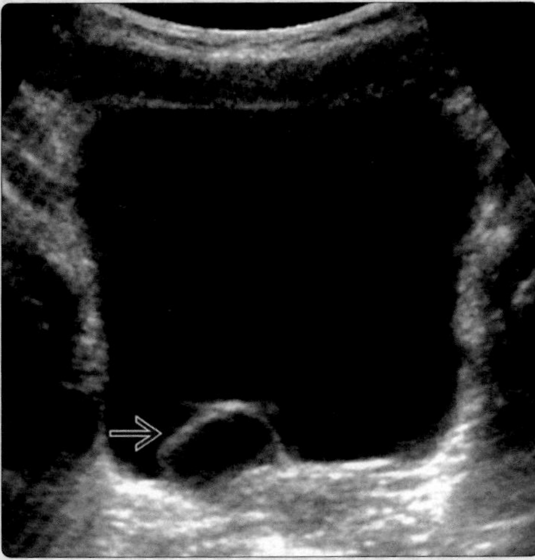

(Left) *Upper graphic shows orthotopic ureterocele ➡ at the trigone in a single system. Lower graphic shows ectopic ureterocele ➡ with hydroureter ➡ of the upper moiety, inserting inferior and medial to the lower moiety ureter ➡ in duplex system.* **(Right)** *Transabdominal transverse ultrasound of the pelvis shows typical ureterocele ➡ as a balloon-like cyst within the urinary bladder.*

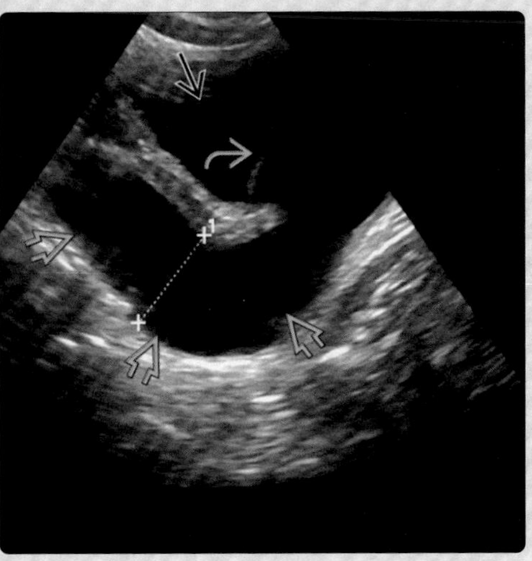

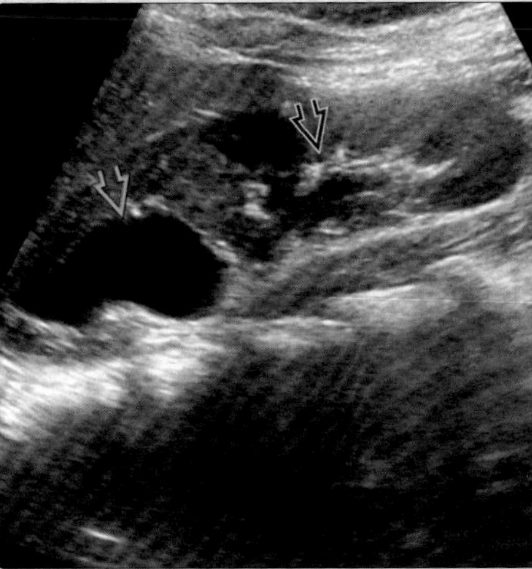

(Left) *Transabdominal longitudinal oblique ultrasound shows a typical ureteric duplex system associated with a ureterocele ➡ within the bladder ➡ at the distal end of the upper pole moiety ureter. The ureter is dilated ➡.* **(Right)** *Transabdominal longitudinal ultrasound through the right kidney in the same patient shows duplex collecting system with dilated upper moiety ➡ and nondilated lower moiety ➡.*

Bladder Diverticulum

KEY FACTS

TERMINOLOGY

- Saccular outpouching from herniation of bladder mucosa and submucosa through muscular wall of bladder

IMAGING

- Most commonly near ureterovesical junction
- Anechoic outpouching from bladder with narrow or wide neck, may empty with micturition

TOP DIFFERENTIAL DIAGNOSES

- Urachus
- Everted ureterocele
- Paraovarian cysts in female
- Pelvic cysts in male

PATHOLOGY

- Acquired: Most common secondary to chronic bladder outlet obstruction (60%)
- Congenital: Hutch diverticulum (40%)
- Vesicoureteral reflux

CLINICAL ISSUES

- Narrow-neck diverticula: Urinary stasis → complications such as infection, stone, and ureteral obstruction
- Secondary inflammation predisposes to development of carcinoma within diverticulum
- Complications
  - Carcinoma
  - Vesicoureteral reflux
  - Ureteral obstruction

SCANNING TIPS

- Look for debris, calculi, or solid masses in diverticula, which can indicate complication
- Color Doppler may show jet to and from diverticulum to bladder; do not mistake for ureteral jet

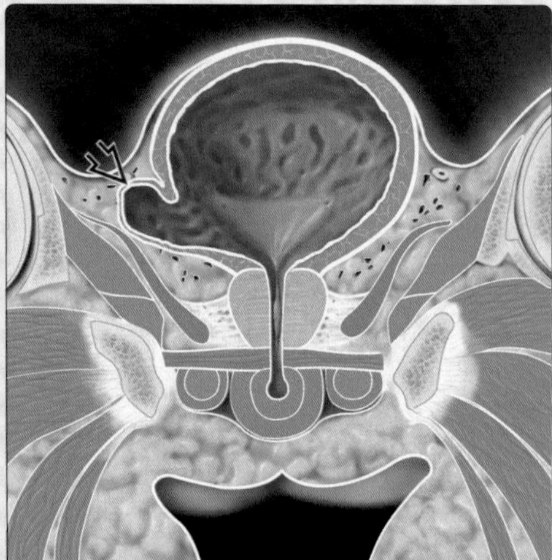

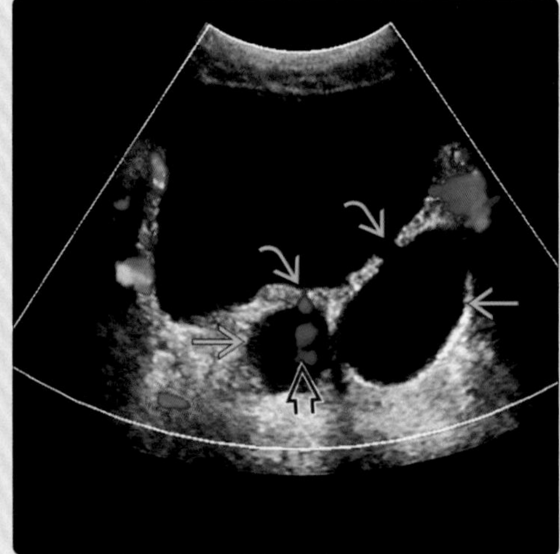

(Left) *Graphic shows a diverticulum ➡ arising from the lateral bladder wall, due to herniation of the mucosa and submucosa through the muscular wall.* **(Right)** *Transabdominal transverse oblique ultrasound of the urinary bladder shows 2 left posterolateral diverticula ➡ with narrow necks ➡. One of the diverticula shows a urinary jet as Doppler signal into the diverticulum ➡.*

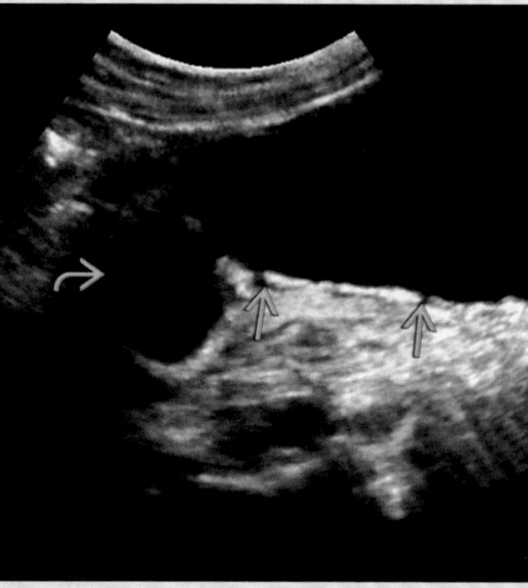

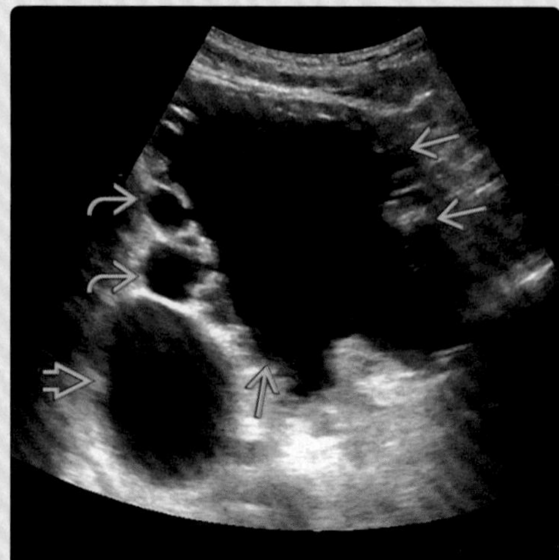

(Left) *Transabdominal longitudinal oblique ultrasound of the urinary bladder shows a posterior wall diverticulum ➡. Note mild wall trabeculation of the bladder ➡ in this patient with prostatomegaly resulting in chronic bladder outlet obstruction.* **(Right)** *Transabdominal transverse oblique ultrasound in a patient with neurogenic urinary bladder shows a trabeculated bladder wall ➡ with multiple small ➡ and 1 large diverticula ➡.*

Bladder Calculi

KEY FACTS

TERMINOLOGY

- Concretions of mineral salts/crystal within bladder lumen

IMAGING

- Mobile avascular echogenic focus/foci in bladder with posterior acoustic shadowing on US
- May see associated twinkling artifact on color Doppler
- Smooth, round or ovoid lamellated calcification in bladder region on plain radiograph
- May see associated bladder wall thickening, internal echoes, or debris

TOP DIFFERENTIAL DIAGNOSES

- Bladder neoplasm
- Blood clot
- Fungal ball
- Prostatomegaly

PATHOLOGY

- Stasis: Bladder outlet obstruction, neurogenic bladder, bladder diverticula
- Infection, especially proteus mirabilis

CLINICAL ISSUES

- Most asymptomatic
- May present with hematuria, suprapubic pain, or UTI
- Complication: Increased risk of developing malignant bladder tumors due to chronic irritation

SCANNING TIPS

- Examine with color Doppler to exclude underlying vascularity, which can be seen with neoplasm
  - Pulsed wave Doppler may help confirm real flow vs. twinkling artifact or motion
- Roll patient or ask patient to cough to see if calcification is mobile

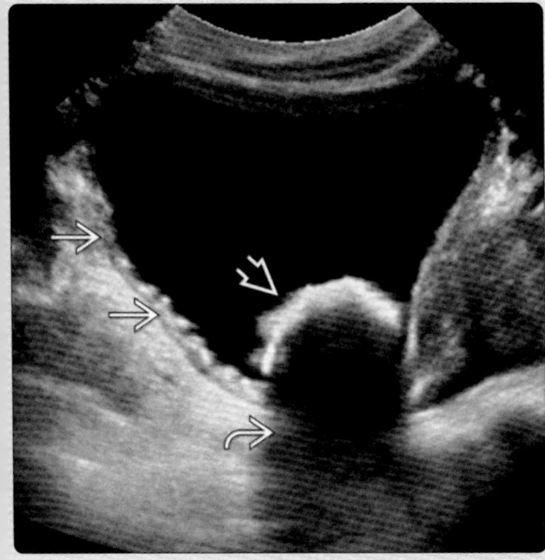

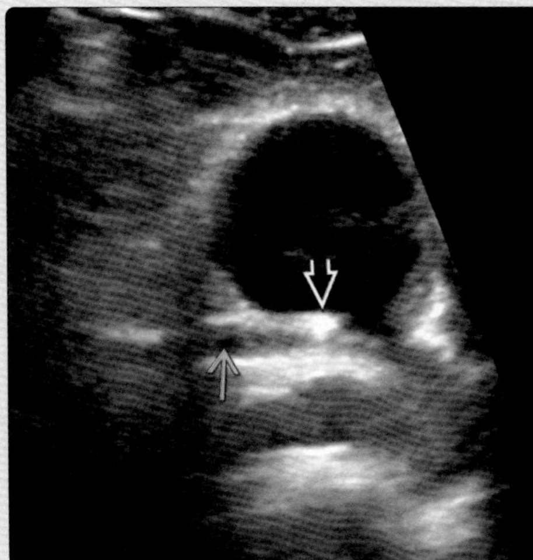

(Left) *Longitudinal transabdominal US shows a large, echogenic stone ➡ within the urinary bladder. The stone is lobulated in contour and associated with posterior acoustic shadowing ↪. Note the diffuse bladder wall thickening ➡ related to chronic bladder outlet obstruction, a known risk factor for development of bladder calculi.* **(Right)** *Transverse oblique transabdominal US of the bladder shows a partly obstructing stone ➡ at the right UVJ and mildly dilated upstream ureter ➡.*

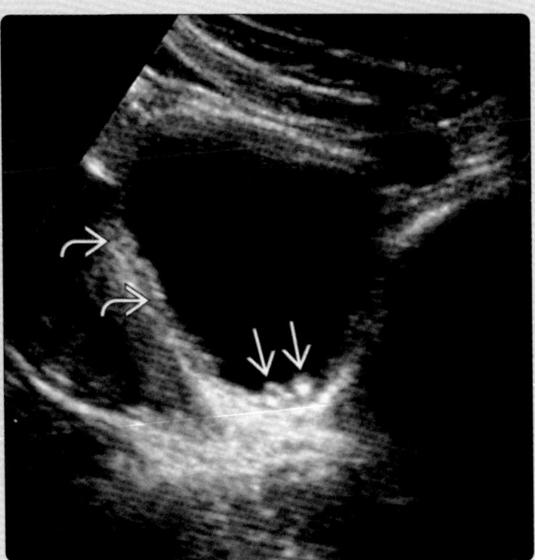

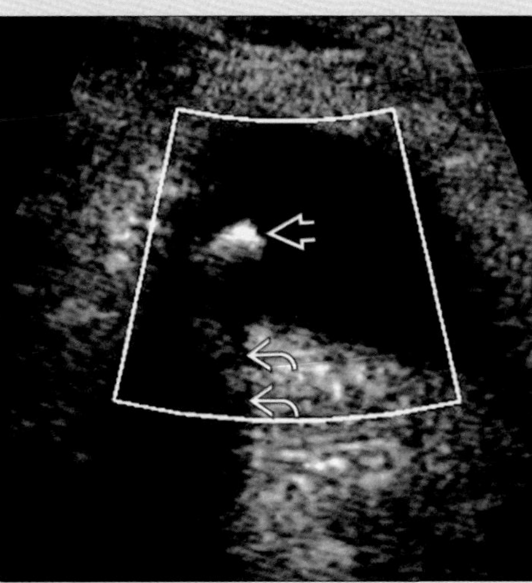

(Left) *Longitudinal transabdominal US shows multiple tiny, layering echogenic stones ➡ within the urinary bladder. Note the mild bladder wall thickening ↪.* **(Right)** *Longitudinal oblique transabdominal US shows a small, echogenic stone ➡ with posterior acoustic shadowing ↪ seen adherent to the bladder wall.*

PART I
SECTION 6
Kidney Transplant

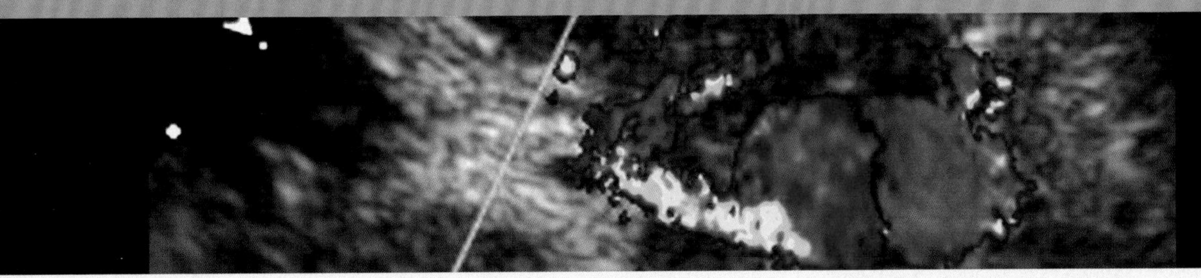

Renal Transplant Complications

Perigraft Fluid Collections

KEY FACTS

TERMINOLOGY

- Perigraft fluid collections include hematomas, seromas, urinomas, lymphoceles, and abscesses

IMAGING

- US is 1st-line modality for evaluating renal transplants; excellent for fluid collections
- Collections of variable size and echogenicity, typically walled off due to extraperitoneal placement of kidney
- Anechoic fluid suggests seroma, lymphocele, or urinoma
- Fluid with internal echoes or septations suggests hematoma or abscess
- Definitive diagnosis established by US-guided needle aspiration as well as therapeutic drainage
- Aspirate should be tested for creatinine, which is markedly elevated in urine leak, and for infection

TOP DIFFERENTIAL DIAGNOSES

- Ovarian and renal cysts
- Penile prosthesis reservoir
- Peritoneal inclusion cyst

CLINICAL ISSUES

- Large collections may compress transplant ureter resulting in hydronephrosis or may compress kidney, causing graft dysfunction
- Small hematomas and seromas are common and usually resolve spontaneously
- Lymphoceles occur in 5-15% patients, usually after 4 weeks; majority are asymptomatic but can be slow growing
- Urinomas occur in 2-5% of patients; within first 2 weeks, secondary to anastomotic leak or ureteric ischemia
    - Pain, swelling, discharge from wound, and elevated serum creatinine; intervention required
- Abscesses: Fever, abdominal pain, raised white cell count

SCANNING TIPS

- Color Doppler to assess for active bleeding

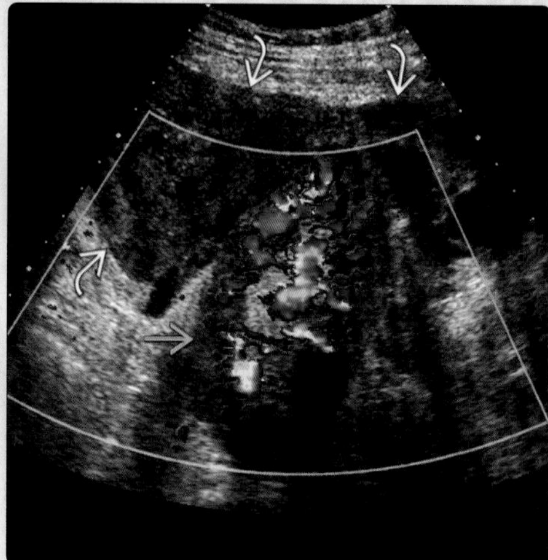
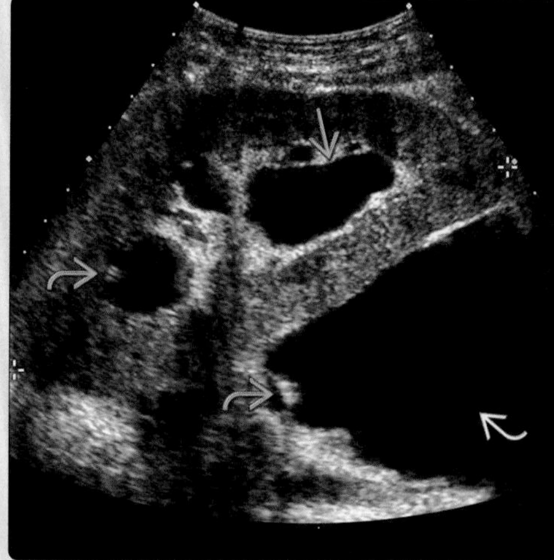

(Left) *Longitudinal color Doppler US shows a right lower quadrant renal allograft ➡. The allograft is well perfused despite a large, acute, echogenic perinephric hematoma ➡.* **(Right)** *Longitudinal US shows a renal allograft with moderate hydronephrosis ➡. The transplant ureter was compressed by a large lymphocele ➡, and a ureteral stent is present ➡.*

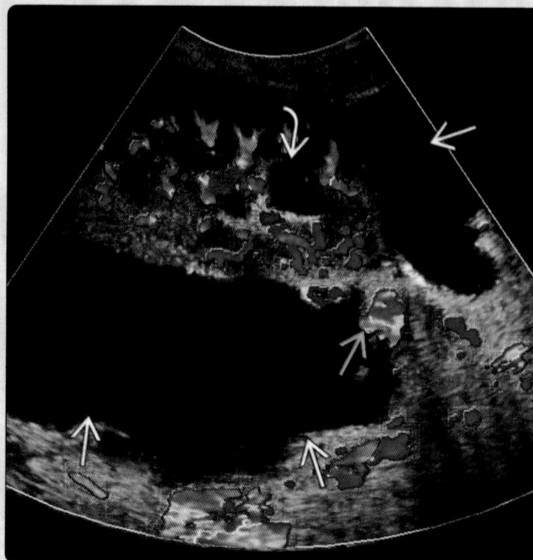
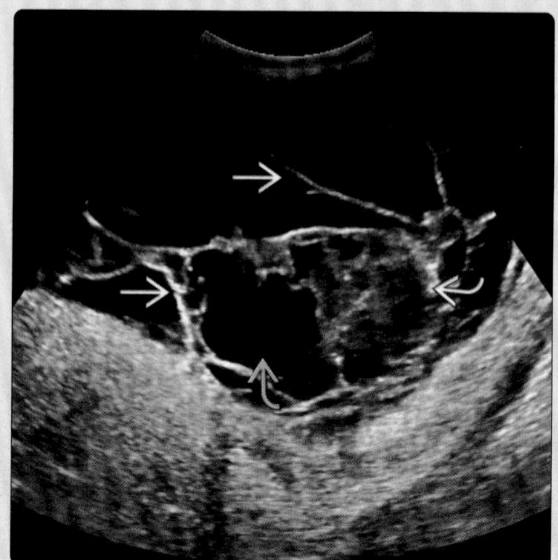

(Left) *Longitudinal color Doppler US shows a renal transplant with mild hydronephrosis ➡. There was a large lymphocele ➡ anterior and posterior to the transplant, encircling vessels ➡.* **(Right)** *Longitudinal ultrasound shows a chronic hematoma in the right pelvis. There are multiple thick and irregular septations ➡ with more solid, avascular areas ➡. Some loculi contain echogenic fluid ➡.*

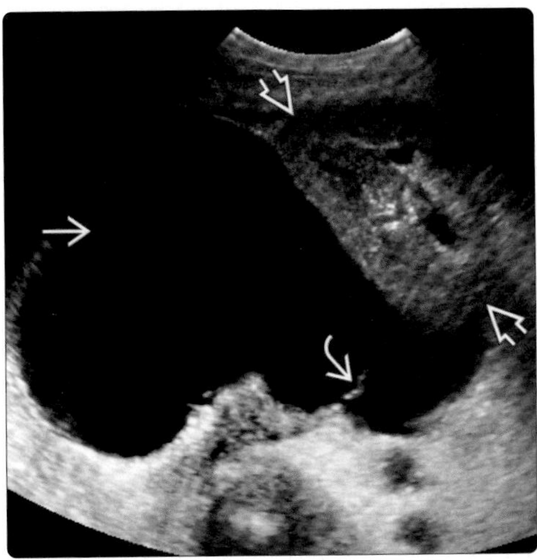

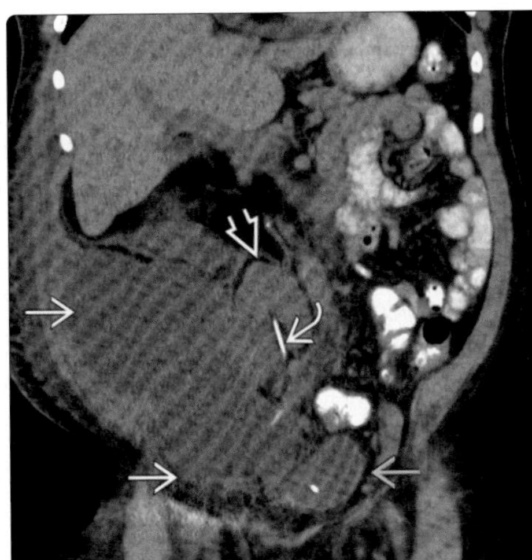

(Left) *Transverse ultrasound of the right pelvis shows a large fluid collection ➡ with a thin septation ↪, displacing a renal transplant ⇨.* **(Right)** *Unenhanced CT of the same patient shows the extent of the large collection ➡ that displaces the renal transplant ⇨ and the bladder ➡. There is a stent ↪ in the ureter. Collections of this size are drained.*

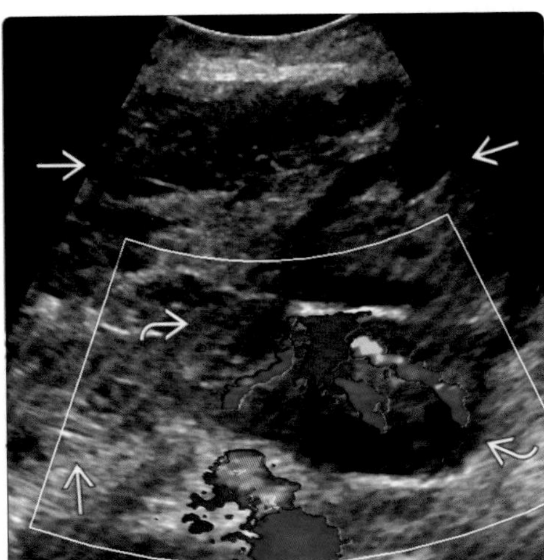

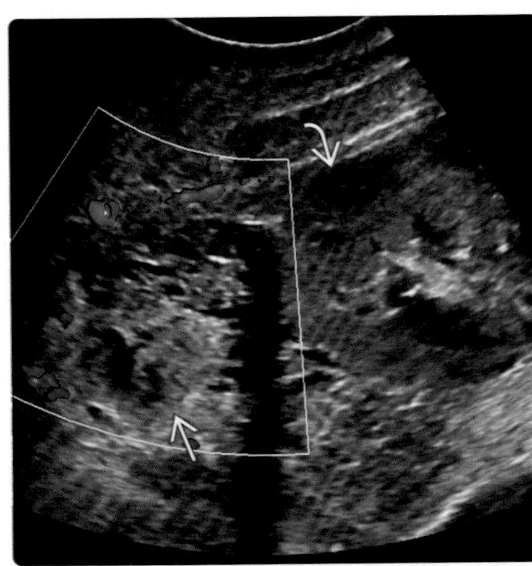

(Left) *Longitudinal color Doppler ultrasound shows a large perinephric hematoma ➡ compressing a renal transplant ↪. A hematoma this size is usually treated by surgical evacuation.* **(Right)** *Longitudinal color Doppler ultrasound shows a small perinephric hematoma ➡ superior to the renal transplant ↪. There is no mass effect.*

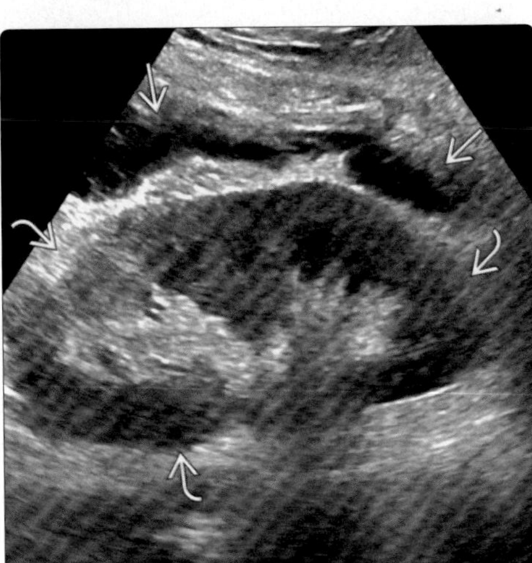

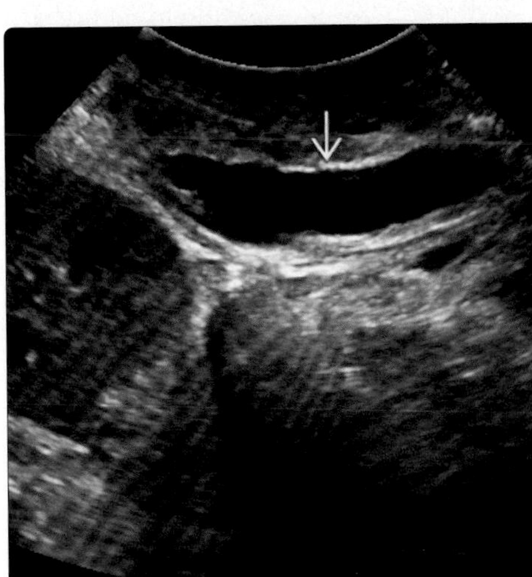

(Left) *Longitudinal ultrasound shows a small perinephric seroma ➡ anterior to a normal renal transplant ↪.* **(Right)** *Longitudinal ultrasound shows an elongated perinephric simple fluid collection ➡ away from the transplant ureter and vascular pedicle.*

Renal Transplant Hydronephrosis

KEY FACTS

IMAGING

- Dilated renal pelvis and calyces ± dilated ureter
- Distended bladder may cause functional obstruction or reflux resulting in hydronephrosis
- Low-level echoes within lumen suggest pus (pyonephrosis) or blood (hemonephrosis)
- Highly echogenic shadowing intraluminal structures represent stones, twinkling artifact on color Doppler
- Urothelial thickening suggests infection or rejection
- Ultrasound is sensitive and specific for hydronephrosis but may be limited for site of obstruction

TOP DIFFERENTIAL DIAGNOSES

- Nonobstructive dilatation, early postoperative edema
- Functional obstruction from overdistended bladder
- Prominent hilar vessels
- Renal sinus cysts (more common in native kidneys)

PATHOLOGY

- Causes include ischemic stricture, rejection, clot, calculus, extrinsic compression, infection, and tumor
- Reflux, infection, and decreased ureteral tone may cause nonobstructive dilatation

CLINICAL ISSUES

- Ureteral obstruction occurs in 3-6% of renal allografts
- Most common in first 6 months after transplantation
- Over 90% of strictures at ureterovesical anastomosis and distal 1/3 of ureter

SCANNING TIPS

- Look for transition zone and cause for obstruction
- Use color Doppler to distinguish hilar vessels from dilated renal pelvis and to distinguish clot or debris from solid tumor
- Use color Doppler to look for ureteral jet
- If bladder is distended, rescan with empty bladder

(Left) *Longitudinal ultrasound shows mild to moderate hydronephrosis ⇨ in a renal transplant. The ureter ➡ is dilated secondary to obstruction by a fluid collection ⮊, which wrapped around the ureter.* **(Right)** *Longitudinal ultrasound shows severe hydronephrosis with ballooned calyces ➡ and thinned echogenic cortex ⇨. This was secondary to a proximal ureteral stricture, which required ureteral reconstruction.*

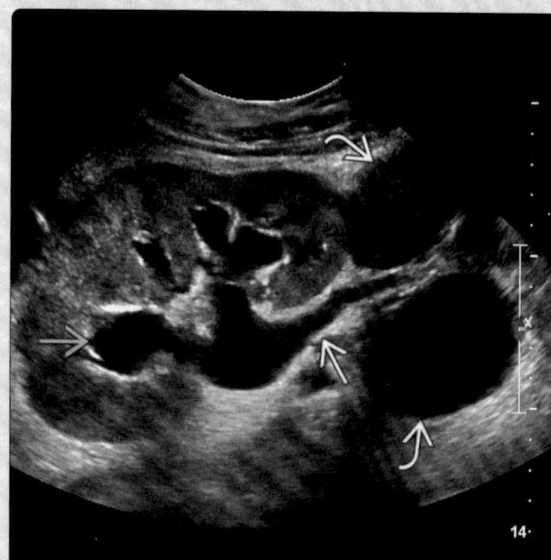

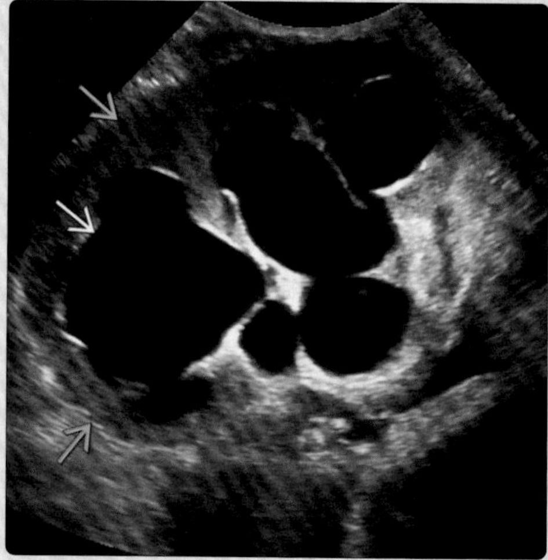

(Left) *Longitudinal ultrasound shows mild to moderate hydronephrosis ⇨ secondary to a shadowing calculus ➡ in the transplant ureter.* **(Right)** *Longitudinal color Doppler ultrasound shows a dilated renal pelvis ⮊ containing avascular hypoechoic clot ➡. This bleeding followed a renal transplant biopsy.*

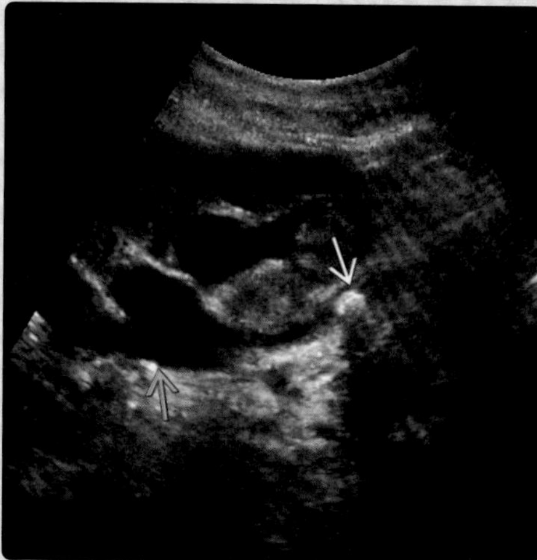

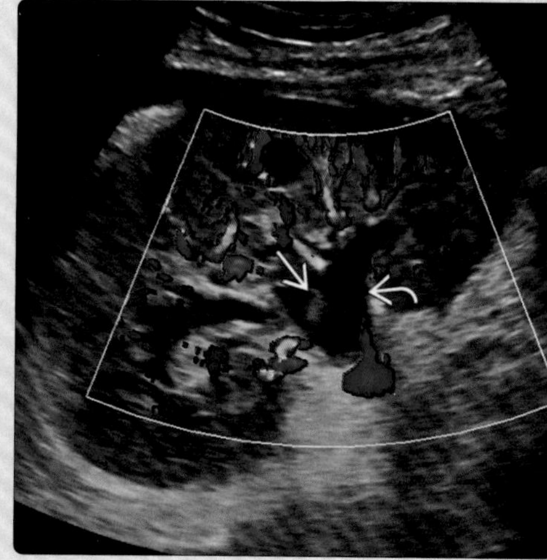

Transplant Renal Artery Stenosis

KEY FACTS

IMAGING

- Color, power, spectral Doppler US is screening modality for transplant renal artery stenosis
- Stenosis occurs most commonly at arterial anastomosis but can occur along length of artery
- Focal elevation of peak systolic velocity (PSV) > 250-300 cm/s at stenosis with poststenotic turbulence
- Color aliasing and soft tissue vibration at area of stenosis
- Renal artery to Iliac PSV ratio > 1.8-3.5
- Secondary sign: Tardus parvus **intrarenal** waveforms = slow systolic upstroke and decreased peak velocity
  - Decreased acceleration index < 3 m/s^2 and increased acceleration time > 0.1 s in segmental arteries
  - Low resistive index (RI) < 0.5
- Catheter angiography is gold standard for diagnosis and allows treatment with angioplasty or stenting

TOP DIFFERENTIAL DIAGNOSES

- Abrupt renal artery curves and kinks
- Pseudorenal artery stenosis from iliac stenosis
- Systemic hypotension may cause low RI

PATHOLOGY

- Surgical injury during harvesting or transplantation
- Immune-mediated vascular damage from rejection
- Older donors and recipients, atherosclerosis, diabetes

CLINICAL ISSUES

- 2-10% of transplants
- Present with hypertension, acute renal failure or progressive decline in renal function, bruit

SCANNING TIPS

- Careful attention to Doppler angle to ensure accurate PSV measurements
- Compare highest peak renal artery velocity to iliac artery velocity
- Curves and kinks may elevate velocities, mimicking stenosis

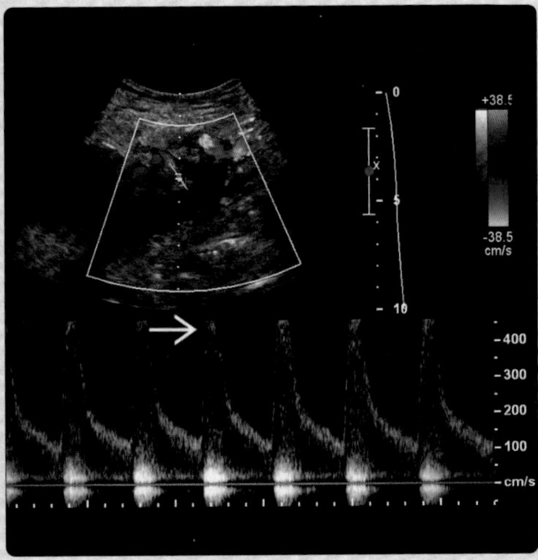

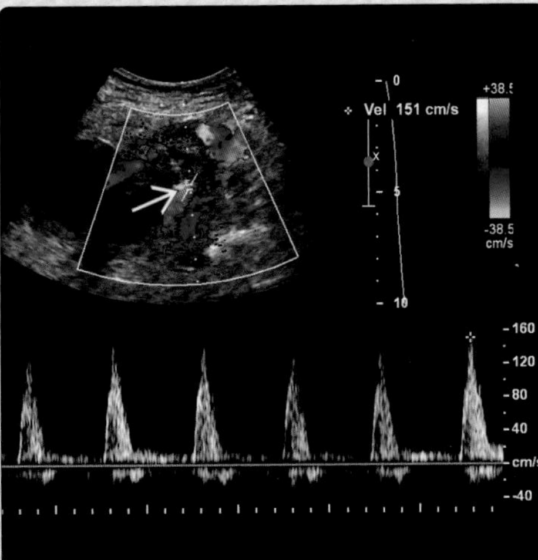

(Left) *Longitudinal spectral Doppler ultrasound shows the main renal artery 3 weeks after cadaveric renal transplant in an 82-year-old man. The peak systolic velocity* ➡ *in the main renal artery exceeds 400 cm/s with aliasing of the Doppler spectrum indicating a significant artery stenosis. Renal function was poor.* **(Right)** *Longitudinal spectral Doppler ultrasound of the same patient with renal artery stenosis shows the peak systolic velocity of the external iliac artery* ➡ *was 151 cm/s with a renal artery to iliac artery ratio > 2.6.*

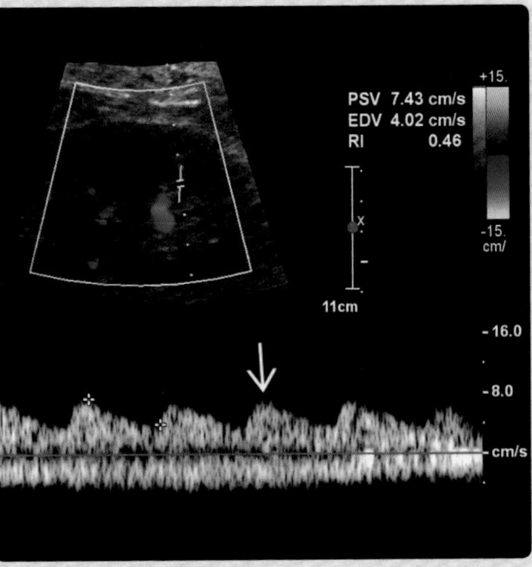

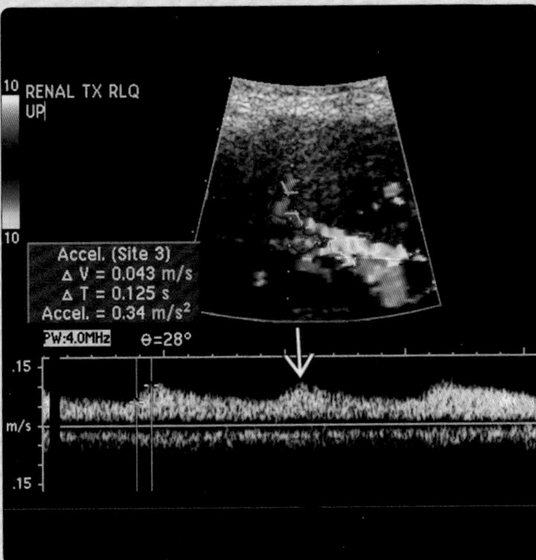

(Left) *Doppler ultrasound of an interlobar artery in a renal transplant with renal artery stenosis shows tardus parvus* ➡ *with a low resistive index of 0.46.* **(Right)** *Doppler ultrasound of a segmental artery in transplant renal artery stenosis shows tardus parvus* ➡ *with increased acceleration time of 0.125 s and decreased acceleration index of 0.34 m/s^2.*

Transplant Renal Artery Thrombosis

KEY FACTS

TERMINOLOGY

- Occlusion of transplant renal artery secondary to thrombus

IMAGING

- Edematous hypoechoic kidney if total thrombosis
- Absence of blood flow in main renal artery
- Diffuse absence of parenchymal perfusion on color or power Doppler
- Blunted low-resistance waveforms in ischemic areas from collateral flow
- If involving accessory renal artery
  - Segmental wedge-shaped peripheral area of decreased color flow and altered echogenicity
- Color, power, spectral Doppler US 1st-line imaging modality for complications of renal transplantation
- Optimize color and spectral Doppler settings for slow flow

TOP DIFFERENTIAL DIAGNOSES

- Transplant renal vein thrombosis
- Acute rejection/acute on chronic rejection
- Hyperacute rejection

CLINICAL ISSUES

- Rare (< 1%)
- Abrupt onset of oliguria, decreased function, pain and swelling of allograft
- Poor prognosis; graft loss typical when single main artery thrombosed
  - Transplant nephrectomy
  - Thrombectomy or thrombolysis rarely successful unless diagnosis made early
- Accessory or segmental arterial thrombosis → ischemia and subsequent atrophy

DIAGNOSTIC CHECKLIST

- Severe acute rejection or tubular necrosis may cause propagating small vessel thrombosis resulting in infarction and mimicking transplant renal artery thrombosis
- Urgent finding requiring prompt communication

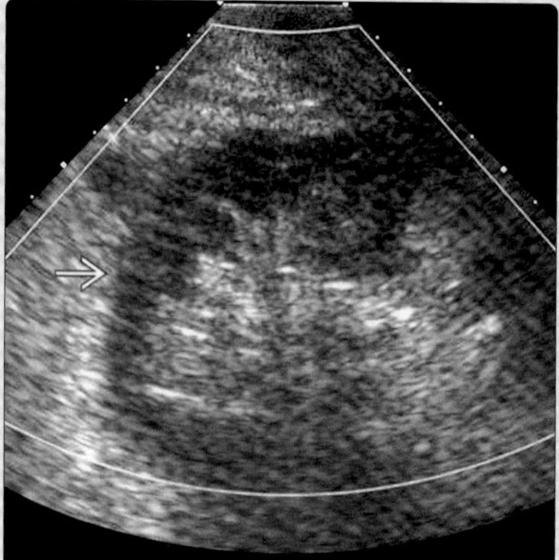

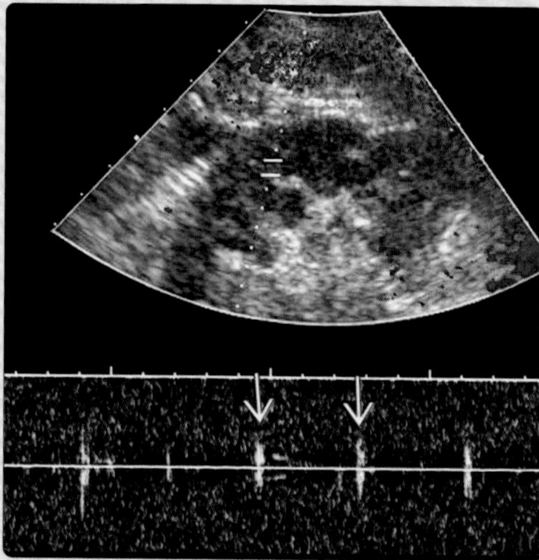

(Left) *Longitudinal color Doppler ultrasound on 1st day after renal transplant shows no color flow in the allograft ➡ secondary to early thrombosis in a hypercoagulable patient.* **(Right)** *Longitudinal pulsed Doppler ultrasound of the same patient shows no intrarenal arterial flow. Noise ➡ was transmitted to the kidney.*

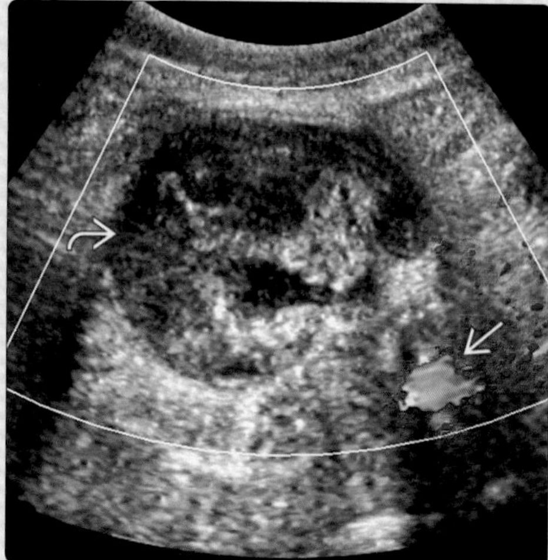

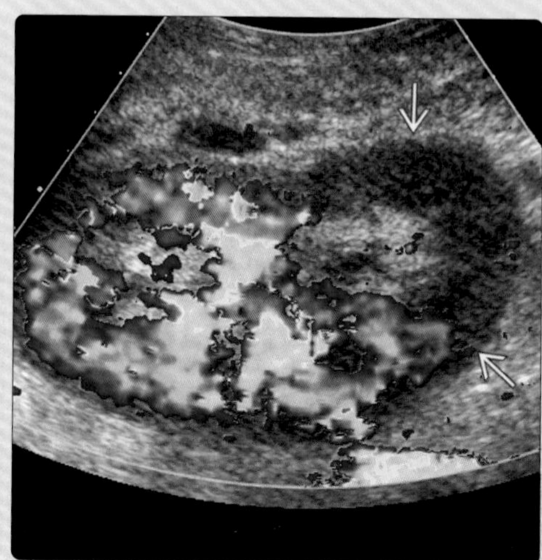

(Left) *Transverse color Doppler ultrasound of a thrombosed recent renal transplant shows an edematous allograft ➡ with no internal color flow. The iliac artery ➡ is patent.* **(Right)** *Longitudinal color Doppler ultrasound shows a renal allograft with segmental ischemia of the lower pole ➡ secondary to thrombosis of an accessory renal artery. Absence of color flow is noted in the lower 1/2 of the allograft.*

Transplant Renal Vein Thrombosis

KEY FACTS

IMAGING

- Enlarged, edematous, hypoechoic kidney due to outflow obstruction
- Absence or decreased color flow in renal vein at hilum
- Patent renal artery early, later renal artery will thrombose also
- High systolic arterial peaks with flow reversal in diastole
- Color, power, spectral Doppler US is 1st-line imaging modality for complications of renal transplantation

TOP DIFFERENTIAL DIAGNOSES

- Acute, severe rejection or delayed graft function
- Iliac vein thrombosis or renal vein compression

PATHOLOGY

- Surgical injury or technical problem
- Compression by fluid collection
- Hypovolemia, hypercoagulable state
- Thrombus propagation from common femoral/external iliac vein

CLINICAL ISSUES

- Abrupt onset of graft tenderness and swelling, decreased function
- Usually within 1st week, most commonly within 48 hours of transplantation
- ≤ 4% of transplants
- Poor prognosis even with prompt diagnosis and thrombectomy/surgical revision
- May progress to rupture with hemorrhage and hypovolemia

DIAGNOSTIC CHECKLIST

- Consider renal vein thrombosis when there is sudden drop in urine output in early postoperative period
- Reversal of arterial diastolic flow and absence of venous flow confirms this diagnosis

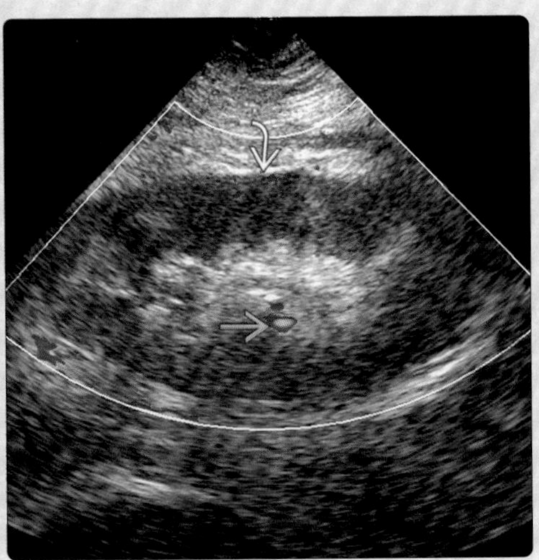

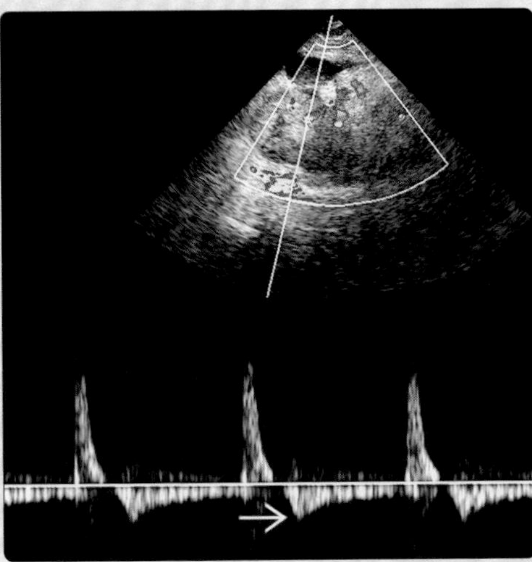

(Left) *Longitudinal power Doppler ultrasound of the renal allograft in a patient who developed pain and anuria is shown. Minimal color flow ⇨ is seen in the allograft ➡, which is edematous.* **(Right)** *Longitudinal Doppler of the same patient shows abnormal segmental arterial waveform with narrow systolic peaks and reversal of flow ➡ in diastole. The renal vein was thrombosed.*

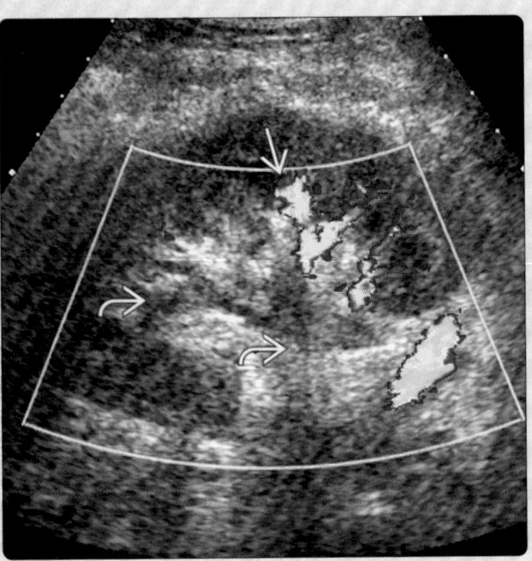

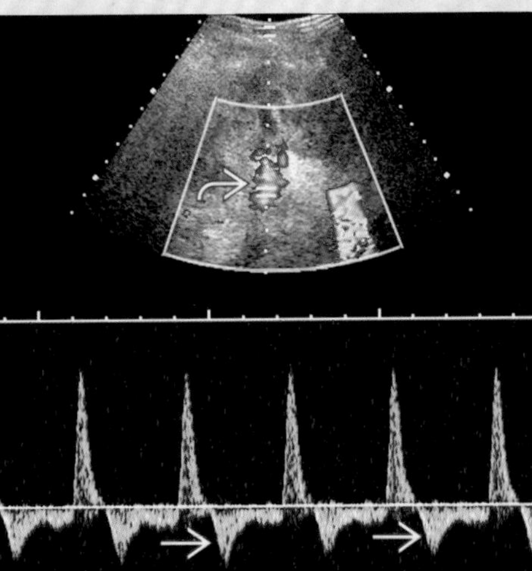

(Left) *Longitudinal color Doppler ultrasound shows renal vein thrombosis in a renal allograft. Thrombus can be seen in the main renal vein ➡ extending into segmental veins. Arterial flow ➡ was still detected in the lower pole.* **(Right)** *Longitudinal color Doppler ultrasound of the same patient is shown. The main renal artery ➡ was patent, but the waveform is abnormal with reversal of diastolic flow ➡.*

Renal Transplant Arteriovenous (AV) Fistula

KEY FACTS

TERMINOLOGY

- Abnormal direct communication between artery and vein

IMAGING

- Usually in renal parenchyma; may be extrarenal
- Not usually visible when small
- Large arteriovenous fistulas: Dilated serpiginous vessels
- Feeding artery shows high-velocity, low-resistance waveform with spectral broadening
- Pulsatile arterialized flow in draining vein when large
- Perivascular tissue vibration producing color in adjacent tissues on color Doppler
- Catheter angiography is gold standard for diagnosis, allows endovascular treatment

TOP DIFFERENTIAL DIAGNOSES

- Pseudoaneurysm
- Renal artery stenosis

PATHOLOGY

- Complication of percutaneous transplant biopsy or insertion of nephrostomy

CLINICAL ISSUES

- Postbiopsy incidence: 1-18%
- Most asymptomatic or present with hematuria
- 50% disappear within 48 hours; 70% resolve spontaneously within 1-2 years
- 30% symptomatic and persistent
- Observation in majority with serial ultrasound
- Treated with superselective embolization of feeding artery if hematuria persists or renal function impaired

SCANNING TIPS

- Look for arteriovenous fistula when patients develop hematuria after renal transplant biopsy
- Best detected when background normal color flow is suppressed by using higher Doppler scale

(Left) *Longitudinal ultrasound of the lower pole of a renal allograft shows a tubular, serpiginous, anechoic structure extending from the sinus to the cortex.* **(Right)** *Longitudinal color Doppler ultrasound of the same patient shows that the serpiginous structure fills in with color, representing an intrarenal arteriovenous fistula. This was confirmed with spectral Doppler.*

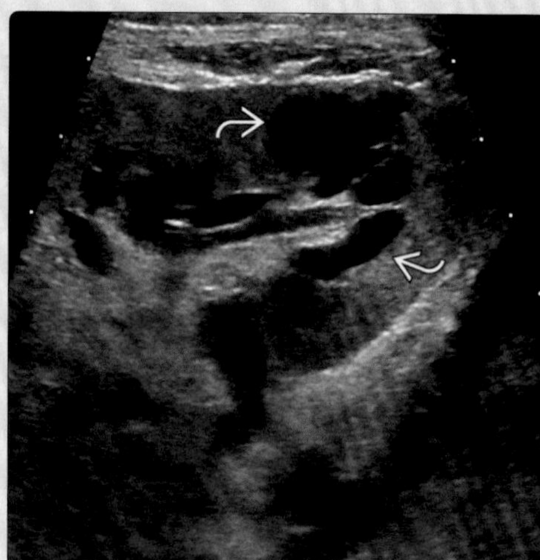

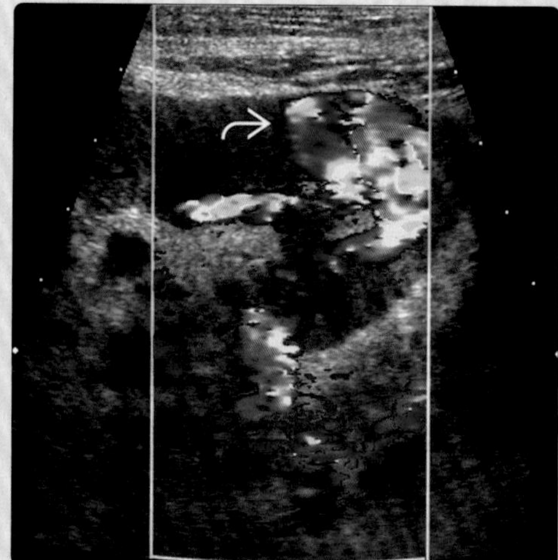

(Left) *Longitudinal color Doppler ultrasound of a renal allograft with a lower pole arteriovenous fistula is shown. There is pronounced perivascular tissue vibration producing color signal.* **(Right)** *Longitudinal spectral Doppler of the same arteriovenous fistula is shown. There is a characteristic high-velocity, low-resistance turbulent waveform. The color scale has been increased to suppress normal flow and the artifact.*

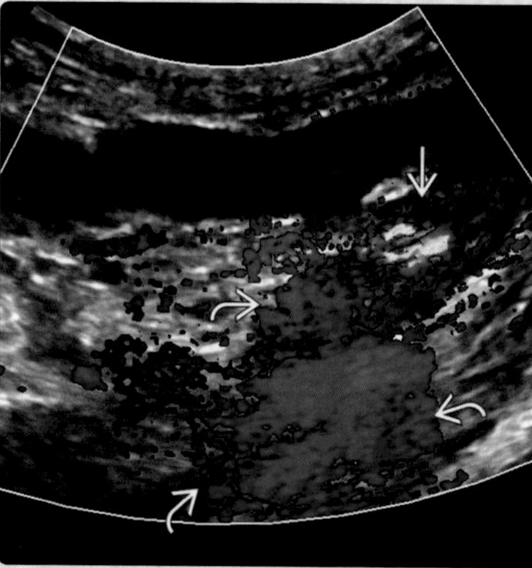

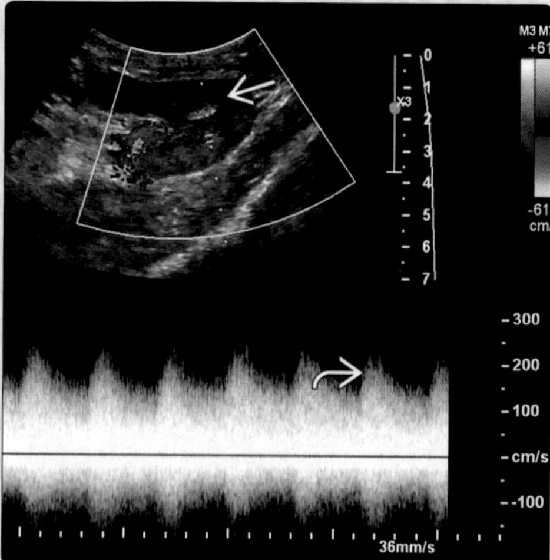

KEY FACTS

TERMINOLOGY

- Contained rupture secondary to defect in artery wall

IMAGING

- Usually in renal parenchyma, rarely extrarenal
- Usually ≤ 1 cm
- Extrarenal pseudoaneurysm may be larger
- Saccular, round or ovoid lesion
- Mimics simple or complex renal cyst on grayscale but with pulsations or swirling internal echoes
- Doppler: High-velocity jet into sac with internal turbulent flow
  - Swirling yin-yang internal flow
  - To-and-fro waveform in neck
- Internal clot when large
- CTA/MRA are confirmatory tests, which provide additional information about entire arterial tree

TOP DIFFERENTIAL DIAGNOSES

- Cyst
- Arteriovenous fistula, may coexist with pseudoaneurysm
- Perinephric collection (extra renal pseudoaneurysm)

PATHOLOGY

- Intrarenal: Iatrogenic injury during biopsy or percutaneous procedure

CLINICAL ISSUES

- Most asymptomatic
- Hematuria, abnormal renal function
- Pain, bleeding/hypotension from rupture
- Increased risk of rupture when extrarenal and > 2 cm

SCANNING TIPS

- Always turn on color Doppler when evaluating renal cystic lesions
- Look for characteristic to-and-fro flow in neck

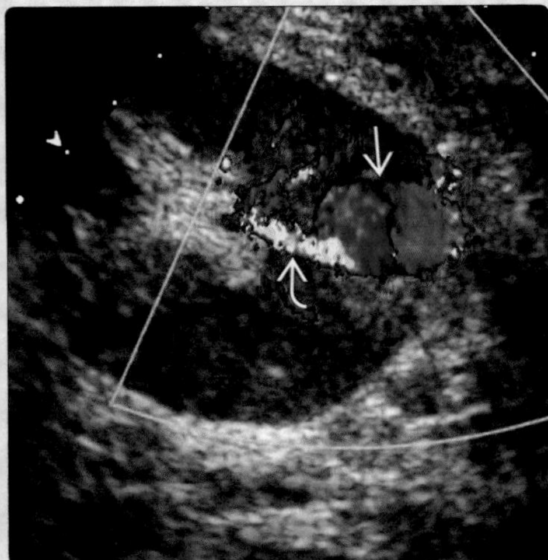

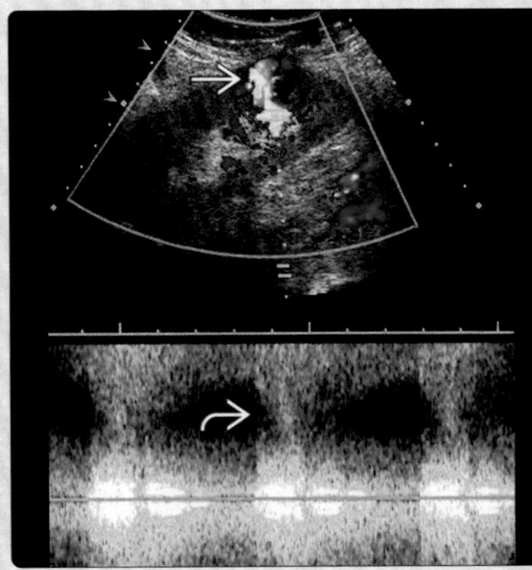

(Left) *Longitudinal color Doppler ultrasound shows a pseudoaneurysm ➡ in the lower pole of a renal transplant. Yin-yang internal swirling flow is present. Color aliasing is noted in the feeding artery ➡.* **(Right)** *Longitudinal spectral Doppler ultrasound of a pseudoaneurysm ➡ shows disorganized turbulent flow ➡ at the base of the pseudoaneurysm.*

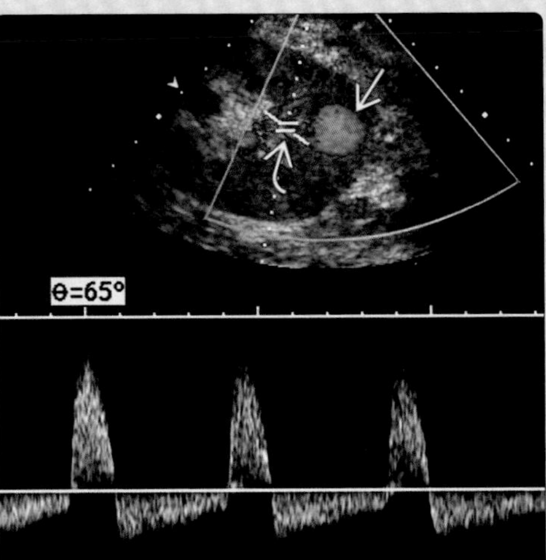

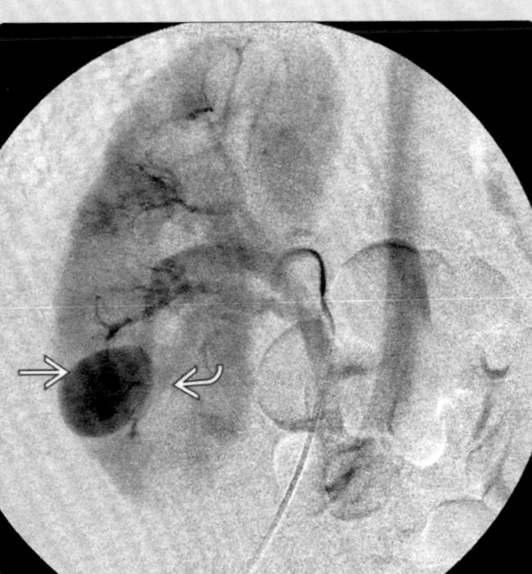

(Left) *Longitudinal Doppler ultrasound shows a pseudoaneurysm ➡ in the lower pole of a renal transplant. To-and-fro flow in the neck ➡ is characteristic.* **(Right)** *Digital subtracted selective renal arteriogram shows a pseudoaneurysm ➡ filling from a lower pole artery ➡. This was embolized.*

Renal Transplant Rejection

KEY FACTS

IMAGING

- No specific imaging characteristics
- Ultrasound-guided renal biopsy is gold standard
- Acute rejection (AR): Nonspecific allograft edema, urothelial thickening
- Resistive index (RI) may be elevated, or there may be loss or reversal of arterial diastolic flow
- Elevated RI > 0.80 in early postoperative period associated with increased risk of graft failure
- Chronic rejection (CR): Cortical atrophy, increased echogenicity, calcification
- Color perfusion may be decreased in both AR or CR

TOP DIFFERENTIAL DIAGNOSES

- Acute tubular necrosis/delayed graft function
- Infection
- Renal vascular thrombosis
- Calcineurin inhibitor toxicity

PATHOLOGY

- AR and CR: Diagnosed and staged pathologically

CLINICAL ISSUES

- 14% in first 3-6 months
- Acute cellular rejection most common after postoperative day 4
- Symptoms and signs include elevation of creatinine, decreased urine output, fever, graft tenderness and swelling

SCANNING TIPS

- Interval graft enlargement and tenderness with normal perfusion are suggestive of AR
- Poor correlation between RI and rejection
  - Small, hypoperfused, hyperechoic renal transplants are compatible with CR

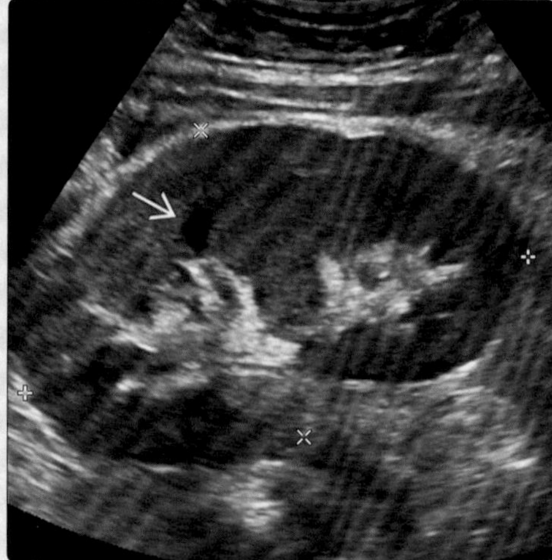

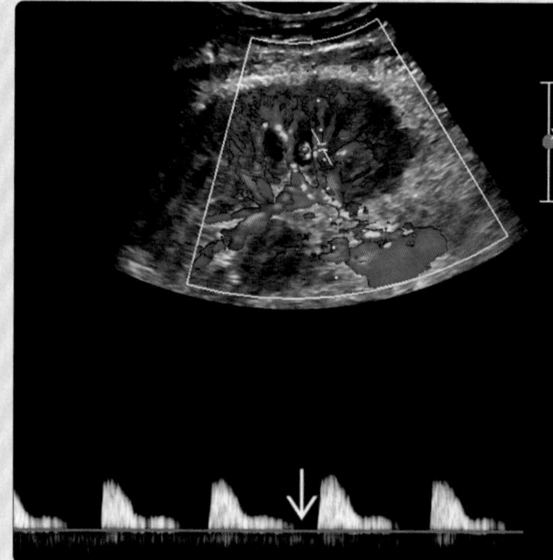

(Left) *Longitudinal ultrasound of a renal transplant with oliguria secondary to acute rejection shows swelling and loss of corticomedullary differentiation. Pyramids ➡ are less conspicuous.* **(Right)** *Longitudinal pulsed Doppler ultrasound of the same renal transplant shows normal color Doppler but absence of flow in diastole ➡.*

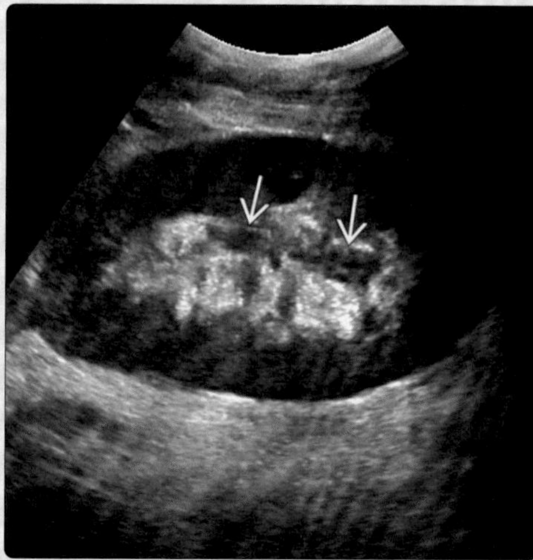

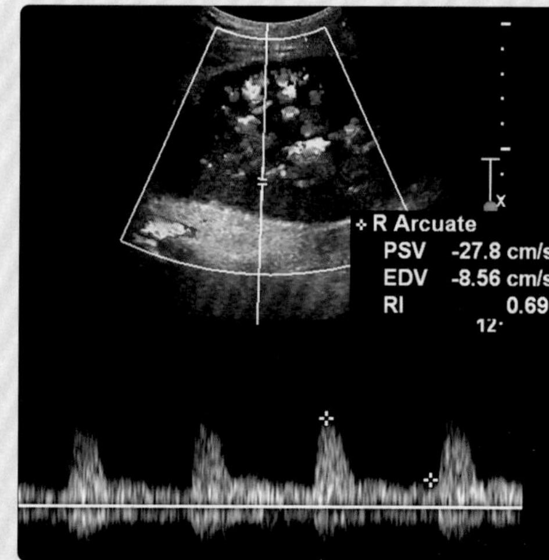

(Left) *Longitudinal ultrasound of a living related renal transplant with biopsy-proven moderate acute cell-mediated rejection is shown. The kidney appears swollen with urothelial thickening ➡.* **(Right)** *Longitudinal pulsed Doppler ultrasound of the same patient shows normal diastolic flow and a resistive index within normal limits at 0.69.*

Delayed Renal Graft Function

KEY FACTS

TERMINOLOGY

- Need for dialysis or failure of serum creatinine to halve in 1st week after transplantation

IMAGING

- Clinical diagnosis with no specific imaging findings
- Renal transplant may be edematous
- Ultrasound with Doppler serves to exclude other causes of renal transplant dysfunction
  - Look for hemorrhage, vascular thrombosis, or hydronephrosis
- Resistive indices may be elevated or there may be absence of diastolic flow

PATHOLOGY

- 21% incidence in deceased donor transplantation
- 2-5% after living donor transplantation
- Most common cause is acute tubular necrosis: 70-90%
- Risk factors
  - Donor age, harvest injury, preservation
  - Injury at procurement, organ preservation methods, warm and cold ischemia time

CLINICAL ISSUES

- Present with oliguria, lack of renal function
- Delayed graft function has significant impact on long-term graft and patient survival
- Increased incidence of acute rejection
- May be complicated by vascular thrombosis
- Treatment is supportive with dialysis as indicated

SCANNING TIPS

- Determine vascular patency, exclude ureteral obstruction and collections
- Use ultrasound to guide renal transplant biopsy

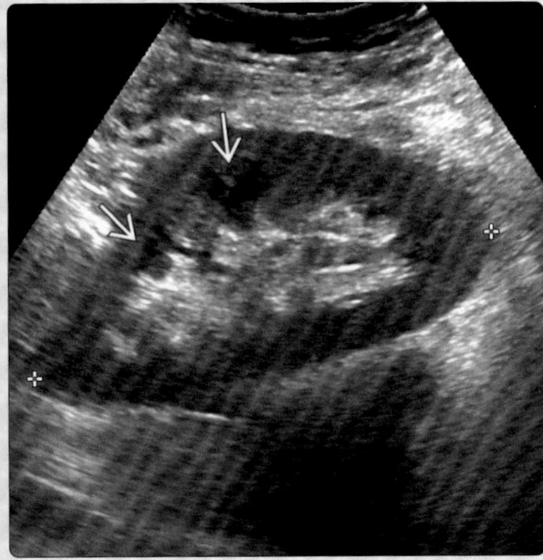

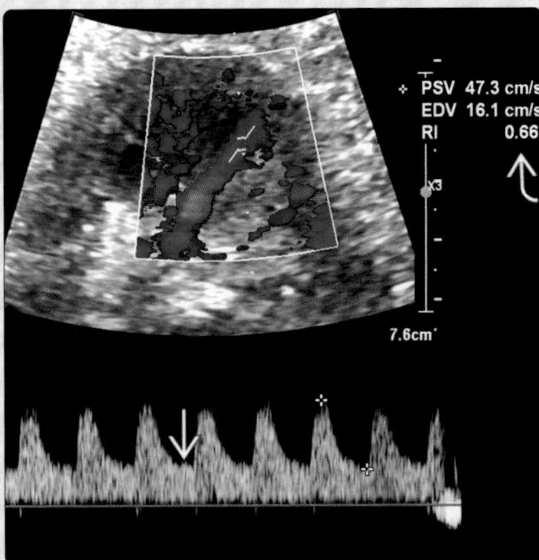

(Left) *Longitudinal ultrasound obtained on postoperative day 1 after cadaver donor renal transplant is shown. The patient had poor urine output, and the serum creatinine was not dropping. The transplant appears normal with visible medullary pyramids ➡.* **(Right)** *Pulsed Doppler ultrasound in the same patient with delayed graft function shows normal diastolic flow ➡ and resistive index ➡.*

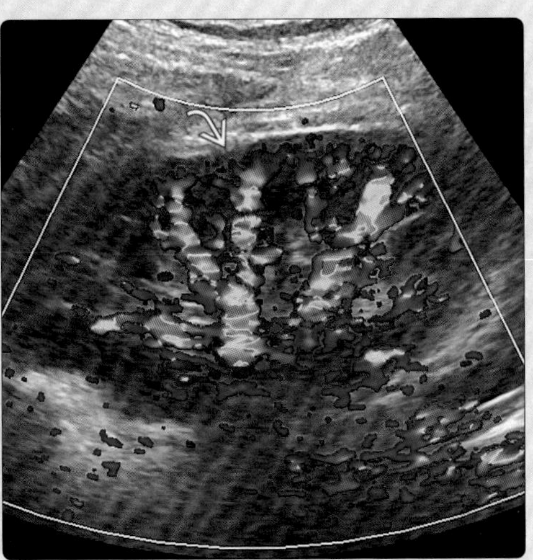

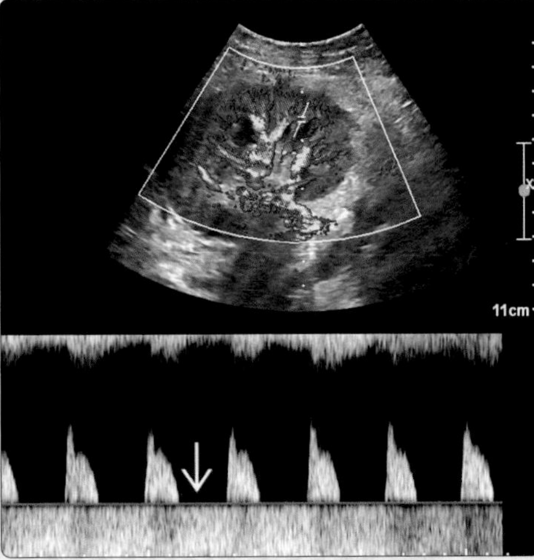

(Left) *Longitudinal color Doppler ultrasound shows a nonfunctioning renal transplant ➡ with delayed graft function. The transplant is perfused, excluding vascular thrombosis as a cause of dysfunction. There was also no hydronephrosis or collection.* **(Right)** *In a 76-year-old woman with delayed graft function after deceased donor renal transplant, color Doppler shows normal perfusion, but there is no diastolic flow ➡. Biopsy showed acute tubular necrosis with mild acute rejection.*

PART I
SECTION 7
Adrenal Gland

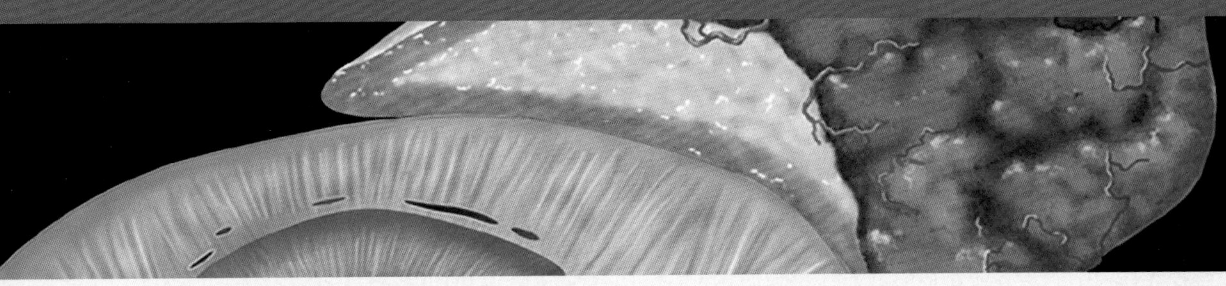

Anatomy and Approach

Adrenal Lesions

GROSS ANATOMY

Overview

- Adrenal (suprarenal) glands are part of both endocrine and nervous systems
- Lie within perirenal space, bounded by perirenal (Gerota) fascia
- **Right adrenal** is more apical in location
  - Lies anterolateral to right crus of diaphragm, medial to liver, posterior to inferior vena cava (IVC)
  - Often pyramidal in shape, inverted V shape on transverse section
- **Left adrenal** is more caudal
  - Lies medial to upper pole of left kidney, lateral to left crus of diaphragm, posterior to splenic vein and pancreas
  - Often crescentic in shape, lambda, tricorn hat, or triangular on transverse section
- **Adrenal cortex**
  - Derived from mesoderm
  - Has important endocrine functions
  - Secretes corticosteroids (cortisol, aldosterone) and androgens
- **Adrenal medulla**
  - Derived from neural crest
  - Part of sympathetic nervous system
  - Chromaffin cells secrete catecholamines (mostly epinephrine) into bloodstream
- Adrenal gland has very rich vascular and nervous connections
- **Arteries**
  - **Superior adrenal arteries**: 6-8 from inferior phrenic arteries
  - **Middle adrenal artery**: 1 from abdominal aorta
  - **Inferior adrenal artery**: 1 from renal arteries
- **Veins**
  - Right adrenal vein drains into IVC
  - Left adrenal vein drains into left renal vein (usually after joining left inferior phrenic vein)

ANATOMY IMAGING ISSUES

Imaging Recommendations

- Transducer: 2-5 MHz for adults
- High-frequency (7.5- to 10.0-MHz) linear transducer used in neonates
- Complex shape requires multiplanar evaluation
  - Sweeps should be taken in both transverse and longitudinal planes
- **Right adrenal gland**
  - Intercostal transverse approach, using liver as acoustic window
  - Direct anterior abdomen scanning is limited by overlying bowel loops and depth to gland
- **Left adrenal gland**
  - Intercostal at midaxillary line, using spleen or left kidney as acoustic window
  - In pediatric subjects and thin adults, direct transabdominal US at epigastrium
    - Stomach may be distended with fluid to serve as acoustic window
- **Sonographic appearance**
  - Relative to body size, adrenal glands are much larger and more easily identified in neonatal population
    - Also makes them more vulnerable to hemorrhage
  - Cortex is hypoechoic with hyperechoic medulla
    - Creates **ice cream sandwich** appearance
  - Adrenal glands often difficult to see and easily overlooked in adult patients (especially if obese) unless specifically targeted
  - Any masses should be documented and measured
    - Pay particular attention to sonographic appearance (e.g., echogenic mass highly suggestive of fat in a myelolipoma)

CLINICAL IMPLICATIONS

Clinical Importance

- Rich blood supply reflects important endocrine function
- Adrenal glands are designed to respond to stress (trauma, sepsis, surgery, etc.) by secreting cortisol and epinephrine
- **Hemorrhage**
  - Most common in neonatal population
    - Associated with many perinatal stressors: Asphyxia, sepsis, birth trauma, coagulopathies
    - Right > left; bilateral in 5-10%
  - Adults
    - Anticoagulation therapy most common cause
    - Overwhelming stress (surgery, sepsis, burns, hypotension) may result in adrenal hemorrhage, acute adrenal insufficiency (addisonian crisis)
      - □ Relatively uncommon condition but potentially catastrophic event
    - Blunt abdominal trauma
      - □ Generally unilateral (right > left)
  - Appearance changes over time
    - Acute: Hemorrhage appears echogenic & mass-like
    - Subacute: Blood products liquefy & contract, creating mixed echotexture mass
    - Chronic: Adrenal resumes normal size, ± Ca^{2+} or cyst
- **Metastases**: Common site for hematologic metastases (lung, breast, melanoma, etc.)
- **Adrenal adenoma**
  - Very common (at least 2% of general population), but most are small, nonfunctioning
  - Functional adenomas
    - **Cushing syndrome (excess cortisol)**: Truncal obesity, hirsutism, hypertension, abdominal striae
    - **Conn syndrome (excess aldosterone)**: Hypertension, hypokalemic alkalosis
- **Myelolipoma**
  - Benign tumor composed of mature adipose tissue and variable amount of hematopoietic elements
  - Characteristic echogenic appearance on US
- **Pheochromocytoma**
  - Catecholamine-secreting tumor from adrenal medulla
  - Location: Adrenal gland (90%), sympathetic chain from neck to bladder (10%)
- **Neuroblastoma**
  - Most common extracranial solid malignancy in children (median age at diagnosis: 15-17 months)
  - Location: Adrenal gland > retroperitoneum > posterior mediastinum

ADRENAL GLANDS

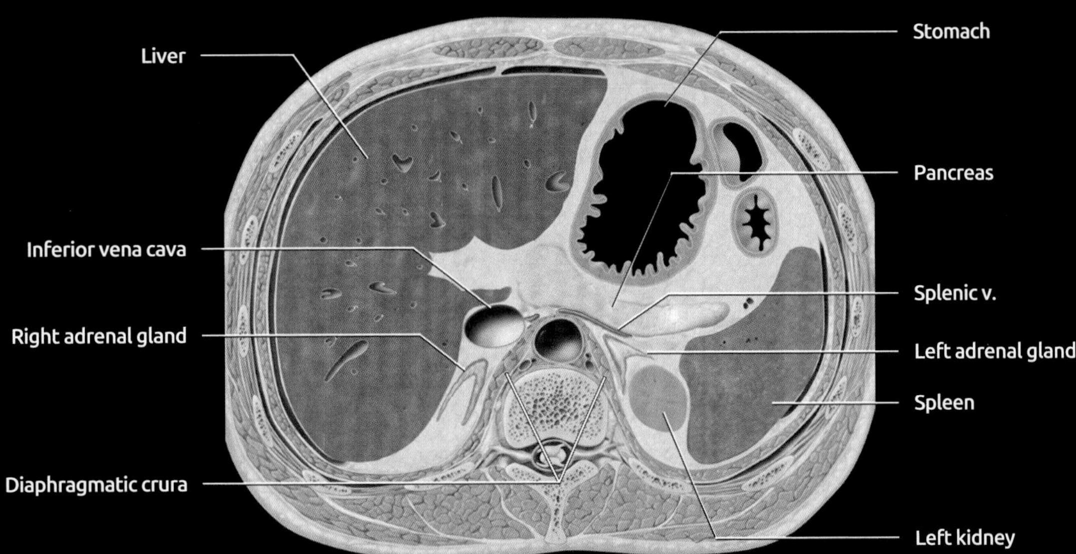

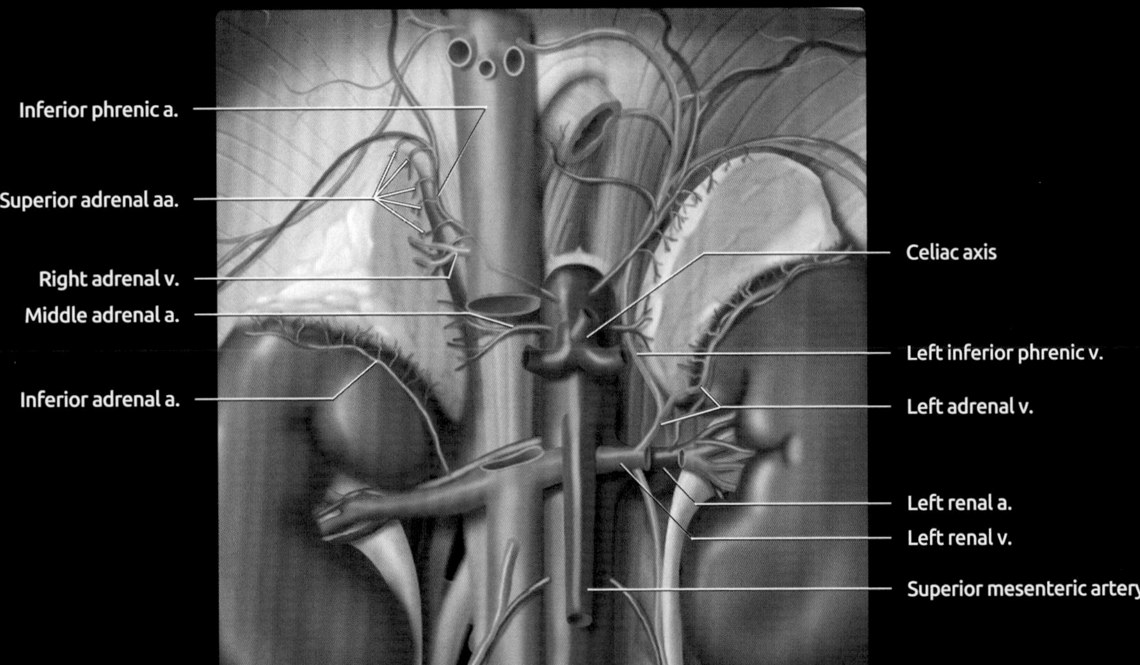

(Top) *Graphic shows the right adrenal gland lying above the right kidney, while the left adrenal gland lies partly in front of the upper pole of the left kidney. The left adrenal gland lies directly posterior to the splenic vein and body of pancreas and lateral to the left crus of the diaphragm. The right adrenal gland lies lateral to the right crus, medial to the liver, and directly behind the inferior vena cava (IVC).* **(Bottom)** *The size of the adrenal glands is exaggerated in this illustration to facilitate demonstration of the vascular anatomy. The adrenal glands have a very rich neural and vascular supply, reflecting their critical role in maintaining homeostasis and responding to stress. The superior adrenal arteries are short branches of the inferior phrenic arteries bilaterally. The middle adrenal arteries are short vessels arising from the aorta. The inferior adrenal arteries are branches of the renal arteries. The left adrenal vein drains into the left renal vein (usually after joining with the inferior phrenic vein), while the right adrenal vein drains directly into the IVC.*

ADRENAL GLANDS, NEONATE

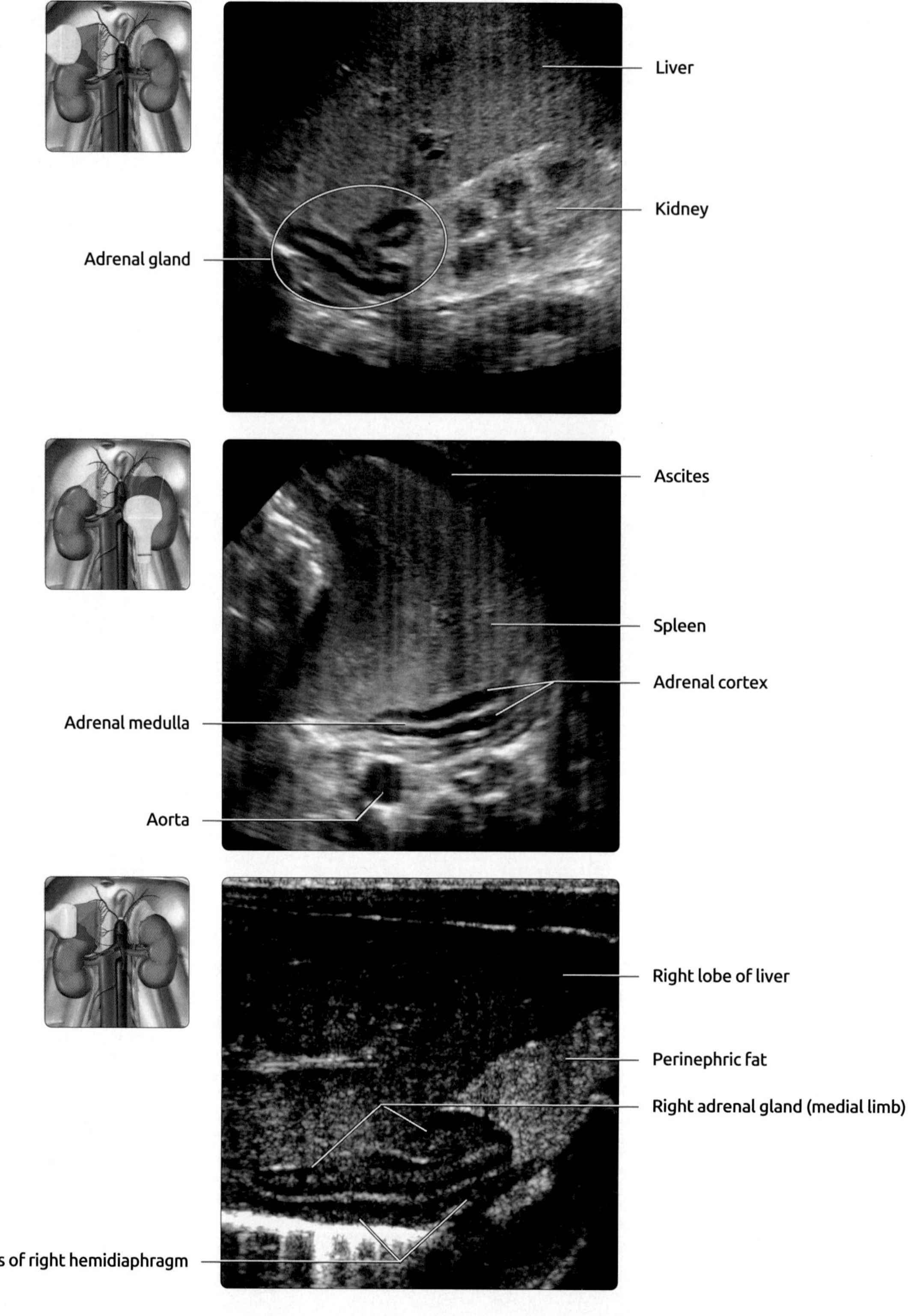

(Top) *Longitudinal US of the right adrenal gland in a neonate shows its folded, triangular morphology and relative large size when compared to the kidney. Relative to body size, adrenal glands are much larger and more easily identified in neonatal population. This also makes them more vulnerable to hemorrhage.* **(Middle)** *Transverse US of the left adrenal gland in a newborn shows the typical trilaminar, ice cream sandwich appearance with a hypoechoic cortex and hyperechoic medulla.* **(Bottom)** *Longitudinal US of the right adrenal gland is shown using the liver as acoustic window. Using a high-frequency linear transducer better demonstrates the adrenal gland in neonates and infants; note the typical trilaminar appearance. Be careful not to confuse the crus of the diaphragm, which has a uniform hypoechoic appearance, with the adrenal gland.*

ADRENAL GLANDS, ADULT

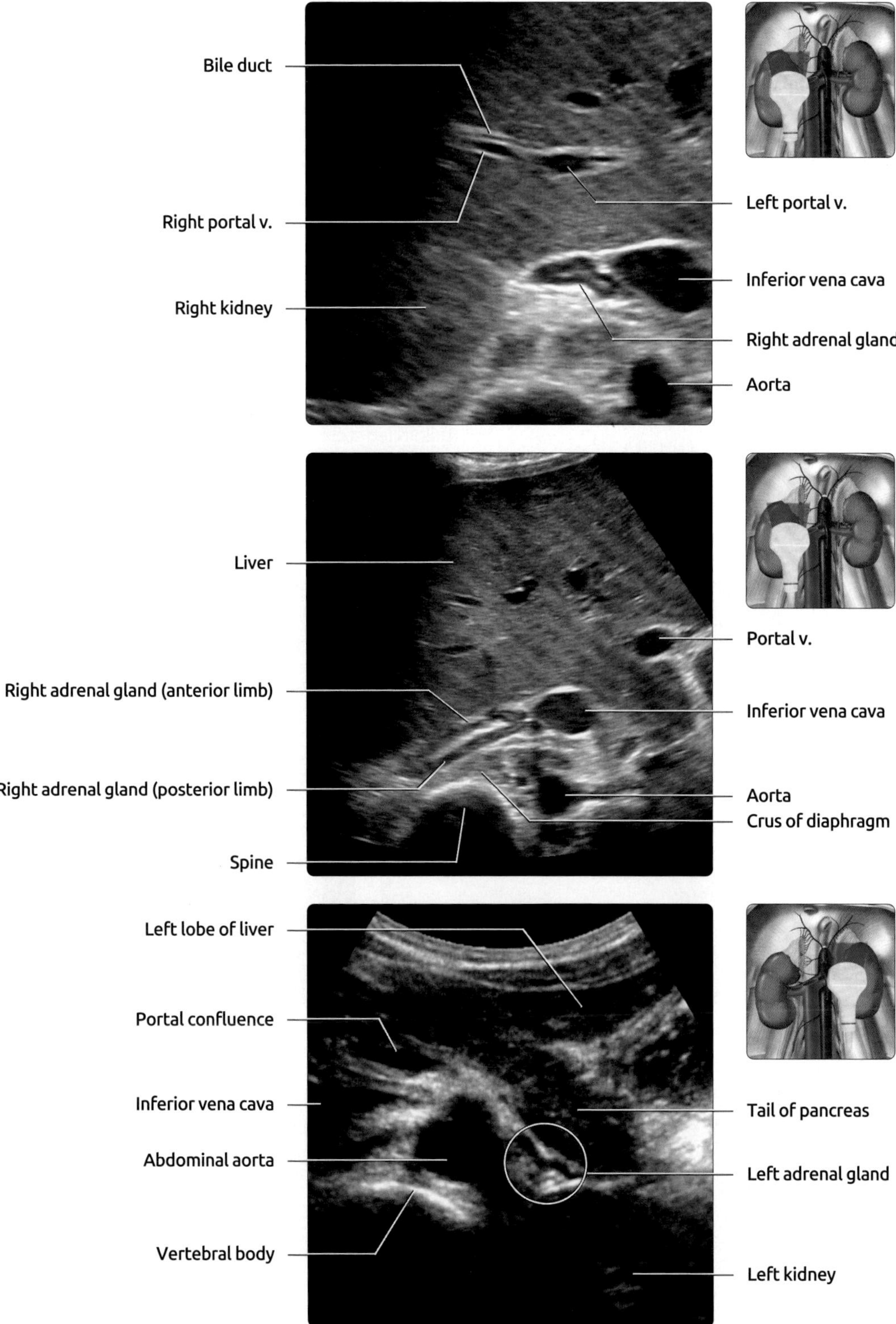

(Top) *Axial US in a 19-year-old woman shows the adrenal gland adjacent to the IVC. Note the trilaminar appearance is still seen in this young adult.* **(Middle)** *Using the liver as an acoustic window, the right adrenal gland is particularly well seen in this thin adult. Two limbs are easily identified.* **(Bottom)** *Subxiphoid transverse grayscale US performed at the epigastrium shows the pancreatic body and tail. The left adrenal gland is seen as a lambda structure and surrounded by hyperechoic perirenal fat. It is anterior to the left kidney and to the left of the abdominal aorta. The adrenal gland can be easily missed if not specifically targeted.*

Adrenal Hemorrhage

KEY FACTS

IMAGING

- Unilateral or bilateral, round or oval, well-defined mass
- Variable echogenicity depending on stage of hemorrhage
- Acute hematoma: Hyperechoic
- Subacute hematoma: Mixed echogenicity ± central hypoechoic area
- Chronic hematoma: Hypo- or anechoic cyst-like lesion
  - Curvilinear calcification, internal echoes/layering debris
- Adreniform enlargement of adrenal gland
- Displacement & mass effect on kidney and IVC
- Avascular on color Doppler

TOP DIFFERENTIAL DIAGNOSES

- Adrenal adenoma
- Pheochromocytoma
- Myelolipoma
- Primary adrenal, metastatic, or adjacent tumors

PATHOLOGY

- Blunt abdominal trauma (right gland > left gland)
- Nontraumatic pathogenesis: Vascular dam of abundant arterial supply and limited venous drainage
  - Anticoagulation therapy, recent surgery, sepsis, burns, hypotension, steroids, pregnancy
  - Hemorrhage in primary adrenal or metastatic tumors: Pheochromocytoma, myelolipoma, adrenal carcinoma

CLINICAL ISSUES

- Relatively uncommon condition but potentially catastrophic event due to adrenal insufficiency
- More common in neonates than children and adults
- Abdominal, flank, or back pain, nausea, and vomiting, fever, tachycardia, hypotension

SCANNING TIPS

- Left adrenal gland can be difficult to image, use spleen or fluid-filled stomach as acoustic window

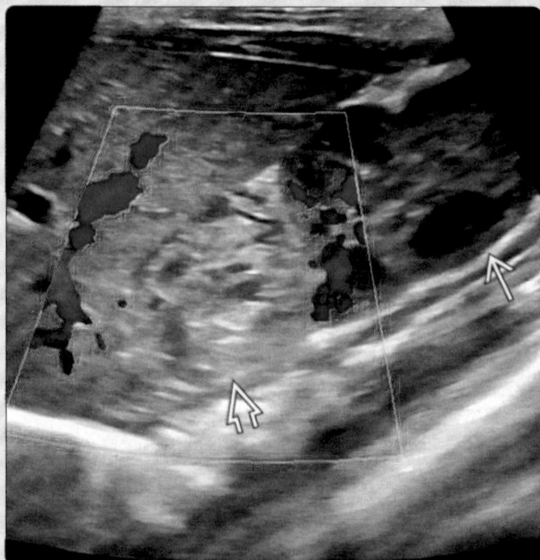
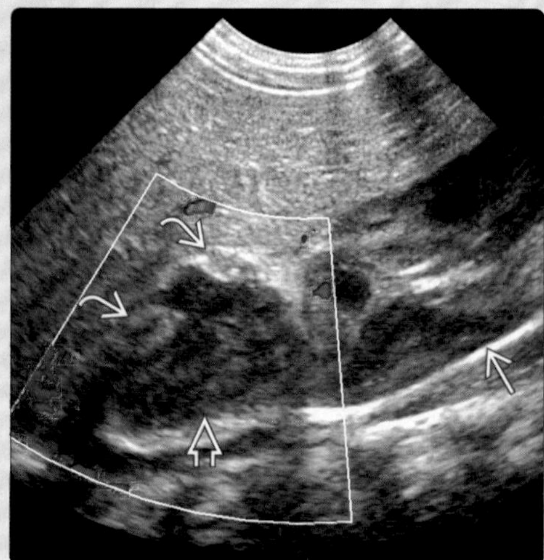

(Left) *Longitudinal color Doppler ultrasound shows an avascular, heterogeneously hyperechoic, right suprarenal lesion ➡. Note right kidney ➡.* **(Right)** *Longitudinal color Doppler ultrasound shows a heterogeneous, avascular right suprarenal lesion with a hypoechoic center ➡ and irregular echogenic components along the periphery ➡. Note right kidney ➡.*

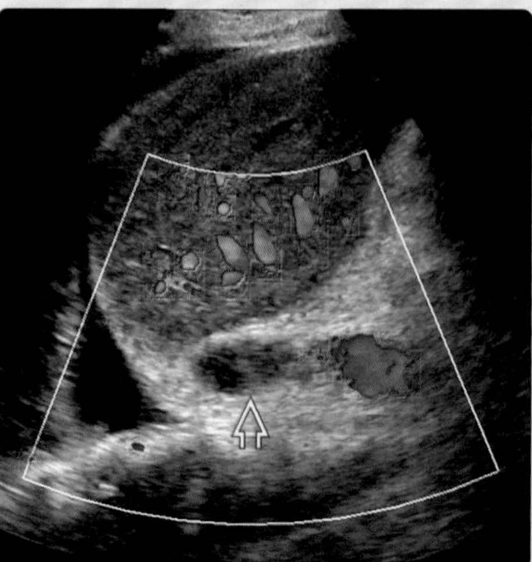
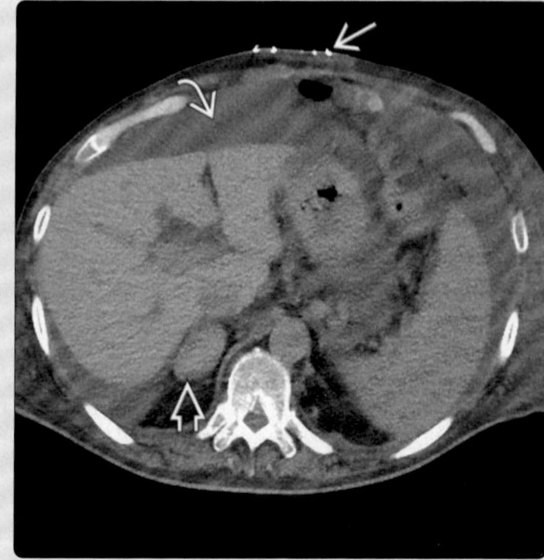

(Left) *Longitudinal color Doppler ultrasound shows a well-defined, hypoechoic lesion in the right adrenal gland with no vascular flow ➡.* **(Right)** *Axial NECT in the same patient demonstrates a well-defined, hyperdense right adrenal hematoma ➡. Note skin staples ➡ in the abdominal wall from recent liver transplantation as well as ascites ➡.*

Myelolipoma

KEY FACTS

TERMINOLOGY

- Definition: Rare benign tumor consisting of macroscopic fat interspersed with hematopoietic elements

IMAGING

- Appearance varies depending on admixture of fatty and myeloid soft tissue components
- Predominantly fatty: Well-defined, homogeneous, hyperechoic suprarenal mass
  - When small, difficult to distinguish from echogenic retroperitoneal fat
- When myeloid cells predominate: Heterogeneous mass, isoechoic or hypoechoic
- Punctate calcification in 25-30% of cases
- Hemorrhage more common when > 4 cm, varied appearance
- Color Doppler: Avascular to hypovascular

TOP DIFFERENTIAL DIAGNOSES

- Adrenal hemorrhage
- Pheochromocytoma
- Liposarcoma
- Renal angiomyolipoma
- Adrenal adenoma
- Adrenal metastases

CLINICAL ISSUES

- Usually in older age group: 50-70 years; M=F
- Usually found incidentally
- Clinical signs are usually absent except in rare cases of hemorrhage and rupture producing acute abdomen
- Pain from necrosis, hemorrhage, or compression of structures

SCANNING TIPS

- Look for acoustic shadowing or propagation speed artifact from fat

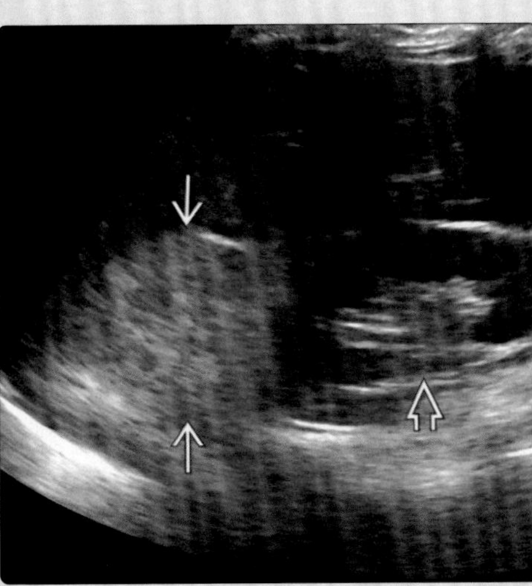

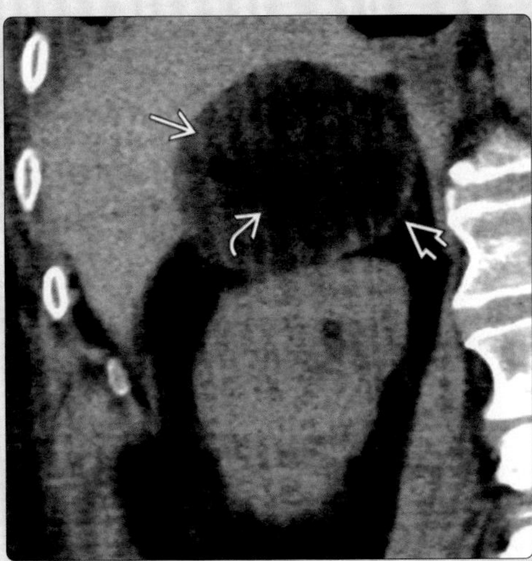

(Left) *Longitudinal ultrasound of a myelolipoma shows a lobulated, well-defined, heterogeneously hyperechoic mass → above the right kidney ⇨.* **(Right)** *Coronal CT demonstrates a heterogeneous, encapsulated, suprarenal mass → containing ill-defined, "smoky" soft tissue elements ↪ and macroscopic fat ⇨.*

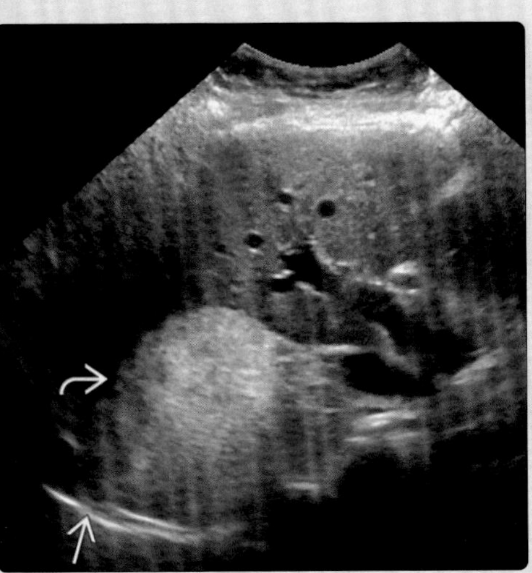

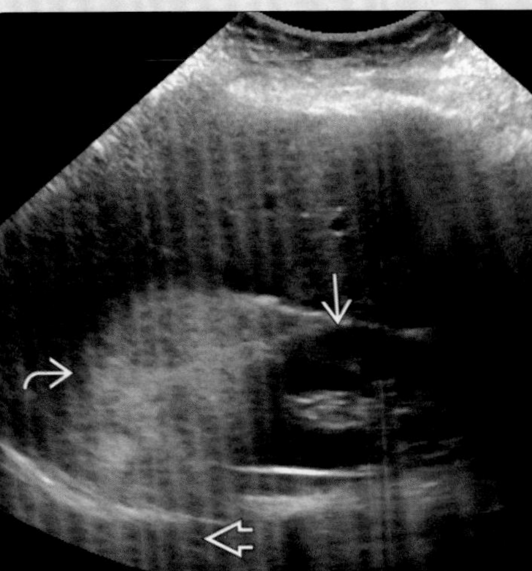

(Left) *Transverse ultrasound of a myelolipoma shows a lobulated, well-defined, heterogeneously hyperechoic mass ↪ posterior to the liver. There is discontinuity of the diaphragm → from propagation speed artifact.* **(Right)** *Longitudinal ultrasound of a myelolipoma ↪ shows the well-defined, hyperechoic mass above the right kidney →. There is posterior shadowing ⇨.*

Adrenal Adenoma

KEY FACTS

TERMINOLOGY

- Synonym: Adrenocortical adenoma

IMAGING

- Varies from 2-5 cm, typically < 3 cm, bilateral in 10%
- Nonspecific sonographic appearance
- Well-circumscribed, solid, oval-shaped mass
- Usually homogeneous and hypoechoic
- Atypically can appear more heterogeneous, but necrosis is rare in small adenomas
- CT and MR: Best imaging modalities to confirm diagnosis
- Hypovascular on color Doppler

TOP DIFFERENTIAL DIAGNOSES

- Adrenal metastases
- Adrenal hemorrhage
- Pheochromocytoma

PATHOLOGY

- Classified as nonfunctioning vs. functioning
- 70% show high intracytoplasmic lipid content: "lipid rich"

CLINICAL ISSUES

- More commonly detected as incidental finding
  - Increased detection in recent years due to greater imaging utilization, > 90% of all incidentalomas
- 15% are functional and produce hormones
- Functioning adenomas: Cushing syndrome, Conn syndrome, or virilization syndromes
- Hypertension and weakness with Cushing and Conn syndrome

SCANNING TIPS

- Size and stability are helpful clues to diagnosis
- CT or MR required for confirmation

(Left) *Graphic shows a small, homogeneous, solid nodule ➡ arising from the peripheral adrenal gland. Note the oval shape and smooth margin typical of an adrenal adenoma. Adenomas have a high cholesterol content similar to adrenal cortex.* **(Right)** *Longitudinal ultrasound shows a well-circumscribed, homogeneous, solid mass ➡ above the right kidney ➡.*

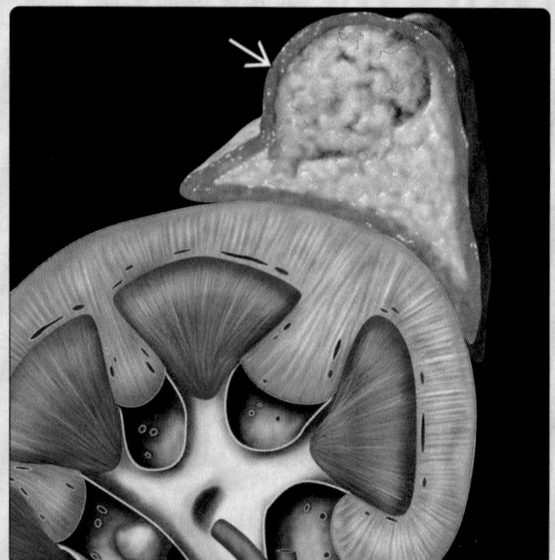

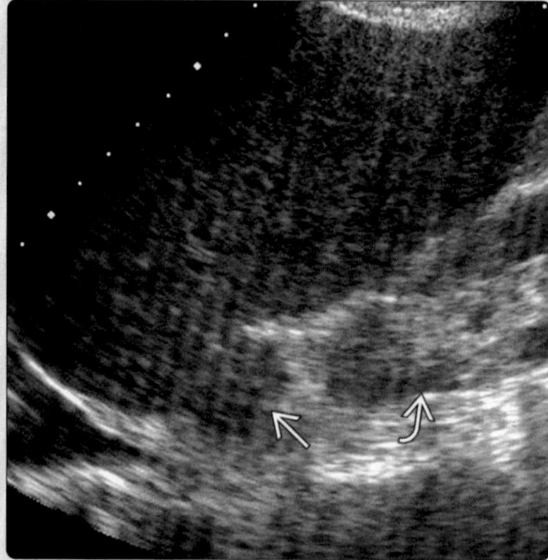

(Left) *Transverse ultrasound shows a well-demarcated, homogeneous right adrenal mass ➡, which is mildly hyperechoic relative to the liver ➡.* **(Right)** *Transverse color Doppler ultrasound in the same patient shows that the lesion ➡ is relatively hypovascular.*

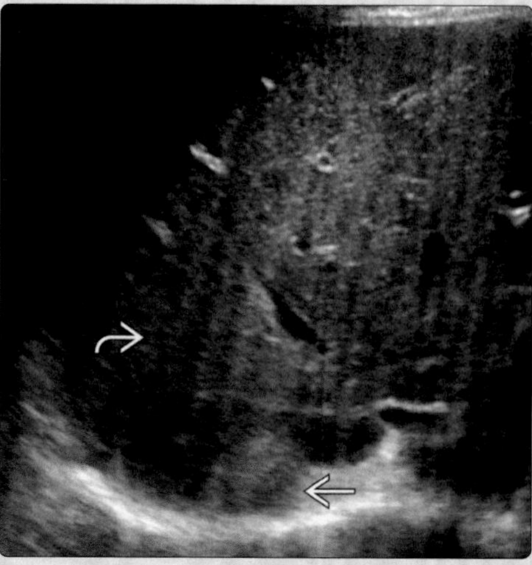

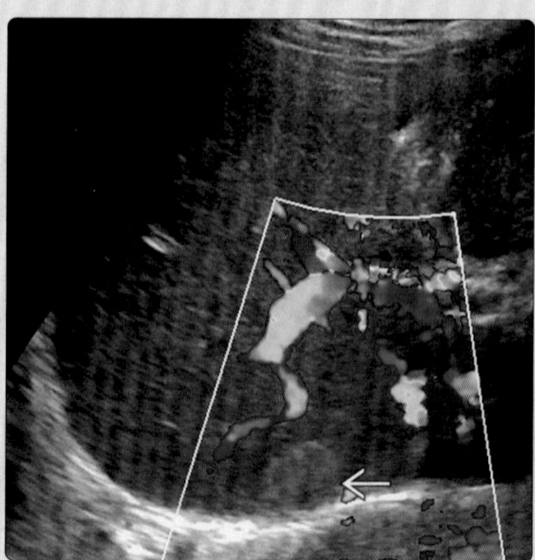

Adrenal Cyst

KEY FACTS

TERMINOLOGY

- Simple or complex cystic lesion in adrenal gland

IMAGING

- Well-defined, round, typically unilocular, thin-walled, suprarenal cyst
- Anechoic or hypoechoic lesion with thin wall and posterior acoustic enhancement
  - Low-level internal echoes, calcification, fluid-fluid levels, and septations suggest recent hemorrhage
- Concerning features: Complicated cyst, ≥ 5 cm, internal echogenicity, or thick wall (≥ 3 mm) → suspect malignancy
- Color Doppler shows no internal flow
- May be initially detected and characterized by ultrasound; ultrasound can be used for follow-up
- CT and MR for further characterization if complex

TOP DIFFERENTIAL DIAGNOSES

- Adjacent cystic lesions
- Adrenal adenoma
- Necrotic adrenal tumor

PATHOLOGY

- Endothelial lining (~ 45%): Lymphangioma (majority) and hemangioma
- Pseudocyst (~ 39%): Prior hemorrhage or infarction
- Epithelial lining (~ 9%): True simple cyst
- Parasitic cyst (~ 7%): Usually due to disseminated *Echinococcus granulosus* infection

CLINICAL ISSUES

- Typically clinically silent
- Abdominal or flank pain due to mass effect or cyst rupture
- Often increases in size over time; not indicative of malignancy

SCANNING TIPS

- Adrenal cysts are avascular; optimize Doppler settings to avoid misdiagnosis

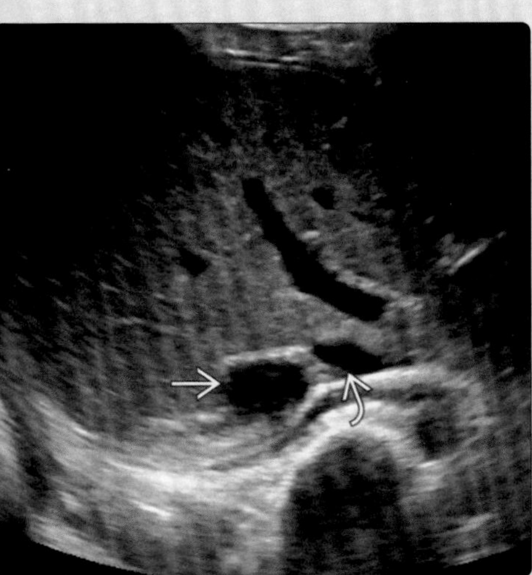

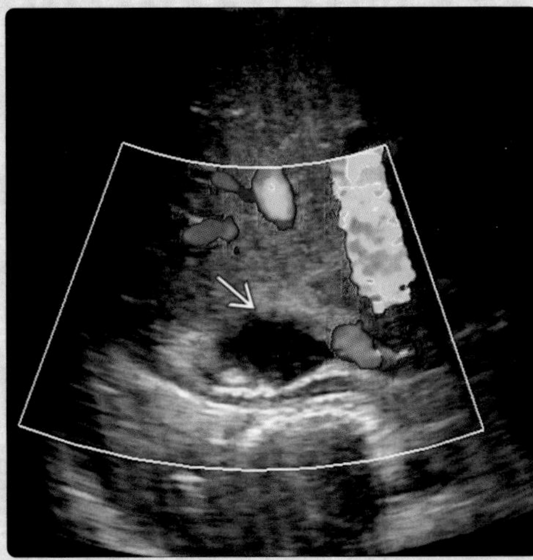

(Left) *Transverse ultrasound of a posttraumatic adrenal cyst ➡ lateral to the vena cava ➡ is shown. The cyst is small and unilocular with low-level internal echoes.* **(Right)** *Transverse color Doppler ultrasound shows the same posttraumatic adrenal cyst ➡. There is no internal color flow.*

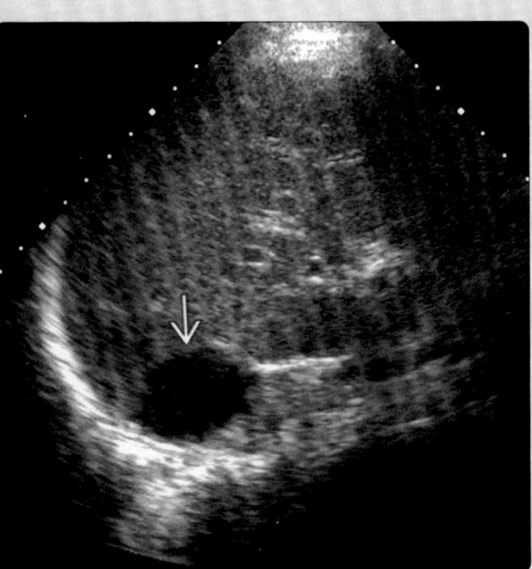

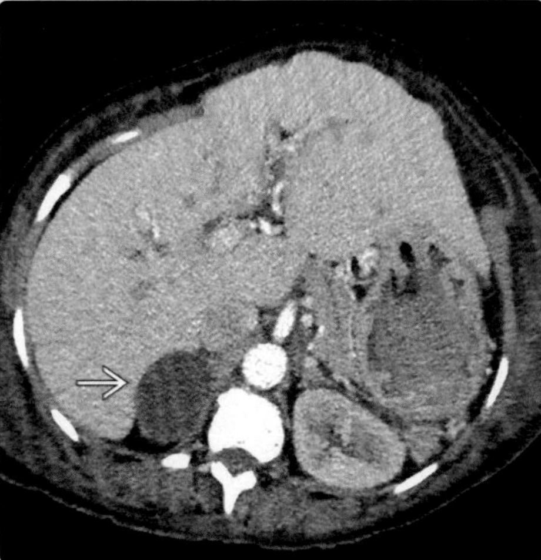

(Left) *Oblique ultrasound shows a well-circumscribed, thin-walled lesion with low-level echoes and posterior acoustic enhancement ➡ in the right adrenal. There was no internal color flow in this adrenal cyst.* **(Right)** *Axial CECT of the same patient shows a nonenhancing right adrenal cyst ➡.*

KEY FACTS

TERMINOLOGY

- Rare catecholamine-secreting tumor arising from chromaffin cells of adrenal medulla
- Termed **paraganglioma** if extraadrenal

IMAGING

- Size: Up to 15 cm (typically 3-5 cm)
- Variable appearance: Solid (75%) > solid/cystic or cystic
- Larger tumors: Solid; homogeneous (46%) or heterogeneous (54%)
- Can be predominantly cystic due to chronic hemorrhage and necrotic debris (fluid-fluid level)
- Hypervascular
- Ultrasound may detect adrenal masses but is limited for extraadrenal disease
- **68Ga-DOTATATE PET/CT** or **I-123 MIBG**: Most specific modalities for localization and detection of metastatic/recurrent disease

TOP DIFFERENTIAL DIAGNOSES

- Adrenal adenoma
- Adrenal metastases or lymphoma
- Adrenocortical carcinoma
- Adrenal neuroblastoma
- Adrenal granulomatous infection

PATHOLOGY

- 25% have autosomal dominant gene mutation

CLINICAL ISSUES

- Classic triad (arises from adrenergic excess): Paroxysmal headache, palpitations, sweating
- Majority are asymptomatic; symptoms may be episodic or paroxysmal
- Hypertensive crisis: Palpitations, tremors, arrhythmias, pain, myocardial infarction
- Hereditary cases (mean age: 25 years)
- Sporadic cases: 3rd and 4th decades (mean age: 44 years)

(Left) *Graphic shows a typical pheochromocytoma ➔, moderate in size, with a well-circumscribed margin and solid appearance. Note hypervascularity ➔ of the mass, which commonly results in necrosis and cystic change.* **(Right)** *Longitudinal transabdominal ultrasound shows a well-demarcated, solid right adrenal mass ➔, which was proven to be a pheochromocytoma. It is hyperechoic to the renal cortex ➔.*

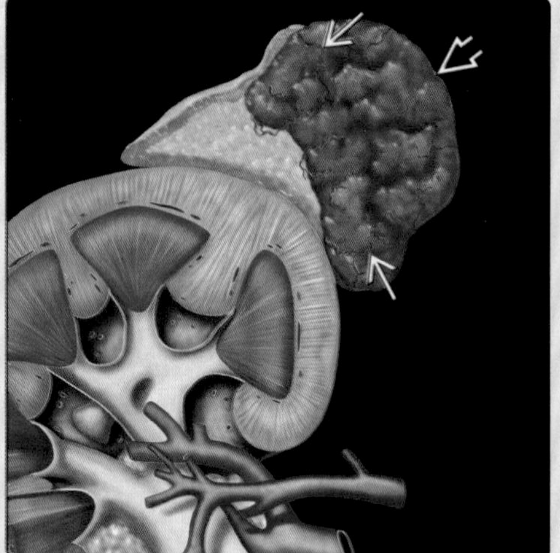

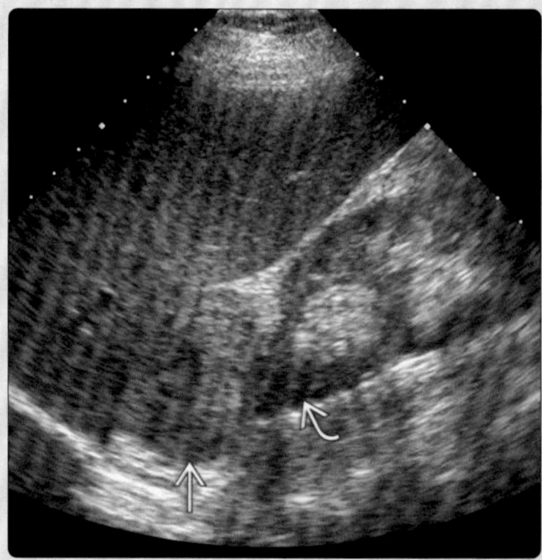

(Left) *Transverse ultrasound of a right adrenal pheochromocytoma shows a well-defined solid mass ➔ with central cystic areas ➔ representing hemorrhage or necrosis.* **(Right)** *Longitudinal ultrasound of a right adrenal pheochromocytoma shows that the mass ➔ is separate from the upper pole of the kidney ➔. This patient had bilateral pheochromocytomas but the left-sided mass was not detected by ultrasound.*

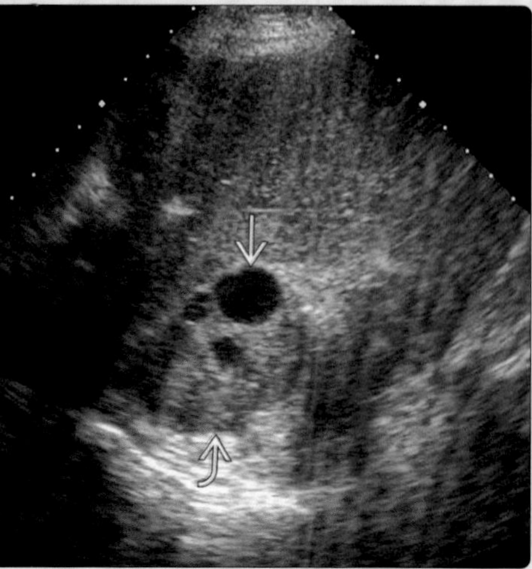

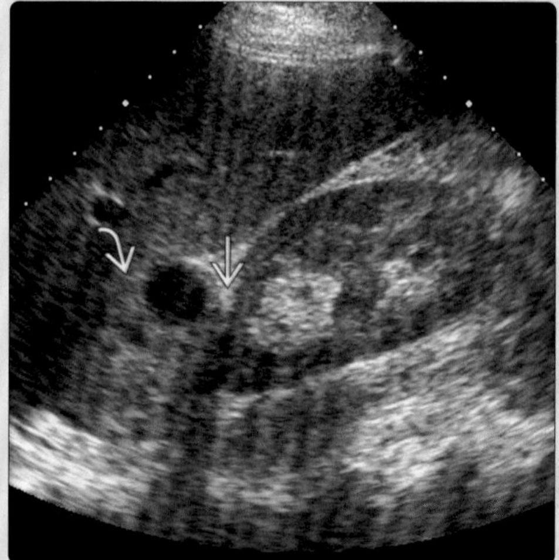

KEY FACTS

TERMINOLOGY

- **Synonyms**: Adrenocortical carcinoma; adrenal cancer

IMAGING

- Ultrasound may be used for initial screening in patients with abdominal pain but offers limited ability to characterize or differentiate from other adrenal masses
- Large masses; average size: 9 cm; 70% > 6 cm
  - Heterogeneous, hypoechoic/anechoic areas (necrosis &/or hemorrhage)
  - Echogenic solid components; ± calcification
  - Local invasion: Inferior vena cava, kidney, liver
- Small tumors: Homogeneous, hypoechoic, similar to renal cortex
- Functioning tumors usually smaller (≤ 5 cm) than nonfunctioning tumors (≥ 10 cm) at presentation
- Invasion/occlusion of adrenal vein, renal vein, and inferior vena cava; ± intraluminal tumor thrombus
- Best imaging tool: CECT or CEMR

TOP DIFFERENTIAL DIAGNOSES

- Pheochromocytoma
- Adrenal metastases
- Neuroblastoma (in children)
- Adrenal hemorrhage
- Other adrenal tumors complicated by hemorrhage

PATHOLOGY

- Rare, aggressive tumor arising from adrenal cortex, often with local invasion
- Metastases to regional lymph nodes, liver, lung, bone

CLINICAL ISSUES

- Rare: < 0.2% of all cancers, slightly more common in women
- Bimodal distribution: < 5 years old (1st peak) and 30-50 years old (2nd peak)
- Associated syndromes: Cushing, female virilization, Conn, male feminization

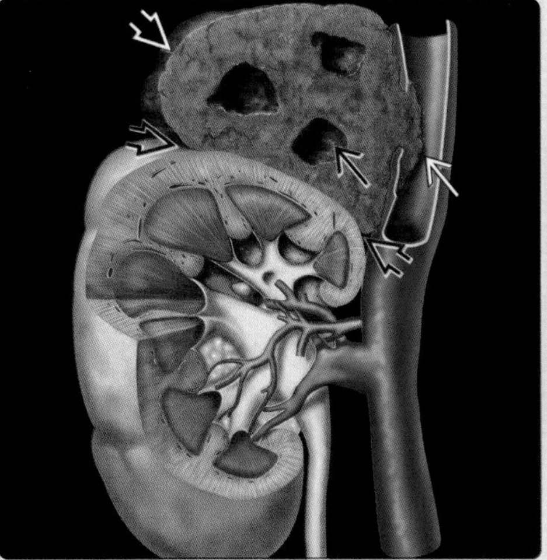

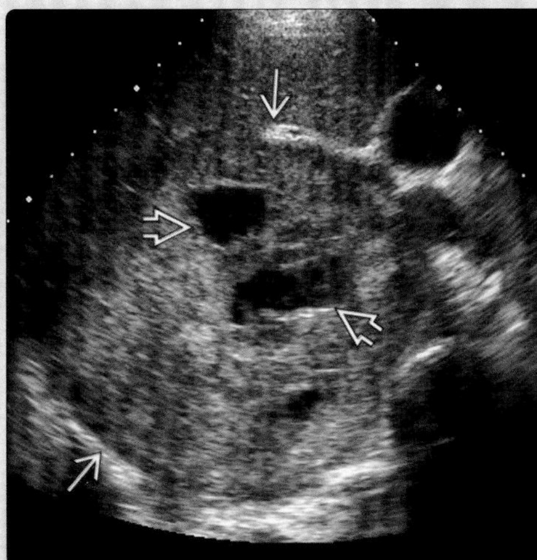

(Left) *Longitudinal graphic shows a large right adrenal carcinoma ➡ with areas of necrosis ➡, tumor invasion into the inferior vena cava (IVC) ➡, and compression of the right renal upper pole ➡.* **(Right)** *Transverse ultrasound of a tender mass in a 15-year-old male patient is shown. A large, predominantly solid mass ➡ represents adrenal cortical carcinoma. There were areas of necrosis ➡.*

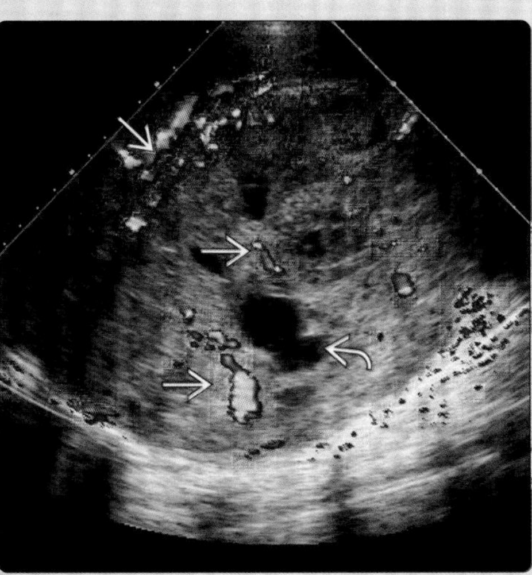

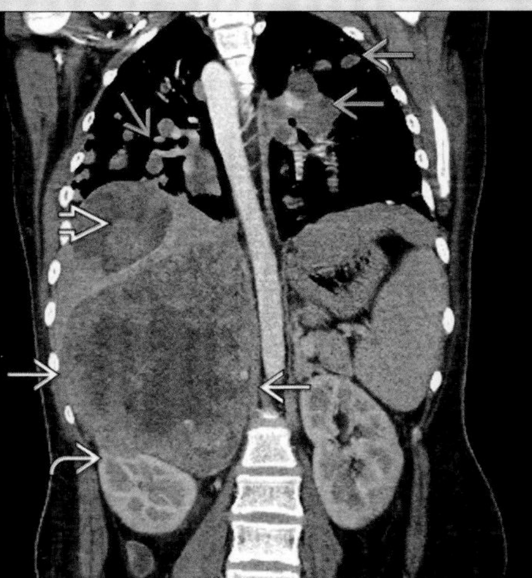

(Left) *Longitudinal color Doppler ultrasound of adrenal cortical carcinoma in a 15-year-old male patient is shown. There is color flow in the solid components of the tumor ➡ but none in the cystic necrotic areas ➡.* **(Right)** *Coronal CECT of adrenal cortical carcinoma in a 15-year-old male patient is shown. The large adrenal mass ➡ invades the right kidney ➡. There were numerous lung ➡ and liver ➡ metastases.*

PART I
SECTION 8
Abdominal Wall/Peritoneal Cavity

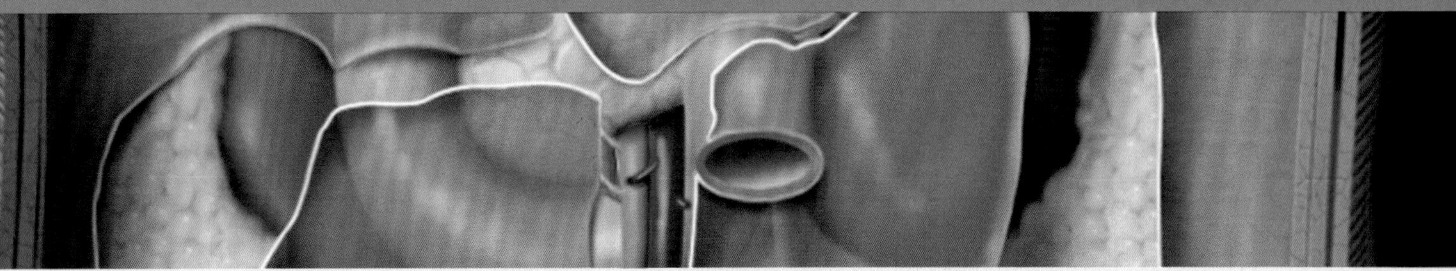

Anatomy and Approach

Abdominal Wall

Peritoneal Cavity

GROSS ANATOMY

Overview

- Major lymphatic vessels and nodal chains lie along major blood vessels (aorta, inferior vena cava, iliac)
- Lymph nodes carry same name as vessel they accompany
- Lymph from alimentary tract, liver, spleen, and pancreas passes along celiac, superior mesenteric chains to nodes
  - Efferent vessels from alimentary nodes form intestinal lymphatic trunks
  - Cisterna chyli (chyle cistern)
    - Formed by confluence of intestinal lymphatic trunks and right and left lumbar lymphatic trunks, which receive lymph from nonalimentary viscera, abdominal wall, and lower extremities
    - May be discrete sac or plexiform convergence
- Thoracic duct: Inferior extent is chyle cistern at L1-L2 level
  - Formed by convergence of main lymphatic ducts of abdomen
  - Ascends through aortic hiatus in diaphragm to enter posterior mediastinum
  - Ends by entering junction of left subclavian and internal jugular veins
- Lymphatic system drains surplus fluid from extracellular spaces and returns it to bloodstream
  - Important function in defense against infection, inflammation, and tumor via lymphoid tissue present in lymph nodes, gut wall, spleen, and thymus
  - Absorbs and transports dietary lipids from intestine to thoracic duct and bloodstream
- Lymph nodes
  - Composed of cortex and medulla
  - Invested in fibrous capsule, which extends into nodal parenchyma to form trabeculae
  - Internal honeycomb structure filled with lymphocytes that collect and destroy pathogens
  - Hilum: In concave side, with artery and vein, surrounded by fat

Abdominopelvic Nodes

- Preaortic nodes
  - Celiac nodes: Drainage from gastric nodes, hepatic nodes, and pancreaticosplenic nodes
  - Superior and inferior mesenteric nodes: Drainage from mesenteric nodes
- Lateral aortic (paraaortic/paracaval) nodes
  - Drainage from kidneys, adrenal glands, ureter, posterior abdominal wall, testes and ovary, uterus, and fallopian tubes
- Retroaortic nodes
  - Drainage from posterior abdominal wall
- External iliac nodes
  - Primary drainage from inguinal nodes
  - Flow into common iliac nodes
- Internal iliac nodes
  - Drainage from inferior pelvic viscera, deep perineum, and gluteal region
  - Flow into common iliac nodes
- Common iliac nodes
  - Drainage from external iliac, internal iliac, and sacral nodes
  - Flow into lumbar (lateral aortic) chain of nodes
- Superficial inguinal nodes
  - In superficial fascia parallel to inguinal ligament, along cephalad portion of greater saphenous vein
  - Receive lymphatic drainage from superficial lower extremity, superficial abdominal wall, and perineum
  - Flow into deep inguinal and external iliac nodes
- Deep inguinal nodes
  - Along medial side of femoral vein, deep to fascia lata and inguinal ligament
  - Receive lymphatic drainage from superficial inguinal and popliteal nodes
  - Flow into external iliac nodes

IMAGING ANATOMY

Overview

- CT is test of choice for cancer staging
- May be supplemented by PET/CT in select cancers
- US may be useful in children or thin adults
  - Normal nodes are elliptical with echogenic fatty hilum and uniform hypoechoic cortex
  - Normal lymph nodes rarely detected on abdominal US
- Normal diameter of lymph node varies depending on location
  - Short-axis diameter
    - Abdominopelvic < 10 mm
    - Hepatogastric ligament < 8 mm
    - Retrocrural < 6 mm

ANATOMY IMAGING ISSUES

Imaging Recommendations

- Transducer: 2-5 MHz or 5-9 MHz for thinner adult patients
- Patient examined in supine position with > 4 hours of fasting to decrease bowel gas
- Graded compression technique to clear overlying bowel loops

CLINICAL IMPLICATIONS

Clinical Importance

- Nodal enlargement is nonspecific, may be neoplastic, inflammatory, or reactive
- Normal-sized lymph nodes may harbor metastatic malignancy
- Node morphology is more specific for pathology
  - Abnormal nodes have replacement or loss of fatty hilum
  - Look for central necrosis, cystic change, or calcification
- Lymphoma
  - Multiple enlarged hypoechoic or anechoic nodes
- Metastatic lymphadenopathy
  - More echogenic and heterogeneous nodes compared to lymphomatous nodes
- Infectious/reactive lymphadenopathy
  - Nonspecific sonographic features
  - May contain necrotic centers in mycobacterial infection

RETROPERITONEAL LYMPH NODES

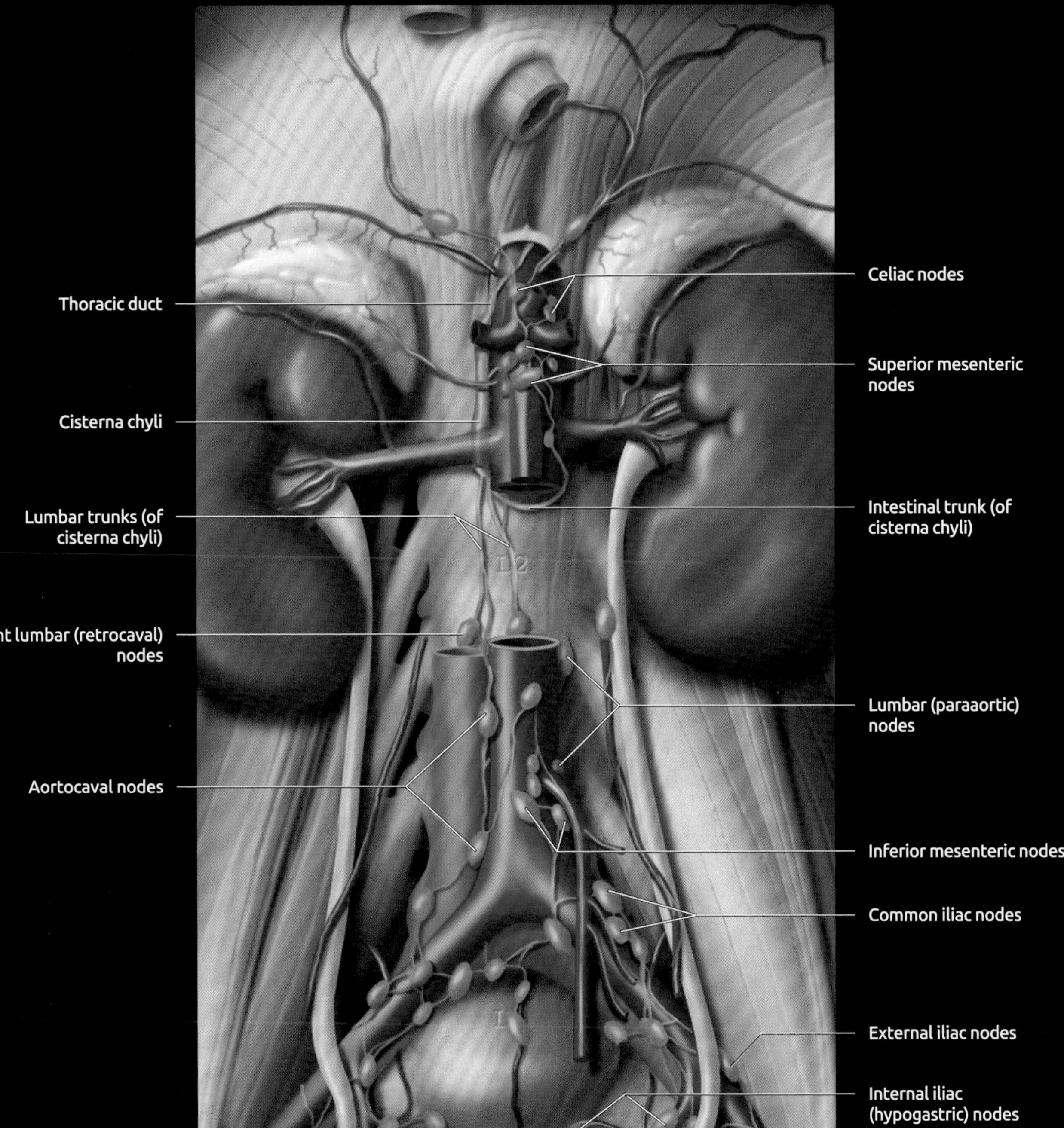

Graphic shows that the major lymphatics and lymph nodes of the abdomen are located along and share the same name as the major blood vessels, such as the external iliac nodes, celiac, and superior mesenteric nodes. The paraaortic and paracaval nodes are also referred to as the lumbar nodes and receive afferents from the lower abdominal viscera, abdominal wall, and lower extremities; they are frequently involved in inflammatory and neoplastic processes. The lumbar trunks join with an intestinal trunk (at ~ the L1 level) to form the cisterna chyli, which may be a discrete sac or a plexiform convergence. The cisterna chyli and other major lymphatic trunks join to form the thoracic duct, which passes through the aortic hiatus to enter the mediastinum. After picking up additional lymphatic trunks within the thorax, the thoracic duct empties into the left subclavian or innominate vein.

NONENLARGED NODES AND PATHOLOGIC NODES

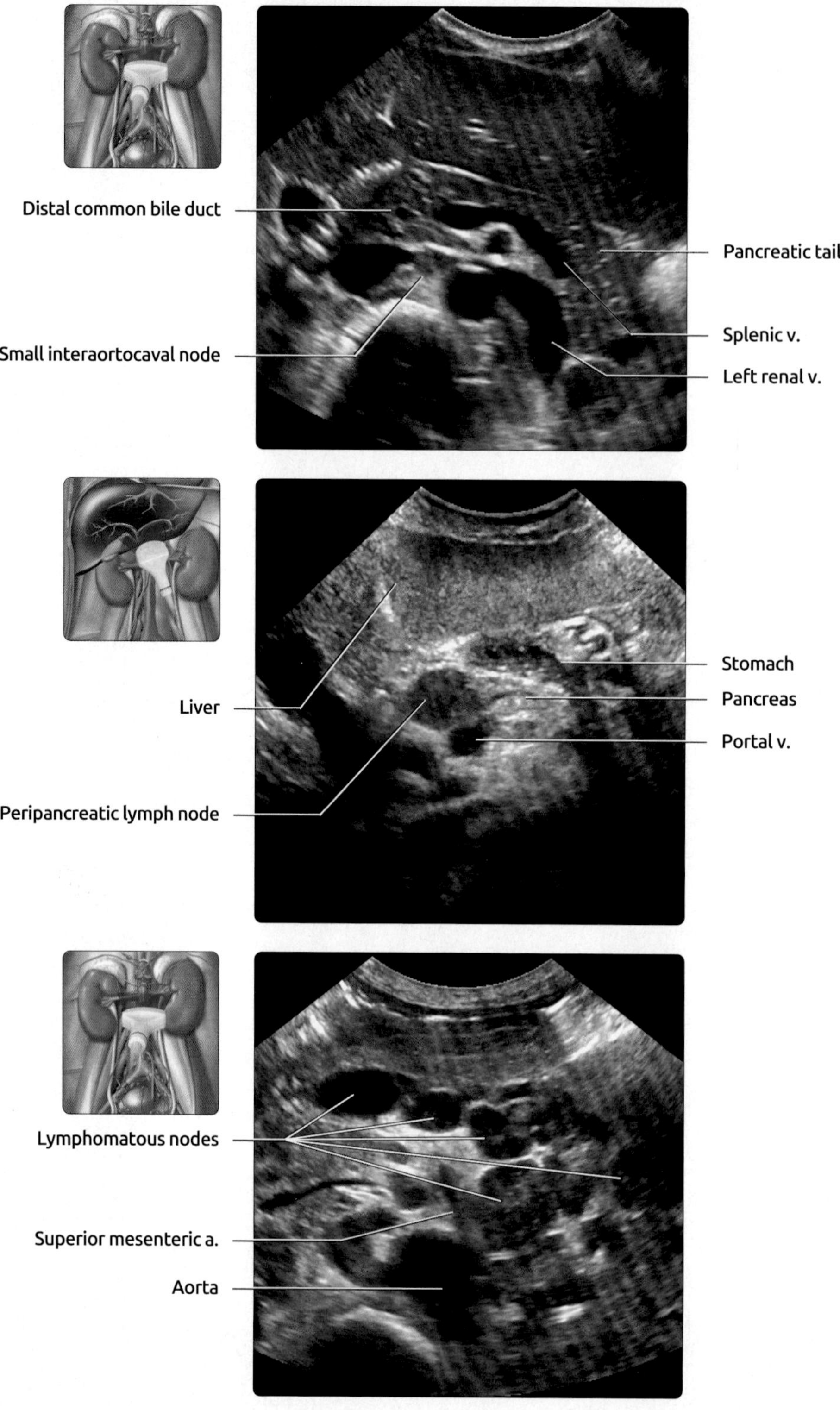

(Top) *Transverse US at the level of the pancreas and splenic vein shows a small interaortocaval node.* **(Middle)** *Transverse US of the epigastric region shows an enlarged hypoechoic peripancreatic lymph node anterior to the portal vein in a patient with hepatitis C. Normal-sized lymph nodes are rarely seen in adult abdominal US.* **(Bottom)** *Transverse US of the upper midline abdomen in a patient with lymphoma shows multiple, abnormal, enlarged hypoechoic lymph nodes around the superior mesenteric artery.*

LYMPHOMA

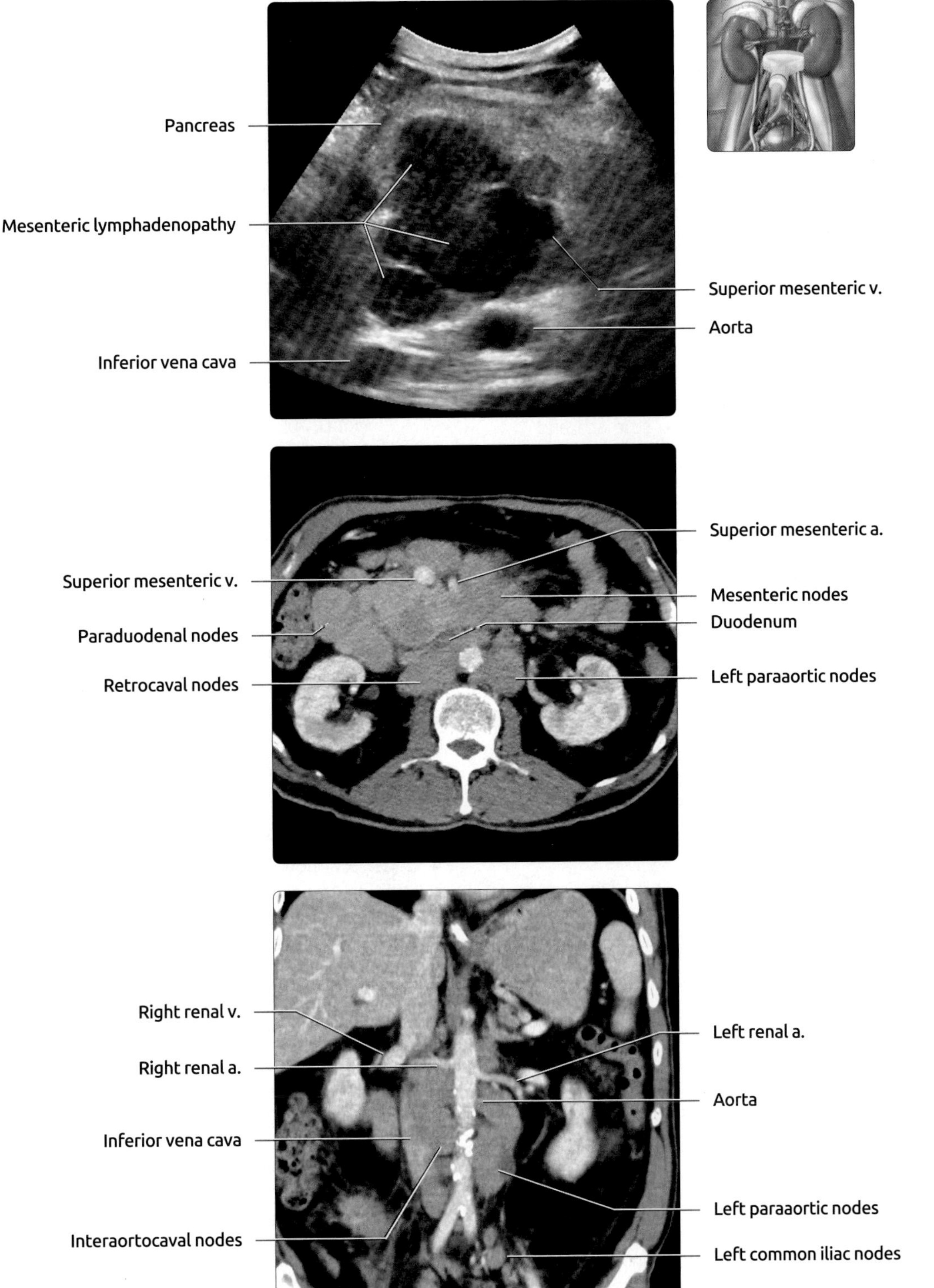

(Top) *Transverse ultrasound through the upper abdomen shows markedly enlarged lymph nodes anterior to the aorta and inferior vena cava. Nodes are usually hypoechoic in lymphoma.* **(Middle)** *Axial CECT at a lower level than the preceding image shows multiple pathologic lymph node groups in the mesentery and retroperitoneum.* **(Bottom)** *Coronal CECT through the retroperitoneum in the same patient shows rows of enlarged lymph nodes extending to the pelvis.*

TERMINOLOGY

Definitions

- Peritoneal cavity: Potential space in abdomen between visceral and parietal peritoneum, usually containing only small amount of peritoneal fluid (for lubrication)
- Abdominal cavity: Not synonymous with peritoneal cavity
    - Contains all of abdominal viscera (intra- and retroperitoneal)
    - Limited by abdominal wall muscles, diaphragm, and (arbitrarily) pelvic brim

GROSS ANATOMY

Divisions

- Greater sac of peritoneal cavity
- Lesser sac (omental bursa)
    - Communicates with greater sac via epiploic foramen (of Winslow)
    - Bounded anteriorly by caudate lobe, stomach, and greater omentum
        - Posteriorly by pancreas, left adrenal, and kidney
        - On left by splenorenal and gastrosplenic ligaments
        - On right by epiploic foramen and lesser omentum

Compartments

- Supramesocolic space
    - Divided into right and left supramesocolic spaces, which are separated by falciform ligament
        - Right supramesocolic space: Composed of right subphrenic space, right subhepatic space, and lesser sac
        - Left supramesocolic space: Divided into left perihepatic spaces (anterior and posterior) and left subphrenic (anterior perigastric and posterior perisplenic)
- Inframesocolic compartment
    - Divided into right inframesocolic space, left inframesocolic space, paracolic gutters, and pelvic cavity
    - Pelvic cavity is most dependent part of peritoneal cavity in erect and supine positions

Peritoneum

- Thin serous membrane consisting of single layer of squamous epithelium (mesothelium)
    - Parietal peritoneum lines abdominal wall
    - Visceral peritoneum (serosa) lines abdominal organs

Mesentery

- Double layer of peritoneum that encloses organ and connects it to abdominal wall
- Covered on both sides by mesothelium and has core of loose connective tissue containing fat, lymph nodes, blood vessels, and nerves passing to and from viscera
- Most mobile parts of intestine have mesentery, while ascending and descending colon are considered retroperitoneal (covered only by peritoneum on anterior surface)
- Root of mesentery is its attachment to posterior abdominal wall
- Root of small bowel mesentery is ~ 15 cm and passes from left side of L2 vertebra downward and to right
    - Contains superior mesenteric vessels, nerves, and lymphatics
- Transverse mesocolon crosses almost horizontally in front of pancreas, duodenum, and right kidney

Omentum

- Multilayered fold of peritoneum that extends from stomach to adjacent organs
- Lesser omentum joins lesser curve of stomach and proximal duodenum to liver
    - Hepatogastric and hepatoduodenal ligament components contain common bile duct, hepatic and gastric vessels, and portal vein
- Greater omentum
    - 4-layered fold of peritoneum hanging from greater curve of stomach like apron, covering transverse colon and much of small intestine
        - Contains variable amounts of fat and abundant lymph nodes
        - Mobile and can fill gaps between viscera
        - Acts as barrier to generalized spread of intraperitoneal infection or tumor

Ligaments

- All double-layered folds of peritoneum, other than mesentery and omentum, are peritoneal ligaments
- Connect 1 viscus to another (e.g., splenorenal ligament) or viscus to abdominal wall (e.g., falciform ligament)
- Contain blood vessels or remnants of fetal vessels

Folds

- Reflections of peritoneum with defined borders, often lifting peritoneum off abdominal wall (e.g., median umbilical fold covers urachus and extends from dome of urinary bladder to umbilicus)

Peritoneal Recesses

- Dependent pouches formed by peritoneal reflections
- Many have eponyms [e.g., Morison pouch for posterior subhepatic (hepatorenal) recess; pouch of Douglas for rectouterine recess]

ANATOMY IMAGING ISSUES

Imaging Recommendations

- Transducer: Typically 2-5 MHz for abdominal survey and deep recesses, up to 9 MHz for thinner patients
- High-frequency linear transducer 8-15 MHz may be used to evaluate anterior abdominal wall and parietal peritoneum
- Patient examined supine with additional decubitus positions to determine if fluid collection is free or loculated
- Peritoneal cavity and its various mesenteries and recesses are usually not apparent on imaging studies unless distended or outlined by intraperitoneal fluid or air

PERITONEAL CAVITY

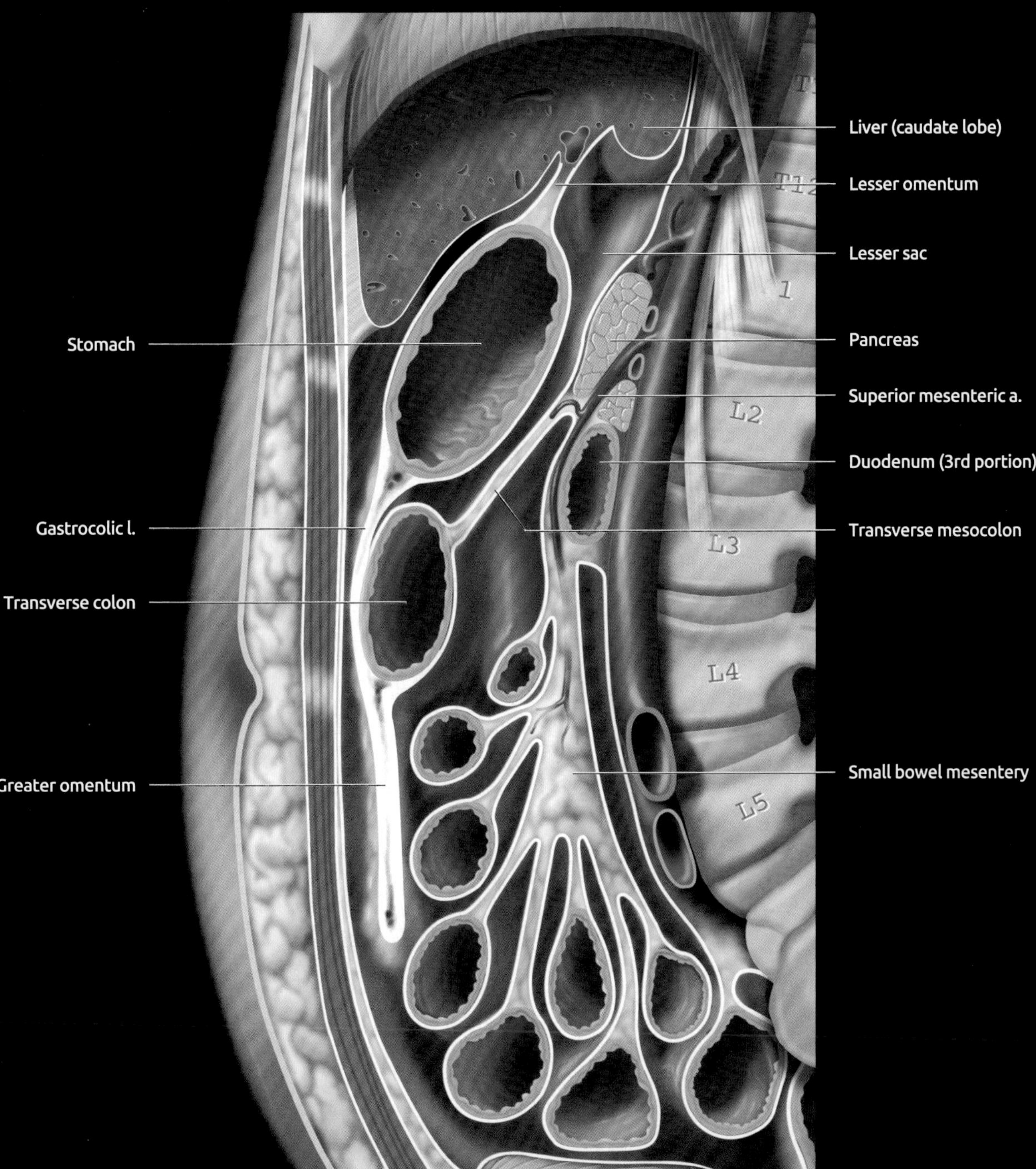

Graphic of a sagittal section of the abdomen shows the peritoneal cavity artificially distended to show anatomy. Note the margins of the lesser sac in this plane, including the caudate lobe of the liver, stomach, gastrocolic ligament anteriorly, and pancreas posteriorly. The hepatogastric ligament is part of the lesser omentum and carries the hepatic artery and portal vein to the liver. The mesenteries are multilayered folds of the peritoneum that enclose a layer of fat and convey blood vessels, nerves, and lymphatics to the intraperitoneal abdominal viscera. The greater omentum is a 4-layered fold of the peritoneum that extends down from the stomach, covering much of the colon and small intestine. The layers are generally fused together caudal to the transverse colon. The gastrocolic ligament is part of the greater omentum.

PERITONEAL DIVISIONS AND COMPARTMENTS

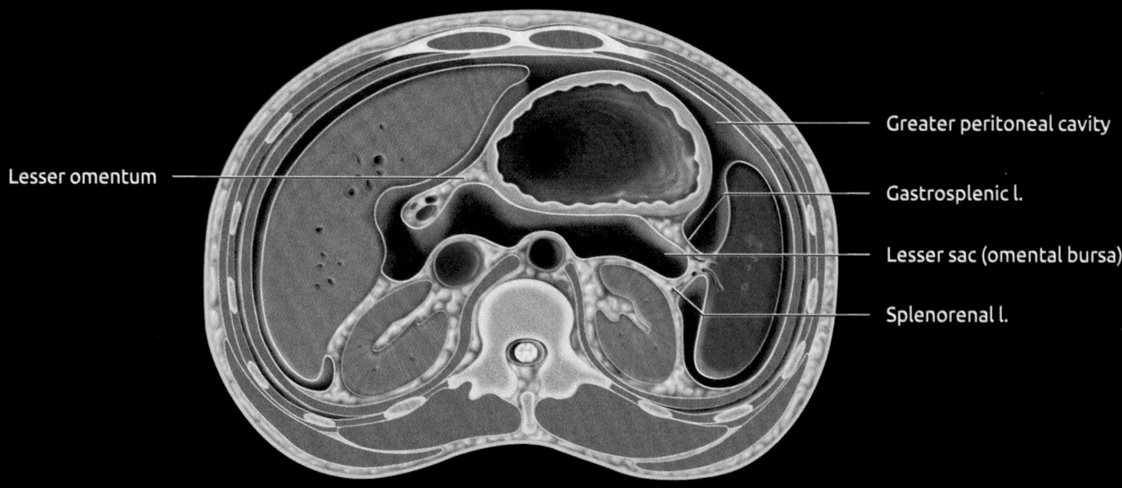

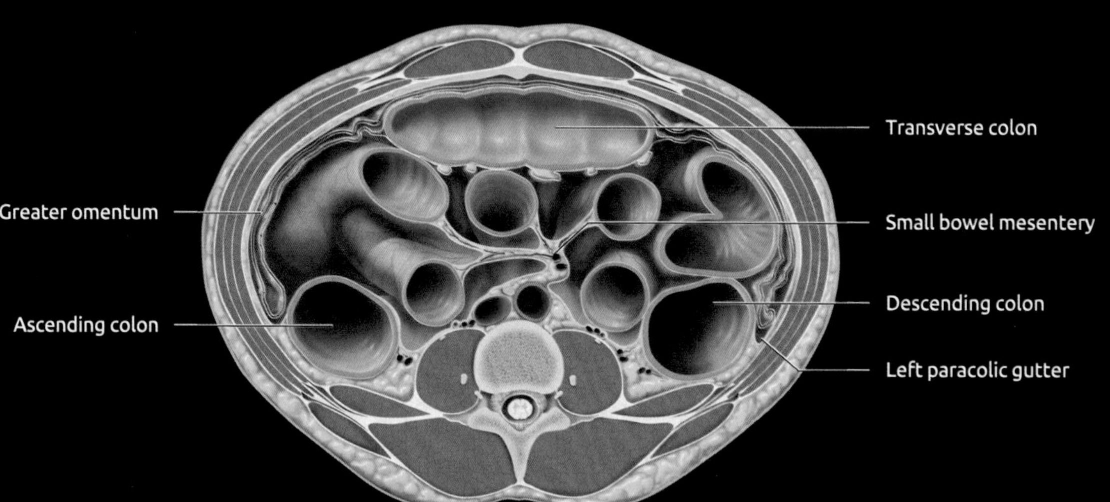

(Top) *The borders of the lesser sac (omental bursa) include the lesser omentum, which contains the common bile duct and hepatic and gastric vessels. The left border includes the gastrosplenic ligament (with short gastric vessels) and the splenorenal ligament (with splenic vessels).* **(Bottom)** *The paracolic gutters are formed by reflections of the peritoneum covering the ascending and descending colon and the lateral abdominal wall. Note the innumerable potential peritoneal recesses lying between the bowel loops and their mesenteric leaves. The greater omentum covers much of the bowel like an apron.*

PERITONEAL DIVISIONS AND COMPARTMENTS

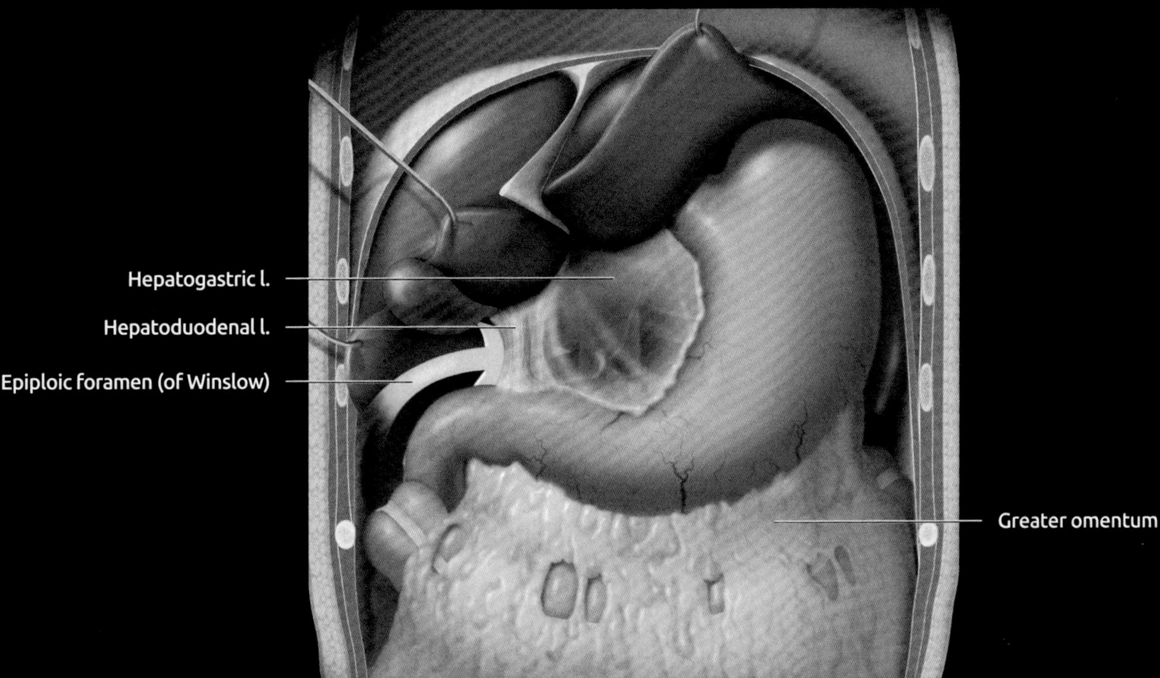

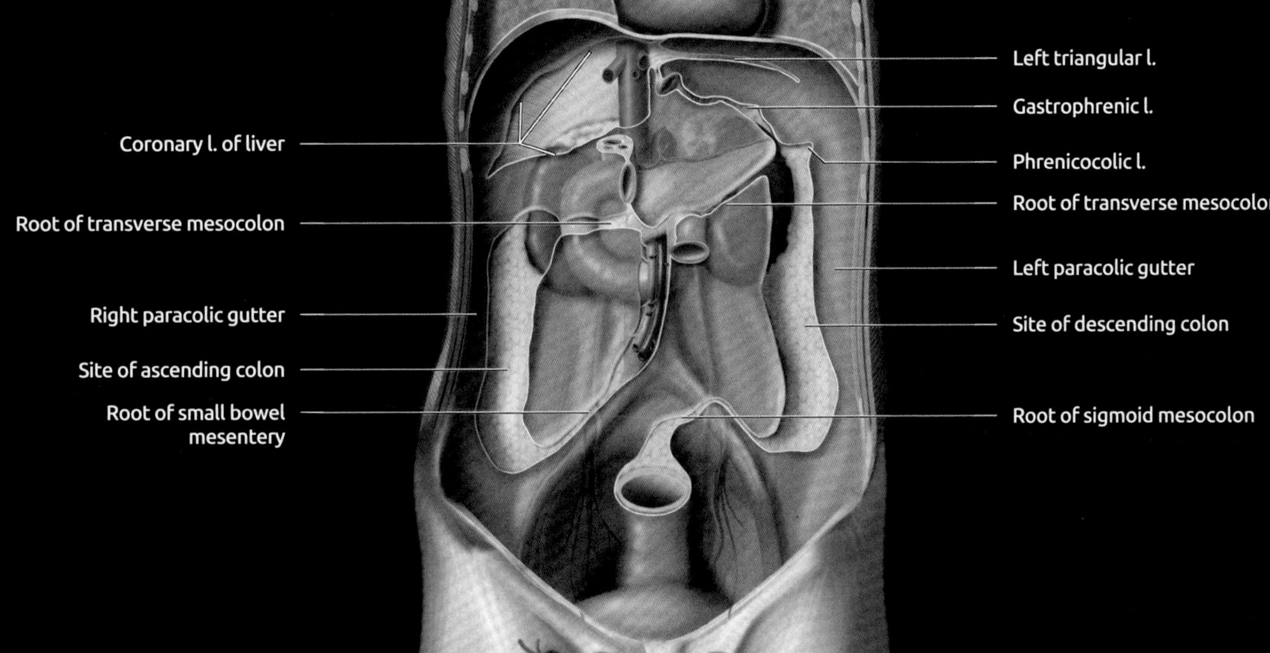

(Top) *In this graphic, the liver has been retracted upward. The lesser omentum is comprised of the hepatoduodenal and hepatogastric ligaments. It forms part of the anterior wall of the lesser sac and contains the common bile duct, hepatic and gastric vessels, and portal vein. The aorta and celiac artery can be seen through the lesser omentum, as they lie just posterior to the lesser sac.* **(Bottom)** *Frontal view of the abdomen, with all of the intraperitoneal organs removed, shows the root of the transverse mesocolon divides the peritoneal cavity into supramesocolic and inframesocolic spaces that communicate only along the paracolic gutters. The coronary and triangular ligaments suspend the liver from the diaphragm. The superior mesenteric vessels traverse the small bowel mesentery, whose root crosses obliquely from the upper left to the lower right posterior abdominal wall.*

RIGHT SUPRAMESOCOLIC SPACE

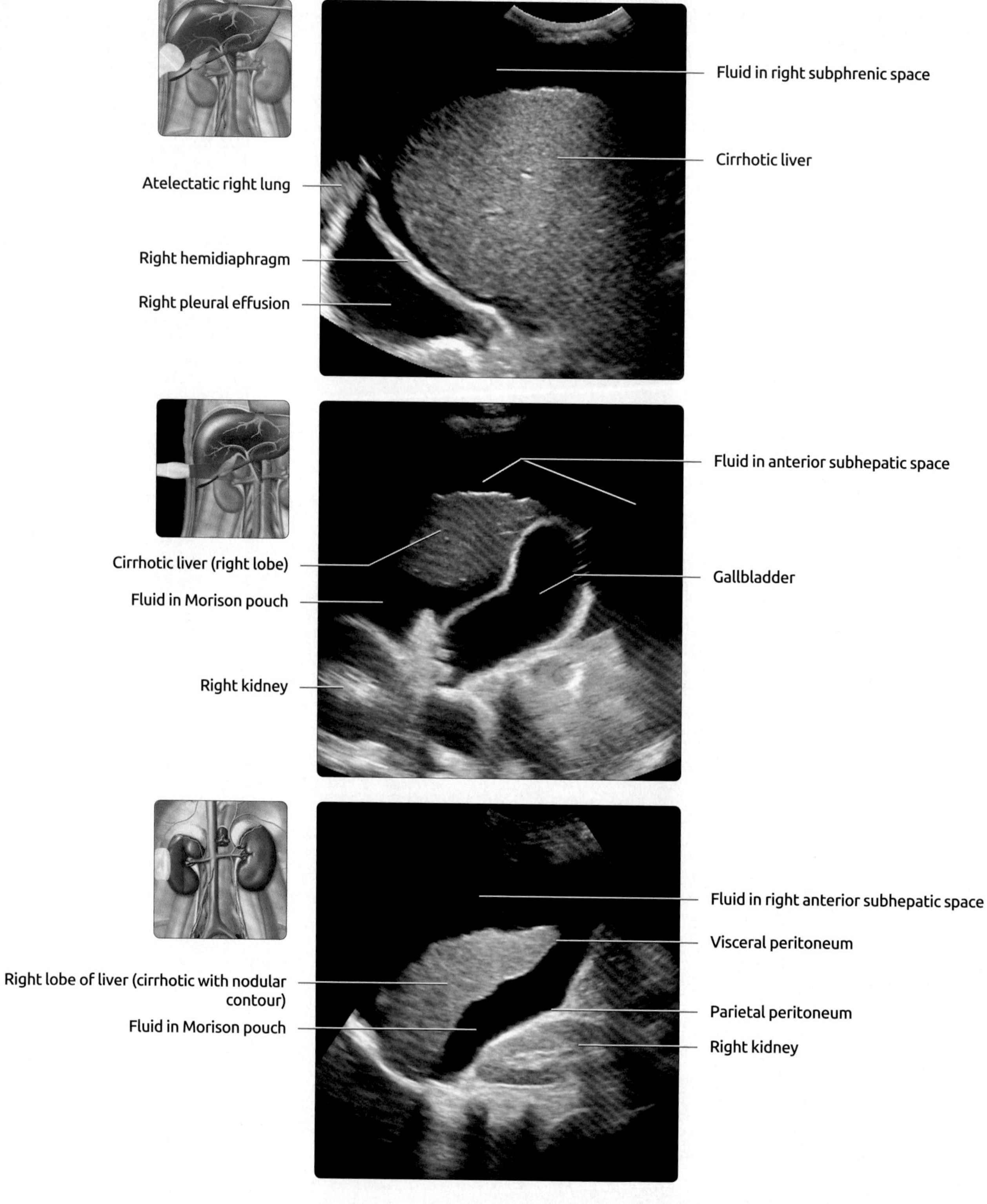

(Top) *Intercostal oblique grayscale ultrasound (in a patient with cirrhosis) shows the dome of the right lobe of the liver and moderate fluid in the right subphrenic region extending anterior to the liver. The fluid is separated from the right-sided pleural effusion by the right diaphragmatic leaf.* **(Middle)** *Subcostal oblique transverse ultrasound of the right upper quadrant shows fluid in the right anterior subhepatic space and in the hepatorenal space. The ascites are secondary to hepatic cirrhosis, and the gallbladder is physiologically distended.* **(Bottom)** *Longitudinal transabdominal grayscale ultrasound shows fluid in the right posterior subhepatic space, also known as the Morison pouch, and hepatorenal fossa. This space is continuous with the right anterior subhepatic space and right paracolic gutter.*

RIGHT SUPRAMESOCOLIC SPACE: LESSER SAC

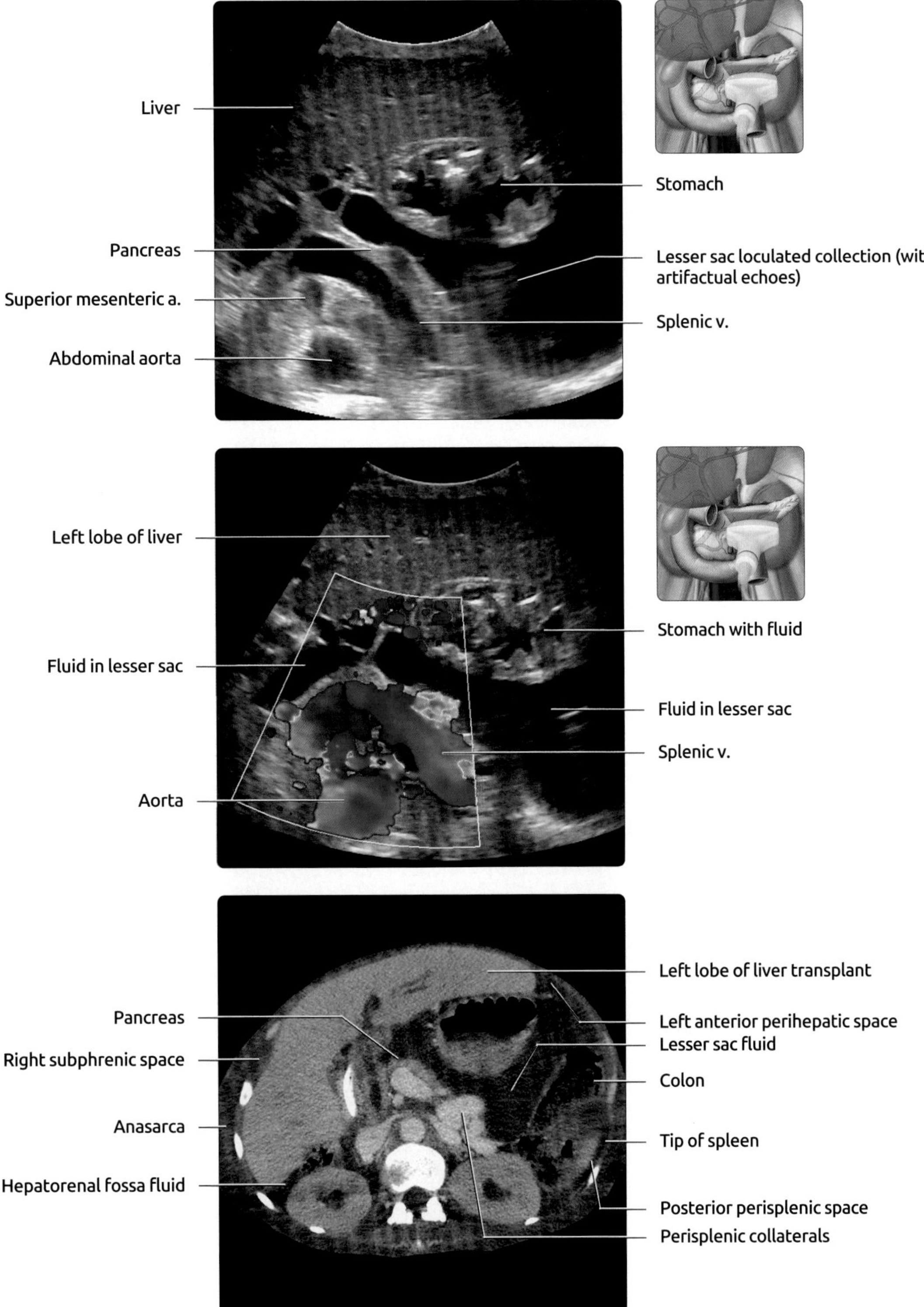

(Top) *Subxiphoid transverse grayscale ultrasound shows a fluid collection in the lesser sac, which extends to the left, behind the stomach and anterior to the pancreas. The lesser sac is part of the right supramesocolic space and communicates with the rest of the peritoneal cavity through the epiploic foramen (of Winslow).* **(Middle)** *Subxiphoid transverse color Doppler ultrasound of the same patient shows moderate fluid in the lesser sac posterior to the stomach. The splenic vein was dilated in this patient with portal hypertension status post liver transplant.* **(Bottom)** *Axial CECT of the same patient shows fluid in the lesser sac and peritoneal cavity as well as diffuse anasarca.*

LEFT SUPRAMESOCOLIC SPACE

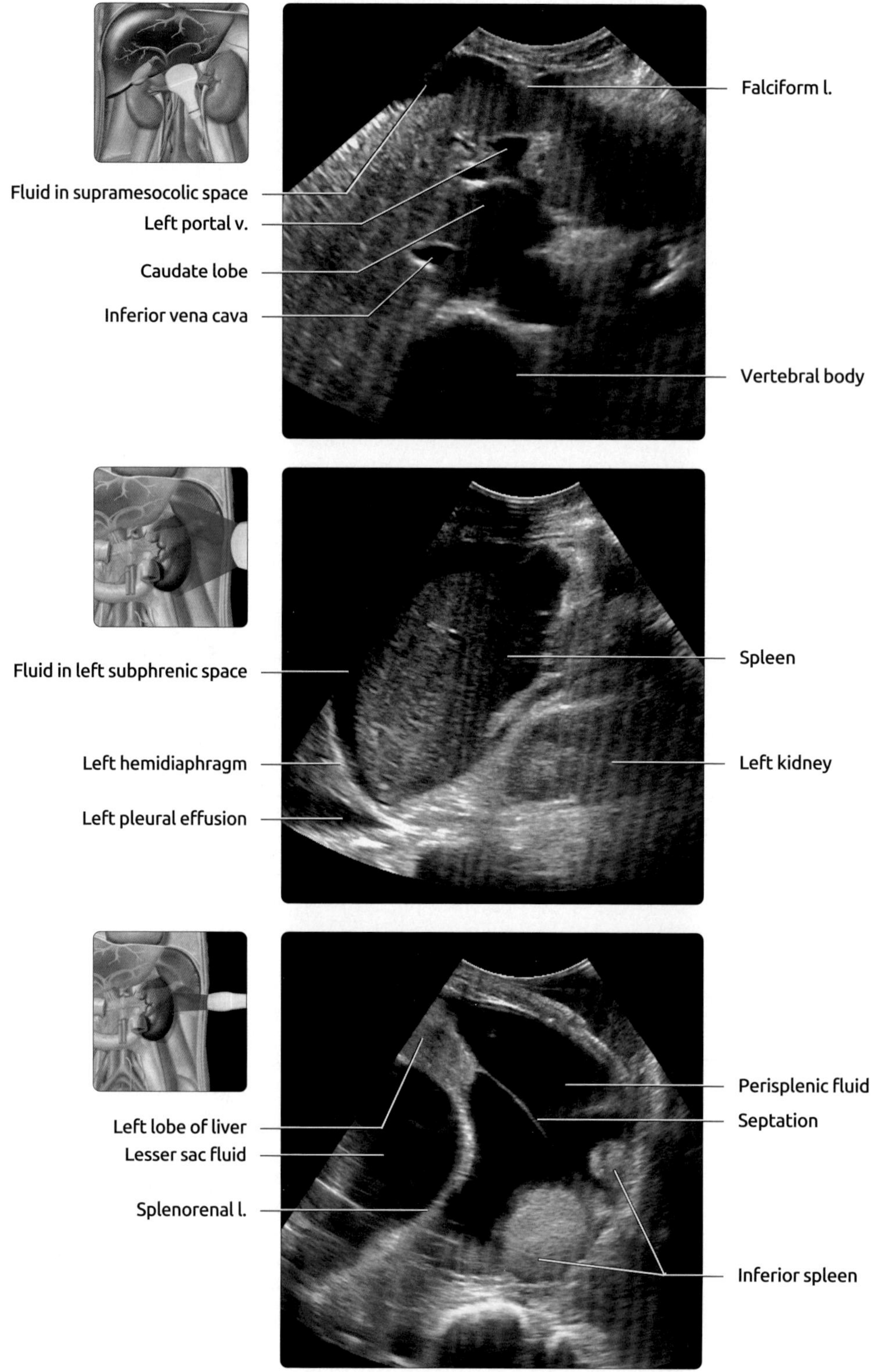

(Top) *Subxiphoid transverse grayscale ultrasound shows fluid anterior to the left lobe of the liver that is localized to the left posterior subhepatic space. Incidental calculi are seen within a dilated intrahepatic biliary duct.* **(Middle)** *Longitudinal grayscale ultrasound of the left upper quadrant shows a small amount of perisplenic fluid extending under the left hemidiaphragm. The left subphrenic space is separated from the right subphrenic space by the falciform ligament.* **(Bottom)** *Transverse grayscale ultrasound of the left upper quadrant reveals fluid in the perisplenic space and lesser sac.*

INFRAMESOCOLIC SPACE

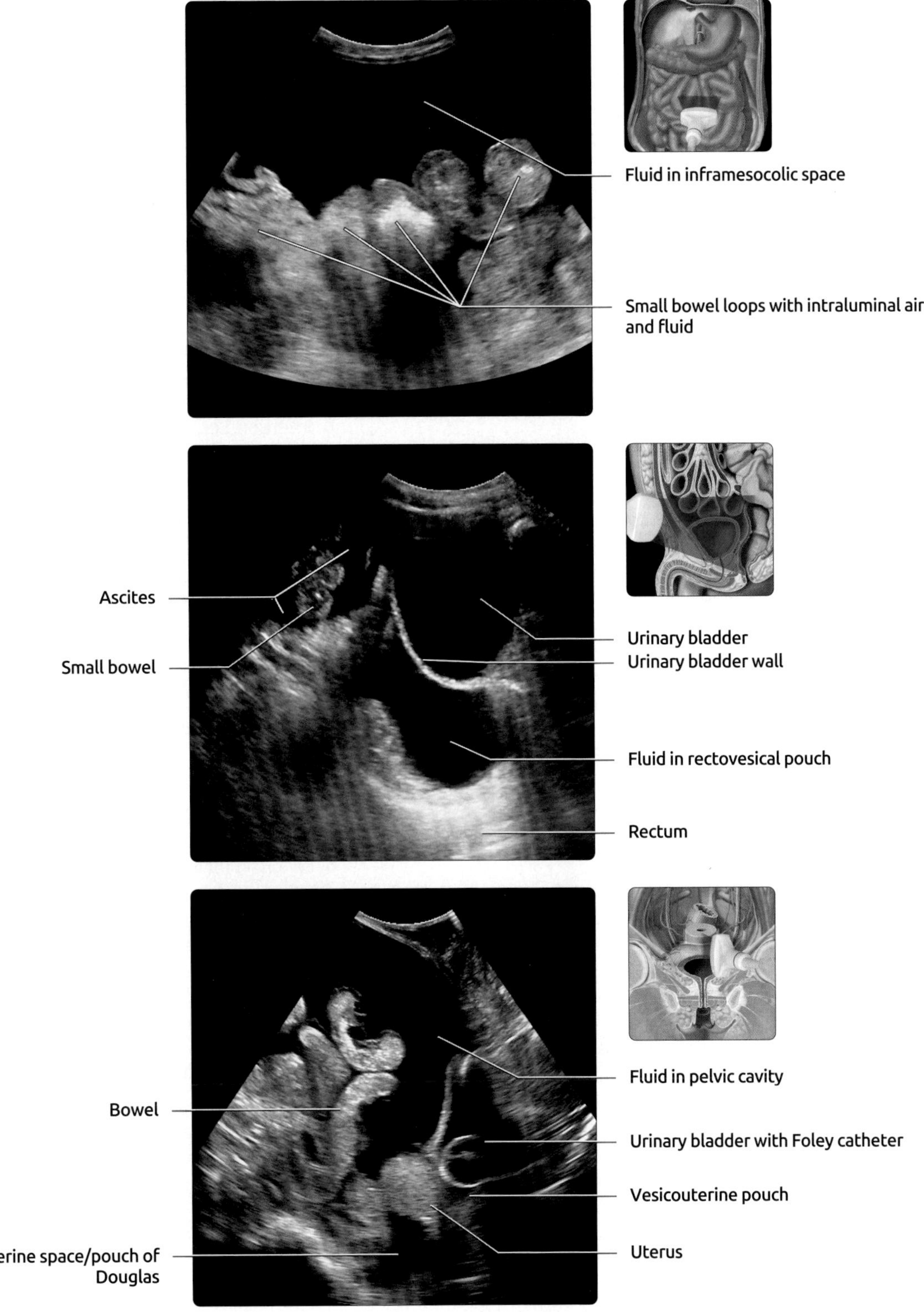

(Top) *Transverse transabdominal ultrasound of the central abdomen reveals moderate to large ascites with floating small bowel loops. The left inframesocolic space is larger compared to the right and communicates directly with the pelvic cavity.* **(Middle)** *Longitudinal ultrasound of the midline suprapubic region in a male patient demonstrates intraperitoneal fluid between bowel loops and extending into the dependent rectovesical pouch. There is a distended urinary bladder.* **(Bottom)** *Longitudinal grayscale ultrasound of the female pelvis shows free fluid. The uterus divides the pelvic cavity into the vesicouterine and rectouterine (pouch of Douglas) spaces. In this case, the vesicouterine space contains minimal fluid.*

TERMINOLOGY

Definitions

- Abdomen: Region between diaphragm and pelvis

GROSS ANATOMY

Anatomic Boundaries of Anterior Abdominal Wall

- Superiorly: Xiphoid process and costal cartilages of 7th-10th ribs
- Inferiorly: Iliac crest, iliac spine, inguinal ligament, and pubis
- Inguinal ligament is inferior edge of aponeurosis of external oblique muscle

Muscles of Anterior Abdominal Wall

- Consist of 3 flat muscles (external oblique, internal oblique, and transverse abdominal), and 1 strap-like muscle (rectus)
- Combination of muscles and aponeuroses (sheet-like tendons) act as corset to confine and protect abdominal viscera
- Linea alba is fibrous raphe stretching from xiphoid to pubis
    - Forms central anterior attachment for abdominal wall muscles
    - Formed by interlacing fibers of aponeuroses of oblique and transverse abdominal muscles
    - Rectus sheath also formed by these aponeuroses as they surround rectus muscle
- Linea semilunaris is vertical fibrous band at lateral edge of rectus sheath bilaterally
    - Aponeuroses of internal and transversus abdominis join in linea semilunaris before forming rectus sheath
- External oblique muscle
    - Largest and most superficial of 3 flat abdominal muscles
    - Origin: External surfaces of ribs 5-12
    - Insertion: Linea alba, iliac crest, pubis via broad aponeurosis
- Internal oblique muscle
    - Middle of 3 flat abdominal muscles
    - Runs at right angles to external oblique
    - Origin: Posterior layer of thoracolumbar fascia, iliac crest, and inguinal ligament
    - Insertion: Ribs 10-12 posteriorly, linea alba via broad aponeurosis, pubis
- Transversus abdominis (transversalis) muscle
    - Innermost of 3 flat abdominal muscles
    - Origin: Lowest 6 costal cartilages, thoracolumbar fascia, iliac crest, inguinal ligament
    - Insertion: Linea alba via broad aponeurosis, pubis
- Rectus abdominis muscle
    - Origin: Pubic symphysis and pubic crest
    - Insertion: Xiphoid process and costal cartilages 5-7
    - Rectus sheath: Strong, fibrous compartment that envelops each rectus muscle
        - Contains superior and inferior epigastric vessels
- Actions of anterior abdominal wall muscles
    - Support and protect abdominal viscera
    - Help flex and twist trunk, maintain posture
    - Increase intraabdominal pressure for defecation, micturition, and childbirth
    - Stabilize pelvis during walking, sitting up
- Transversalis fascia
    - Lies deep to abdominal wall muscles and lines entire abdominal wall
    - Separated from parietal peritoneum by layer of extraperitoneal fat

Muscles of Posterior Abdominal Wall

- Consist of psoas (major and minor), iliacus, and quadratus lumborum
- Psoas: Long, thick, fusiform muscle lying lateral to vertebral column
    - Origin: Transverse processes and bodies of vertebrae T12-L5
    - Insertion: Lesser trochanter of femur (passing behind inguinal ligament)
    - Action: Flexes thigh at hip joint; bends vertebral column laterally
- Iliacus: Large triangular sheet of muscle lying along lateral side of psoas
    - Origin: Superior part of iliac fossa
    - Insertion: Lesser trochanter of femur (after joining with psoas tendon)
    - Action: "Iliopsoas muscle" flexes thigh
- Quadratus lumborum: Thick sheet of muscle lying adjacent to transverse processes of lumbar vertebrae
    - Invested by lumbodorsal fascia
    - Origin: Iliac crest and transverse processes of lumbar vertebrae
    - Insertion: 12th rib
    - Actions: Stabilizes position of thorax and pelvis during respiration, walking; bends trunk to side

Paraspinal Muscles

- Also called erector spinae muscles
    - Invested by lumbodorsal fascia
- Composed of 3 columns
    - Iliocostalis: Lateral
    - Longissimus: Intermediate
    - Spinalis: Medial
- Origins: Sacrum, ilium, and spines of lumbar and 11th-12th thoracic vertebrae
- Insertions: Ribs and vertebrae with additional muscle slips joining columns at successively higher levels
- Action: Extends vertebral column

ANATOMY IMAGING ISSUES

Imaging Recommendations

- High-frequency (5-12 MHz) linear transducer for anterior abdominal wall and paraspinal muscles
- 3-5 MHz for posterior abdominal wall muscles
- Supine position for examination of anterior and lateral abdominal wall
    - Image during Valsalva maneuver and in standing position to increase abdominal pressure and elicit hernias
    - Prone position for ultrasound of paraspinal muscles
- Compare with contralateral side to check for symmetry
- Panoramic/extended field-of-view techniques are very useful to demonstrate muscles and soft tissue

ANTERIOR ABDOMINAL WALL

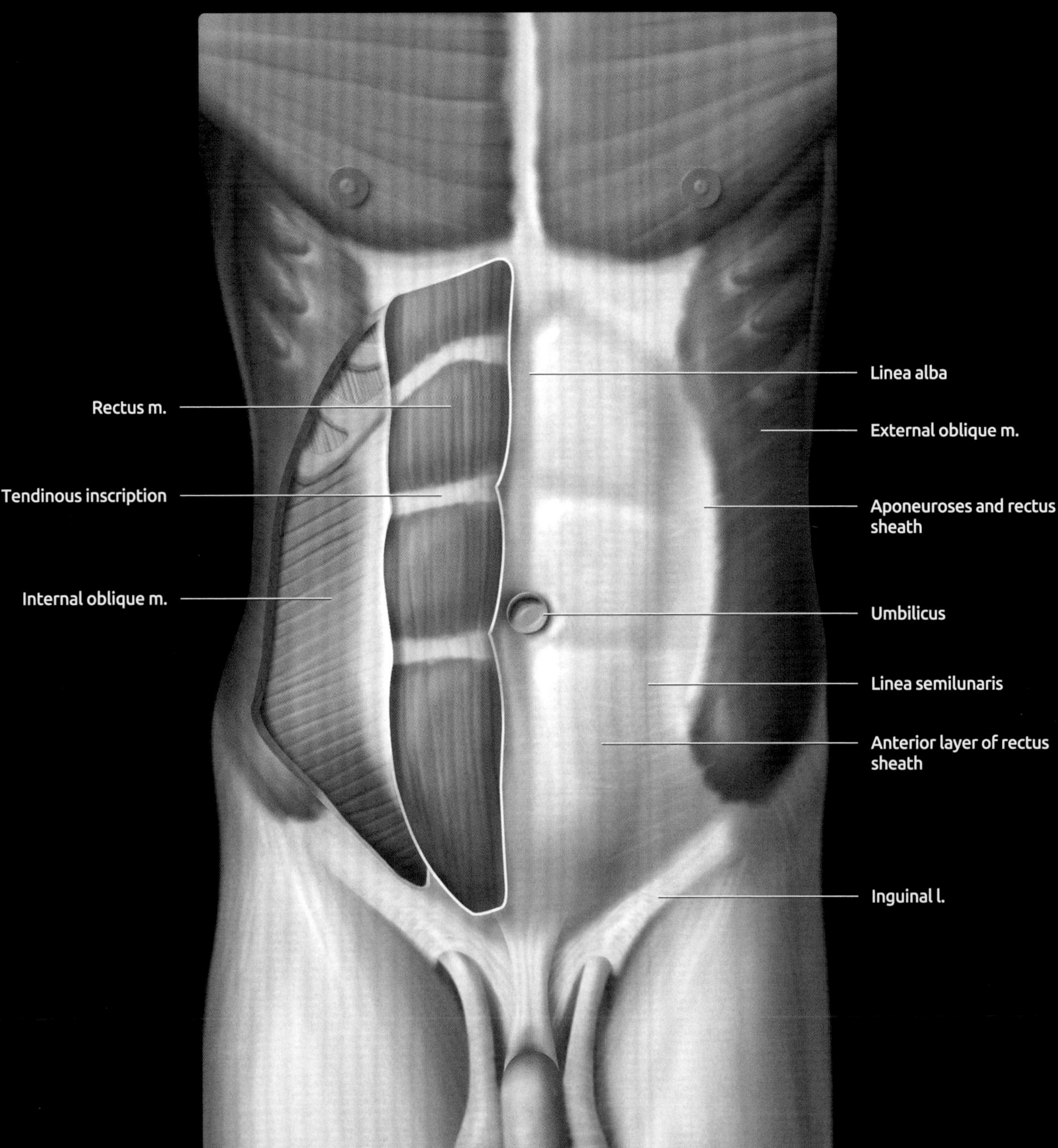

Graphic shows the aponeuroses of the internal and external oblique and transverse abdominal muscles are 2 layered and interweave with each other, covering the rectus muscle, constituting the rectus sheath and linea alba. About midway between the umbilicus and symphysis, at the arcuate line, the posterior rectus sheath ends (arcuate line), and the transversalis fascia is the only structure between the rectus muscle and parietal peritoneum.

POSTERIOR ABDOMINAL WALL

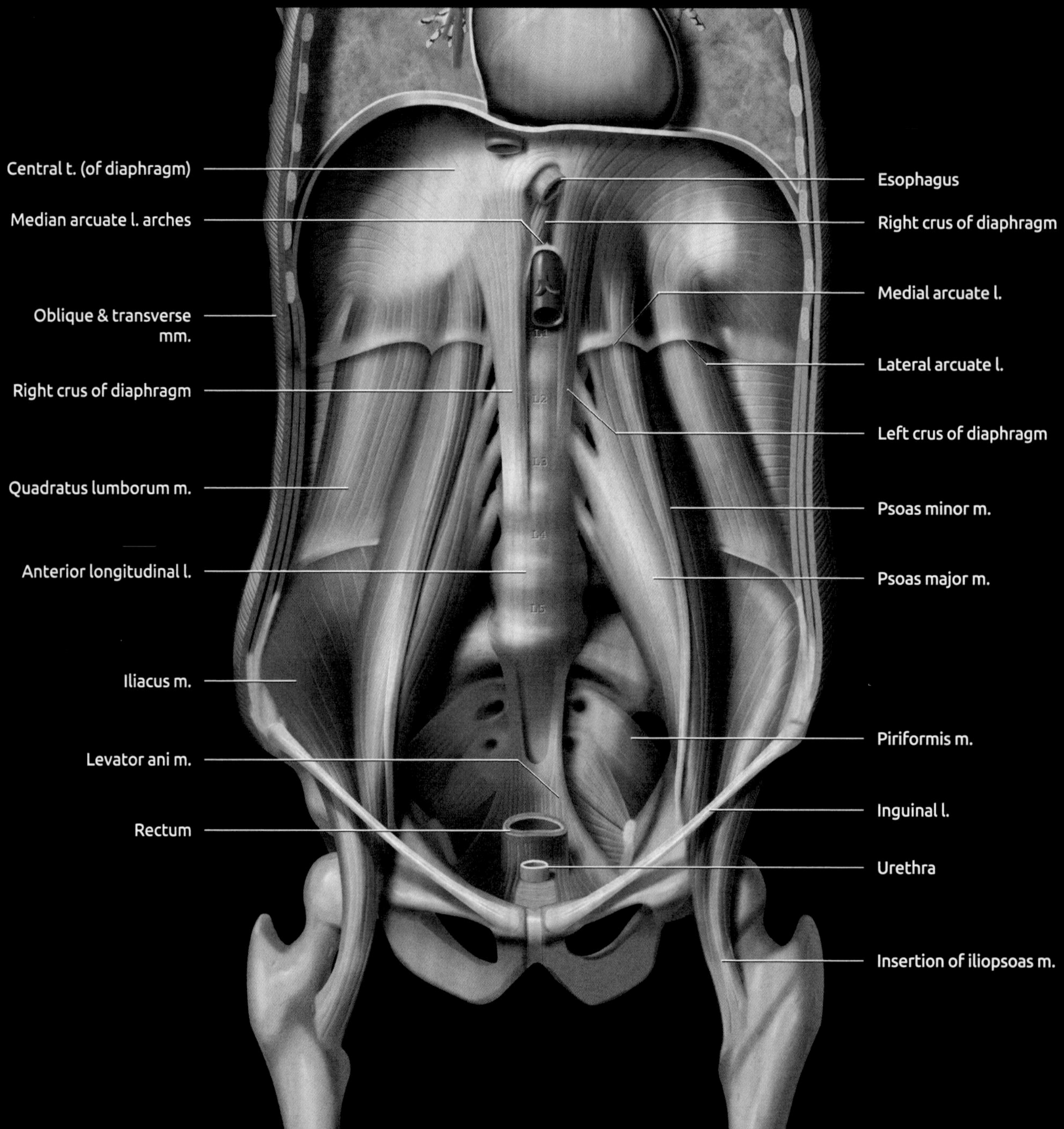

Graphic shows the lumbar vertebrae are covered and attached by the anterior longitudinal ligament, and the diaphragmatic crura are closely attached to it, as are the origins of the psoas muscles, which also arise from the transverse processes. The iliacus muscle arises from the iliac fossa of the pelvis and inserts into the tendon of the psoas major, constituting the iliopsoas muscle, which inserts onto the lesser trochanter. The quadratus lumborum arises from the iliac crest and inserts onto the 12th rib and transverse processes of the lumbar vertebrae. The diaphragmatic and transverse abdominal fibers interlace. The psoas and quadratus lumborum pass behind the diaphragm under medial and lateral arcuate ligaments.

MUSCLES OF BACK IN SITU

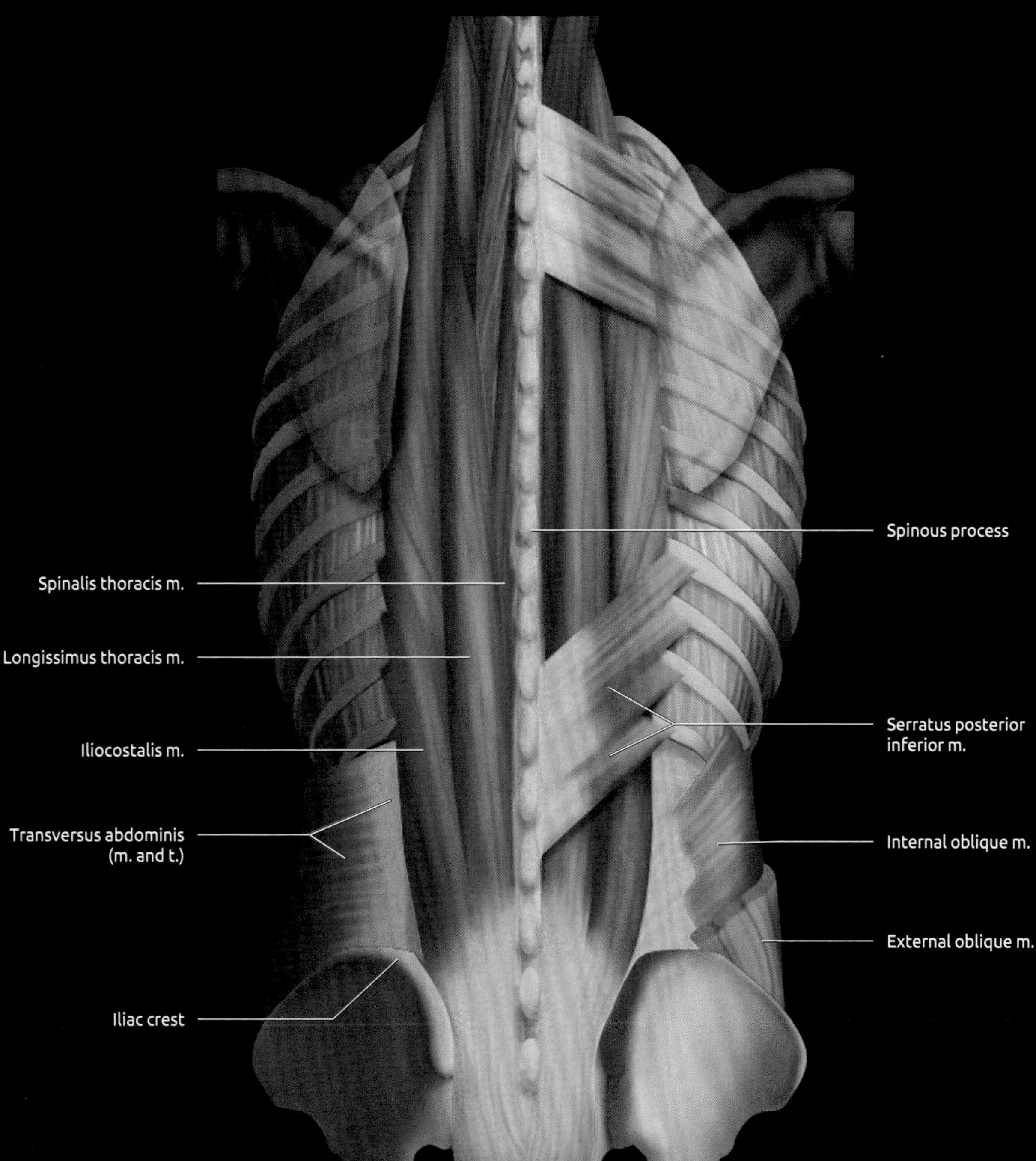

Graphic shows the paraspinal muscles and muscles of the back. The latissimus dorsi muscles are not included. The erector spinae have thick, tendinous origins from the sacral, iliac crests, the lumbar, and 11th to 12th thoracic spinous processes. Superiorly, the muscle becomes fleshy, and in the upper lumbar region subdivides to become the iliocostalis, longissimus, and spinalis muscles (from lateral to medial), tapering as they insert into the vertebrae and ribs. The erector muscles flank the spinous processes and span the length of the posterior thorax and abdomen. They are responsible for extension of the vertebral column.

ANTERIOR ABDOMINAL WALL

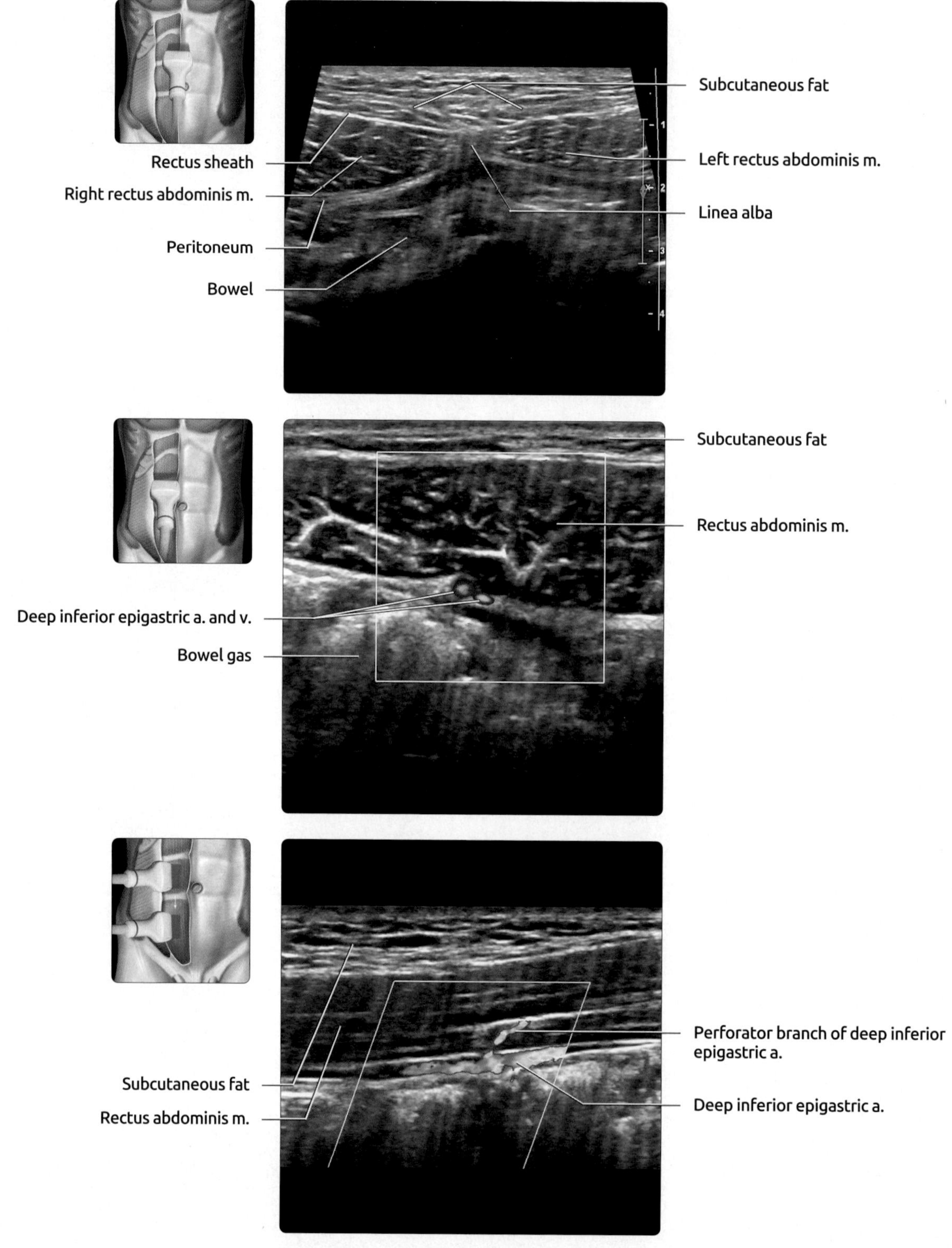

(Top) *Transverse grayscale ultrasound of the midline anterior abdominal wall shows the paired rectus abdominis muscles separated by the linea alba. The rectus abdominis muscles are comparable in echogenicity and thickness. The surrounding rectus sheath is seen as a fine, thin, echogenic structure around the muscles.* **(Middle)** *Transverse power Doppler ultrasound of a rectus abdominis muscle in the lower abdomen shows the deep inferior epigastric artery and vein. Branches of the superior epigastric artery that arise in the upper abdomen anastomose with branches of the inferior epigastric artery at the umbilicus.* **(Bottom)** *Longitudinal color Doppler ultrasound shows a perforating branch of the deep inferior epigastric artery extending into the rectus muscle. These perforators are important for breast reconstruction with abdominal wall flaps.*

ANTEROLATERAL ABDOMINAL WALL

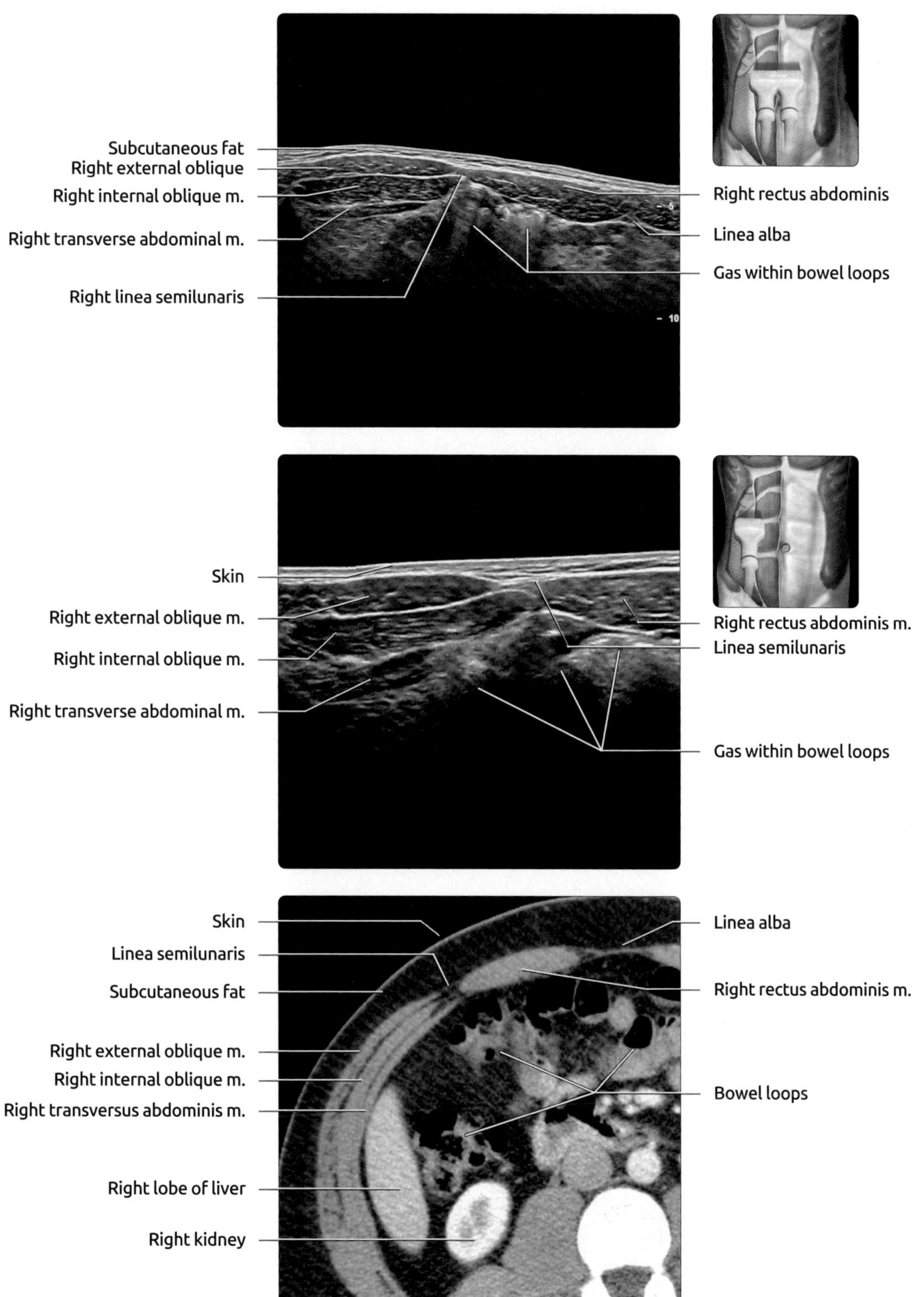

(Top) *Transverse extended field-of-view (FOV) grayscale ultrasound shows the relationship of the medially located rectus abdominis and the laterally located oblique and transverse abdominal muscles. Medially, the external and internal oblique and the transversus abdominal muscles form aponeuroses that compose the rectus sheath with the muscles thinning at the linea semilunaris. The linea alba is thin in the lower abdomen.* **(Middle)** *Transverse grayscale ultrasound at the right anterolateral abdominal wall shows the relationship of the lateral abdominal wall muscles in better detail. Note the oblique and transverse abdominal muscles taper medially as they become aponeuroses.* **(Bottom)** *Correlative axial CECT illustrates the muscles of the abdominal wall. The rectus abdominis muscle in the anterior abdominal wall is shown, along with the oblique and transverse abdominal muscles in the anterolateral abdominal wall and their aponeuroses.*

POSTERIOR ABDOMINAL WALL

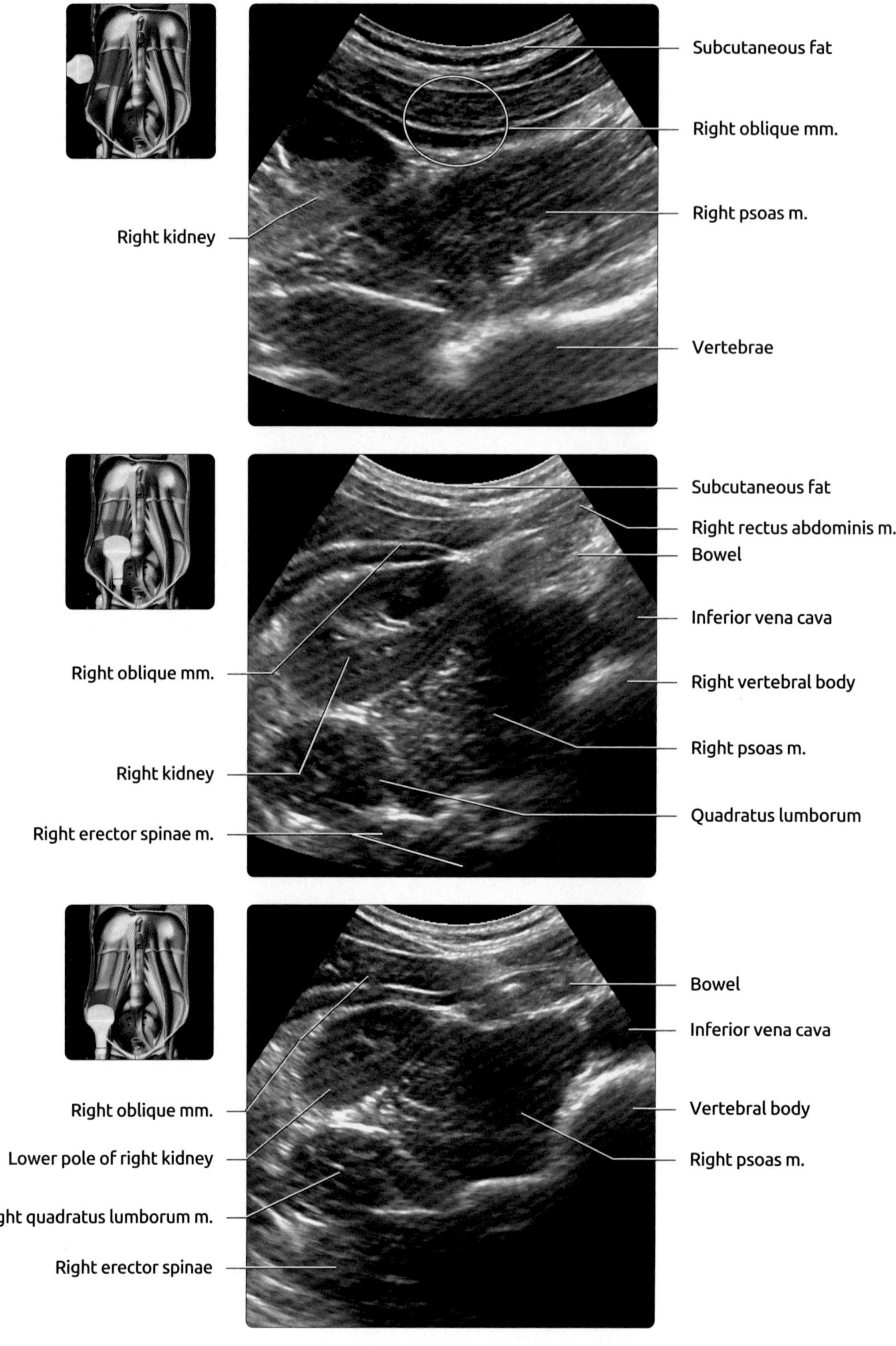

(Top) *Longitudinal oblique grayscale ultrasound through the lower right abdomen shows the right psoas muscle, which originates from the lumbar spine and inserts into the proximal femur.* **(Middle)** *Transverse grayscale ultrasound of right midabdomen using the kidney as an acoustic window is shown. The kidney is anterior and lateral to the psoas and anterior to the quadratus lumborum. The psoas runs along the paravertebral region in its entire abdominal course. The quadratus lumborum originates from the iliolumbar ligament and iliac crest to insert into the last rib and lumbar transverse processes. It is easily identified as the muscle on which the kidney rests.* **(Bottom)** *Transverse grayscale ultrasound of the right upper abdomen, continuing the scan inferiorly, shows the relationship of the posterior abdominal wall muscles are maintained.*

POSTERIOR ABDOMINAL WALL, CT CORRELATION

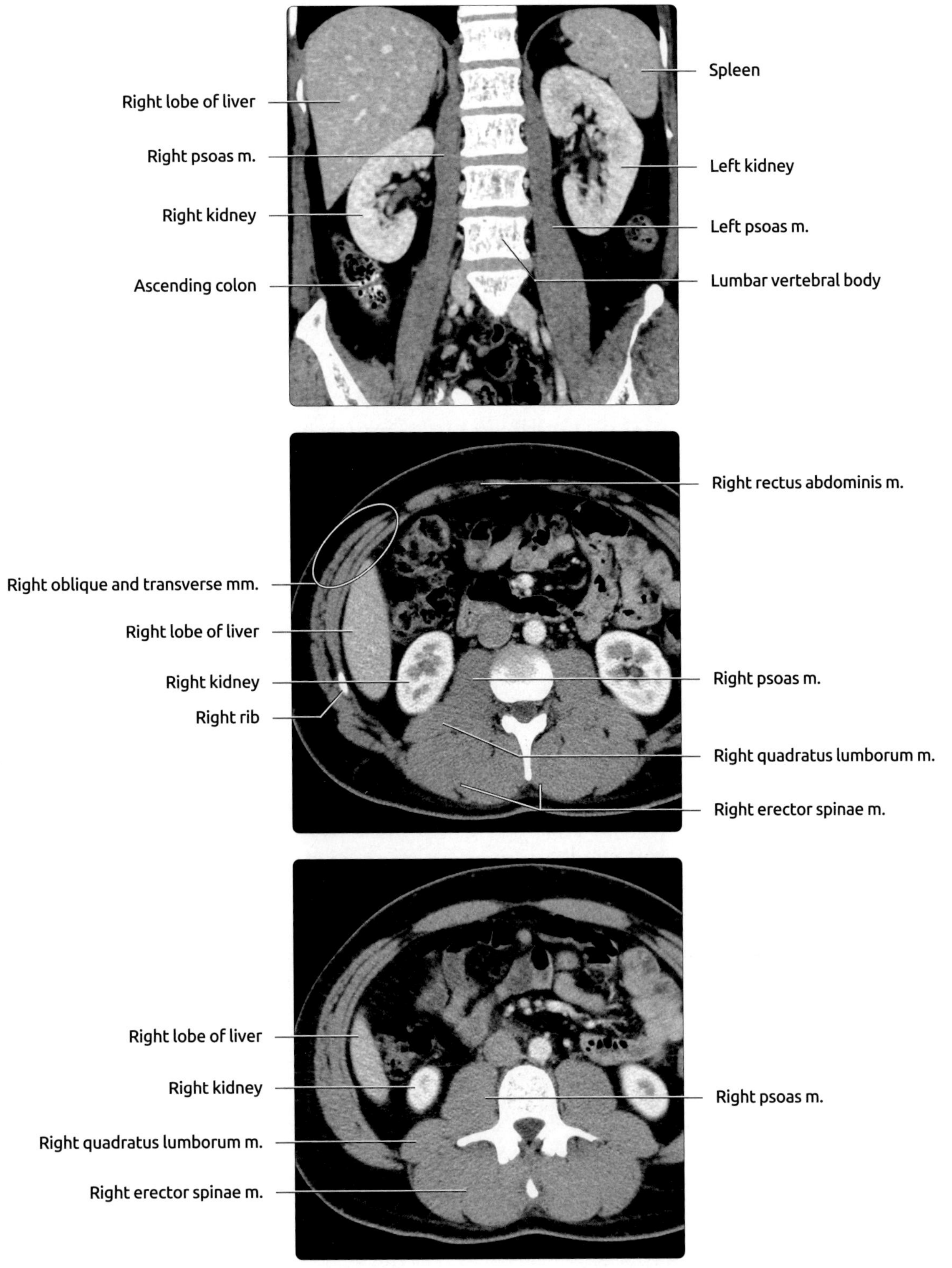

(Top) *Correlative coronal CECT shows the paralumbar location of the psoas muscles and their medial location relative to the kidneys. The psoas muscles originate from the lumbar and 12th thoracic vertebral bodies and their transverse processes and run past the pelvic brim, where they course inferolaterally to be joined by the iliacus muscle.* **(Middle)** *Correlative axial CECT better illustrates the anatomic relationships of the kidney with the posterior abdominal wall muscles. The kidney is lateral to the psoas muscle and rests upon the quadratus lumborum muscle. The erector spinae muscles are immediately posterior to the quadratus lumborum, and the 2 muscles are invested by the lumbodorsal fascia.* **(Bottom)** *Correlative axial CECT at the level of the inferior pole of the right kidney is shown. The psoas muscle and quadratus lumborum muscles, seen in their midsections, are now thicker.*

POSTERIOR ABDOMINAL WALL

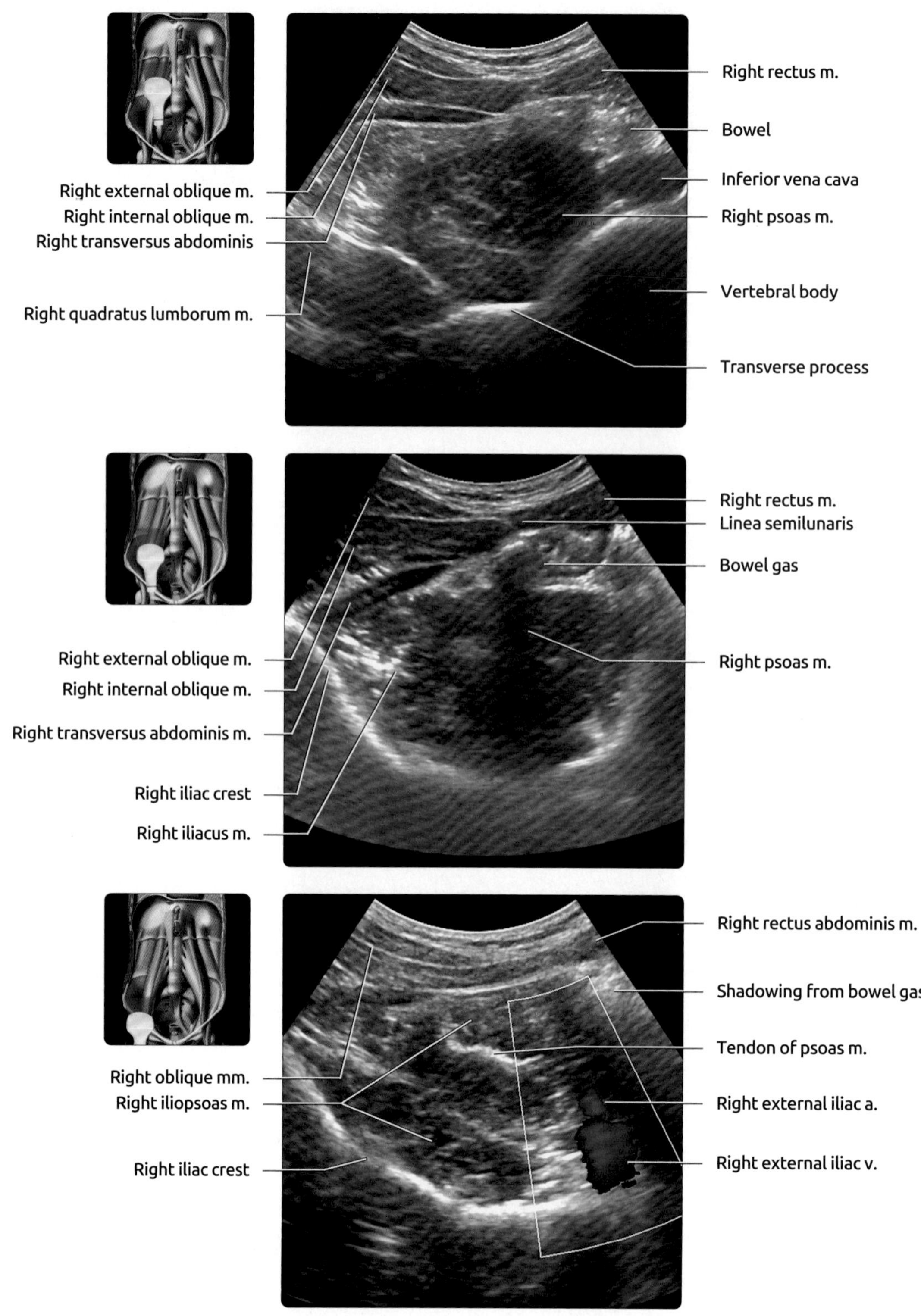

(Top) *Transverse grayscale ultrasound in the lower abdominal region shows the right psoas muscle composed of the psoas minor, which rests upon the psoas major. The 2 muscles cannot be separated clearly on ultrasound. Because of their depth, the paraspinal muscles cannot be demonstrated in detail.* **(Middle)** *Transverse grayscale ultrasound of the right lower abdomen in the same patient shows that the distal psoas muscle has diminished in size. It rests on the medial portion of the iliacus muscle; the latter is a flat muscle that fills the iliac fossa. Both continue inferiorly together.* **(Bottom)** *Distally, the fibers from the iliacus muscle converge and insert into the lateral side of the psoas muscle to form the iliopsoas muscle. Common iliac vessels can be seen medially.*

POSTERIOR ABDOMINAL WALL, CT CORRELATION

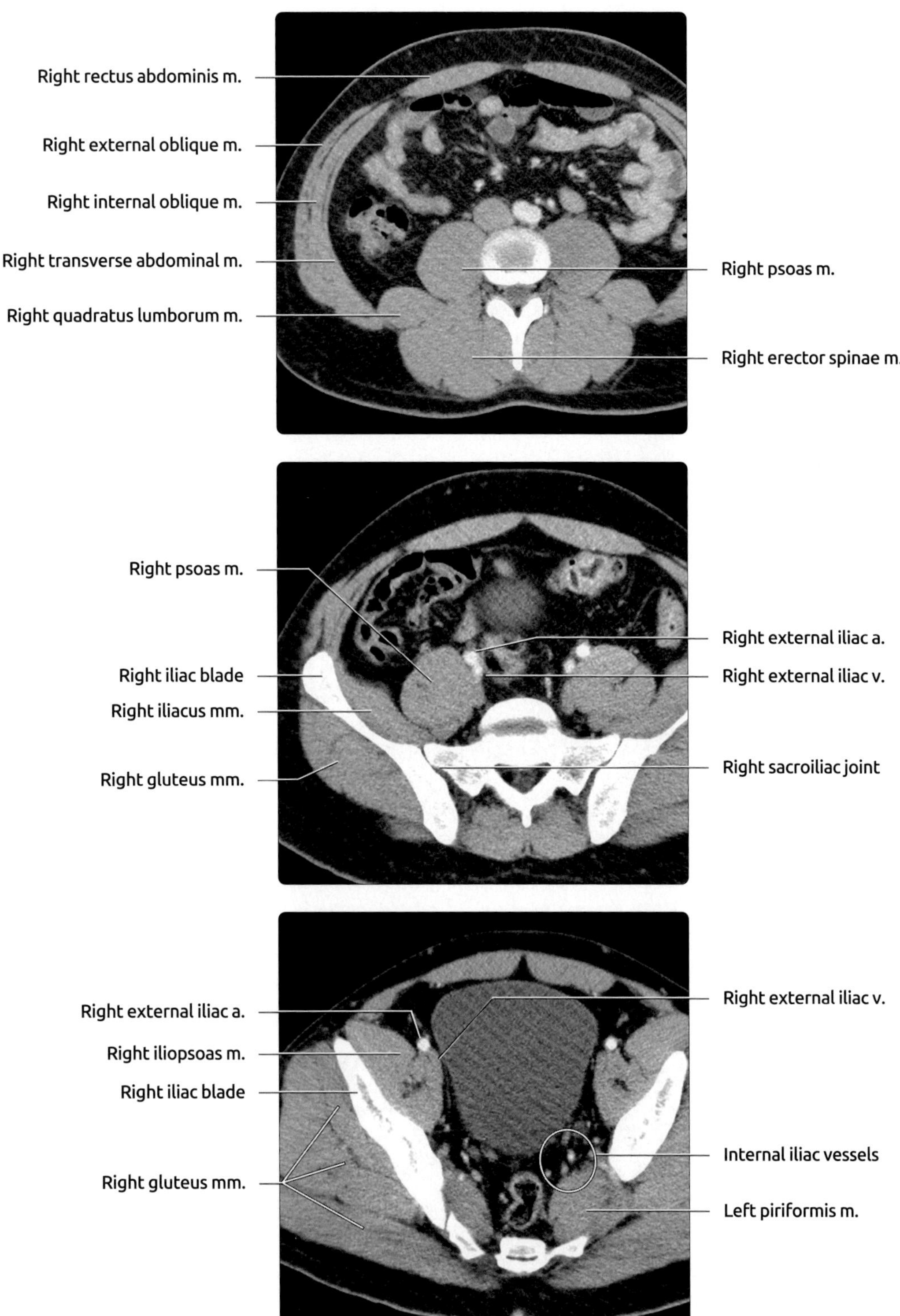

(Top) *Correlative axial CECT below the kidneys shows the quadratus lumborum muscle is more laterally located, and the psoas muscle is directly anterior to the erector spinae muscle.* **(Middle)** *Axial correlative CECT shows the psoas muscle has begun its dorsolateral course and is now anterior to the iliacus muscle. The iliacus muscle is easily identified as a flat muscle filling the iliac fossa, arising from the upper 2/3 of the iliac fossa, inner lip of the iliac crest, anterior sacroiliac and the iliolumbar ligaments, and base of the sacrum.* **(Bottom)** *Correlative axial CECT shows the psoas and iliacus muscles have converged and are now indistinguishable from one another. The resultant iliopsoas muscle passes beneath the inguinal ligament and becomes tendinous as it inserts into the lesser trochanter of the femur.*

PARASPINAL MUSCLES

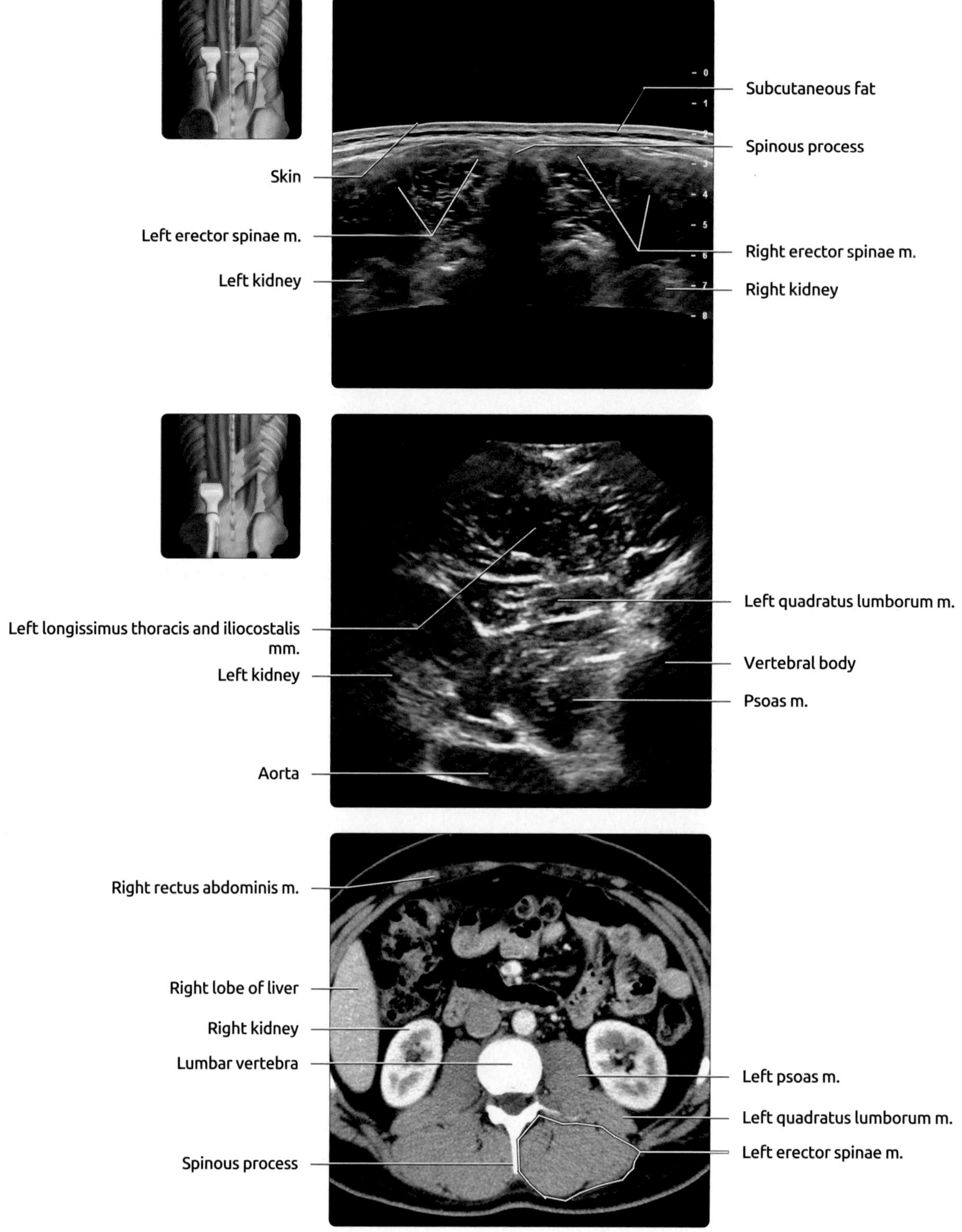

(Top) *Transverse extended FOV grayscale ultrasound of the back (with the patient prone) shows the erector spinae muscles flanking the spinous process. They are invested by the lumbodorsal fascia, which also invests the anteriorly located quadratus lumborum muscle. The kidneys are partially demonstrated.* **(Middle)** *Transverse oblique grayscale ultrasound shows the left erector spinae muscle (with the patient prone). The 3 columns (iliocostalis, longissimus, and spinalis muscles, from lateral to medial) comprising the erector spinae are not clearly separated from one another on ultrasound. They are identified collectively as a thick, fleshy muscle lateral to the spinous process.* **(Bottom)** *Correlative axial CECT of the paraspinal muscles at the level of the kidneys shows the erector spinae muscles originate from a broad and thick tendon, which originates from the sacrum and iliac crest, lumbar, and 11th and 12th thoracic spinous processes.*

MR

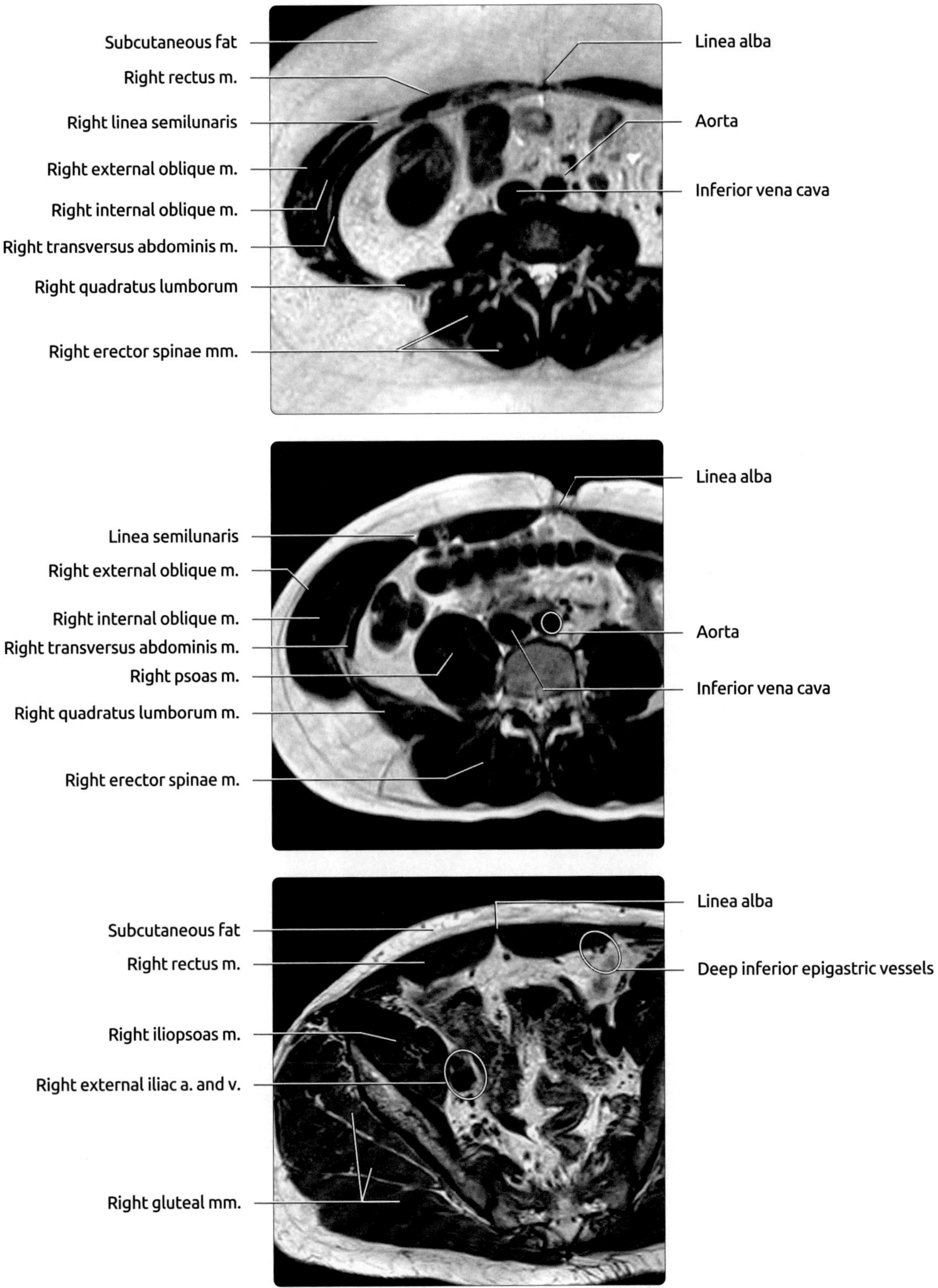

(Top) *Axial T2 HASTE MR in an older patient with muscle atrophy shows fat in between the individual muscles of the anterior and posterior abdominal wall.* **(Middle)** *Axial T2 HASTE MR in a younger male patient shows more bulky abdominal wall musculature with little intermuscular fat.* **(Bottom)** *Axial T1 MR at a lower level shows the iliopsoas as 1 muscle bundle.*

KEY FACTS

TERMINOLOGY

- Hernia: Weakness or defect in fibromuscular wall with protrusion of organ or tissue through defect

IMAGING

- Midline hernias
  - Epigastric: Between xiphisternum and umbilicus
  - Umbilical: Umbilical or immediate paraumbilical region
  - Hypogastric: Between umbilicus and pubic symphysis
- Lateral hernias
  - Spigelian
  - Lumbar: Occur in 2 potentially weak areas of flank
- Incisional hernia: Located at surgical incisional site
- Ultrasound 1st-line imaging for smaller hernias or children
  - Dynamic, real-time examination; using maneuvers such as Valsalva or standing position to improve detection
- Localize site/size of abdominal wall defect and content
  - Bowel: "Target" echo pattern with visible peristalsis
  - Omental fat: Echogenic/hypoechoic nonperistalsing
- Document with cine clips
- Complications: Incarceration, strangulation, bowel obstruction

TOP DIFFERENTIAL DIAGNOSES

- Abdominal wall tumor
- Abdominal wall abscess or seroma
- Abdominal wall or rectus sheath hematoma
- Divarication (diastasis) of rectus abdominis muscles

CLINICAL ISSUES

- Most common abdominal wall lesion seen in ultrasound practice; discomfort, pain, intermittent intestinal obstruction
- Reducible/enlarging abdominal wall swelling

SCANNING TIPS

- High-resolution linear transducer for abdominal wall; curvilinear lower frequency and extended field of view (panoramic) for diastasis recti/large hernias/overview

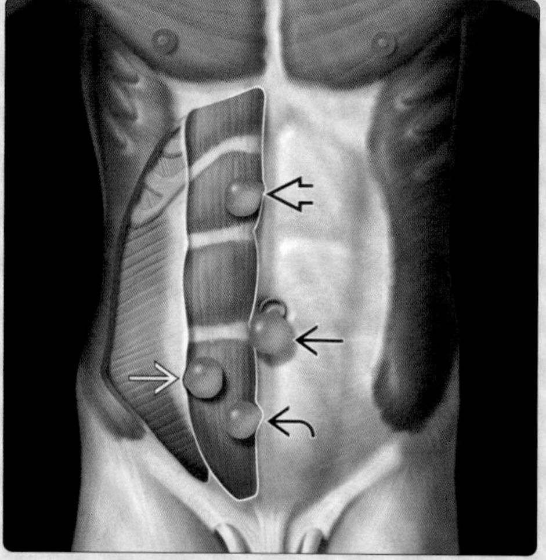

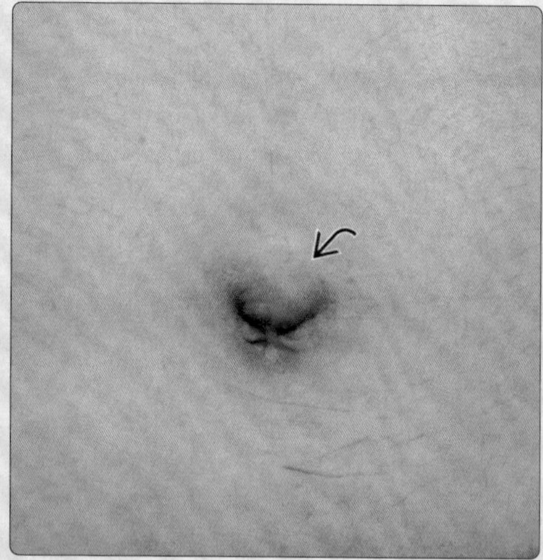

(Left) *Graphic shows a paraumbilical hernia ⇒ arising from around the umbilicus. The locations of epigastric ⇒, spigelian ➡, and hypogastric ⇒ hernias are also shown for reference.* **(Right)** *Clinical photograph shows a typical appearance of a small paraumbilical hernia in an adult with swelling ⇒ at the superior aspect of the umbilicus.*

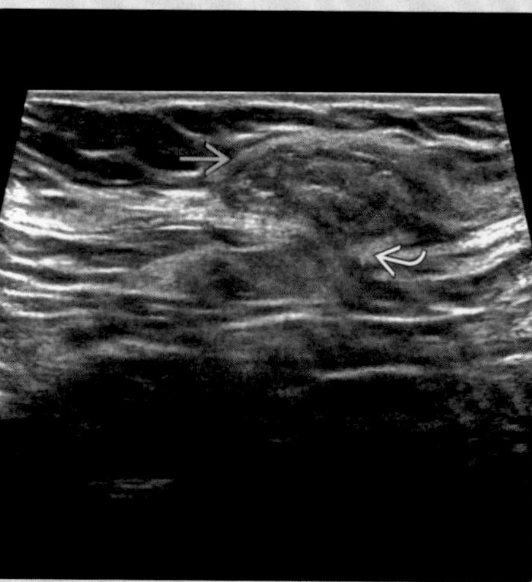

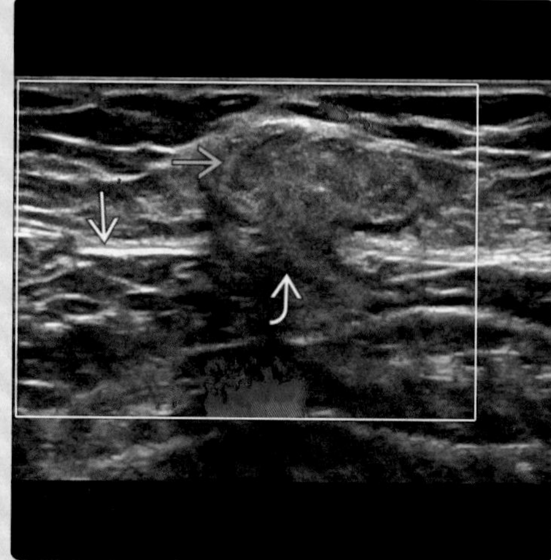

(Left) *Longitudinal ultrasound of a recurrent periumbilical hernia in a young woman following 2 pregnancies is shown. Omental fat ⇒ protrudes through a narrow defect ➡ in the linea alba, accentuated by the Valsalva maneuver.* **(Right)** *Longitudinal color Doppler ultrasound shows the same recurrent periumbilical hernia. The linea alba is better seen as a thin echogenic line ➡ with a small defect ➡. No color flow is seen in the herniated omentum ⇒, not necessarily indicative of strangulation, as fat is usually hypovascular.*

KEY FACTS

TERMINOLOGY

- Hernia: Weakness or defect in fibromuscular wall with protrusion of organ or part of organ through defect

IMAGING

- US accurate at detecting hernia sac and contents as well as fascial defect
  - Increase in hernia size during cough, Valsalva maneuver, or standing
- Direct inguinal hernia passes through transversalis fascial defect in Hesselbach triangle
- Indirect inguinal hernia passes through deep inguinal ring, extends along inguinal canal, and emerges at superficial inguinal ring, extending to scrotal sac
- Femoral hernia passes through femoral canal into superomedial thigh, accompanying femoral vessels
- Color Doppler helps identify inferior epigastric artery and its relationship to hernia neck for inguinal hernias

TOP DIFFERENTIAL DIAGNOSES

- Lipoma of spermatic cord
- Encysted hydrocele canal of Nück
- Inguinal canal lesions

CLINICAL ISSUES

- Hernia repair is most common surgical procedure in US
- Indirect inguinal hernia: Young to middle aged, 5-10x more common in males
  - Children = patent processus vaginalis
- Direct inguinal hernia nearly always in males, ↑ with ↑ age
- Femoral hernia: More common in female, older patients
- Groin lump or discomfort with positive cough impulse, constant or intermittent
- Obstruction or strangulation more common with femoral hernias due to narrow neck

SCANNING TIPS

- Localize inferior epigastric artery, provoke hernia

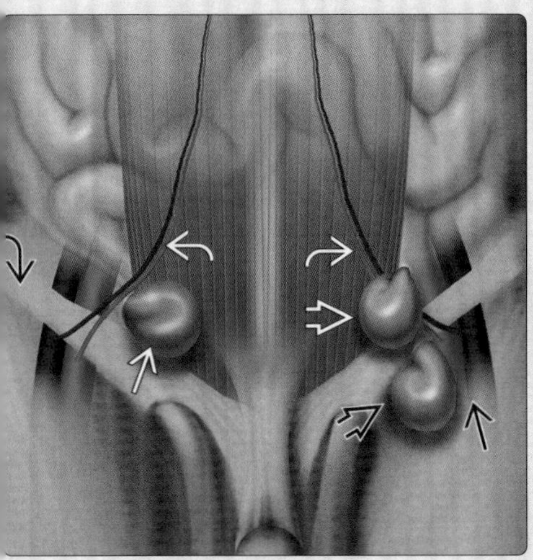

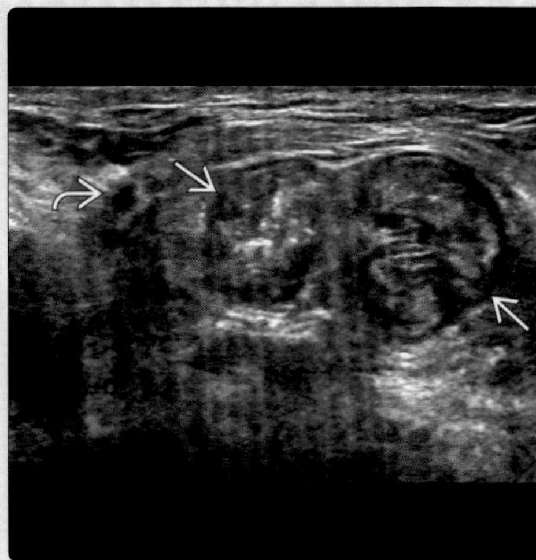

(Left) *Graphic shows 3 types of groin hernia: Direct and indirect inguinal hernias arise above the inguinal ligament, medial and lateral to the inferior epigastric vessels, respectively; femoral hernias arise below the inguinal ligament medial to femoral vessels.* **(Right)** *Transverse US of the right groin shows a direct inguinal hernia containing small bowel. The hernia neck was medial to the inferior epigastric vessels. The small bowel was only seen during Valsalva or while standing.*

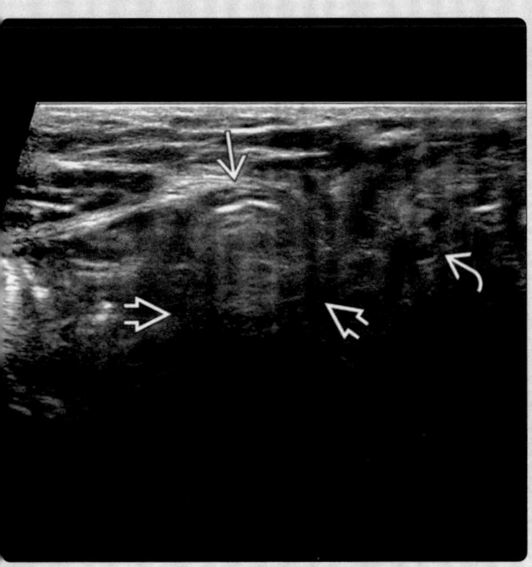

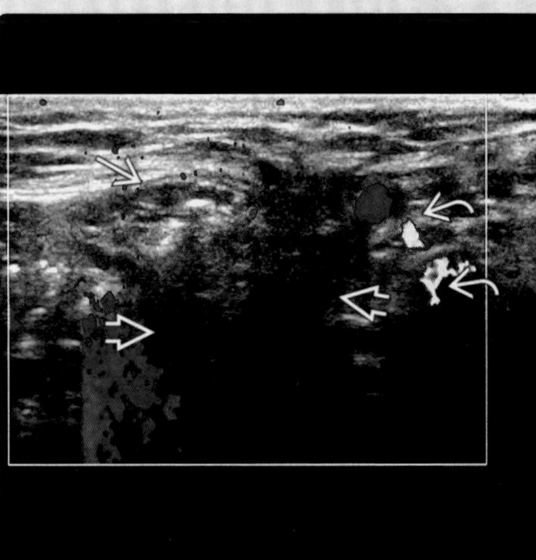

(Left) *Transverse US shows a left direct-type inguinal hernia containing bowel. The neck of the hernia lies medial to the inferior epigastric vessels.* **(Right)** *Transverse color Doppler US of the same left direct inguinal hernia during Valsalva maneuver is shown. The hernia sac is larger. The hernia neck is medial to the inferior epigastric vessels. Direct inguinal hernias rarely obstruct.*

Ascites

KEY FACTS

TERMINOLOGY

- Abnormal accumulation of fluid within peritoneal cavity

IMAGING

- Free-flowing fluid insinuates itself between organs & is shaped by surrounding structures
- Fluid collects in most dependent locations, such as pouch of Douglas, Morison pouch, & bilateral flanks, unless there are loculations
- Ultrasound accurate at detecting, localizing, & characterizing ascites; quantification more subjective
- Simple: Anechoic; homogeneous, freely mobile, deep acoustic enhancement
- Complicated: Echogenic fluid with coarse or fine internal echoes, layering debris or particulate material, septa
- Small free fluid in cul-de-sac is physiologic in women
- Look for associated hepatic disease, peritoneal masses, or adherent bowel

TOP DIFFERENTIAL DIAGNOSES

- Hemoperitoneum
- Malignant ascites
- Peritoneal inclusion cyst
- Pseudomyxoma peritonei
- Large cyst (ovarian, mesenteric)
- Other fluids, such as bile, urine
- Phsyiologic free fluid

PATHOLOGY

- Most common causes: Acute & chronic liver disease, heart & kidney failure, pancreatitis, nephrotic syndrome, cancer

SCANNING TIPS

- Paracentesis is required for protein content, cell count, culture, & cytology
- Soft tissue nodules along peritoneal surfaces suggest tumor
- Peritoneal thickening suggests tumor or infection

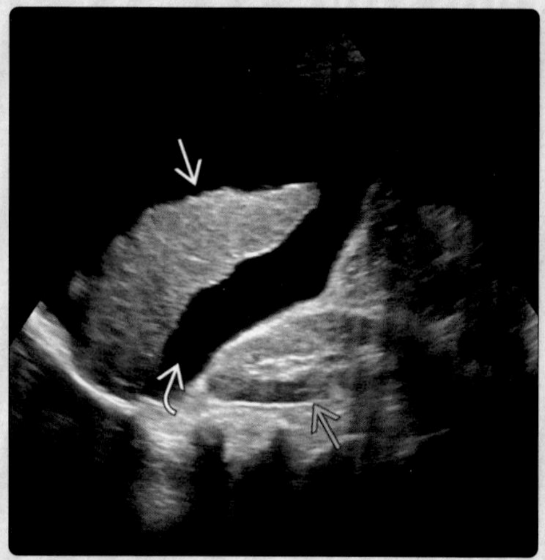

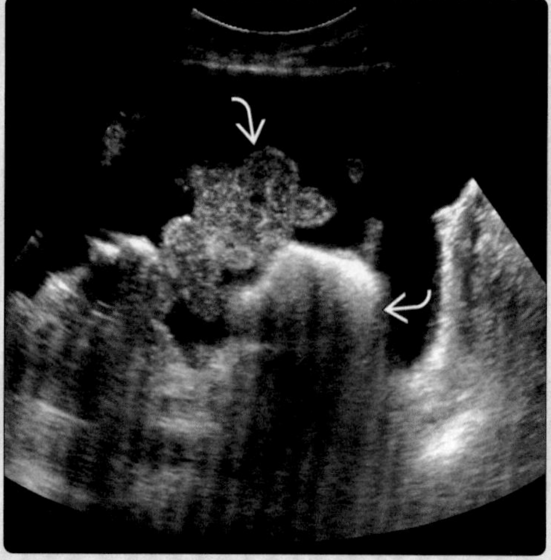

(Left) *Longitudinal ultrasound shows the right upper quadrant in a patient with cirrhosis and ascites. The liver contour is nodular ➡. Ascites surrounds the liver and fills Morison pouch ➡. The right kidney ➡ appears echogenic secondary to acoustic enhancement.* **(Right)** *Transverse ultrasound shows the left lower quadrant in a patient with end-stage liver disease. There is free fluid surrounding the bowel ➡ with no mass effect.*

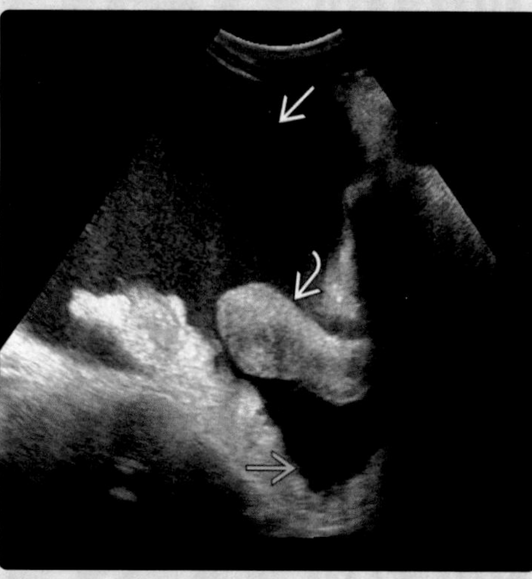

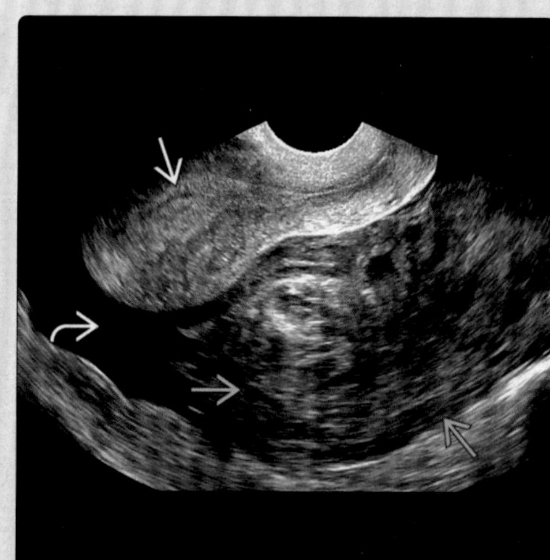

(Left) *Longitudinal ultrasound of the pelvis in a patient with cirrhosis shows a large volume of complex ascites ➡ containing low-level echoes. Paracentesis showed hemorrhage. Ascites extends into the cul-de-sac ➡. The uterus ➡ is normal.* **(Right)** *Longitudinal transvaginal ultrasound shows the pelvis in a ruptured ectopic pregnancy. There is free anechoic fluid in the upper pelvis ➡ with clotted blood ➡ in the dependent pouch of Douglas. Endometrial thickening is noted in the uterus with no intrauterine sac ➡.*

KEY FACTS

TERMINOLOGY

- Peritoneal spread of tumor from epithelial malignancy resulting in peritoneal thickening, omental infiltration, serosal implants, and ascites

IMAGING

- Implants develop where peritoneal fluid collects: Dome of liver, omentum, paracolic gutters, and pelvic recesses
- Peritoneal masses may be solid, cystic, or mixed, depending on primary neoplasm
- Hypoechoic rind-like thickening of peritoneum or discrete irregular nodular masses along peritoneum
- Omental involvement may be nodular or diffuse, producing an omental cake
    - Thickened and hypoechoic or heterogeneous with preserved islands of echogenic fat
- Ascites: Complex with septations or internal echoes (jiggle with transducer pressure)
- Thickening of mesenteric leaves due to desmoplastic reaction; typically mesenteric side of terminal ileum
- Color Doppler flow in solid omental/peritoneal deposits

TOP DIFFERENTIAL DIAGNOSES

- Pseudomyxoma peritonei
- Peritoneal mesothelioma
- Peritoneal tuberculosis
- Peritoneal sarcomatosis
- Peritoneal lymphomatosis

CLINICAL ISSUES

- Present with abdominal distension and pain, weight loss, malaise, fever
- May have elevated tumor markers such as CA125 or CEA
- Prognosis variable depending on primary tumor but generally poor prognosis

SCANNING TIPS

- Use linear transducers to evaluate anterior peritoneum

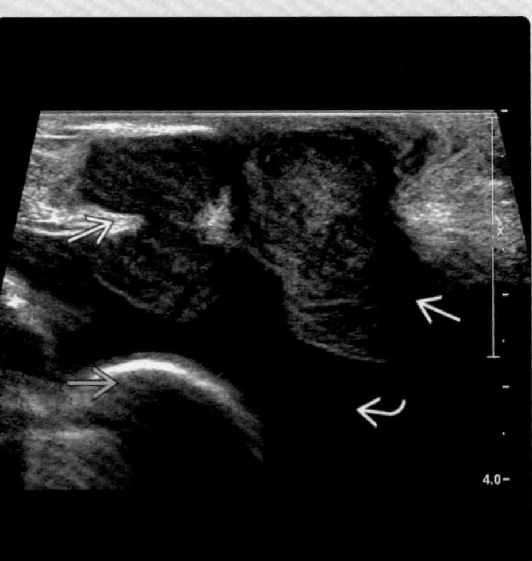

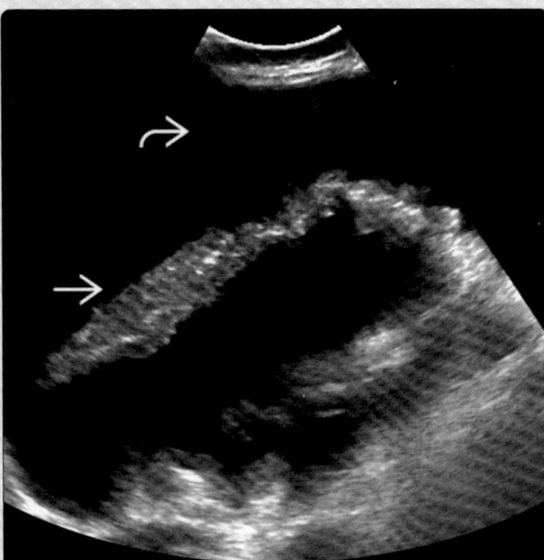

(Left) *Longitudinal ultrasound of the midline anterior abdominal wall in a patient with metastatic pancreatic neuroendocrine carcinoma shows 2 peritoneal soft tissue implants growing through the anterior abdominal wall ➡ with adjacent ascites ➡ and bowel ➡.* **(Right)** *Longitudinal ultrasound of the right upper quadrant inferior to the liver shows ascites ➡ and a thick lobular omental cake ➡ from pancreatic carcinomatosis.*

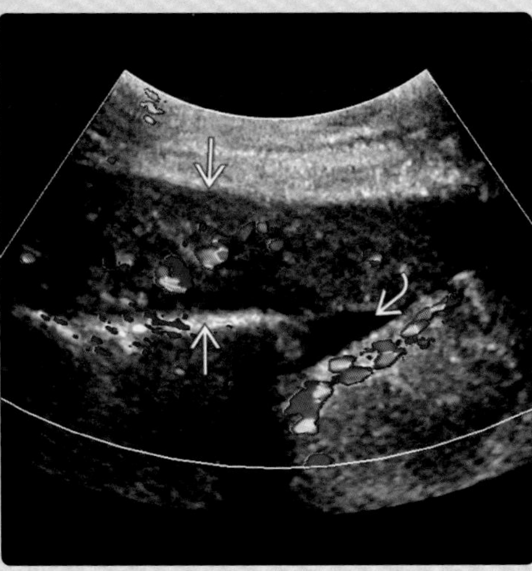

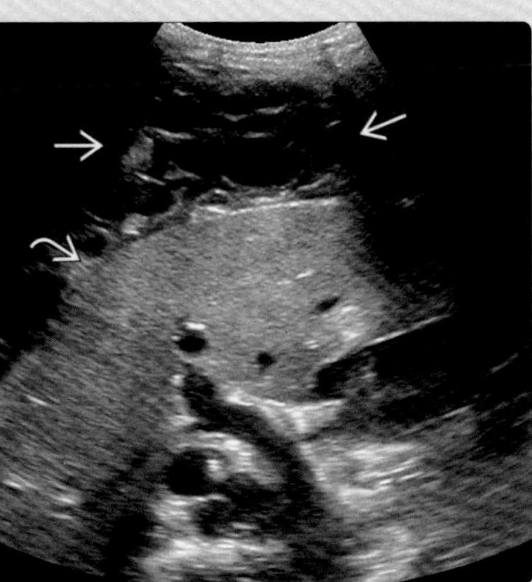

(Left) *Transverse color Doppler ultrasound of the midline anterior abdominal wall shows ovarian carcinomatosis and an omental cake ➡. Color flow is present within the omentum. A small amount of ascites ➡ is noted.* **(Right)** *Transverse ultrasound of the right upper quadrant shows complex septated ascites ➡ anterior to the liver ➡, representing mucinous carcinomatosis from appendiceal carcinoma.*

  - Continuous with muscularis propria of rectum
  - Forms incomplete ring in females
- External anal sphincter
  - Thick ring of skeletal muscle around internal anal sphincter
  - Under voluntary control
  - 3 parts from superior to inferior: Deep, superficial, and subcutaneous
- Longitudinal muscle
  - Thin muscle between internal and external anal sphincters
  - Conjoined muscle from muscularis propria of rectum and levator ani

Histology

- Bowel wall throughout GI tract has uniform general histology, comprised of 4 layers
  - Mucosa
    - Functions for absorption and secretion
    - Composed of epithelium and loose connective tissue
    - Lamina propria
    - Muscularis mucosa (deep layer of mucosa)
  - Submucosa
    - Consists of fibrous connective tissue
    - Contains Meissner plexus
  - Muscularis externa
    - Muscular layer responsible for peristalsis or propulsion of food through gut
    - Contains Auerbach plexus
  - Serosa
    - Epithelial lining continuous with peritoneum

IMAGING ANATOMY

Overview

- GI tract extends from mouth to anus
- Esophagus, which is intrathoracic, is difficult to visualize with external ultrasound due to rib cage and air-containing lungs
  - Endoluminal ultrasound performed to assess mural pathology
- Stomach to rectum lie within abdomen and pelvis
- Stomach, 1st part of duodenum, jejunum, ileum, transverse colon, and sigmoid colon suspended within peritoneal cavity by peritoneal folds and are mobile
- 2nd-4th parts of duodenum, ascending colon, descending colon, and rectum typically extraperitoneal/retroperitoneal
  - Retroperitoneal structures have more fixed position and are easy to locate
- Stomach located in left upper quadrant
  - Identified by presence of rugae/mural folds
  - Prominent muscular layer facilitates identification of pylorus
- Small bowel loops are located centrally within abdomen
  - Abundant valvulae conniventes helps identify jejunal loops
  - Jejunalization of ileum seen in celiac disease to compensate for atrophy of folds in proximal small bowel
  - Contents of jejunal loops usually liquid and appear hypoechoic/anechoic
- Cecum and colon identified by haustral pattern
  - Located peripherally in abdomen
  - Contain feces and gas
  - Haustra seen as prominent curvilinear echogenic arcs with posterior reverberation
  - Cecum identified by curvilinear arc of hyperechogenicity (representing feces and gas) in right lower quadrant blind ending caudally
  - Not uncommonly, cecum high lying and may be horizontally placed
  - Sigmoid colon variable length and mobile
  - Junction of left colon with sigmoid colon identified in left iliac fossa by tracing descending colon
  - Rectosigmoid junction has fixed position and is identified with full bladder, which acts as acoustic window
- Appendicular base normally located in right lower quadrant
  - Length and direction of tip vary
  - Retrocecal appendix and pelvic appendix can be difficult to locate transabdominally
    - Transvaginal ultrasound examination useful to identify pelvic appendix
- Normal measurements of bowel caliber
  - Small bowel < 3 cm
  - Large bowel
    - Cecum < 9 cm
    - Transverse colon < 6 cm
- Stratified appearance of bowel wall on histology is depicted by 5 distinct layers on ultrasound as **alternating echogenic/sonolucent (hypoechoic) appearance (gut signature)**
  - Interface of lumen and mucosa: Echogenic
  - Muscularis mucosa: Hypoechoic
  - Submucosa: Echogenic
  - Muscularis propria/externa: Hypoechoic
  - Serosa: Echogenic
- Normal bowel wall thickness < 3 mm

Imaging Recommendations

- Ultrasound is the initial study of choice for gastrointestinal conditions in children and young adults and for select indications in adults
  - Focused survey for acute appendicitis, pyloric stenosis, intussusception, and malrotation
  - Extended systematic survey in Crohn disease
- 5- to 8-MHz curvilinear probe for wider field of view and deeper penetration
- 7- to 12-MHz linear probe for higher resolution
- 12- to 18-MHz linear probe for delineation of 5 bowel layers
- Fixed points of bowel easy to assess with transabdominal ultrasound: Pylorus, "C loop" of duodenum, and ileocecal junction
- Abnormal bowel identified as thickened or dilated segments, ± disturbance of gut signature
  - Thickened bowel demonstrates reduced peristalsis, which stands out among normally peristalsing loops of normal bowel
- Optimize settings, evaluate abnormal bowel in 2 planes
- Slow, graded compression
- Evaluate surrounding tissues for secondary signs: Echogenic fat, fluid, enlarged lymph nodes, tracts
- Color Doppler: Increased vascularity in acute inflammation, may be helpful in malrotation

GASTROINTESTINAL TRACT IN SITU

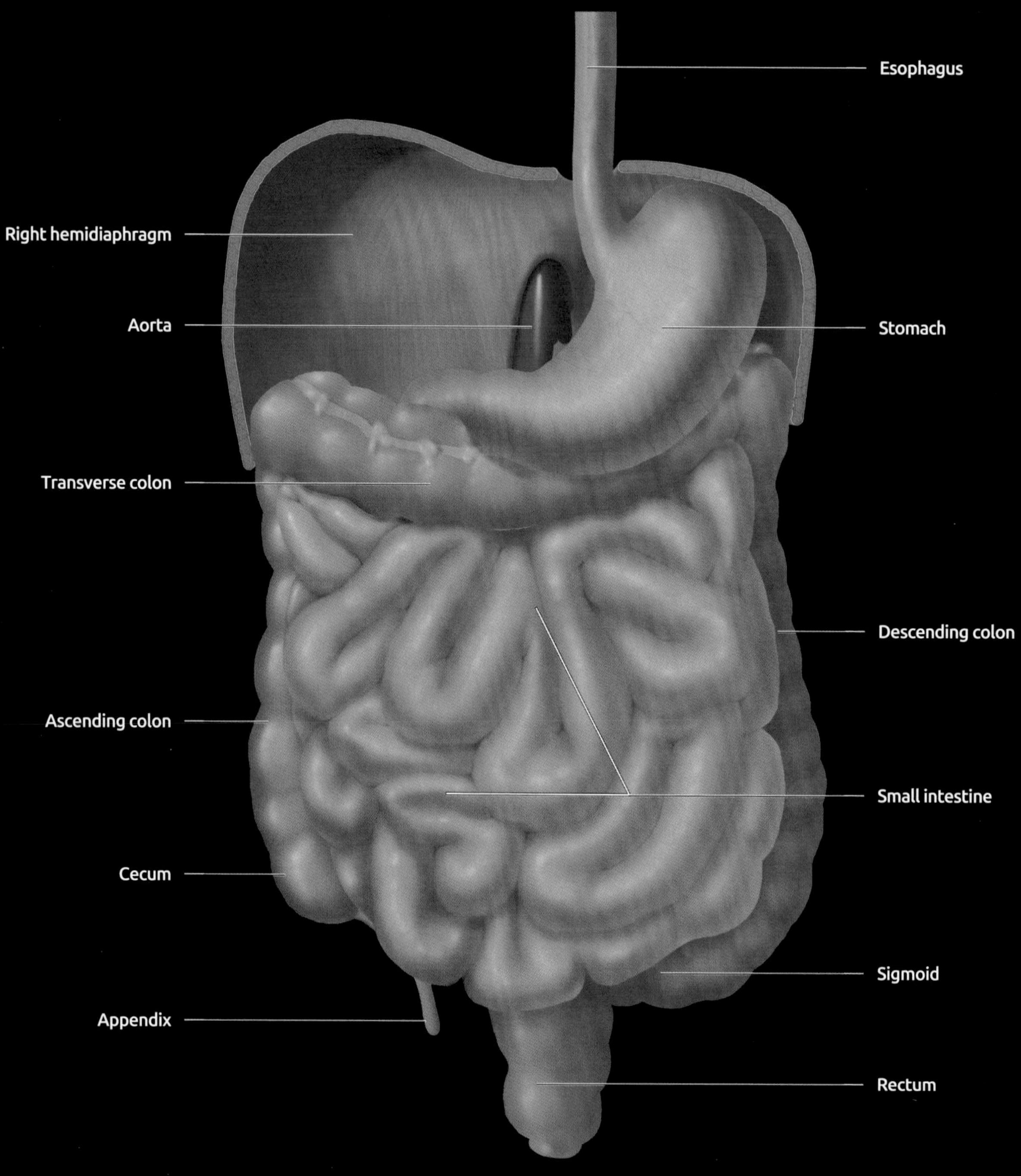

Graphic shows the gastrointestinal tract in situ. The liver and the greater omentum have been removed. Note the relatively central location of the small intestine compared with the peripherally located large intestine. Most of the bowel segments are intraperitoneal, apart from the 2nd-4th parts of the duodenum, the ascending and descending colon, and the middle 1/3 of the rectum, which are retroperitoneal. The distal 1/3 of the rectum is extraperitoneal.

STOMACH AND DUODENUM IN SITU

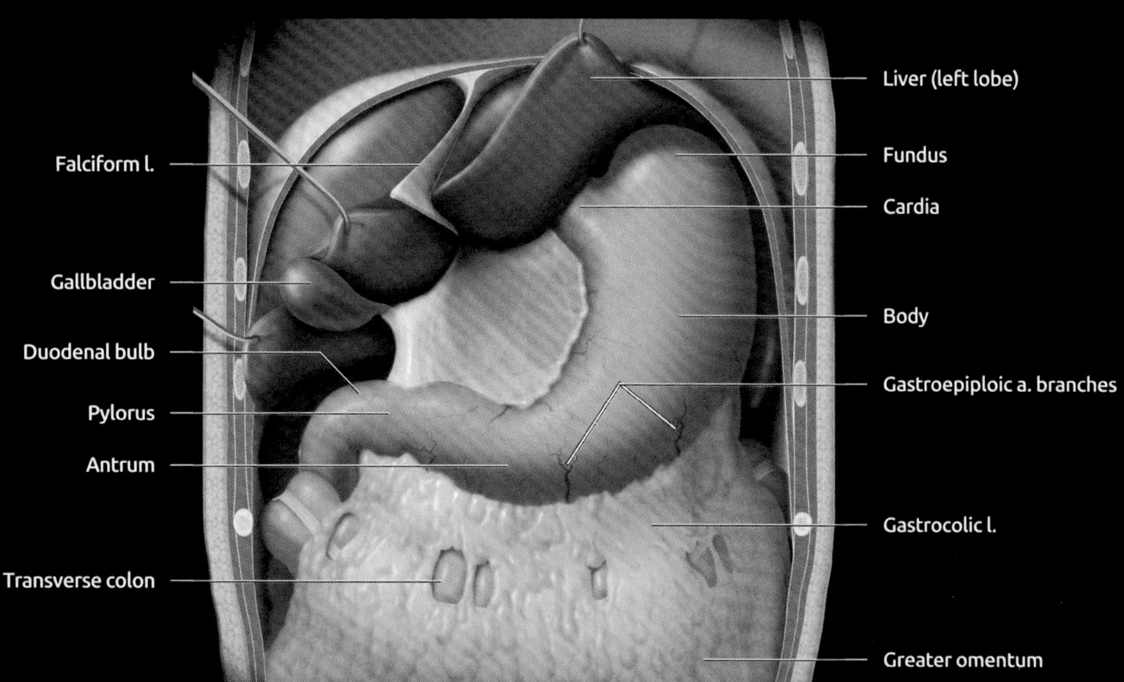

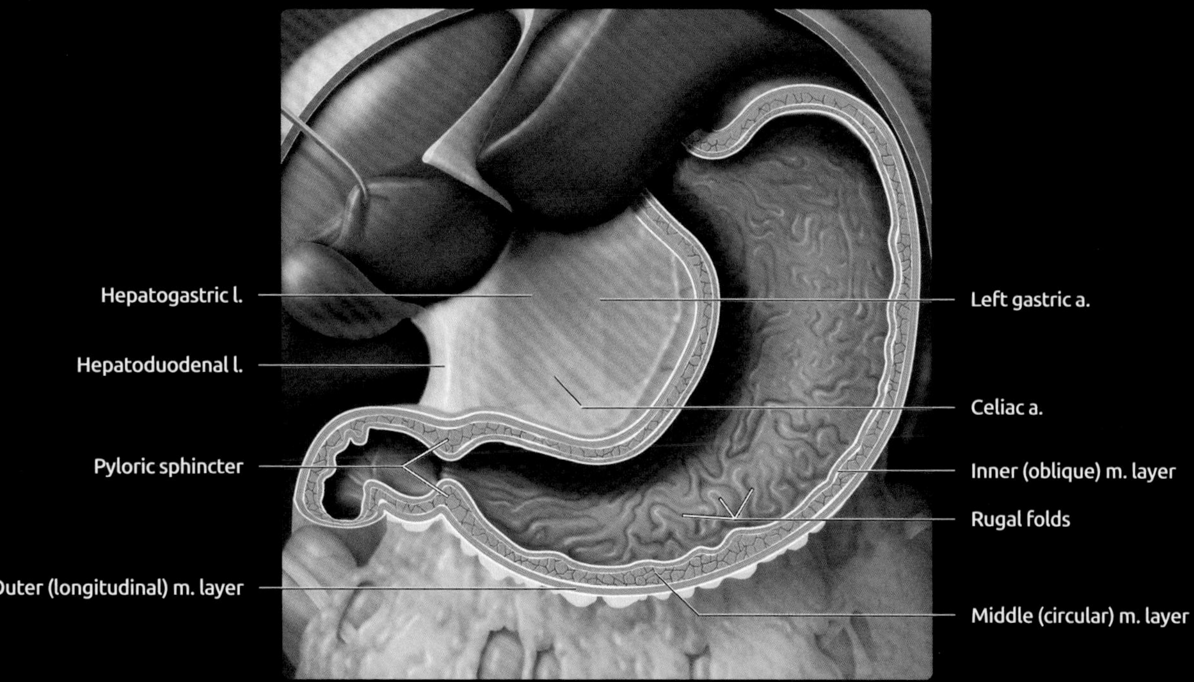

(Top) *Graphic shows the stomach and proximal duodenum in situ. The liver and gallbladder have been retracted upward. Note that the lesser curvature and anterior wall of the stomach touch the underside of the liver, and the gallbladder abuts the duodenal bulb. The greater curvature is attached to the transverse colon by the gastrocolic ligament, which continues inferiorly as the greater omentum, covering most of the colon and small bowel.* **(Bottom)** *Graphic shows the lesser omentum extending from the stomach to the porta hepatis, divided into the broader and thinner hepatogastric ligament and the thicker hepatoduodenal ligament. The lesser omentum carries the portal vein, hepatic artery, common bile duct, and lymph nodes. The free edge of the lesser omentum forms the ventral margin of the epiploic foramen. Note the layers of gastric muscle; the middle circular layer is thickest.*

DUODENUM

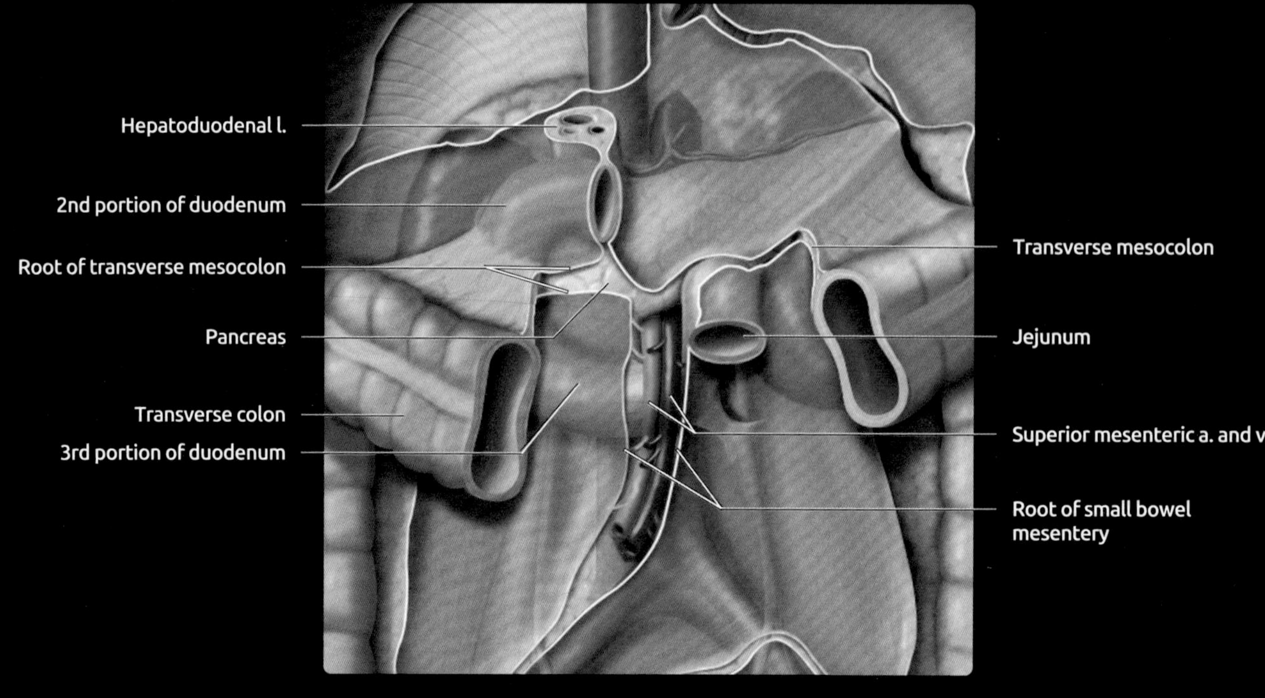

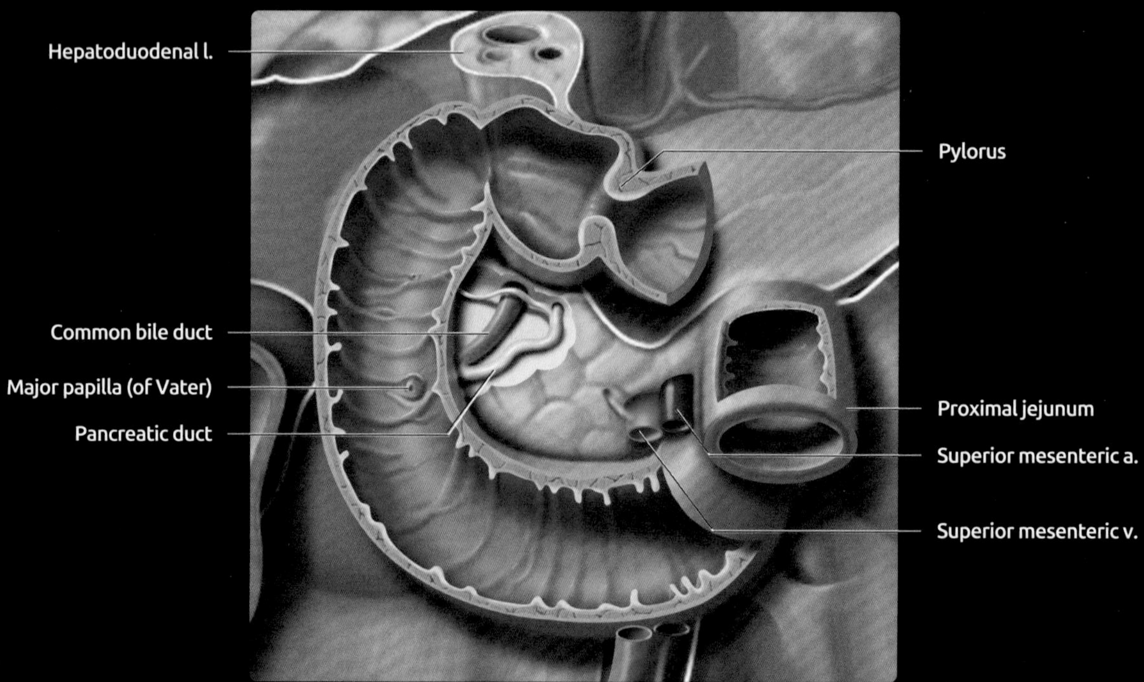

(Top) *The duodenum is retroperitoneal, except for the bulb (1st part). The proximal jejunum is intraperitoneal. The hepatoduodenal ligament attaches the duodenum to the porta hepatis and contains the portal triad (bile duct, hepatic artery, portal vein). The root of the transverse mesocolon and mesentery both cross the duodenum. The 3rd portion of the duodenum crosses in front of the aorta and inferior vena cava (IVC) and behind the superior mesenteric vessels. The 2nd portion of the duodenum is attached to the pancreatic head and lies close to the hilum of the right kidney.* **(Bottom)** *Graphic shows the duodenal bulb suspended by the hepatoduodenal ligament. The duodenal-jejunal flexure is suspended by the ligament of Treitz, an extension of the right crus. The major pancreaticobiliary papilla enters the medial wall of the 2nd portion of the duodenum.*

SMALL INTESTINE

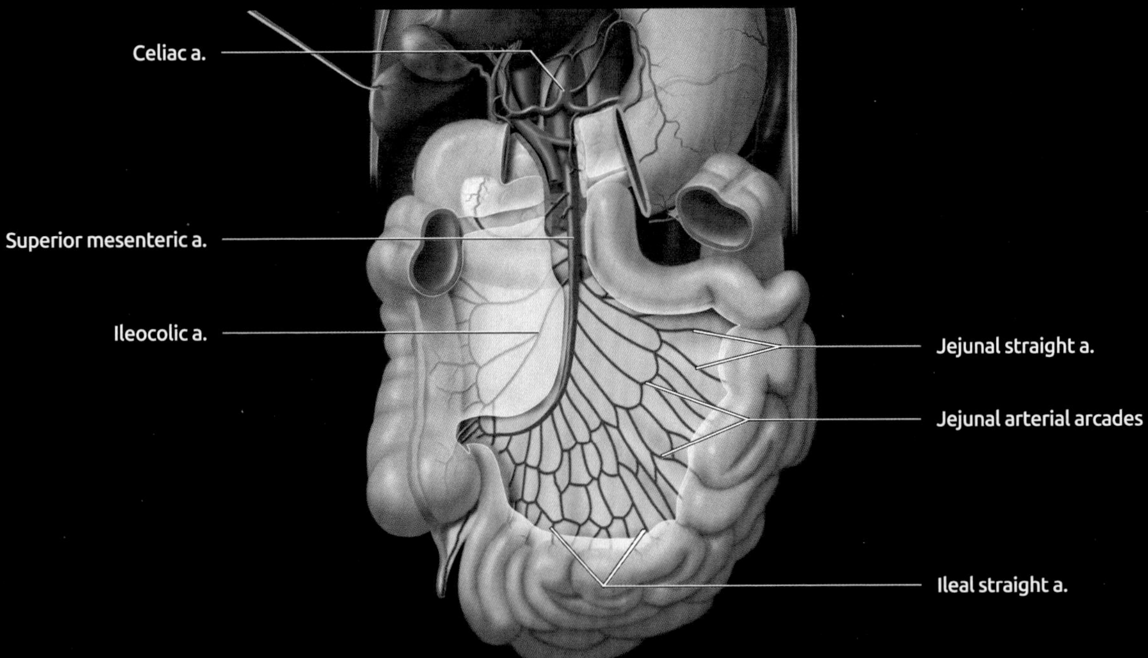

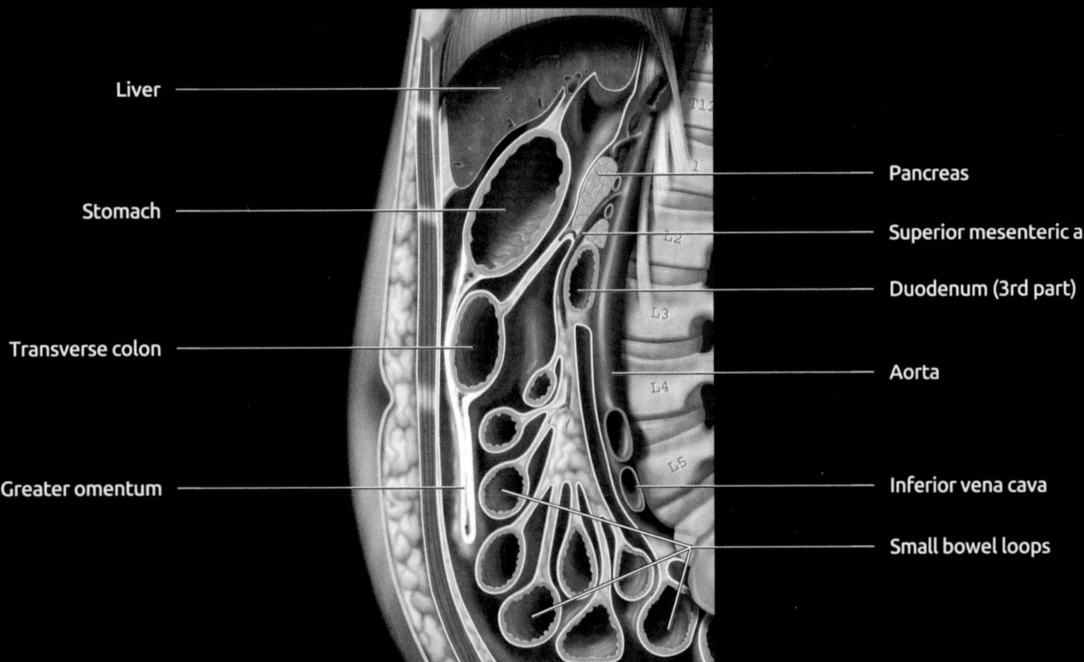

(Top) *Graphic shows the vascular supply of the entire small intestine from the superior mesenteric artery (SMA). The small bowel segments are displaced inferiorly. The SMA arises from the anterior abdominal aorta and gives off the inferior pancreaticoduodenal branch that supplies the duodenum and pancreas. Arising from the left side of the SMA are numerous branches to the jejunum and ileum. Jejunal arteries are generally larger and longer than those of the ileum. After a straight course, the arteries form multiple intercommunicating, curvilinear arcades.* **(Bottom)** *Graphic shows the sagittal section of the central abdomen, revealing the jejunum and ileum suspended in a radial pattern by the mesentery. Note the overlying greater omentum attached from the inferior portion of the stomach to drape the small bowel segments and transverse colon.*

COLON, RECTUM, AND ANUS

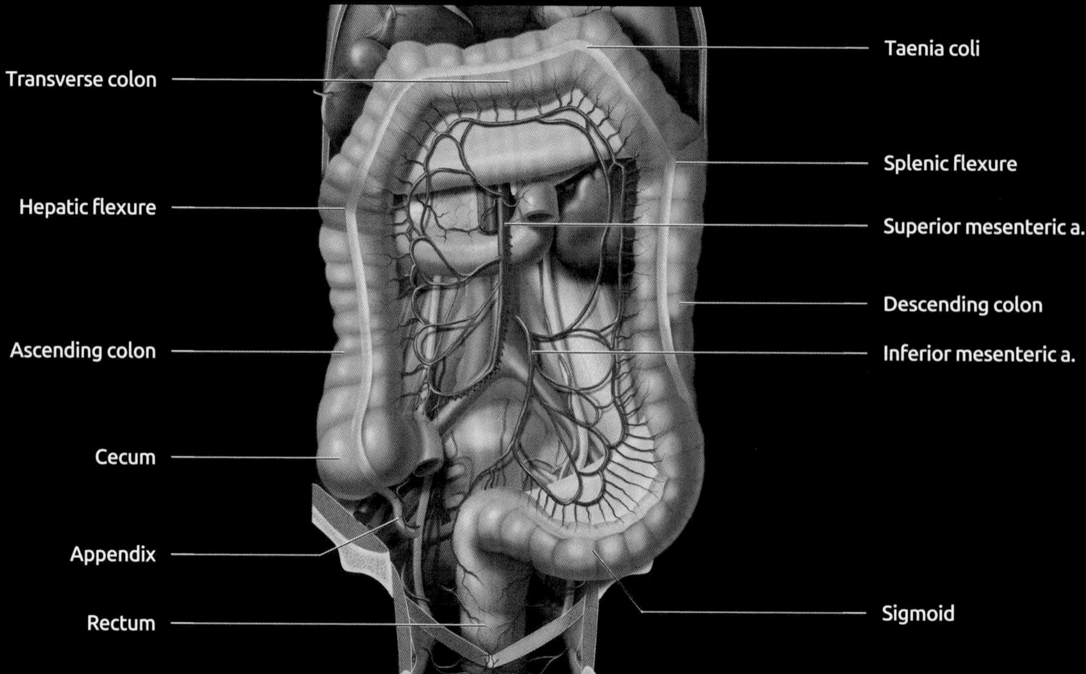

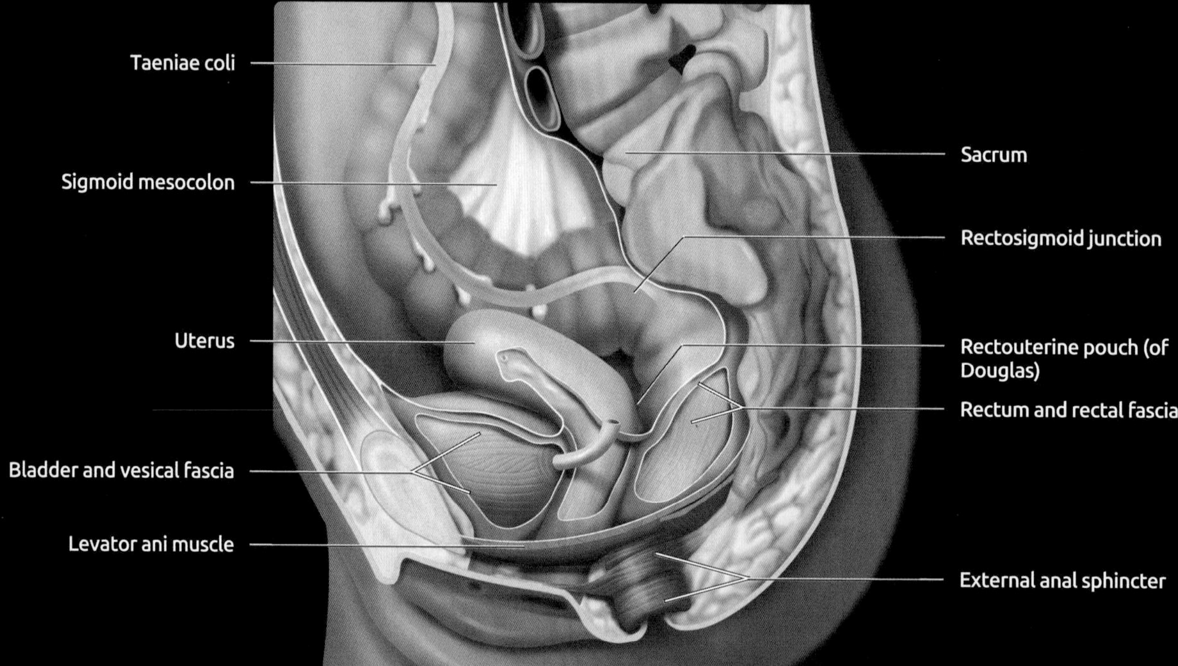

(Top) *Graphic shows the colon in situ. The transverse colon has been retracted upward to demonstrate the arterial supply of the colon from the SMA and inferior mesenteric artery (IMA). The SMA supplies the colon from the appendix through the splenic flexure, and the IMA supplies the descending colon through the rectum. Note the band of smooth muscle (taenia coli) running along the length of the intestine, which terminates in the vermiform appendix; these result in sacculations/haustrations along the colon, giving it a segmented appearance.* **(Bottom)** *The sigmoid colon is on a mesentery, while the rectum is retroperitoneal. The anterior surface of the rectum has a peritoneal covering, which extends deep in the pelvis in women, forming the rectouterine pouch (of Douglas) as it is reflected along the posterior surface of the uterus. The rectum is narrowed as it passes through the pelvic diaphragm and then enters the anal canal with 3 levels of the anal sphincter (deep, superficial, and subcutaneous). The rectum has a continuous external longitudinal coat of muscle, unlike the colon with its discontinuous rows of taeniae.*

STOMACH

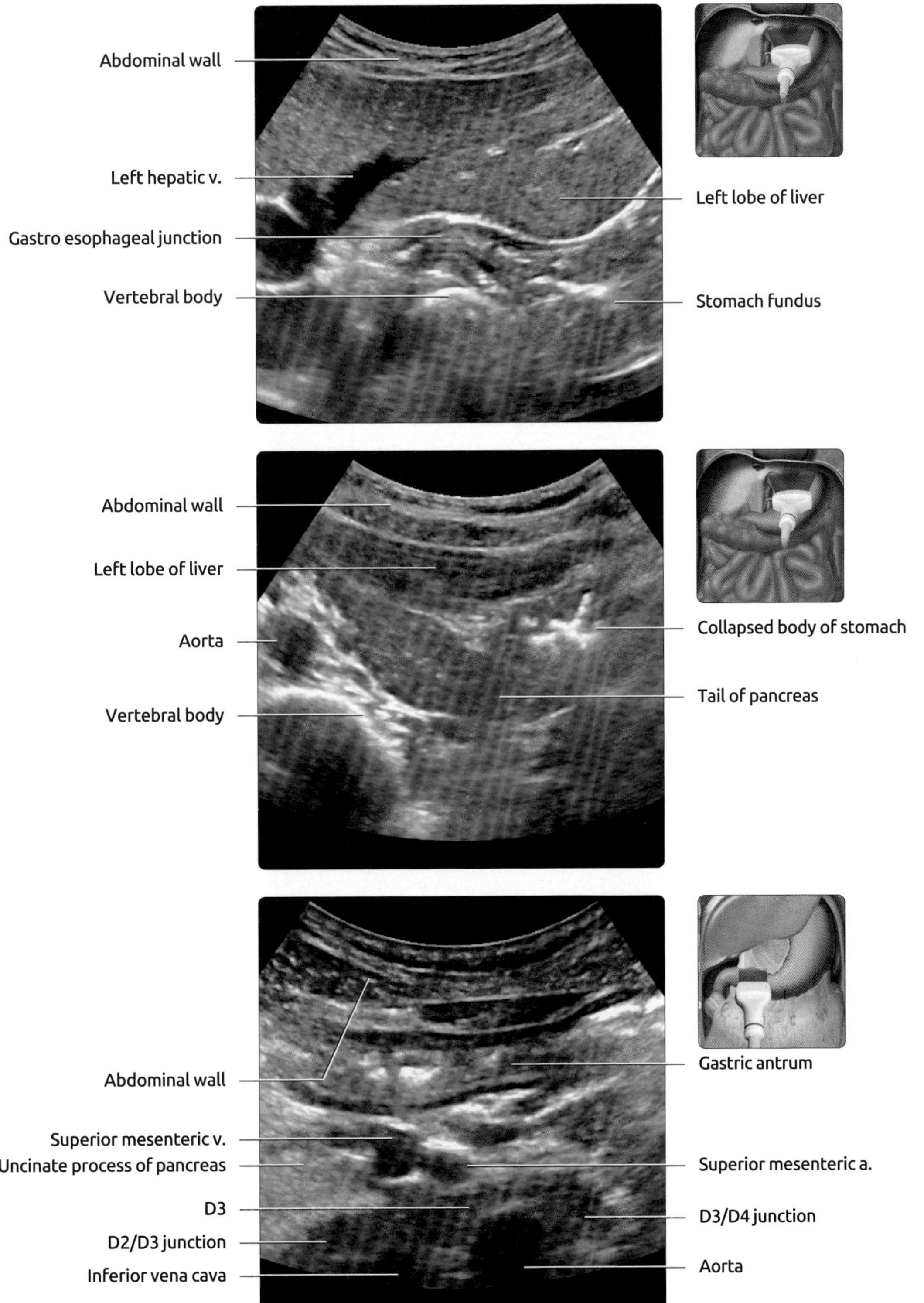

(Top) *Transverse oblique ultrasound at the epigastric region shows the gastroesophageal junction, which can be traced to the fundus of the stomach. Note the relationship to the adjacent structures.* **(Middle)** *Transverse oblique ultrasound through the left upper quadrant shows the collapsed stomach body with the rugal folds. Echogenic gas is seen between the rugae. The tail of the pancreas is seen posterior to the stomach, and the left lobe of the liver is anterior to the stomach.* **(Bottom)** *Transverse ultrasound through the upper abdomen shows the gastric antrum anteriorly compressed by the curvilinear probe and collapsed 3rd part of the duodenum (D3) posteriorly. The SMA and the superior mesenteric vein are seen in the plane in between. The IVC and aorta are seen posterior to the D3.*

DUODENUM/SMALL BOWEL

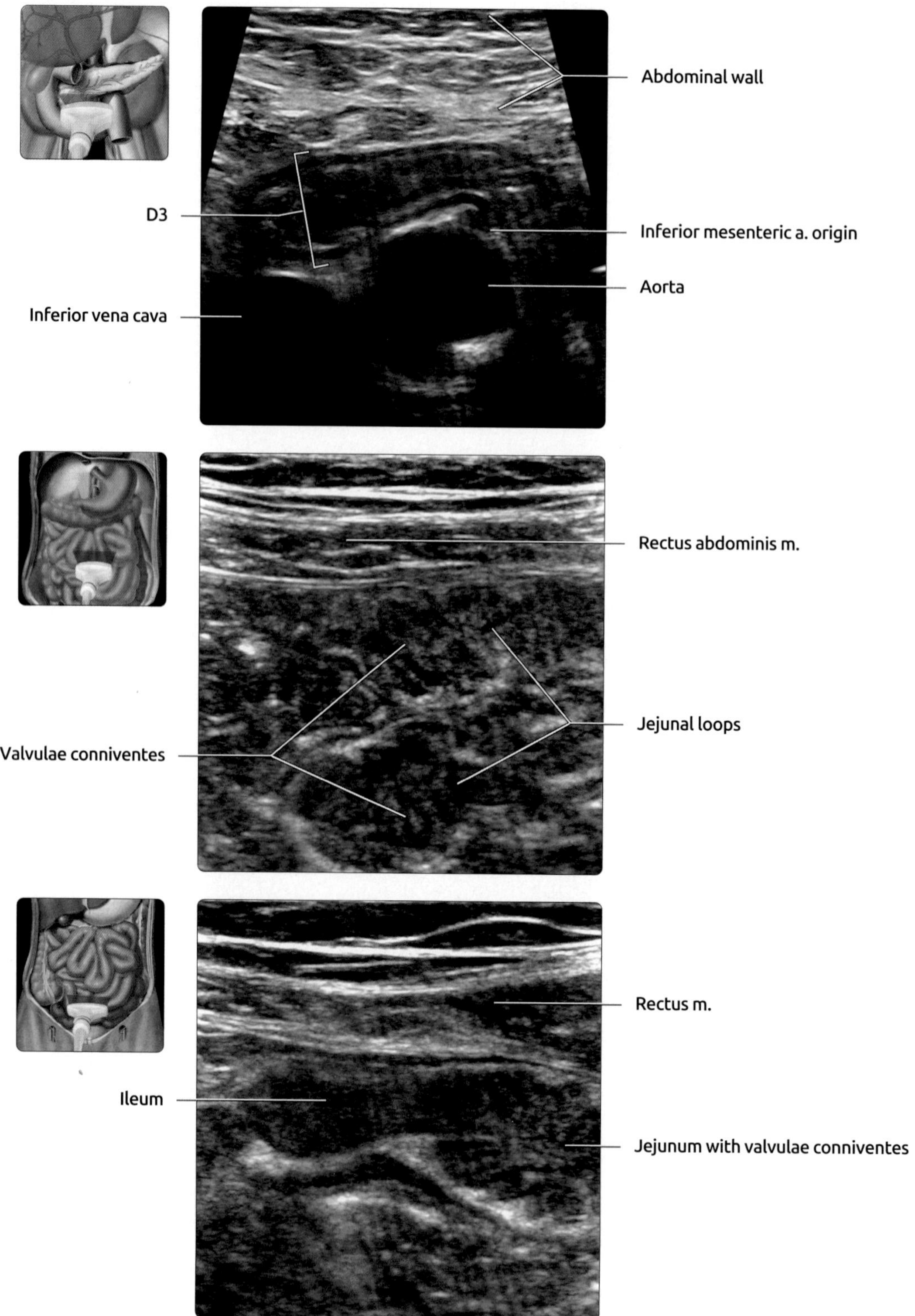

(Top) *Axial midline high-resolution ultrasound through the upper abdomen shows fluid distended in the D3 located across, in the upper retroperitoneum. Note the aorta and IVC posterior to the D3. Gut signature is seen in the wall of the D3.* **(Middle)** *Transverse oblique ultrasound through the left midabdomen shows jejunal loops with mucosal folds, valvulae conniventes.* **(Bottom)** *Transverse ultrasound through the lower abdomen close to midline shows jejunal ileal transition from a segment with folds to a segment with no folds.*

ILEUM, APPENDIX AND LARGE BOWEL

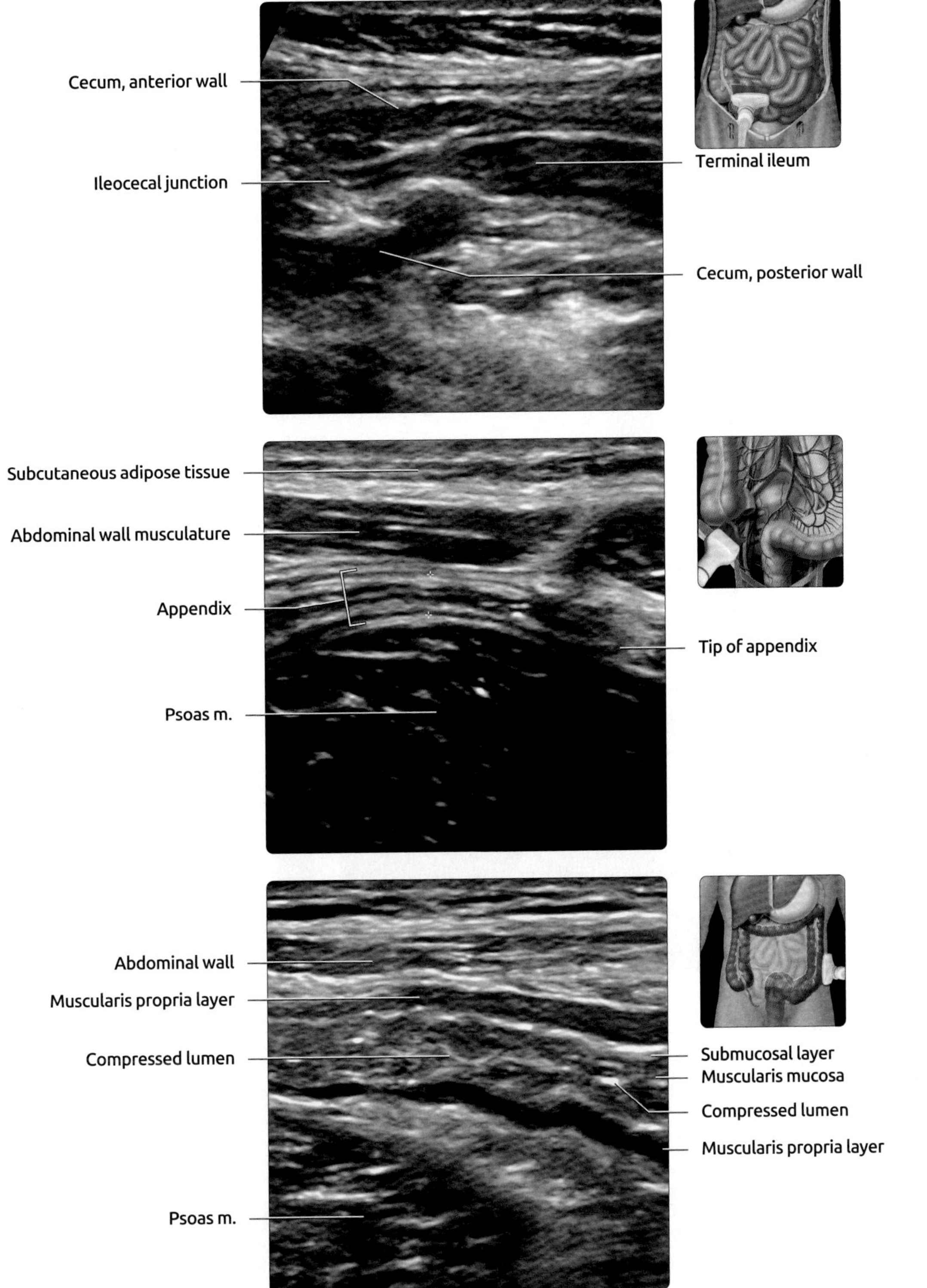

(Top) *Transverse high-resolution ultrasound through the right iliac fossa shows the ileocecal junction and the ileocecal valve.* **(Middle)** *Coronal oblique ultrasound through the right iliac fossa shows a long-axis normal appendix with a stratified mural appearance. Note the absence of periappendiceal inflammatory changes.* **(Bottom)** *High-resolution left sagittal ultrasound obtained with a higher frequency linear probe shows the collapsed descending colon with gut signature. The hypoechoic outer layer represents the muscularis propria layer.*

Appendicitis

KEY FACTS

IMAGING

- Blind-ended, aperistaltic, thick-walled tubular structure with gut signature
- Length ranges between 2-20 cm; base between ileocecal valve and cecal apex
- Noncompressible appendix with outer diameter ≥ 7 mm; single wall thickness > 3 mm
    - Increased caliber alone is not reliable indicator
- Mural stratification seen in early stages, absent in gangrenous appendicitis
- Periappendiceal edema seen as echogenic fat
- Additional findings: Appendicolith, periappendiceal fluid
- Perforated appendicitis: Periappendiceal abscess or phlegmon, free appendicolith
- Increased vascularity on color Doppler
- US: 1st choice in children, thin young adults, and pregnancy

TOP DIFFERENTIAL DIAGNOSES

- Appendiceal mucosal lymphoid hyperplasia
- Appendicular mucocele
- Cecal diverticulitis/ileocolitis
- Appendiceal/cecal carcinoma
- Pelvic inflammatory disease
- Meckel diverticulitis

PATHOLOGY

- Can be obstructive (appendicolith) or nonobstructive

CLINICAL ISSUES

- All ages affected, M = F
- Periumbilical pain migrating to RLQ; peritoneal irritation at McBurney point; atypical signs in 1/3 of patients
- Anorexia, nausea, vomiting, diarrhea, fever

SCANNING TIPS

- Scan over area of pain, use graded compression and color/power Doppler, consider decubitus positioning
- Use combination of linear and curved transducers
- Transvaginal US: For visualization of pelvic appendix

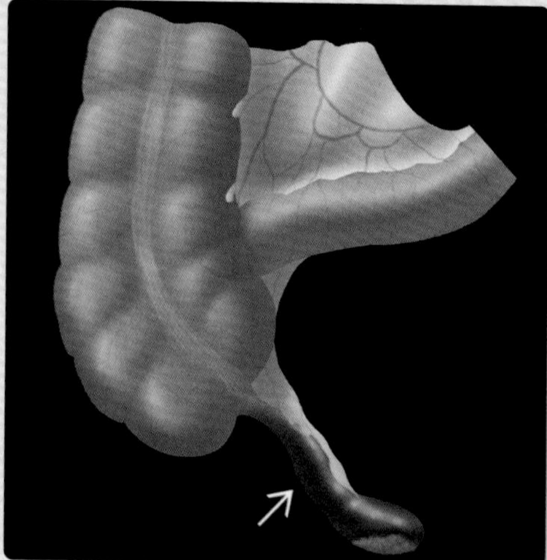

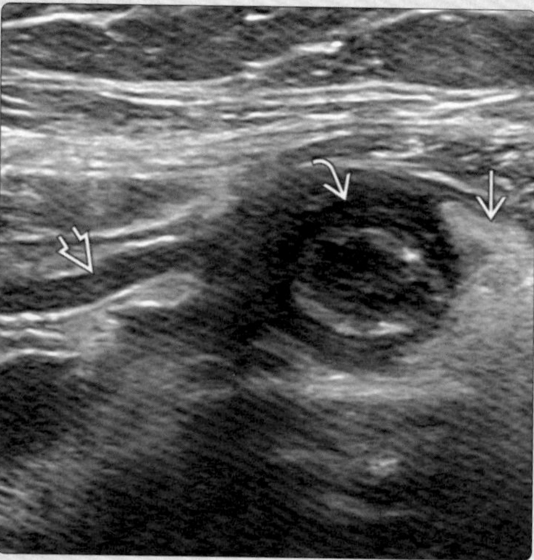

(Left) *Graphic shows the typical location and morphology of an inflamed appendix* ➔. *The direction of the tip of the appendix and length can vary.* **(Right)** *Axial ultrasound through an inflamed appendix demonstrates a target-like* ➔ *appearance due to the preservation of mural stratification. Note the surrounding echogenic, inflamed fat* ➔ *and a thickened, inflamed parietal layer* ➔ *of the peritoneum, which is in contact with the inflamed appendix.*

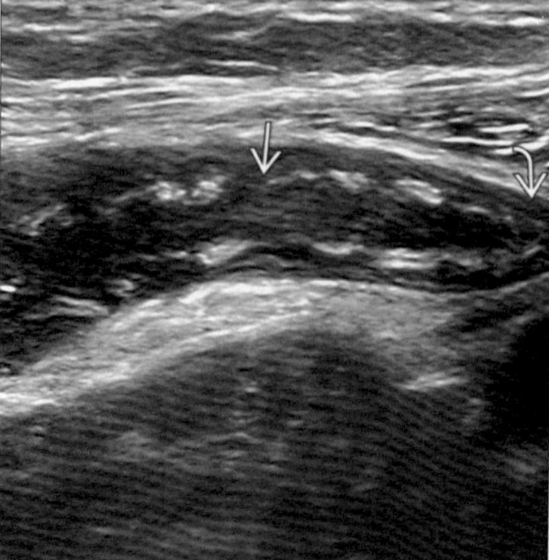

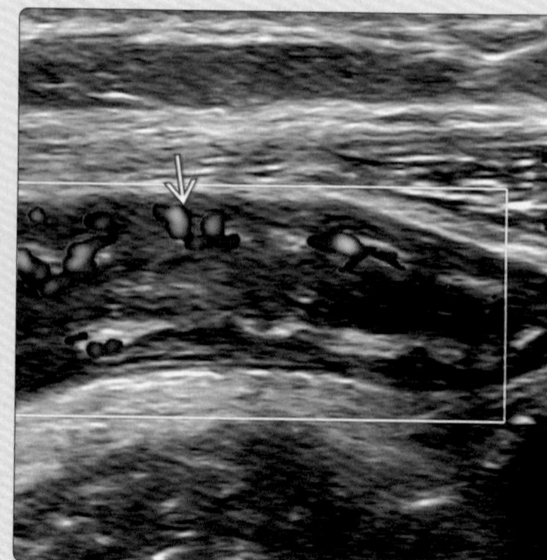

(Left) *In this axial oblique ultrasound of the same patient, note the blind-ending tip* ➔ *and mural stratification* ➔. **(Right)** *Power Doppler ultrasound of the inflamed appendix shows increased vascular flow* ➔.

KEY FACTS

TERMINOLOGY

- Distension of appendiceal lumen as result of mucin accumulation from epithelial proliferation or obstruction

IMAGING

- Distended tubular or pear-shaped cystic structure in right lower quadrant with low-level internal echoes
- Connects with medial wall of cecal pole
- Presence of calcification in wall strongly supports diagnosis of appendicular mucocele
- Concentric layering of dense mucoid material gives onion skin appearance
- Fecalith or appendicolith may be visible in obstructive type
- Hypovascular
- Soft tissue thickening and irregularity of mucocele wall suggest malignancy
- Contrast-enhanced CT scan is best imaging modality for characterization and staging

TOP DIFFERENTIAL DIAGNOSES

- Appendiceal carcinoma or acute appendicitis
- Hydrosalpinx
- Cystic ovarian neoplasm
- Tuboovarian abscess
- Duplication cyst/mesenteric cyst

PATHOLOGY

- Benign > malignant

CLINICAL ISSUES

- Most commonly: Right lower quadrant pain/palpable mass
- Frequently discovered incidentally
- Preoperative differentiation of benign and malignant mucoceles challenging

SCANNING TIPS

- Transvaginal ultrasound improves image quality and helps to differentiate from ovarian cystic masses

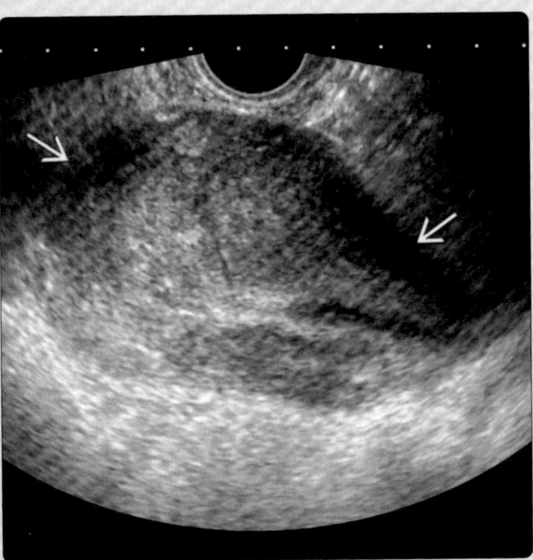

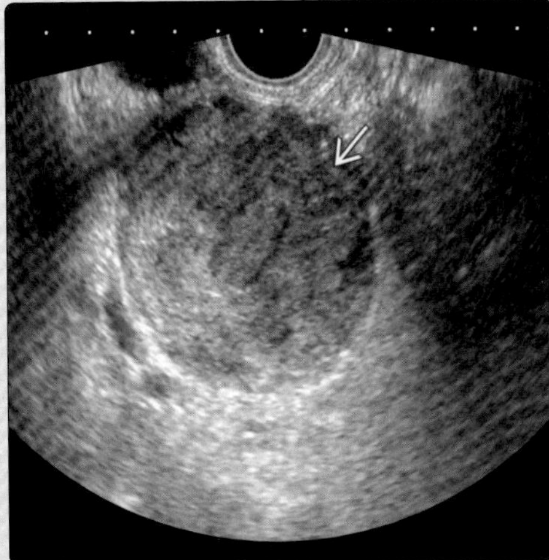

(Left) *Longitudinal transvaginal ultrasound shows a well-marginated, pear-shaped cystic mass ➡ in the right pelvis, containing echogenic mucoid material.* **(Right)** *Transvaginal coronal ultrasound shows the central echogenic, inspissated mucoid material ➡.*

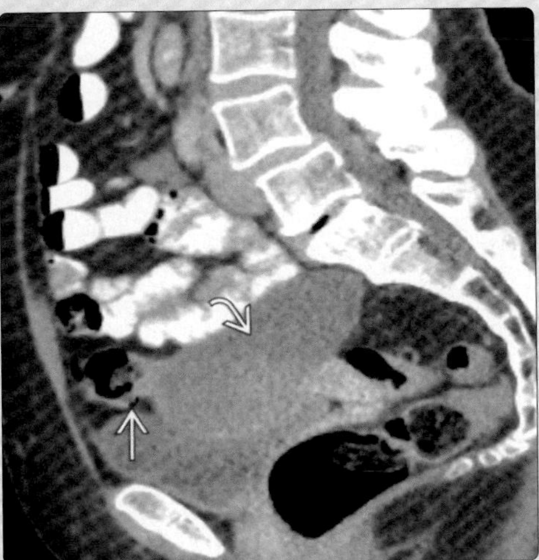

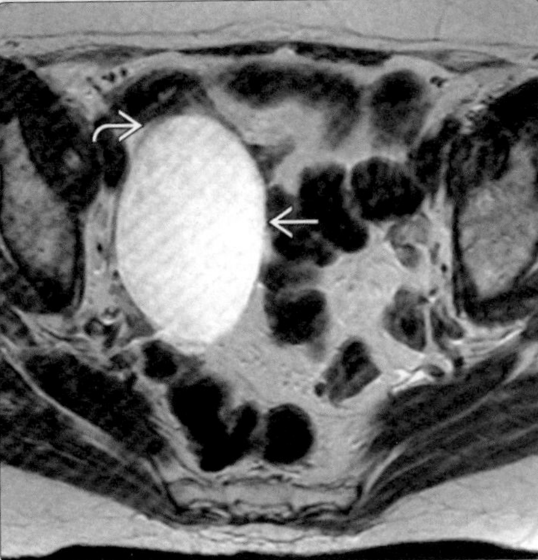

(Left) *Sagittal MPR from a CECT of the same patient shows a tubular, cystic structure with the base ➡ attached to the cecal pole. Note the central homogeneous low attenuation ➡.* **(Right)** *Axial T2 MR in the same patient shows the cystic mass ➡ with contents of uniform high signal intensity. The base ➡ can be traced to the cecal pole.*

Intussusception

KEY FACTS

TERMINOLOGY

- Invagination or telescoping of 1 segment of gastrointestinal tract and its mesentery (intussusceptum) into lumen of adjacent distal segment (intussuscipiens)

IMAGING

- Bowel within bowel appearance: Concentric parallel rings of bowel wall (target, doughnut, or bull's-eye sign)
- Echogenic crescent of intussuscepted mesenteric fat (crescent within doughnut sign)
- Central lead point lesion or lymph nodes
- Layering of fluid trapped between compressed bowel segments
- Mesenteric vessels trapped between entering and returning limbs of intussusceptum
- Reduced or absent mural vascularity of intussusceptum indicative of vascular compromise → ischemia with risk of infarction and perforation
- Ultrasound: 1st line in children

TOP DIFFERENTIAL DIAGNOSES

- Tumor, inflammation, infection

PATHOLOGY

- Occurs anywhere from stomach to rectum
- Children: Idiopathic in 95%; enlarged lymphoid tissue post infection; rare before 3 months of age
- Adults: Identifiable etiology in 90%

CLINICAL ISSUES

- Children (95%): Most common abdominal surgical emergency
  - Acute pain, palpable mass, "red currant jelly" stools
- Adults (5%): Insidious, vague abdominal symptoms, vomiting, red blood in stool
- Complications: Obstruction, bowel ischemia, or infarction

SCANNING TIPS

- Large-volume ascites, debris, and free gas are suggestive of perforation

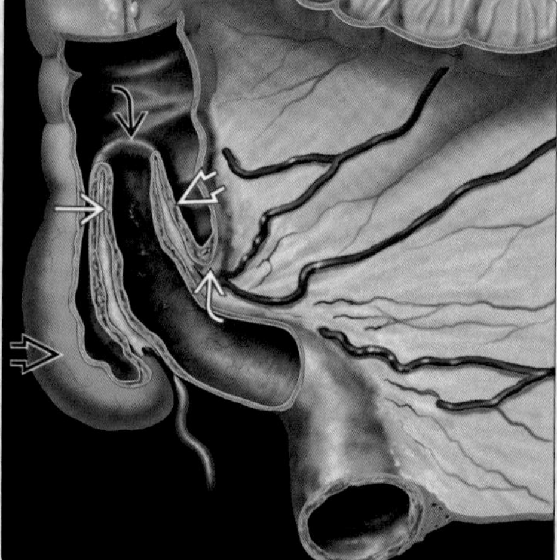

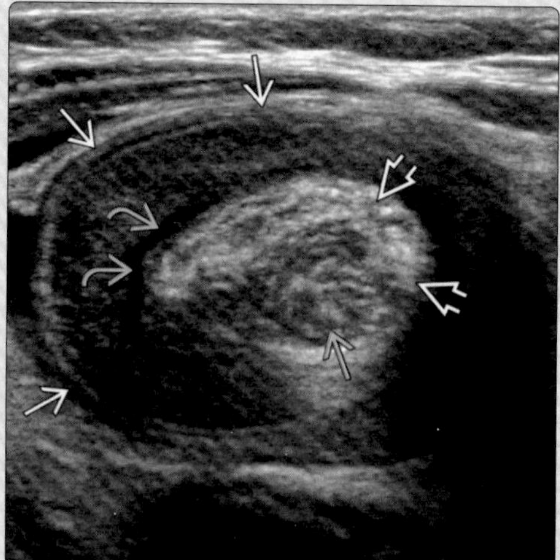

(Left) *Graphic shows ileocolic intussusception. Note entering layer ➡, returning layer ➡, and apex ➡ of intussusceptum (terminal ileum). Intussuscipiens (cecum) ➡ and neck of intussusception ➡ are noted.* **(Right)** *Transverse transabdominal ultrasound shows the classic bowel within bowel appearance of ileocolic intussusception. Note the inner intussusceptum (ileum ➡ and mesentery ➡) and outer intussuscipiens (hypoechoic layer of edematous bowel ➡) and intervening fluid ➡.*

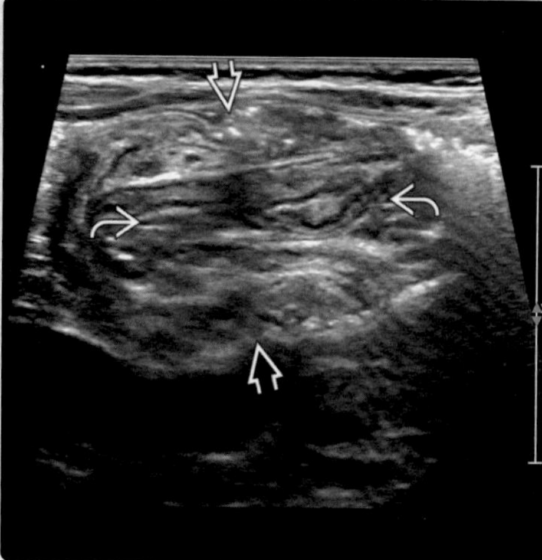

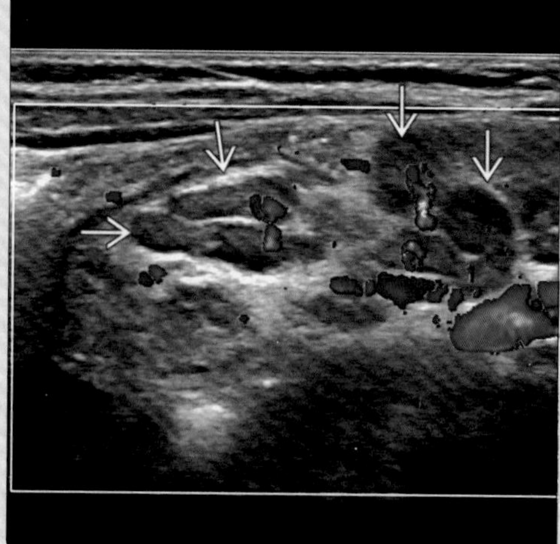

(Left) *Longitudinal ultrasound shows the layers of bowel wall involved in the intussusception. Outer layer of edematous bowel wall ➡ (intussuscipiens) and compressed inner layers ➡ (intussusceptum) are noted.* **(Right)** *Longitudinal color Doppler ultrasound shows multiple lymph nodes ➡ at the apex of the intussusceptum, acting as lead point.*

Epiploic Appendagitis

KEY FACTS

TERMINOLOGY

- Ischemic infarction of epiploic appendages (small pouches filled with fat, located along colon)

IMAGING

- Noncompressible, hyperechoic oval mass, adjacent to colon, deep to region of maximal tenderness
- Adjacent absent or minimal bowel wall thickening with local mass effect
- Hypoechoic rim of inflamed visceral peritoneum (93%)
- ± central hypoechoic areas of hemorrhagic change
- Color Doppler: Absence of central blood flow
- Contrast-enhanced ultrasound
  - Rim of peripheral arterial hyperenhancement
  - Central, nonenhancing hypoechoic regions

TOP DIFFERENTIAL DIAGNOSES

- Segmental omental infarction
- Diverticulitis
- Appendicitis
- Sclerosing mesenteritis
- Pelvic inflammatory disease

PATHOLOGY

- Torsion of epiploic appendage along its long axis with impairment of its vascular supply and subsequent necrosis
- Rectosigmoid junction is most common site

CLINICAL ISSUES

- 4th-5th decades of life; male predominance (M:F = 4:1)
- Abrupt onset of very localized abdominal pain, most frequently left lower quadrant, gradually resolving over 3-10 days, palpable mass (10-30%)
- Mild or absent systemic symptoms and signs
- Conservatively managed

SCANNING TIPS

- Use combination of linear and curved transducers over area of maximal pain and tenderness

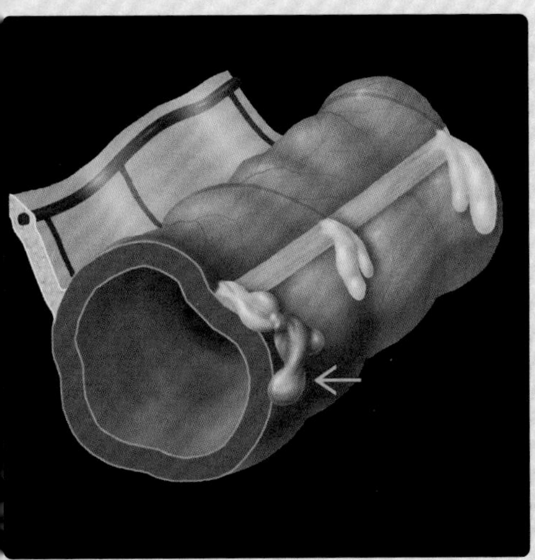

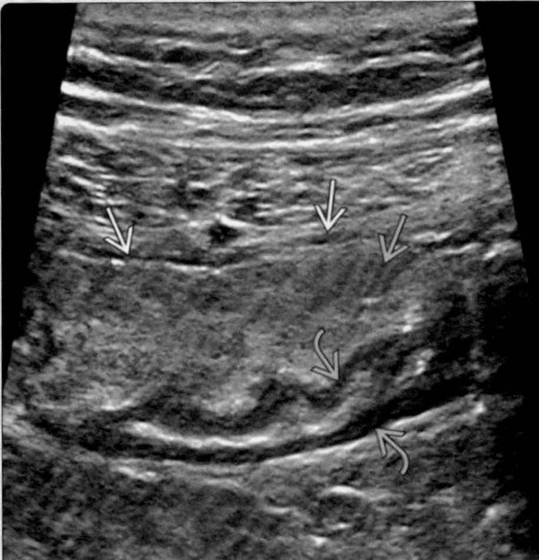

(Left) *Graphic shows a torsed and infarcted epiploic appendage ⇨ and 2 adjacent normal appendages.* **(Right)** *Grayscale ultrasound shows a well-defined, echogenic mass ⇨ with a hypoechoic rim of visceral peritoneal thickening ➡ and central, ill-defined, hypoechoic foci. Note the normal hypoechoic layers representing the muscularis propria of the sigmoid colon ⇨.*

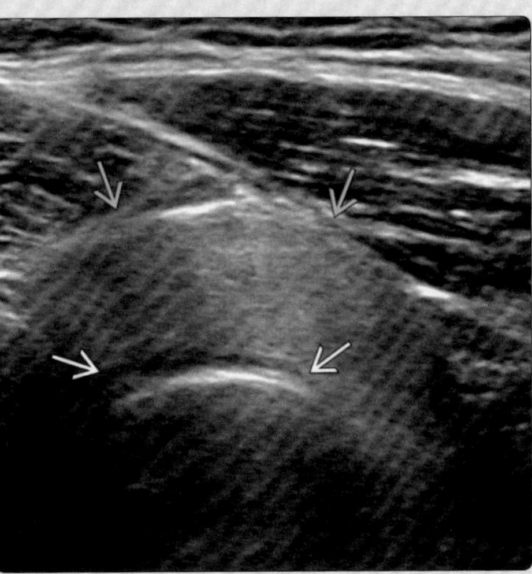

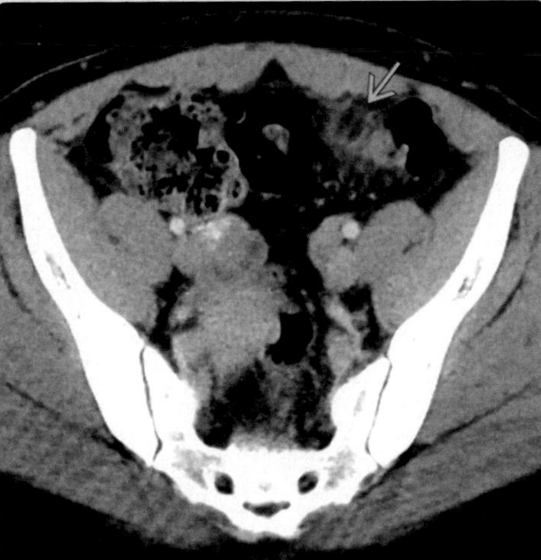

(Left) *Grayscale transabdominal ultrasound at the point of maximal tenderness in a patient with clinically suspected ovarian torsion shows an ovoid, hyperechoic mass ⇨ adherent to the colonic wall ➡.* **(Right)** *Axial CECT of the same patient demonstrates an ovoid, fat-density lesion with a hyperattenuating rim and surrounding inflammation ⇨ abutting the sigmoid colon, consistent with epiploic appendagitis.*

KEY FACTS

TERMINOLOGY

- Diverticulum: Focal sac-like outpouching off colon
- Diverticulosis: Presence of uncomplicated diverticula
- Diverticulitis: Inflammation of colonic diverticulum

IMAGING

- Diverticulosis with adjacent inflamed echogenic pericolic fat ± gas in diverticulum
- Localized tenderness at site of inflamed pericolic fat
- Thickened bowel wall
- Hyperemia on color Doppler assessment
- Complications: Abscess, fistula, stricture, obstruction, perforation with purulent or fecal peritonitis

TOP DIFFERENTIAL DIAGNOSES

- Colon cancer
- Colitis
- Acute appendicitis
- Epiploic appendagitis and segmental omental infarction

PATHOLOGY

- Due to localized microperforation of inflamed colonic diverticulum secondary to impacted fecalith

CLINICAL ISSUES

- Prevalent in Western society, low dietary fiber intake
- Diverticulosis increases with age; < 5% before 40 years to > 65% by 80 years
- Most common in sigmoid and left colon; right-sided diverticulum is more common in young adults
- Acute lower abdominal pain, local tenderness, fever, diarrhea, and rectal bleeding
- Majority settle with conservative management

SCANNING TIPS

- Optimally evaluated with combination of linear, curved, and endoluminal transducers
- Scan over area of tenderness, look for complications
- CT or MR for complications

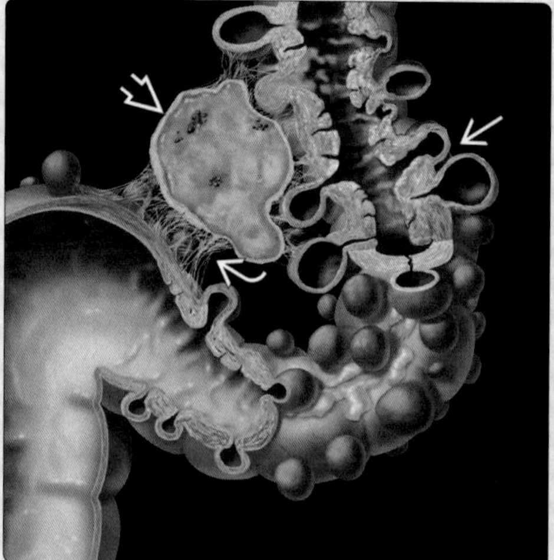

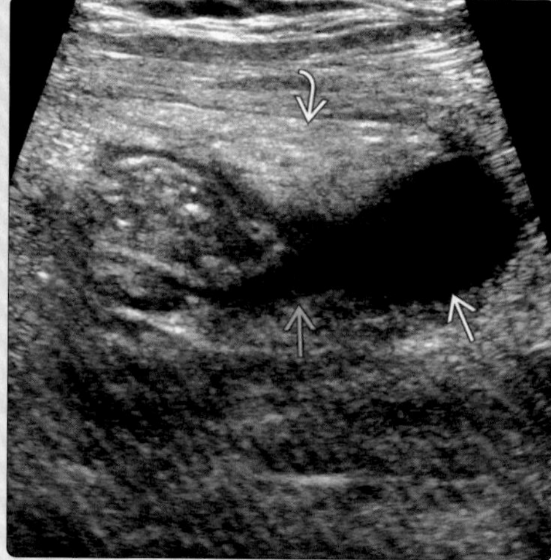

(Left) *Acute sigmoid diverticulitis with pericolonic abscess is shown by the thick-walled sigmoid colon ➡ containing multiple diverticula. Localized fat stranding ➡ and pericolic abscess ➡ can also be seen.* **(Right)** *Transverse ultrasound of acute sigmoid diverticulitis with an abscess ➡ is shown. The bowel wall is absent at the site of the perforated diverticulum ➡. The pericolic fat ➡ is inflamed.*

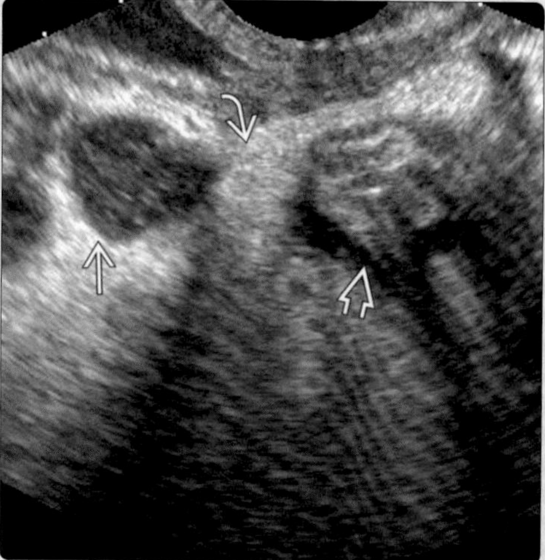

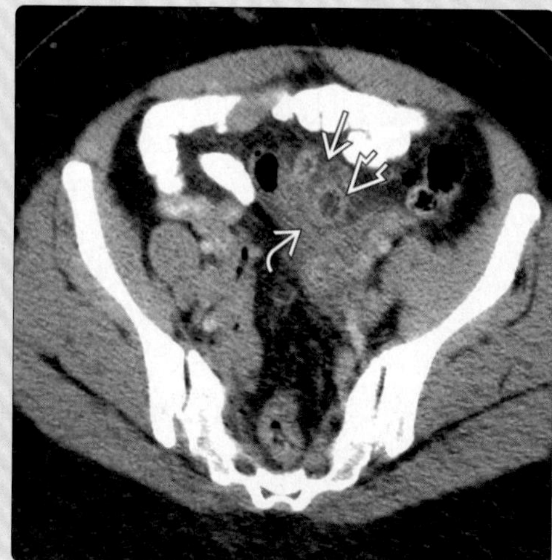

(Left) *Coronal transvaginal ultrasound performed for evaluation of left pelvic pain is shown. Inflamed tender pericolic fat ➡ surrounds an inflamed diverticulum ➡. There was a pericolonic abscess ➡.* **(Right)** *Axial CECT in the same patient confirms the inflamed pericolic fat ➡, multiple diverticula ➡, and the pericolonic abscess ➡. The degree of inflammation is easier to appreciate on CT.*

KEY FACTS

TERMINOLOGY

- Chronic, relapsing granulomatous inflammatory disease with predominant involvement of gastrointestinal tract

IMAGING

- Bowel wall thickening
  - Adults: > 3 mm
  - Children: Small bowel thickness > 2.5 mm and large bowel wall thickness > 2 mm
- Loss of normal bowel wall stratification
- Hyperemia of bowel wall correlates with disease activity
- Thickening/increased echogenicity of mesentery
- Anywhere from mouth to anus: Terminal ileum (95%), colon (22-55%), rectum (14-50%)
- Look for skip lesions
- Complications: Phlegmon and abscess, fistulas (enteroenteric, enteromesenteric, enterocutaneous, enterovesical, enterovaginal), bowel dilatation
- Undiagnosed or suspected patients stratified into high or low risk based on symptoms, laboratory values, physical exam, and family history

TOP DIFFERENTIAL DIAGNOSES

- Infectious colitis
- Ulcerative colitis
- Lymphoma
- Appendicitis

CLINICAL ISSUES

- 18-25 years, 20-30% < 20 years; M = F
- More common in Caucasian, Jewish populations
- Recurrent abdominal pain and diarrhea, weight loss, fatigue, poor growth/weight gain, anemia, anorexia, nutritional deficiencies, and bowel obstruction

SCANNING TIPS

- Best evaluated with combination of linear and curved transducers, including endoluminal transducers

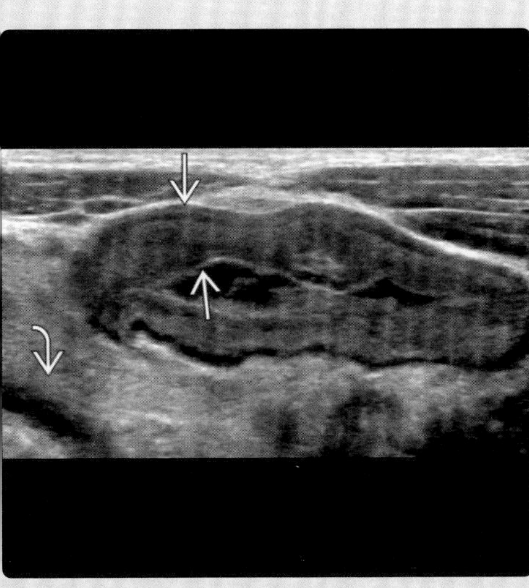

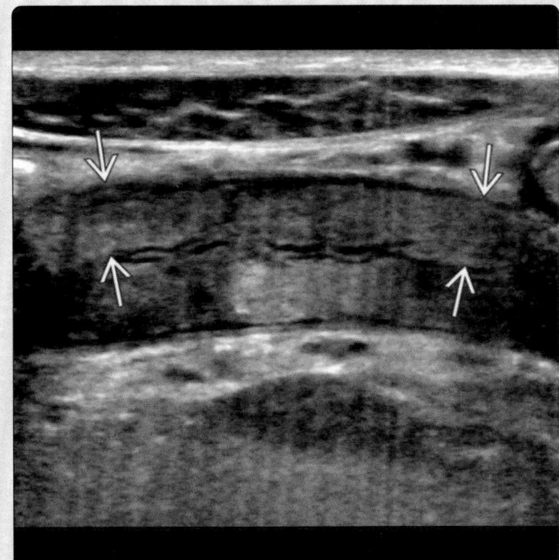

(Left) *Short-axis ultrasound of the sigmoid colon shows marked thickening ➡ of the wall and loss of normal stratification. There is adjacent inflamed mesenteric fat ➡.* **(Right)** *Long-axis ultrasound shows marked thickening ➡, loss of bowel wall stratification, and luminal narrowing in this 17 year old with Crohn disease.*

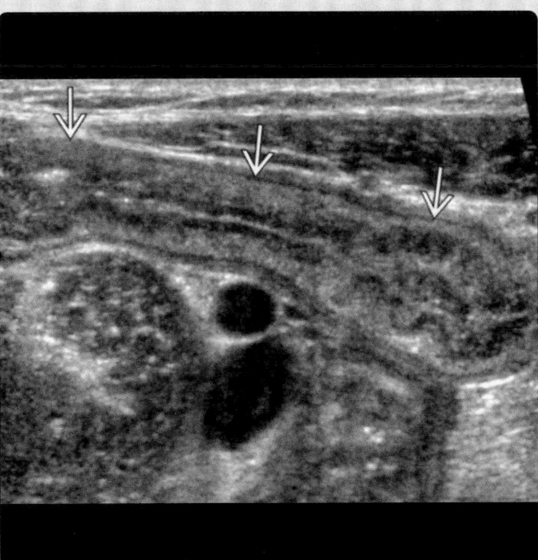

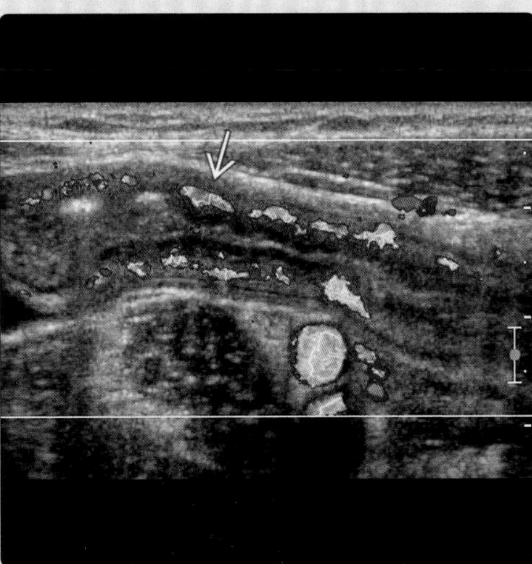

(Left) *Grayscale long-axis oblique ultrasound shows a thickened terminal ileum ➡.* **(Right)** *Color Doppler ultrasound in the same patient shows hyperemia ➡ in the terminal ileum compatible with active inflammation.*

PART II
SECTION 1
Male Pelvis

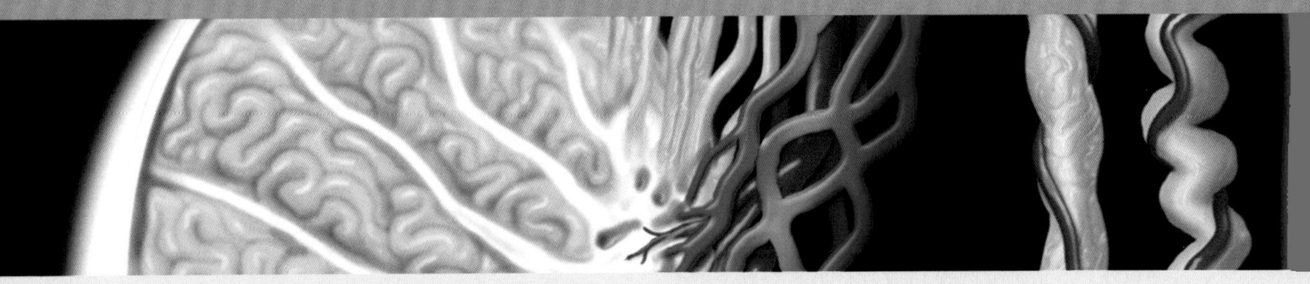

Anatomy and Approach

Scrotal Lesions

GROSS ANATOMY

Prostate

- Walnut-sized gland beneath bladder and in front of rectum
  - Normal prostate in young male ~ 3-cm length x 4-cm width x 2-cm depth
- Inverted conical shape
  - **Base**: Superior portion, continuous with bladder neck
  - **Apex**: Inferior portion, continuous with striated urinary sphincter
- Main function is to add nutritional secretions to sperm to form semen during ejaculation
- Also plays role in controlling flow of urine; prostate muscle fibers are under control of involuntary nervous system and contract to slow and stop urine
- **Urethra** traverses prostate
  - **Verumontanum** midway between base and apex where urethra makes ~ 35° bend anteriorly
    - Openings of prostatic utricle and ejaculatory ducts
    - Divides prostatic urethra into proximal (preprostatic) and distal (prostatic) segments
  - **Urethral crest**: Narrow longitudinal ridge on posterior wall with small openings draining prostatic ducts
- **Neurovascular bundles**
  - Lie posterolaterally to prostate at 5- and 7-o'clock positions
  - Carry nerves and vascular supply to corpora cavernosa of penis (necessary for normal erection)
- **Seminal vesicles**
  - Sac-like structures superolateral to prostate
  - Secrete fructose-rich fluid (energy source for sperm)
- **Ejaculatory ducts** located on either side of midline
  - Formed by union of seminal vesicle duct and vas deferens
  - Start at base of prostate and run forward and downward through gland to verumontanum

Zonal Anatomy

- Prostate is histologically composed of ~ 70% glandular and 30% nonglandular elements
- **Central zone (CZ)**: ~ 25% glandular tissue; cone-shaped zone around ejaculatory ducts with widest portion making majority of prostatic base
- **Peripheral zone (PZ)**: ~ 70% glandular tissue, covers posterolateral aspects of gland
  - Surrounds CZ and distal prostatic urethra
  - Zone where cancer most commonly occurs
- **Transition zone (TZ)**: 2 separate lobules surround urethra proximal to verumontanum
  - ~ 5-10% glandular tissue in young males; can be very large in older males with **benign prostatic hypertrophy (BPH)**
- **Anterior fibromuscular stroma** is nonglandular tissue
  - Runs anteriorly from bladder neck to striated urinary sphincter
- **Prostate pseudocapsule ("surgical capsule")**
  - Visible boundary between TZ and PZ representing compressed tissue
  - Frequently, calcified corpora amylacea (laminated bodies formed of secretions and degenerate cells) highlight plane between PZ and TZ

Zonal Distribution of Prostatic Disease

- **Prostate adenocarcinomas**
  - Up to 80% of prostatic cancers occur in PZ
    - Most appear as hypoechoic lesions
  - 20% in TZ, 5% in CZ and are often indistinguishable from BPH
  - Signs of extraprostatic extension of prostatic carcinoma include asymmetry of neurovascular bundles and irregular bulge in prostatic contour
- **BPH**: Benign nodular hyperplasia in periurethral glands and TZ
  - Can cause bladder outlet obstruction from urethral compression &/or increased smooth muscle tone along bladder neck and urethra
  - Compresses PZ posteriorly
  - Periurethral gland hypertrophy creates what has been termed **median lobe**, which can be seen projecting into bladder on transabdominal scans

IMAGING ANATOMY

Ultrasound Technique

- Transabdominal ultrasound can assess size, but **transrectal ultrasound (TRUS)** is required for detailed assessment
  - Transducer
    - 3.5- to 6.0-MHz curved transducer for transabdominal ultrasound
    - 7- to 10-MHz rectal transducer (end firing or transverse panoramic)
  - Patient position
    - Transabdominal ultrasound: Supine, using urinary bladder as acoustic window (transvesical)
    - TRUS: Left lateral decubitus with flexed hips and knees or in lithotomy position
  - Transrectal biopsy of prostate
    - Transrectal transducers have needle guidance system
      - □ May be directed at lesion or in grid pattern covering prostate for random sampling
    - Complications include hematuria, hematochezia, hematospermia, and infection
  - Color/power Doppler nonspecific; may see increased flow in hypertrophy, inflammation, and cancer
    - Useful for directing biopsy
- Normal PZ is typically uniformly more echogenic than inner gland
  - May be compressed in setting of BPH
- TZ may appear heterogeneous and nodular in setting of BPH
- Look for pseudocapsule (often with small calcifications) separating TZ from PZ
- Seminal vesicles have cystic appearance on TRUS, should be symmetric
- Prostate volume measurement
  - Perform in at least 2 orthogonal planes (axial and sagittal)
  - Prolate ellipse volume for 3 unequal axes: Width x height x length x 0.523
  - 1 cc of prostate tissue weighs ~ 1 g; prostate weighs ~ 20 g in young men
  - Prostatic enlargement when gland is > 40 g

PROSTATE

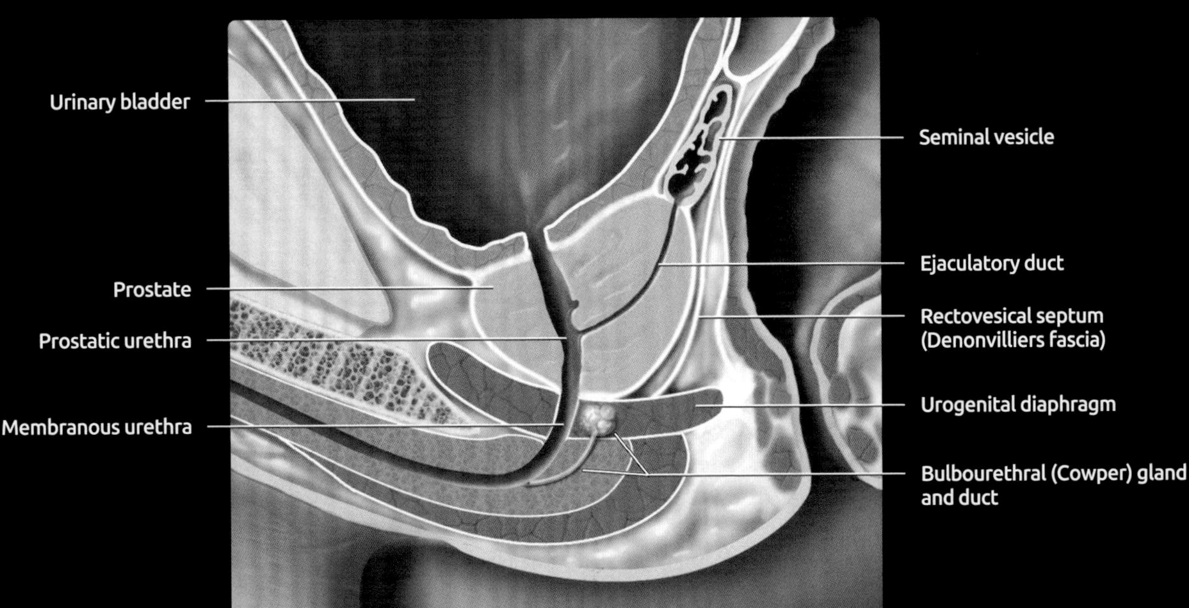

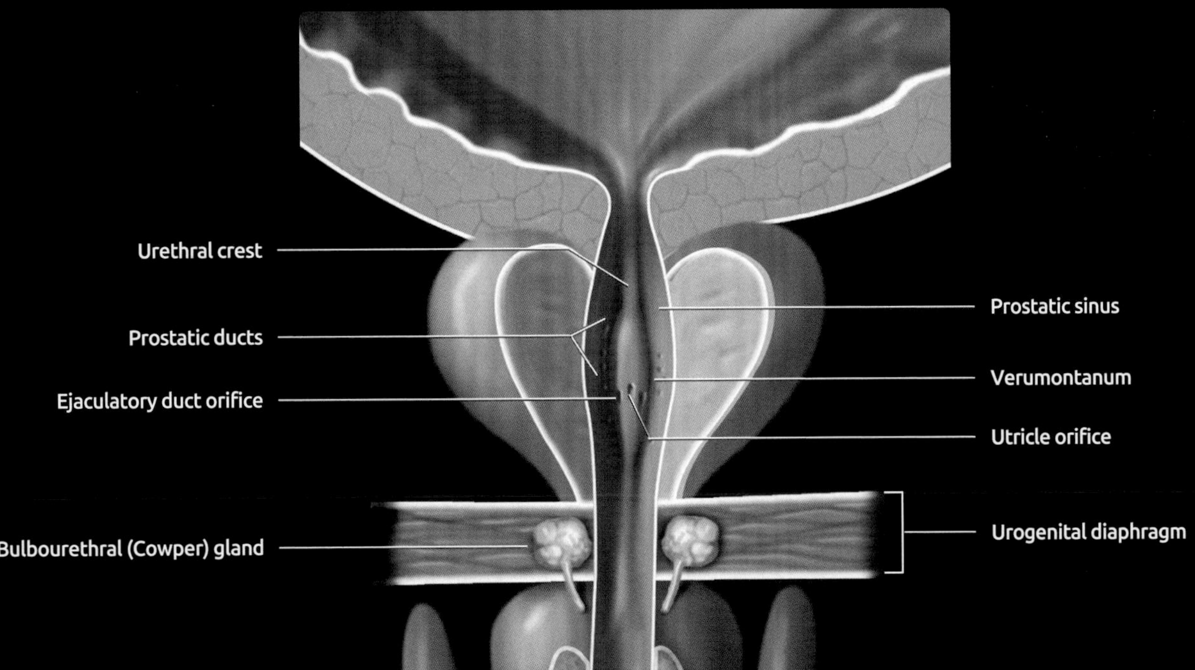

(Top) *Graphic illustrates the relationship between the prostate and the male pelvic organs. The prostate surrounds the upper part of the urethra (prostatic urethra). The base of the prostate is continuous with the bladder neck, and its apex is continuous with the external sphincter. The posterior surface is separated from the rectum by the rectovesical septum (Denonvilliers fascia).* **(Bottom)** *Graphic shows the topography of the posterior wall of the prostatic urethra. The urethral crest is a mucosal elevation along the posterior wall with the verumontanum being a mound-like elevation in the midportion of the crest. The utricle opens midline onto the verumontanum with the ejaculatory ducts opening on either side. The prostatic ducts are clustered around the verumontanum and open into the prostatic sinuses, which are depressions along the sides of the urethral crest.*

VAS DEFERENS AND SEMINAL VESICLES

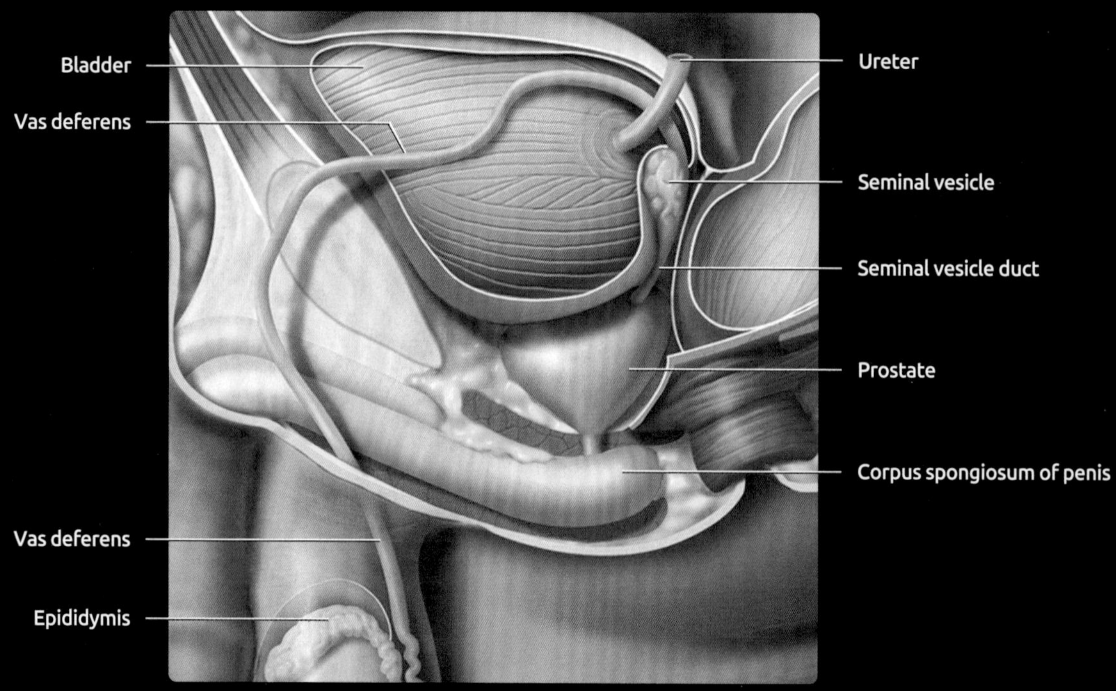

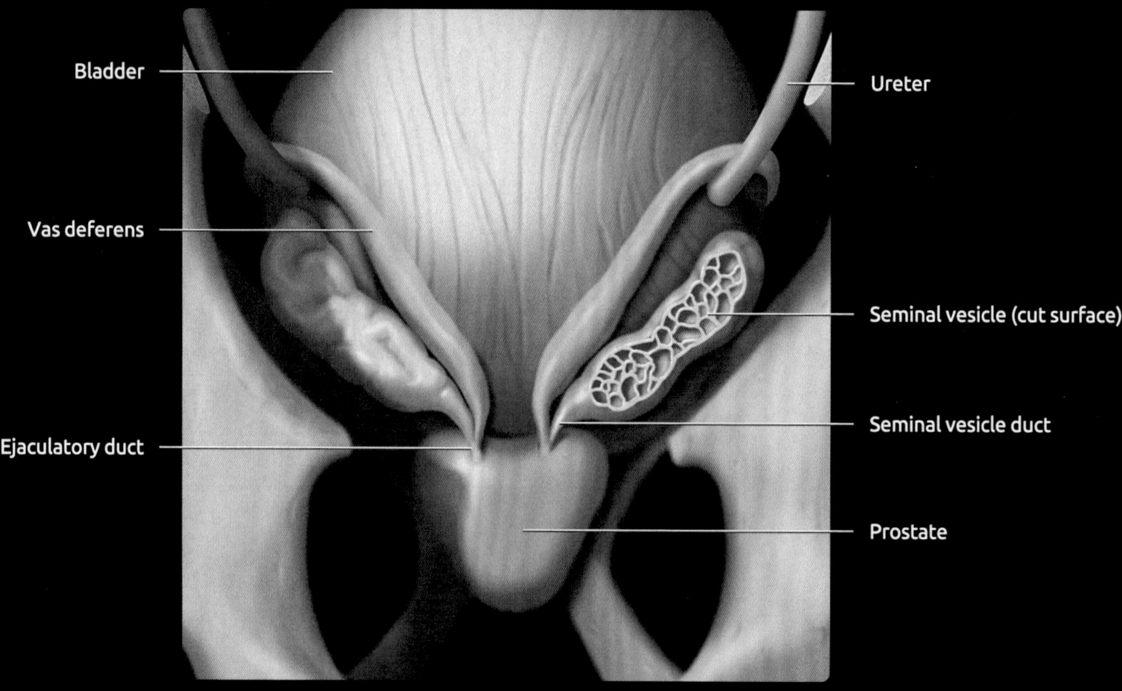

(Top) *This lateral view shows the position of the prostate deep in the pelvis. The vas deferens leaves the scrotum as a component of the spermatic cord, which courses through the inguinal canal into the pelvis.* **(Bottom)** *Posterior view of the prostate gland and seminal vesicles is shown. The cut surface of the seminal vesicle shows its highly convoluted fold pattern. The vas deferens crosses superior to the ureterovesical junction and continues along the posterior surface of the urinary bladder medial to the seminal vesicle. In the base of the prostate, it is directed forward and joined at an acute angle by the duct of the seminal vesicle to form the ejaculatory duct. The ejaculatory ducts course anteriorly and downward through the prostate to slit-like openings on either side of the orifice of the prostatic utricle.*

ZONAL ANATOMY OF THE PROSTATE

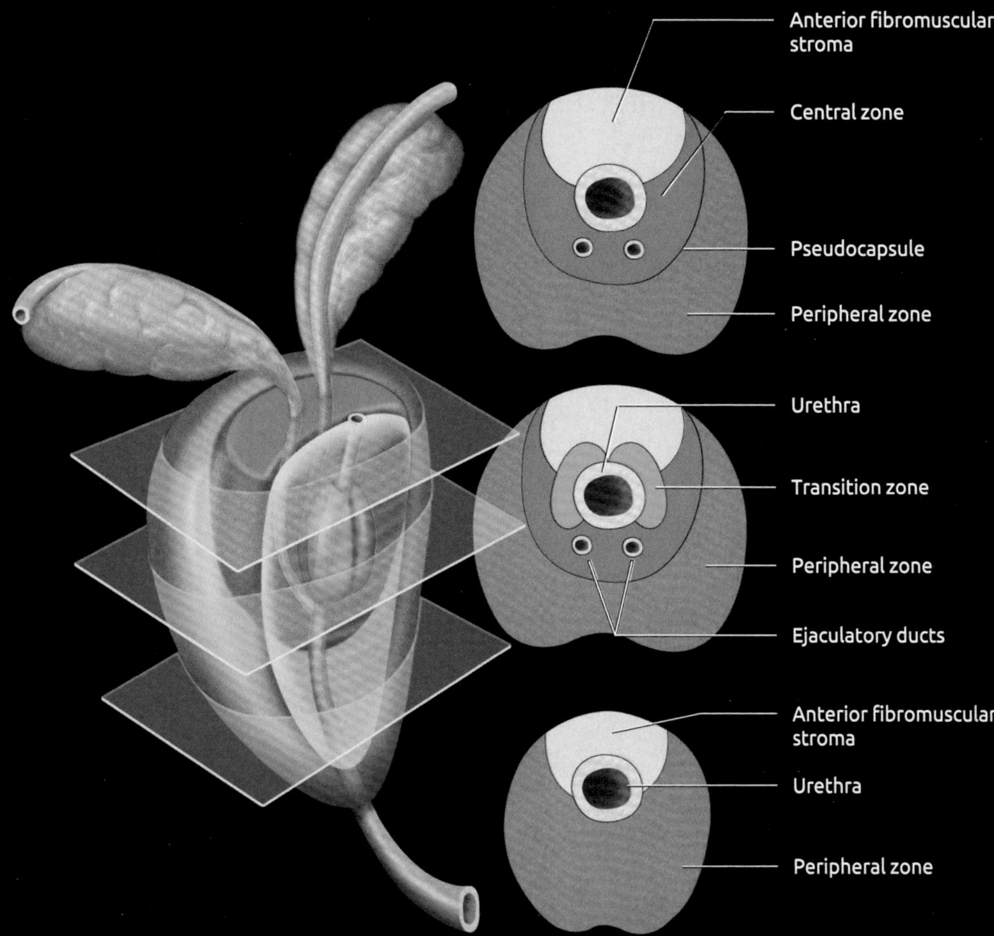

Graphic depiction of the prostate with axial drawings of the zonal anatomy at 3 different levels is shown. The transition zone (TZ) (in blue) is anterolateral to the verumontanum. The central zone (CZ) (in orange) surrounds the ejaculatory ducts and encloses the periurethral glands and the TZ. It is conical in shape and extends downward to about the level of the verumontanum. The peripheral zone (PZ) (in green) surrounds the posterior aspect of the CZ in the upper 1/2 of the gland, and it surrounds the urethra in the lower 1/2, below the verumontanum. The prostatic pseudocapsule is a visible boundary between the CZ and PZ. The anterior fibromuscular stroma (in yellow) covers the anterior part of the gland and is thicker superiorly and thins inferiorly in the prostatic apex.

ZONAL ANATOMY OF THE PROSTATE

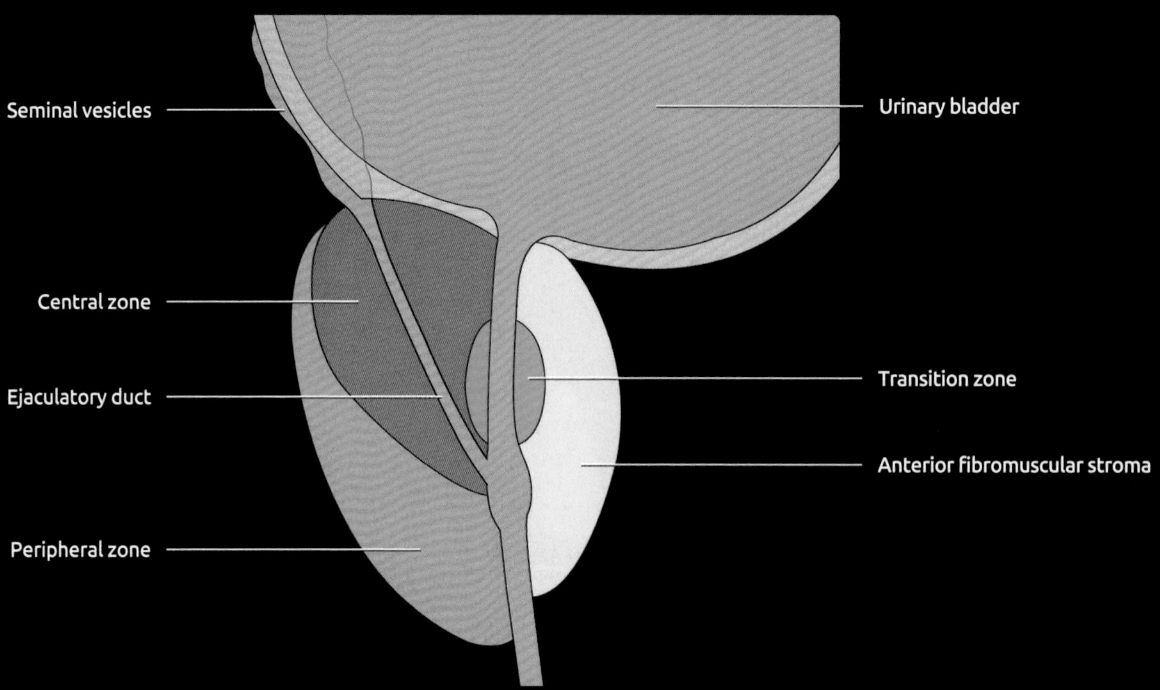

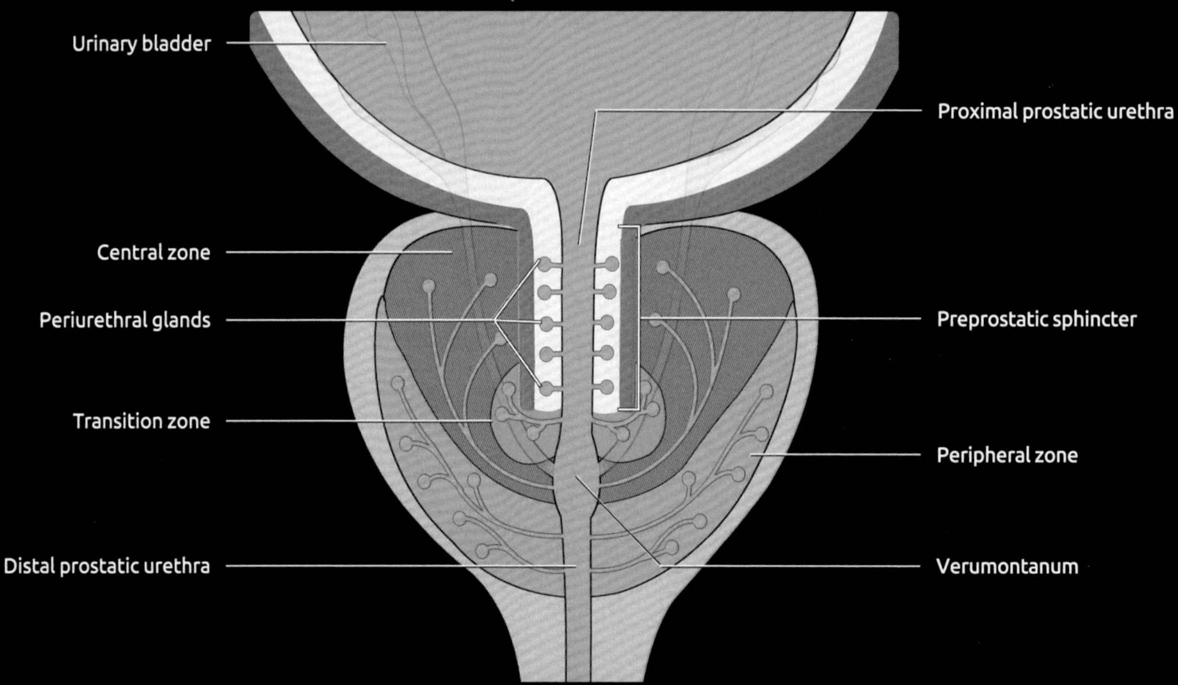

(Top) *Graphic illustrates the zonal anatomy of the prostate in the sagittal plane. The CZ surrounds the proximal urethra posterosuperiorly, enclosing both the periurethral glands and the TZ. It forms most of the prostatic base. The PZ surrounds both the CZ and the distal prostatic urethra.* **(Bottom)** *The proximal 1/2 of the prostatic urethra is surrounded by the preprostatic sphincter, which extends inferiorly to the level of the verumontanum and encloses the periurethral glands. The preprostatic sphincter is thought to function during ejaculation to prevent retrograde flow and may also contribute to resting tone. The TZ is a downward extension of the periurethral glands around the verumontanum. Periurethral glands are < 1% of the normal prostate but are one of the sites of origin for benign prostatic hyperplasia (BPH) and can enlarge significantly.*

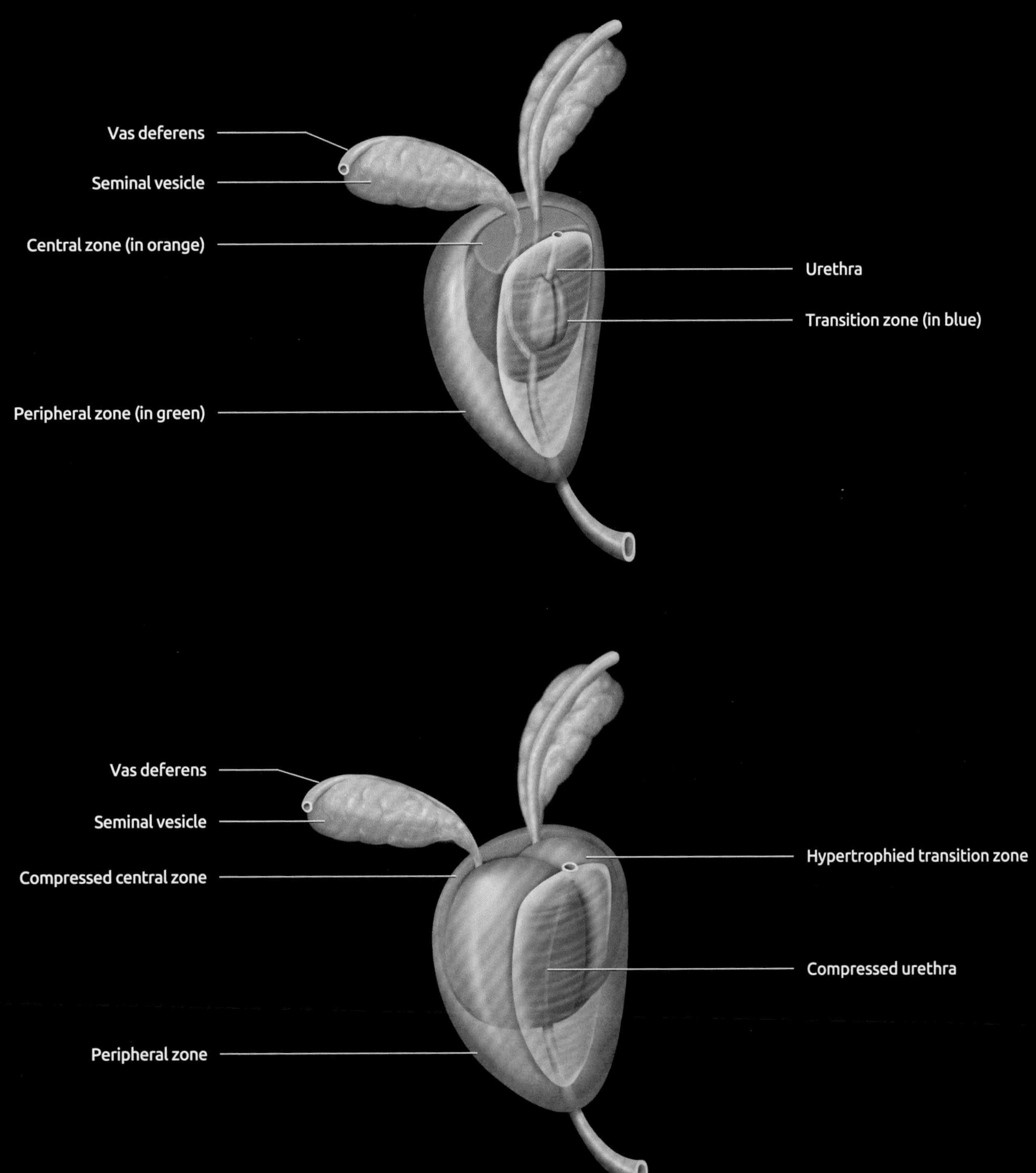

(Top) *First of 2 graphics comparing zonal anatomy in a young man to an older man with BPH is shown. The TZ in young men is small in size, comprising 5% of the volume of the glandular tissue of the prostate. It surrounds the anterolateral aspect of the urethra at the level of verumontanum in a horseshoe fashion.* **(Bottom)** *With the development of BPH, there is enlargement of the TZ (in blue). This causes enlargement of the prostate and compression of the CZ (in orange) and PZ (in green). BPH mainly involves the TZ, though other zones may also be involved. The enlarged TZ causes compression of the prostatic urethra, the primary reason for development of urinary obstructive symptoms in patients with BPH.*

PROSTATE

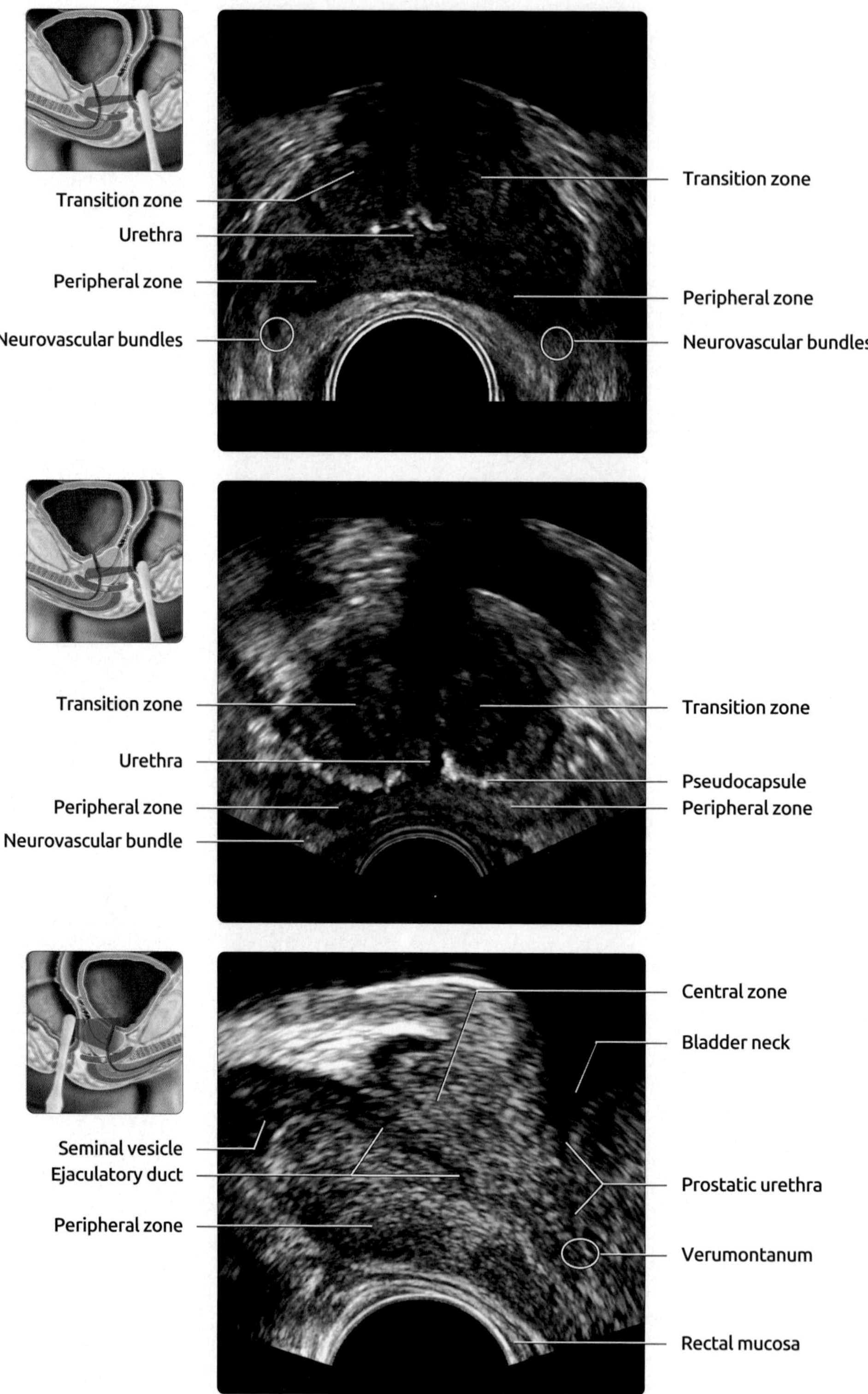

(Top) *Transverse TRUS at the level of the midprostate shows the 2 lobes of the TZ on either side of the urethra. The more homogeneous PZ is along the posterolateral aspects of the prostate. The neurovascular bundles course through the retroprostatic fat at the 5- and 7-o'clock positions but are usually not identified as discrete structures. Note the periurethral calcifications.* **(Middle)** *Transverse TRUS of the midprostate gland demonstrates an enlarged TZ in a patient with BPH. The pseudocapsule separates the TZ from the PZ. Frequently, the pseudocapsule will be outlined by calcifications, which represent calcified corpora amylacea (laminated bodies formed by secretions and degenerate cells).* **(Bottom)** *Sagittal TRUS in a patient without significant BPH shows the course of the proximal prostatic urethra anterior to the CZ. The ejaculatory ducts start at the base of the prostate and run forward and downward through the CZ. They terminate at the verumontanum on either side of the utricle orifice. The verumontanum is the boundary between the proximal and distal segments of the prostatic urethra.*

PROSTATE

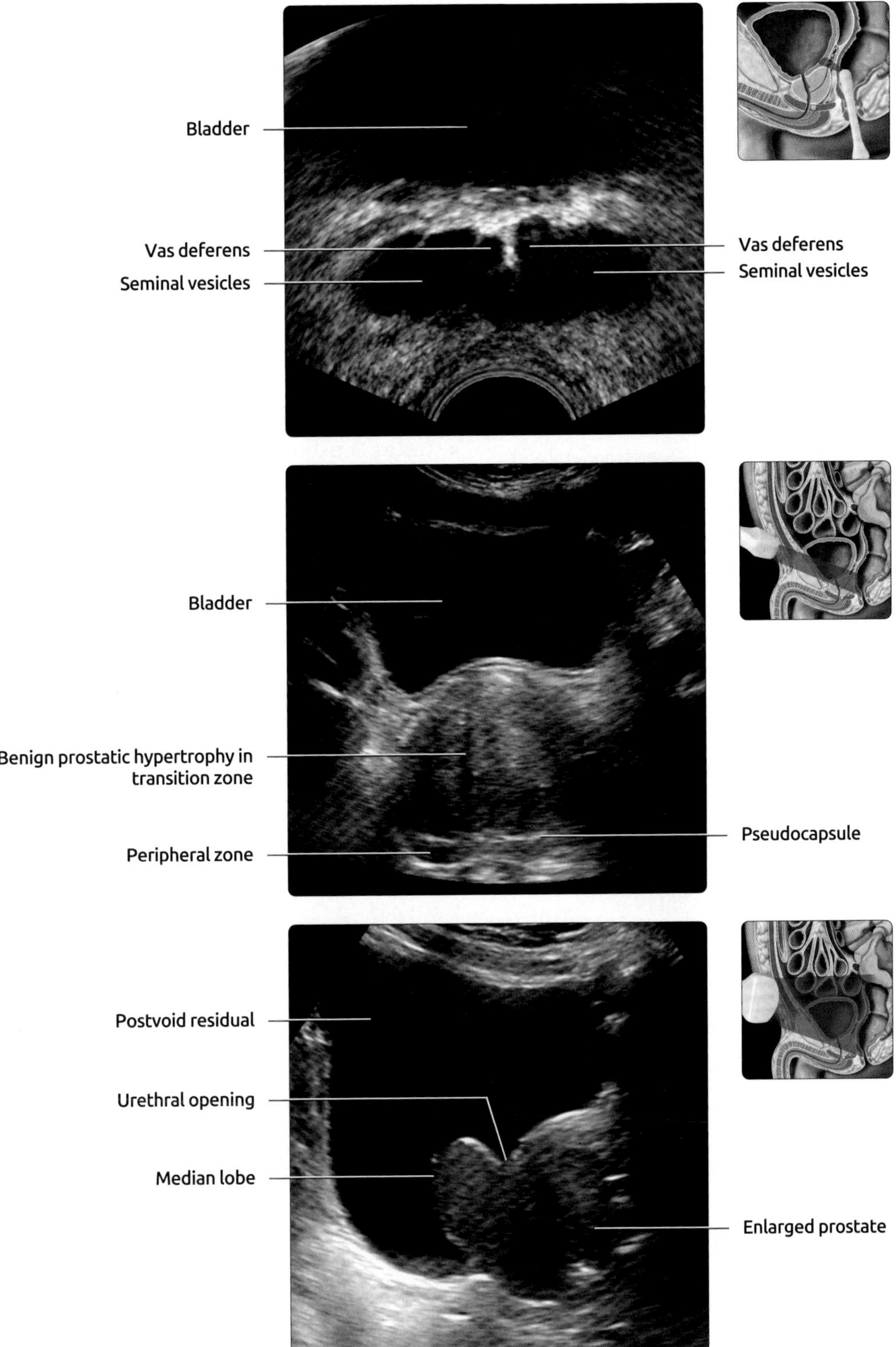

(Top) *Transverse TRUS shows the vas deferens converging with the seminal vesicles. Their union will form the ejaculatory ducts, which enter the prostate base and course within the prostate enclosed within the CZ. The ejaculatory ducts empty into the urethra at the verumontanum.* **(Middle)** *Transverse transabdominal ultrasound of the midprostate in a patient with BPH shows a markedly enlarged TZ and hyperechoic pseudocapsule. The PZ is compressed posterolaterally.* **(Bottom)** *This longitudinal transabdominal postvoid image shows a markedly enlarged prostate with a hypertrophied median lobe projecting into the bladder. The median lobe represents hyperplasia of the periurethral glands and is common with BPH. It typically projects cephalad into the bladder and can be associated with significant urinary retention. There is a large postvoid residual in this case.*

GROSS ANATOMY

Testes

- Densely packed seminiferous tubules separated by thin, fibrous septa
- Seminiferous tubules join to form **rete testis**, which converge posteriorly into efferent ductules
  - Penetrate posterior tunica albuginea at mediastinum to form head of epididymis
  - May become dilated, but tubular appearance and location should differentiate from mass
- **Tunica albuginea** forms thick, fibrous capsule around testis
- **Mediastinum testis** is thickened area of tunica albuginea where ducts, nerves, and vessels enter and exit testis
- **Testicular descent**: Testis develop in retroperitoneum and descend through inguinal canal to scrotum
  - Failure of descent results in cryptorchidism
- **Tunica vaginalis**: Mesothelial-lined sac around anterior and lateral sides of testis formed during descent
  - Fluid (**hydrocele**) may accumulate between parietal and visceral layers (hydrocele)
- **Appendix testis**: Embryologic remnant, which forms small, nodular protuberance from surface of testis

Epididymis

- Crescent-shaped structure along posterior border of testis
- Efferent ductules from testis form **epididymal head**, which coalesce to form a single, long, convoluted tubule in epididymal body
- Tubule continues inferiorly to form epididymal tail, which is attached to lower pole of testis by loose areolar tissue
- Tubule emerges at acute angle from tail as vas deferens, which continues cephalad within spermatic cord
  - Eventually merges with duct of seminal vesicle to form ejaculatory duct
- **Appendix epididymis**: Small, nodular protuberance from surface of epididymis similar to appendix testis
  - Both appendages can undergo torsion and form scrotal calculi

Spermatic Cord

- Contains vas deferens, nerves, lymphatics, and vessels
- Begins at internal (deep) inguinal ring and exits through external (superficial) inguinal ring into scrotum
- **Testicular artery** is primary blood supply to testis
- **Pampiniform plexus** is interconnected network of small veins, which can dilate resulting in **varicocele**
  - This plexus merges to form testicular veins
    - Right testicular vein drains to inferior vena cava
    - Left testicular vein drains to left renal vein
- Lymphatic drainage follows testicular veins
  - Right side drains to interaortocaval chain
  - Left side drains to left paraaortic nodes near renal hilum
- Layers of spermatic cord and scrotum form during testicular descent through abdominal wall

IMAGING ANATOMY

Imaging Recommendations

- High-frequency (10- to 15-MHz) linear transducer
- Patient in supine position with penis positioned on anterior abdominal wall and draped with towel
  - Folded towel placed between thighs to elevate scrotum
- Use copious gel; may need stand-off pad for superficial lesions
- Image in both longitudinal and transverse planes
  - Size and echogenicity of both testes and epididymitides should be symmetric
- Always evaluate asymptomatic side 1st to adjust settings
  - Serves as standard to compare with symptomatic side
  - Color Doppler should be optimized for low-flow state
    - Power Doppler may be needed if flow is difficult to document; this is particularly true in children
- Doppler particularly important in setting of acute pain
  - Obtain "buddy shot" (both testes on same image) for easy comparison of flow between sides
- Additional imaging during Valsalva maneuver and upright positioning important when evaluating for varicocele or inguinal hernia

Sonographic Anatomy

- **Testes**: Ovoid, homogeneous, medium-level, granular echotexture
  - **Mediastinum testis** may appear as prominent echogenic line emanating from posterior testis
  - **Blood flow**
    - Testicular artery pierces tunica albuginea and arborizes over periphery of testis
    - Multiple radially arranged vessels travel along septa
    - May have prominent **transmediastinal artery**
    - **Tunica vasculosa**: Vascular plexus in periphery of testis, beneath tunica albuginea
    - Low-velocity, low-resistance waveform on Doppler imaging with continuous forward flow in diastole
- **Epididymis**: Iso- to slightly hyperechoic compared with testis
  - Best seen in longitudinal plane
  - Head has rounded or triangular configuration
  - Head: 10-12 mm; body and tail often difficult to visualize
    - May be helpful to follow in transverse plane if difficult to visualize in longitudinal plane
- **Spermatic cord**
  - Scan along course of inguinal canal; may be difficult to differentiate from surrounding soft tissues
  - Slow flow in pampiniform plexus may make identification on color Doppler difficult
    - Use provocative maneuvers (Valsalva, standing), especially when looking for varicocele

Key Questions

- **Is pain acute?**
  - Torsion vs. epididymitis/orchitis
  - Color Doppler is key to diagnosis
- **Is there palpable mass?**
  - Intratesticular masses are overwhelming malignant
  - Extratesticular masses typically benign
    - Cystic-appearing extratesticular masses include: Hydrocele, varicocele, spermatocele, epididymal cyst, tunica albuginea cyst
    - Solid extratesticular masses include: Scrotal calculi, inguinal hernia with bowel &/or omentum, or, more rarely, epididymal adenomatoid tumor or fibrous pseudotumor

TESTIS AND EPIDIDYMIS

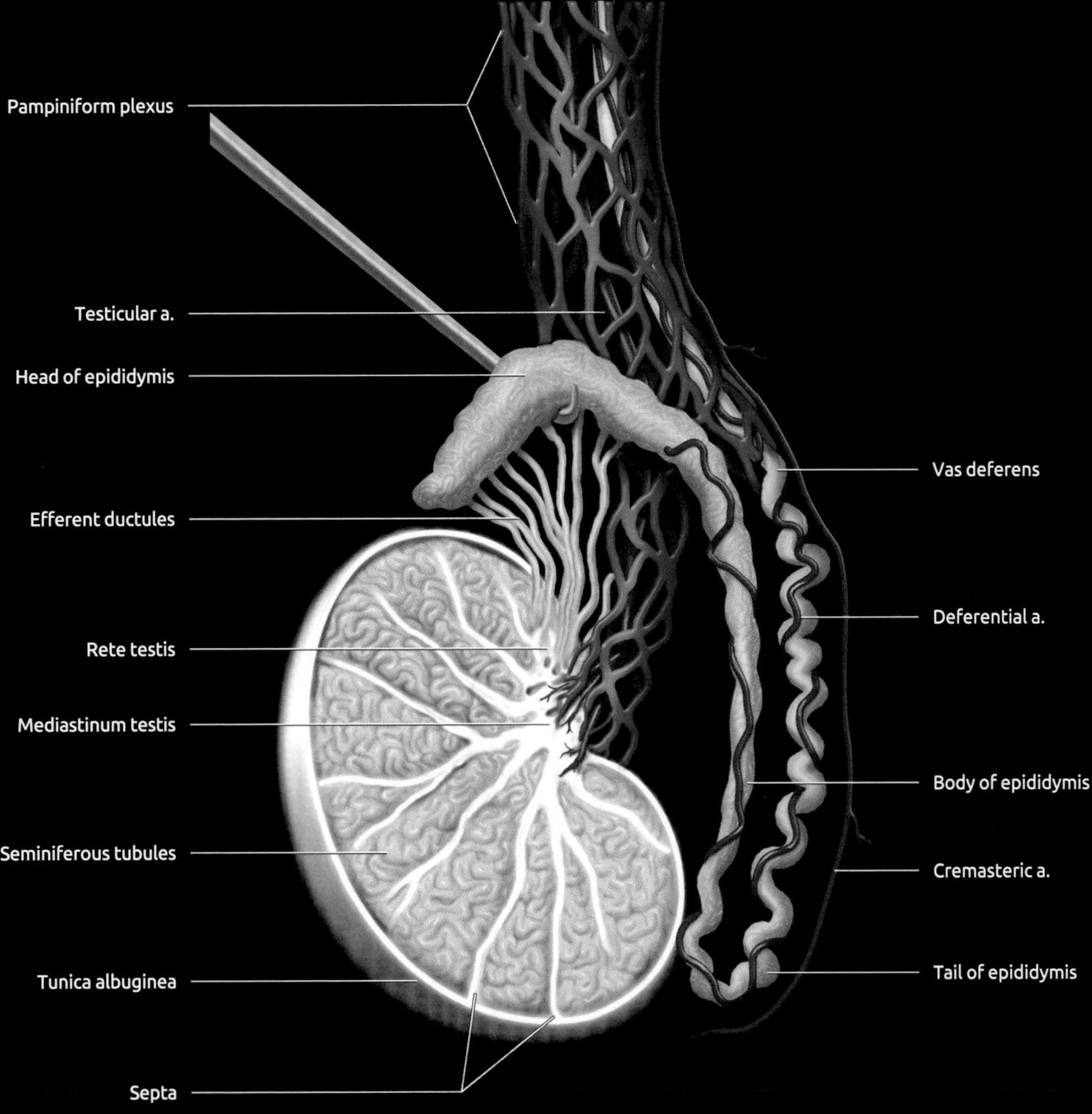

Graphic shows the testis is composed of densely packed seminiferous tubules, which are separated by thin, fibrous septa. These tubules converge posteriorly, eventually draining into the rete testis. The rete testis continues to converge to form the efferent ductules, which pierce through the tunica albuginea at the mediastinum testis and form the head of the epididymis. Within the epididymis these tubules unite to form a single, highly convoluted tubule in the body, which finally emerges from the tail as the vas deferens. In addition to the vas deferens, other components of the spermatic cord include the testicular artery, deferential artery, cremasteric artery, pampiniform plexus, lymphatics, and nerves.

EPIDIDYMIS AND INGUINAL CANAL

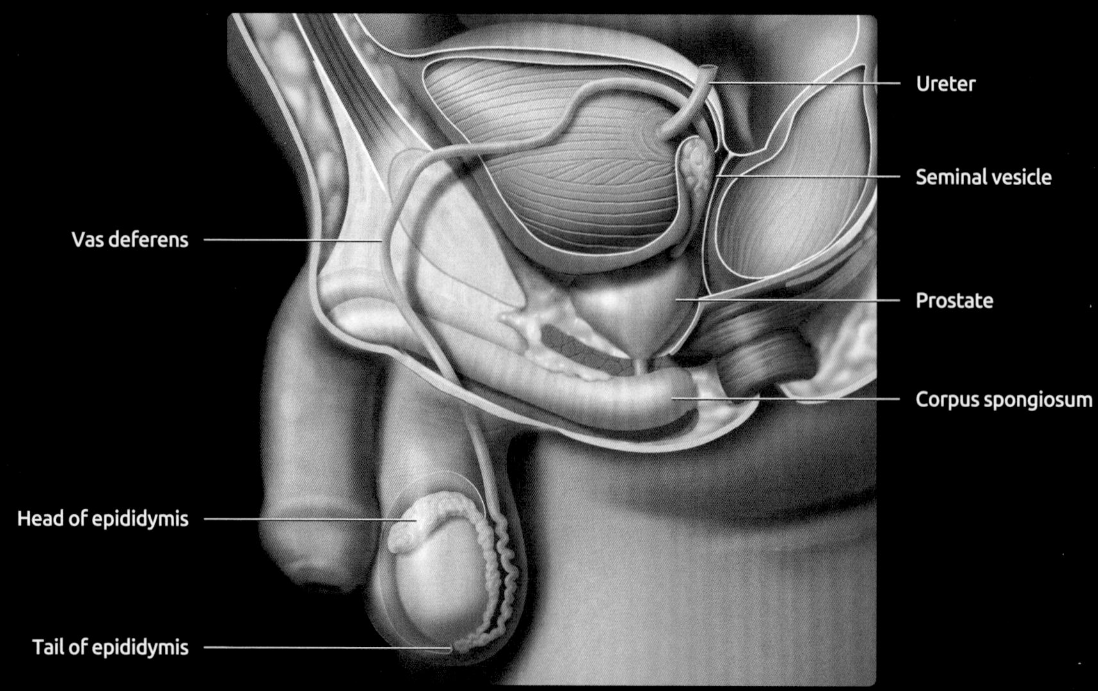

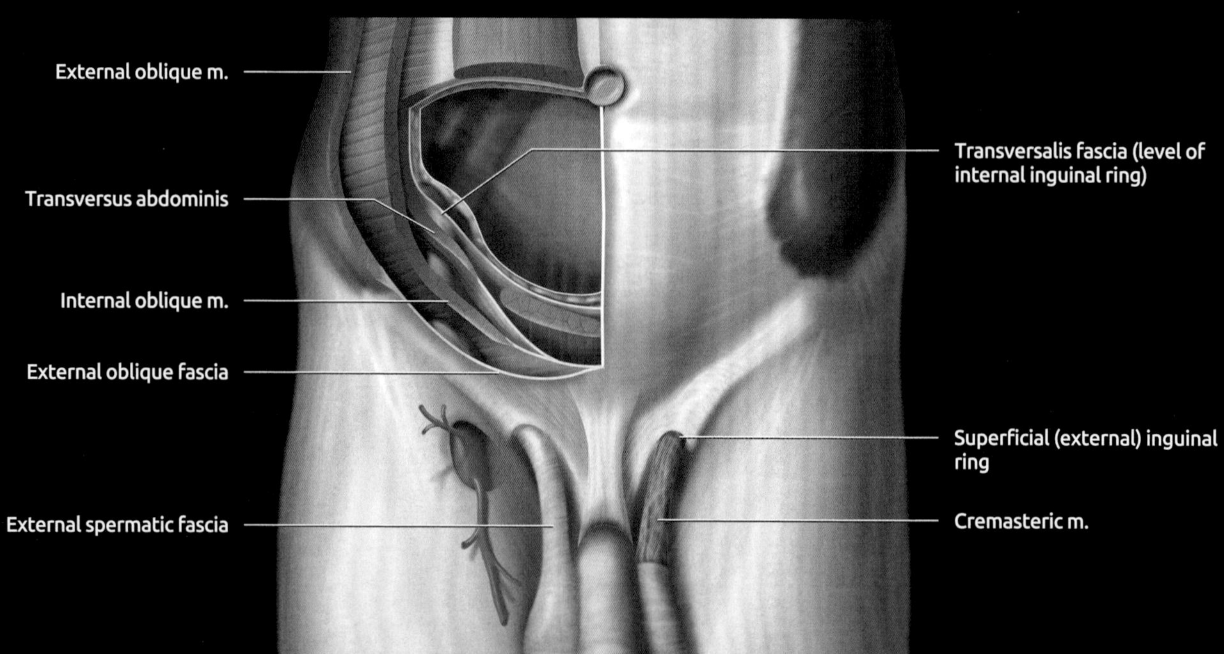

(Top) *Graphic shows that the tail of the epididymis is loosely attached to the lower pole of the testis by areolar tissue. The vas deferens (also referred to as the ductus deferens) emerges from the tail at an acute angle and continues cephalad as part of the spermatic cord. After passing through the inguinal canal, the vas deferens courses posteriorly to unite with the duct of the seminal vesicle to form the ejaculatory duct. These narrow ducts have thick, muscular walls composed of smooth muscle, which reflexly contract during ejaculation and propel sperm forward.* **(Bottom)** *The muscle layers of the pelvic wall have been separated to show the spermatic cord as it passes through the inguinal canal. The cremasteric muscle is derived from the internal oblique muscle, while the external spermatic fascia is formed by the fascia of the external oblique muscle.*

SCROTUM AND TESTES

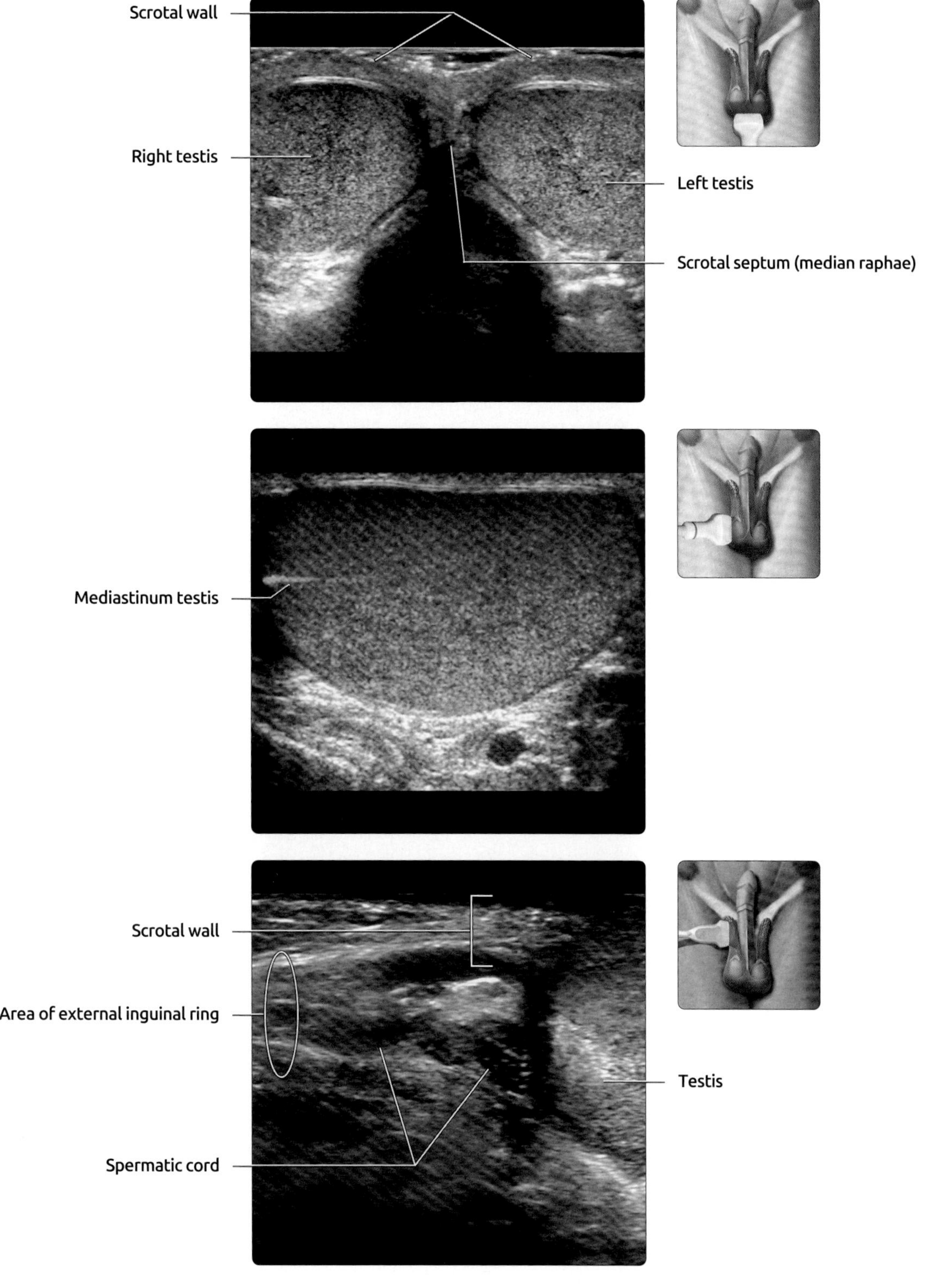

(Top) *Transverse grayscale ultrasound shows both testes. This is a useful approach for comparing the appearance of the testes, which should have similar, homogeneous, medium-level, granular echotexture.* **(Middle)** *Longitudinal ultrasound shows the ovoid shape. The tunica albuginea may form an echogenic linear band where it invaginates at the mediastinum testis. The mediastinum testis has a craniocaudal linear course and is where the efferent ductules, vessels, and lymphatics pierce through the capsule.* **(Bottom)** *Longitudinal scan at the superior pole of the testis shows the spermatic cord as it is entering the inguinal canal. It is important to look at the spermatic cord for a twist (whirlpool sign) in cases of suspected torsion.*

TUNICA VAGINALIS, ALBUGINEA, AND VASCULOSA

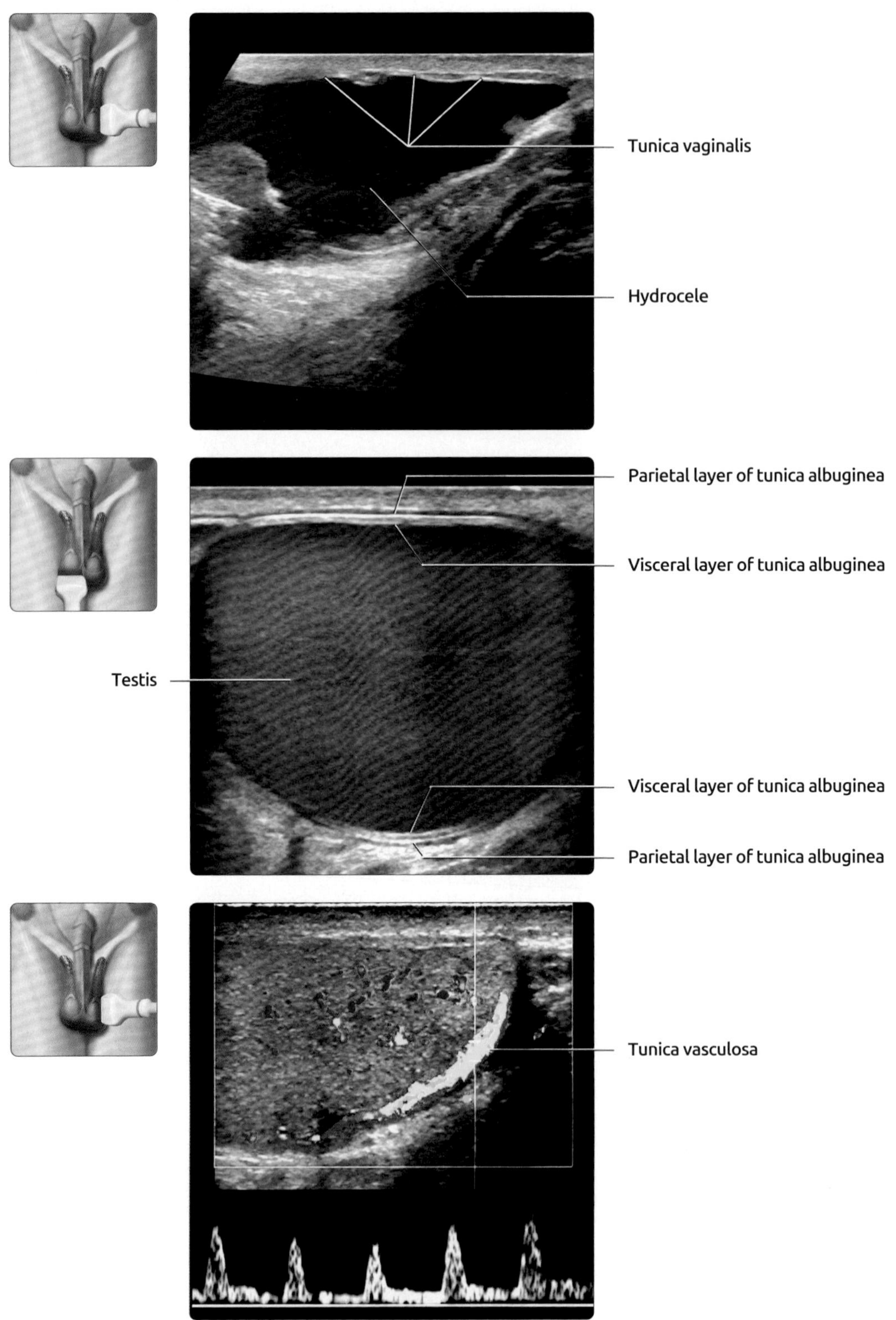

(Top) *Sagittal grayscale ultrasound of the left side of the scrotum shows the outermost serous membrane covering the testis and epididymis, the tunica vaginalis. A small amount of fluid is present within the tunica vaginalis (hydrocele).* **(Middle)** *Transverse grayscale ultrasound of the right testis shows 2 thin, echogenic layers covering the testis, representing the parietal and visceral layers of tunica albuginea, which is the fibrous covering of the testis.* **(Bottom)** *Sagittal color Doppler ultrasound shows the vascular plexus (tunica vasculosa) along the outermost layer of the testis, just beneath the tunica albuginea.*

SCROTAL DOPPLER

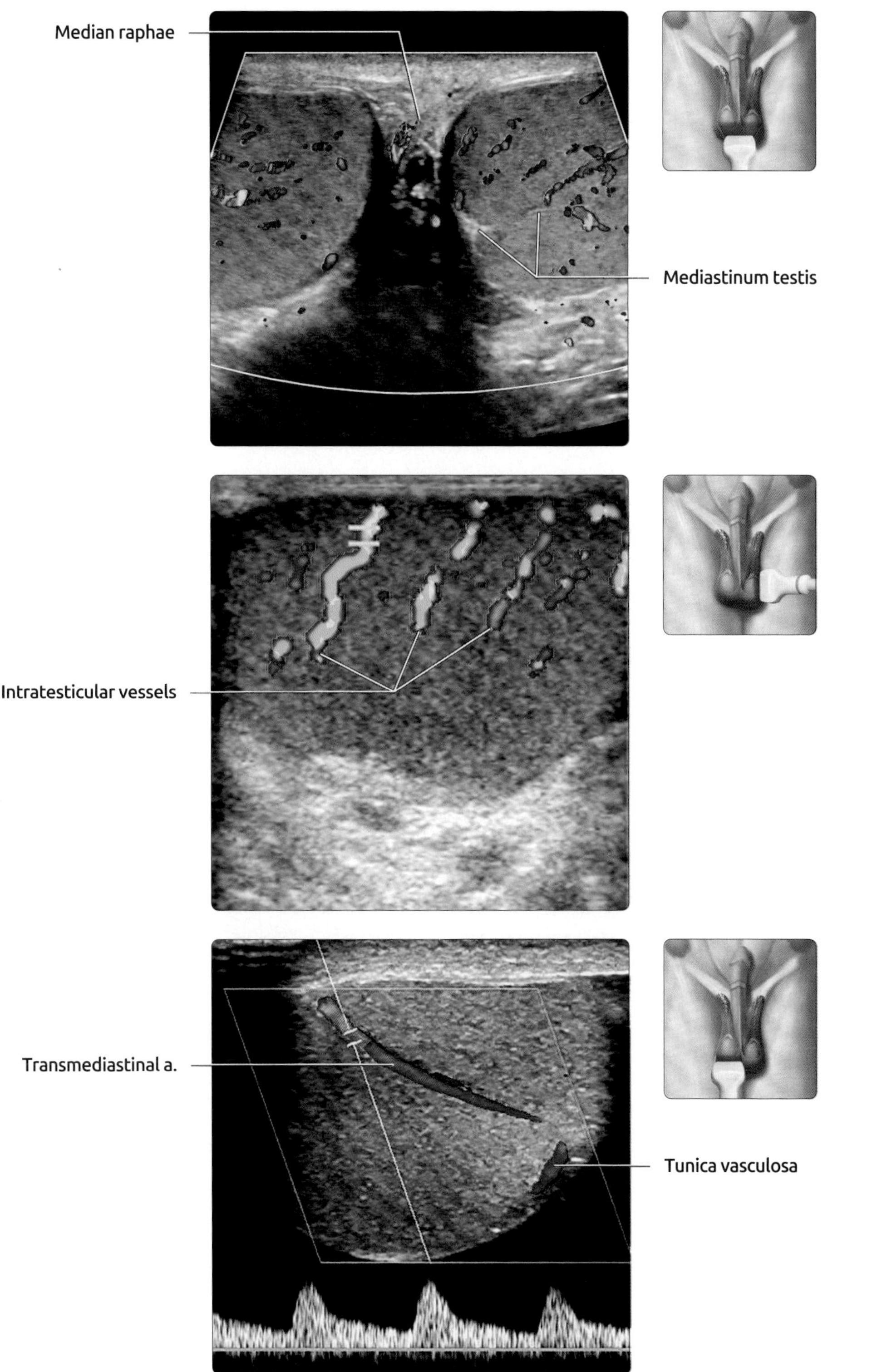

(Top) *Transverse color Doppler ultrasound shows normal symmetric blood flow in the testes. It is important to compare flow between testes to determine if the symptomatic side has increased or decreased flow when compared to the asymptomatic side.* **(Middle)** *Longitudinal color Doppler ultrasound shows prominent, radially arranged vessels within the testis.* **(Bottom)** *Color Doppler ultrasound shows a prominent transmediastinal artery; pulsed Doppler ultrasound shows normal low-resistance arterial flow. Also shown is the tunica vasculosa, a vascular plexus that runs beneath the tunica albuginea.*

SCROTAL DOPPLER

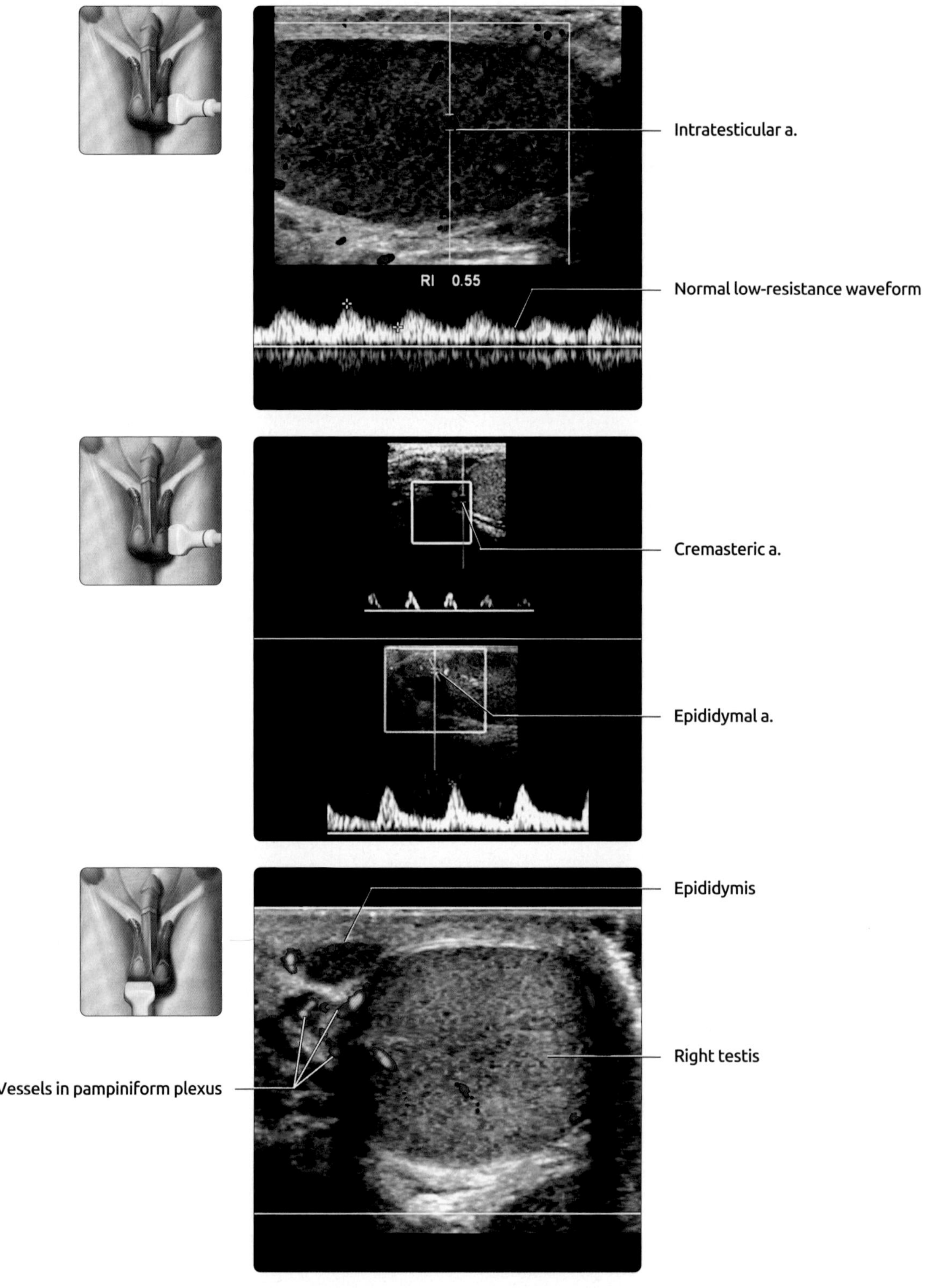

(Top) *Sagittal color Doppler ultrasound of a normal left testis shows normal blood flow with a normal spectral waveform of an intratesticular artery. The artery should have a low-resistance waveform and the resistive index (RI) should be between 0.48-0.75 (mean RI: 0.62).* **(Middle)** *Color Doppler ultrasound shows the epididymal arterial supply. The upper image demonstrates the normal cremasteric artery with a low-flow, high-resistance pattern. The lower image shows the normal epididymal artery, a branch of the testicular artery with a low-resistance waveform.* **(Bottom)** *Transverse power Doppler ultrasound shows flow within the pampiniform plexus of the spermatic cord. If looking for a varicocele, it is important to use provocative maneuvers, including Valsalva and scanning in the standing position, to distend the veins.*

EPIDIDYMIS

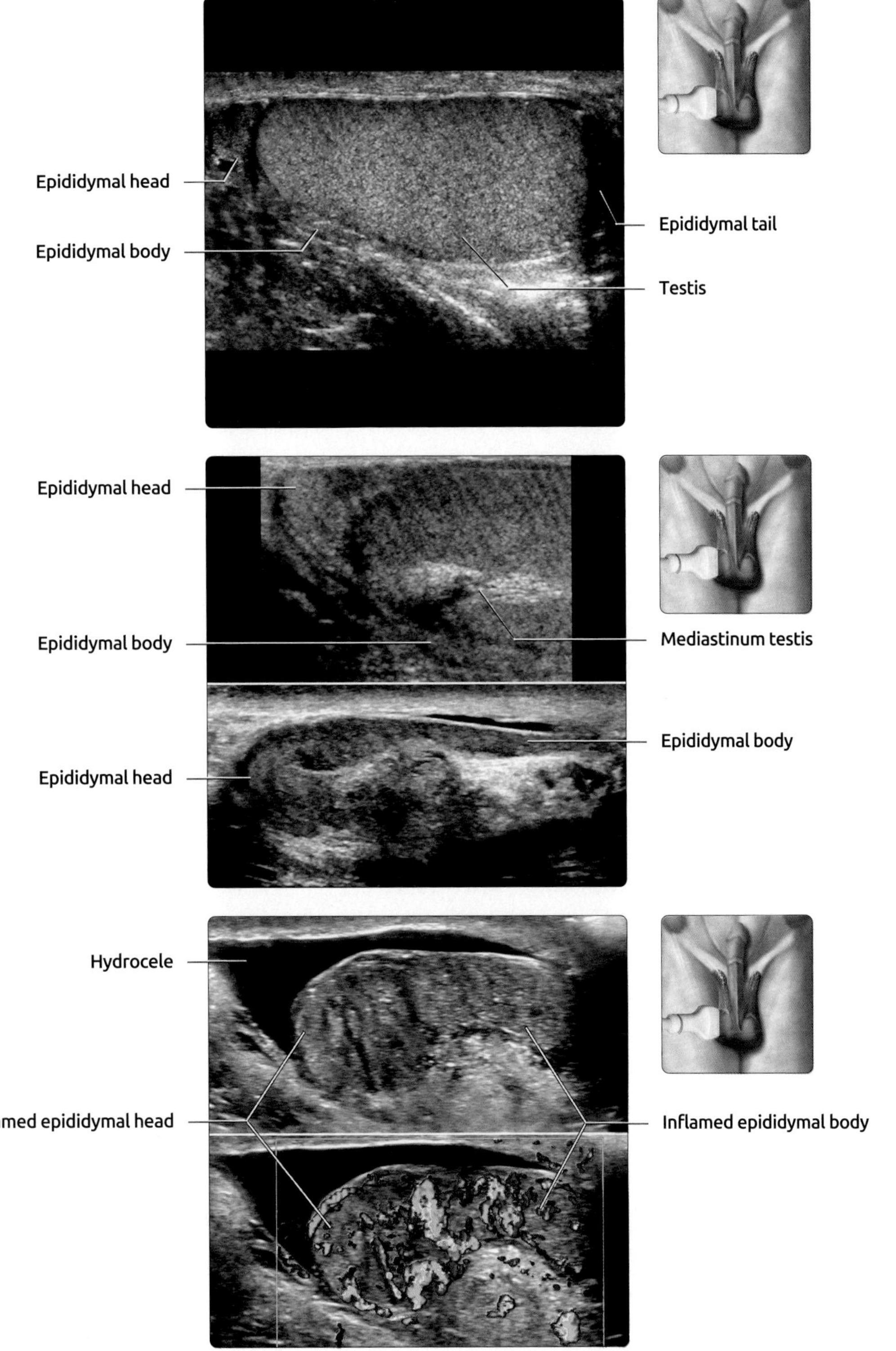

(Top) *Longitudinal ultrasound shows both the epididymal head (globus major) and tail (globus minor). The epididymal head measures ~ 10-12 mm and is iso- to slightly hyperechoic compared to the testis. The body and tail are often more difficult to visualize and may be slightly less echogenic than the head.* **(Middle)** *Composite image shows the normal epididymal head and body. The body may be difficult to visualize from an anterior scanning plane (above), but by moving the transducer more posteriorly (below), it is often better visualized.* **(Bottom)** *Composite image of a longitudinal grayscale ultrasound (above) and a color Doppler ultrasound (below) in a patient with acute epididymitis shows enlargement and hyperemia of both the epididymal head and body.*

RETE TESTIS AND TUBULAR ECTASIA

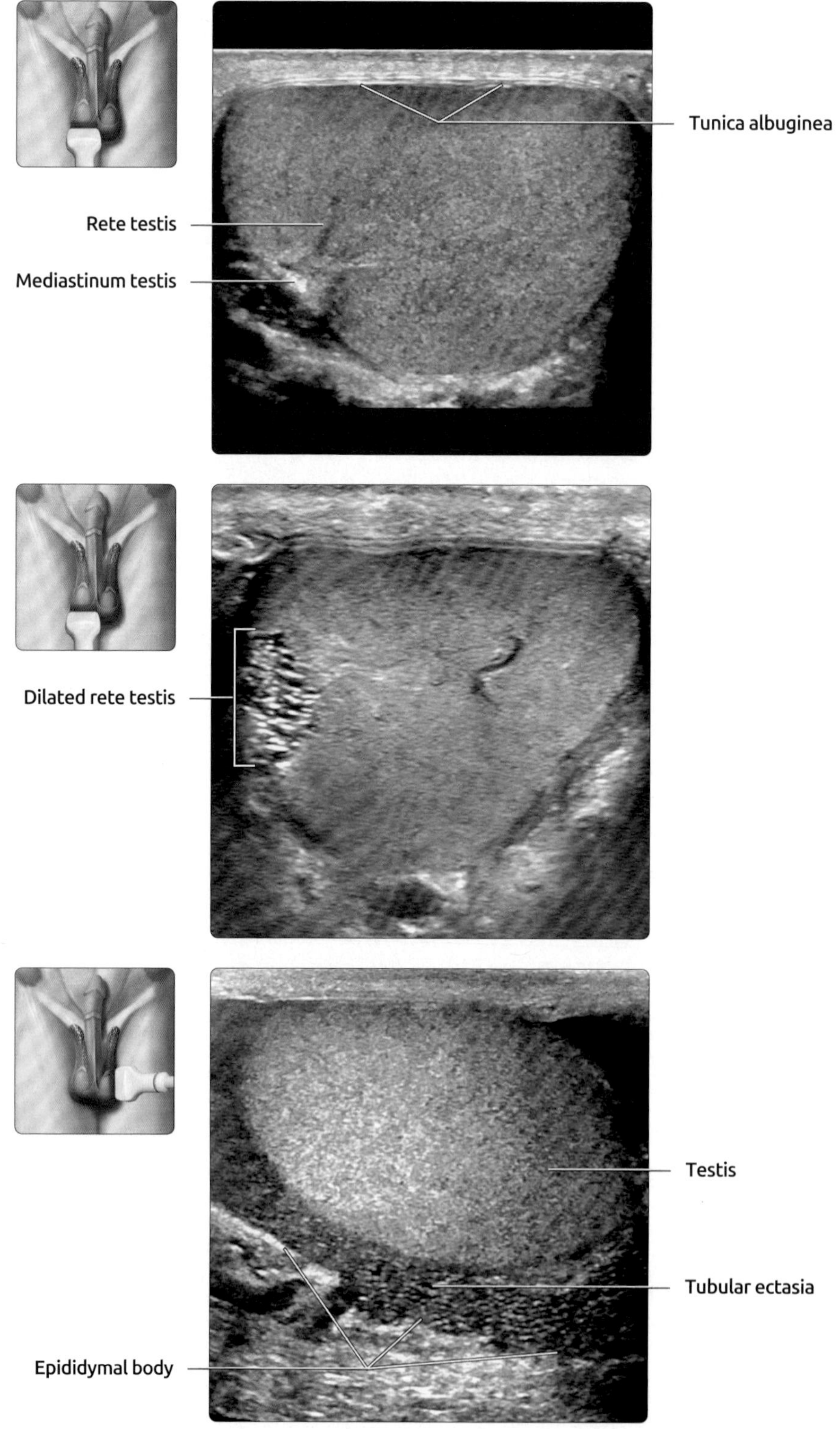

(Top) *Transverse grayscale ultrasound of the normal testis shows diffuse low-level internal echoes in the parenchyma, an echogenic mediastinum testis, and the striated pattern of the rete testis as it converges to the mediastinum. The testis is covered with 2 thin, echogenic layers of tunica albuginea.* **(Middle)** *Transverse ultrasound of the the right testis shows tubular ectasia of the rete testis. Tubular ectasia is located posteriorly by the mediastinum and is frequently bilateral. It may give an impression of a mass, but careful scanning shows the "mass" is actually a series of dilated tubules and is a "do not touch" lesion.* **(Bottom)** *Sagittal grayscale ultrasound of the epididymis demonstrates tubular ectasia within the epididymis.*

TESTICULAR AND EPIDIDYMAL APPENDAGES

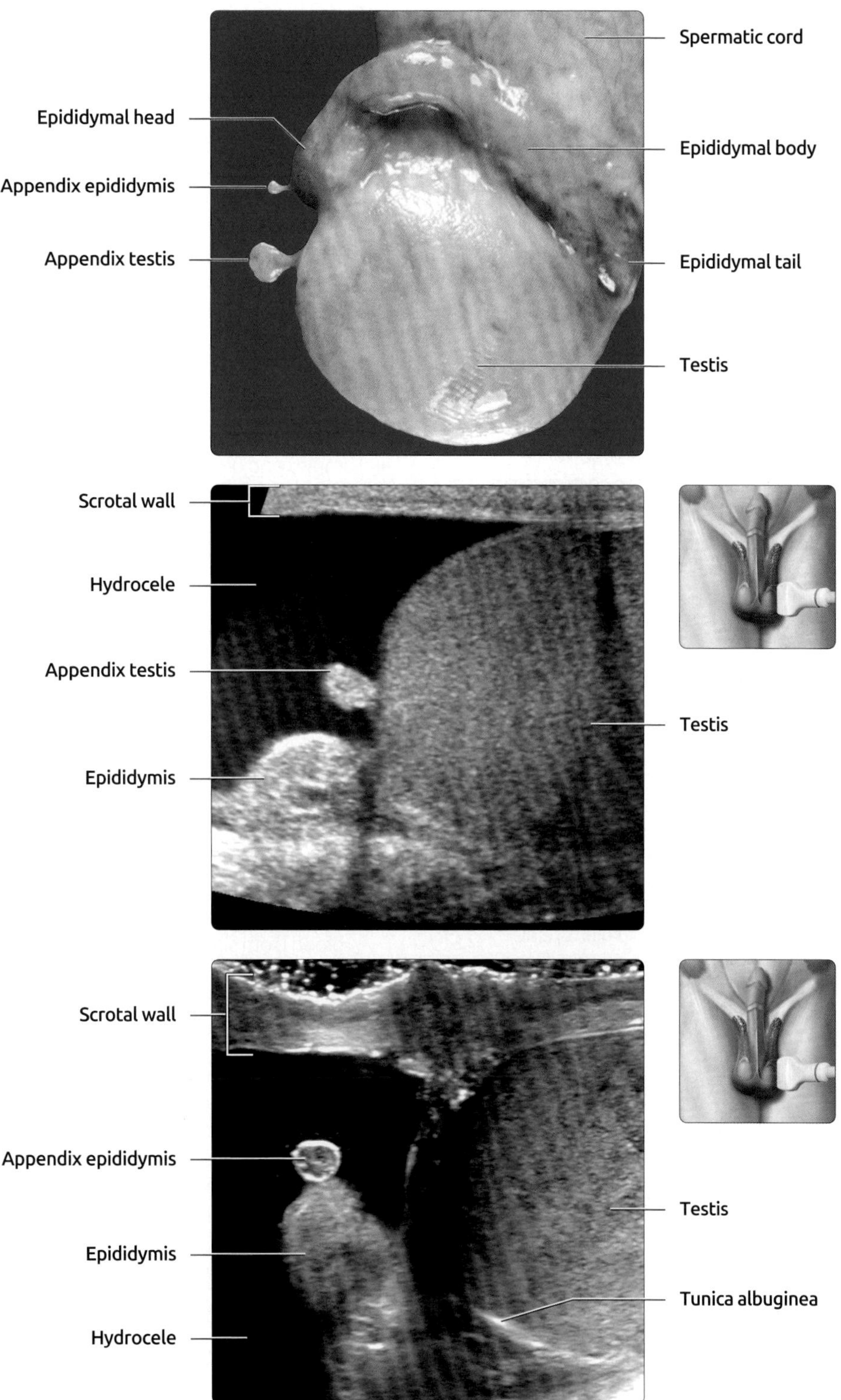

(Top) *Gross specimen shows the the testis, epididymis, and spermatic cord. Two embryologic remnants form small appendages from the testis and epididymis.* **(Middle)** *Ultrasound of the testis in a patient with a hydrocele shows a small, nodular protuberance from the surface of the testis. This is the appendix testis, which is a remnant of the embryologic müllerian system.* **(Bottom)** *Longitudinal ultrasound of the upper testis and epididymis shows a small "tag" of tissue projecting from the epididymis. This is an appendix epididymis, which is an embryologic remnant of the wolffian system. Both the appendix testis and appendix epididymis are usually not visible sonographically unless there is a hydrocele. They are usually of no clinical significance; however, they can undergo torsion and be a cause of scrotal pain. Once separated, they are freely mobile and calcify (scrotal calculi).*

IMAGING ANATOMY

Penis

- **Composed of 3 cylindrical shafts**
  - **2 corpora cavernosa**: Main erectile bodies
    - On dorsal surface of penis
    - Diverge at root of penis (**crura**) and are invested by **ischiocavernosus muscles**
    - Chambers traversed by numerous trabeculae, creating sinusoidal spaces
    - Multiple fenestrations between corpora, creating multiple anastomotic channels
  - **1 corpus spongiosum**: Contains urethra
    - On ventral surface, in groove created by corpora cavernosa
    - Becomes **penile bulb** at root and is invested by **bulbospongiosus muscle**
    - Forms **glans penis** distally
    - Also erectile tissue but of far less importance
- **Tunica albuginea** forms capsule around each corpora
  - Thinner around spongiosum than cavernosa
- All 3 corpora surrounded by deep fascia (**Buck fascia**) and superficial fascia (**Colles fascia**)
- Main arterial supply from internal pudendal artery
  - **Cavernosal artery** runs within center of each corpus cavernosum
    - Gives off **helicine arteries**, which fill trabecular spaces
    - Primary source of blood for erectile tissue
  - **Paired dorsal penile arteries** run between tunica albuginea of corpora cavernosa and Buck fascia
    - Supplies glans penis and skin
- **Venous drainage** of corpora cavernosa
  - Emissary veins in corpora pierce through tunica albuginea → circumflex veins → deep dorsal vein of penis → retropubic venous plexus
  - Superficial dorsal vein drains skin and glans penis

Normal Erectile Function

- Neurologically mediated response eliciting smooth muscle relaxation of cavernosal arteries, helicine arteries, and cavernosal sinusoids
- Blood flows from helicine arteries into sinusoidal spaces
- Sinusoids distend, eventually compressing emissary veins against rigid tunica albuginea
  - Venous compression prevents egress of blood from corpora, which maintains erection

Urethra: 4 Segments

- Prostatic urethra: Traverses prostate
- Membranous urethra: Short course through urogenital diaphragm (level of external urethral sphincter)
  - Contains bulbourethral glands (Cowper glands)
- Bulbous urethra: Below urogenital diaphragm to suspensory ligament of penis at penoscrotal junction
- Penile urethra: Pendulous portion, distal to suspensory ligament

ANATOMY IMAGING ISSUES

Imaging Recommendations

- Transducer: High-frequency (7.5- to 10.0-MHz) linear transducer
- Patient is supine with penis positioned on anterior abdominal wall
  - Use towels for padding, forming "nest" to keep penis in appropriate position
- Transducer placed on ventral side of penis
  - Corpus spongiosum easily compressed, so use ample gel and gentle pressure
- For erectile dysfunction studies, vasodilating agent is injected into dorsal 2/3 of shaft
- Urethra may also be examined by ultrasound
  - Imaging of anterior urethra is optimal with distension
    - Gel may be injected retrograde or patient may be asked to void during scan
  - Posterior urethra is best imaged by transrectal ultrasound of prostate

CLINICAL IMPLICATIONS

Erectile Dysfunction

- Complex and often multifactorial, including vascular, neurogenic, and psychologic factors
- **Arteriogenic impotence** affects inflow
  - Usually internal pudendal and penile arteries
  - Blockage may be as high as distal aorta (Leriche syndrome)
  - **Cavernosal artery evaluation**
    - In flaccid state, there is little diastolic flow
    - At onset of erection, there is dilatation with increase in both systolic and diastolic flow
    - At maximum erection, venous drainage is blocked
      - Waveform changes to high resistance with reversal of diastolic flow
      - Peak systolic velocity > 30 cm/s
      - Cavernosal artery diameter increase > 75%
- **Venogenic impotence** affects outflow
  - Ineffective venoocclusion with continuous outflow of blood from sinusoids
  - At peak erection end, diastolic flow is reversed or absent
    - End diastolic velocity > 5 cm/s indicative of venous insufficiency

Penile Trauma

- Penile fractures occur by forceful bending of erect penis, typically during intercourse
  - Results in rupture of corpus cavernosum with tearing of tunica albuginea
  - Patients often report "snap" followed by immediate pain
  - Expanding hematoma; if Buck fascia also disrupted, may extend to perineum and scrotum
- Need to carefully evaluate tunica albuginea for any areas of disruption
- Document location and extent of hematoma

Peyronie Disease

- Localized, benign, connective tissue disorder with fibrotic plaque formation on tunica albuginea
  - Causes painful erections with shortening and curvature of penis
- Scan tunica albuginea carefully looking for areas of hyperechoic thickening ± calcifications

PENIS AND URETHRA

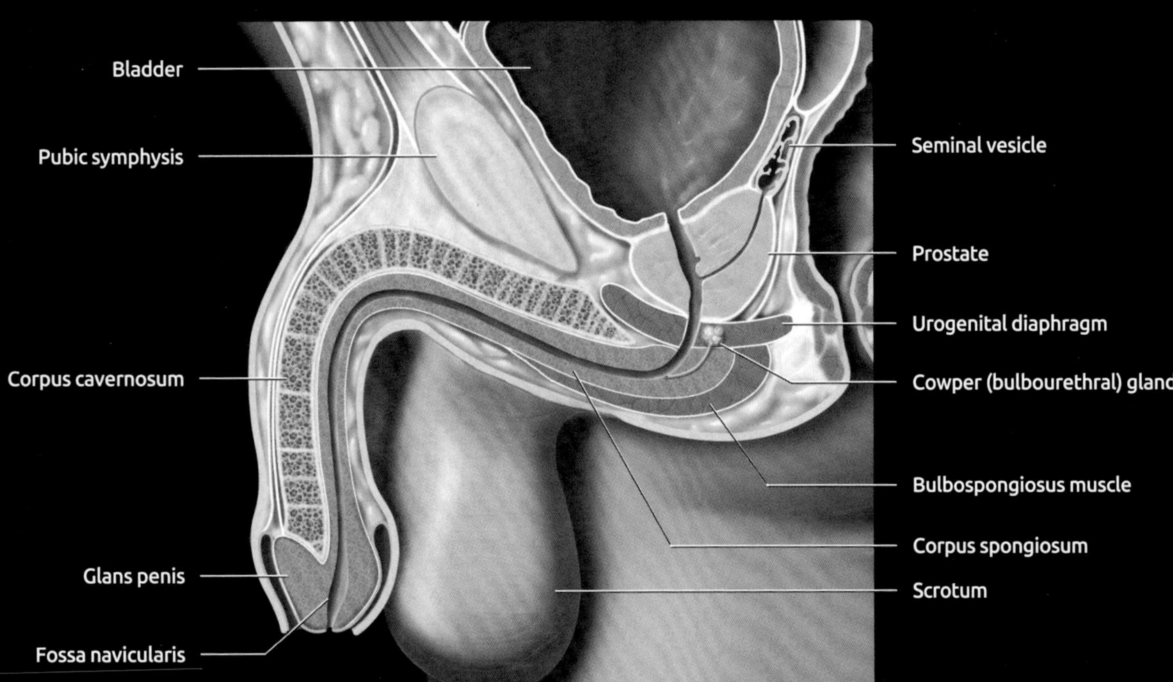

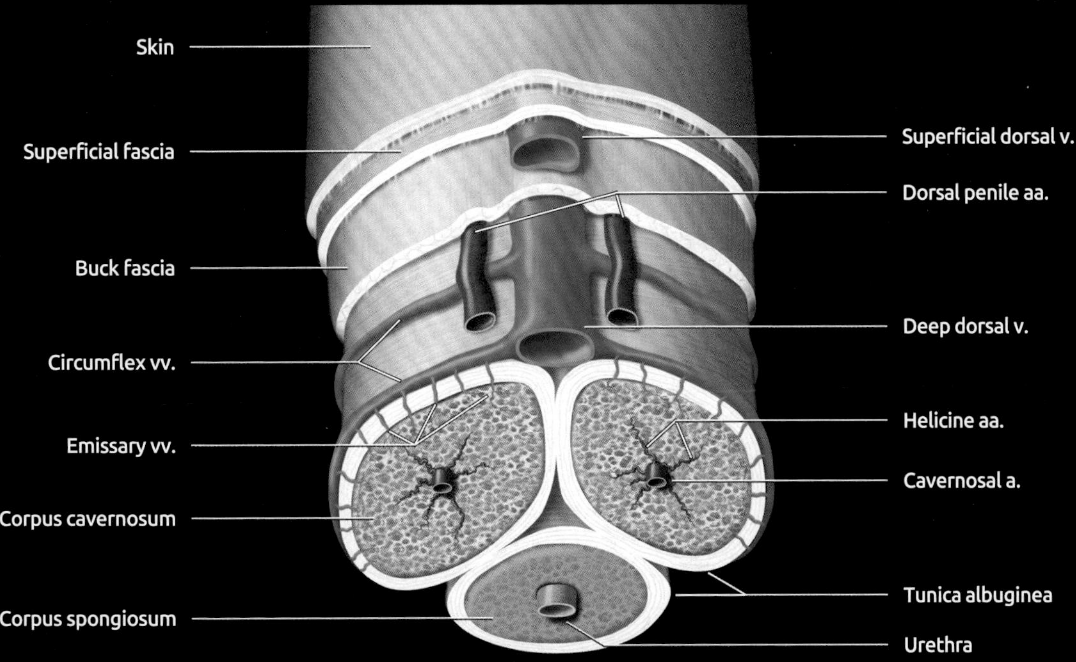

(Top) *Sagittal midline graphic shows the course of the urethra. The posterior portion traverses the prostate and urogenital diaphragm. The anterior urethra runs within the corpus spongiosum. The external (pendulous) portion of the penis begins below the pubic symphysis at the penoscrotal junction.* **(Bottom)** *Cross section of the penis viewed from above shows the 3 corpora, each of which is invested by a tunica albuginea. The 3 corpora are surrounded by Buck fascia. The cavernosal arteries run within the corpora cavernosa and give rise to the helicine arteries, which fill the sinusoids. Normal drainage is via the emissary veins → circumflex veins → deep dorsal vein of penis. With an erection, the emissary veins are compressed against the strong tunica albuginea, occluding venous drainage. The dorsal penile arteries and deep dorsal vein run beneath the Buck fascia. The penile arteries supply the glans and skin, but there are significant anastomoses between both the arterial and venous systems.*

NORMAL ERECTILE FUNCTION

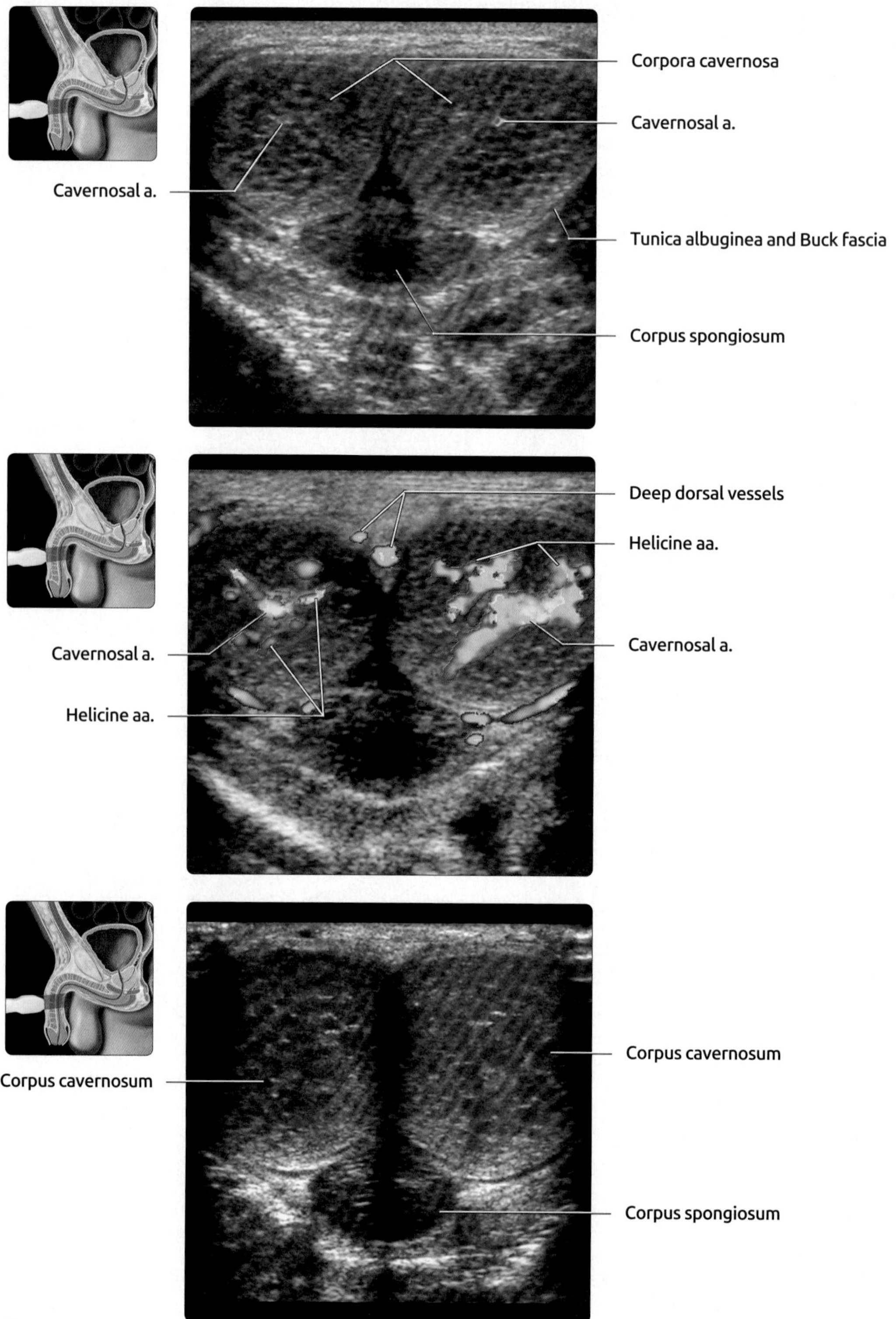

(Top) *The 1st of 3 cross-sectional ultrasounds of the penis shows the changing appearance during a normal erection. The paired corpora cavernosa are the primary erectile bodies. They are composed of a complex network of trabeculae, which creates the sinusoids and give a sponge-like appearance on ultrasound. Each corpus is surrounded by a tough tunica albuginea that appears as a thin, echogenic line. Buck fascia, which surrounds all 3 corpora, is intimately associated with the tunica and cannot be distinguished as a separate structure.* **(Middle)** *Color Doppler ultrasound at the onset of an erection shows arterial inflow. There is dilation of the cavernosal and helicine arteries as they begin to fill the sinusoidal spaces.* **(Bottom)** *With continued arterial inflow and compressed venous outflow, the corpora become maximally distended and rigid.*

NORMAL ERECTILE FUNCTION

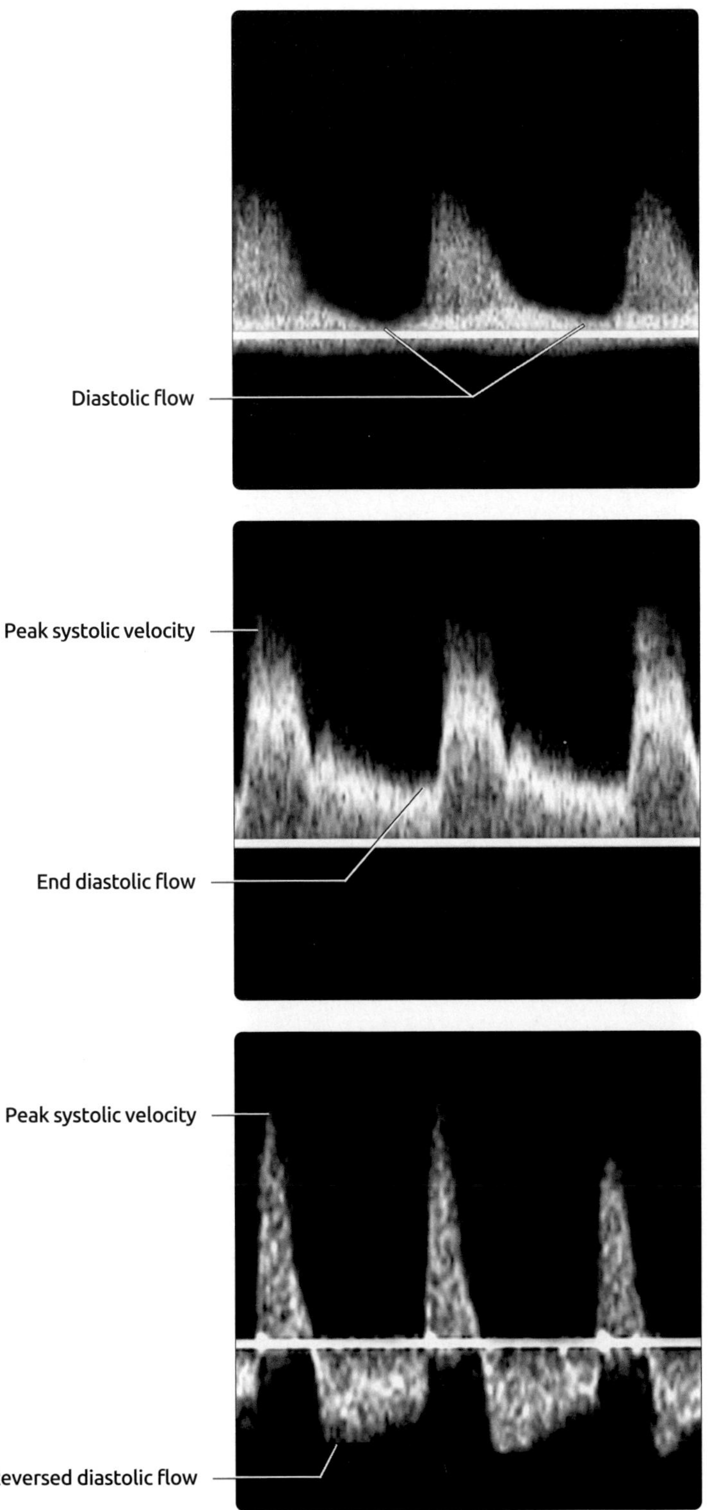

(Top) *The 1st of 3 Doppler tracings shows the changing flow patterns during a normal erection. In the flaccid state, there is little to no diastolic flow.* **(Middle)** *At onset of erection, there is vasodilation of the cavernosal and helicine arteries (increased inflow) and smooth muscle relaxation within the sinusoids (decreased resistance). This causes a marked increase in both the peak systolic velocity (PSV) and end diastolic flow.* **(Bottom)** *In the fully erect state, the emissary veins are compressed against the rigid tunica albuginea, preventing outflow of blood. This dramatically increases the arterial resistance, resulting in absent or reversed diastolic flow. A PSV > 30 cm/s is considered normal, while < 25 cm/s is strong evidence of arteriogenic impotence (25-30 borderline). Venogenic impotence is due to failure of draining vein occlusion. The Doppler tracing would show continuous forward flow in diastole with a velocity > 5 cm/s.*

NORMAL ERECTILE FUNCTION

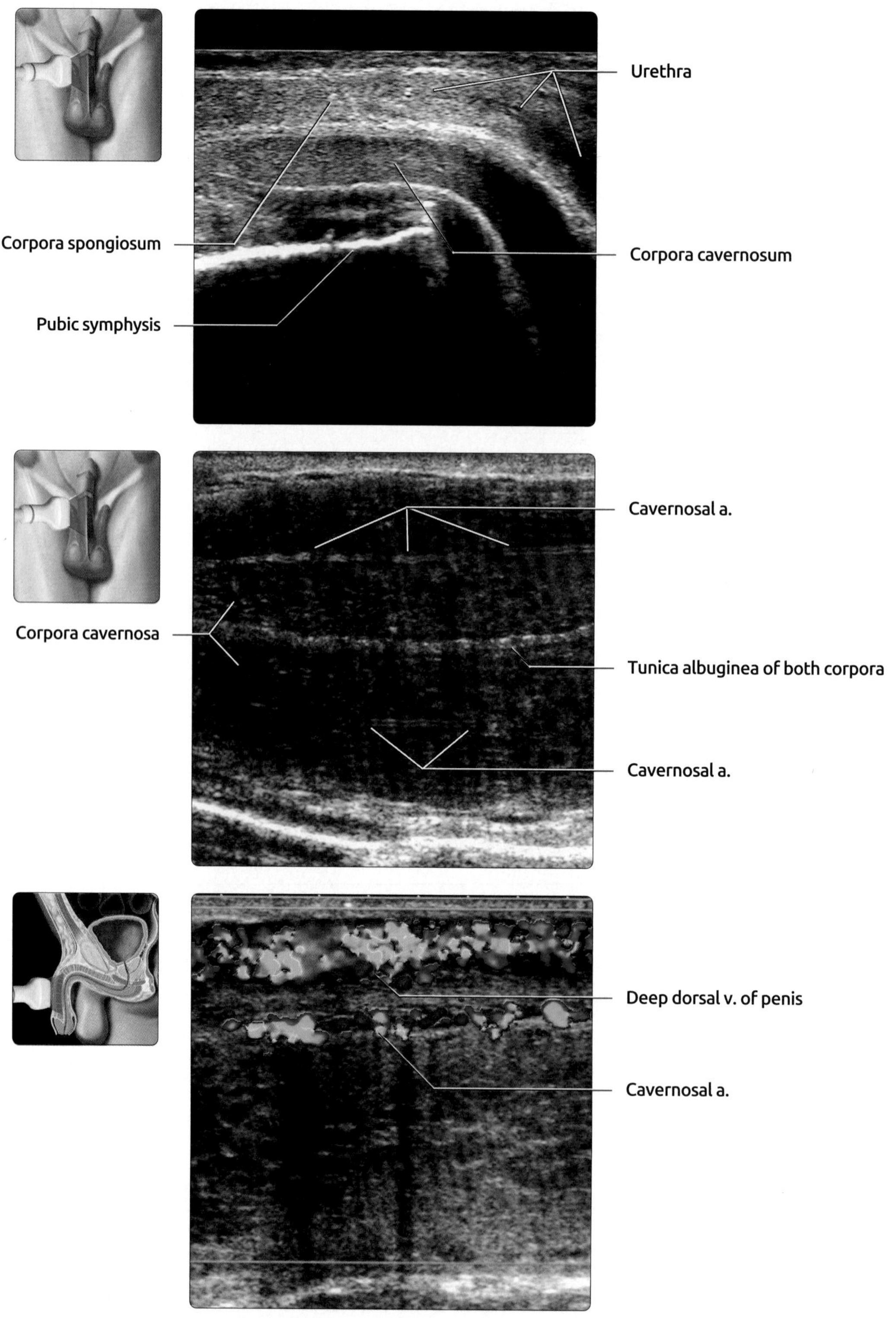

(Top) *Longitudinal scan shows the penis positioned on the anterior abdominal wall and scanned on the ventral side. The urethra is identified within the substance of the corpora spongiosum. One of the paired corpora cavernosa, which is more hypoechoic relative to the spongiosum, is shown.* **(Middle)** *In the erect state, the cavernosal arteries assume a straighter course and can be easily imaged. Magnified views of the cavernosal artery should be obtained to measure vessel diameter. Most measure < 1 mm in the flaccid state. The diameter should increase by 75% with an erection. Failure to increase in size, coupled with an abnormal Doppler waveform, is strong evidence of arteriogenic impotence. The thick, echogenic line is formed where the 2 tunica albuginea abut.* **(Bottom)** *Color Doppler shows flow in both the cavernosal artery and deep dorsal vein of the penis. As an erection starts to wane, or in venogenic impotence, significant flow is seen in the draining vein.*

PATHOLOGY

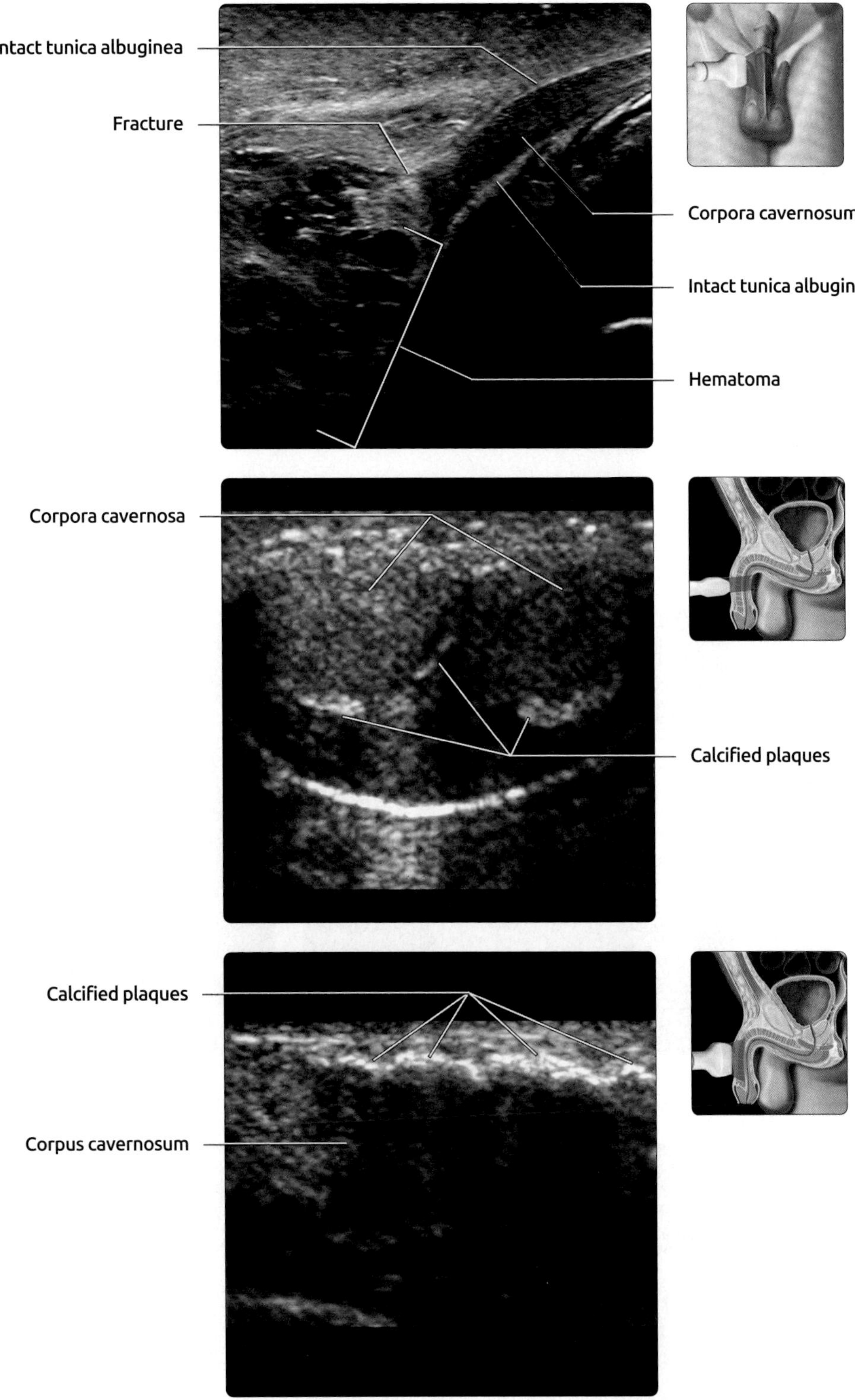

(Top) *Longitudinal ultrasound along the base of the penis shows a fracture of the corpora cavernosum with a large hematoma. It is important to carefully scan all along the tunica albuginea, both in the longitudinal and transverse planes, looking for the site of disruption.* **(Middle)** *Transverse ultrasound of the penis in a patient with Peyronie disease shows scattered hyperechoic plaques within the tunica albuginea of the corpora cavernosa. The plaques hinder normal expansion of the corpora during an erection and cause shortening and curvature of the penis.* **(Bottom)** *Longitudinal ultrasound of one corpus cavernosum shows densely calcified plaques with significant posterior shadowing in a more severe case of Peyronie disease.*

KEY FACTS

IMAGING

- Discrete, solid, intratesticular mass on grayscale ultrasound with abnormal intrinsic vessels on color Doppler
- Most common neoplasm in males aged 15-34
- Seminoma is most common pure germ cell tumor of testis
- Tumors < 1.5 cm commonly hypovascular, and tumors > 1.6 cm more often hypervascular
- US used to identify and characterize scrotal mass; CT or MR for metastatic staging; PET to evaluate posttreatment residual masses
- Lymph nodes < 1 cm suspicious if located in typical drainage areas; left renal hilus and right retrocaval in location

TOP DIFFERENTIAL DIAGNOSES

- Lymphoma
  - Older male > 60
- Hematoma
  - Pain after trauma and avascular on color Doppler
- Segmental infarct
  - Present with acute pain rather than painless palpable mass
- Focal orchitis
  - Present with acute pain and fever
- Epidermoid cyst
  - Characteristic "onion ring" concentric layers, avascular on color Doppler, well-defined rim

PATHOLOGY

- Associated with testicular maldescension, previous contralateral cancer, infertility, and family history of tumor

SCANNING TIPS

- Document whether lesion is palpable
- Look for lymph nodes
  - Along right side of IVC for right-sided tumors
  - Along left renal vein for left-sided tumors

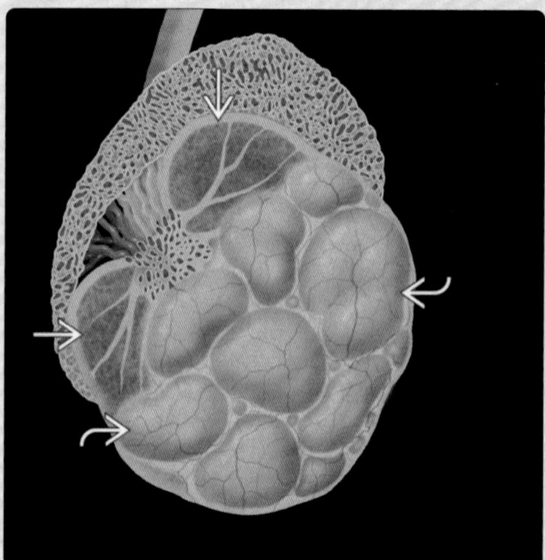

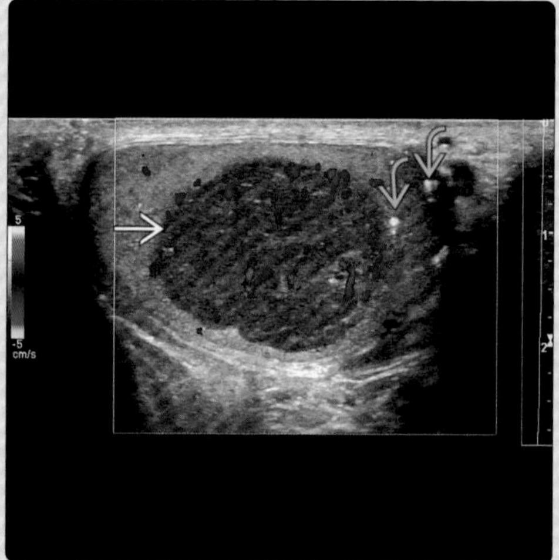

(Left) *Graphic shows a multilobulated testicular mass. Note the compressed and near-complete replacement of normal testicular parenchyma.* **(Right)** *Longitudinal color Doppler US of the right testis demonstrates a well-defined, hypoechoic, solid mass with mild internal vascularity. Imaging features are classic for seminoma. A few scattered microliths are also seen in the noninvolved portion of the testicle.*

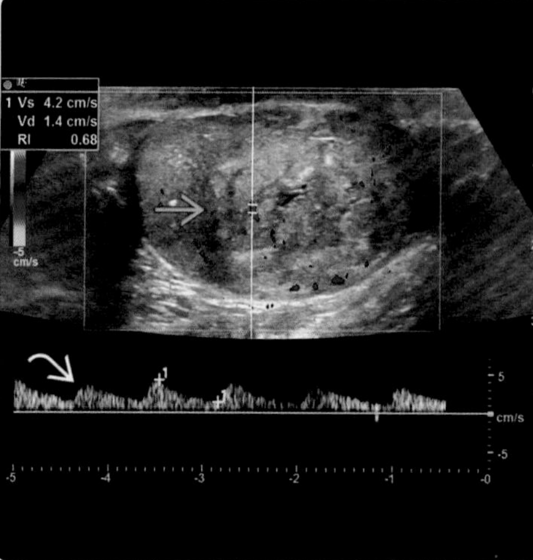

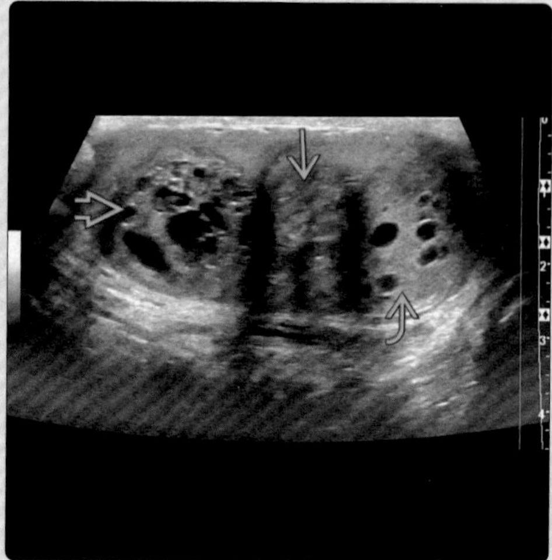

(Left) *Sagittal spectral Doppler US of the right testicle shows a predominantly solid, heterogeneous mass with internal arterial vascularity. Pathology revealed a mixed germ cell tumor with 95% embryonal component and 5% teratoma.* **(Right)** *Sagittal grayscale US of the left testicle shows multifocal masses with 3 different sonographic patterns including solid, multiple cystic spaces, and solid and cystic spaces. Pathology revealed MGCT with 55% embryonal, 35% teratoma, and 10% yolk sac.*

KEY FACTS

TERMINOLOGY

- Gonadal stromal tumors arise from nongerm cell elements

IMAGING

- Leydig cell tumors
  - Small, solid, hypoechoic intratesticular mass
  - May occasionally show cystic change
- Sertoli cell tumors
  - Small, hypoechoic mass with occasional hemorrhage, which may lead to heterogeneity and cystic components
  - ± punctate calcification; large, calcified mass in large-cell calcifying Sertoli cell tumor
  - May produce estrogen/müllerian inhibiting factor
- Gonadoblastoma
  - Stromal tumor in conjunction with germ cell tumor, usually mixed sonographic features

CLINICAL ISSUES

- 30% of patients with gonadal stromal tumors have endocrinopathy secondary to testosterone or estrogen production by tumor presenting with
  - Precocious virilization in children
  - Gynecomastia, impotence, ↓ libido in adults
- Majority of these tumors are benign
- Orchidectomy is preferred treatment

DIAGNOSTIC CHECKLIST

- Consider stromal tumor in any patient with endocrinopathy and testicular mass

SCANNING TIPS

- May be indistinguishable from germ cell tumors on grayscale ultrasound but typically smaller in size
- High-frequency transducer (9-15 MHz) best imaging tool for detection of gonadal stromal neoplasms

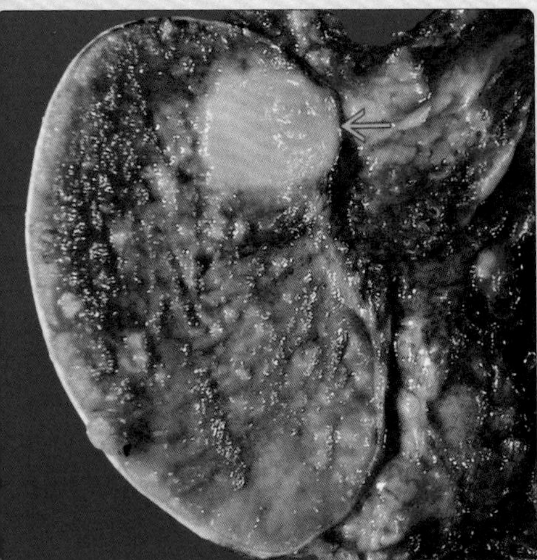

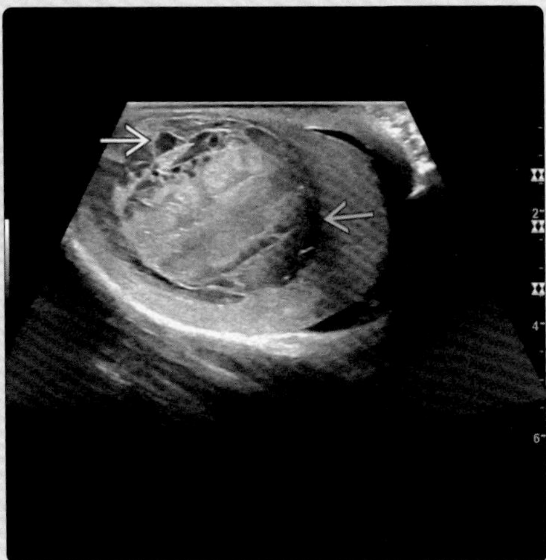

(Left) *Granulosa cell tumor shows a well-circumscribed, homogeneous, tan-white nodule ⇨. The tumor is small and, like many sex cord stromal tumors, does not extensively involve the testis. Hemorrhage and necrosis are lacking.* **(Right)** *Sagittal grayscale ultrasound in a 16-year-old male demonstrates a well-defined, predominantly solid mass ⇨ with some interspersed cystic areas ➡. Pathology confirmed it to be a granulosa cell tumor (adult type).*

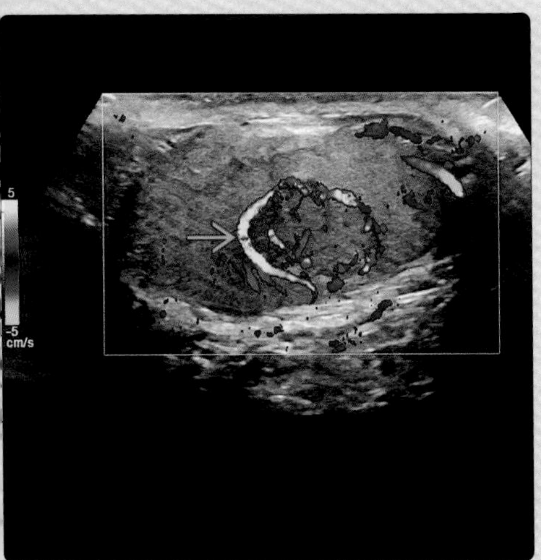

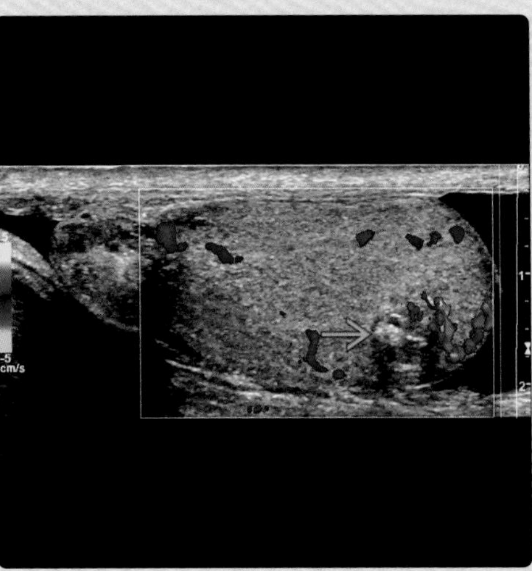

(Left) *Sagittal color Doppler ultrasound of the right testis in a 33-year-old man demonstrates a well-defined, hypoechoic, solid mass with marked internal vascularity ⇨. Pathology confirmed it to be a Leydig cell tumor.* **(Right)** *Sagittal color Doppler ultrasound shows the right testis with a partially calcified mass ⇨ and minimal to no internal vascularity. Pathology confirmed a Sertoli cell tumor.*

Testicular Lymphoma/Leukemia

KEY FACTS

TERMINOLOGY

- Infiltrative neoplasm of testis in which tumor cells surround and compress seminiferous tubules and normal testicular vessels

IMAGING

- Bilateral, solid, hypoechoic, hypervascular nodules/masses
- Diffuse hypoechoic testis with hypervascularity
- Striated pattern
- Testicular shape not altered
- Normal testicular vessels with straight course crossing through lesions

PATHOLOGY

- Most commonly secondary lymphomatous involvement of testis; rarely primary
- Lymphoma behaves similar to leukemia with abnormal cells diffusely infiltrating interstitium with compression of seminiferous tubules without causing their destruction
- Testis is "sanctuary organ": Blood gonad barrier limits accumulation of chemotherapeutic agents

CLINICAL ISSUES

- Stages IE and IIE: Orchidectomy
- Stages IIIE and IVE: Systemic chemotherapy using cyclophosphamide, doxorubicin, vincristine, and prednisolone
- Radiation in symptomatic and bulky deposits
- Lymphoma accounts for ~ 5% of all testicular tumors
- Most common bilateral testicular tumor

SCANNING TIPS

- Side-by-side comparison of both testes in single image with both grayscale and color Doppler is essential to assess for symmetry in size, echogenicity, and vascularity
  - Do not use dual image/split screen because scan parameters, such as TGC or color Doppler scale, may be altered between windows

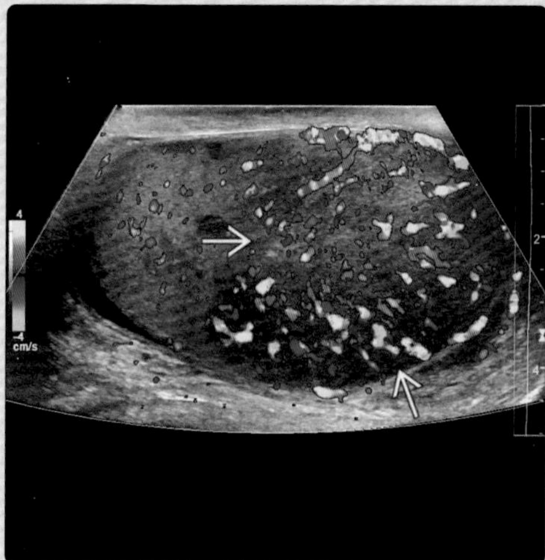

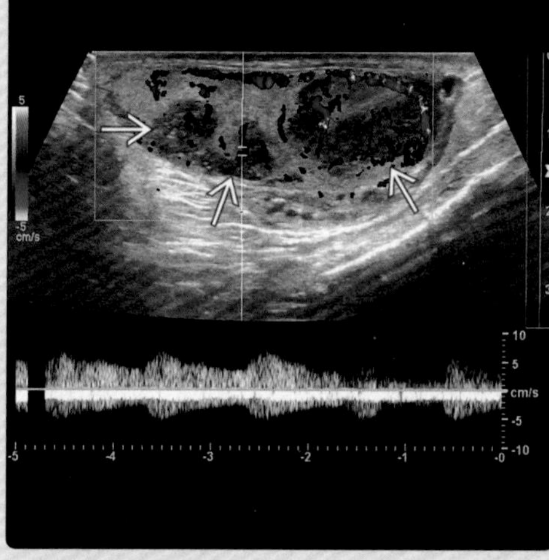

(Left) *Sagittal color Doppler ultrasound of the right testis in a 56-year-old man with non-Hodgkin lymphoma shows a hypervascular focal mass ➡ in the inferior pole with focal enlargement of the testis. Note that the shape of the testis is maintained. Pathology confirmed lymphoma.* **(Right)** *Sagittal color Doppler ultrasound of the left testis in a 65-year-old man shows multiple hypervascular hypoechoic masses ➡ in the testis. Pathology confirmed lymphoma.*

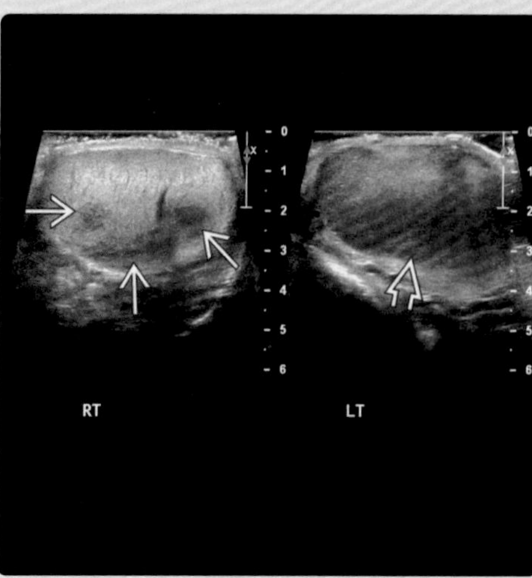

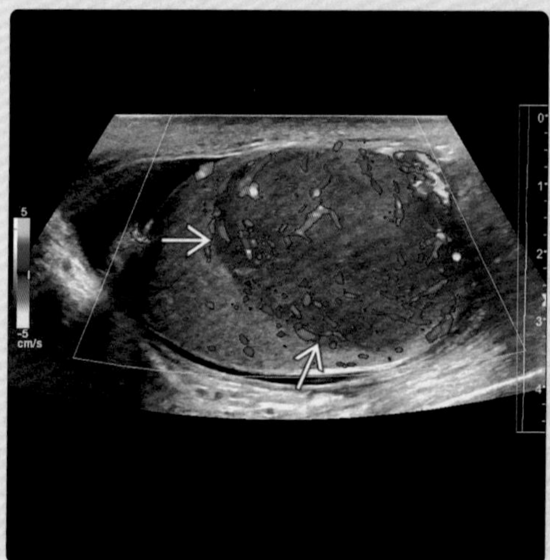

(Left) *Sagittal grayscale ultrasound of the testes in a 60-year-old man with non-Hodgkin lymphoma shows bilateral hypoechoic masses, multifocal on the right ➡ and diffuse infiltrative on the left ➡.* **(Right)** *Sagittal color Doppler ultrasound of the right testis in a 51-year-old man with known history of acute myeloid leukemia shows a hypervascular focal hypoechoic mass ➡ in the inferior pole. Pathology confirmed acute myeloid leukemia.*

Epidermoid Cyst

KEY FACTS

TERMINOLOGY

- Rare, benign, keratin-containing lesion of controversial origin

IMAGING

- High-resolution ultrasound (≥ 10 MHz) is imaging modality of choice
- **Grayscale ultrasound**
  - Characteristic onion skin, concentric rings, or target/bull's-eye appearance of testicular mass
  - Unilocular cyst containing keratin; fibrous wall
  - Sharply circumscribed, encapsulated round "mass"
- **Color Doppler ultrasound**
  - Avascular, no blood flow demonstrable
- Most commonly intratesticular but rarely may be extratesticular

TOP DIFFERENTIAL DIAGNOSES

- Tunica albuginea cyst
  - Located within tunica, solitary, unilocular, and anechoic
- Germ cell tumor
  - Heterogeneous mass with vascularity seen on Doppler
- Testicular granuloma
  - Most probably due to TB, usually multiple

CLINICAL ISSUES

- May occur at any age; 2nd-4th decades most common
- 1-2% of all testicular tumors
- No malignant potential
- Enucleate 1st if lesion < 3 cm with characteristic ultrasound appearance and no color flow; testis can be spared if
  - Frozen sections of lesion are consistent with epidermoid cyst
  - No evidence of malignancy within or surrounding lesion
  - Negative tumor markers (AFP, β-HCG)

SCANNING TIPS

- Lesion should be avascular on color Doppler

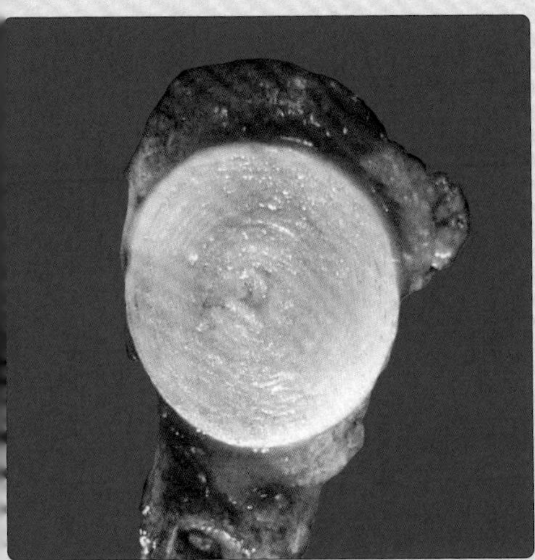

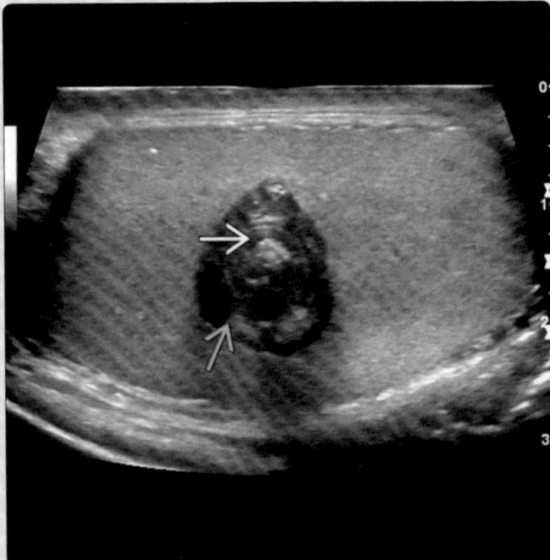

(Left) *Gross pathologic specimen of an epidermoid cut in half shows the numerous concentric keratin layers that leads to the characteristic onion skin or target appearance of an epidermoid.* **(Right)** *Sagittal grayscale ultrasound of the testis demonstrates a unilocular, well-demarcated intratesticular epidermoid cyst ⇨. The central hyperechoic focus ➡ corresponds to keratin. The surrounding testicular parenchyma is normal in echogenicity.*

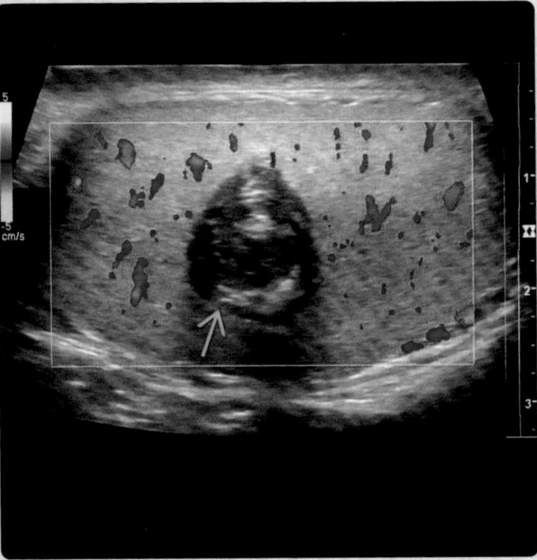

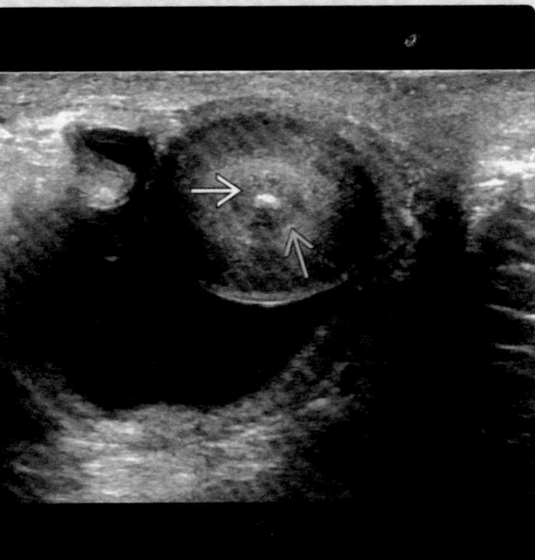

(Left) *Color Doppler ultrasound of the same lesion ⇨ demonstrates no internal vascularity, which further supports the diagnosis of epidermoid cyst.* **(Right)** *Sagittal ultrasound of a patient with a painless scrotal lump demonstrates a circumscribed, oval, extratesticular epidermoid cyst with a classic onion skin appearance ⇨ and central echogenic focus ➡.*

Tubular Ectasia of Rete Testis

KEY FACTS

TERMINOLOGY

- Dilated rete testis
- Cystic transformation of rete testis

IMAGING

- Frequently bilateral
  - Usually asymmetric involvement
- Branching tubules converging at mediastinum testis
  - Dilated tubules create lace-like or fishnet appearance
- Adjacent parenchyma is normal
- Associated ipsilateral spermatoceles are common
- Tubules are avascular and fluid filled
  - No flow on color Doppler imaging
- MR performed for confirmation if cystic malignant neoplasm cannot be ruled out

TOP DIFFERENTIAL DIAGNOSES

- Testicular carcinoma
  - Mixed germ cell tumors with teratomatous components will often have cystic areas
  - Does not form network of tubules
- Intratesticular varicocele
  - Characteristic color flow on Doppler
- Testicular infarct
  - Avascular wedge-shaped area with sharp borders

CLINICAL ISSUES

- Generally nonpalpable and asymptomatic
- May be found when doing ultrasound for related issue, such as epididymal cyst
- Often seen in setting of prior vasectomy

SCANNING TIPS

- Check with color or power Doppler to ensure lesion is avascular

(Left) *Transverse grayscale ultrasound of the testes demonstrates bilateral tubular ectasia of the rete testis, which is slightly asymmetric, right ➡ > left ➡.* **(Right)** *Sagittal grayscale ultrasound of the left testis demonstrates cystic areas ➡ within the mediastinum testis, consistent with tubular ectasia of the rete testis.*

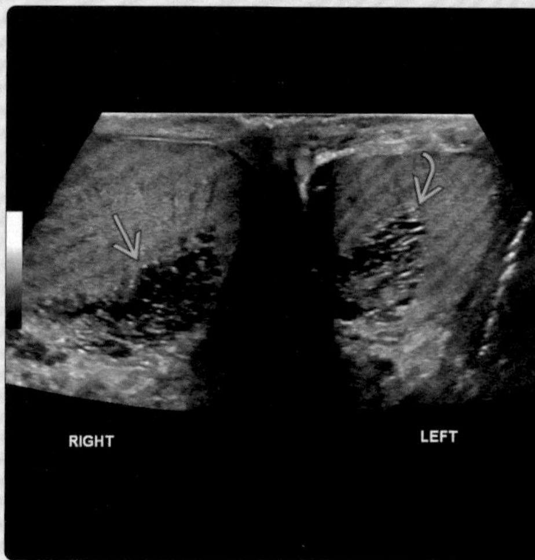

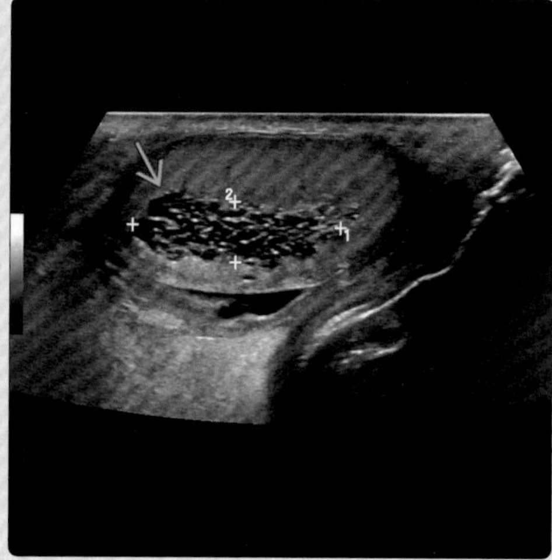

(Left) *Transverse color Doppler ultrasound of the right testicle demonstrates avascular cystic areas within the testis ➡ with a cystic area within the epididymal head ➡. These findings are consistent with tubular ectasia of the rete testis with associated spermatocele.* **(Right)** *Sagittal grayscale ultrasound of the epididymal head demonstrates large spermatoceles ➡ with partially visualized tubular ectasia ➡.*

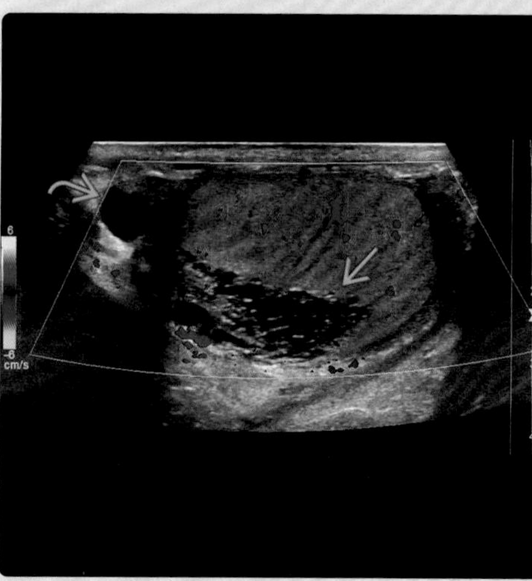

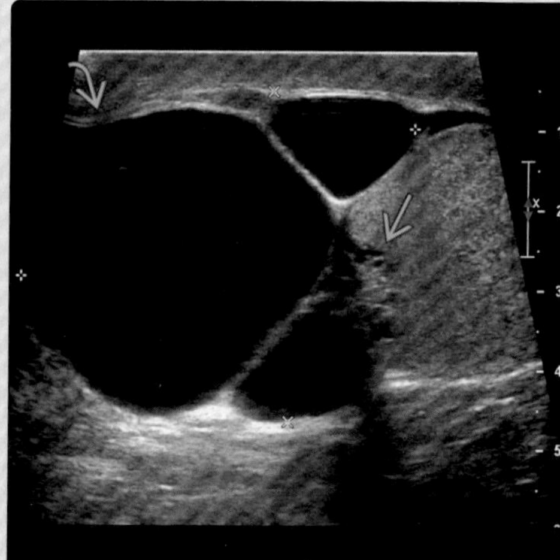

KEY FACTS

TERMINOLOGY

- Testicular microlithiasis (TML): Presence of 5 or more microliths or microcalcifications in whole testis or 5 or more microliths per field of view
- Limited TML: Presence of < 5 microcalcifications per field of view
- Microcalcifications composed of hydroxyapatite, located within spermatic tubules

IMAGING

- On US, seen as discrete, punctate, nonshadowing echogenic foci scattered within testicular parenchyma
- Majority are idiopathic; previous infection or trauma may also be responsible
- May occasionally see comet-tail artifact
- May occasionally see twinkling artifact on color Doppler

TOP DIFFERENTIAL DIAGNOSES

- Scrotal pearls (scrotoliths)
- Large-cell calcifying Sertoli cell tumor
- Testicular granuloma

PATHOLOGY

- Testicular neoplasia in 18-75%, intratubular germ cell neoplasia, germ cell version of carcinoma in situ

CLINICAL ISSUES

- Microlithiasis in absence of other risk factors is not indication for further sonographic screening or biopsy
- Follow-up US recommended in patients with risk factors, including personal/family history of GCT, maldescent or undescended testes, orchidopexy, testicular atrophy

SCANNING TIPS

- If TML is seen, check bilateral testes carefully for any focal solid lesion
- Scan carefully from medial to lateral in longitudinal plane and superior to inferior in transverse plane to detect limited TML

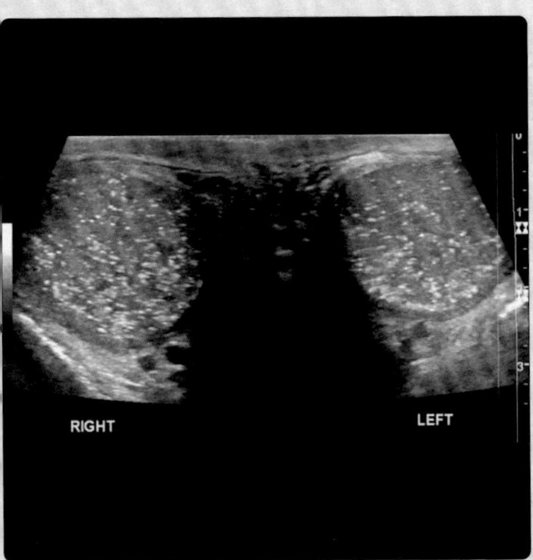

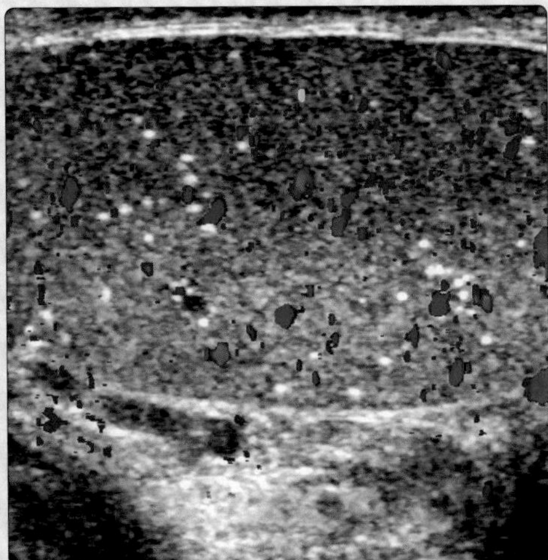

(Left) *Transverse grayscale ultrasound of bilateral testes demonstrates extensive microlithiasis.* **(Right)** *Oblique color Doppler ultrasound of testicular microlithiasis demonstrates no specific vascularity.*

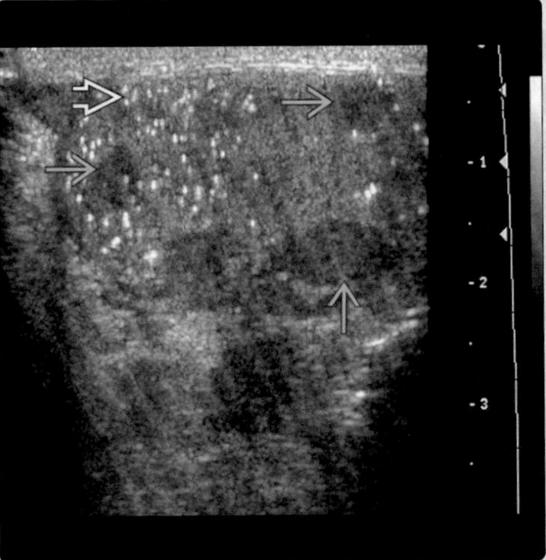

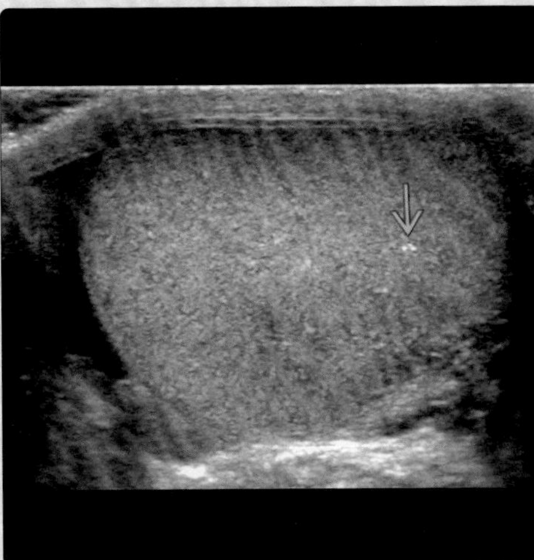

(Left) *Sagittal grayscale ultrasound of the right testis demonstrates multifocal hypoechoic masses ➙ in a background of microlithiasis with clustering at the superior pole ➡. Pathology after orchiectomy confirmed multifocal seminoma.* **(Right)** *Transverse grayscale ultrasound of the left testis demonstrates an isolated microlith ➙ in the parenchyma. This does not meet the definition of testicular microlithiasis and is likely a sequela of prior infection or trauma.*

Testicular Torsion/Infarction

KEY FACTS

TERMINOLOGY

- Spontaneous or traumatic twisting of testis & spermatic cord within scrotum, resulting in vascular occlusion/infarction

IMAGING

- Absent or decreased abnormal testicular blood flow on color Doppler US
- Findings vary with duration and degree of rotation of cord
- Unilateral in 95% of patients
- Role of spectral Doppler is limited; may be helpful to detect partial torsion; in partial torsion of 360° or less, spectral Doppler may show diminished diastolic arterial flow
- Spiral twist of spermatic cord cranial to testis and epididymis causing torsion knot or whirlpool pattern of concentric layers

PATHOLOGY

- Varying degrees of ischemic necrosis & fibrosis depending on duration of symptoms
- Undescended testes have increased risk of torsion
- Intravaginal torsion: Common type, most frequently occurs at puberty

SCANNING TIPS

- Scan testes side-by-side in single image
    - Side-by-side color and power Doppler to demonstrate asymmetry in blood flow to affected side
    - Side-by-side grayscale to demonstrate asymmetry in orientation of testicle
- Must document which side is symptomatic

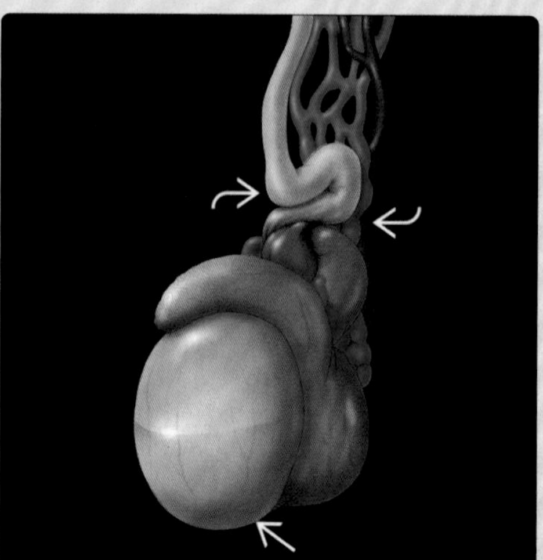

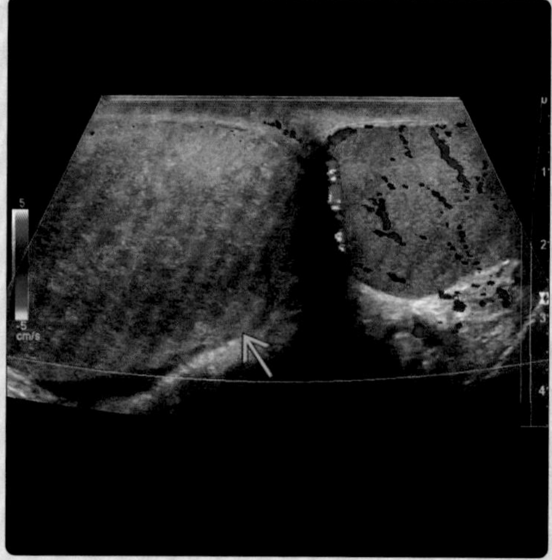

(Left) *Graphic shows spiral twist ➔ of the spermatic cord with torsion, leading to venous congestion and compromised blood supply to the testis ➔.* **(Right)** *Transverse color Doppler ultrasound of both testes side-by-side shows an enlarged heterogeneous avascular right testis ➔ with an abnormal orientation. Patient was symptomatic for 24 hours; testis could not be salvaged after detorsion.*

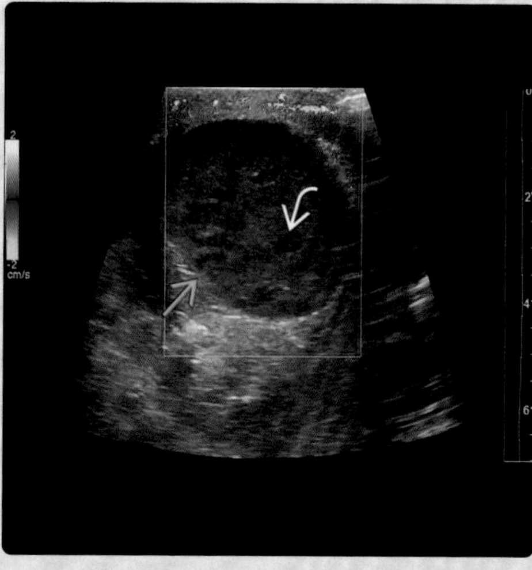

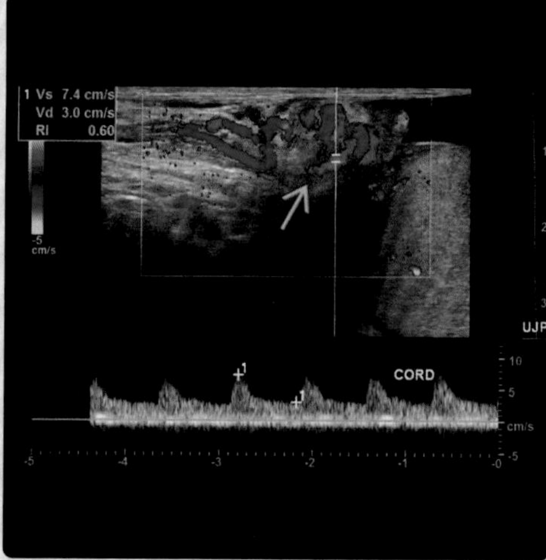

(Left) *Transverse color Doppler ultrasound of the testis in a young male with an acute painful scrotum for 48 hours shows a heterogeneous avascular testis ➔ with cystic areas ➔, consistent with an infarcted testis with necrosis secondary to torsion.* **(Right)** *Sagittal spectral Doppler ultrasound superior to the left testis in a young male with acute painful scrotum shows a whirlpool sign ➔ secondary to a twisted spermatic cord. Patient was manually detorsed followed by bilateral orchidopexy.*

Undescended Testis

KEY FACTS

TERMINOLOGY

- Cryptorchidism, cryptorchism
- Definition: Incomplete descent of testis into base of scrotum

IMAGING

- Unilateral or bilateral absence of testis in scrotum
- Located anywhere from kidney to inguinal canal, inguinal canal most common (80%)
  - Bilateral in 10%
- Ultrasound features: Ovoid homogeneous, hypoechoic, well-circumscribed structure smaller than normal descended testis

TOP DIFFERENTIAL DIAGNOSES

- Inguinal lymphadenopathy
- Inguinal hernia
- Anorchia: Absent testis

PATHOLOGY

- Undescended testis: Arrest of testis along normal path of descent
- Ectopic testis: Testis outside normal path of descent

CLINICAL ISSUES

- Complications: Increased risk of testicular cancer (1:1,000-1:2,500), torsion, atrophy, infertility, and trauma
- Treatment
  - Orchiopexy before age 2 to preserve fertility
  - Orchiectomy: Consider in patients aged 12-50 years

SCANNING TIPS

- Start in high scrotal location and ask patient if palpable mass is present in inguinal region (most common location)
- If still not found: (1) Follow spermatic cord upward: (2) Next, using transverse approach, check lower abdominal region near groin, iliac fossa, and pelvis and in abdominal region near kidneys

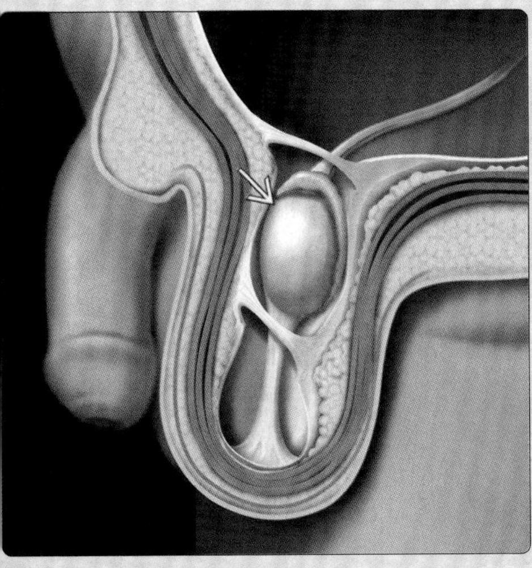

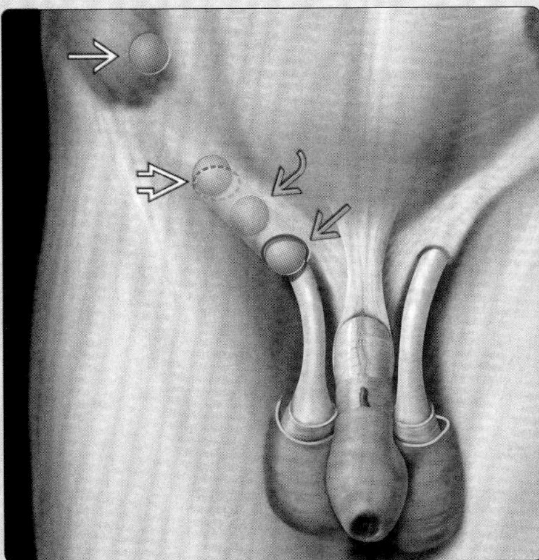

(Left) *Graphic shows a testis at a high scrotal location due to incomplete descent. An undescended testis may be located anywhere from the kidney to the inguinal canal.* **(Right)** *Undescended testes can be located anywhere along the normal path of testicular descent: Intraabdominal, internal inguinal ring, in the inguinal canal, or at the external inguinal ring.*

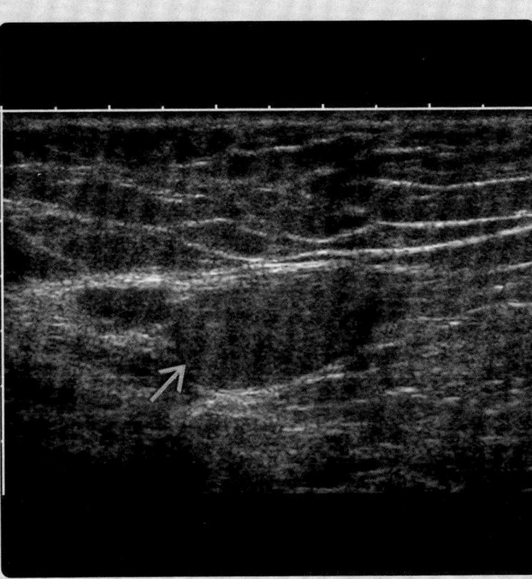

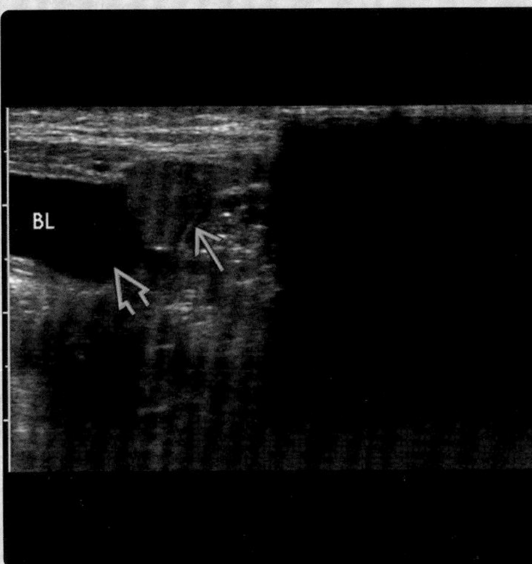

(Left) *Sagittal grayscale ultrasound demonstrates a shrunken, hypoechoic, atrophic testicle within the inguinal canal.* **(Right)** *Grayscale ultrasound demonstrates an intraabdominal testis in the left paravesical location. Note that BL stands for bladder.*

Epididymitis/Orchitis

KEY FACTS

TERMINOLOGY

- Inflammation of epididymis &/or testis

IMAGING

- Grayscale US
  - Epididymis enlarged and hypoechoic
  - Testes mildly heterogeneous
- Color Doppler US
  - Diffuse or focal hyperemia in body and tail of epididymis ± increased vascularity of testis
  - In severe cases can cause vascular compromise and ischemia or infarction
  - Reversal of arterial diastolic flow of testis is ominous finding associated with testicular infarction

TOP DIFFERENTIAL DIAGNOSES

- Testicular torsion
- Testicular lymphoma
- Testicular trauma

CLINICAL ISSUES

- Commonest cause of acute scrotal pain in adolescent boys and adults (15-35 years)
- Scrotal swelling, erythema; fever; dysuria
  - Scrotal pain due to epididymitis is usually relieved after elevation of testes (scrotum) over symphysis pubis (Prehn sign)
  - Associated lower urinary tract infection and its symptoms, urethral discharge

SCANNING TIPS

- Compare side by side with contralateral asymptomatic side with both color and power Doppler in single image
  - Avoid using dual image for side-by-side comparison
  - Suggested setting for color Doppler: 5 cm/s
- Head, body, and tail of epididymis should be carefully evaluated
- Use high-frequency transducers (9-15 MHz)

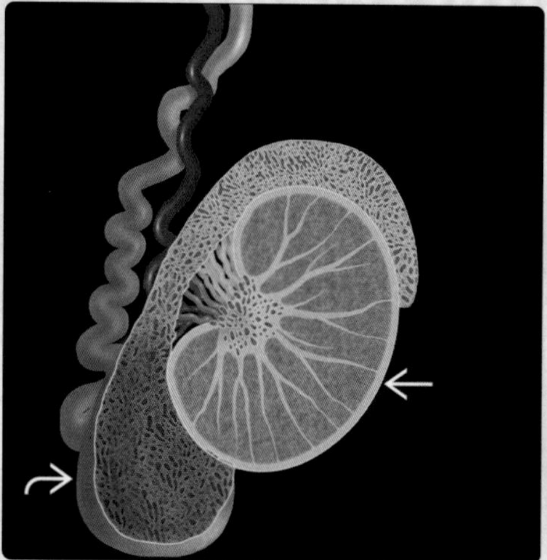

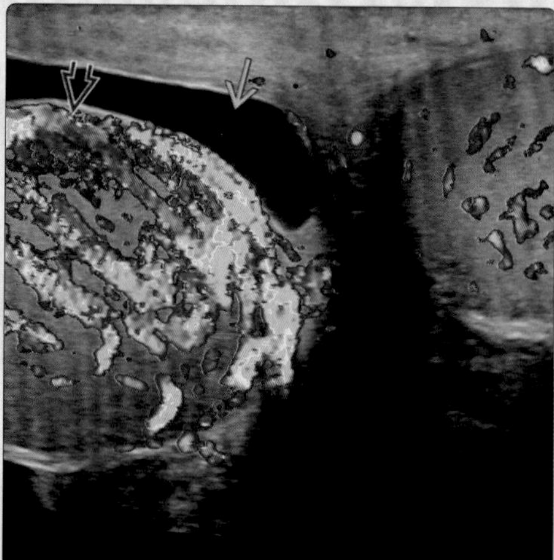

(Left) *Graphic shows an enlarged and inflamed epididymis ➡ enveloping the testis posteriorly. Note that the testis ➡ appears normal in size and configuration.* **(Right)** *Transverse side-by-side color Doppler view of the testes in a patient with right-sided epididymo-orchitis shows the right testicle is markedly hypervascular ➡ compared to the left, and there is a small right hydrocele ➡.*

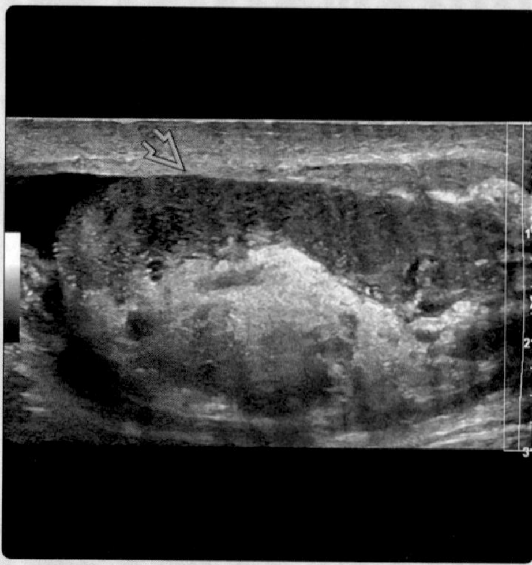

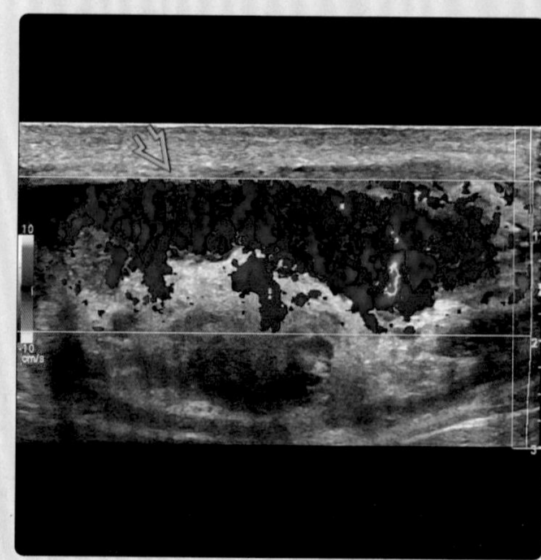

(Left) *Sagittal grayscale US of the right scrotum demonstrates a thickened heterogeneous and hypoechoic epididymis ➡.* **(Right)** *Color Doppler US of the epididymis in the same patient reveals marked hyperemia ➡ of the epididymis consistent with acute epididymitis.*

KEY FACTS

IMAGING

- Heterogeneous testicular parenchyma or contour abnormality of testis in setting of scrotal trauma
  - Disruption of tunica albuginea very specific for testicular rupture
- Extratesticular hematocele: Most common finding in scrotum after blunt injury
- US appearance of hematoma depends on time elapsed since trauma
- Intra- or extratesticular air in scrotum, missile track &/or foreign bodies (bullet/pellet) indicative of penetrating injury
- Spermatic cord hematoma appears as heterogeneous, avascular mass superior to testis
- Color Doppler useful to determine viable portions of testis

PATHOLOGY

- Sports injuries (> 50%), vehicular and ballistic trauma, and iatrogenic

CLINICAL ISSUES

- Unless repaired within 72 hours, salvage rate only 45%
- Follow-up of conservatively treated testicular hematomas essential due to increased risk of infection, which may result in orchiectomy
- Orchiectomy (total or partial) performed for nonviable testis in testicular rupture
- Surgical exploration and drainage must be performed for large, intratesticular hematomas

SCANNING TIPS

- Focal disruption of tunica albuginea = testicular rupture in setting of trauma

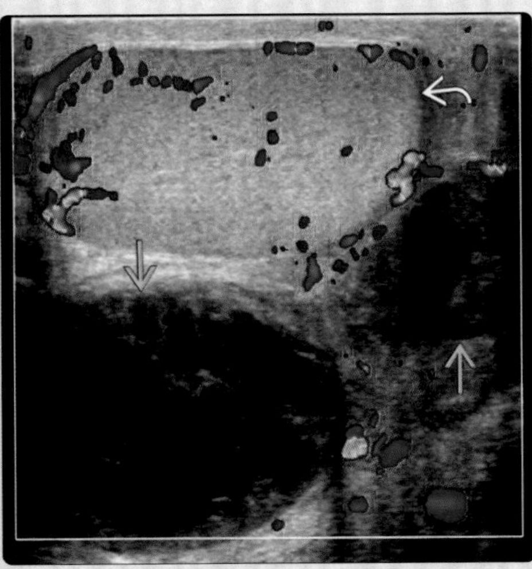

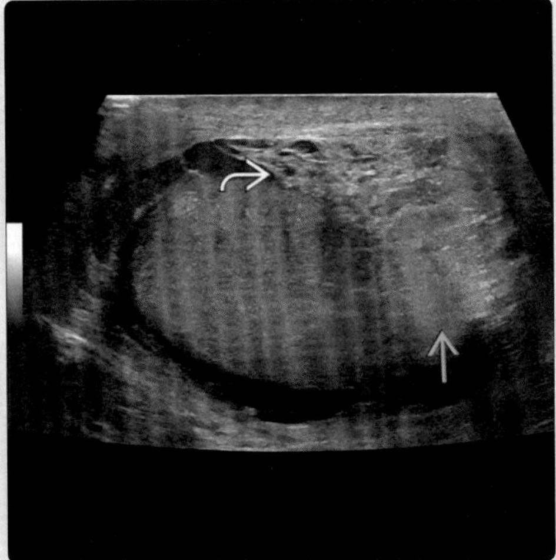

(Left) *Transverse color Doppler ultrasound of the scrotum demonstrates 2 large, extratesticular, avascular fluid collections (hematomas) ➡ in the scrotal cavity. The patient was status post recent vasectomy with new-onset scrotal swelling. Testis ➡ is normal.* **(Right)** *Sagittal ultrasound of the right testis after a MVC demonstrates heterogeneous testicular parenchyma ➡ with indistinct tunica albuginea and adjacent hematocele ➡. Surgery confirmed a testicular rupture.*

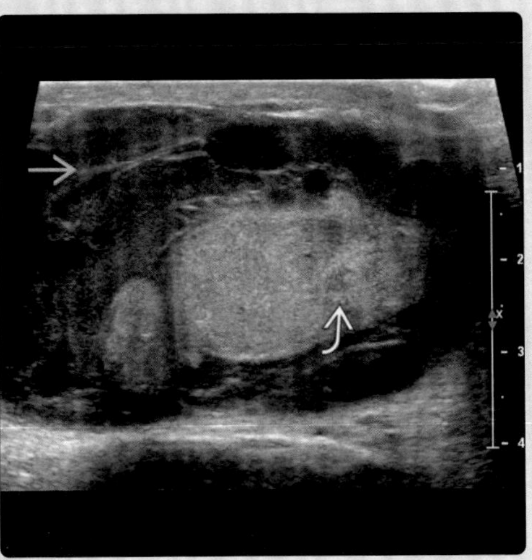

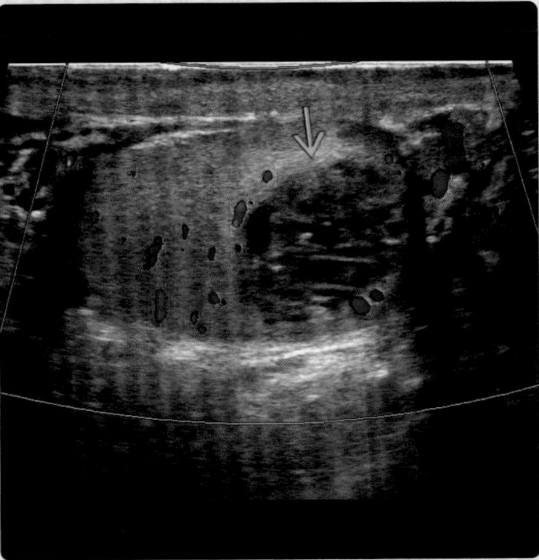

(Left) *Sagittal grayscale ultrasound of the right scrotal cavity shows a large, complex extratesticular fluid collection ➡, consistent with hematocele. Mildly heterogeneous testis ➡ is suggestive of contusion/hematoma.* **(Right)** *Color Doppler ultrasound of the right testis shows an avascular, complex fluid collection ➡, consistent with an intratesticular hematoma. The patient was continually followed until resolution of this hematoma.*

Hydrocele

KEY FACTS

TERMINOLOGY

- Congenital or acquired serous fluid contained within layers of scrotal tunica vaginalis

IMAGING

- Scrotal fluid surrounding testis, except for "bare area" where tunica vaginalis does not cover testis and is attached to epididymis
- Intrascrotal, external to testis and epididymis
- Specific anatomic location: Tunica vaginalis
- Simple or complex avascular fluid
- High-resolution US (9-15 MHz) is modality of choice

PATHOLOGY

- Congenital or communicating hydrocele is due to failure of processus vaginalis to close
- Secondary occurrence in adults due to epididymitis, trauma, surgery, or tumor
- Simple fluid collection within tunica vaginalis
- Chronic cases show thickened tunica with septation
- Complex fluid may be seen in acute infection or afterward
- Scrotal hematoma may be slow to resolve and manifest as complex collection

CLINICAL ISSUES

- Congenital hydroceles usually resolve by 18 months of age
- 25-50% of acquired hydroceles are associated with trauma
- 10% of testicular tumors have associated hydrocele

SCANNING TIPS

- Look for hydroceles along anterolateral aspect of testis
- Cholesterol crystals cause low-level mobile echoes and cannot be distinguished from inflammatory debris; beware of artifacts on color Doppler
- Scan with minimal pressure to visualize fluid overlying testis; too much pressure may compress scrotum and lead to underestimation of size of hydrocele

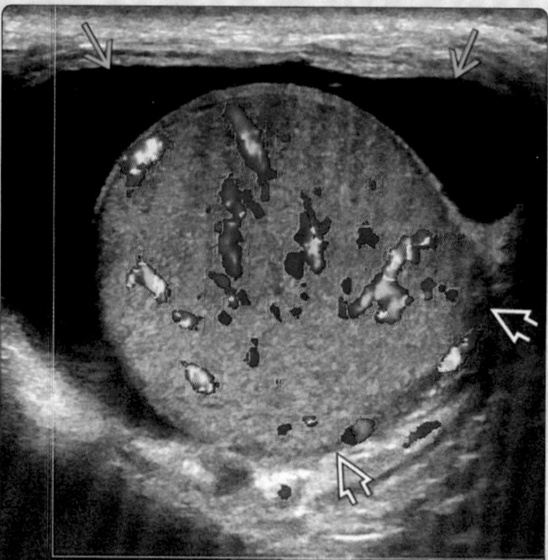

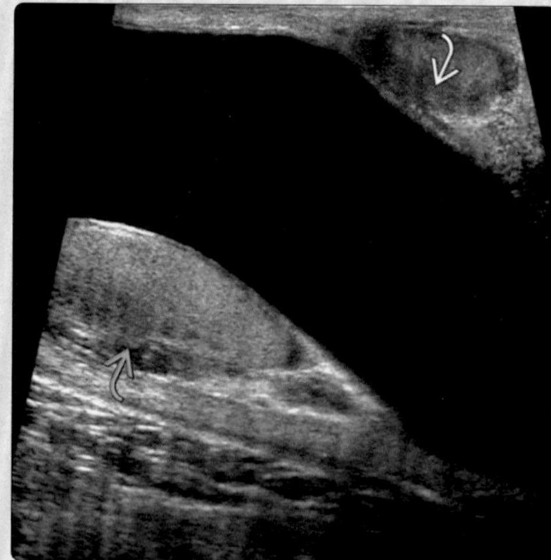

(Left) *Transverse color Doppler ultrasound shows simple-appearing fluid ➙ in a small hydrocele. Note that the fluid does not surround the testicle along the bare area ➙ where the tunica vaginalis does not cover the testicle and is attached to the epididymis.* **(Right)** *Massive simple hydrocele in a 90-year-old man compresses the right testis ➙ along the scrotal wall. The left testis ➙ is also visible in this image.*

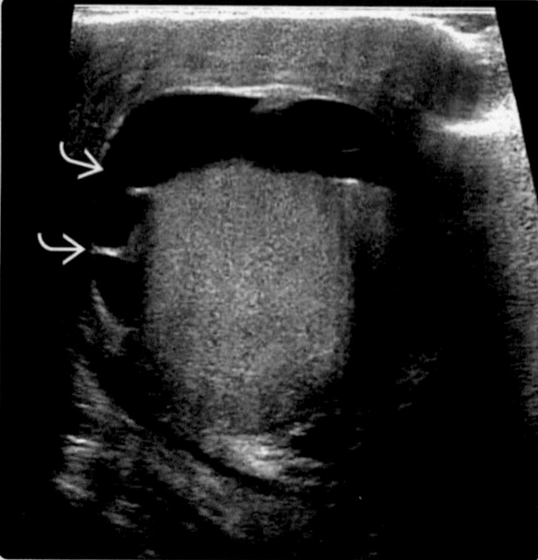

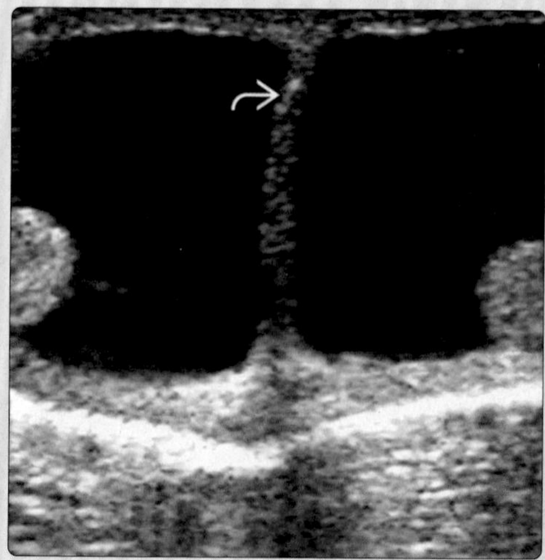

(Left) *Thin septations ➙ are shown within a minimally complex hydrocele in a patient with epididymo-orchitis.* **(Right)** *Transverse ultrasound in a newborn boy shows symmetrical hydrocele in both hemiscrotums with clear separation ➙ between right and left scrotal sac, characteristic of neonatal hydrocele.*

KEY FACTS

TERMINOLOGY

- Spermatocele: Retention cyst of rete testis or epididymis containing nonviable spermatozoa
- Epididymal head cyst: Collection of simple fluid

IMAGING

- Spermatoceles may contain linear septations and internal debris; low-level echoes due to spermatozoa
  - Falling snow sign: Mechanically moving particulate material within cyst due to acoustic radiation force from color Doppler
- Epididymal head cysts are anechoic, thin walled, and avascular

PATHOLOGY

- Etiology: Unknown, may reflect scarring secondary to either epididymitis, trauma, or vasectomy
- Associated abnormalities: Dilation of rete testis within mediastinum of testis

CLINICAL ISSUES

- Most common signs/symptoms: Painless scrotal mass
  - Rare hypofertility or torsion
- Treatment: Most can be observed if asymptomatic
  - Surgery (spermatocelectomy) only if sufficiently large to cause discomfort

DIAGNOSTIC CHECKLIST

- Cystic extratesticular lesions almost always benign; if no vascularized soft tissue elements, not neoplasm

SCANNING TIPS

- Look for acoustic streaming of nonviable spermatazoa in spermatoceles with both grayscale and color or power Doppler to elicit falling snow sign

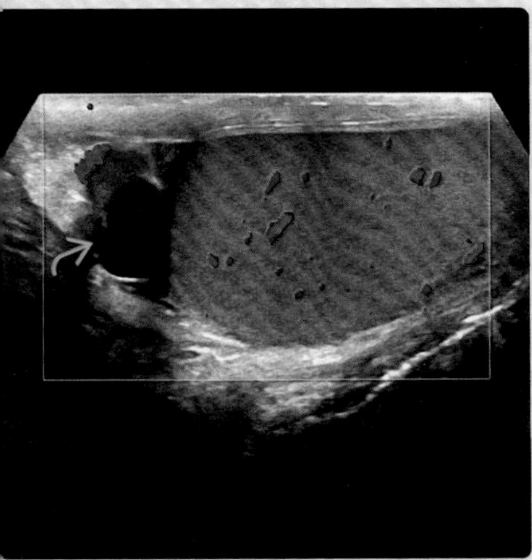

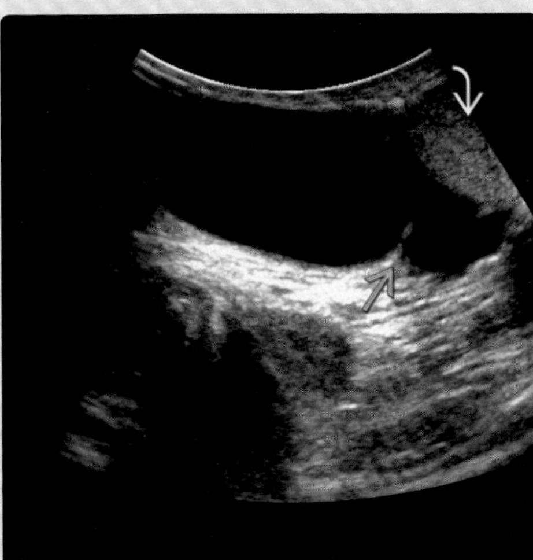

(Left) *Typical appearance of an incidentally discovered and clinically unimportant epididymal cyst is shown. Note the well-circumscribed, anechoic, avascular lesion* ➢ *in the epididymal head.* **(Right)** *Large epididymal cyst (calipers) is shown with a single thin septation* ➢ *in the right hemiscrotum, displacing the testis* ➡ *inferiorly. Note that the abdominal probe, rather than the high-frequency linear probe, was needed to capture this large lesion.*

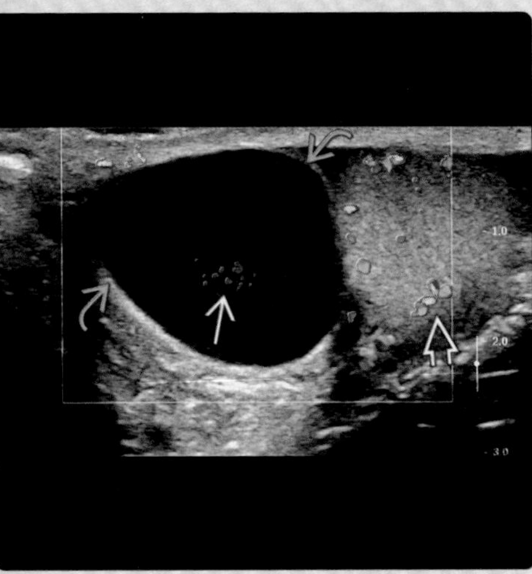

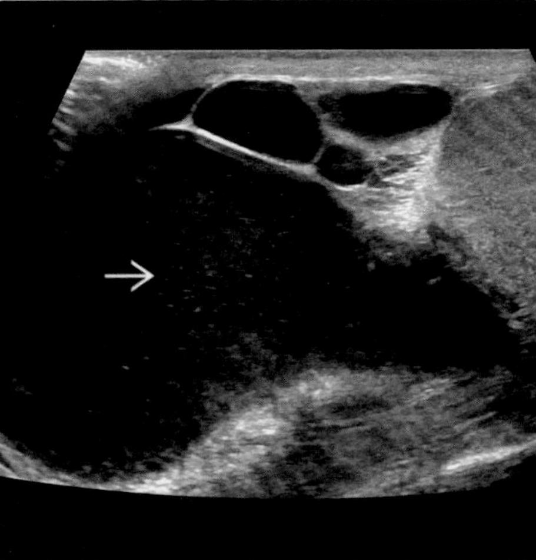

(Left) *Large spermatocele* ➢ *superior to the right testis* ➡ *contains punctate low-level echoes with corresponding Doppler artifact* ➡*. These punctate foci were mobile in real time.* **(Right)** *Longitudinal grayscale ultrasound demonstrates a complex, multiseptate cystic mass with numerous locules containing debris* ➡*, characteristic findings for a spermatocele.*

Adenomatoid Tumor

KEY FACTS

TERMINOLOGY

- Benign, solid paratesticular tumor of mesenchymal origin

IMAGING

- Solid intrascrotal mass, usually extratesticular
- Rounded or oval, well circumscribed, varying echogenicity
- Size: 5 mm to 5 cm
- Hypovascular or avascular on color Doppler US
- Location
  - Epididymis: Most common location overall
  - May arise in tunica albuginea
  - Rarely intratesticular or other locations, such as spermatic cord and prostate

TOP DIFFERENTIAL DIAGNOSES

- Leiomyoma
- Lipoma
- Cystadenoma

CLINICAL ISSUES

- Most common solid mass in epididymis
  - 36% of all paratesticular tumors
- Slowly enlarges over years
- Most surgically excised to confirm diagnosis
- Some urologists and patients elect surveillance
- Age: 20 years and older
  - Mean: 36 years
  - Rarely seen in boys

SCANNING TIPS

- Gentle transducer pressure may show mass can move independently of testis
- Small adenomatoid tumors of epididymis may be easily missed and, therefore, full visualization of head, body, and tail of epididymis is important on all routine scrotal exams

(Left) *This palpable hypoechoic adenomatoid tumor ➔ located in the in tail of the epididymis in a 41-year-old man has no demonstrable internal vascularity.* **(Right)** *This 50-year-old man had 5 years of ultrasound surveillance for a presumed adenomatoid tumor. This ovoid, well-circumscribed mass ➔ in the tail of the epididymis is isoechoic to testis and shows minimal internal vascularity ➔. Note the very different echogenicity compared to the otherwise similar patient shown previously.*

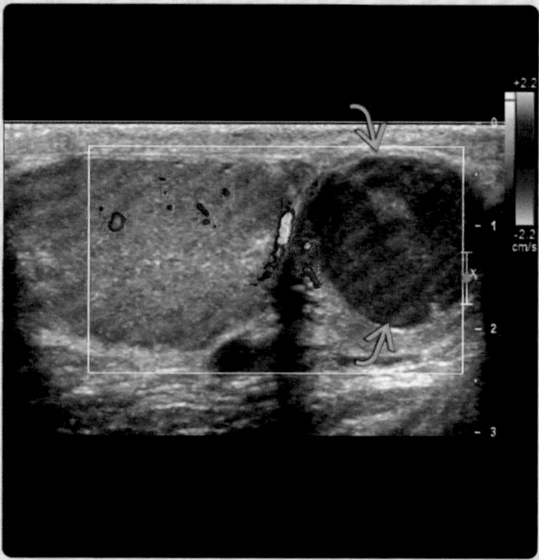

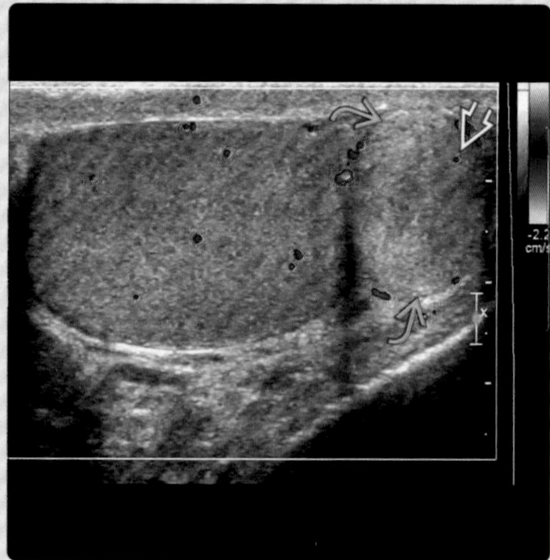

(Left) *This hyperechoic ovoid adenomatoid tumor ➔ in the tail of the epididymis was an incidental finding in a 37-year-old man.* **(Right)** *This adenomatoid tumor of the tunica albuginea ➔ was incidentally noted on a pelvic MR in a 12-year-old boy. The lesion is equally endophytic and exophytic to the testis, as it is centered in the tunica. Note minimal internal vascularity.*

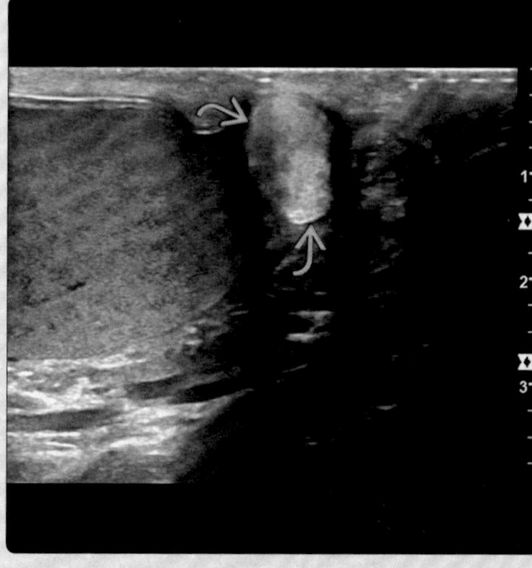

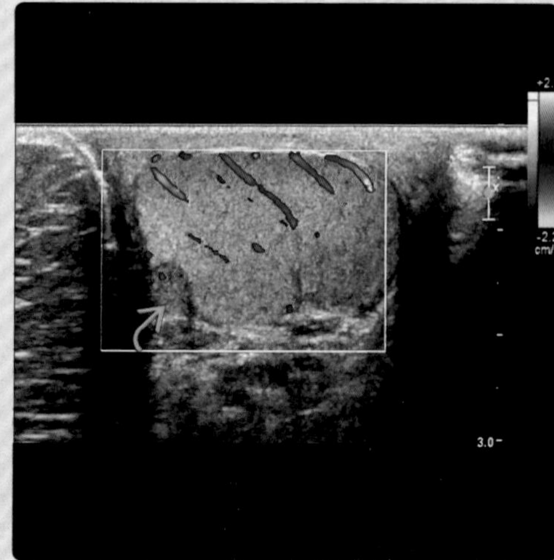

Varicocele

KEY FACTS

TERMINOLOGY

- Dilatation of pampiniform plexus > 2-3 mm due to congestion and retrograde flow in internal spermatic vein

IMAGING

- Dilated serpiginous veins at superior pole of testis
- "Flash" of color Doppler with Valsalva
- Left (78%), right (6%), bilateral (16%)
- Varicose veins > 2-3 mm diameter, increase in size with Valsalva

PATHOLOGY

- Primary: Incompetent venous valve near junction of left renal vein (LRV) and IVC
- Secondary: Obstruction of LRV by renal or adrenal tumor, nodes or rarely SMA compression

CLINICAL ISSUES

- Most frequent cause of male infertility
- Vague scrotal discomfort or pressure when standing
- 10-15% of men in USA have varicoceles
- Subclinical varicocele in 40-75% of infertile men
- Emerging research suggests even subclinical varicoceles should be treated

SCANNING TIPS

- Unilateral and left-sided varicoceles common; isolated right-sided varicoceles uncommon and should prompt evaluation along IVC to exclude mass
- Valsalva with color Doppler essential for diagnosis of small varicoceles
- Measure diameter of vein on grayscale; blooming artifact on color Doppler will obscure true diameter and lead to overestimation of diameter
- Measure vein from inner wall to inner wall
- Avoid mistaking vas deferens as dilated vein
- Varicoceles usually lie superior to testicle but may lie posterior or lateral to testicle

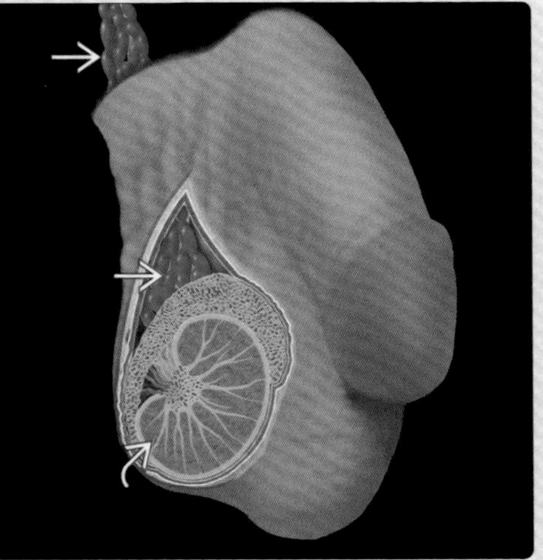

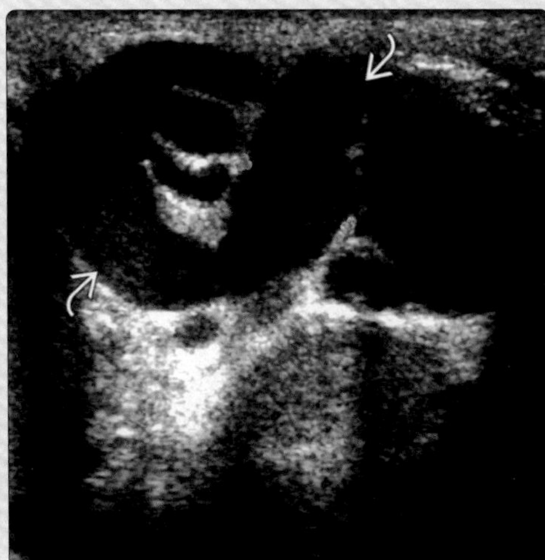

(Left) *Graphic shows dilated, tortuous varicose veins of the pampiniform plexus ➡ in the spermatic cord and along the posterosuperior aspect of the testis ➡.* **(Right)** *Oblique grayscale ultrasound through cord, in supine position with normal respiration, shows a dilated, tortuous principal vein ➡ in pampiniform plexus measuring 7.5 mm in caliber.*

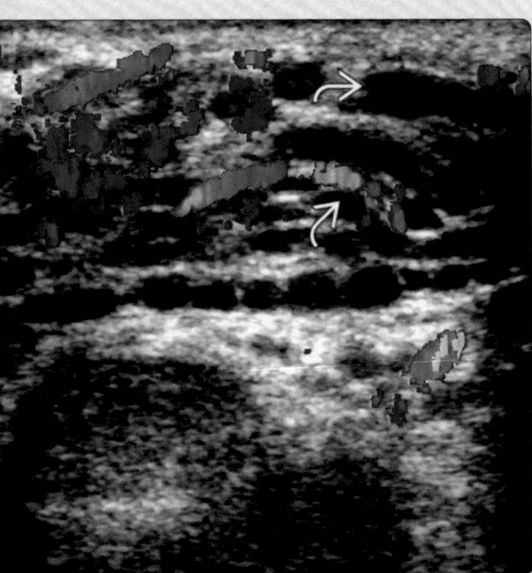

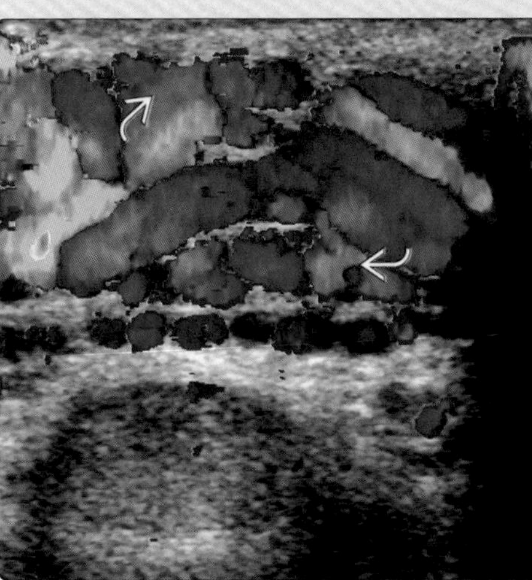

(Left) *Longitudinal color Doppler ultrasound shows multiple serpiginous, dilated veins ➡ in the pampiniform plexus of the cord, along the posterosuperior aspect of testis in supine position during normal respiration.* **(Right)** *Longitudinal color Doppler ultrasound in the same patient shows flow ➡ in these dilated veins during Valsalva, indicative of moderate varicocele. Blood flow in the varicocele is slow and may be detected only with low Doppler settings.*

Prostatic Hyperplasia

KEY FACTS

TERMINOLOGY

- Benign prostatic hyperplasia (BPH)
  - Term reserved for histopathologic pattern of smooth muscle and epithelial cell proliferation
  - Hyperplasia correct term since BPH is characterized by increased number of epithelial stromal cells in periurethral area of prostate (not hypertrophy, which means increase in size)

IMAGING

- Sonographic appearance of BPH variable, depending on histopathologic changes
- Ultrasound cannot reliably differentiate BPH from prostate cancer
- Ultrasound may be used to measure prostate size and PVR as well as evaluate for upper tract obstruction in men with BPH and renal insufficiency
- Estimated prostate volume: Prolate ellipsoid formula: Width x height x length x π/6 = W x H x L x 0.52

TOP DIFFERENTIAL DIAGNOSES

- Prostate, bladder carcinoma
- Prostatitis

PATHOLOGY

- Bladder outlet obstruction from BPH may occur from urethral constriction from increased smooth muscle tone and resistance (dynamic component) &/or urethral compression from gland enlargement (static component)
- Possible bladder sequelae: Trabeculation, diverticula, calculi, detrusor muscle failure
- Possible upper tract changes: Ureterectasis, hydronephrosis
  - Can be from 2° vesicoureteral reflux, obstruction from muscular hypertrophy or angulation at ureterovesical junction, sustained high-pressure bladder storage

SCANNING TIPS

- Avoid including seminal vesicles in transabdominal prostate measurements

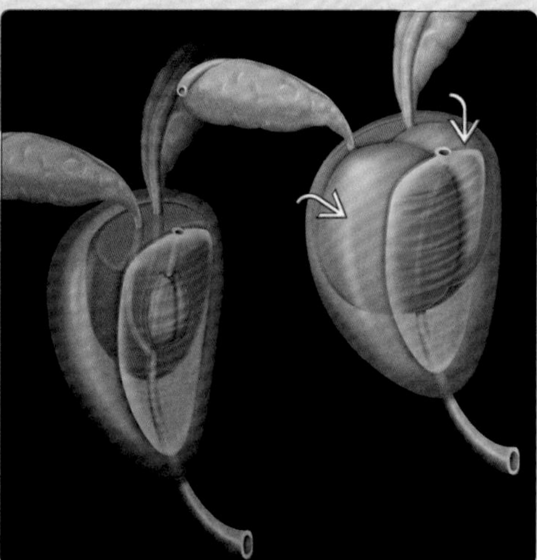

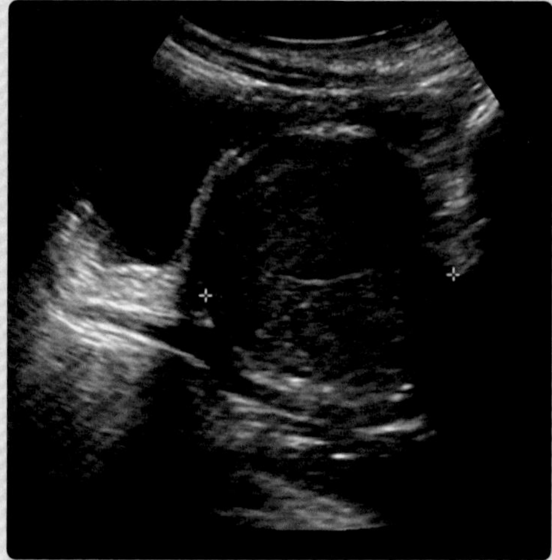

(Left) *Graphic shows a normal (left) and hyperplastic (right) prostate gland with enlargement of the transition zone (TZ) (blue ➔) surrounding the urethra. Central zone is in orange, peripheral zone is in green, and anterior fibromuscular stroma is in yellow.* **(Right)** *Sagittal transabdominal ultrasound of the enlarged prostate shows nodular enlargement of the TZ and compressed, more hyperechoic TZ.*

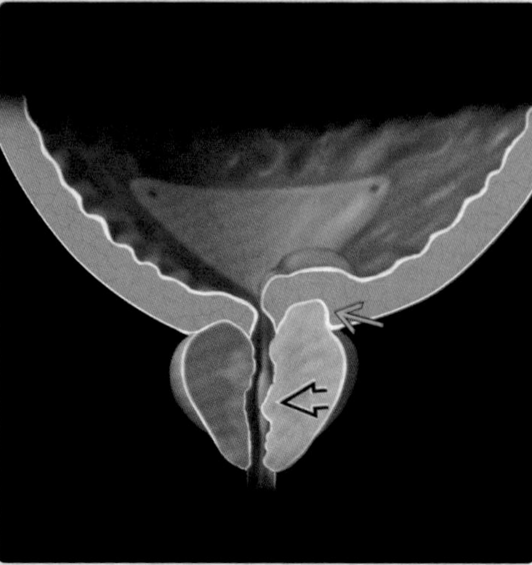

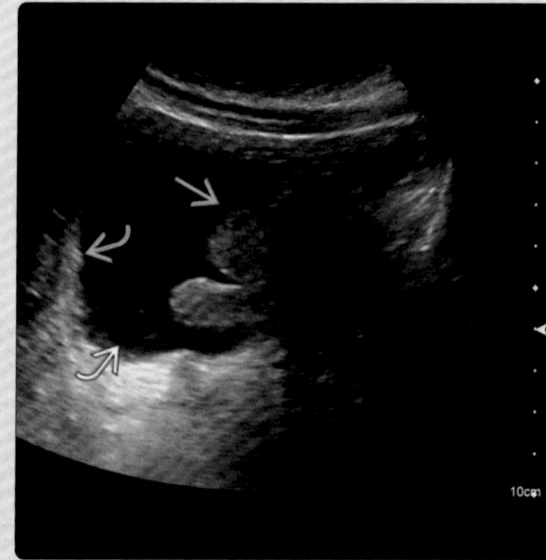

(Left) *Nodular enlargement of the periurethral glands and TZ cause external compression of the prostatic urethra ➔ and elevation of the bladder base ➔. Nodular protrusion into the bladder (a.k.a. enlarged "median lobe") can ball-valve into the urethra and cause severe obstructive symptoms.* **(Right)** *Sagittal US shows the "median lobe" of BPH protruding into the bladder base lumen ➔, which may simulate a polypoid bladder mass. Thickening of bladder wall ➔ and low-level intraluminal echoes ➔ are due to urinary tract infection.*

KEY FACTS

IMAGING

- Grayscale US
  - Prostate carcinoma (PCa) can appear as hypoechoic (60-70%), isoechoic/invisible (30-40%), rarely hyperechoic ± asymmetric capsular bulging or irregularity
- Color Doppler US
  - PCa may be hypervascular; however, absence does not exclude cancer, and other benign entities (e.g., prostatitis) may also be hypervascular
- Transrectal US (TRUS) is imaging of choice to guide biopsy in evaluation for PCa but performs poorly in cancer detection and staging
- Calculate prostate volume using largest cross-sectional image in transverse and mid sagittal planes: Transverse x AP x long x 0.52
- MR imaging
  - Most sensitive imaging technique for PCa diagnosis and staging
  - Peripheral zone (PZ): T2 dark lesion with restricted diffusion; transition zone (TZ): Erased charcoal sign on T2WI
  - Targeted MR-guided and MR/US fusion-guided biopsy is promising for increasing detection of high-risk prostate cancer while reducing detection of low-risk cancer compared with standard biopsy

PATHOLOGY

- Most common noncutaneous malignancy in western world, 2nd most common cause of cancer deaths among men
- 95% of tumors are acinar adenocarcinoma
- Staging based on tumor-node-metastasis staging, prostate specific antigen at time of diagnosis, and Gleason score
- Location of prostate cancer: PZ: 70-80%, TZ: 20%, central zone: 1-5%

SCANNING TIPS

- Although classically PCa is hypoechoic on grayscale US, > 30-40% PCa may be invisible on TRUS

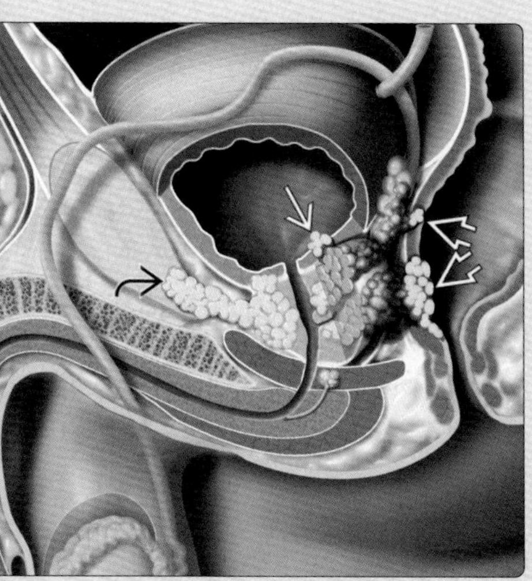

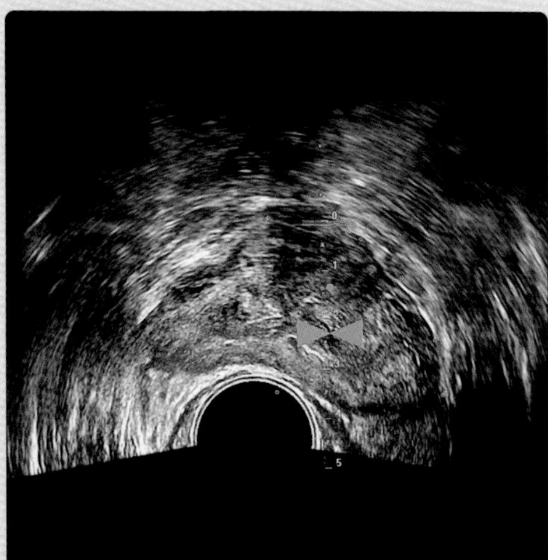

(Left) *Longitudinal graphic shows advanced prostatic carcinoma (PCa) with extracapsular spread to the adjacent pelvic structures, such as the bladder ➡, rectal wall ➡, and symphysis pubis ➡.* **(Right)** *Transverse transrectal US (TRUS) shows a hypoechoic lesion (outlined in red) within the left transition zone. Pathology from a targeted MR/US fusion biopsy showed Gleason 4 + 5 adenocarcinoma.*

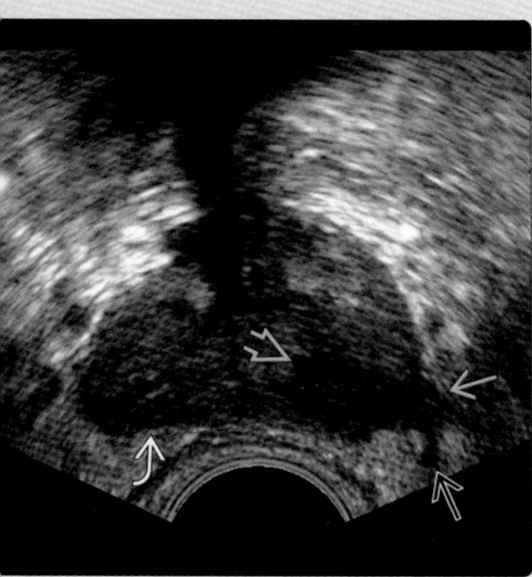

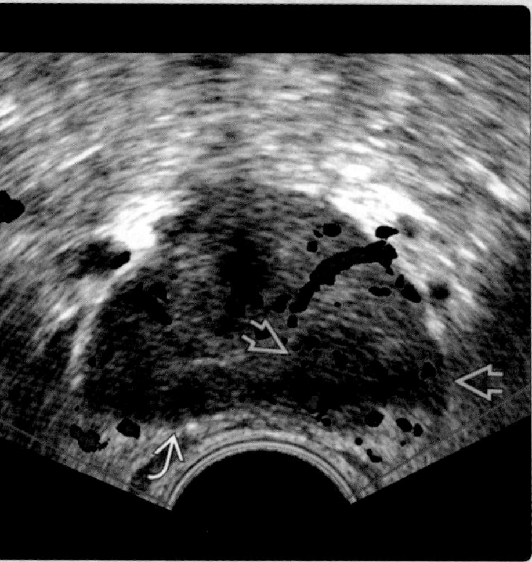

(Left) *Transverse TRUS shows a hypoechoic left PZ lesion ➡ with capsular bulging and nodularity extending into the adjacent fat ➡ and left neurovascular bundle ➡. A smaller hypoechoic lesion is seen in the right PZ ➡.* **(Right)** *Corresponding Doppler US shows focal hypervascularity ➡ in the left PZ lesion. The right PZ lesion is mildly hypervascular ➡. Prostatectomy revealed multifocal PCa, including Gleason 5 + 5 adenocarcinoma with left extraprostatic extension and lymphovascular and perineural invasion.*

PART II

SECTION 2

Female Pelvis

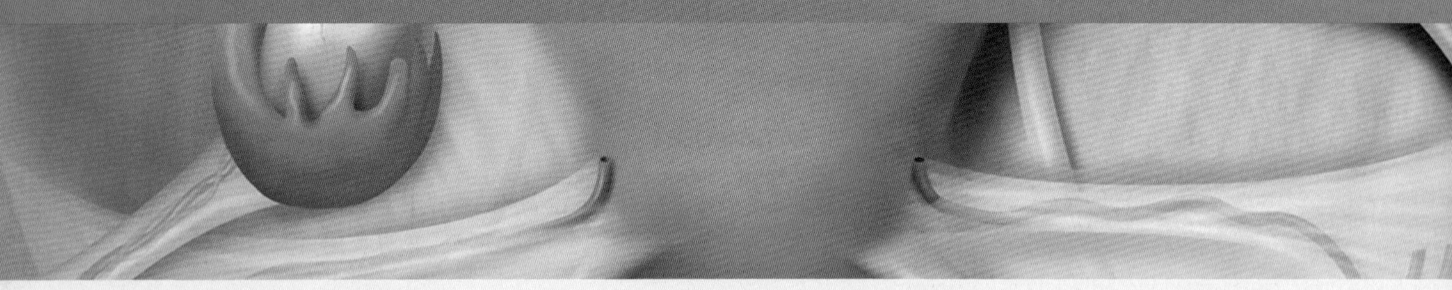

Anatomy and Approach

Cervical and Myometrial Pathology

Endometrial Disorders

Ovarian Cysts and Cystic Neoplasms

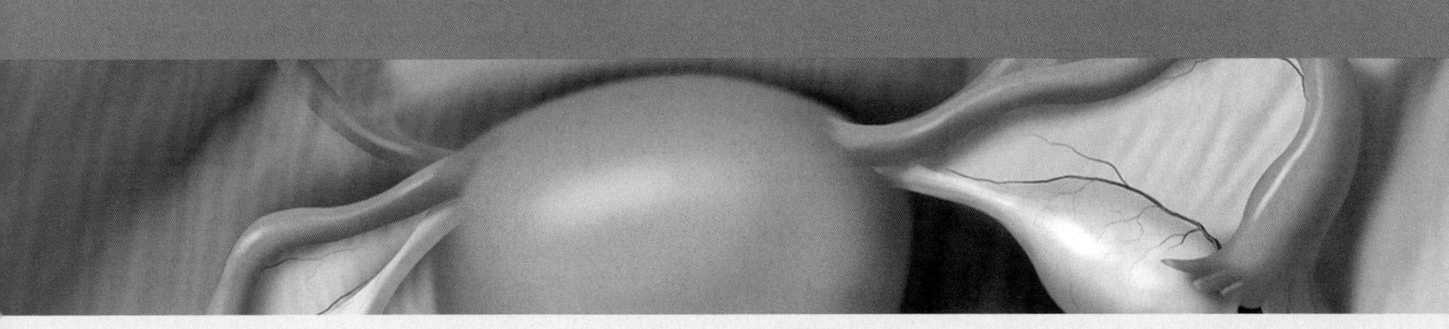

Nonovarian Cystic Masses

Vaginal and Vulvar Cysts

Miscellaneous Ovarian Masses

GROSS ANATOMY

Overview

- **Body (corpus)**: Upper 2/3 of uterus
  - Fundus: Superior to ostia of fallopian tubes
- **Cervix**: Lower 1/3 of uterus
  - Isthmus: Junction of body and cervix
- **Parametrium**: Tissue immediately surrounding uterus
- **Myometrium**: Smooth muscle forming bulk of uterus
- **Endometrium**: Composed of 2 layers
  - Stratum basalis attached to myometrium, does not change
  - Stratum functionalis: Thicker, varies with cycle
- Uterus is extraperitoneal in midline of true pelvis
- Uterine position
  - **Flexion** is axis of uterine body relative to cervix
  - **Version** is axis of cervix relative to vagina
  - Anteversion ± anteflexion is most common
- Peritoneum extends over bladder dome anteriorly and rectum posteriorly
  - **Vesicouterine pouch (anterior cul-de-sac)**: Anterior recess between uterus and bladder
  - **Rectouterine pouch of Douglas (posterior cul-de-sac)**: Posterior recess between vaginal fornix and rectum; most dependent portion of peritoneum in female pelvis
- **Supporting ligaments**
  - Broad ligaments: Extend laterally to pelvic wall and form supporting mesentery for uterus
  - Round ligaments: Arise from uterine cornu and course through inguinal canal to insert on labia majora
  - Uterosacral ligaments (posteriorly), cardinal ligaments (laterally), and vesicouterine ligaments (anteriorly) form from connective tissue thickening by cervix
- **Fallopian tubes** connect uterus to peritoneal cavity
  - 4 segments: Interstitial (portion going through myometrium at cornua), isthmus, ampulla, infundibulum
- **Arteries**: Dual blood supply
  - Uterine artery (UA) arises from internal iliac artery, anastomoses with ovarian artery
    - UA crosses over the ureter and enters uterus just above cervix
  - Arcuate arteries arise from UAs; seen in outer 1/3 of myometrium → radial arteries → spiral arteries (endometrium)

Uterine Variations With Age

- Neonatal: Prominent size secondary to effects of residual maternal hormone stimulation
- Infantile: Corpus < cervix (1:2)
- Prepubertal: Corpus = cervix (1:1)
- Reproductive: Corpus > cervix (2:1)
  - 7.5-9.0 cm (length); 4.5-6.0 cm (width); 2.5-4.0 cm (thickness)
- Postmenopausal: Overall reduction in size, similar to prepubertal uterus

IMAGING ANATOMY

Myometrium

- Inner layer (junctional zone): Thin and hypoechoic, < 12 mm
- Middle layer: Thick, homogeneously echogenic
- Outer layer: Thin, hypoechoic layer peripheral to arcuate vessels

Endometrium

- **Proliferative phase (follicular phase of ovary)**
  - Cessation of menses to ovulation (up to day 14)
  - Estrogen induces proliferation of functionalis layer
  - Early: Thin, single echogenic line
  - Progressive hypoechoic thickening (4-8 mm), classic trilaminar appearance
- **Secretory phase (luteal phase of ovary)**
  - Ovulation to beginning of menstrual phase (days 14-28)
  - Increased echogenicity and progressive thickening up to 16 mm
- **Menstrual phase**
  - Early: Cystic areas within echogenic endometrium indicating endometrial breakdown
  - Progressive heterogeneity with mixed cystic (blood) and hyperechoic (clot or sloughed endometrium) regions

Imaging Recommendations

- Start with transabdominal exam, typically using curved low-frequency transducer
  - Gives "lay of the land"
    - Large lesions, particularly exophytic fibroids, may be much better seen transabdominally
  - Bladder should be partially full to push small bowel away and create an acoustic window
- With rare exception (young virginal females), **transvaginal exam** should be performed for more detail
  - Sweep completely through uterus in both longitudinal and transverse planes
  - Angle probe posteriorly to evaluate cul-de-sac
    - Most dependent portion so free fluid and other peritoneal pathology implants in this area
  - Gently push on probe to show uterus slides easily over bowel (**sliding sign**)
    - Adhesions (e.g., endometriosis) causes organs to be fixed
- Measure uterus in all 3 dimensions and document all myometrial lesions
- Entire length of endometrium needs to be evaluated in sagittal (longitudinal) plane
  - Measure thickest point perpendicular to endometrial stripe
  - If fluid is in the canal, measure each side separately and add measurements together
- Color and pulsed-wave Doppler should be performed on any suspicious lesions
- 3D ultrasound additive in many cases, particularly müllerian duct (duplication) anomalies and intrauterine device evaluation
  - 3D volume data sets are acquired and can be manipulated to show optimal projection
  - May also slice through data set creating individual images similar to CT
  - Perform at beginning of transvaginal scan before bladder starts to refill
- Sonohysterography, with infusion of saline into endometrial cavity, may be used to evaluate endometrial pathology
  - Polyps vs. submucosal fibroid, hyperplasia, carcinoma

UTERUS

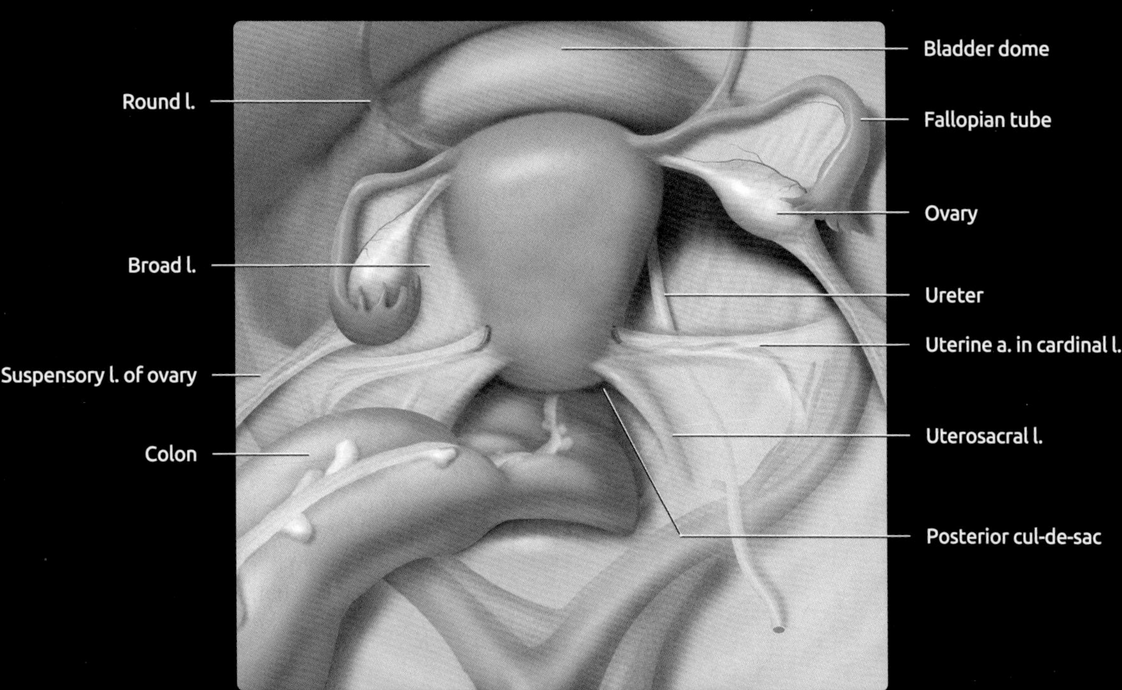

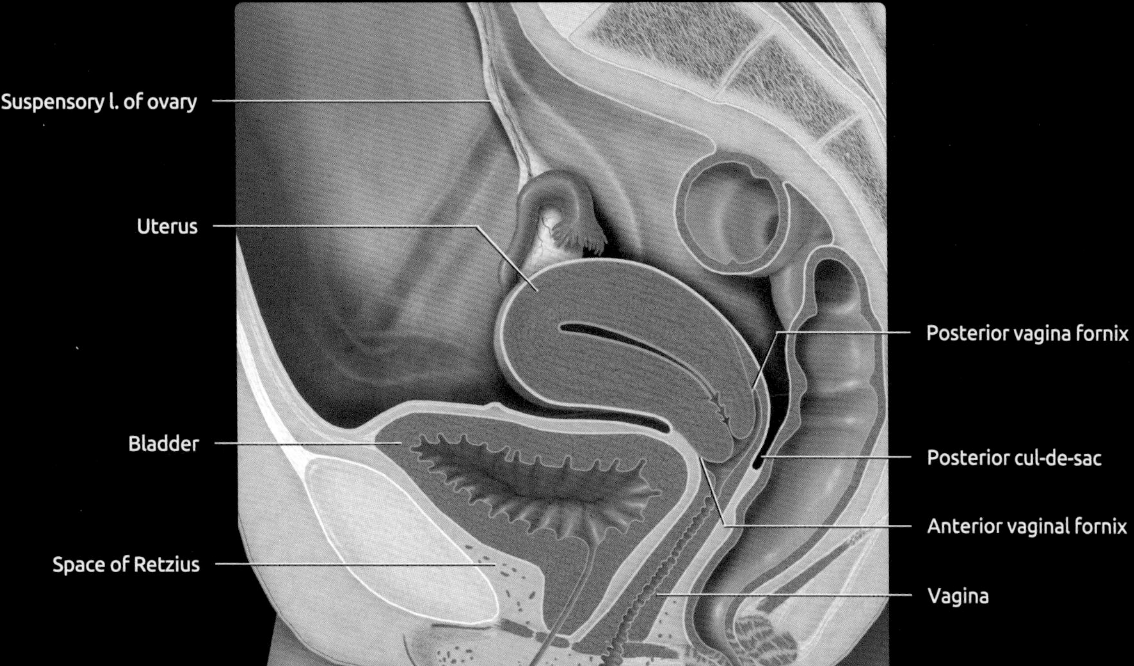

(Top) *Uterus viewed in situ from above and behind shows its positioning and major ligaments. The uterus is covered by a sheet of peritoneum, creating a double layer (the broad ligament), which sweeps laterally to attach to the pelvic wall. Areas of thickening at its base are the cardinal ligaments, which attach to the lateral pelvic wall, and the uterosacral ligaments, which attach to the sacrum. The uterosacral ligaments form the lateral borders of the posterior cul-de-sac (rectouterine pouch or pouch of Douglas). The round ligaments arise from the cornu of the uterus and course anteriorly to pass through the inguinal canal and insert on the labia majora.* **(Bottom)** *Sagittal graphic of the female pelvis shows the bladder, uterus, and rectum, all of which are extraperitoneal. Note the posterior vaginal fornix extends more cephalad than the anterior vaginal fornix, and the posterior cul-de-sac is the most dependent portion of the peritoneal cavity. Always look in the cul-de-sac for free fluid or masses from intraperitoneal pathology.*

NORMAL VARIATIONS, UTERINE POSITION

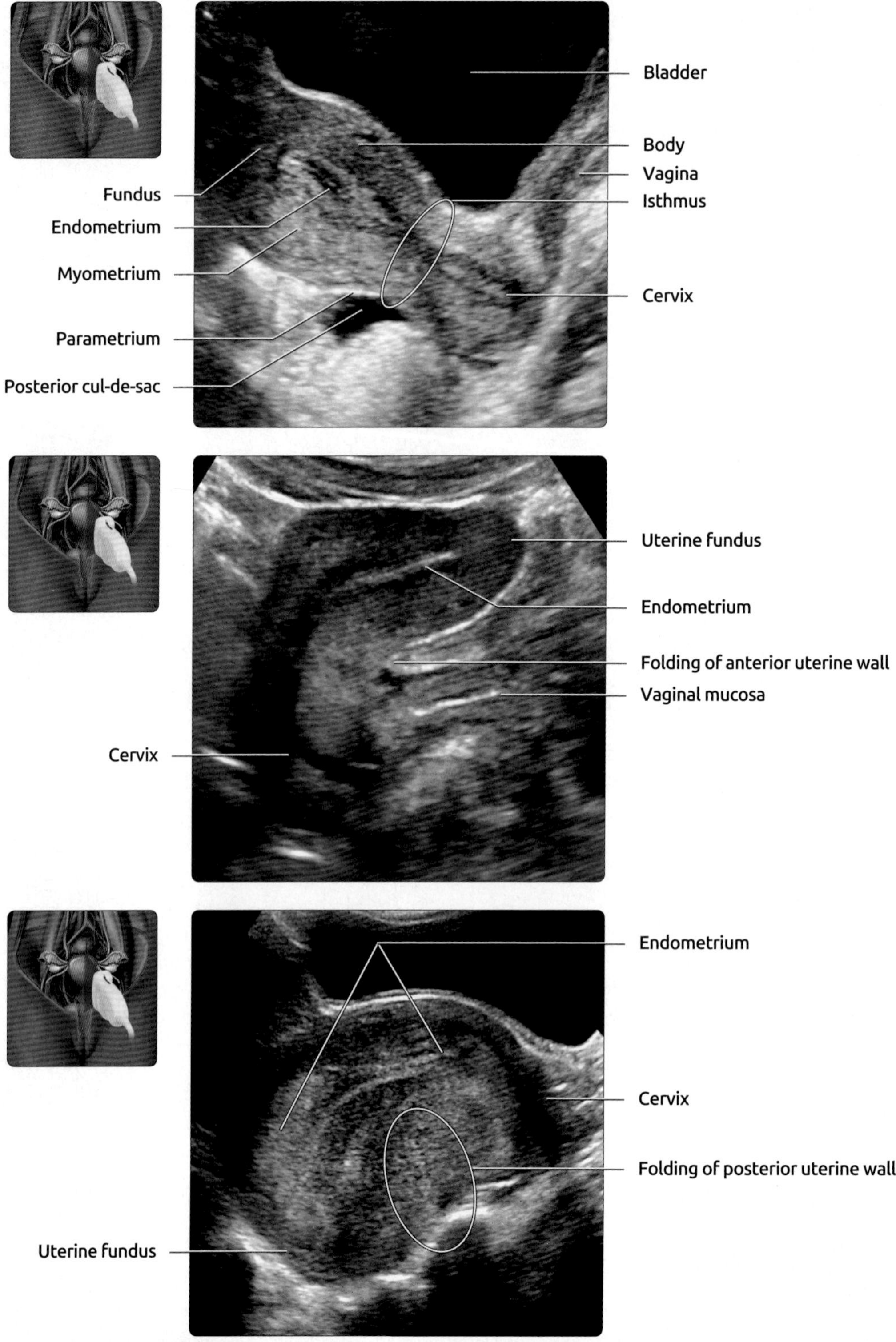

(Top) *Longitudinal transabdominal (TA) ultrasound shows a normal anteverted uterus. Version refers to the angle the cervix makes with the vagina. In this case, the cervix is angled anteriorly, and the uterus continues in a straight line with the cervix. This is the most common position found in the female pelvis.* **(Middle)** *Longitudinal TA ultrasound of an anteverted, anteflexed uterus shows the uterine cervix is angled forward with respect to the vagina, and the uterine body is angled forward with respect to the cervix. Version refers to the angle of the cervix relative to the vagina. Flexion refers to the angle of the uterine body relative to the cervix, i.e., the uterus and the cervix are not in a straight line.* **(Bottom)** *Uterine retroflexion is shown. This is an anteverted uterus with exaggerated retroflexion in which the uterus resembles a boxing glove. Folding of the posterior uterine wall may be confused with an intramural fibroid.*

3D UTERUS

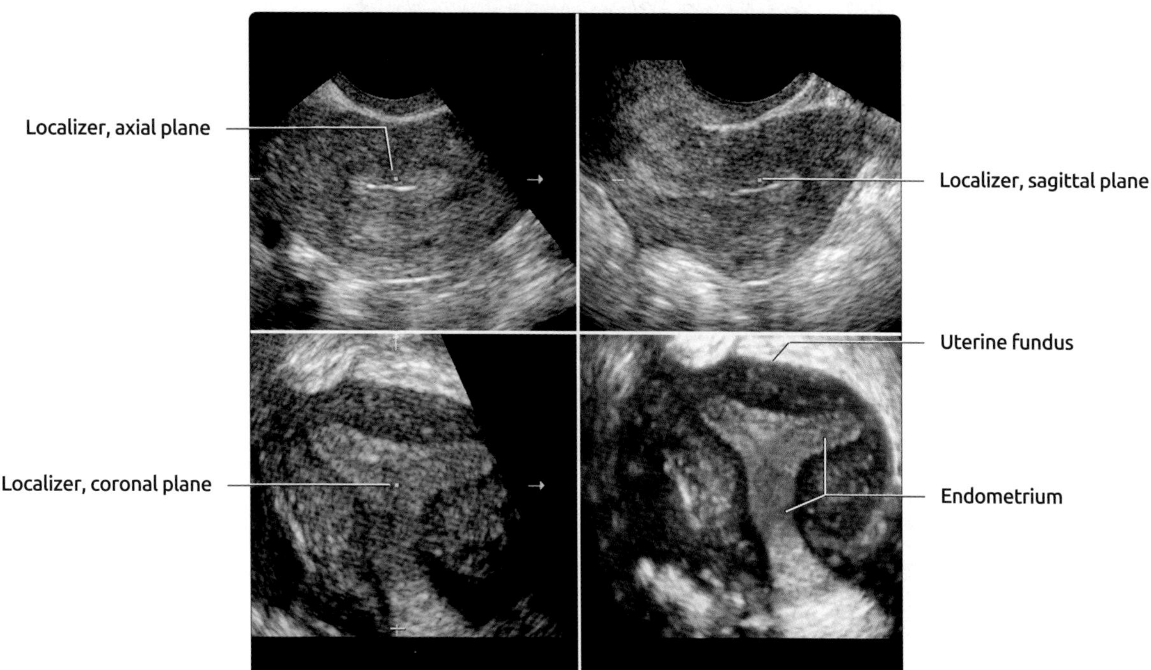

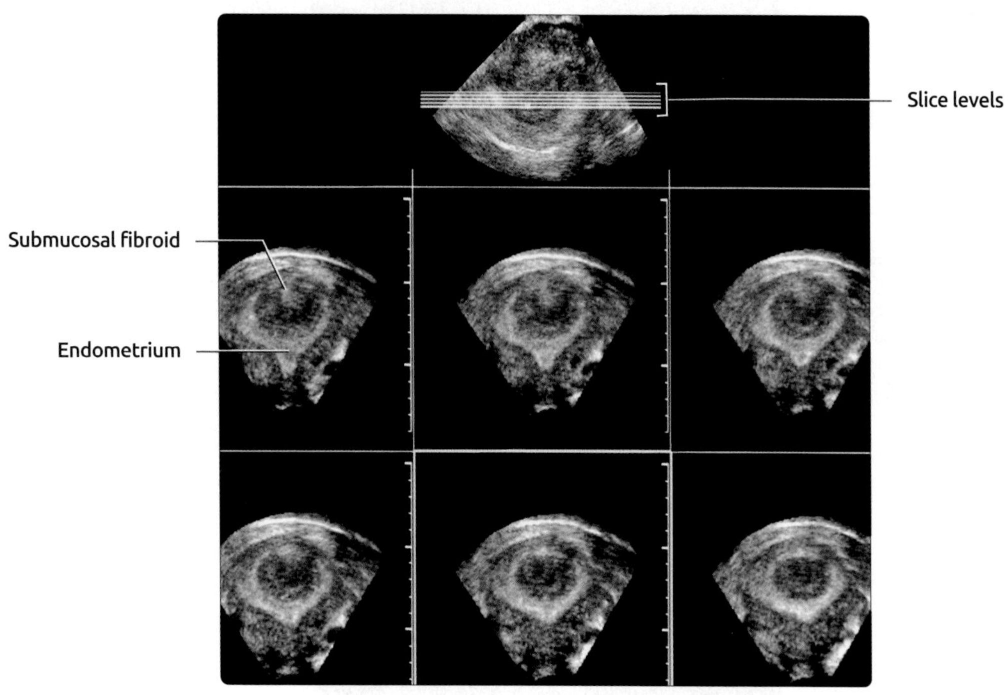

(Top) *This set of images shows a 3D data set of a normal uterus. A dedicated 3D ultrasound probe provides automated acquisition of a volume data set. This data is displayed in 3 simultaneous orthogonal planes. A central localizer point on each image allows the operator to know the precise location in all 3 planes and manipulate the image to the optimal projection. In the coronal image, the entire endometrial and fundal contours are displayed. This has particular utility in evaluating müllerian duct anomalies.* **(Bottom)** *3D data sets can be manipulated and sliced through like a CT or MR. This shows a set of 6 slices through a submucosal fibroid, which is projecting into the endometrial cavity. The lines on the localizer image on top correspond to slices below (the yellow line indicates the level of the image in the yellow box).*

CYCLIC CHANGES OF ENDOMETRIUM

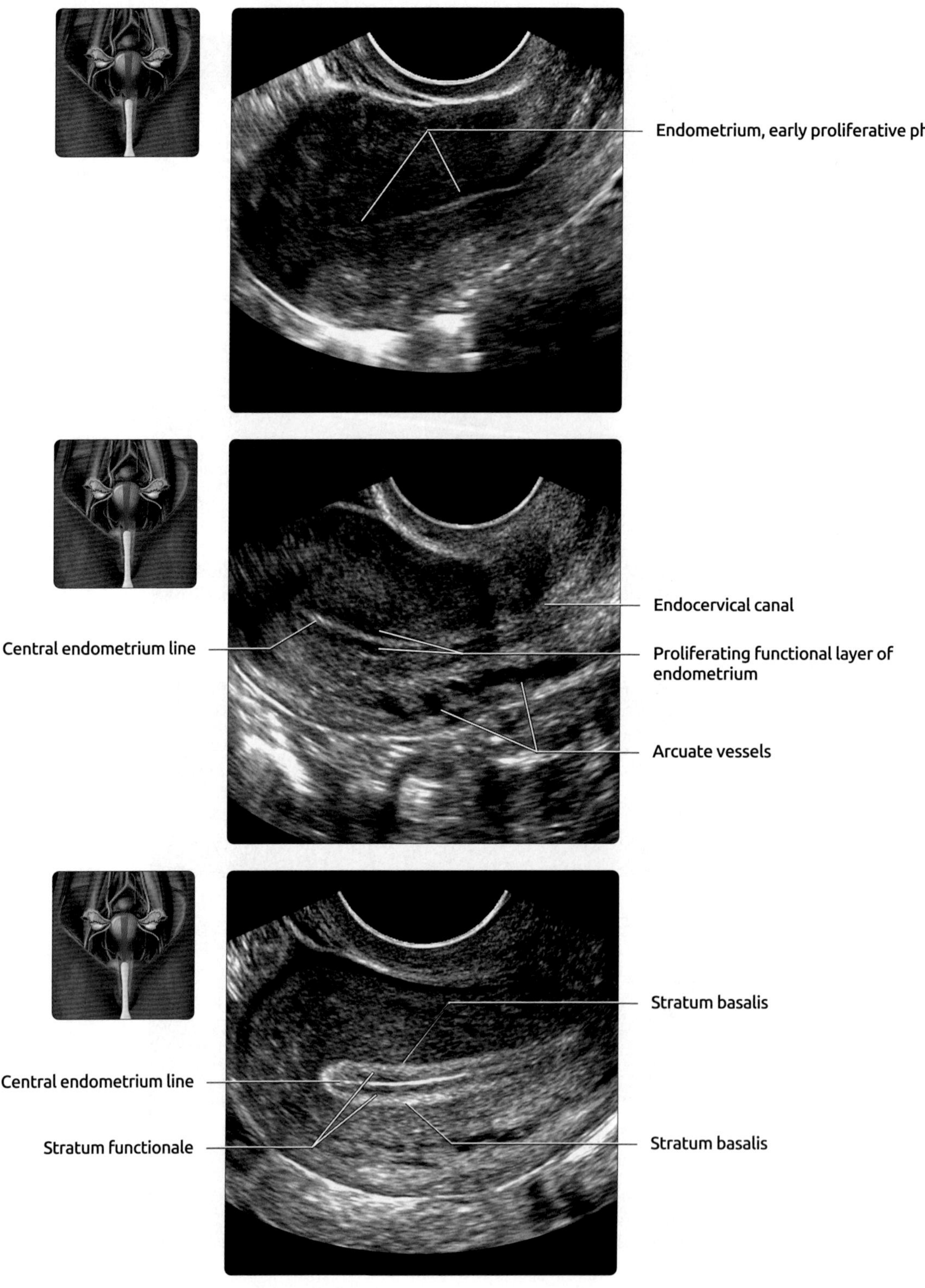

(Top) *Longitudinal transvaginal (TV) ultrasound shows the endometrium in the immediate postmenstrual, early proliferative phase. Note the endometrium is thin and echogenic.* **(Middle)** *Longitudinal TV ultrasound of the endometrium during mid proliferative phase shows the endometrium progressively thickened and slightly more echogenic.* **(Bottom)** *Longitudinal image of the endometrium in the periovulatory phase shows thickening of the stratum functionalis with an echogenic central line where the 2 walls coapt and a more echogenic basalis layer where the endometrium attaches to the myometrium. This classic layered, trilaminar appearance is seen around ovulation (~ day 14 of cycle).*

CYCLIC CHANGES OF ENDOMETRIUM

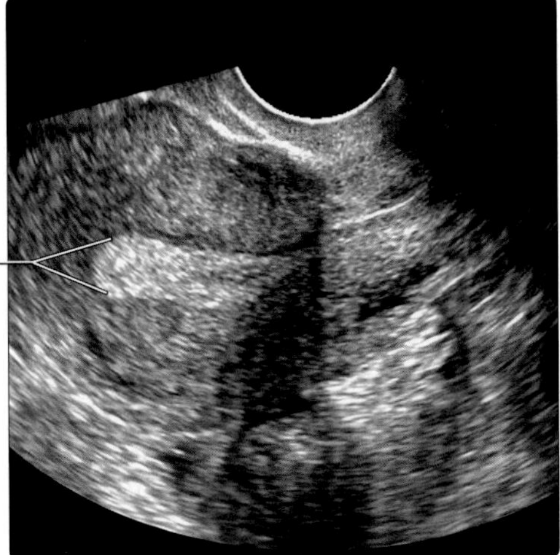

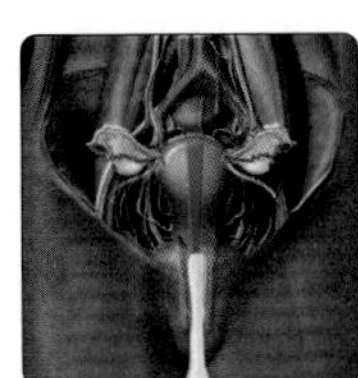

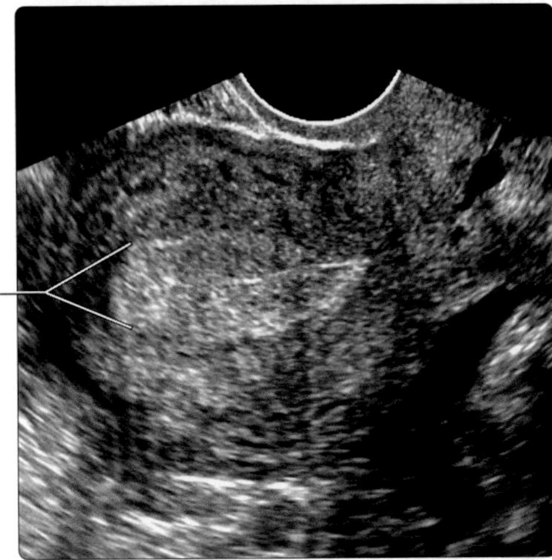

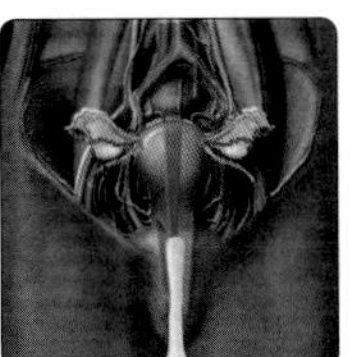

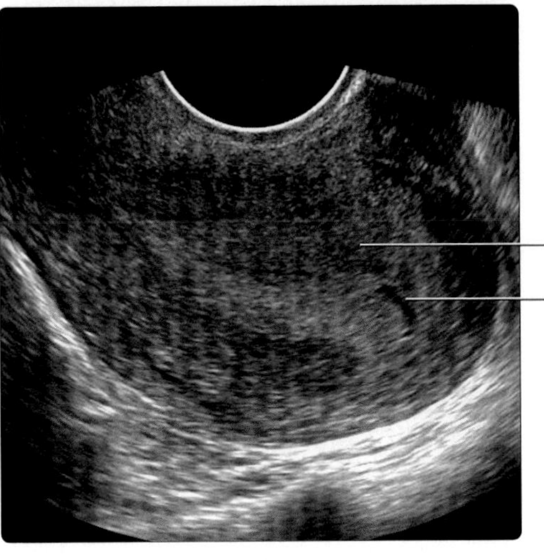

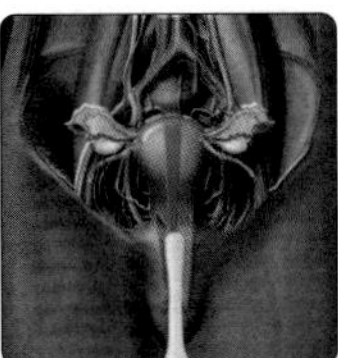

(Top) *Longitudinal TV ultrasound shows the endometrium during the early secretory phase. The endometrium becomes progressively thickened and more echogenic with loss of the trilaminar appearance.* **(Middle)** *Longitudinal TV ultrasound in the late secretory phase shows the endometrium is uniformly thickened and echogenic. The normal maximal endometrial thickness should not exceed 1.6 cm, through transmission can sometimes be visualized secondary to the mucus-filled glands.* **(Bottom)** *Longitudinal TV ultrasound shows a thickened endometrium just prior to menstruation. Echogenicity has decreased and is more heterogeneous than in the secretory phase. A small amount of fluid can be seen within the endometrial cavity.*

UTERINE VARIATIONS WITH AGE

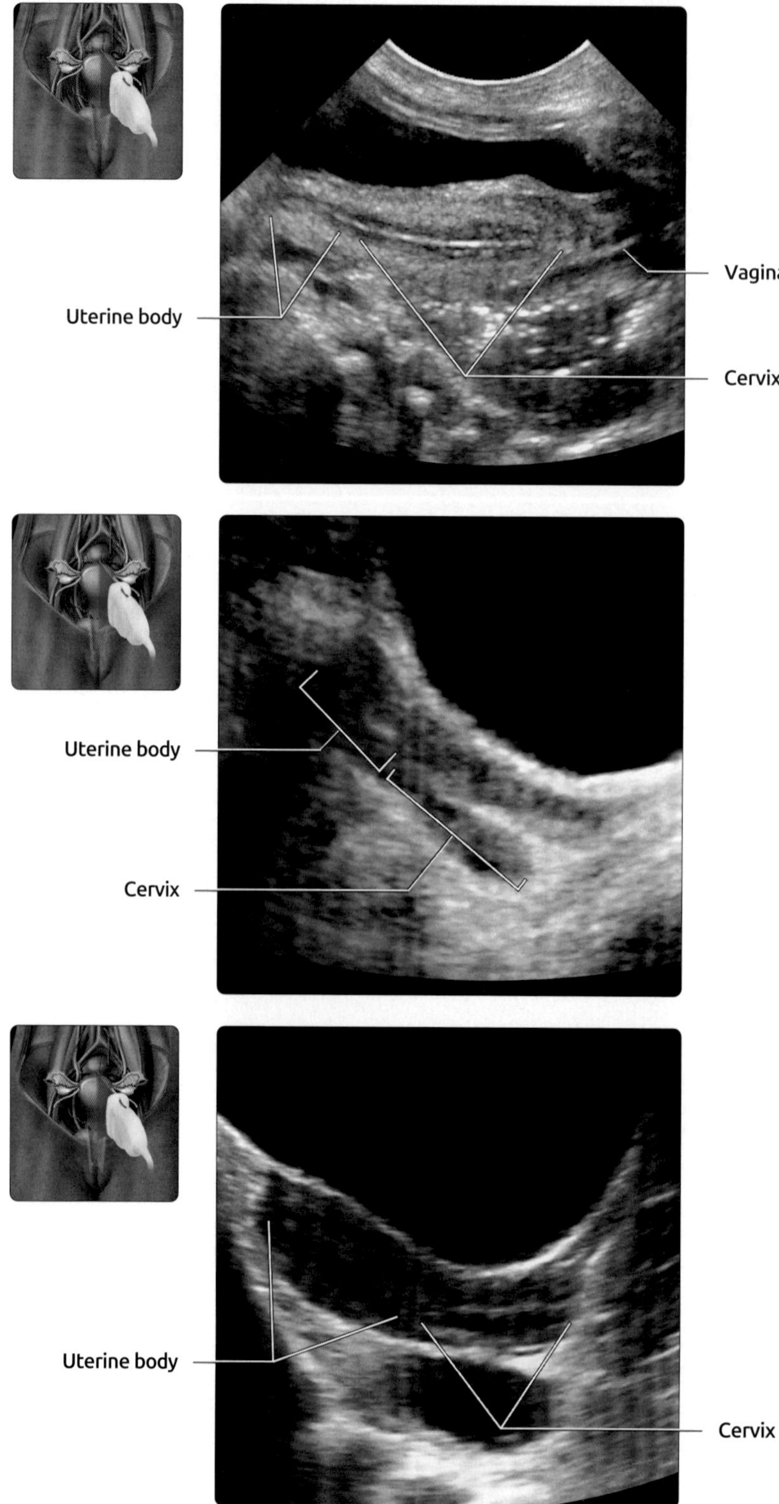

(Top) *Longitudinal TA ultrasound shows neonatal uterus on day 2 of life. The uterus is often well visualized secondary to the stimulation by the residual maternal hormones. The cervix is long and bulbous with a small uterine body. The endometrium is seen as a thin, echogenic line.* **(Middle)** *Longitudinal TA ultrasound shows a prepubertal uterus in an 8-year-old girl. The uterus demonstrates a tubular appearance with the length of the cervix nearly double that of the uterine body.* **(Bottom)** *Longitudinal TA ultrasound shows an early pubertal uterus in a 12-year-old girl. The body length of the uterus approximates the cervical length with the endometrium, changing in appearance and thickness during the menstrual cycle. At this time, the uterine body grows dramatically until it reaches the adult size.*

UTERINE VARIATIONS WITH AGE

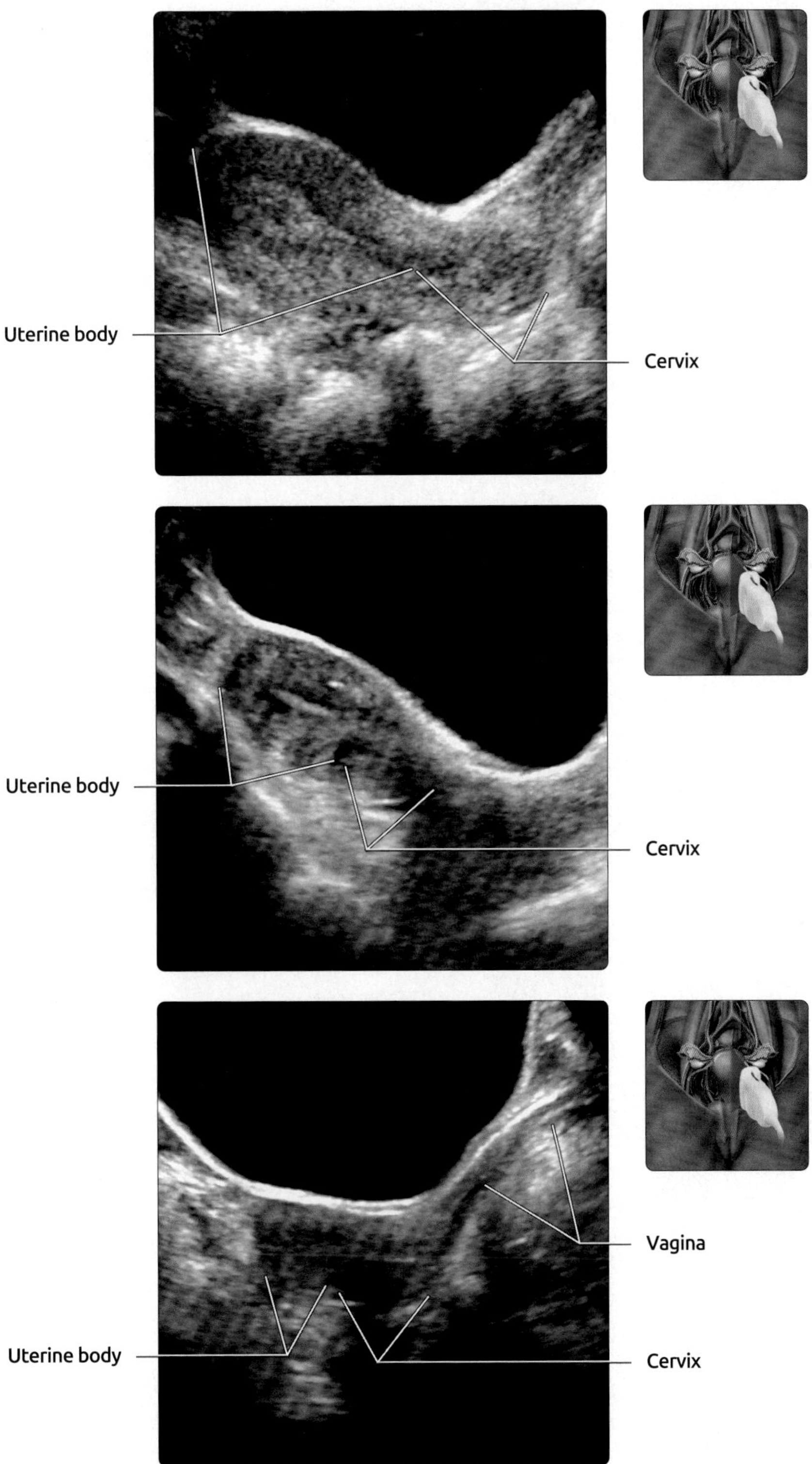

(Top) *Longitudinal TA ultrasound shows a nulliparous uterus. The normal adult uterus should attain a pear-shaped or hourglass appearance with the length of the uterine body double that of the cervix. The size of a nulliparous uterus is usually smaller than that of a parous uterus.* **(Middle)** *Longitudinal TA ultrasound shows an early postmenopausal uterus, which is undergoing atrophy with prominent reduction in body size relative to the cervix.* **(Bottom)** *Longitudinal TA ultrasound shows a later postmenopausal uterus. Note that the cervix:body ratio is similar to that of a prepubertal uterus.*

UTERINE VASCULAR SUPPLY

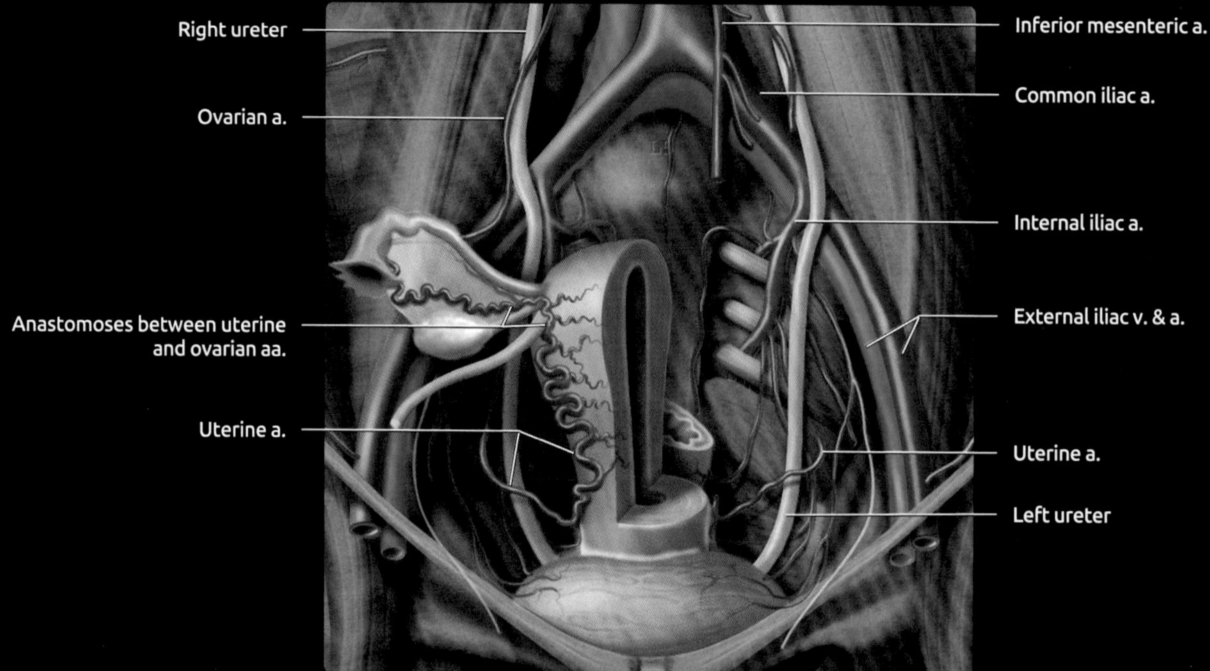

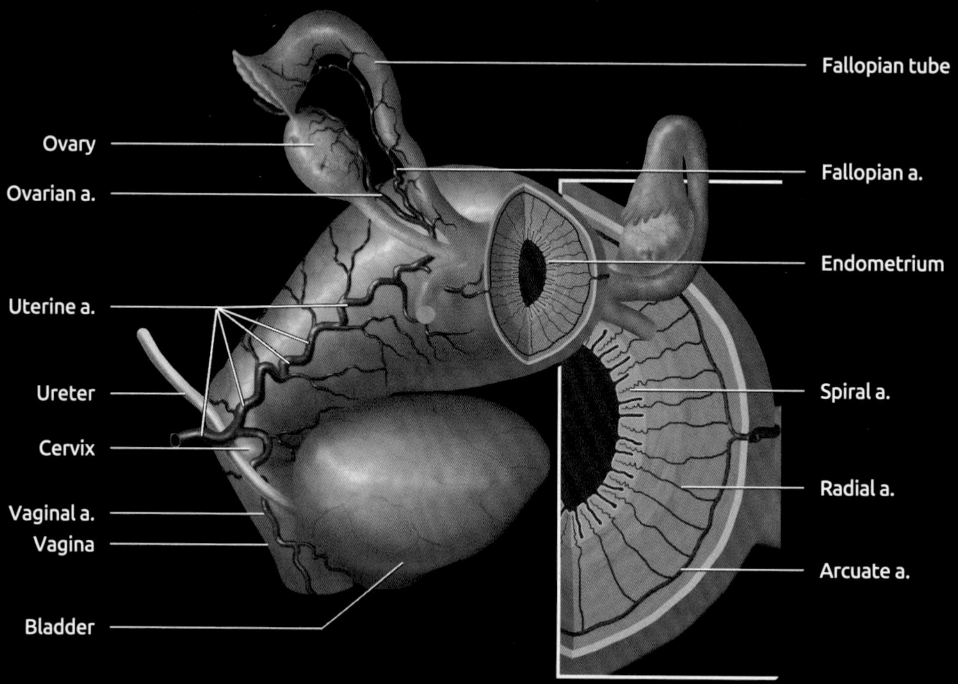

(Top) *Frontal graphic shows the arterial supply to the pelvis. The uterus has a dual blood supply with contributions from both the uterine and ovarian arteries. The ovarian artery originates from the aorta, and the uterine artery is a branch off the anterior trunk of the internal iliac artery.* **(Bottom)** *Graphic shows a more detailed vein of the uterine arterial supply. The uterine artery passes over the ureter to the uterus near the cervix. It ascends along the lateral margin of the uterus, giving off the arcuate arteries, and forms anastomoses with the ovarian artery near the fundus. The arcuate arteries and the their accompanying veins travel in the outer third of the myometrium and may be quite prominent on ultrasound. The arcuate arteries give rise to the radial arteries, which penetrate the myometrium and run vertically, terminating as the spiral arteries of the endometrium.*

UTERINE VASCULAR SUPPLY

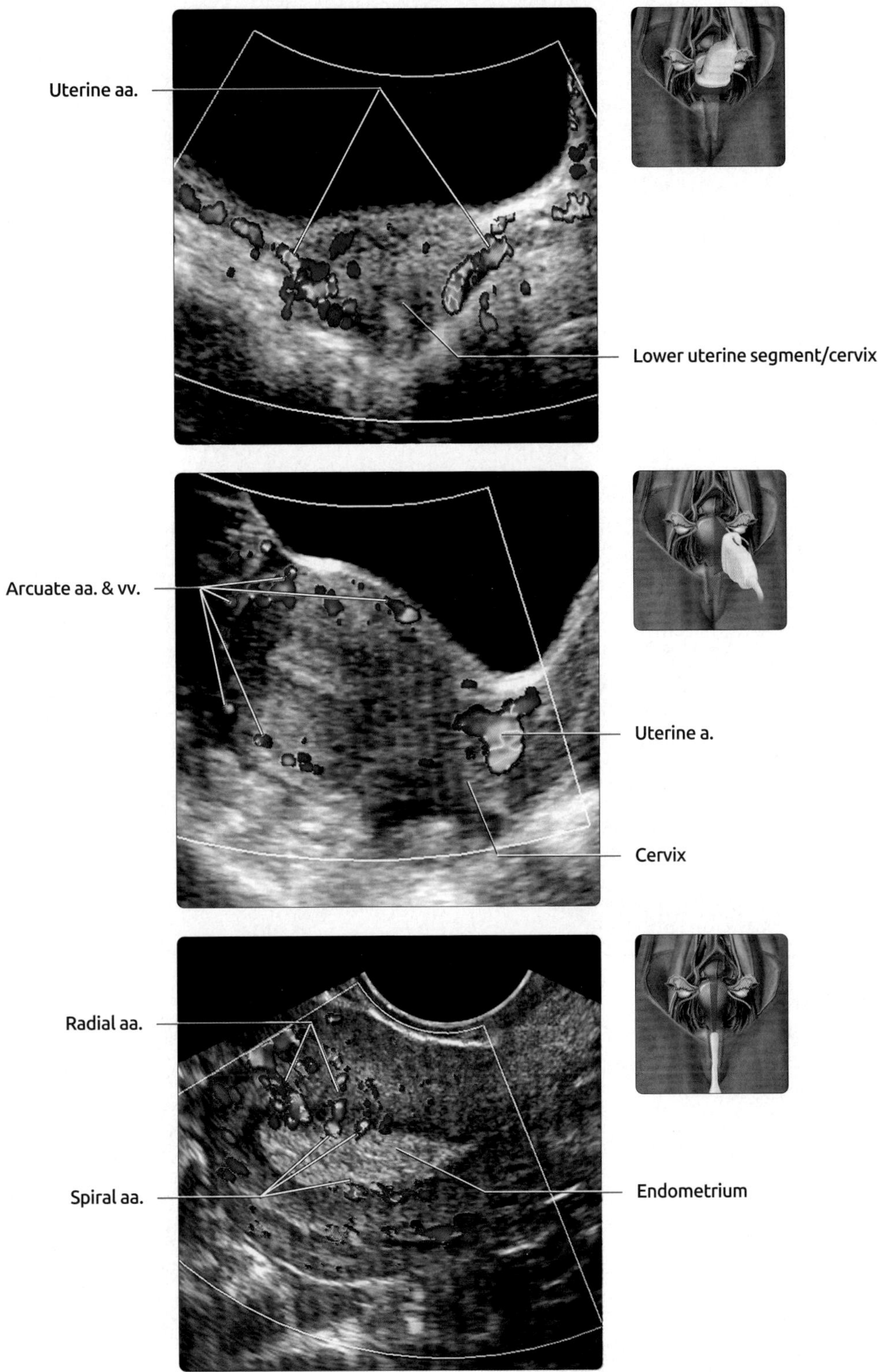

(Top) *Transverse TA color Doppler ultrasound shows both uterine arteries running medially at the level of the cervix. Care must be taken not to confuse these with the iliac arteries, which lie more laterally.* **(Middle)** *Longitudinal TA color Doppler ultrasound shows the uterine artery as it enters the uterus by the cervix. Arcuate arteries and veins are located in the outer 3rd of the myometrium and can be quite prominent. The arcuate arteries commonly calcify with advancing age and should not be confused with a calcified mass.* **(Bottom)** *Longitudinal TV color Doppler ultrasound shows arcuate arteries branching into radial arteries, which run vertically in the myometrium. These in turn give rise to the spiral arteries, which supply the endometrium.*

FALLOPIAN TUBES

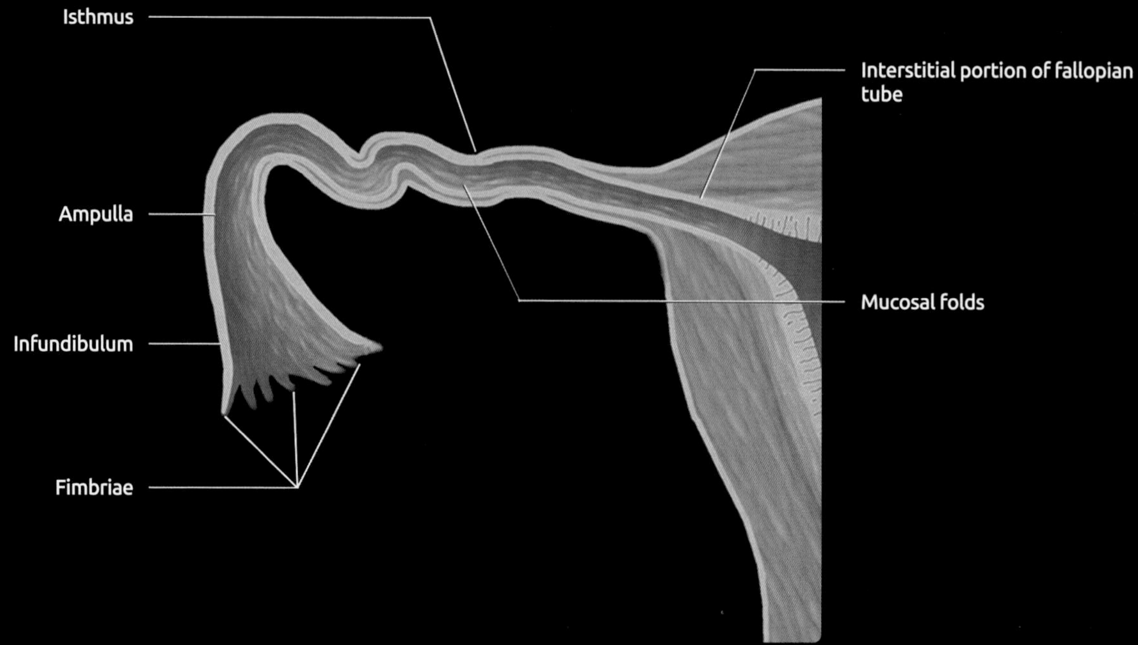

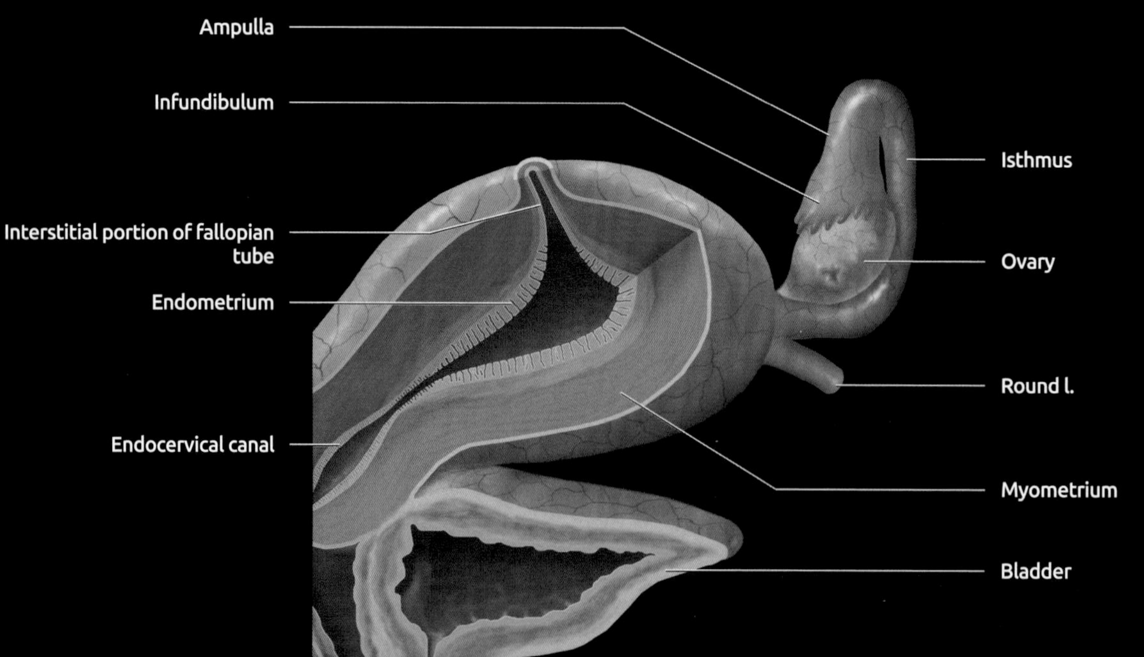

(Top) *Graphic of the right fallopian tube shows the 4 segments, including the interstitial (intramural) portion, isthmus, ampulla, and infundibulum, which is ringed by the fimbriae. The fallopian tubes connect the uterus to the peritoneal cavity. The interstitial portion traverses the uterine wall and is ~ 1 cm in length. The isthmus is the longest and narrowest portion of the tube, which widens into the ampulla and infundibulum.* **(Bottom)** *Graphic cut-away view at the cornua shows the interstitial (intramural) portion of the fallopian tube as it crosses the myometrium. The infundibular end has a funnel-shaped opening which "cradles" the posterior surface of the ovary allowing it to capture the ovum following ovulation. Fertilization usually occurs in the ampullary portion of tube. This is also the most common site of an ectopic pregnancy.*

FALLOPIAN TUBES

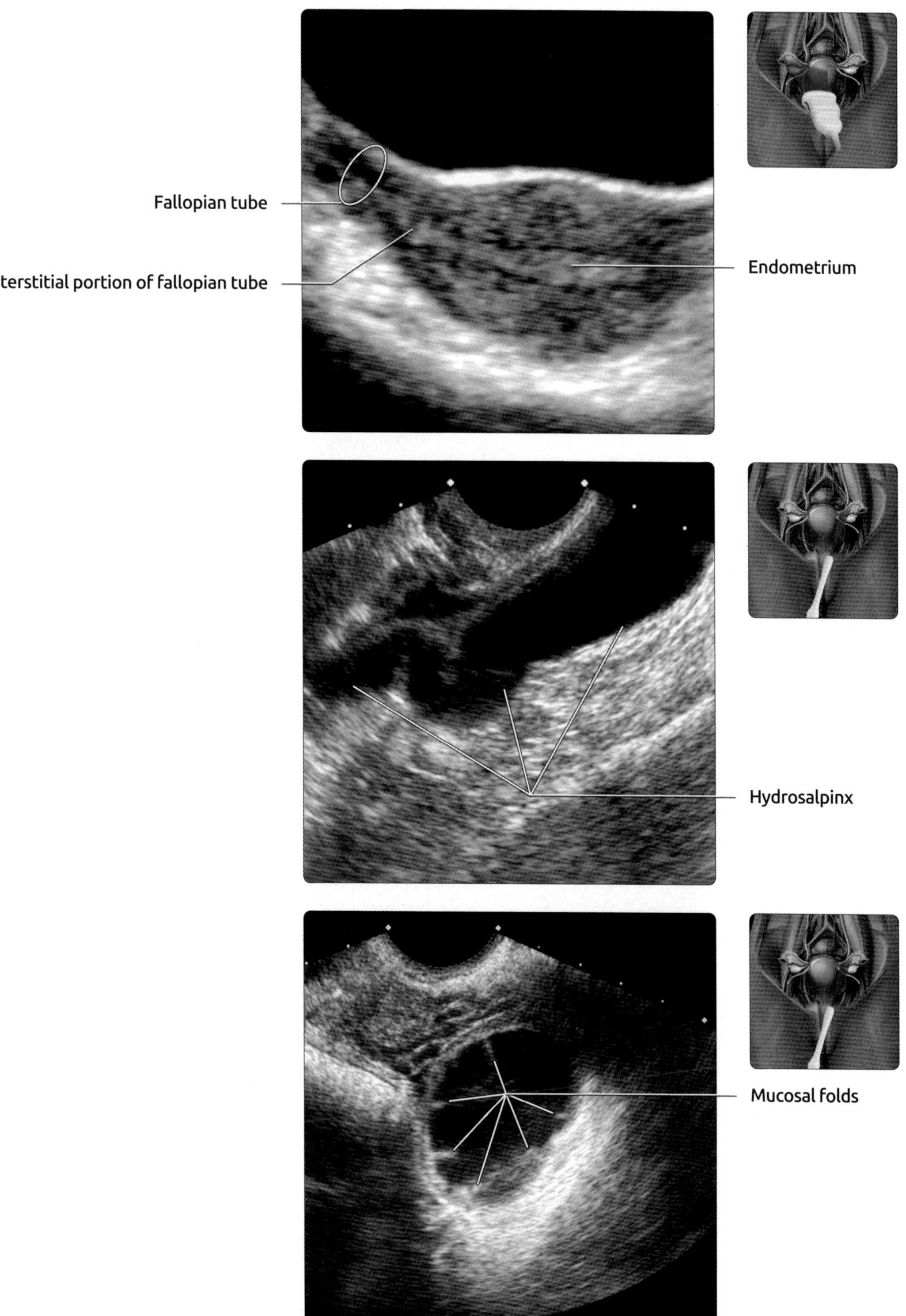

(Top) *Transverse TA ultrasound of the uterus shows the level where the fallopian tube opens into the endometrial cavity. The fallopian tube has 4 segments, including interstitial, isthmus, ampulla, and infundibulum. This image shows the interstitial portion of the tube traversing the myometrial wall at the cornu.* **(Middle)** *First of 2 TV ultrasound images of a left-sided hydrosalpinx is shown. During real-time scanning, it is important to try to elongate the tube, as in this image. This allows differentiation from a cystic ovarian mass.* **(Bottom)** *In the cross-sectional plane, a hydrosalpinx will often display a cogwheel appearance. The mucosal folds of the fallopian tube project into the lumen. As the hydrosalpinx becomes more chronic, these folds will become thick and nodular.*

GROSS ANATOMY

Overview

- Begins at inferior narrowing of uterus (isthmus)
  - Supravaginal portion: Endocervix
  - Vaginal portion: Ectocervix
- Endocervical canal: Spindle-shaped cavity communicates with uterine body and vagina
- Internal os: Opening into uterine cavity
- External os: Opening into vagina
- Largely fibrous stroma with high proportion of elastic fibers interwoven with smooth muscle
- Endocervical canal lined by mucus-secreting columnar epithelium
  - Epithelium in series of small, V-shaped folds (plicae palmatae)
- Ectocervix lined by stratified squamous epithelium
- Squamocolumnar junction near external os but exact position variable
- Nabothian cysts commonly seen
  - Represent obstructed mucus-secreting glands
- Entire cervix is extraperitoneal
  - Anterior: Peritoneum reflects over dome of bladder above level of internal os
  - Posterior: Peritoneum extends along posterior vaginal fornix, creating rectouterine pouch of Douglas (cul-de-sac)
- Arteries, veins, nerves, and lymphatics
  - Arterial supply
    - Descending branch of uterine artery from internal iliac artery
  - Venous drainage
    - To uterine vein and drains into internal iliac vein
  - Lymphatics
    - Drain into internal and external iliac lymph nodes
  - Innervation
    - Sympathetic and parasympathetic nerves from branches of inferior hypogastric plexuses
- Variations with pregnancy
  - Nulliparous: Circular external os, arterial waveform shows high resistivity index (RI)
  - During pregnancy: Changes become apparent by ~ 6 weeks of gestation
    - Softened and enlarged cervix due to engorgement with blood with decreased RI of uterine artery
    - Hypertrophy of mucosa of cervical canal: Increased echogenicity of mucosal layer
    - Increased secretion of mucous glands: Increased volume of mucus ± mucus plug in cervical canal
  - Parous: Larger vaginal part of cervix, external os opens out transversely with anterior and posterior lips
- Variations with age: Cervix grows less with age than uterus
  - Neonatal: Adult configuration due to residual maternal hormonal stimulation
  - Infantile: Cervix predominant with cervix:corpus length ratio ~ 2:1
  - Prepubertal: Cervix:corpus length ratio ~ 1:1
  - Reproductive: Uterus predominant, cervix:corpus length ratio ≥ 1:2
  - Postmenopausal: Overall reduction in size

Anatomy Relationships

- Anterior
  - Supravaginal cervix: Superior aspect of posterior bladder wall
  - Vaginal cervix: Anterior fornix of vagina
- Posterior
  - Supravaginal cervix: Rectouterine pouch of Douglas
  - Vaginal cervix: Posterior fornix of vagina
- Lateral
  - Supravaginal cervix: Bilateral ureters
  - Vaginal cervix: Lateral fornices of vagina
- Ligamentous support: Condensations of pelvic fascia attached to cervix and vaginal vault
  - Transverse cervical (cardinal) ligaments
    - Fibromuscular condensations of pelvic fascia
    - Pass to cervix and upper vagina from lateral walls of pelvis
  - Pubocervical ligaments
    - 2 firm bands of connective tissue
    - Extend from posterior surface of pubis, position on either side of neck of bladder and then attach to anterior aspect of cervix
  - Sacrocervical ligaments
    - Fibromuscular condensations
    - Attach posterior aspect of cervix and upper vagina from lower end of sacrum
    - Form 2 ridges, 1 on either side of rectouterine pouch of Douglas

IMAGING ANATOMY

Ultrasound

- Transabdominal scan
  - Mucus within endocervical canal usually creates echogenic interface
  - In periovulatory phase, cervical mucus becomes hypoechoic due to high fluid content
  - Mucosal layer: Echogenic
    - Thickness and echogenicity show cyclical changes similar to endometrium
  - Submucosal layer: Hypoechoic
  - Cervical stroma: Intermediate to echogenic
- Transvaginal scan
  - Angle of insonation should be optimized for best visualization
  - Imaging may be improved with withdrawal of probe into midvagina
- Transperineal scan
  - Useful for evaluation of cervical shortening and incompetence after premature rupture of membranes or preterm labor
  - Useful when transvaginal scan cannot be tolerated

GRAPHICS OF CERVIX ANATOMY

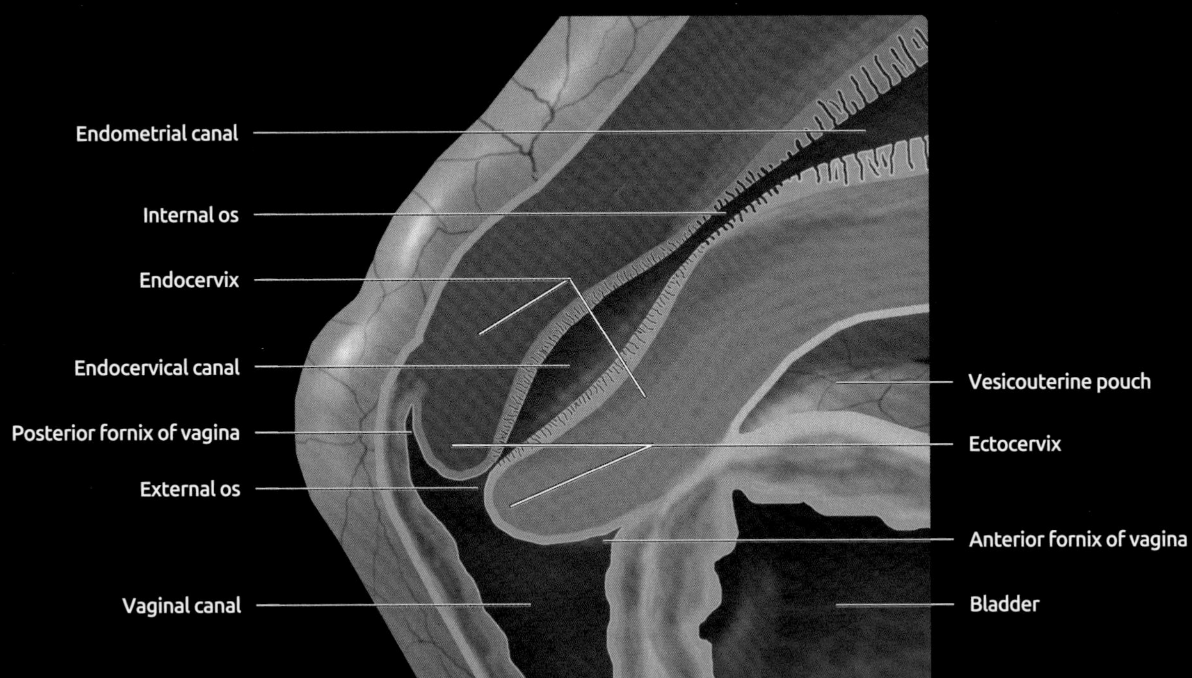

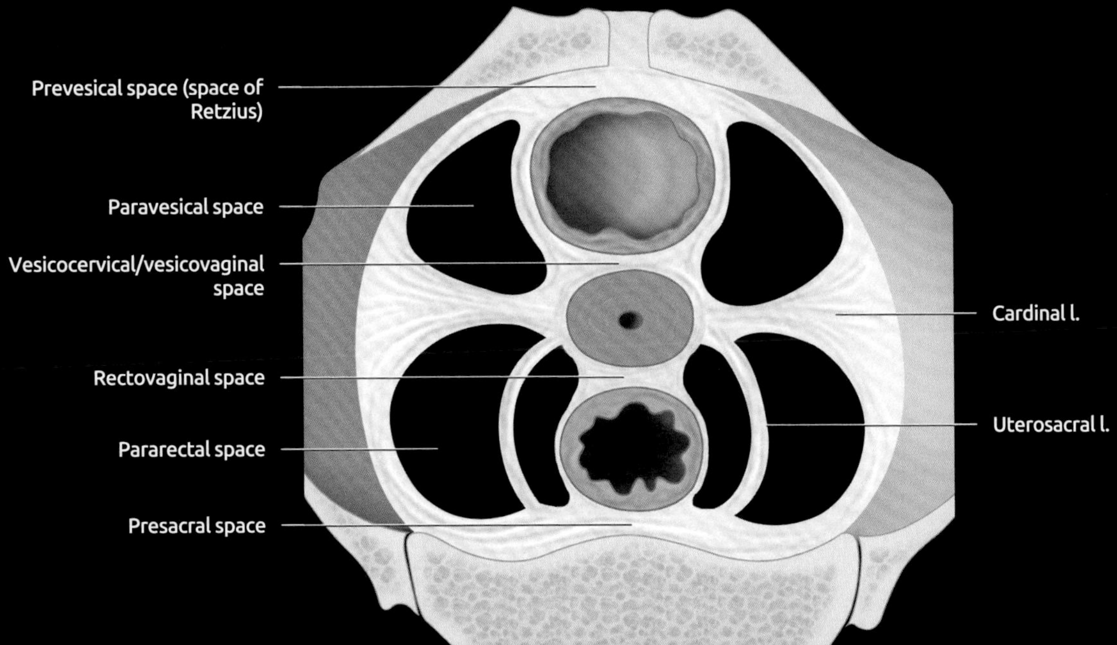

(Top) *Median sagittal graphic shows the cervix, which begins at the isthmus, the inferior narrowing portion of the uterus. It has a supravaginal portion (endocervix) and a vaginal portion (ectocervix), which divides the vagina into shallow anterior fornix, deep posterior, and lateral fornices.* **(Bottom)** *Graphic shows the female pelvic ligaments and spaces at the cervical/vaginal junction. The ligaments are visceral ligaments, which are composed of specialized endopelvic fascia and contain vessels, nerves, and lymphatics. Some of the main supporting ligaments for the uterus are attached to the cervix, which are cardinal and uterosacral ligaments. The spaces are largely filled with loose connective tissue and are used as dissection planes during surgery.*

TRANSVAGINAL ULTRASOUND OF CERVIX

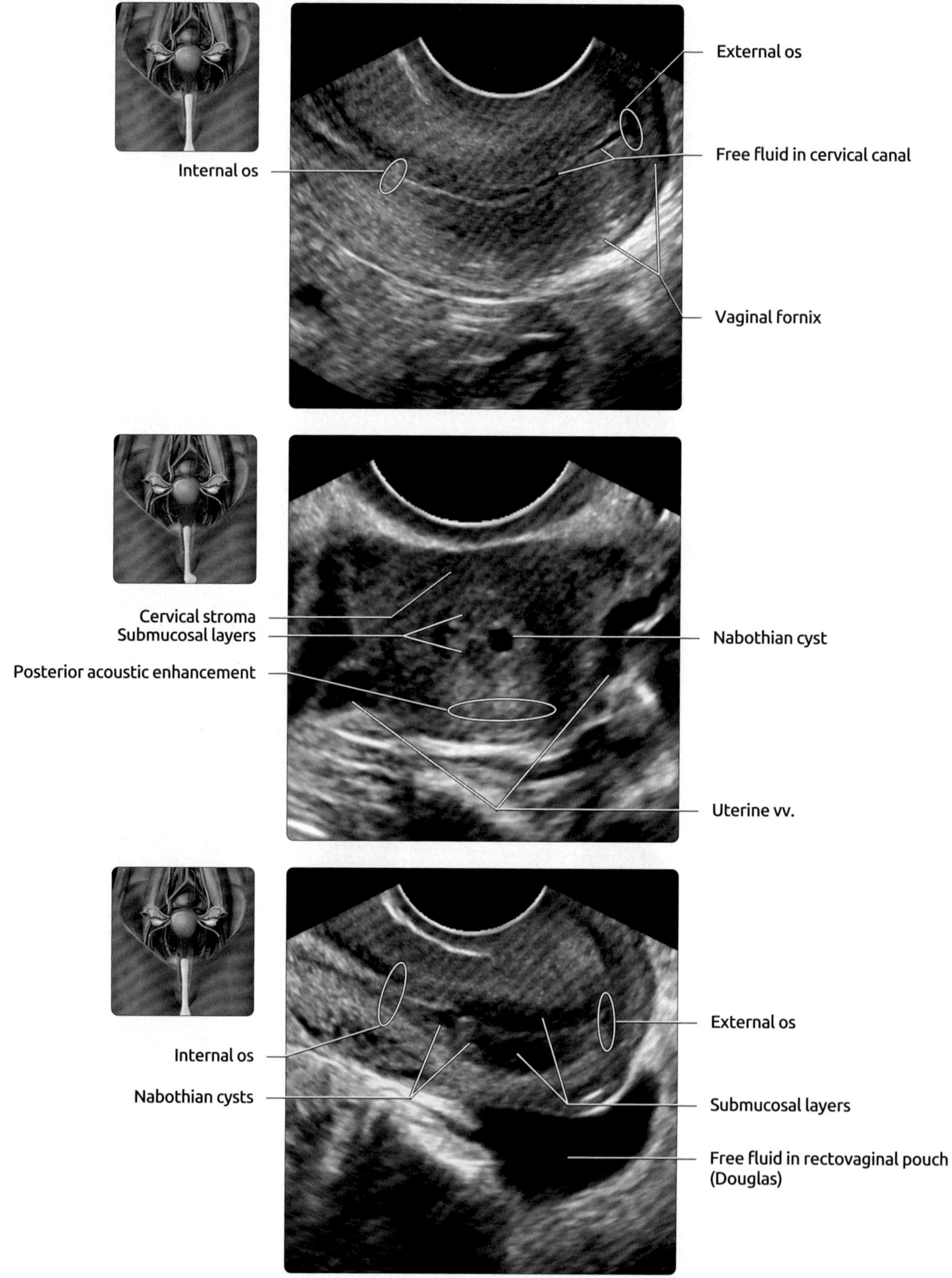

(Top) *Sagittal transvaginal ultrasound of the cervix shows hypoechoic fluid present in the endocervical canal. The endocervical canal is rich in mucus-secreting glands. The mucus secreted is usually slightly echogenic but becomes hypoechoic during periovulatory phase. As the transducer abuts the anterior lip of the cervix, the posterior wall of the vaginal fornix can be seen to cover the external os and extend along the posterior lip of the cervix.* **(Middle)** *Transverse transvaginal ultrasound of the cervix at the midendocervical canal shows the echogenic mucosal layers and thickened submucosal layers. A simple nabothian cyst is present with minimal posterior acoustic enhancement. The submucosal layer is filled with mucus-secreting glands leading to its hypoechoic appearance and posterior acoustic enhancement.* **(Bottom)** *Longitudinal transvaginal ultrasound shows the transducer abutting the anterior lip of the external os. The submucosal layer is thickened with typical low echogenicity.*

DILATED CERVIX

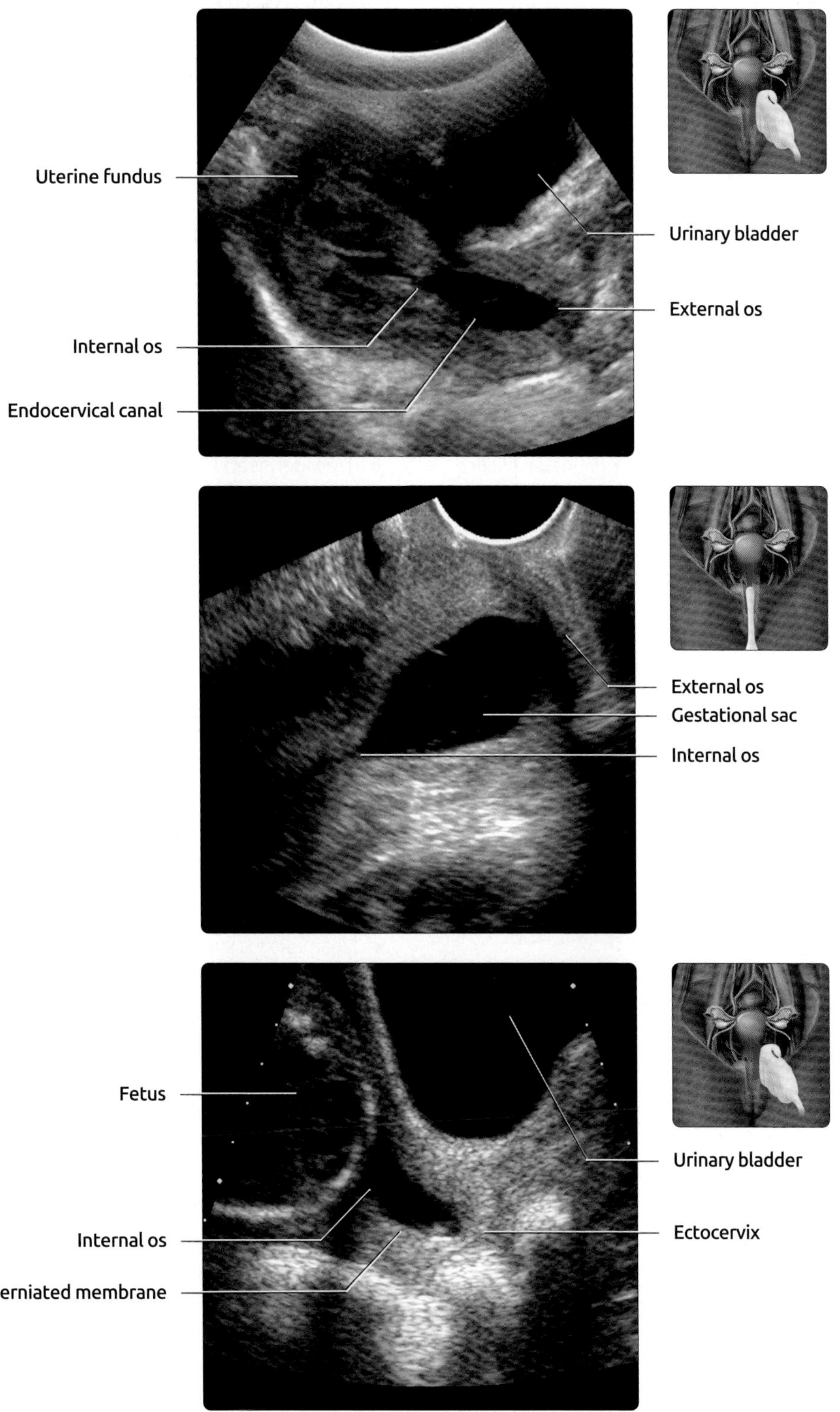

(Top) *Longitudinal transabdominal ultrasound in a failed 1st-trimester pregnancy shows an abnormal position of the gestational sac, herniating into the open cervix.* **(Middle)** *Longitudinal transvaginal ultrasound in the same patient shows the abnormal sac protruding into the cervical canal and reaching the external os, an inevitable abortion.* **(Bottom)** *Longitudinal transabdominal ultrasound during pregnancy shows shortening of the cervix with an open internal os.*

TERMINOLOGY

Abbreviations

- Vaginal artery (VA), uterine artery (UA)

GROSS ANATOMY

Overview

- Muscular tube formed by smooth muscle and elastic connective fibers
- Serves as excretory duct for uterus, female organ for copulation, and part of birth canal
- Extends up and back from vestibule of external genitalia to surround cervix of uterus
- Has anterior and posterior walls, normally in apposition, with longer posterior wall
- Superiorly, cervix projects downward and backward into vagina and divides vagina into shallow anterior, deep posterior, and lateral fornices
- Upper 1/2 of vagina lies above pelvic floor, lower 1/2 lies within perineum
- Lined with stratified squamous epithelium
- Inner mucosal surface of wall form rugae when collapsed
- Thin mucosal fold called hymen surrounds entrance to vaginal orifice
- Outer surface (adventitial coat) is thin fibrous layer continuous with surrounding endopelvic fascia
- Vasculature
  - Arterial supply
    - VA: Can branch directly from internal iliac artery (anterior trunk) or sometimes from inferior vesical artery or UA
    - Vaginal branches of UA
    - Branches of VA and UA anastomose to form 2 median longitudinal vessels: Azygos arteries, 1 in front and 1 behind vagina
  - Venous drainage
    - Form venous plexus around vagina
    - Eventually drains to internal iliac veins
- Variations with age
  - Menarche: 7-10 cm long
  - Postmenopausal: Shrinks in length and diameter; fornices virtually disappear

Anatomic Relationships

- Anterior
  - Superior: Bladder base
  - Inferior: Urethra
- Posterior
  - Upper 1/3: Rectouterine pouch of Douglas
  - Middle 1/3: Ampulla of rectum
  - Lower 1/3: Perineal body
- Lateral
  - Upper 1/3: Ureters
  - Middle 1/3: Levator ani and pelvic fascia
  - Lower 1/3: Bulb of vestibule, urogenital diaphragm, and bulbospongiosus muscles
- Ligamentous supports
  - Upper 1/3: Levator ani muscles, transverse cervical (cardinal), pubocervical, and sacrocervical ligaments
  - Middle 1/3: Urogenital diaphragm
  - Lower 1/3: Perineal body

IMAGING ANATOMY

Ultrasound

- Transabdominal US with distended bladder is standard imaging technique
  - Caudal angulation on both longitudinal and transverse scans
  - Commonly found at/near sagittal midline of pelvis
  - Length and wall thickness vary in response to bladder and rectal filling
  - Combined thickness of anterior and posterior vaginal walls should not exceed 1 cm for transabdominal scan with distended bladder
  - Characteristic appearance of 3 parallel lines
    - Highly echogenic mucosa centrally, may be difficult to visualize if stretched by distended bladder
    - Moderately hypoechoic muscular walls
- Transperineal US with nondistended bladder for assessment of uterine prolapse or for difficult cases
  - Vagina, especially vaginal canal, is less well defined
- Transvaginal US may require withdrawal of transducer so as not to compress pathology

EMBRYOLOGY

Embryologic Events

- Uterus and upper vagina are formed from paired müllerian (paramesonephric) ducts
- Paired ducts meet in midline and fuse, forming uterovaginal canal
- Lower vagina is formed from urogenital sinus

CLINICAL IMPLICATIONS

Uterine Prolapse

- Ligamentous support of pelvic organs may be damaged or become lax, leading to uterine prolapse or prolapse of vaginal walls
- Cystocele: Sagging of bladder with bulging of anterior vaginal wall
- Rectocele: Sagging of ampulla of rectum with bulging of posterior vaginal wall
- Best to be investigated by transperineal US supplemented with 3D

Müllerian Duct Anomalies

- Failure of müllerian duct development ± fusion
- Vagina most commonly affected in uterus didelphys (class III anomaly); vaginal septum seen in ~ 75% of cases
- Hematocolpos from imperforate hymen or vaginal septum may be evaluated by transperineal US

Pelvic Abscess

- Common site: Rectouterine pouch of Douglas
- Transvaginal approach allows US-guided drainage of pelvic abscess without surgery

Infertility

- Transvaginal US is used for egg retrieval in assisted reproduction

VAGINA IN SITU AND ARTERIAL SUPPLY

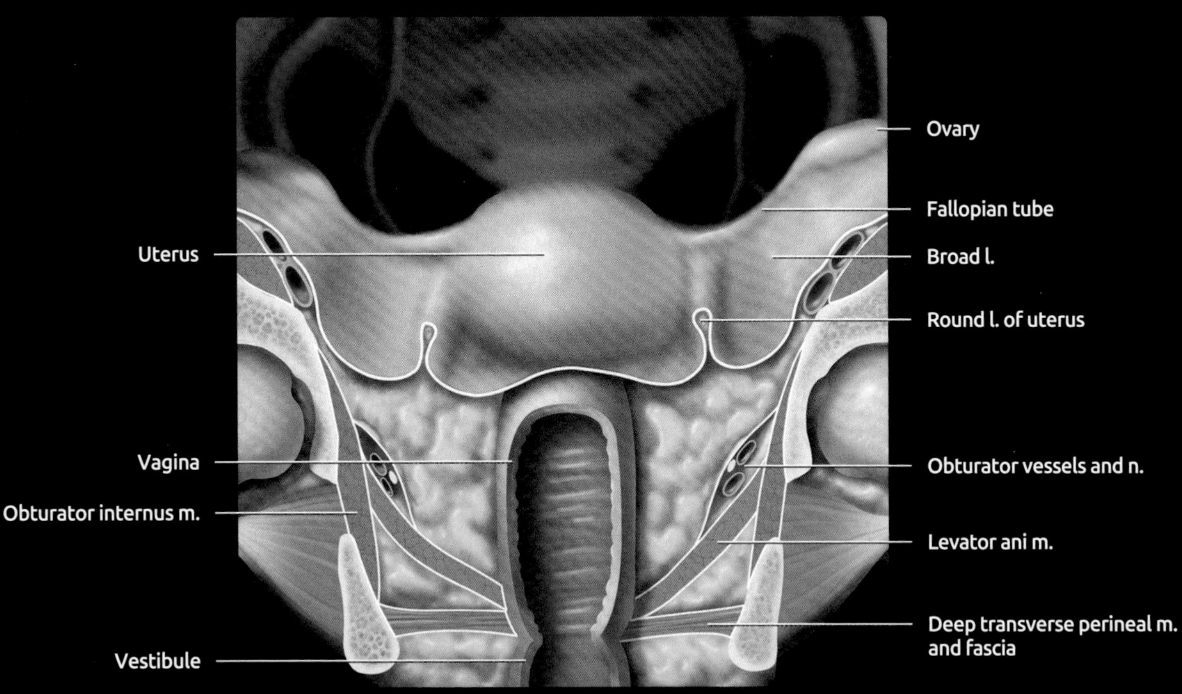

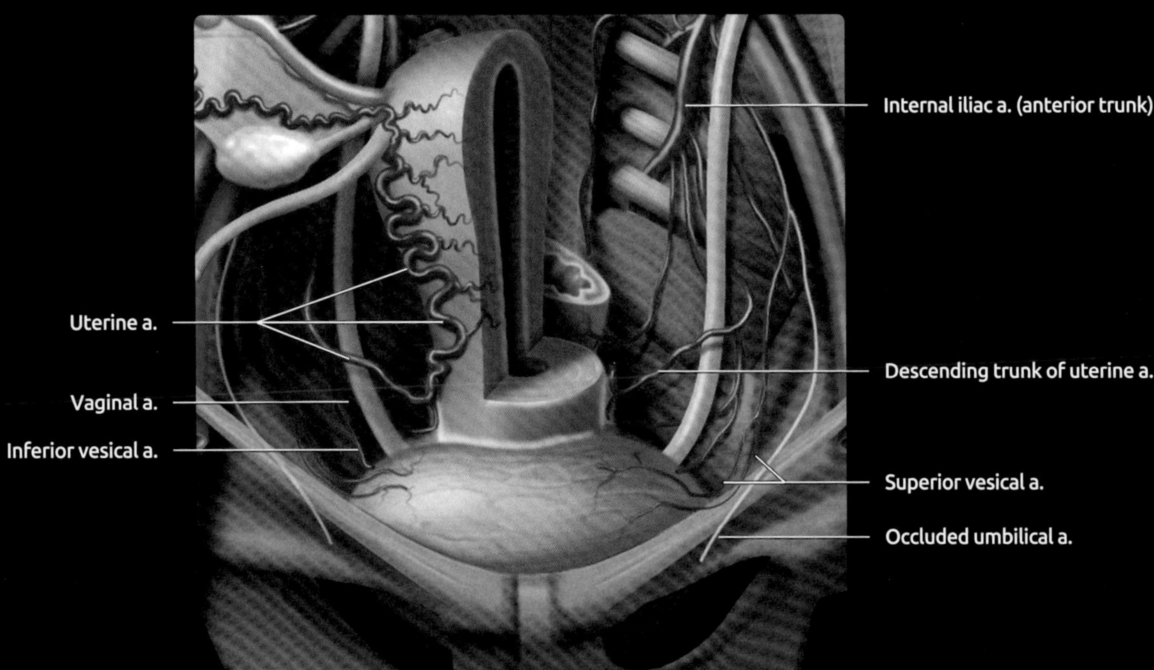

(Top) *Coronal view shows the pelvic floor at the level of the vagina. The levator ani muscles form the pelvic floor through which the urethra, vagina, and rectum pass and are the main support for the pelvic organs. The deep transverse perineal muscle and fascia, along with the urethral sphincter, form the urogenital diaphragm, which is the main support of the lower vagina.* **(Bottom)** *Frontal graphic shows the iliac vessels. The internal iliac artery divides into an anterior trunk and posterior trunk. The vaginal artery (VA) can branch off directly from the anterior trunk of the internal iliac artery or sometimes from the inferior vesical artery or uterine artery (UA). The arterial supply of the vagina includes the VA and vaginal branch of the descending trunk of UA.*

VAGINAL IMAGING BY VARIOUS TECHNIQUES

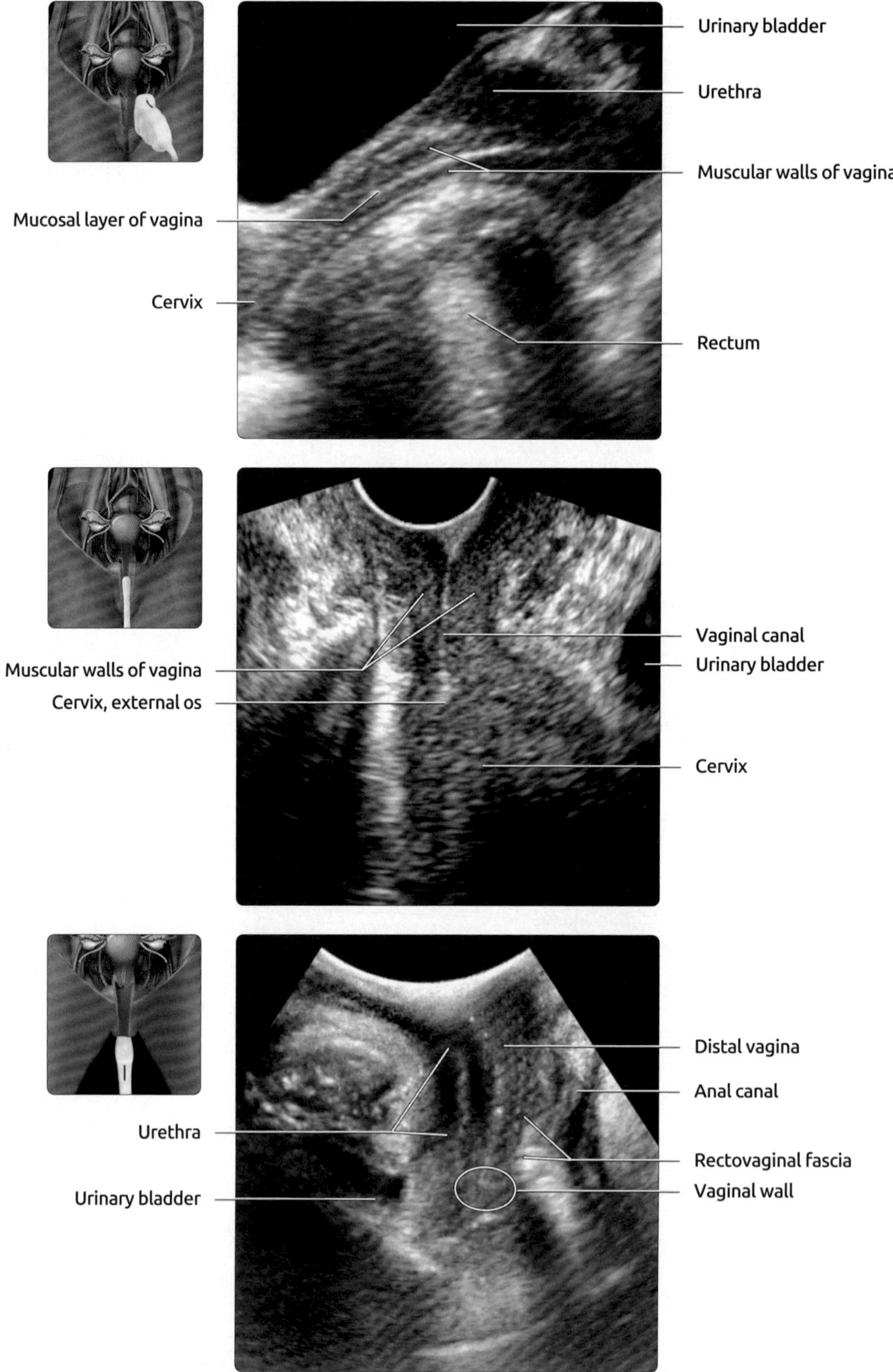

(Top) *Transabdominal midline sagittal US of the vagina shows characteristic triple-line echoes, i.e., hypoechoic muscular walls interfaced by echogenic mucosa. When looking for the vagina using transabdominal US, it is best to view with a distended bladder, starting at the midline near the cervical level and tilting the transducer further caudally.* **(Middle)** *Longitudinal transvaginal US of the vagina again shows the characteristic triple-line echo pattern. Using transvaginal US, gradually withdraw the high-frequency vaginal transducer so as to outline the vaginal canal.* **(Bottom)** *Transperineal sagittal US shows the vagina sandwiched between the urethra anteriorly and the rectum posteriorly. Note that the vaginal canal is barely visible in the absence of intraluminal acoustic jelly or fluid.*

TRANSVERSE US OF VAGINA

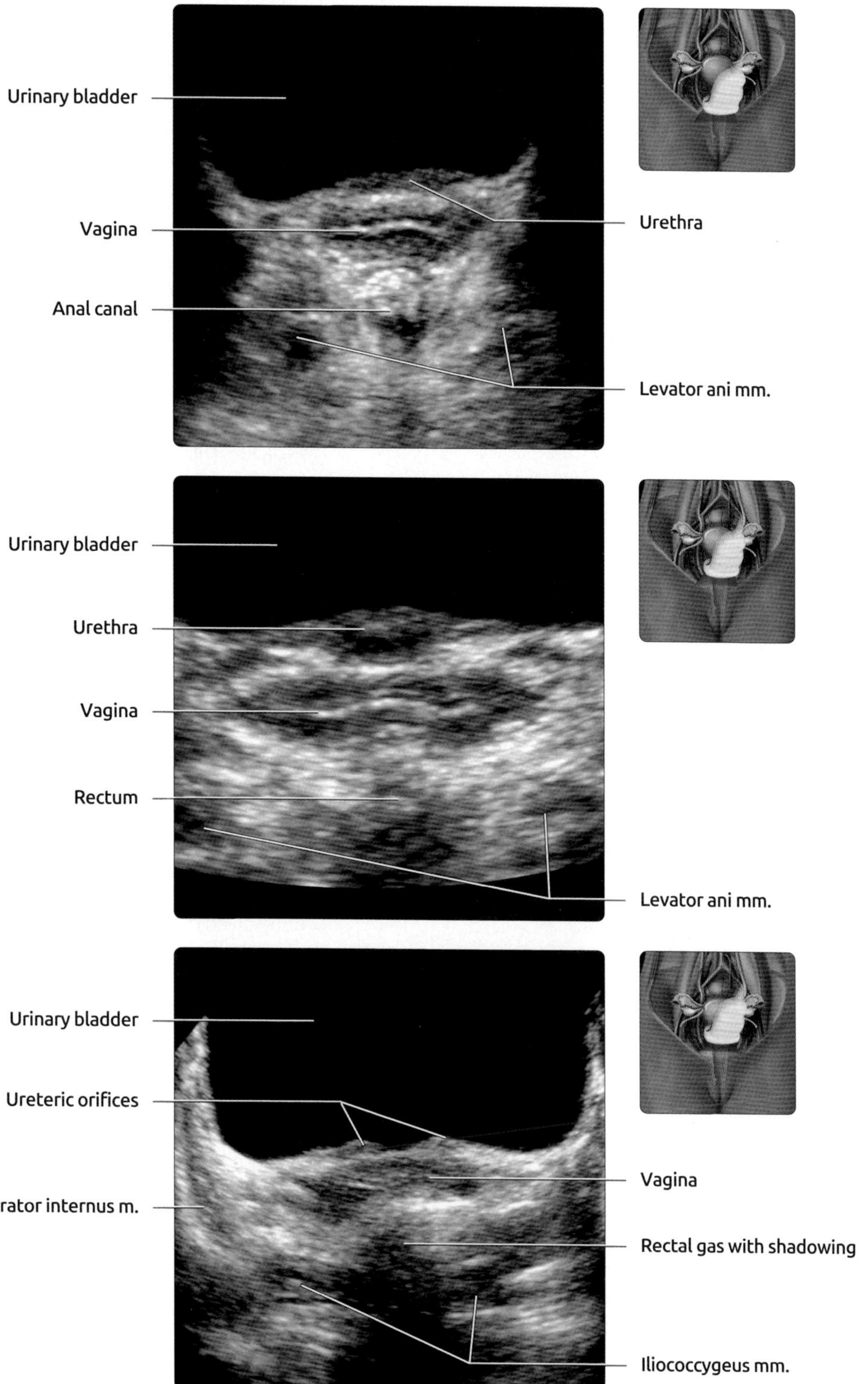

(Top) *Transverse transabdominal US shows the mid- to lower vagina at the level of anal canal. For transabdominal US of the vagina, caudal angulation of the US probe is needed on both longitudinal and transverse scans. Note that the vaginal canal is better demonstrated on transabdominal US because the angle of insonation is more favorable, when approaching a perpendicular angle.* **(Middle)** *Transverse transabdominal US of the midvagina shows the levator ani muscles adjacent to the posterolateral aspect of the vagina.* **(Bottom)** *The upper vagina is shown at the level of the ureteric orifices. The ureters run lateral to the lateral fornices of the vagina, cross anteriorly, and then enter into the posterior wall of the bladder. This is a useful plane for investigation of the ureteric jets.*

GROSS ANATOMY

Overview

- Ovaries located in true pelvis, although exact position variable
  - Only pelvic organ entirely inside peritoneal sac
  - Laxity in ligaments allows some mobility
  - Location affected by parity, bladder filling, ovarian size, and uterine size/position
  - Located within ovarian fossa in nulliparous women
    - Lateral pelvic sidewall below bifurcation of common iliac vessels
    - Anterior to ureter
    - Posterior to broad ligament
  - Position more variable in parous women
    - Pregnancy displaces ovaries, seldom return to same spot
- Fallopian tube drapes over much of surface
  - Partially covered by fimbriated end
- Composed of medulla and cortex
  - Vessels enter and exit ovary through medulla
  - Cortex contains follicles in varying stages of development
  - Surface covered by specialized peritoneum called germinal epithelium
- Ligamentous supports
  - Suspensory ligament of ovary (infundibulopelvic ligament)
    - Attaches ovary to lateral pelvic wall
    - Contains ovarian vessels and lymphatics
    - Positions ovary in craniocaudal orientation
  - Mesovarium
    - Attaches ovary to broad ligament (posterior)
    - Transmits nerves and vessels to ovary
  - Proper ovarian ligament (uteroovarian ligament)
    - Continuation of round ligament
    - Fibromuscular band extending from ovary to uterine cornu
  - Mesosalpinx
    - Extends between fallopian tube and proper ovarian ligament
  - Broad ligament
    - Below proper ovarian ligament
- Arterial supply: Dual blood supply
  - Ovarian artery is branch of aorta, arises at L1/L2 level
    - Descends to pelvis and enters suspensory ligament
    - Continues through mesovarium to ovarian hilum
    - Anastomoses with uterine artery
- Drainage via pampiniform plexus into ovarian veins
  - Right ovarian vein drains to inferior vena cava
  - Left ovarian vein drains to left renal vein
- Lymphatic drainage follows venous drainage to preaortic lymph nodes at L1 and L2 levels

Physiology

- ~ 400,000 follicles present at birth, but only 0.1% (400) mature to ovulation
- Variations in menstrual cycle
  - Follicular phase (days 0-14)
    - Several follicles begin to develop
    - By days 8-12, dominant follicle develops, while remainder start to regress
  - Ovulation (day 14)
    - Dominant follicle, typically 2.0-2.5 cm, ruptures and releases ovum
  - Luteal phase (days 14-28)
    - Luteinizing hormone induces formation of corpus luteum from ruptured follicle
    - If fertilization occurs, corpus luteum maintains and enlarges to corpus luteum cyst of pregnancy

Variations With Age

- At birth: Large ovaries ± follicles due to influence of maternal hormones
- Childhood: Volume < 1 cm^3, follicles < 2-mm diameter
- Above 8 year old: ≥ 6 follicles of > 4-mm diameter
- Adult, reproductive age: Mean volume: ~ 10 ± 6 cm^3; max: 22 cm^3
- Postmenopausal: Mean: ~ 2-6 cm^3; max: 8 cm^3 and may contain few follicle-like structures

IMAGING ANATOMY

US

- Scan between uterus and pelvic sidewall
  - Ovaries often seen adjacent to internal iliac vessels
- Medulla mildly hyperechoic compared to hypoechoic cortex
- Dominant follicle around time of ovulation
  - Cumulus oophorus: Nodule or cyst along margin of dominant follicle represents mature ovum
- Corpus luteum may have thick, echogenic ring
  - Doppler: Vascular wall or "ring"
  - Hemorrhage common
- Echogenic foci common
  - Nonshadowing, 1-3 mm
  - Represent specular reflectors from walls of tiny unresolved cysts or small vessels in medulla
- Doppler: Low-velocity, low-resistance arterial waveform
- Volume (0.523 x length x width x height) more accurate than individual measurements

ANATOMY IMAGING ISSUES

Imaging Recommendations

- Transabdominal (TA) US with full bladder is good for overview of pelvic organs
  - Detects ovaries and masses superior or lateral to uterus that may be missed by transvaginal (TV) US
- TVUS is excellent in assessing detail of ovaries and characterizing lesions compared to TAUS
  - Lesions higher in pelvis can be missed because of limited field of view
  - TVUS should be performed with empty bladder
- Piriformis muscle or exophytic fibroids may mimic ovary
- Knowledge of last menstrual period is useful for not mistaking normal physiology for pathology
- Postmenopausal ovaries can be difficult to detect because of atrophy, paucity of follicles, and surrounding bowel

LIGAMENTOUS SUPPORT AND ANATOMY OF OVARY

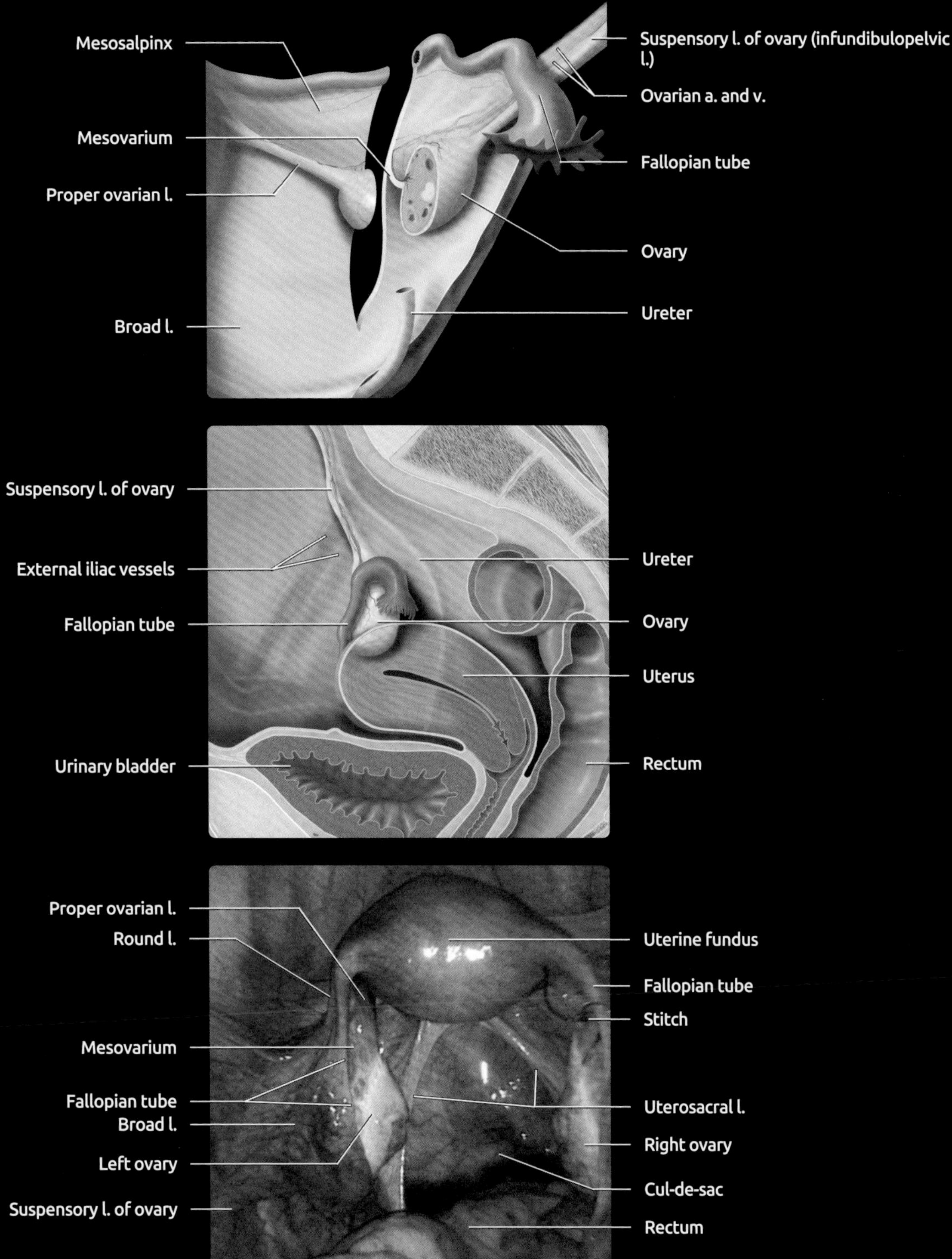

(Top) *Posterior view of the ligamentous attachment of the ovary is shown. The ovary is attached to the pelvic sidewall by the suspensory ligament (infundibulopelvic ligament) of the ovary, which transmits the ovarian artery and vein. These vessels enter the ovary through the mesovarium, a specialized ligamentous attachment between the ovary and broad ligament. The ovary is attached to the uterus by the proper ovarian ligament, which divides the mesosalpinx above from the broad ligament below.* **(Middle)** *Sagittal graphic of the female pelvis shows the location of the ovary, which lies in the ovarian fossa, the area below the iliac bifurcation, posterior to the external iliac vessels, and anterior to the ureter.* **(Bottom)** *Photograph during laparoscopy viewing the uterine fundus from above demonstrates the ligamentous structures of the ovary and uterus.*

NORMAL OVARY, VARIATIONS WITH AGE

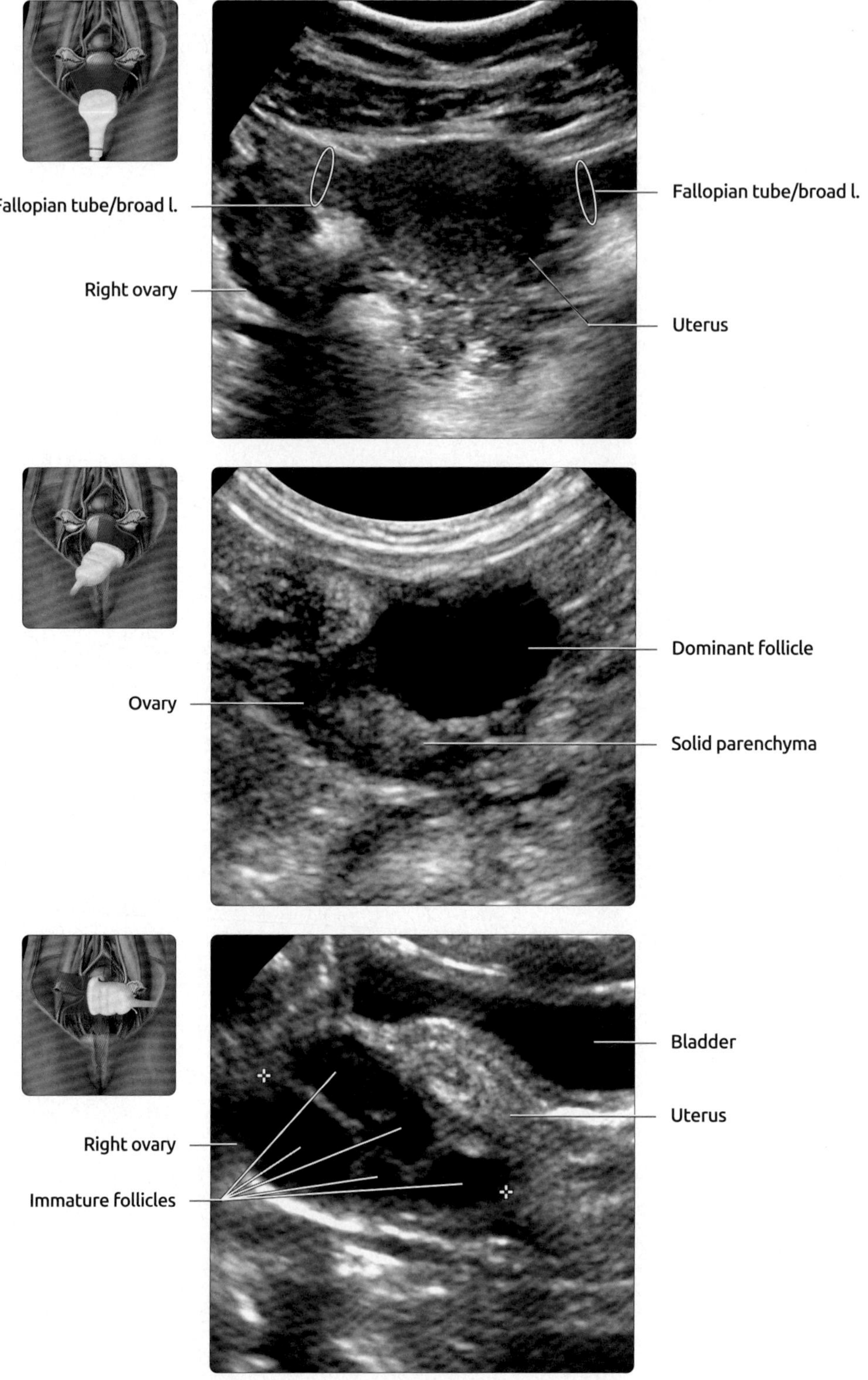

(Top) *Transverse transabdominal (TA) US at the level of the uterine fundus in a 23-year-old woman shows the right ovary in the typical position of the ovarian fossa. The fallopian tube and broad ligament can sometimes be seen as a band of tissue connecting the ovary to the uterine horn. Ovarian ligaments can be lax, making ovarian position quite variable from above the fundus to the posterior rectouterine pouch of Douglas.* **(Middle)** *Transverse TAUS of the ovary in a neonate is shown. The size of the ovary is enlarged with a dominant follicle related to stimulation from residual maternal gonadotrophins. Visible follicles may persist until 9 months of age or longer.* **(Bottom)** *Longitudinal TAUS of the ovary of a 5-month-old girl is shown. The ovary is slightly prominent due to stimulation from maternal hormones. The ovary is small (total volume of 1.7 cc) with immature follicles of variable size (usually < 0.9 cm). The size of the ovaries change very little in the first 6 years of life.*

NORMAL OVARY, VARIATIONS WITH AGE

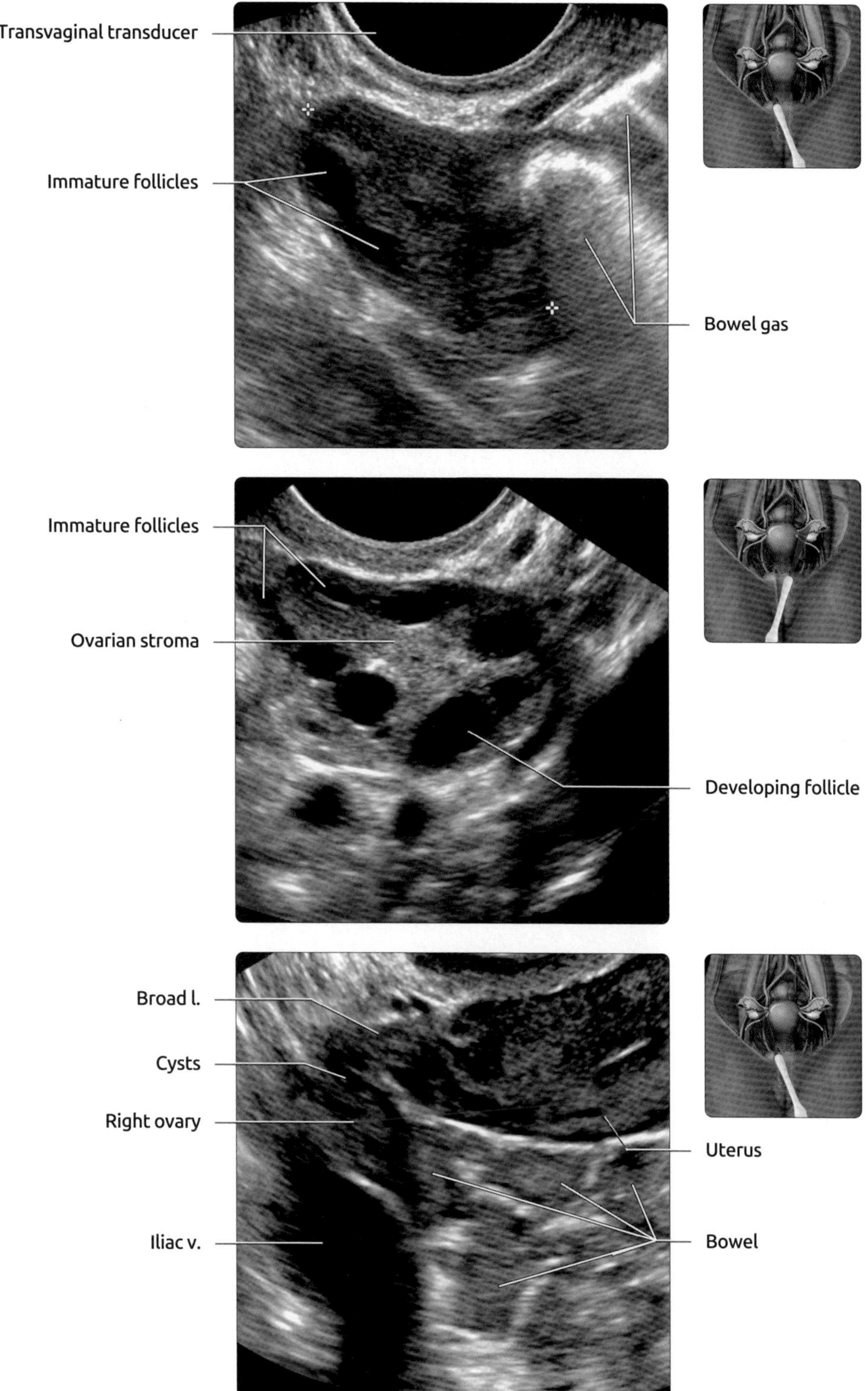

(Top) *Transverse transvaginal (TV) US of the right ovary in an 18-year-old woman shows an oval ovary with immature follicles. This US also demonstrates the superior resolution of TVUS, from the ability to bring the ovary to the near field, as well as the higher frequencies used.* **(Middle)** *Transverse TVUS of an adult ovary is shown. There are multiple developing follicles of variable size around the echogenic ovarian stroma (medulla) where the ovarian vessels and lymphatics enter and exit. Ovulation usually occurs when the follicle enlarges to be between 2.0 and 2.5 cm.* **(Bottom)** *TVUS in a 74-year-old postmenopausal woman demonstrates atrophic right ovary containing tiny cysts. Normal ovaries are variably detected in the postmenopausal woman because of their small size, lack of follicles, and surrounding bowel loops.*

COLOR DOPPLER IMAGING OF OVARIAN ARTERY

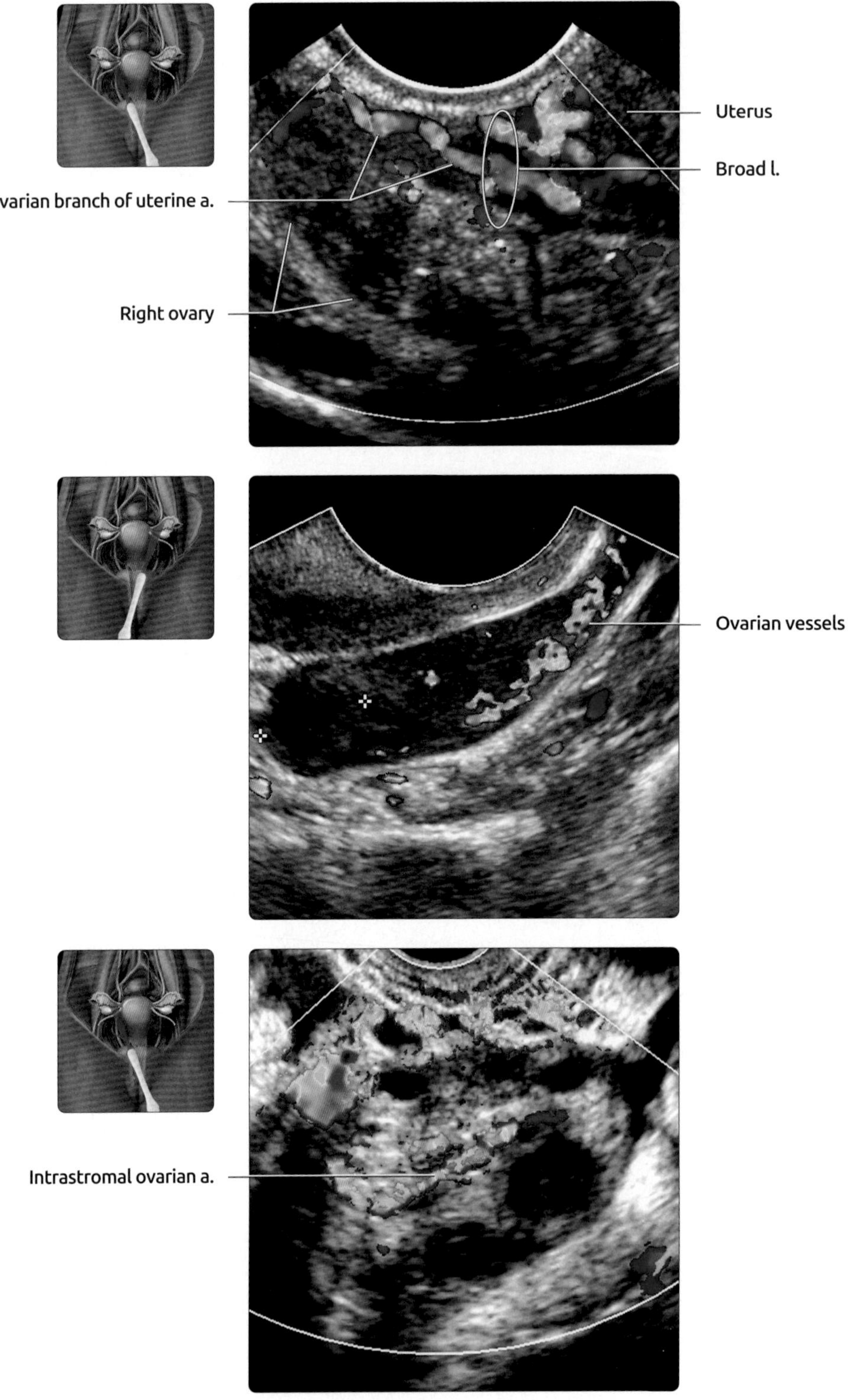

(Top) *Transverse TVUS shows the ovarian branch of the uterine artery running in the broad ligament. It begins at the uterine horn and goes to the ovary through the proper ovarian ligament/mesovarium anastomosing with the ovarian artery.* **(Middle)** *Transverse TVUS of the left ovary demonstrates involuting corpus luteum (calipers). The ovarian vessels are seen entering the ovary from the suspensory ligament of the ovary.* **(Bottom)** *Longitudinal color Doppler TVUS shows an intrastromal ovarian artery running in the ovarian medulla. Note the ovarian vascularity will progressively increase after menstruation and approach a maximum in the luteal phase.*

SPECTRAL WAVEFORM OF OVARIAN ARTERY

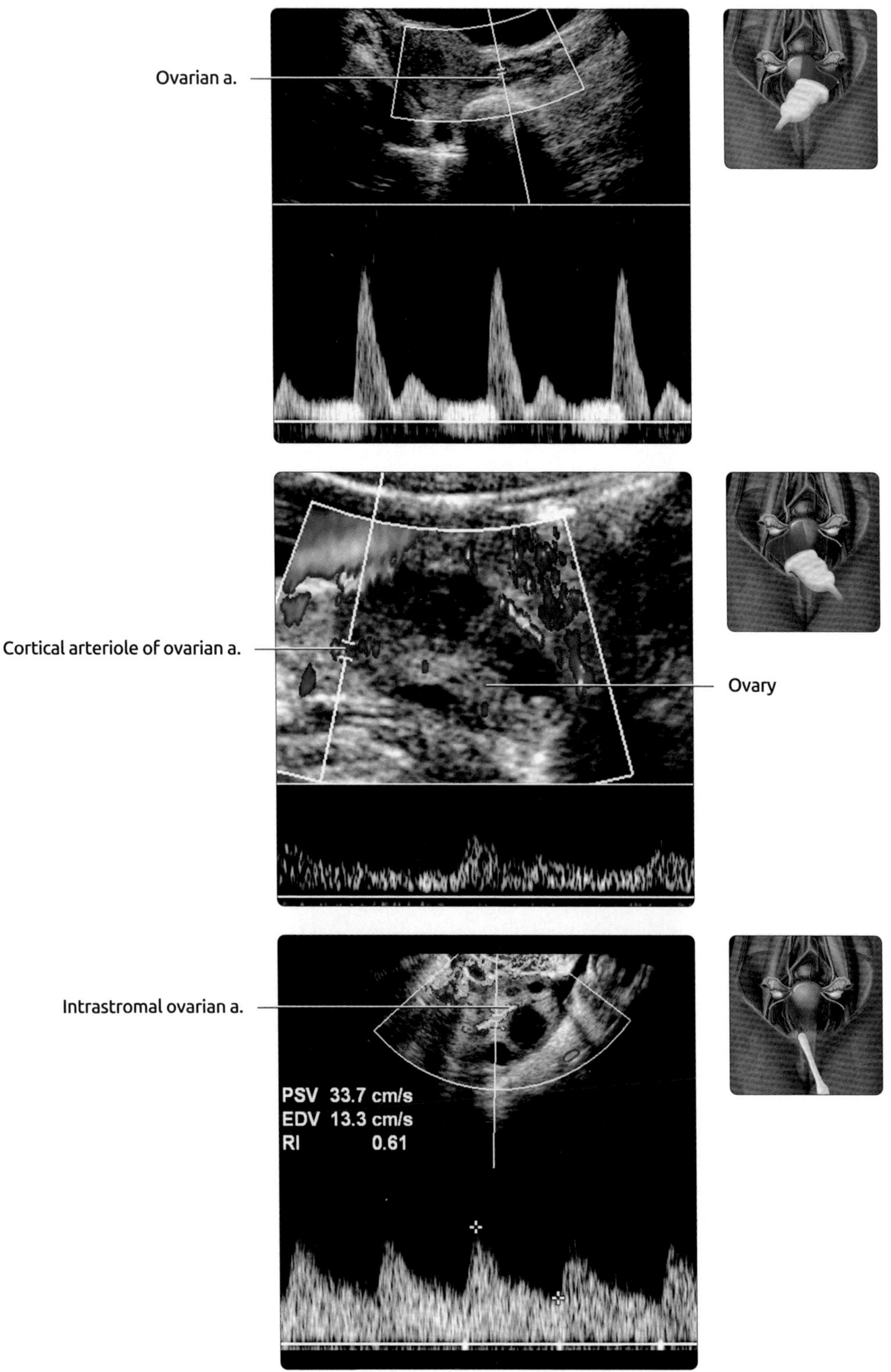

(Top) *Transverse spectral Doppler TAUS shows a normal ovarian artery with a high-resistance flow pattern suggestive of an inactive state of the ovary.* **(Middle)** *Transverse spectral Doppler TAUS shows the waveform of the cortical arteriole of the ovarian artery.* **(Bottom)** *Transverse spectral Doppler TVUS of the intrastromal ovarian artery as a continuation of the straight cortical arteriole shows a typical low-resistance, low-velocity waveform during the luteal phase.*

CYCLIC CHANGES OF OVARY

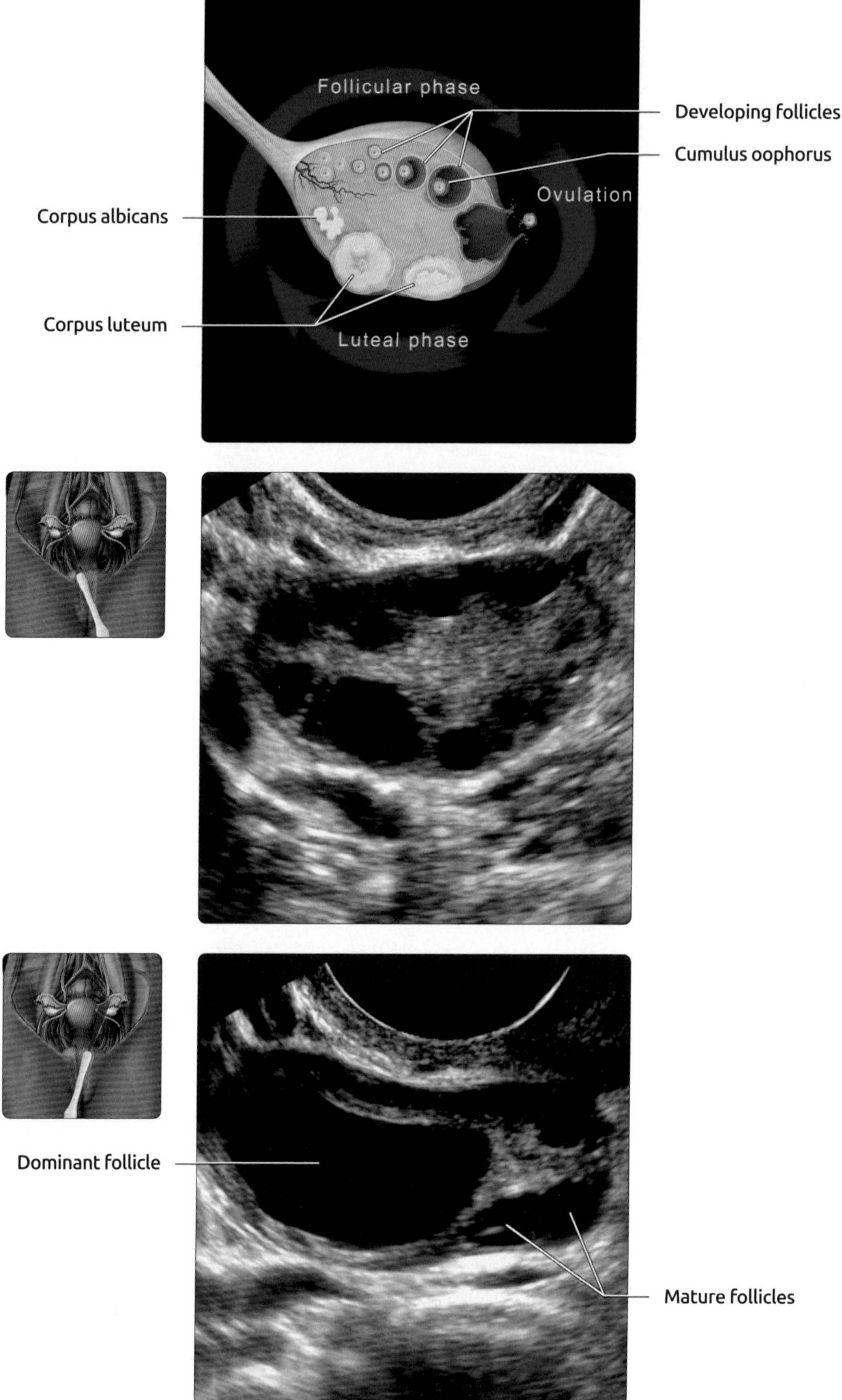

(Top) *During the follicular phase of the menstrual cycle, several follicles begin to develop, but by days 8-12, a dominant follicle has formed, and the remainder begin to regress. On day 14, the follicle ruptures, and the egg is released. After ovulation, a corpus luteum forms, and if fertilization does not occur, the corpus luteum degenerates into a corpus albicans.* **(Middle)** *Longitudinal TVUS of the ovary at the early follicular phase is shown. Note the developing follicles of variable size at the periphery of the ovary.* **(Bottom)** *TVUS shows a dominant follicle developed in the late follicular phase days before ovulation. This should not be confused for a pathologic cyst.*

CYCLIC CHANGES OF OVARY

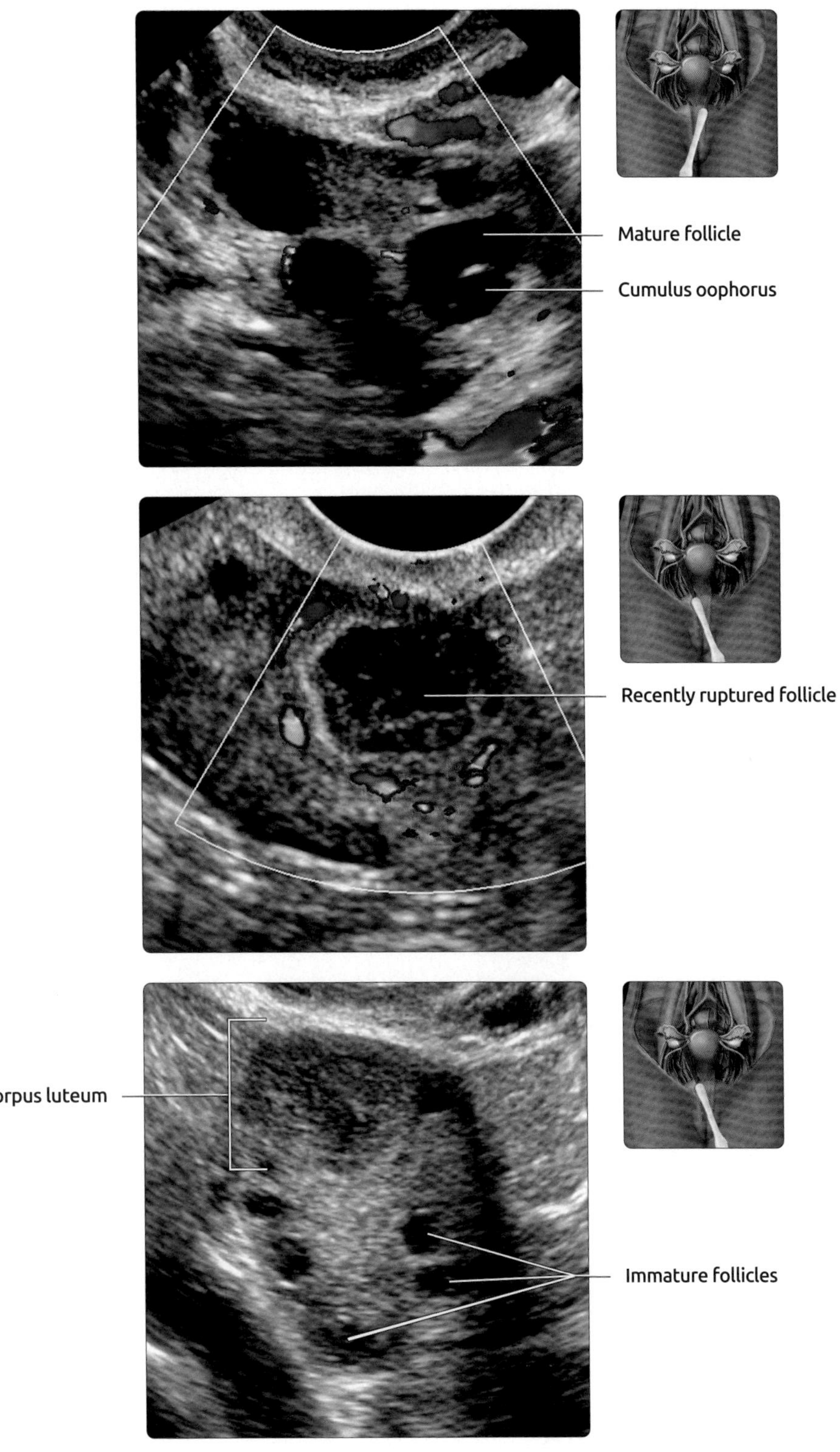

(Top) *Transverse color Doppler TVUS of the ovary demonstrates a large, mature follicle with a small cyst on its wall representing a cumulus oophorus. The size of a mature follicle can reach up to 25 mm before ovulation.* **(Middle)** *Longitudinal color Doppler TVUS of the ovary shows a dominant follicle immediately after its rupture at ovulation. Note the partially collapsed wall resulting from loss of part of the liquor folliculi and the hypoechoic internal contents representing blood.* **(Bottom)** *Transverse TVUS of the ovary shows a regressing corpus luteum with a typical hypoechoic, thick, crenulated wall and echogenic internal contents representing blood.*

CYCLIC CHANGES OF INTRAOVARIAN ARTERY

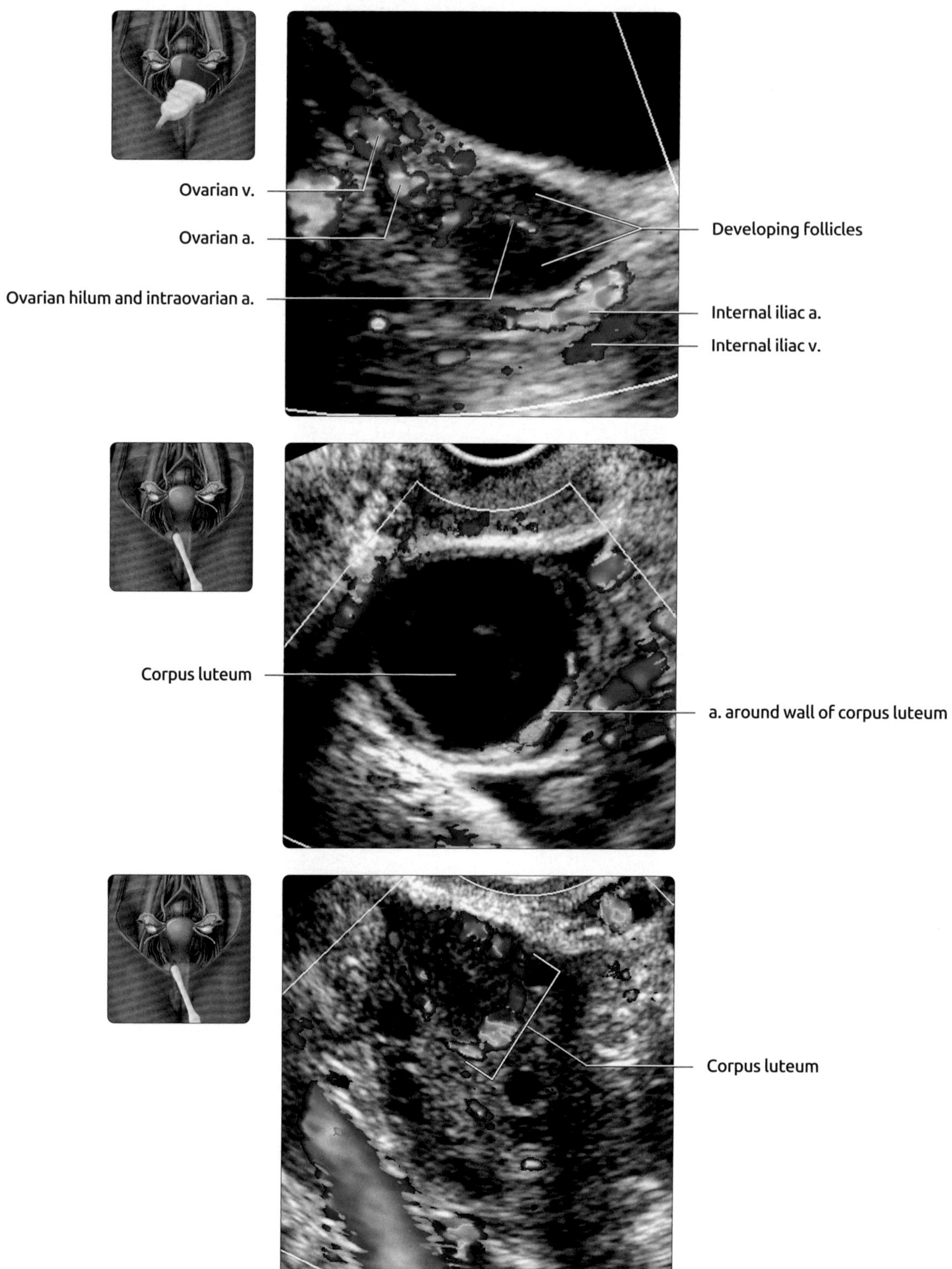

(Top) *Color Doppler TAUS shows an inactive ovary. The ovary demonstrates a hilar artery surrounded by small developing follicles in the early follicular phase. Note the nondominant ovary may show a similar appearance as an inactive ovary.* **(Middle)** *Longitudinal TVUS of the ovary in the early luteal phase is shown. A corpus luteum with low-level internal echoes is seen following ovulation. The wall of the corpus luteum usually displays the most intense color pattern.* **(Bottom)** *Transverse TVUS in midluteal phase is shown. The ovary shows a regressing corpus luteum with typical peripheral color Doppler vascularity.*

CYCLIC CHANGES OF INTRAOVARIAN ARTERY

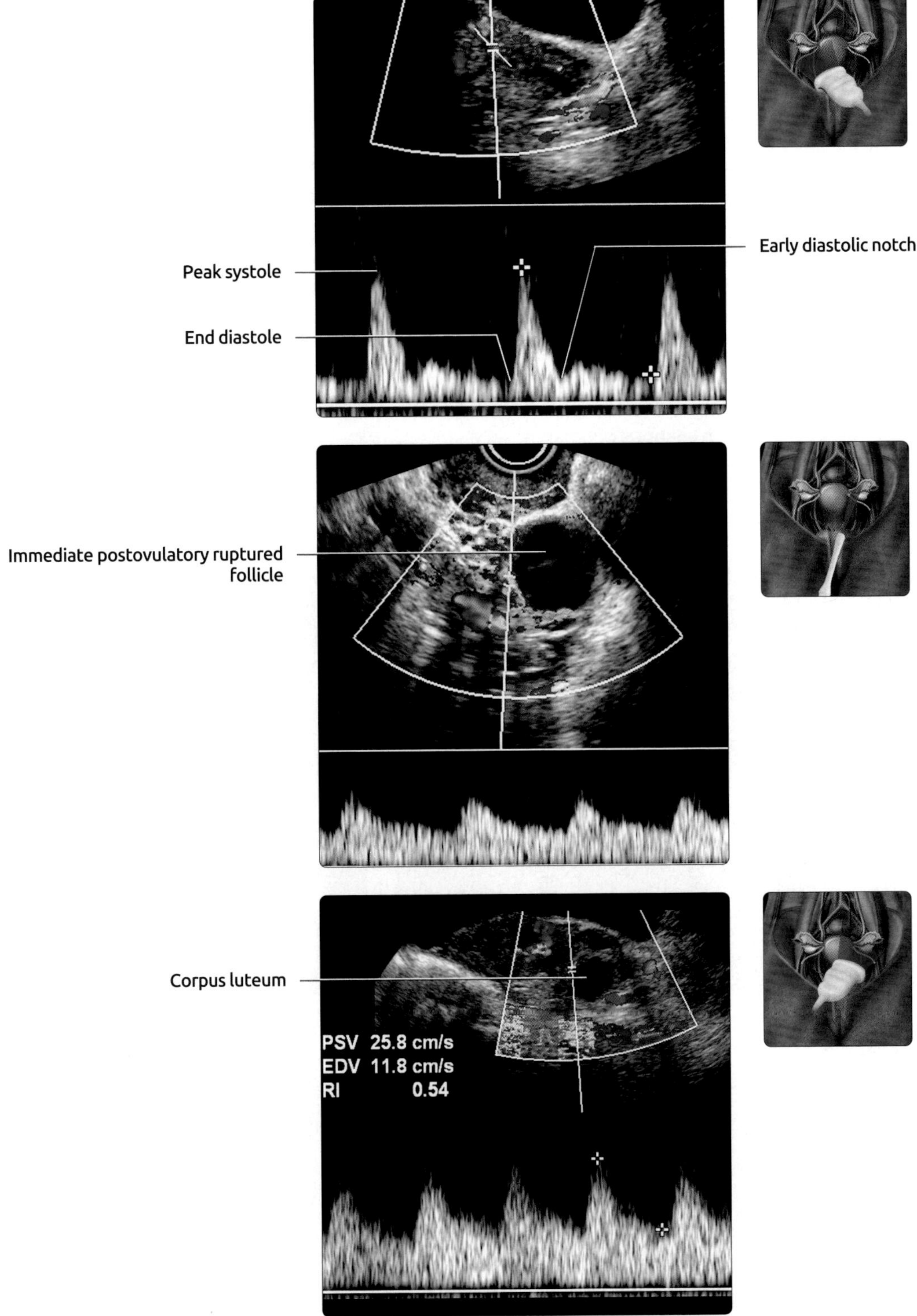

(Top) *Transverse spectral Doppler TAUS of the ovarian artery is shown. The ovarian artery blood flow shows a high-resistance flow pattern with low end-diastolic velocity and an early diastolic notch. This notch indicates initial resistance to forward flow through the ovarian parenchyma. The flow resistance is at its maximum during the first 8 days of the cycle.* **(Middle)** *Spectral Doppler TVUS of the intraovarian artery in early luteal phase is shown. The ovarian artery has a low-resistance flow, which reaches the lowest level in early luteal phase. At this time, the intraovarian vascularity is easily detectable.* **(Bottom)** *Spectral Doppler of TAUS of the intraovarian artery in midluteal phase is shown. The ovarian arterial flow is of medium resistance, and the flow resistance will gradually increase through to the regenerative phase.*

Nabothian Cyst

KEY FACTS

TERMINOLOGY

- Mucus-filled cystic dilatation of endocervical gland
- Tunnel cluster: Type of nabothian cyst characterized by complex multicystic dilatation of endocervical glands

IMAGING

- Circumscribed, superficial, simple unilocular cyst in cervix
  - Imperceptible thin wall
  - Posterior acoustic enhancement
- Average size: 10-15 mm, rarely > 4 cm
- Often multiple
- May distort endocervical canal or enlarge cervix
- Can have proteinaceous debris producing low-level echoes
- Rare septations
- Can mimic multicystic mass when multiple
- Absence of internal or peripheral flow on color Doppler

TOP DIFFERENTIAL DIAGNOSES

- Adenoma malignum (minimal deviation adenocarcinoma)
- Endocervical hyperplasia
- Uterine cervicitis
- Cystic endometrial polyp
- Abortion in progress
- Cervical ectopic pregnancy
- Cervical cancer

PATHOLOGY

- Most common pathologic process of cervix: Healing process of chronic cervicitis

CLINICAL ISSUES

- Incidental finding on imaging or examination, rarely symptomatic from infection or mass effect
- More common in women who have had children

SCANNING TIPS

- Use color Doppler if cyst appears potentially solid

(Left) *Transverse transvaginal ultrasound through the cervix shows a well-circumscribed, simple nabothian cyst ➡ with posterior acoustic enhancement ⇨, separate from the endocervical canal ↪.* **(Right)** *Coronal transvaginal ultrasound shows a simple nabothian cyst ➡ at the lateral margin of the cervix. Real-time imaging helped confirm the location within the cervical stroma; however, this image demonstrates the potential for misdiagnosis as an ovarian follicle.*

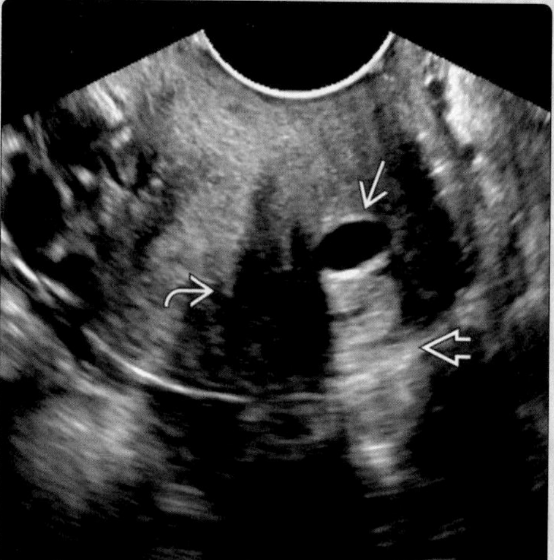

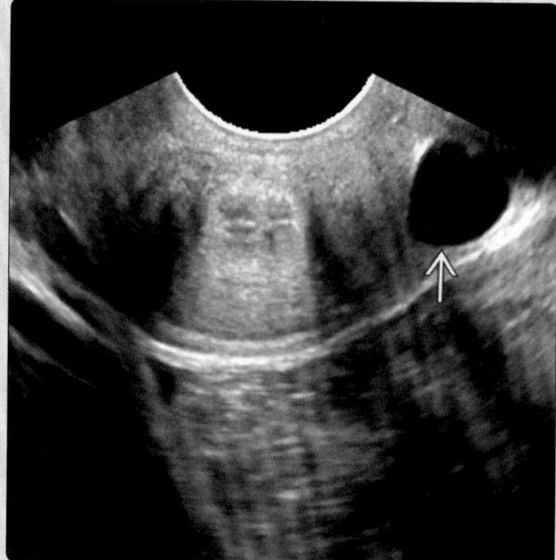

(Left) *Transverse transvaginal ultrasound through the cervix shows a well-circumscribed nabothian cyst ➡ with internal debris. There is posterior acoustic enhancement ⇨. Tiny nabothian cysts ↪ are noted near the endocervical canal ↪.* **(Right)** *Longitudinal transvaginal ultrasound shows a large, complex nabothian cyst ➡ with homogeneous internal echoes, in addition to multiple smaller nabothian cysts ↪. The cervical canal is minimally displaced but remains visible ⇨.*

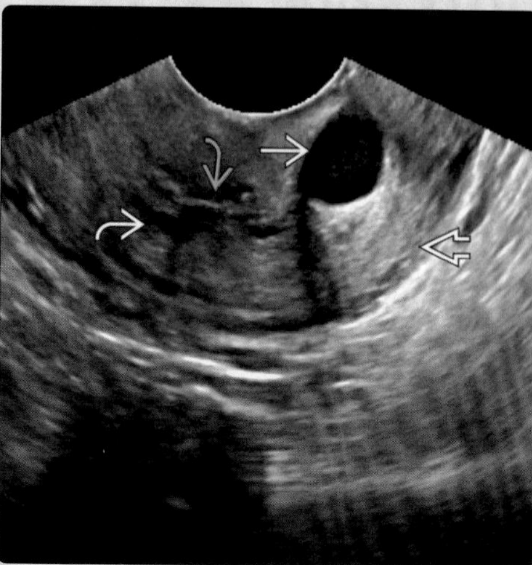

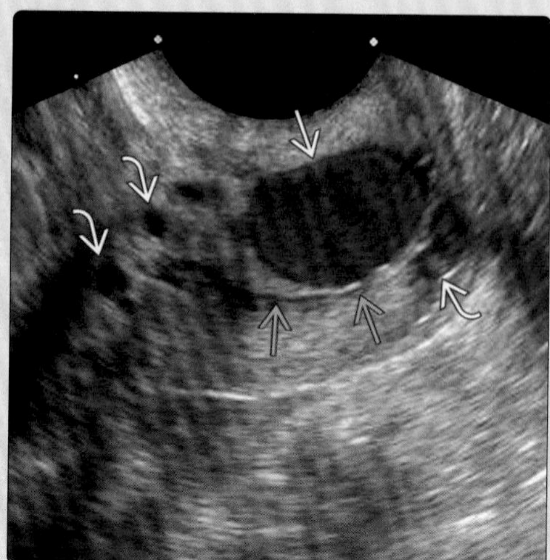

Cervical Carcinoma

KEY FACTS

IMAGING

- Soft tissue mass in cervix: Hypoechoic or isoechoic ± necrosis
- Hydro- or hematometra from cervical obstruction
- Mass extending into upper vagina
- Invasion of posterior bladder wall, anterior rectal wall, ureters
  - Hydronephrosis implies stage IIIB disease
- Enlarged lymph nodes
- Abundant internal color flow on color Doppler
- 3D US may be used to assess tumor volume before/after therapy
- Ultrasound may be used to guide placement of radiotherapy instruments

TOP DIFFERENTIAL DIAGNOSES

- Cervical fibroid
- Cervical polyp
- Endometrial cancer invading cervix
- Adenoma malignum/minimal deviation adenocarcinoma
- Rarer cervical tumors: Lymphoma, neuroendocrine/small cell carcinoma

PATHOLOGY

- ~ 80-90% are squamous carcinoma
- Arise at squamocolumnar junction from precursor lesions

CLINICAL ISSUES

- Abnormal bleeding, pain, or discharge
- Detected by screening cytology from Pap smear
  - ± testing for high-risk HPV
- 3rd most common gynecologic malignancy in USA and most common gynecologic malignancy worldwide
- Risk factors: HPV infection most important, early-onset sexual activity, multiple partners, smoking, immunosuppression, HIV infection

SCANNING TIPS

- Look for disruption of normal cervical morphology

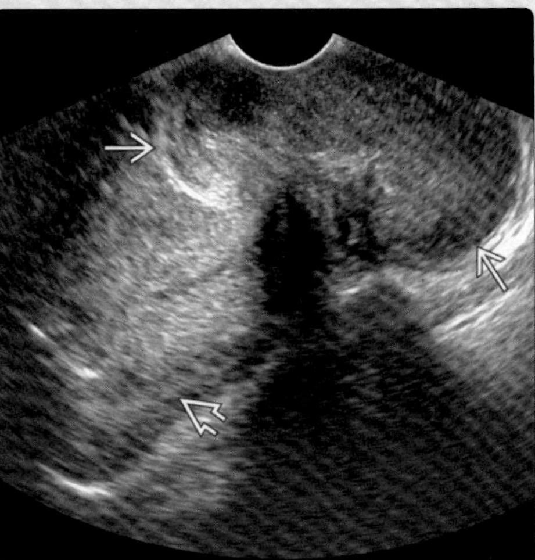

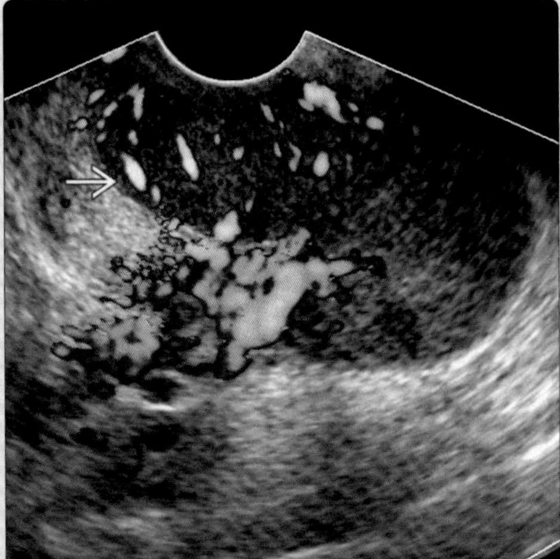

(Left) *Sagittal transvaginal ultrasound shows a bulky soft tissue mass in the cervix, proven to be squamous cell carcinoma. The body of the uterus was unremarkable.* **(Right)** *Parasagittal transvaginal power Doppler ultrasound shows abundant vascularity within the anterior portion of the cervical carcinoma.*

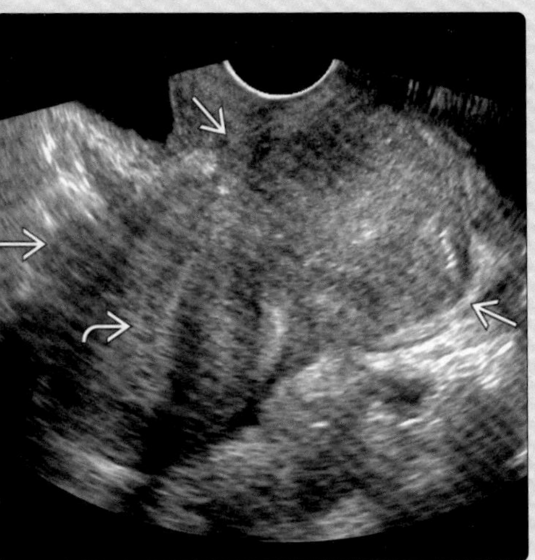

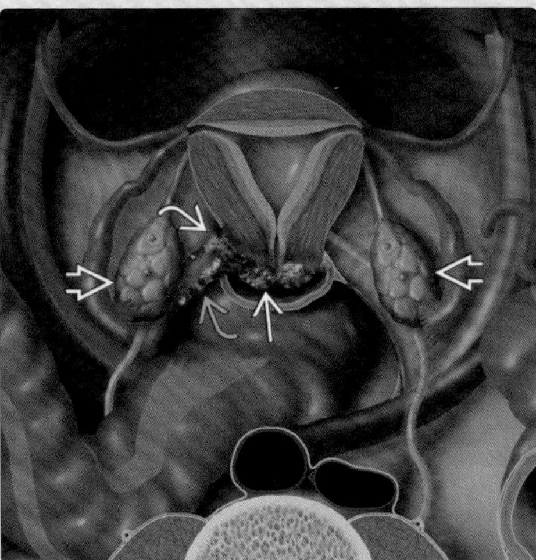

(Left) *Longitudinal transvaginal ultrasound demonstrates a large cervical carcinoma. Local staging cannot be determined. There is no hematometra.* **(Right)** *Graphic shows locally invasive cervical carcinoma, extending onto the right parametrium and growing along ligaments. Bilateral ovaries are not usually involved.*

Adenomyosis

KEY FACTS

TERMINOLOGY

- Ectopic endometrial tissue within myometrium with adjacent smooth muscle hyperplasia

IMAGING

- Globular uterine enlargement, asymmetric myometrial thickening
- Poor definition of endometrial-myometrial interface/thickening of junctional zone
- Heterogeneous myometrial echotexture
  - Echogenic linear striations due to endometrial extension into myometrium
- Focal mass (adenomyoma): Less common
  - Emanates from endomyometrial junction, difficult to differentiate from leiomyoma
- Myometrial cysts in up to 50%: Highly specific for diagnosis
  - Anechoic, usually subendometrial
- Disordered or uncircumscribed myometrial vascular pattern on color Doppler
- Hysterosonography: Saline and bubbles may fill linear tracks in myometrium, producing "myometrial cracks"

TOP DIFFERENTIAL DIAGNOSES

- Leiomyoma
- Diffuse myometrial hypertrophy due to parity
- Endometrial cancer
- Endometrial hyperplasia

CLINICAL ISSUES

- Pre- or perimenopausal, most commonly multiparous
- Often presents with dysmenorrhea, menorrhagia, chronic pelvic pain, dyspareunia, infertility
- Commonly coexists with endometriosis and leiomyomas
- Association with cesarean sections

SCANNING TIPS

- Cine clips with slow sweep are helpful for subtle findings, such as streaky shadowing and small myometrial cysts
- Evaluate for uterine tenderness

(Left) *Longitudinal transvaginal ultrasound demonstrates asymmetric, posterior > anterior linear bands of echogenicity and shadowing* ➡ *without a focal mass, consistent with adenomyosis.* **(Right)** *Transverse transabdominal ultrasound demonstrates poor delineation of the endomyometrial border* ➡ *and diffuse myometrial thickening with areas of band-like shadowing* ➡*.*

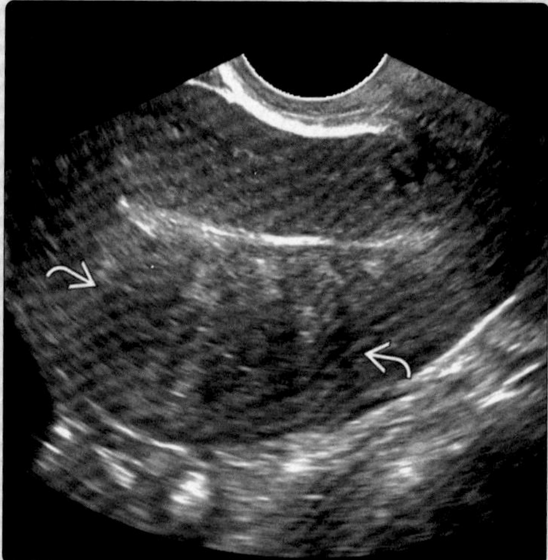

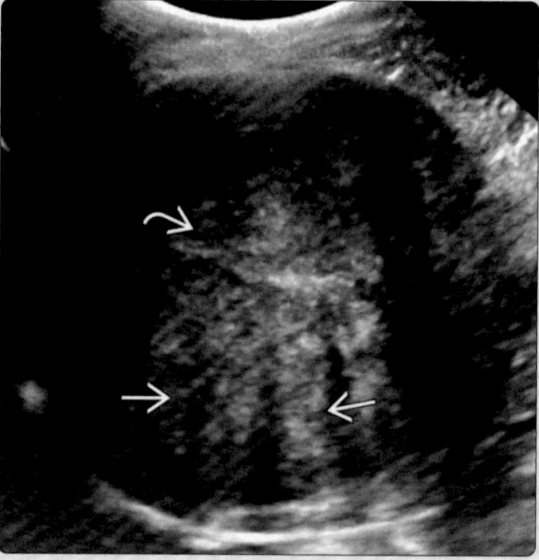

(Left) *Sagittal transabdominal ultrasound of a first trimester pregnancy demonstrates a normal gestational sac* ➡ *with asymmetric anterior myometrial thickening* ➡*. Unlike a fibroid, there is no edge definition to the anterior adenomyosis which contains tiny cysts* ➡*.* **(Right)** *Longitudinal transvaginal ultrasound demonstrates subtle invaginations of the endometrium into the myometrium* ➡*, diagnostic of adenomyosis. Presence of a subendometrial cyst* ➡ *is also highly specific.*

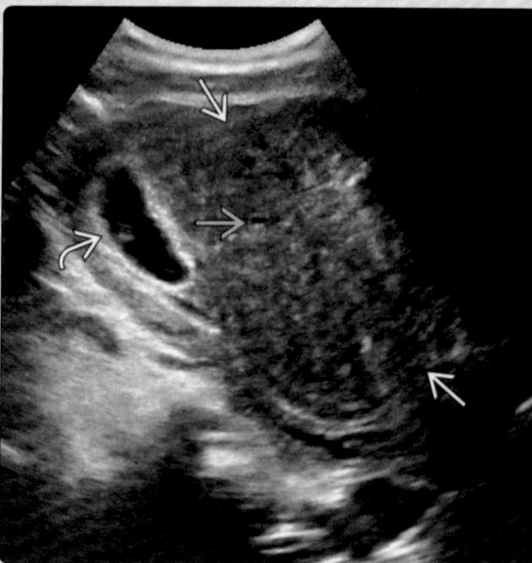

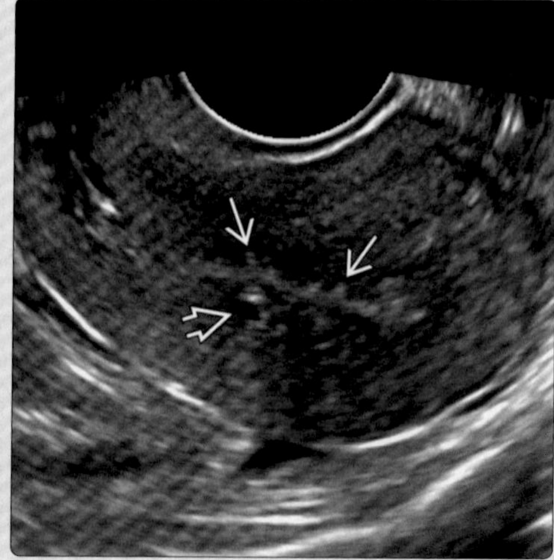

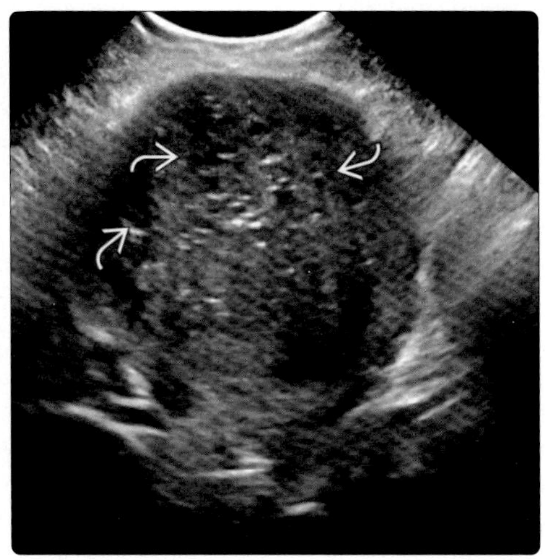

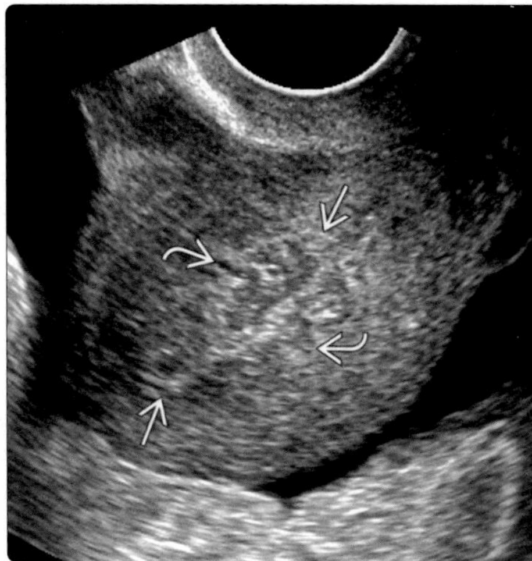

(Left) *Transverse transabdominal ultrasound demonstrates multiple tiny cystic lesions ➔ in the anterior myometrium representing diffuse adenomyosis. The uterus is globular.* **(Right)** *Longitudinal transvaginal ultrasound shows linear striations in the myometrium ➔ without a focal mass. The endomyometrial border is obscured ➔.*

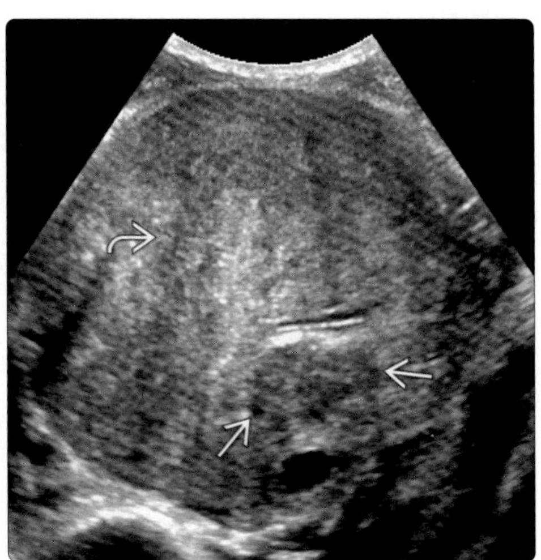

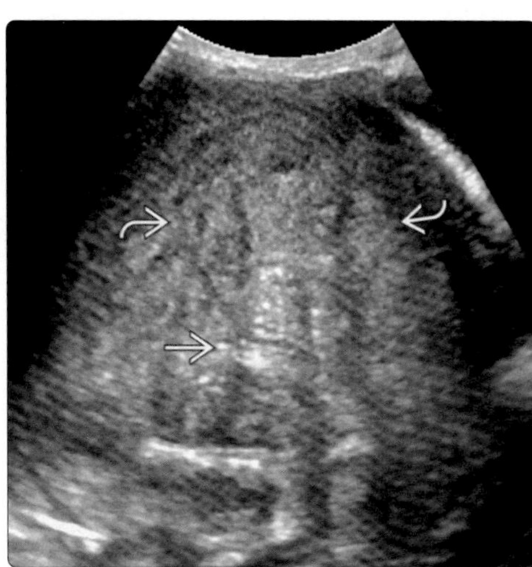

(Left) *Transabdominal ultrasound shows anterior myometrial thickening and linear refractive shadows ➔, consistent with adenomyosis. A well-defined hypoechoic mass with posterior shadowing in the posterior fundus ➔ is an intramural fibroid.* **(Right)** *Transabdominal ultrasound shows a heterogeneous thickened anterior myometrium with linear shadowing ➔, consistent with adenomyosis. The endometrium is barely visible ➔.*

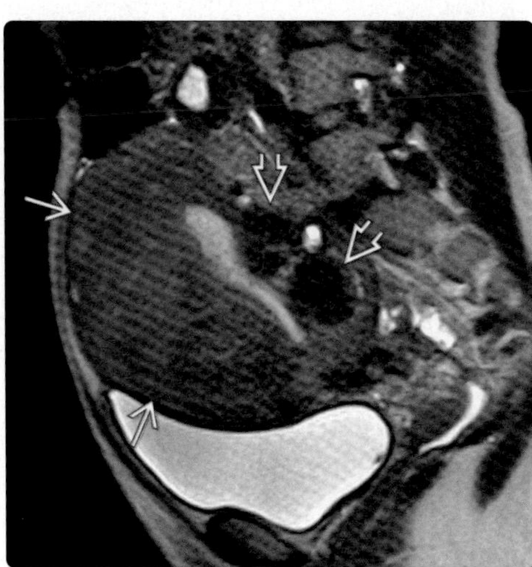

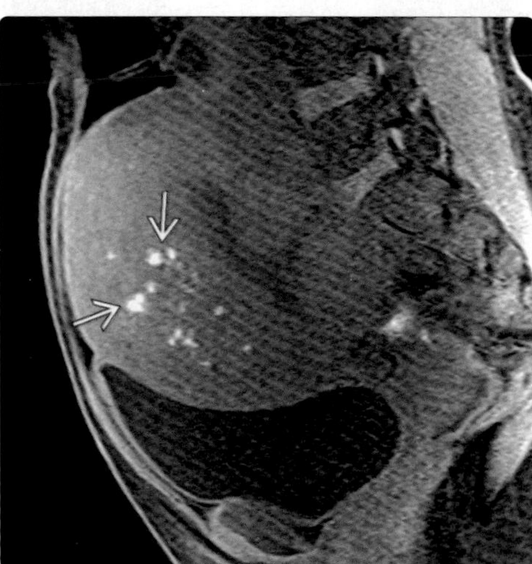

(Left) *Sagittal T2 HASTE MR in the same patient better demonstrates the anterior junctional zone thickening ➔. Multiple low-signal fibroids are seen in the posterior uterus ➔. Fibroids and adenomyosis commonly occur together.* **(Right)** *Sagittal T1 MR in the same patient demonstrates multiple hyperintense foci within the anterior uterus ➔ reflecting hemorrhage, also highly specific for adenomyosis.*

KEY FACTS

TERMINOLOGY

- Benign smooth muscle neoplasm of uterus
- Synonym: Fibroid

IMAGING

- Ultrasound (transabdominal and transvaginal): Study of choice; supplemented by 3D US and saline-infused sonohysterography
- Circumscribed mass, hypoechoic to myometrium
- Posterior acoustic shadowing, even without associated calcifications
- Variable location: Submucosal, intramural, subserosal, intracavitary, pedunculated, cervical, or broad ligament
- Bulky uterine enlargement from large or multiple leiomyomas
- Masses appear heterogeneous when there is cystic degeneration or hemorrhage
- Size: Extremely variable, subcentimeter to > 10 cm
- Color Doppler: Peripheral vascularity
    - Ischemia/degeneration: Decreased or absent color flow
- Vascular stalk helps characterize pedunculated leiomyoma

TOP DIFFERENTIAL DIAGNOSES

- Adenomyosis
- Focal myometrial contraction
- Leiomyosarcoma
- Uterine duplication

CLINICAL ISSUES

- Increase in size and frequency with age
- 25-30% incidence in United States
- Symptoms primarily related to leiomyoma location, size, &/or growth: Heavy bleeding, pelvic pressure, pain
- Degeneration can cause acute pelvic pain
- Can undergo rapid growth during pregnancy

SCANNING TIPS

- Cine clips are useful to differentiate from adenomyosis

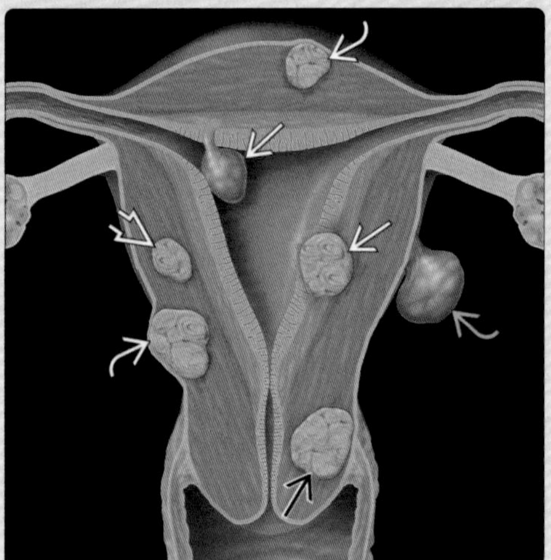

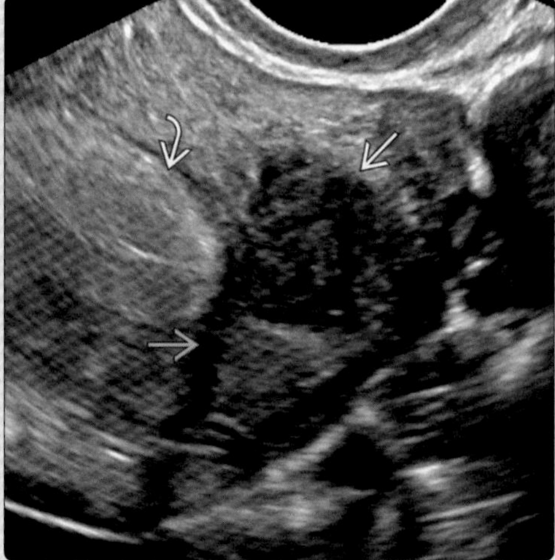

(Left) *Coronal graphic shows various leiomyoma locations, including submucosal and endocavitary ➡, subserosal ➡ and pedunculated ➡, and mural ➡ and cervical ➡. Note the whorled consistency.* **(Right)** *Transvaginal ultrasound demonstrates a lobulated hypoechoic intramural leiomyoma ➡ abutting the endometrium ➡ without any distortion. Note the refractive acoustic shadowing ➡.*

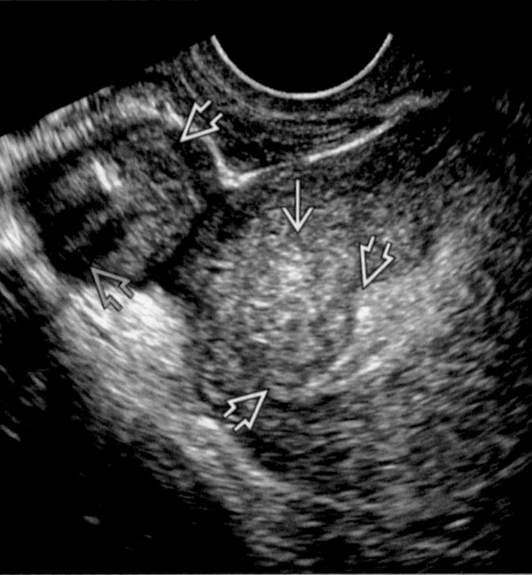

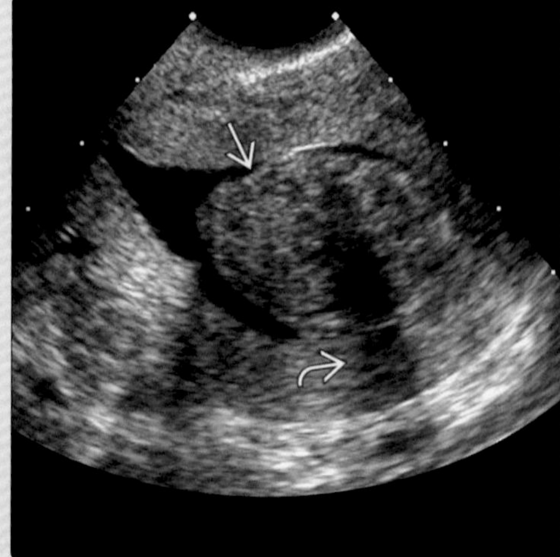

(Left) *Transvaginal ultrasound demonstrates a hypoechoic subserosal pedunculated leiomyoma ➡ with posterior acoustic shadowing ➡. An isoechoic submucosal leiomyoma ➡ causes distortion of the endometrium.* **(Right)** *Saline-infused sonohysterography clearly demonstrates the intracavitary location of a hypoechoic submucosal leiomyoma ➡. Posterior shadowing ➡ is the result of fibrous tissue, not calcifications.*

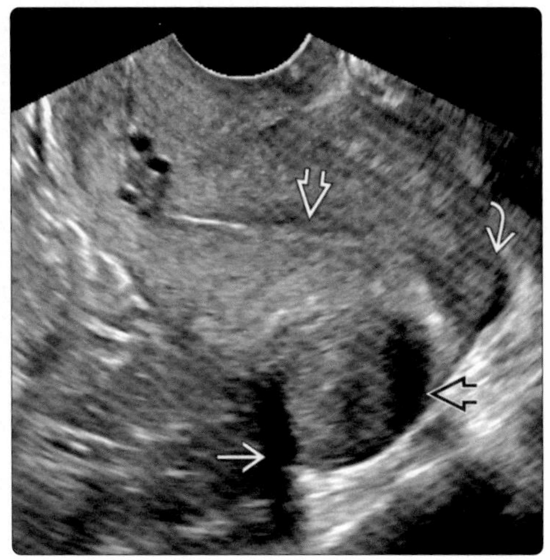

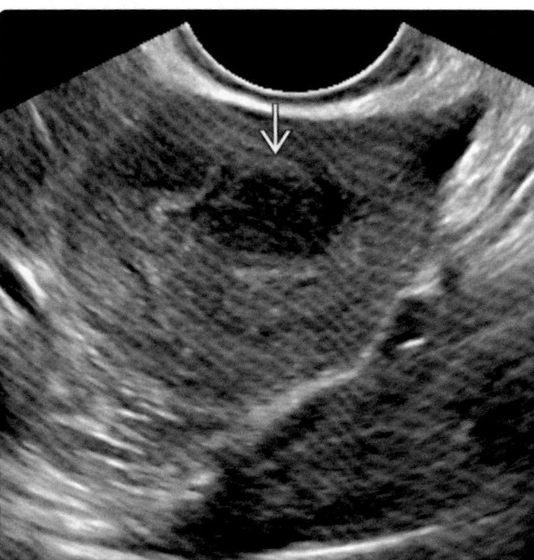

(Left) *Longitudinal transvaginal ultrasound of a retroverted uterus shows a hypoechoic subserosal leiomyoma ➡ with posterior acoustic shadowing ➡. A smaller submucosal leiomyoma ➡ does not shadow. The endometrium ➡ is normal.* **(Right)** *Longitudinal transvaginal ultrasound shows a small, well-marginated, nonshadowing intramural leiomyoma ➡.*

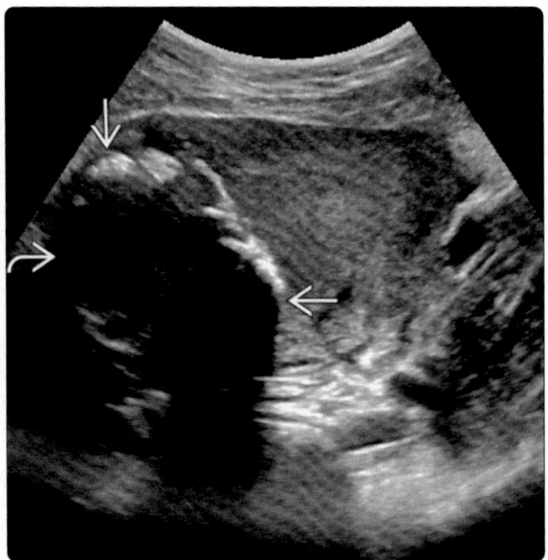

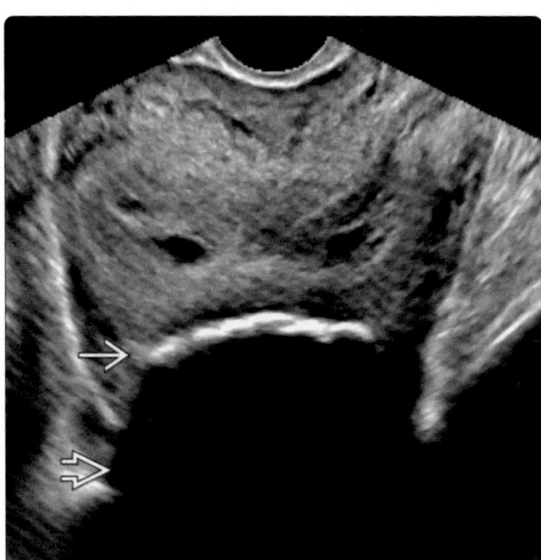

(Left) *Transverse transabdominal ultrasound of the uterus in early pregnancy shows a peripherally calcified large intramural/subserosal leiomyoma ➡. The shadowing ➡ obscures posterior structures.* **(Right)** *Sagittal transvaginal ultrasound of the same patient shows the markedly calcified subserosal leiomyoma ➡ with clean posterior acoustic shadowing ➡.*

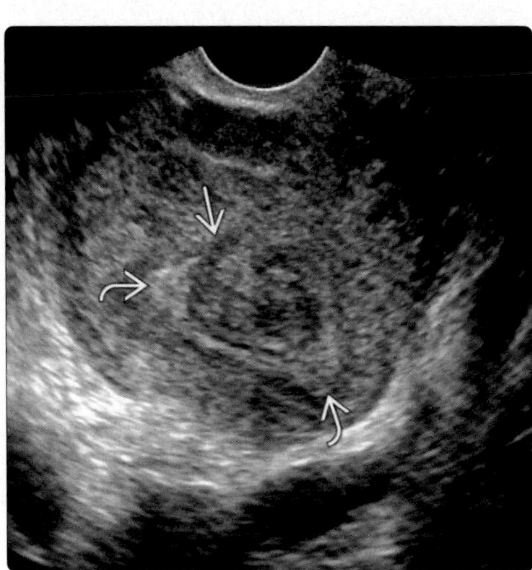

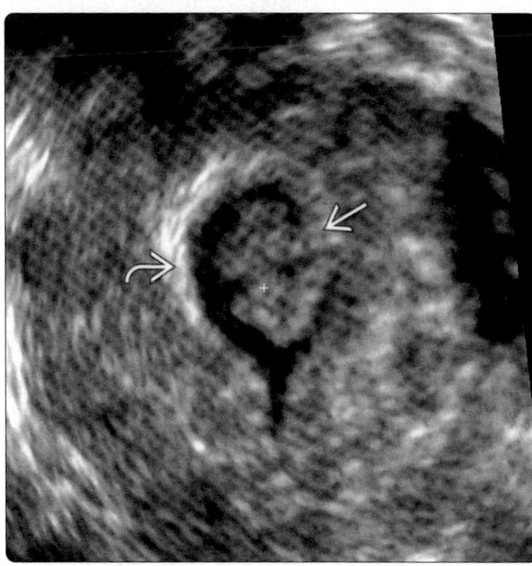

(Left) *Coronal transvaginal ultrasound shows a central well-marginated submucosal leiomyoma ➡ almost completely surrounded by endometrium ➡.* **(Right)** *Coronal 3D reformation from saline-infused sonohysterogram confirms the submucosal leiomyoma ➡ that is attached to the wall but is less echogenic than endometrium ➡. Saline-infused sonohysterography is very useful to determine degree of intramural extension prior to surgery.*

KEY FACTS

TERMINOLOGY

- Müllerian duct anomalies (MDA): Series of uterine malformations resulting from abnormal development, fusion, or resorption of müllerian ducts

IMAGING

- Abnormal configuration of endometrial cavity ± abnormal external contour of uterus
- 3D ultrasound is vital for correct diagnosis, as it enables evaluation of fundus in true coronal plane
- Arcuate uterus
  - Normal external uterine contour
- Septate uterus
  - 2 endometrial cavities, fibrous or muscular septum of variable length and thickness
  - Convex outer uterine contour or cleft < 1 cm
- Bicornuate uterus
  - 2 symmetric uterine horns, fused inferiorly; deep fundal cleft > 1 cm
- Unicornuate uterus
  - Curved and elongated, banana-shaped single uterine horn and endometrium
- Uterus didelphys
  - 2 separate noncommunicating, divergent uterine horns with 2 cervices; deep fundal cleft
- Müllerian agenesis or hypoplasia
  - Absent or small rudimentary uterus

CLINICAL ISSUES

- 1-5% prevalence in general population
- May present with primary amenorrhea or dysmenorrhea at menarche, cyclical pelvic pain and pressure or with obstetric-/fertility-related complications
- Renal anomalies in 30-50%: renal agenesis (most common)

SCANNING TIPS

- Image outer uterine contour
- Image renal fossae to assess for renal agenesis

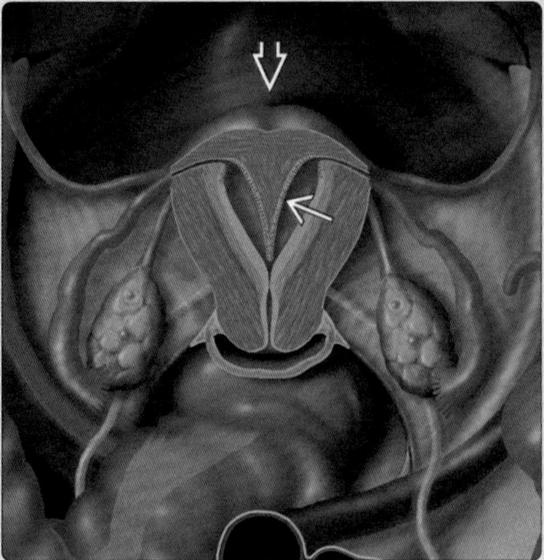

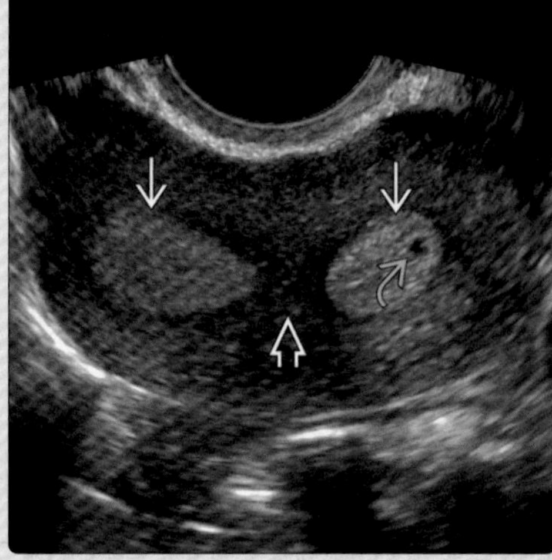

(Left) *Graphic of a septate uterus shows minimal indentation on the uterine fundus ⇨. The cavity is divided with myometrium in the superior aspect of the septum, although normal zonal anatomy is not present in this portion ➡.* **(Right)** *Transverse ultrasound shows 2 endometrial cavities ➡ separated by myometrial tissue ⇨. An early gestational sac ↪ is present on the left side. Evaluation of the external uterine contour was necessary to confirm this as a septate uterus.*

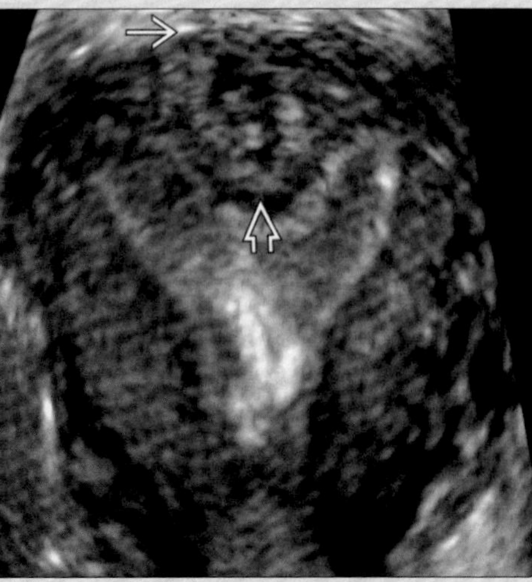

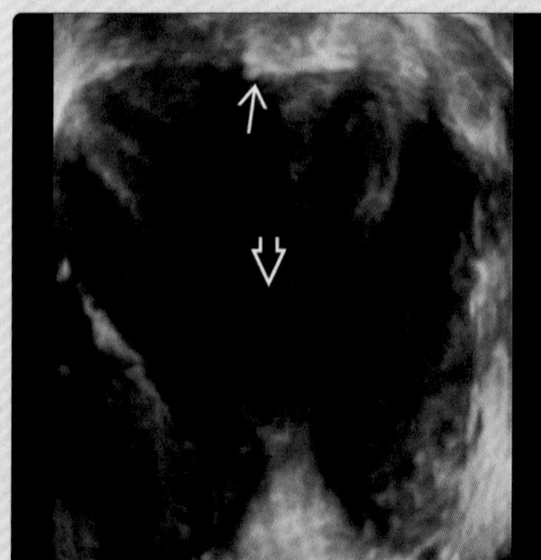

(Left) *3D ultrasound with coronal MIP rendering shows a muscular septum ⇨ indenting the fundal endometrium. The coronal reconstruction readily depicts the normal convex outer uterine contour ➡ of this septate uterus.* **(Right)** *3D ultrasound with volume rendering shows a deep muscular septum ⇨ extending into the fundal endometrium with a normal convex outer uterine contour ➡, consistent with septate uterus.*

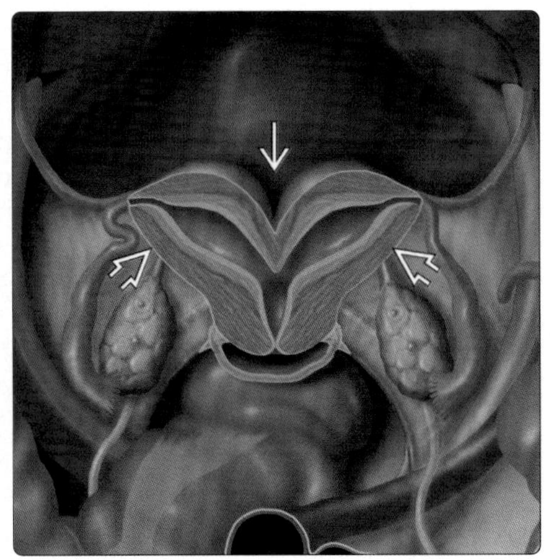

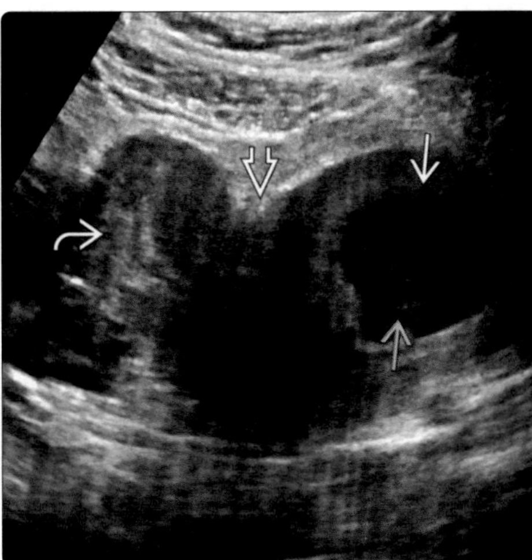

(Left) *Graphic of a bicornuate uterus demonstrates a deep external fundal cleft ➡ and 2 symmetric cornua ➡ that are fused inferiorly.* **(Right)** *Transverse transabdominal ultrasound shows wide separation ➡ of the uterine horns with a 9-week pregnancy ➡ in the left horn ➡ and endometrial thickening in the right horn ➡. There was a single cervix (not shown) confirming a bicornuate unicollis uterus.*

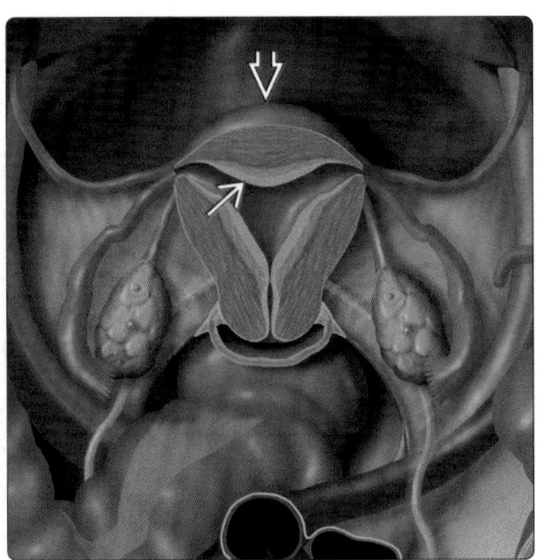

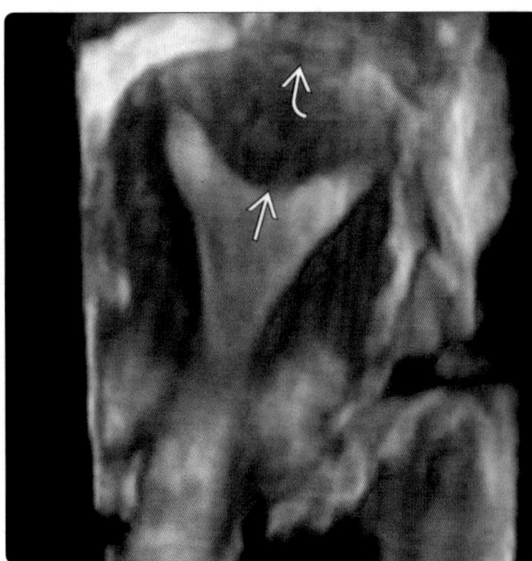

(Left) *Graphic of an arcuate uterus shows normal convex contour of the uterine fundus ➡. There is indentation of the fundal endometrium < 1 cm without a true septum ➡.* **(Right)** *3D ultrasound with volume rendering shows an arcuate uterus with indentation of the fundal endometrium < 1 cm without a true septum ➡. The outer surface of the fundus is convex outward ➡.*

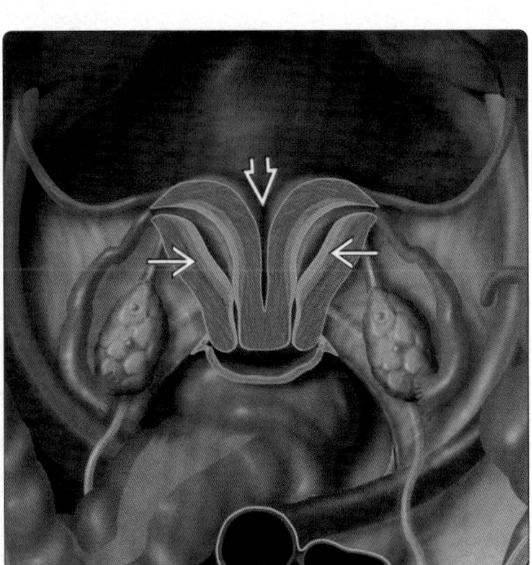

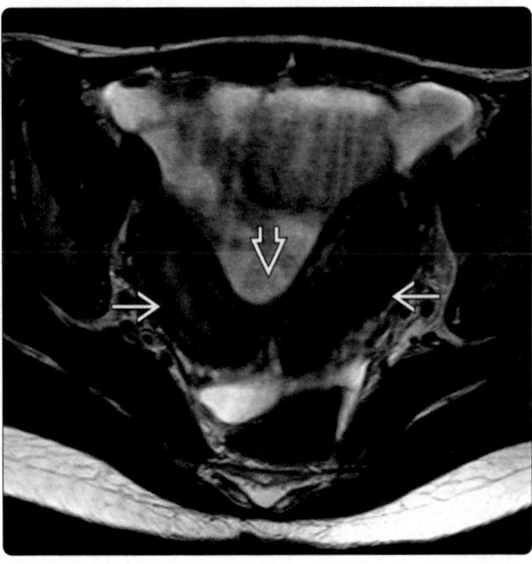

(Left) *Graphic of a uterus didelphys shows complete duplication of uterine horns and cervices with no communication of the endometrial cavities ➡. There is a deep cleft ➡.* **(Right)** *Axial T2 HASTE MR through the pelvis shows widely separated uterine horns ➡ with a deep intervening cleft ➡, representing uterine didelphys.*

Hematometrocolpos

KEY FACTS

TERMINOLOGY

- Hematometrocolpos: Distension of uterus and vagina by accumulated blood secondary to obstruction

IMAGING

- US best for initial evaluation of pelvic mass or primary amenorrhea
- Distended uterine &/or vaginal cavities
- Hematometrocolpos appears thick-walled superiorly due to surrounding myometrium with thinner wall where surrounded by vagina
- Mixed echogenicity material within uterine &/or vaginal cavities: Blood products of varying age
- No color flow
- 3D US allows better evaluation of uterine fundal contour

TOP DIFFERENTIAL DIAGNOSES

- Pyometra
- Endometritis
- Muco-/hydrometrocolpos
- Gestational trophoblastic disease

PATHOLOGY

- Congenital causes present earlier than acquired obstruction
- Congenital: Imperforate hymen (most frequent cause), müllerian duct anomaly, cloacal malformation
- Acquired cervical/vaginal stenosis: Cancer, post surgery or radiation
- Associated with renal anomalies and endometriosis

CLINICAL ISSUES

- Cyclical pelvic pain/pressure, low back pain
- Primary amenorrhea at puberty from imperforate hymen
- Urinary retention, constipation

SCANNING TIPS

- Use combination of transabdominal, transvaginal, and transperineal approaches
- Evaluate renal fossae for associated renal abnormality

(Left) *Longitudinal transabdominal US in a patient with an imperforate hymen shows a markedly distended cervical canal ➡ containing blood, consistent with hematocolpos. There is less severe distension of the uterine cavity ➡ where there is a thicker wall made of myometrium.* **(Right)** *Longitudinal transabdominal US in a patient with vaginal atresia shows a distended vagina with thin walls ➡ containing blood ➡, consistent with hematocolpos. Note the thicker walls of the distended uterine cavity ➡.*

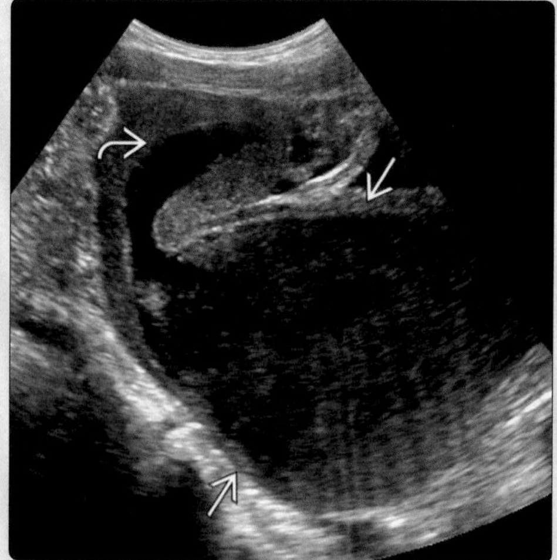

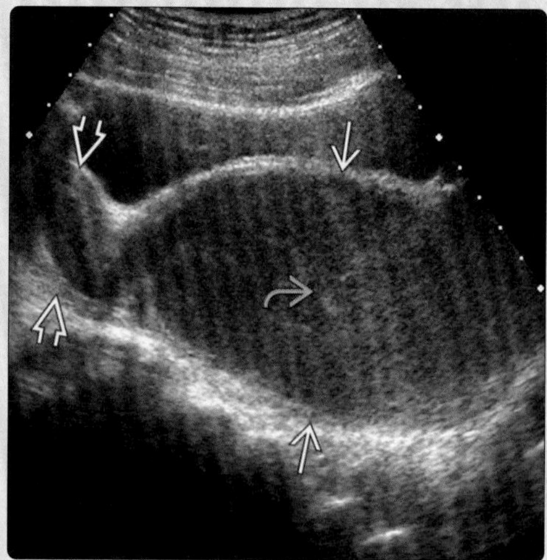

(Left) *Longitudinal transabdominal US of the uterus shows distention of the uterine ➡ and cervical ➡ cavities with blood ➡, consistent with hematometros in this patient who had amenorrhea from cervical stenosis post cone biopsy.* **(Right)** *Longitudinal transvaginal US of the same patient on a different machine shows hematometros ➡ secondary to cervical stenosis post cone biopsy.*

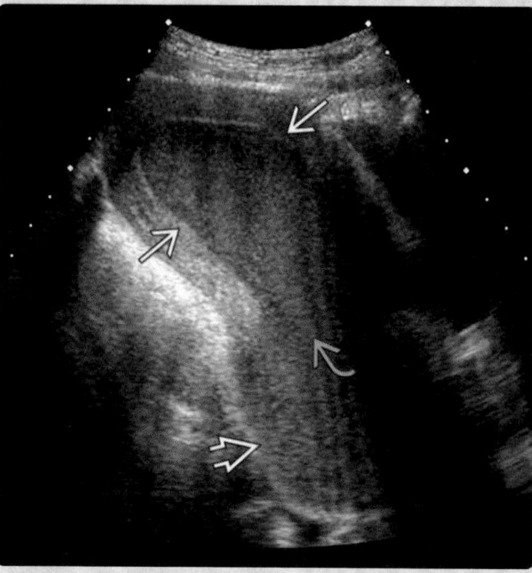

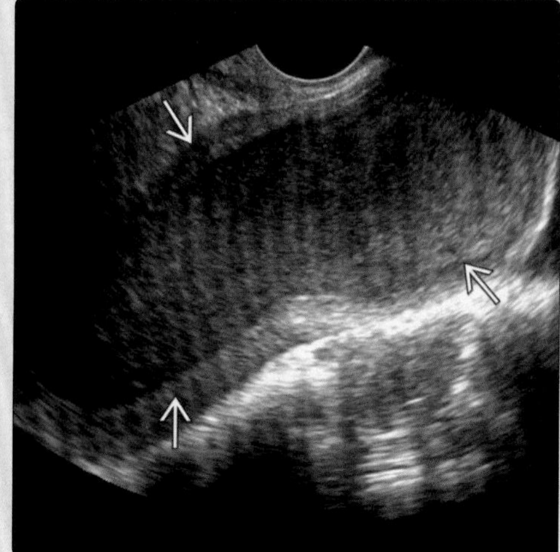

KEY FACTS

ERMINOLOGY

- Focal hyperplastic overgrowth of endometrial tissue

MAGING

- Pedunculated or sessile endometrial lesion, solitary or multiple (20%)
- Echogenic lesion during proliferative phase
- May be less conspicuous during secretory phase as entire endometrium is more echogenic
- Variable size: May be tiny or large enough to fill entire uterine cavity
- May prolapse into cervical canal
- Small "cystic" areas due to dilated endometrial glands
- Hyperechoic line sign: Full/partial echogenic rim around area of endometrial thickening highly specific for endocavitary mass
- Color Doppler: Single feeding vessel in stalk
- Saline infusion sonohysterography (SIS): Best technique to differentiate focal from diffuse endometrial thickening
- Schedule US/SIS within first 10 days of menstrual cycle
- 3D US shows multiple polyps better than 2D
  - Useful during SIS (especially if multiple lesions)

TOP DIFFERENTIAL DIAGNOSES

- Endometrial carcinoma
- Endometrial hyperplasia
- Submucosal fibroid
- Gestational trophoblastic disease
- Retained products of conception

CLINICAL ISSUES

- Often asymptomatic
- Abnormal bleeding: Intermenstrual, post coital, post menopausal (up to 30% of postmenopausal bleeding)
- Polyp site/number/diameter do not correlate with symptomatology

SCANNING TIPS

- Timing of ultrasound and SIS optimizes detection

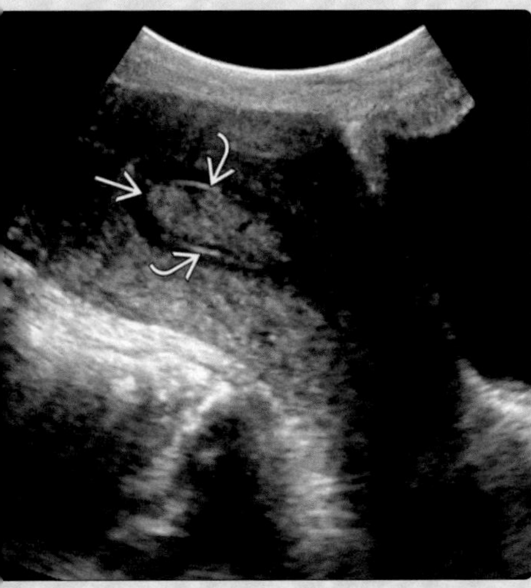

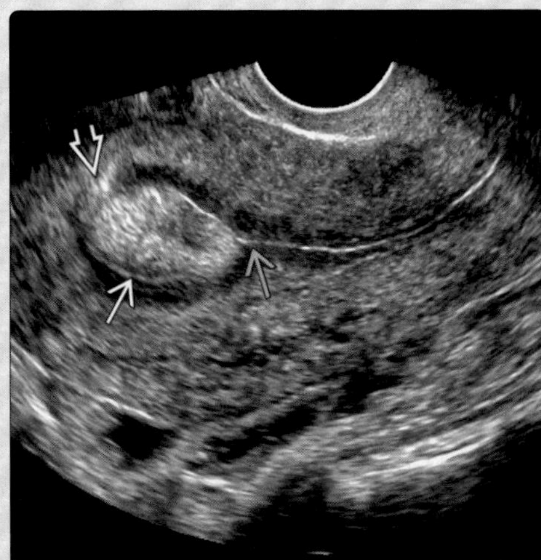

(Left) *Transabdominal pelvic ultrasound in a patient with menorrhagia shows an echogenic endometrial mass → with the hyperechoic line sign →.* **(Right)** *Transvaginal longitudinal pelvic ultrasound in the same patient confirms a large endometrial polyp → attached to the fundus →. Notice interrupted mucosa sign at the interface of endometrial stripe and polyp →, another specific sign of an endometrial polyp.*

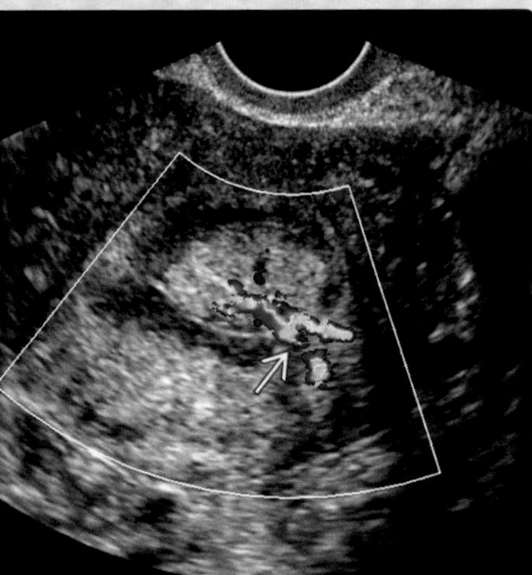

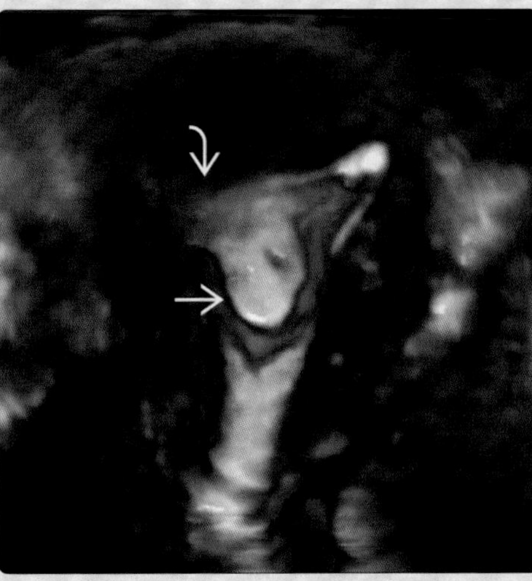

(Left) *Coronal color Doppler ultrasound of the same patient shows the vessels → in the pedicle of the polyp.* **(Right)** *Surface-rendered 3D ultrasound obtained during saline-infused hysterosonography shows an endometrial polyp →, which is broadly attached to the right uterine fundus →.*

Endometrial Carcinoma

KEY FACTS

IMAGING

- Transvaginal sonography study of choice for initial work-up of abnormal vaginal bleeding
- Endometrial thickening: Focal more suspicious than diffuse
- Polypoid masses with internal color flow
- Mixed echogenicity, ± necrosis
- Can invade myometrium, cervix, parametrial structures
- Disruption of endometrial-myometrial interface and subendometrial halo suggests myometrial invasion
- Hematometros if tumor obstructs cavity or cervix
- Multiple feeding vessels on color Doppler
- Saline-infusion sonohysterography useful to differentiate focal from diffuse endometrial pathology

TOP DIFFERENTIAL DIAGNOSES

- Endometrial hyperplasia or polyp
- Submucosal fibroid
- Uterine sarcoma
- Adenomyosis

PATHOLOGY

- Majority are adenocarcinoma, 75% endometrioid type (associated with estrogen stimulation)

CLINICAL ISSUES

- Most common gynecologic malignancy; 75% postmenopausal
- Abnormal bleeding in 90%: Postmenopausal, menorrhagia, intermenstrual bleeding
- Risk factors: Obesity, diabetes, hypertension, chronic anovulation, polycystic ovarian syndrome, unopposed estrogen stimulation, Tamoxifen
- Thickness of endometrium should be correlated with menopausal status and timing in menstrual cycle

SCANNING TIPS

- Both transabdominal and transvaginal probes may be required due to uterine size; evaluate endometrial-myometrial interface carefully

(Left) *Longitudinal transvaginal US performed for irregular vaginal bleeding shows a thickened endometrium in a retroverted uterus. The fundal endometrium is echogenic ➡ with subtle heterogeneity in the lower cavity ➡. Biopsy confirmed endometrioid carcinoma.* **(Right)** *Longitudinal transvaginal US of a retroverted uterus in a patient with postmenopausal bleeding shows a polypoid mass ➡ distending the uterine cavity. Endocervical curettage confirmed endometrioid carcinoma.*

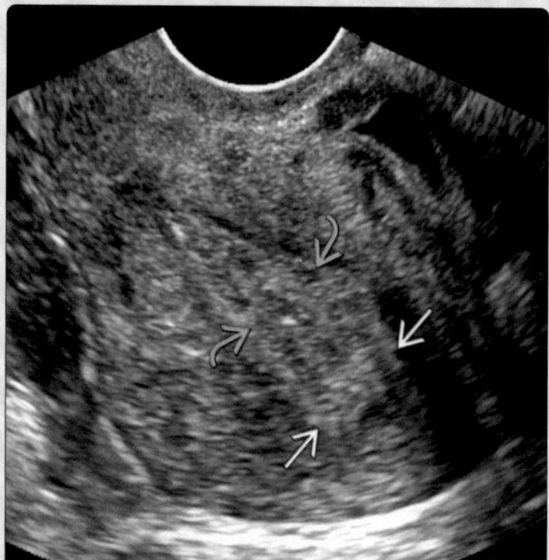

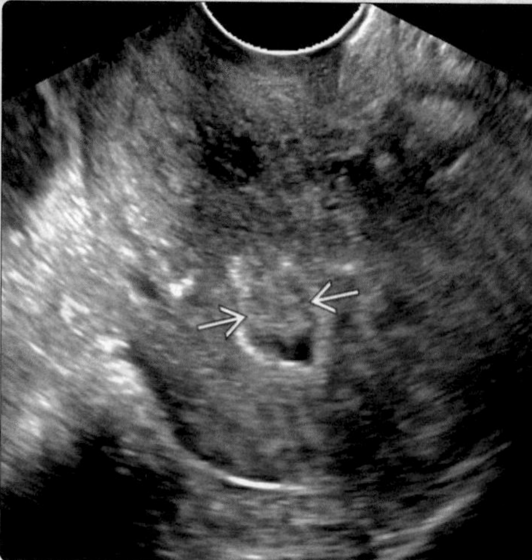

(Left) *Longitudinal transvaginal US shows a large, polypoid mass ➡ within the endometrial cavity with an additional smaller inferior mass ➡, the latter leading to obstructive hematometros ➡. Pathology revealed carcinosarcoma.* **(Right)** *Transabdominal US shows an internally heterogeneous, mixed-echogenicity mass ➡ expanding the uterine cavity, with poorly defined margins and internal calcifications ➡. Pathology confirmed endometrial sarcoma.*

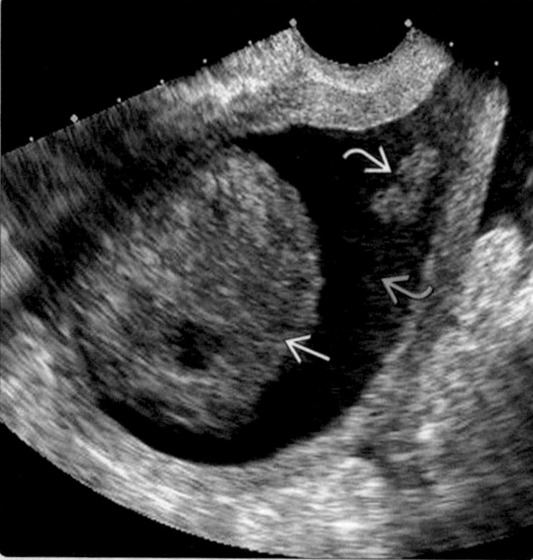

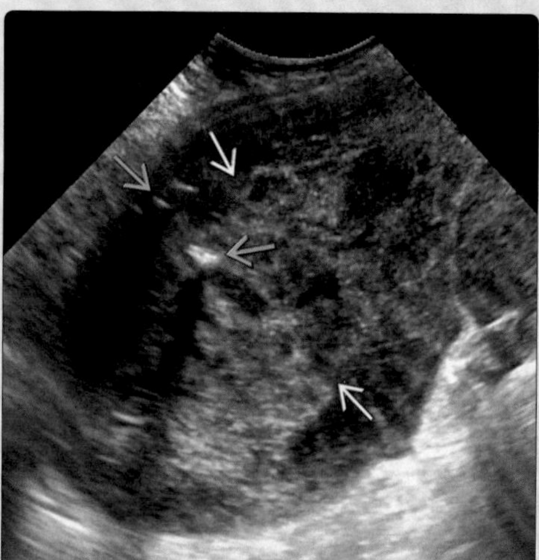

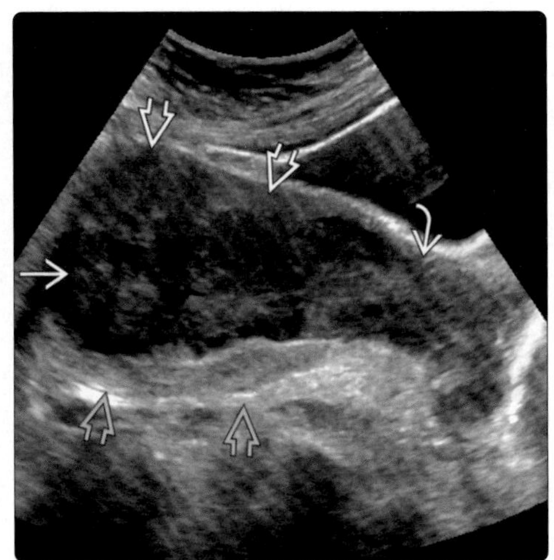

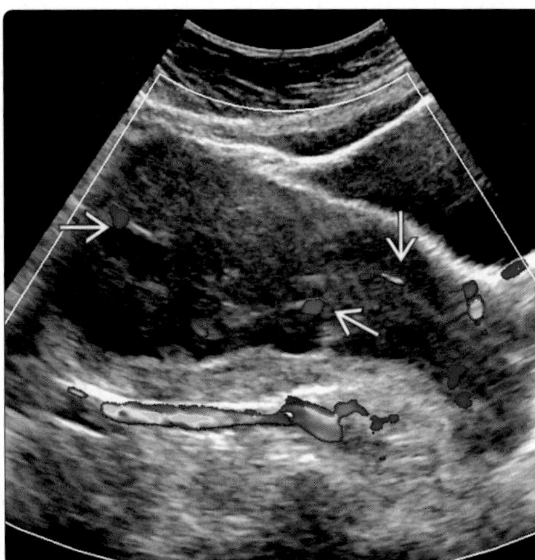

(Left) *Longitudinal transabdominal US performed for postmenopausal bleeding shows an enlarged uterus with heterogeneous tumor invading anterior myometrium and extending into cervix. This was extensive endometrial serous adenocarcinoma. The posterior myometrium is thinned.* **(Right)** *Longitudinal color Doppler US of the same patient shows color flow within the tumor. The size of this tumor usually precludes diagnostic transvaginal US.*

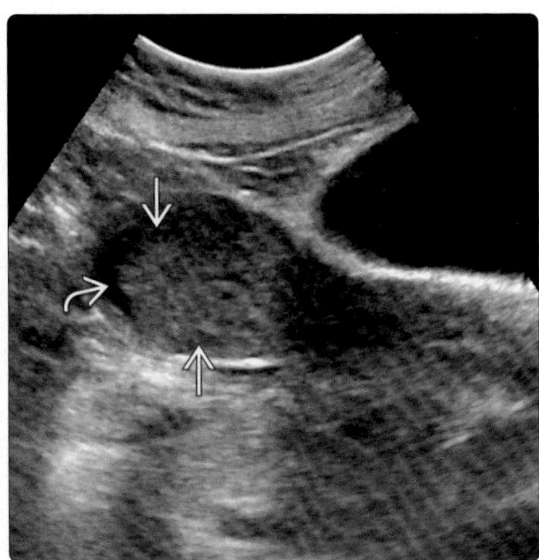

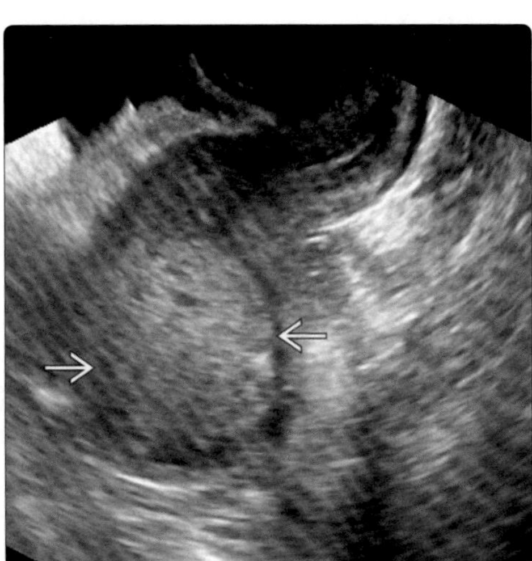

(Left) *Longitudinal transabdominal US performed for postmenopausal bleeding shows an echogenic mass in the endometrial cavity with trace fluid. The interface between the mass and the myometrium is difficult to evaluate in its entirety.* **(Right)** *Longitudinal transvaginal US in the same patient confirms the echogenic mass, but here too the margins are difficult to evaluate. This was endometrial serous carcinoma.*

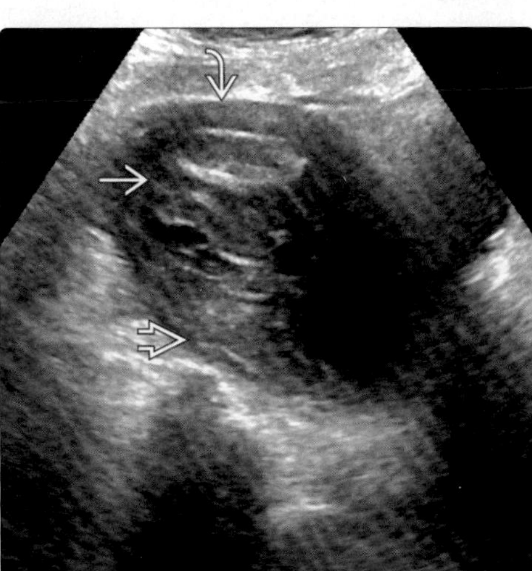

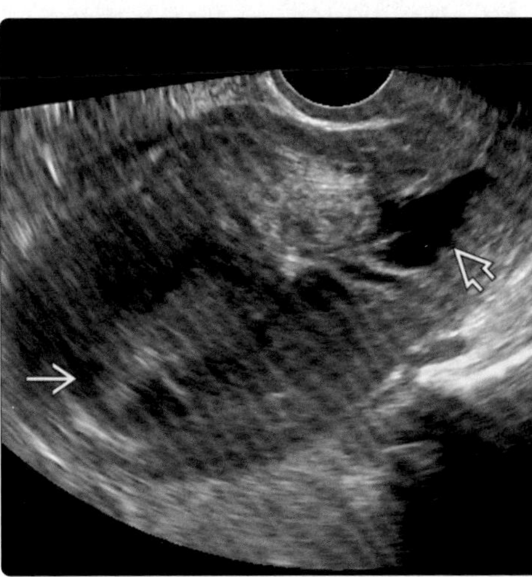

(Left) *Longitudinal transabdominal US performed for postmenopausal bleeding shows an enlarged uterus with a very heterogeneous tumor. Anterior myometrium appears normal, but posterior myometrium appears thin.* **(Right)** *Longitudinal transvaginal US in the same patient shows the heterogeneity of this endometrial sarcoma. There are cystic and necrotic components.*

Endometritis

KEY FACTS

TERMINOLOGY

- Polymicrobial infection resulting from ascending spread of organisms from cervix or from incision into uterus

IMAGING

- Endometritis is predominantly a clinical diagnosis: Postpartum fever and pelvic pain
- Imaging usually ordered to look for complications: Pyometrium, abscess, retained products of conception
- Endometrium may appear normal or be thick and heterogeneous
- Endometrial gas, fluid and inflammatory debris; gas bubbles alone are not diagnostic as gas is normal finding for up to 3 weeks postpartum, present in up to 21% of healthy patients
- Hyperechoic foci within endometrial cavity ± shadowing
- Large amount of echogenic fluid suspicious for pyometra
- May see increased flow on color Doppler
  - Lack of ↑ flow does not rule out endometritis
- Fluid in cul-de-sac

TOP DIFFERENTIAL DIAGNOSES

- Retained products of conception
- Intrauterine blood/clot
- Asymptomatic postpartum endometrial gas
- Endometrial calcifications

CLINICAL ISSUES

- Most common cause of postpartum fever, 1-3% of vaginal deliveries, more common following cesarean section
- Occasionally associated with pelvic inflammatory disease or intrauterine device in nonobstetric patient
- Rarely leads to development of pelvic septic thrombophlebitis

SCANNING TIPS

- Evaluate for color flow in endometrial debris, noting that gas bubbles may produce artifactual signal; confirm with spectral Doppler

(Left) *Graphic shows findings in endometritis, including hyperemia of the endometrium ➡, with associated fluid and gas bubbles ➡ in the endometrial cavity.* **(Right)** *Longitudinal transvaginal ultrasound shows nonspecific endometrial thickening ➡ and echogenic endometrial fluid ➡ in this patient with pelvic inflammatory disease, diagnosed by vaginal discharge and pelvic pain.*

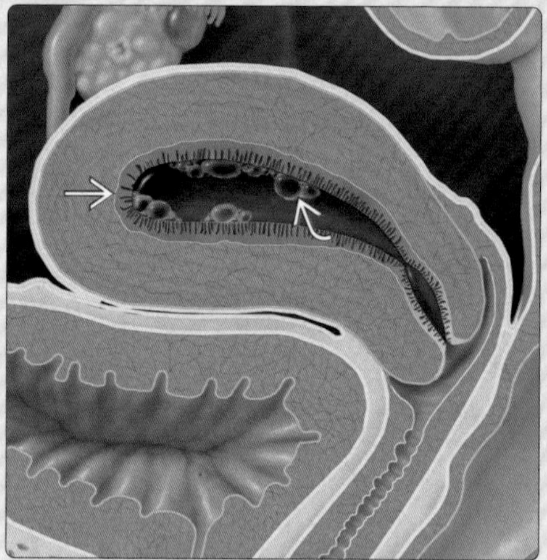

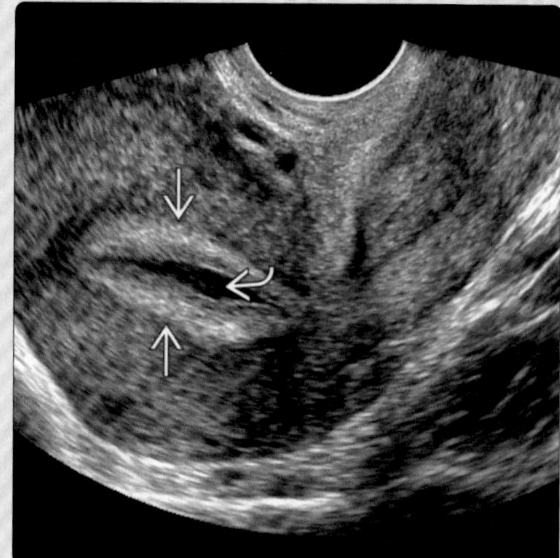

(Left) *Longitudinal transvaginal ultrasound in a patient with fever and pain from endometritis is shown. The endometrium is indistinct and there are multiple punctate and linear echogenicities ➡ at the interface of the myometrium and endometrium.* **(Right)** *Longitudinal transvaginal ultrasound performed for fever 6 weeks after cesarean section shows trace fluid ➡ in the endometrial cavity with nonspecific endometrial thickening ➡. There is no fluid in the cesarean section scar ➡.*

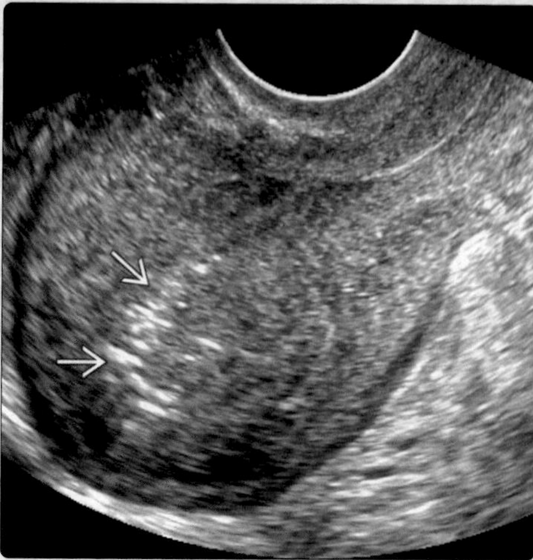

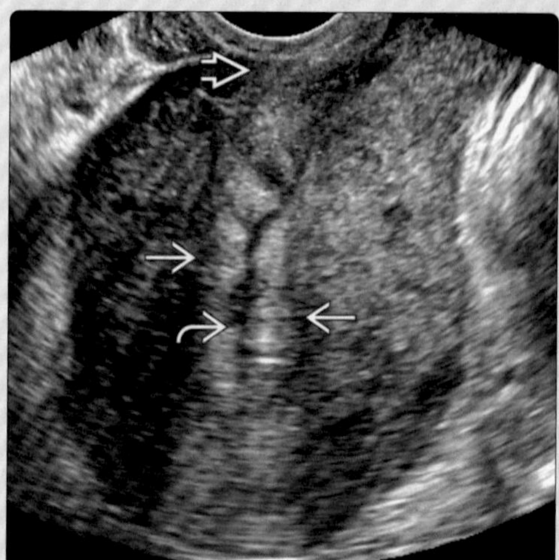

Intrauterine Device

KEY FACTS

ERMINOLOGY

- 2 types of intrauterine devices (IUDs) in USA
  - Copper containing
  - Levonorgestrel releasing
- Device inserted into endometrial cavity to prevent pregnancy
- T-shaped polyethylene frame with polyethylene monofilament string

MAGING

- Transvaginal US is study of choice for IUD position and complications; improved with 3D technique
- IUD stem: Linear bright echo aligned with endometrial cavity
- Arms/cross bars extend laterally at fundus
- ≤ 3 mm between top of IUD and fundal endometrium
- Levonorgestrel-containing IUD is harder to see
- String may be seen as linear bright echo or reverberation in cervix
- Embedment: IUD penetrates endometrium into myometrium without extension through uterine serosa
- Perforation: IUD penetrates through uterine serosa and is partially or completely in peritoneal cavity

CLINICAL ISSUES

- Pain and abnormal bleeding is common within 1st few months of placement
- Later complications, such as prolonged pain/dyspareunia, infection, string, not visualized on exam may result from malpositioned or perforated IUD
- IUD + positive pregnancy test: Assumed to be ectopic until proven otherwise

SCANNING TIPS

- Entire IUD should be visualized within endometrial cavity with arms in appropriate orientation
- 3D US to reconstruct true coronal plane of uterus
- 3D US helpful for diagnosis of embedment and displacement, which may be difficult to identify on 2D US

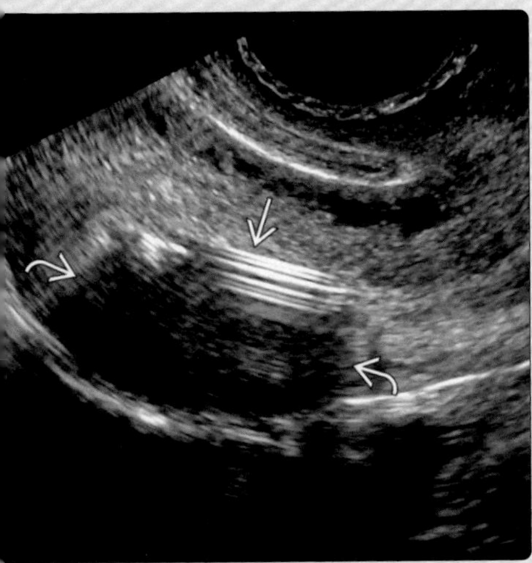

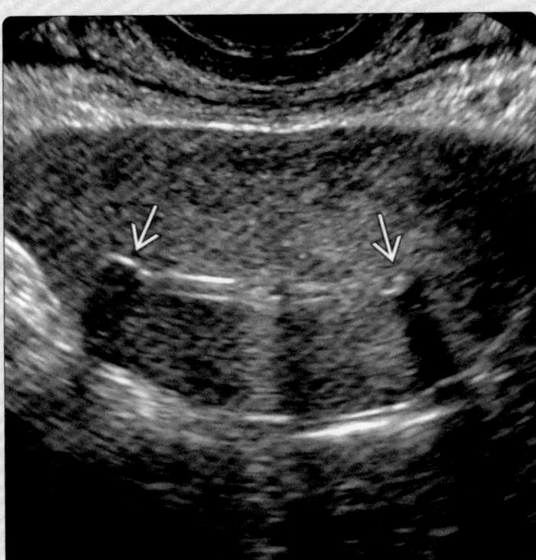

(Left) *Longitudinal endovaginal US shows the typical appearance of a well-positioned intrauterine device (IUD) stem → as an area of reverberation and posterior acoustic shadowing →.* **(Right)** *Transverse US in the same patient shows the normal position of arms/cross bars → extending laterally along the endometrial cavity at the fundus pointing toward the cornua. Note shadowing at the ends that is typical of the levonorgestrel-releasing IUD.*

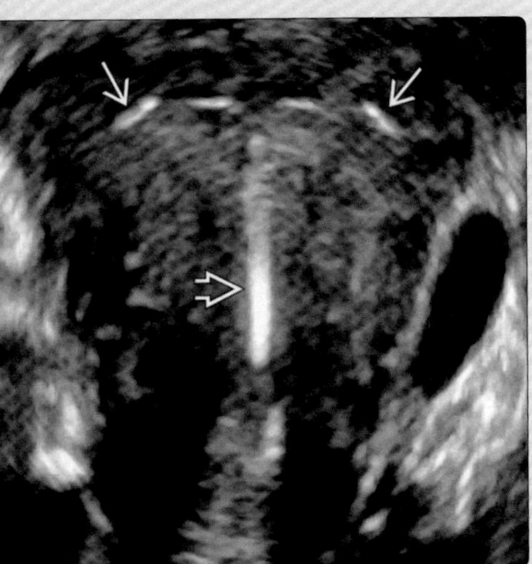

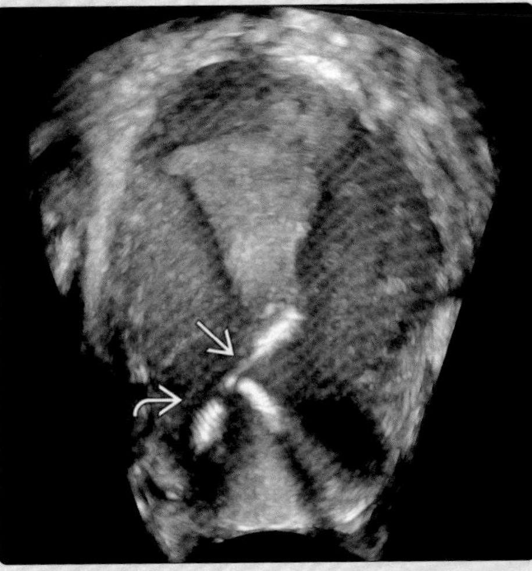

(Left) *3D MPR US shows an IUD in its entirety in the appropriate position with the stem → positioned longitudinally along the canal, the arms → pointing toward the cornua, and the proximal end ≤ 3 mm from the fundal endometrium.* **(Right)** *3D MPR US shows an abnormal IUD →. The right arm is embedded in the lower segment myometrium →.*

Functional Ovarian Cyst

KEY FACTS

TERMINOLOGY

- Follicular cyst (FC) forms from persistent follicle, ovulation does not occur
- Corpus luteum cyst (CLC) forms from graafian follicle following ovulation

IMAGING

- FC: Intraovarian cystic lesion with thin walls
- CLC: Occur after ovulation in latter part of menstrual cycle
  - Thick, hyperechoic wall
  - Central anechoic/hypoechoic cavity
  - Marked vascular flow within CLC wall: "Ring of fire"
  - Commonly complicated by hemorrhage

TOP DIFFERENTIAL DIAGNOSES

- Ectopic pregnancy: "Ring of fire" separate from ovary, usually tubal ectopic
- Ovarian neoplasm

CLINICAL ISSUES

- FC and CLC occur during reproductive years
  - FL and CLC ≤ 5 cm: No follow-up necessary
  - FL and CLC > 5 and ≤ 7 cm: Annual follow-up ultrasound
- Further imaging or surgical evaluation recommended with simple cyst > 7 cm
- CLC may enlarge initially with fertilization and pregnancy
  - Most no longer seen by sonography by early 2nd trimester (16 weeks)
- Malignancy rate in unilocular simple cysts: < 1%

SCANNING TIPS

- Gentle transducer pressure, manual external compression, or scanning while patient coughs may help confirm intraovarian location of CLC vs. tubal ectopic pregnancy, which would be located separate from ovary

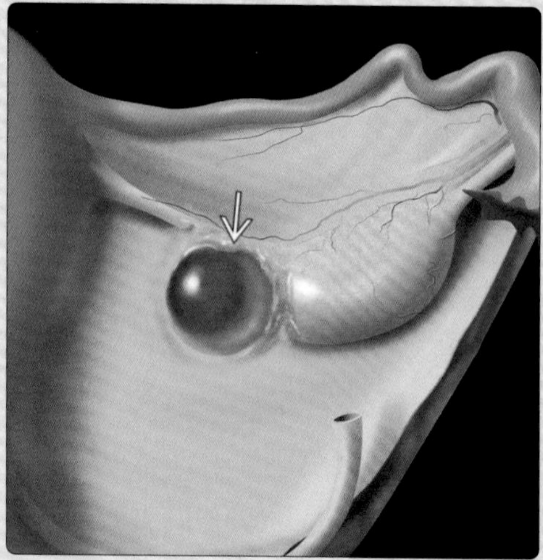

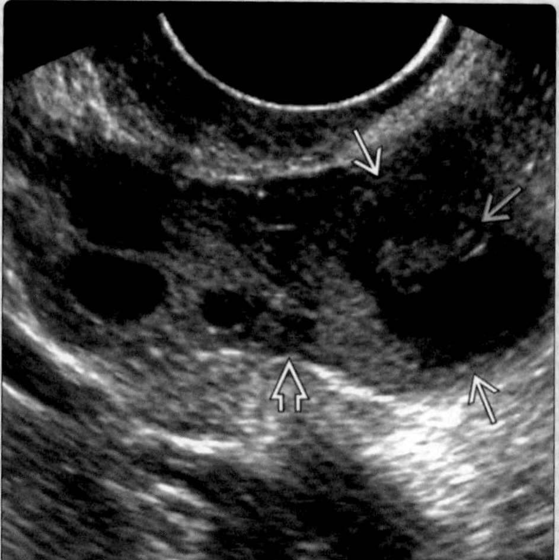

(Left) *Graphic shows a functional ovarian cyst ➡ arising from the left ovary.* **(Right)** *Some corpus luteal cysts (CLC) can have an exophytic appearance arising from the ovary ➡; If in doubt, look for the bridging ovarian parenchyma ➡ in continuity with CLC. Gentle pressure on the ovary with the transducer can also help demonstrate that the CLC arises from the ovary. Small retracted clot is present within this CLC ➡.*

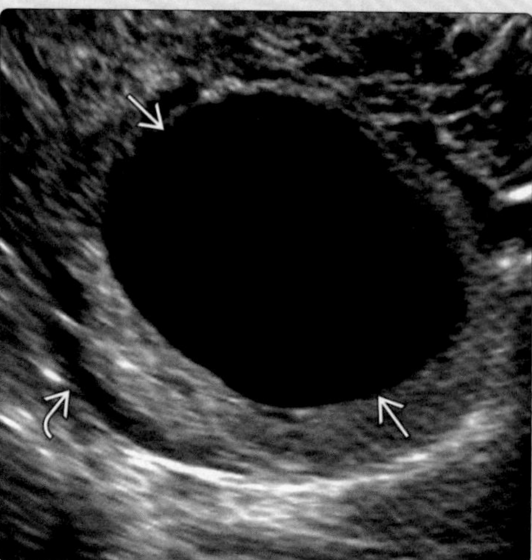

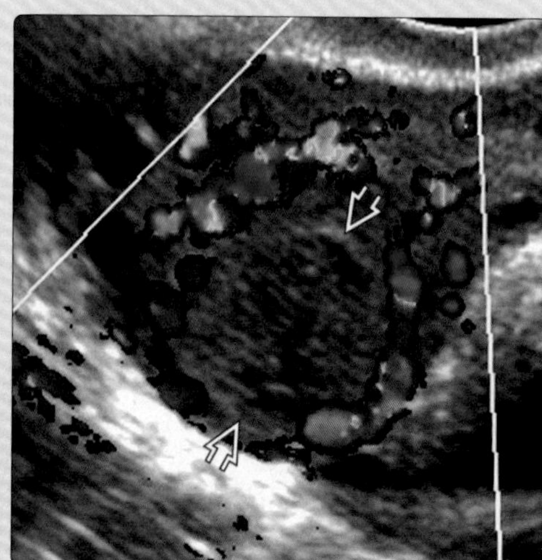

(Left) *Typical appearance of a simple functional ovarian cyst ➡ is shown. The peripheral follicles within the surrounding parenchyma ➡ confirm this is an intraovarian cyst.* **(Right)** *The ring of fire appearance is associated with marked vascular flow within the corpus luteum cyst (CLC) wall on color Doppler. In this case, the CLC is centrally hypoechoic due to internal hemorrhage ➡.*

KEY FACTS

TERMINOLOGY

- Hemorrhage into functional cyst in ovarian parenchyma

IMAGING

- Avascular hypoechoic ovarian "mass" with fine, lacy interstices due to fibrin strands
- May appear as mixed echogenicity mass depending on age of blood
  - Color Doppler shows clot is avascular
- Adjacent echogenic free fluid suggests ruptured hemorrhagic cyst (HC)

TOP DIFFERENTIAL DIAGNOSES

- Endometrioma
  - Uniform, low-level internal echoes from blood breakdown products
  - Will not change much on follow-up
- Solid ovarian mass
  - Internal vascularity on color Doppler
- Ovarian/adnexal torsion

CLINICAL ISSUES

- May be asymptomatic or symptomatic with acute pelvic pain
  - Larger HCs more likely to cause acute pain
- Majority resolve spontaneously
- Rarely, may be associated with significant intraperitoneal hemorrhage requiring surgical treatment

SCANNING TIPS

- Look for stretched ovarian parenchyma around HC
- HC will be avascular on color Doppler
  - Small clot along cyst wall may mimic mural nodule but will be avascular
- Follow-up US in 6-12 weeks if > 5 cm to ensure resolution
  - HC < 5 cm does not require follow-up imaging

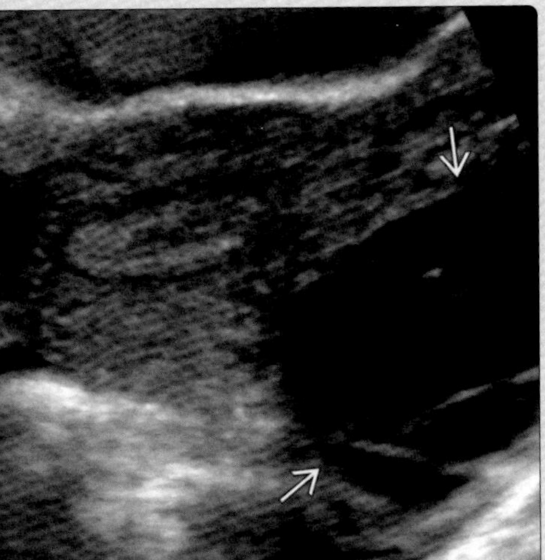

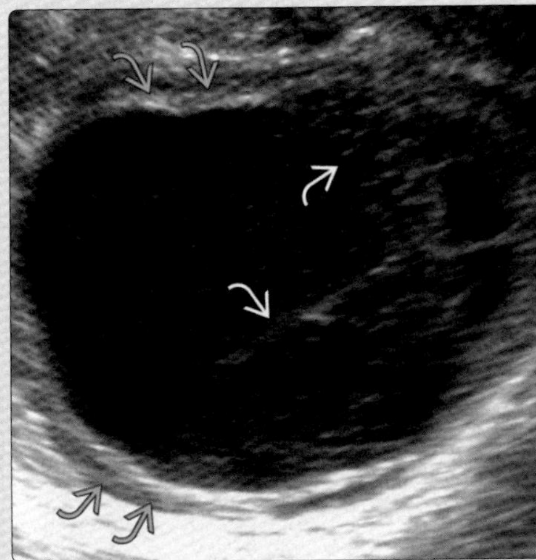

(Left) *In this patient presenting with pelvic pain, there is a septated cystic mass in the left adnexa, which appears anechoic ➡ on transabdominal grayscale US.* **(Right)** *When further evaluated with transvaginal US, the typical hypoechoic and lace-like echoes are seen with retracted clot ➡. Stretched ovarian parenchyma ➡ around the periphery is also characteristic of a hemorrhagic cyst.*

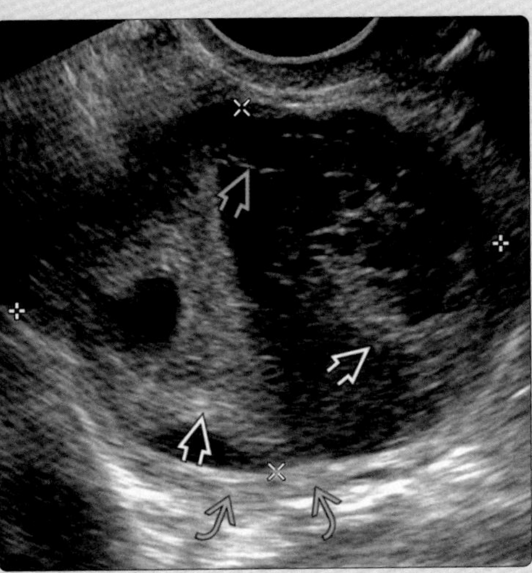

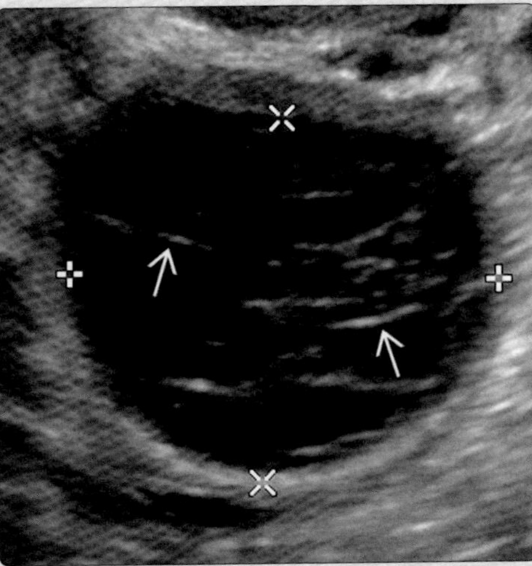

(Left) *Endovaginal US shows a hemorrhagic cyst with areas of more echogenic clot ➡ due to the acute nature of a hemorrhagic cyst. Fibrin strands ➡ and stretched ovarian parenchyma ➡ around the periphery are helpful clues this is a hemorrhagic cyst.* **(Right)** *Endovaginal grayscale US shows typical areas of reticular or lacy internal echoes that are due to fibrin strands within the hemorrhagic cyst ➡.*

Ovarian Hyperstimulation Syndrome

KEY FACTS

TERMINOLOGY

- Ovarian hyperstimulation syndrome (OHSS)
- Clinical syndrome generally associated with ovulation induction

IMAGING

- Bilaterally enlarged, cystic ovaries
  - Heterogeneous complex ovarian cysts with debris and septa if hemorrhagic component present
  - Typical spoke-wheel appearance
- Ascites
  - Occasionally, will find hemorrhagic pelvic fluid
- Pleural effusion

TOP DIFFERENTIAL DIAGNOSES

- Theca lutein cysts
  - Not associated with ascites, pleural effusions, or oliguria
- Hyperreactio luteinalis
  - More mild, indolent course within spectrum of OHSS

PATHOLOGY

- Exaggerated response to ovulation induction
- Relative hemoconcentration due to fluid leaking into peritoneal/pleural spaces

CLINICAL ISSUES

- Typical clinical symptoms
  - Abdominal pain
  - Nausea/vomiting/diarrhea
  - Weight gain
  - Oliguria
- Should be self-limiting as long as supportive care started early in process

SCANNING TIPS

- Avoid aggressive transvaginal imaging, as ovaries can be friable

(Left) *Endovaginal transverse US view of the pelvis shows typical ovarian hyperstimulation syndrome (OHSS), in which decidual reaction is present in the uterus ➡, with anechoic free fluid ➡ and enlarged ovaries containing multiple cysts ➡ (right ovary).* **(Right)** *Transabdominal US of the right upper quadrant shows ascites ➡ and a pleural effusion ➡ in this patient with early OHSS.*

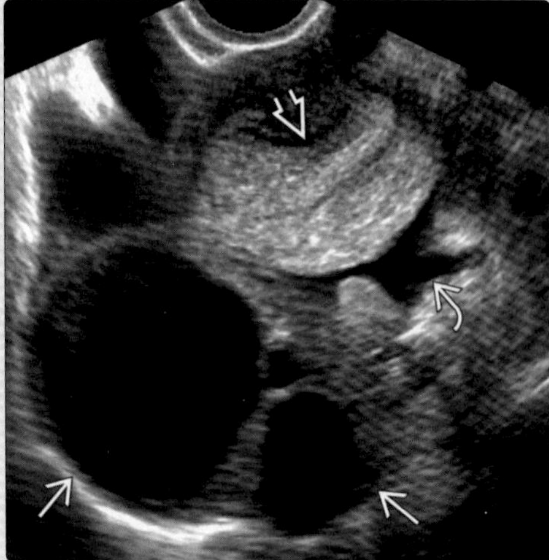

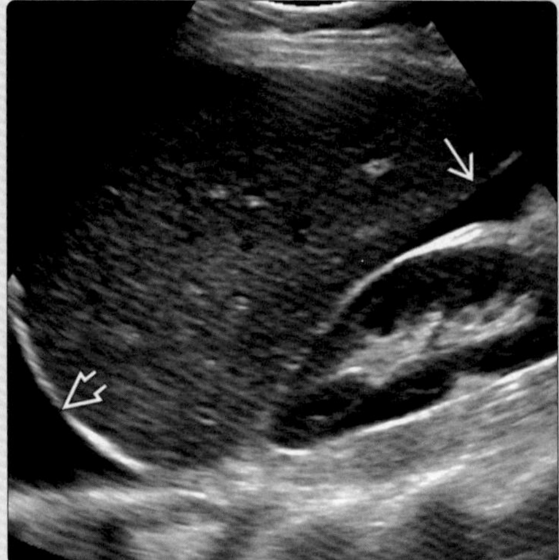

(Left) *Transvaginal US shows a markedly enlarged ovary measuring up to 8 cm (calipers) in diameter with multiple follicles and ascites ➡ in a patient with OHSS.* **(Right)** *Spectral Doppler in the same patient shows normal low-resistance arterial flow in the ovary ➡. Color Doppler and spectral Doppler should be used to evaluate the ovarian parenchyma in patients with OHSS to document good blood flow in patients presenting with pain due to the risk of superimposed adnexal torsion.*

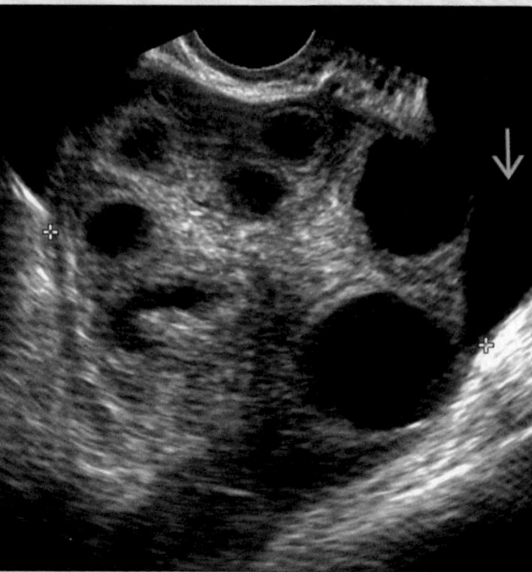

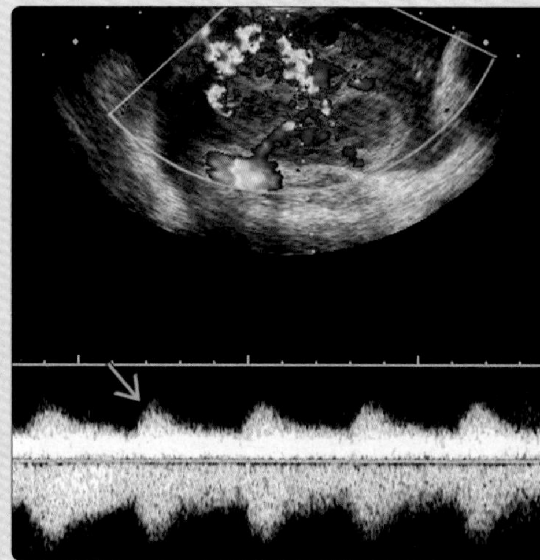

KEY FACTS

ERMINOLOGY

- Serous epithelial neoplasm, which can be benign (serous cystadenoma), borderline (low malignant potential), or malignant (serous cystadenocarcinoma)

MAGING

- Large, thin-walled, unilocular mass ± papillary projections
- Bilateral in 25% of benign and 65% of malignant tumors
- Variable size but often large
- Typically unilocular or with few septations even in malignant tumors
- May see ascites and peritoneal implants in metastatic disease
- Ultrasound for lesion detection and characterization
- CT for tumor staging: Evaluate paracolic gutters and liver capsule for peritoneal disease

OP DIFFERENTIAL DIAGNOSES

- Mucinous cystadenoma/carcinoma

PATHOLOGY

- Metastatic spread
  - Intraperitoneal dissemination most common
  - Direct extension into surrounding organs
  - Lymphatic spread to paraaortic and pelvic nodes

CLINICAL ISSUES

- Pelvic discomfort/pain from large tumors
- 70% of patients with malignant tumors have peritoneal involvement at time of diagnosis
- Serous tumors most common epithelial neoplasm
- Malignant: 25%; borderline: 15%; benign: 60%

SCANNING TIPS

- If ovary displaced superiorly due to mass, use transabdominal approach following iliac vessels with curvilinear probe to locate ovaries then switch to 9-MHz linear probe to interrogate detail

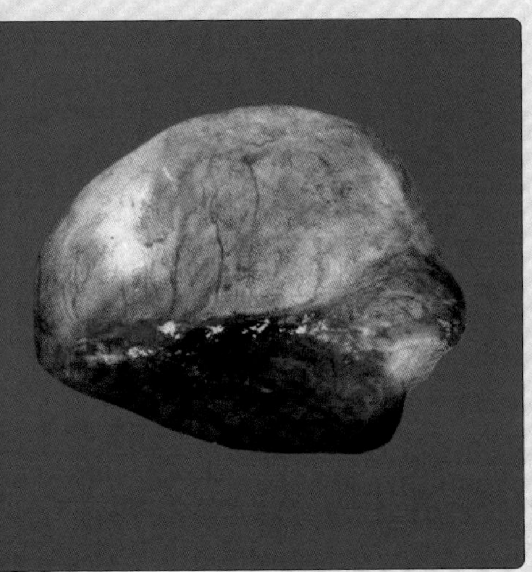

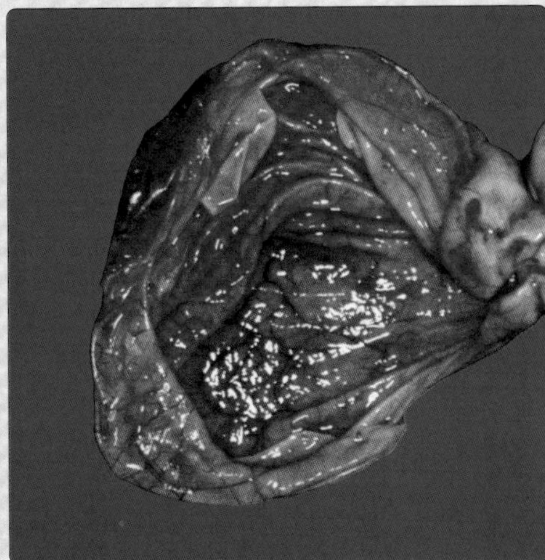

(Left) *In most cases, ovarian masses are removed without rupture of the cyst to prevent contamination of the peritoneum. Typically, soft tissue and node biopsies are obtained at the time of surgery as well as pelvic peritoneal washings for cytology.* **(Right)** *Gross pathology after the fluid has been drained shows the thin wall typical of a serous cystadenoma. They are typically unilocular or have few septations.*

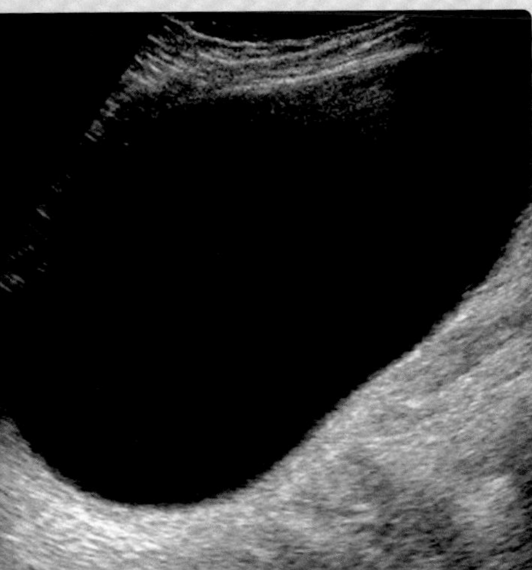

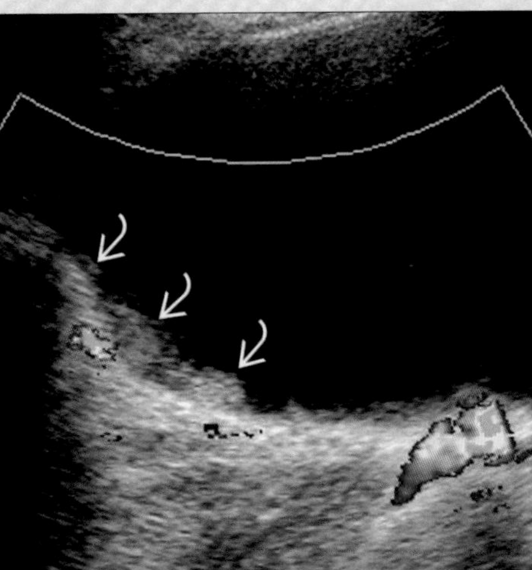

(Left) *Typical serous epithelial neoplasms are large with thin walls and unilocular. This ovarian serous cystadenoma measured up to 18 cm in diameter on this transabdominal grayscale ultrasound.* **(Right)** *Close evaluation of this serous cystadenoma reveals subtle nodularity along the right lateral margin of the wall ➔.*

KEY FACTS

TERMINOLOGY

- Mucinous epithelial neoplasm, which can be benign (mucinous cystadenoma), borderline (low malignant potential), or malignant (mucinous cystadenocarcinoma)

IMAGING

- Multilocular cystic mass with low-level echoes
  - Papillary projections much less common than in serous tumors
  - Solid components increase suspicion for malignancy
- Variable in size but often large; may fill entire pelvis and extend into upper abdomen
- Pseudomyxoma peritonei is potential form of peritoneal spread
  - Amorphous, mucoid material insinuating itself around mesentery, bowel, and solid organs

TOP DIFFERENTIAL DIAGNOSES

- Endometrioma
- Serous cystadenoma/carcinoma

PATHOLOGY

- Method of spread
  - Intraperitoneal dissemination most common (pseudomyxoma peritonei)
  - Direct extension to surrounding organs
  - Lymphatic spread to paraaortic and pelvic nodes

CLINICAL ISSUES

- Massive tumors can cause weight gain and distended abdomen
- Mucinous tumors 2nd most common epithelial neoplasm
- Gelatinous, insinuating nature of pseudomyxoma peritonei makes complete resection difficult

SCANNING TIPS

- Mucinous tumors are less commonly malignant than serous tumors

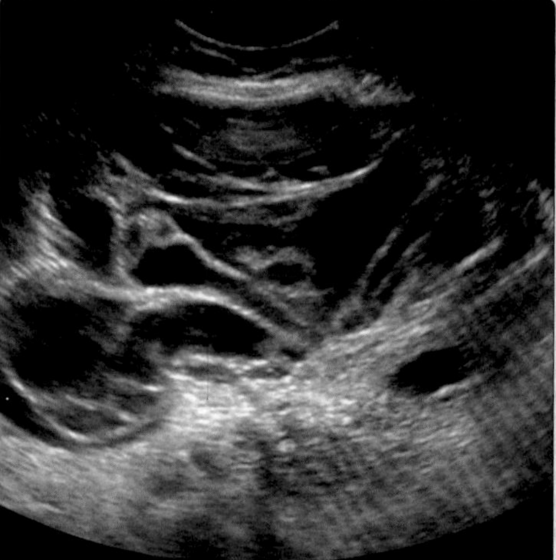

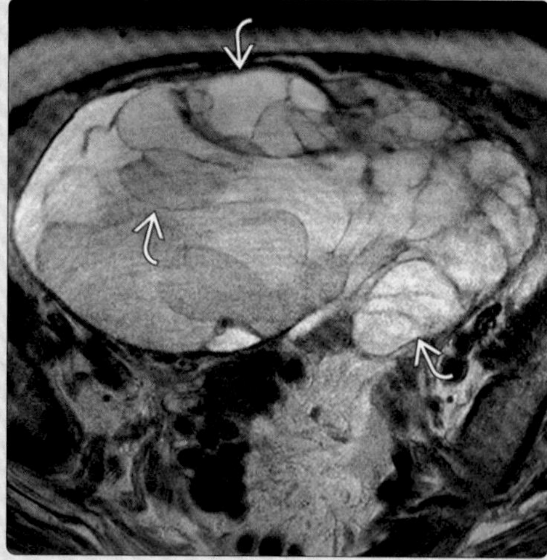

(Left) *Septations within a mucinous tumor are typically thin, creating multiple intervening locules, as seen in this transverse transabdominal ultrasound.* **(Right)** *Axial T2WI MR shows varying signal within the locules of the mass due to differing concentrations of mucin ➲, which creates a stained glass appearance. Loculi with a high concentration of mucin will be higher signal on T1WI and lower signal on T2WI.*

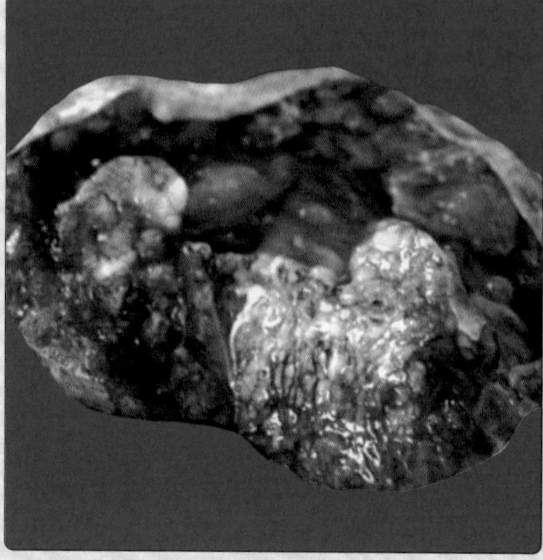

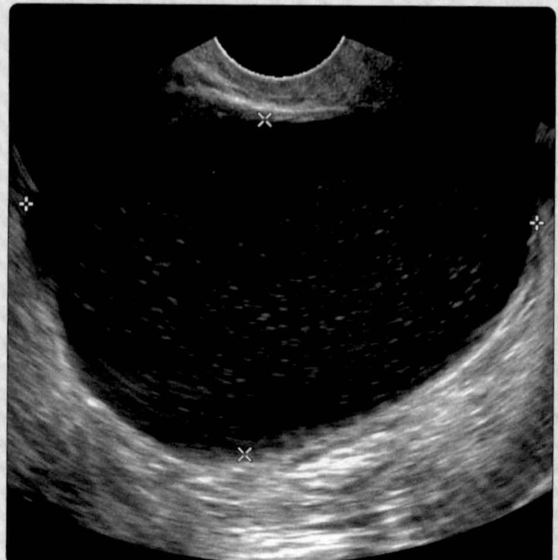

(Left) *Gross pathology of a resected mucinous cystadenocarcinoma shows the solid areas. The greater the amount of solid material, the greater the likelihood of malignancy.* **(Right)** *Transvaginal ultrasound shows low-level echoes within the largest locule (calipers), consistent with mucin.*

KEY FACTS

TERMINOLOGY

- Mature cystic teratoma (MCT) = dermoid cyst
- Immature teratoma
- Monodermal teratoma in which 1 cell line predominates

IMAGING

- **MCTs have variety of appearances**
  - Heterogeneous cystic ovarian mass with echogenic shadowing mural nodule (Rokitansky nodule) on US
  - ± fat-fluid level
  - Highly echogenic focus/foci with distal acoustic shadowing represent teeth
  - Hair within sebum creates characteristic dot-dash-dot appearance
- Fat-containing adnexal mass is diagnostic on CT

TOP DIFFERENTIAL DIAGNOSES

- Hemorrhagic cyst
- Endometrioma
- Bowel

PATHOLOGY

- Mature tissues of endodermal, mesodermal, and ectodermal origin
- 88% unilocular, fat content liquid at body temperature, semisolid at room temperature

CLINICAL ISSUES

- Most common ovarian tumor
- 10-20% bilateral
- Rarely undergo malignant degeneration
- Rupture in < 1% of cases
- May act as lead point for adnexal torsion

SCANNING TIPS

- If dermoid is predominately echogenic in appearance due to predominantly fatty contents, it may mimic bowel and may be difficult to appreciate on transvaginal imaging; these are often better seen on transabdominal view

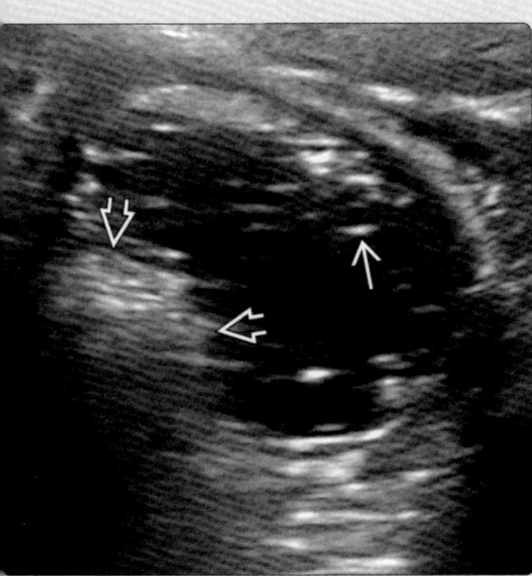

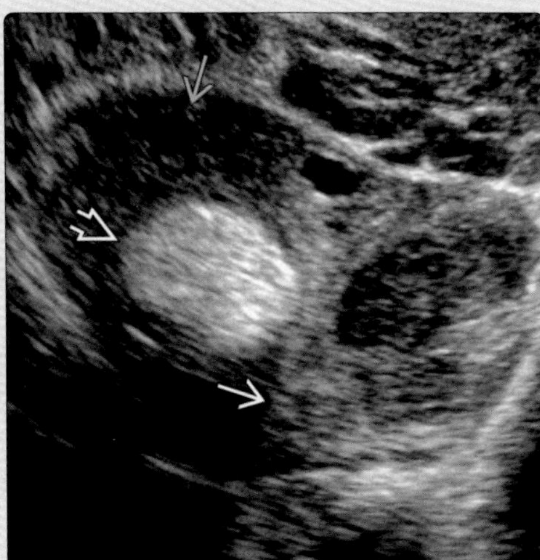

(Left) *Dermoids may be mostly cystic with linear floating echoes consistent with hair ➡. The echogenic shadowing Rokitansky nodule ➡ along the periphery is diagnostic for a dermoid.* **(Right)** *Grayscale ultrasound shows that this dermoid has a more heterogeneous appearance due to differing fat ➡ and echogenic fluid content ➡. A peripheral Rokitansky nodule ➡ is present as well.*

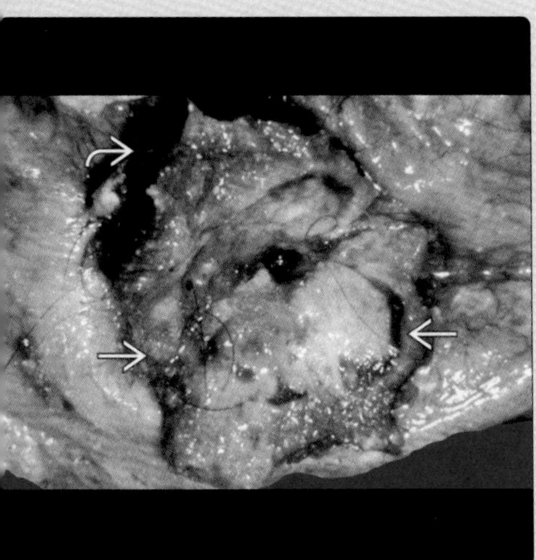

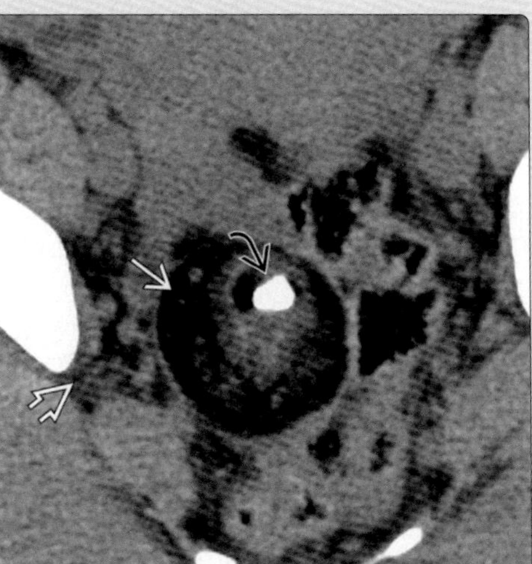

(Left) *Gross pathology shows the typical appearance of a Rokitansky nodule ➡ within the dissected mature cystic teratoma. Hair ➡ arises from nodule.* **(Right)** *Axial CECT of a patient with a dermoid shows a calcified tooth ➡, which is present in ~ 1/3 of cases. Notice the fat ➡ within the dermoid is markedly hypodense even compared to normal extraperitoneal fat ➡.*

Polycystic Ovarian Syndrome

KEY FACTS

TERMINOLOGY

- Complex heterogenous syndrome of ovulatory dysfunction, menstrual irregularity, and androgen excess
- Rotterdam criteria for polycystic ovarian syndrome (PCOS) developed in 2003: 2 of 3 criteria must be present
  - Oligo- or anovulation
  - Hyperandrogenism (clinical or biochemical)
  - Polycystic ovarian morphology (by US)

IMAGING

- Enlarged ovaries with volume > 10 mL **or** ≥ 25 follicles per ovary (updated 2014 criteria) measuring 2-9 mm
  - > 12 follicles per ovary (2003 Rotterdam criteria) use if US transducer frequency < 8 MHz
- Calculate volume using formula for prolate ellipsoid (longitudinal x transverse x AP diameter x 0.5233)
- Ovarian stromal ↑ echogenicity

TOP DIFFERENTIAL DIAGNOSES

- Normal
  - Ovarian morphology alone is insufficient for diagnosis of PCOS
  - Polycystic ovarian **morphology**: Seen in ~ 22% of women, whereas PCOS prevalence is only 5-10%
- Suppressed ovary
- Other causes of hyperandrogenism

CLINICAL ISSUES

- Anovulation → oligo-/amenorrhea
- Hyperandrogenism → hirsutism
- Obesity with associated hyperinsulinemia/insulin resistance

SCANNING TIPS

- If dominant follicle (> 10 mm diameter) or corpus luteum seen, repeat scan during next cycle to avoid false elevation of volume

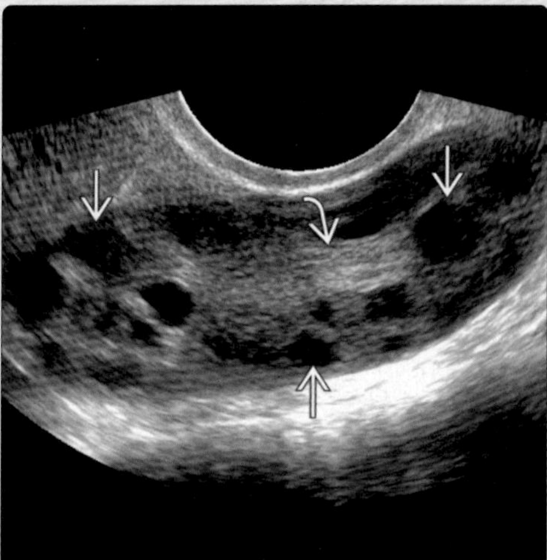

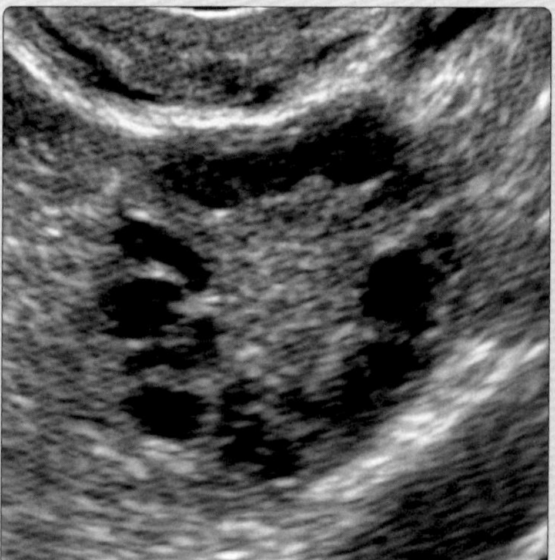

(Left) *Transvaginal US demonstrates an enlarged right ovary with a volume of 19 mL and multiple follicles ➡ between 2-9 mm in size in a patient with polycystic ovarian syndrome (PCOS). Note the echogenic central stroma ➡.* **(Right)** *Transvaginal US demonstrates a normal size ovary with a volume < 10 mL. However, ≥ 25 follicles measuring between 2-9 mL were present in this ovary.*

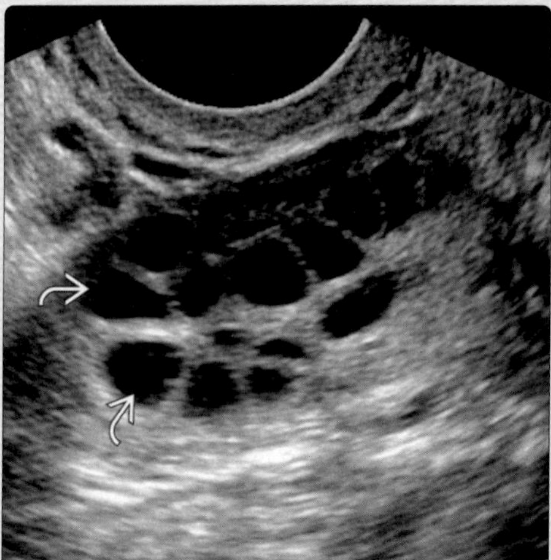

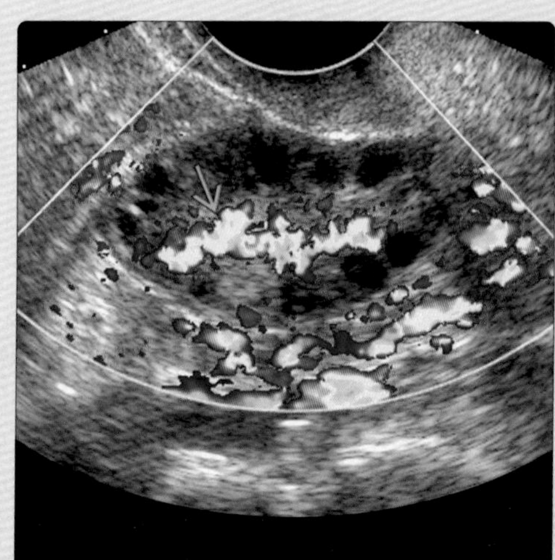

(Left) *Transvaginal US demonstrates the typical appearance of polycystic ovarian morphology with an enlarged ovary containing multiple small follicles ➡.* **(Right)** *Color Doppler longitudinal transvaginal US shows the central stroma of the ovary is well vascularized ➡, which is not a diagnostic criterion but has been noted in polycystic ovarian morphology.*

KEY FACTS

TERMINOLOGY

- Endometriosis: Ectopic endometrial glands outside of uterine cavity
- Endometrioma: Cystic collection of mixed blood products

IMAGING

- Diffuse low-level internal echoes in 95%
  - Homogeneous ground-glass echotexture
  - May see fluid-fluid level in endometrioma
  - Often see increased through transmission
  - Will typically not see acoustic streaming on grayscale or color/power Doppler due to marked viscosity
- Endometrioma may look anechoic transabdominally
- Cyst wall with variable appearance, may see peripheral echogenic foci due to cholesterol crystals
- Avascular on color Doppler
  - Caveat: Decidualization during pregnancy can lead to vascularization

TOP DIFFERENTIAL DIAGNOSES

- Hemorrhagic cyst: Resolves in 4-6 weeks
- Dermoid cyst (mature cystic teratoma)
- Cystic ovarian neoplasm

CLINICAL ISSUES

- Infertility
- Cyclical or chronic pain

SCANNING TIPS

- Use highest possible frequency or coded harmonic imaging to differentiate low-level echoes from near-field artifacts
- Avoid decreasing overall gain or TGC to "clean" real echoes
- Vascularity in peripheral nodules on color Doppler may indicate malignant transformation (except in pregnancy)
- Absence of sliding sign (uterus and bowel slide with gentle EV transducer pressure) suggests adhesions, a common finding in endometriosis

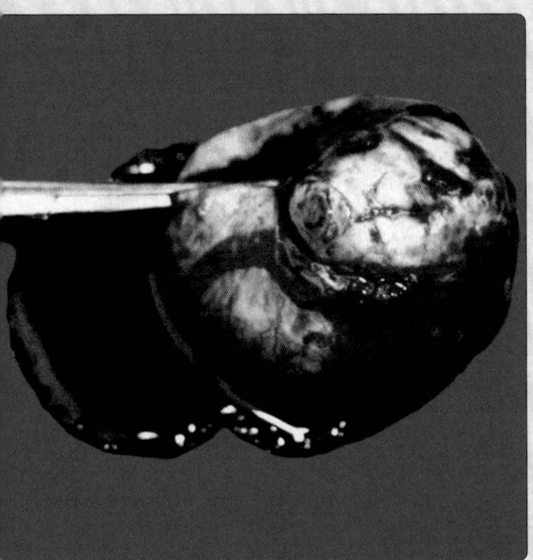

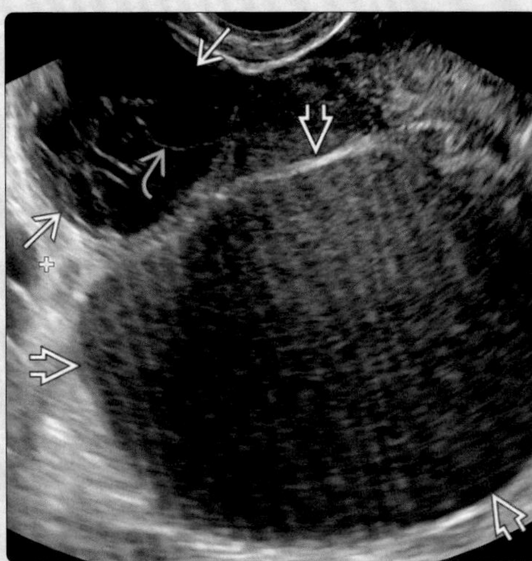

(Left) *Gross pathology of a resected cyst, which has been opened, shows dark brown viscous blood typical of an endometrioma. This appearance has been called a "chocolate cyst."* **(Right)** *Transverse endovaginal US demonstrates a coexistent hemorrhagic cyst ➡ and endometrioma ⇨. Note the homogenous appearance of the echoes in the endometrioma in contradistinction to the fine fibrin strands ↗ and mixed echogenicity of the hemorrhagic cyst.*

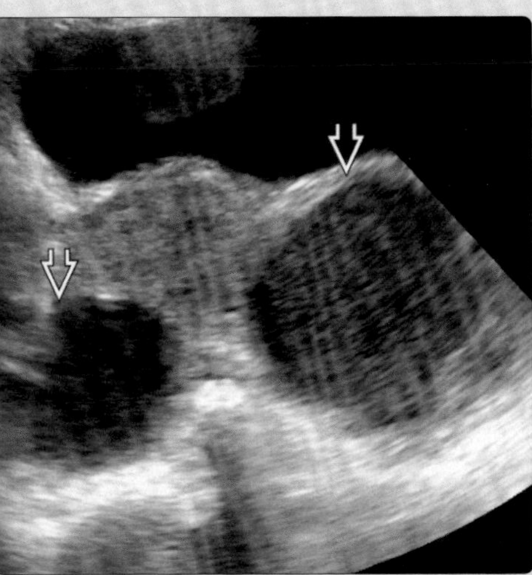

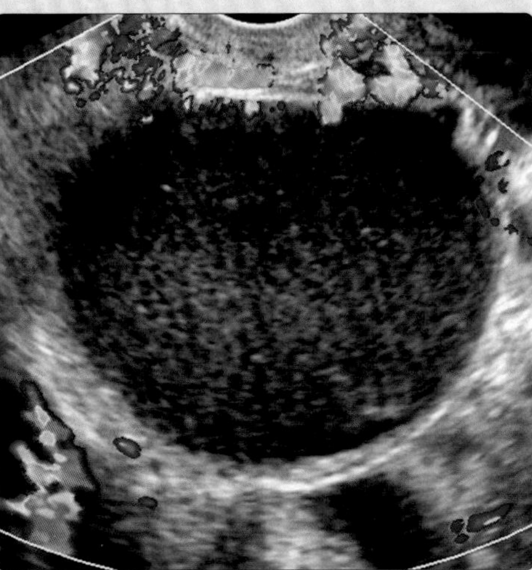

(Left) *Transverse transabdominal US shows bilateral hypoechoic adnexal masses ⇨ with homogeneous low-level internal echoes. Endometriomas are bilateral in up to 50% of cases. Posterior tethering of ovaries is indicative of coexisting endometriosis. When bilateral ovaries touch, this is known as "kissing ovaries," which is pathognomonic for endometriosis.* **(Right)** *Color Doppler endovaginal US demonstrates no internal vascularity of endometrioma.*

Tuboovarian Abscess

KEY FACTS

TERMINOLOGY

- Spectrum of disease, including endometritis, salpingitis, tuboovarian abscess (TOA), and oophoritis

IMAGING

- Transvaginal US is 1st-line modality
- Pyosalpinx: Thickened, dilated fallopian tubes, walls often > 5 mm with internal echoes from pus
- Thickened endosalpingeal folds: Cogwheel sign
- Oophoritis: Enlarged edematous ovary
- TOA: Complex pelvic fluid collection engulfing ovary; may still see components of pyosalpinx
- Tuboovarian complex (TOC): Abscess adherent to tube, distinguishable separate ovary
- Complex peritoneal fluid
- Increased color Doppler in tube, ovary, or abscess

TOP DIFFERENTIAL DIAGNOSES

- Endometrioma ± rupture
- Hemorrhagic cyst ± rupture
- Ovarian neoplasm
- Complicated appendicitis

PATHOLOGY

- Ascending infection crosses endocervical canal and mucus barrier, ascends into upper genital tract, involves endometrium, tubes, and ovaries

CLINICAL ISSUES

- Usually present with pain, fever, vaginal discharge
- Pelvic pain and cervical motion tenderness, positive endocervical smear, elevated WBC, ESR, or CRP
- Infertility, ectopic pregnancy, chronic pelvic pain

SCANNING TIPS

- Transabdominal US may be required to image large/extensive abscesses
- Evaluate for tenderness and mobility of adnexa

(Left) *Longitudinal transabdominal US of a patient with a tuboovarian complex → next to a normal ovary → is shown. There is pus → within the lumen of the dilated tube.* **(Right)** *Coronal transvaginal US shows a tuboovarian abscess → with a pus level →.*

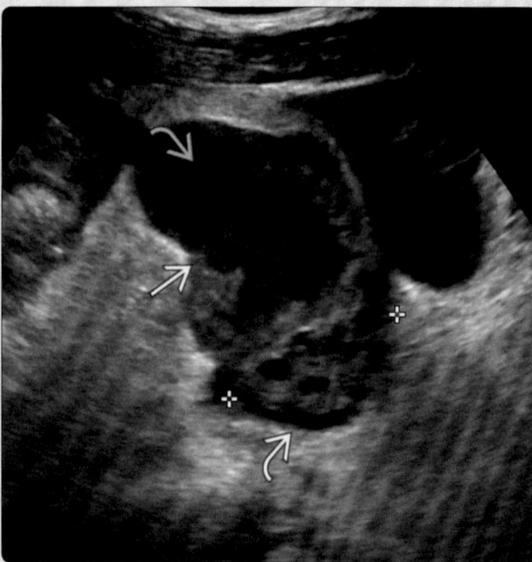

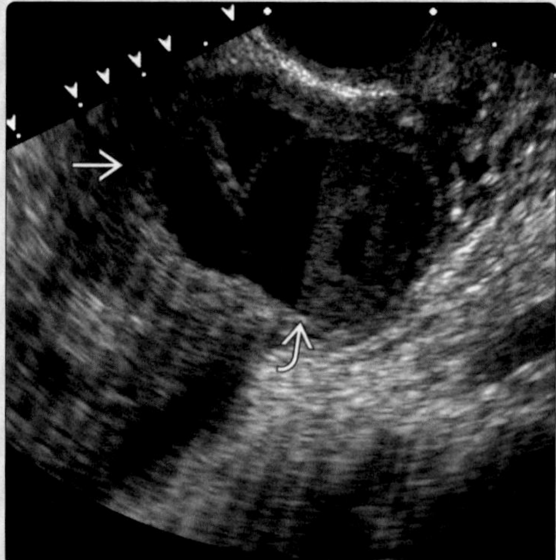

(Left) *Coronal transvaginal US of pelvic inflammatory disease is shown. A thickened, tender fallopian tube → is noted medial to the right ovary →. Complex free fluid is also present →.* **(Right)** *Transverse transabdominal US shows a mixed solid and cystic lesion in the right adnexa →. The right ovary could not be discerned; the uterus → was normal. The patient had a fever and leucocytosis. After antibiotics were initiated, surgery was performed for the tuboovarian abscess.*

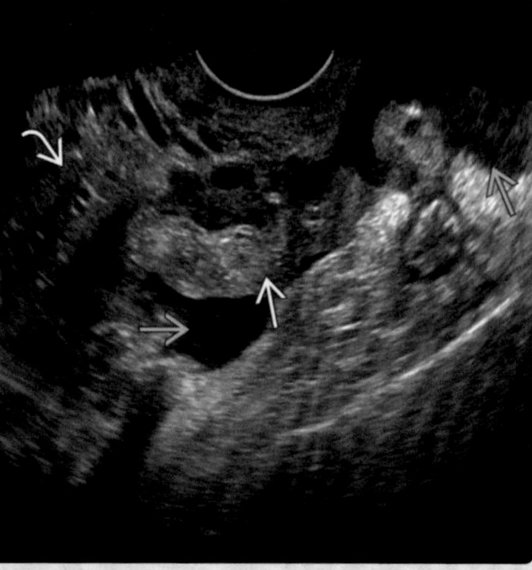

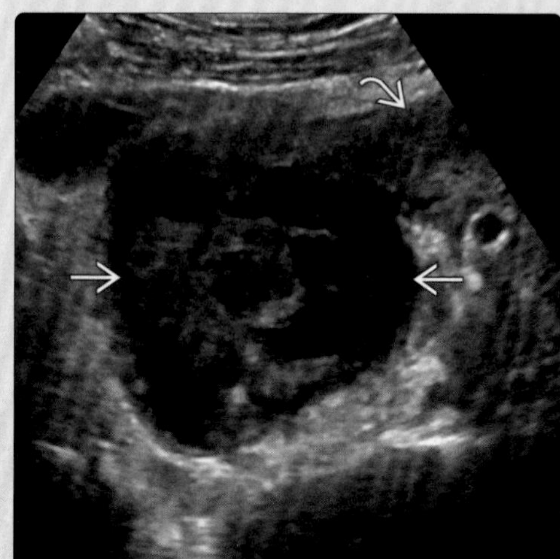

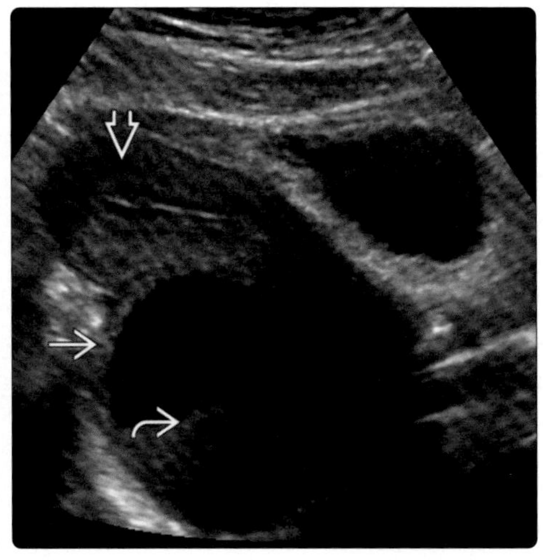

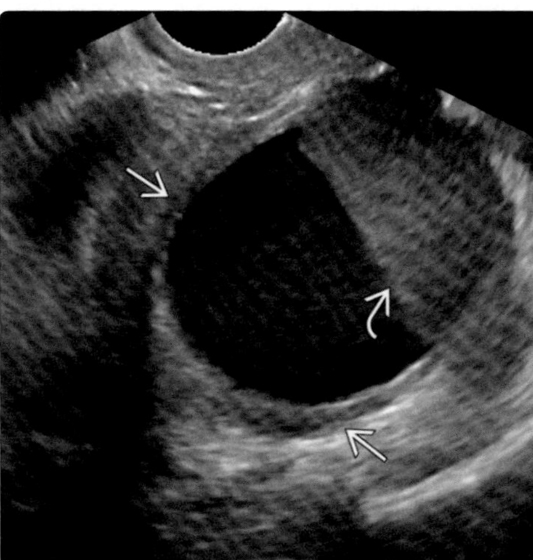

(Left) *Longitudinal transabdominal US of the pelvis in a patient with HIV and recurrent tuboovarian abscesses is shown. There is a large abscess with a debris level posterior to the uterus.* **(Right)** *Longitudinal transvaginal US of the same patient shows the thick-walled tuboovarian abscess with purulent debris.*

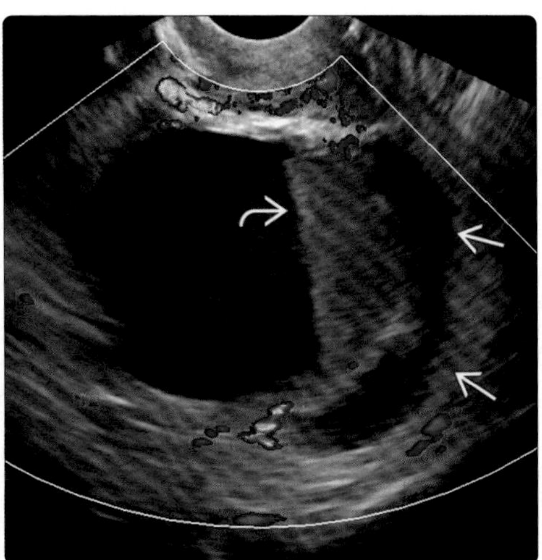

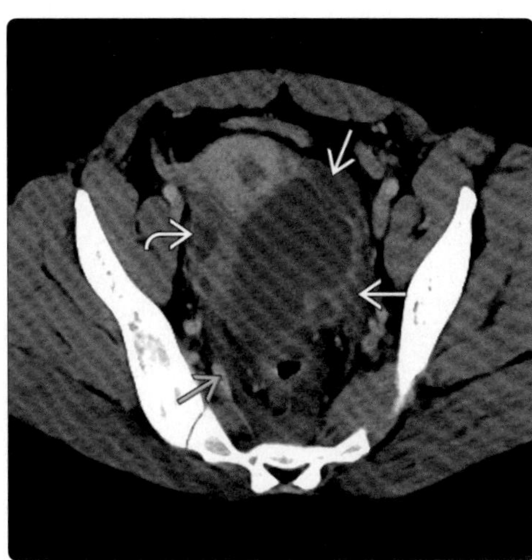

(Left) *Longitudinal color Doppler transvaginal US of the same patient shows the eccentric tubular component to the tuboovarian abscess with purulent debris.* **(Right)** *Axial CT of the same patient is shown. The full extent of the left tuboovarian abscess is easier to image. There is also a smaller right tuboovarian abscess and pelvic fluid.*

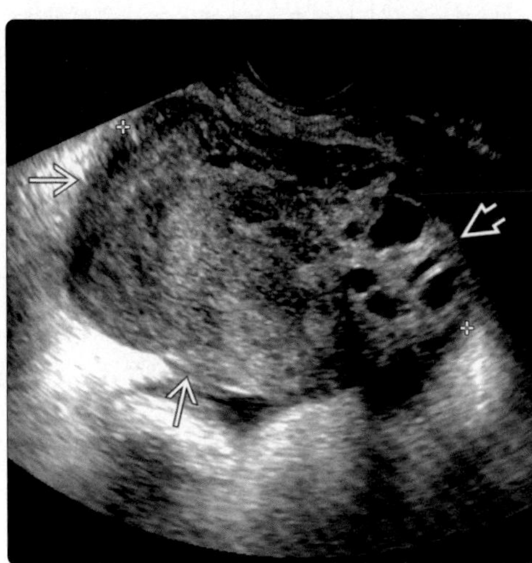

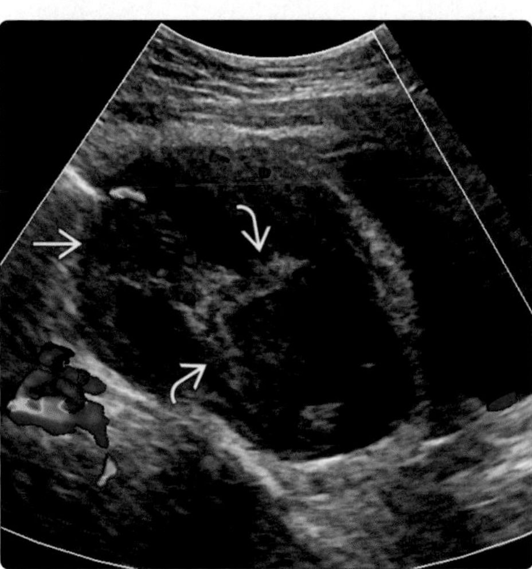

(Left) *Longitudinal US of a left tuboovarian complex is shown. There is complex fluid in the abscess, which is distinct from the ovary.* **(Right)** *Longitudinal transabdominal color Doppler US of a patient with pain, fever, and a pelvic mass is shown. This was surgically proven to be a tuboovarian abscess. There is a multilocular cystic mass with a thick wall and thick septa with color flow in the septa.*

Hydrosalpinx

KEY FACTS

IMAGING

- Thin-walled, distended tube; tube wall < 3 mm
- Convoluted or S-shaped, oval or pear-shaped, more dilated at fimbriated end
- Separate from uterus and ovaries
- Content anechoic; low-level echoes suggest acute pelvic inflammatory disease (PID)
- Thin endosalpingeal folds (~ 2-3 mm) protrude into lumen
- Incomplete septa: Short, linear echogenic projections into lumen from tubal kinking
- Waist sign: Indentation of opposing walls of dilated tubal structure resulting in appearance of waist
- Beads on string sign: Small hyperechoic mural nodules on transverse imaging
- Cogwheel sign: Thicker endosalpingeal folds in acute PID
- No color flow in endosalpingeal folds or wall
- Color flow in thickened tube suggests acute infection (as well as internal debris)

TOP DIFFERENTIAL DIAGNOSES

- Pyosalpinx (acute PID)/tuboovarian complex
- Cystic ovarian neoplasm
- Paraovarian cyst/peritoneal inclusion cyst
- Dilated bowel, acute appendicitis

PATHOLOGY

- Tubal obstruction from PID, endometriosis, appendicitis, or postpelvic surgery

CLINICAL ISSUES

- Usually asymptomatic, can present with pelvic or lower abdominal pain, severe pain may indicate adnexal torsion
- Must be distinguished from pyosalpinx or hematosalpinx based on tubal content and clinical picture
- Can result in infertility or ectopic pregnancy

SCANNING TIPS

- Cine clips are very useful for confirmation of tubular configuration

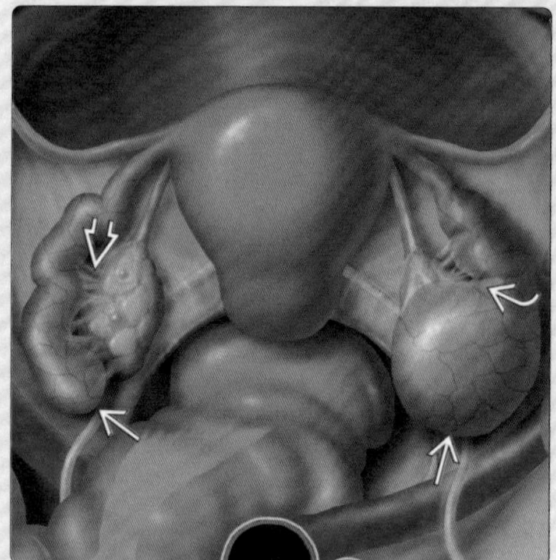

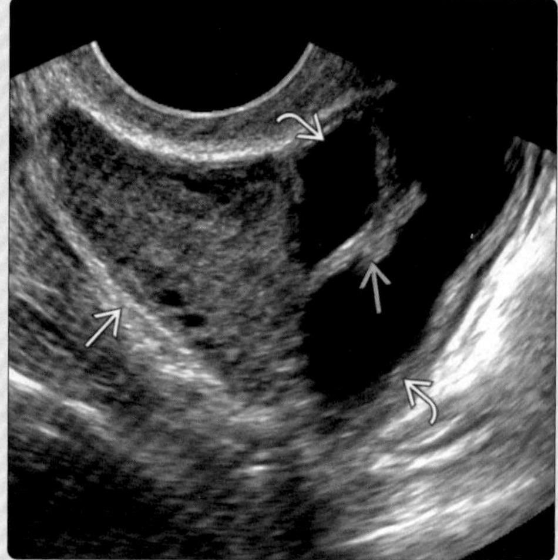

(Left) *Graphic shows bilateral hydrosalpinx. The left tube folds upon itself ➔, which appears as an incomplete septum on US. The fimbriated end ➔ is more dilated. Adhesions ➔ and hydrosalpinx are sequelae of pelvic inflammatory disease (PID).* **(Right)** *Coronal transvaginal US shows a normal ovary ➔ with a dilated fallopian tube ➔. The septa ➔ are the walls of the folded tube.*

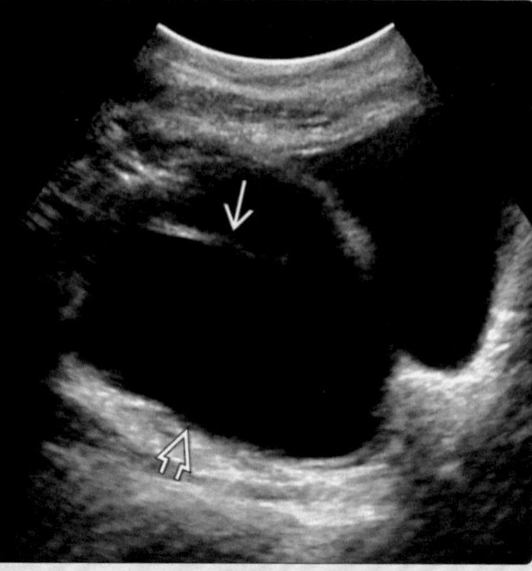

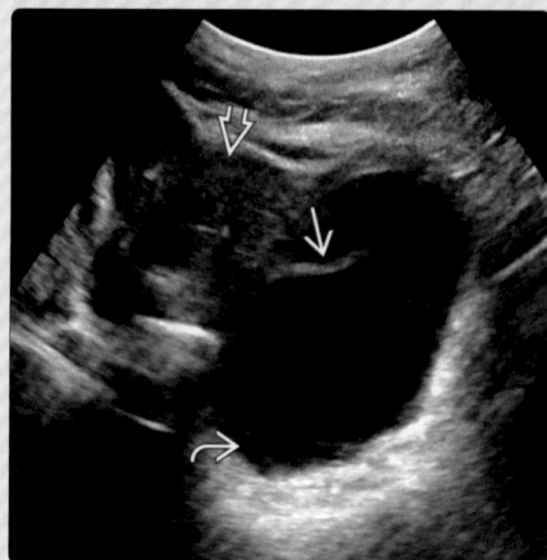

(Left) *Transabdominal longitudinal US shows a markedly dilated, thin-walled hydrosalpinx ➔ with a thin, incomplete septum ➔.* **(Right)** *Transverse transabdominal US of the same patient demonstrates the more dilated distal end of the tube ➔. The uterus ➔ was normal. The incomplete septum ➔ is better seen as a kink in the tube.*

KEY FACTS

TERMINOLOGY

- Cyst originating from wolffian duct in mesosalpinx or broad ligament
- Synonym: Paratubal cyst

IMAGING

- Transvaginal ultrasound is study of choice
- Round or oval cystic structure separate from ovary
- Unilocular in 95%, multilocular in 5%
- Mean diameter: 40 mm (range: 15-120 mm)
- Thin outer wall (< 3 mm)
- Often unilateral
- Lack of follicles distinguishes from ovary; usually does not indent ovary
- Fluid anechoic in 91%
  - Rarely may be complicated by torsion or hemorrhage
- May contain septa that are thin, smooth, complete
- Avascular on color Doppler

TOP DIFFERENTIAL DIAGNOSES

- Peritoneal inclusion cyst
- True ovarian cyst
- Hydrosalpinx

PATHOLOGY

- Benign serous cyst in 98%
- Malignant features in 2%

CLINICAL ISSUES

- 10-20% of all adnexal masses
- Asymptomatic in most women
- Torsion, growth, and malignancy are rare complications

SCANNING TIPS

- Confirm that cyst is separate from ovary by gently pushing with vaginal probe
- Consider torsion if cyst is painful, large, and displaced

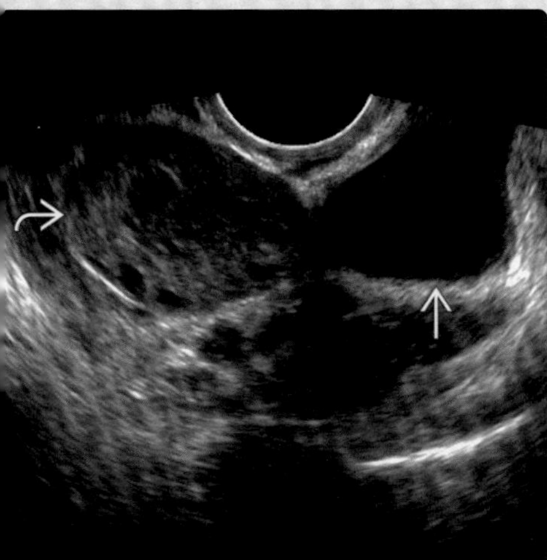

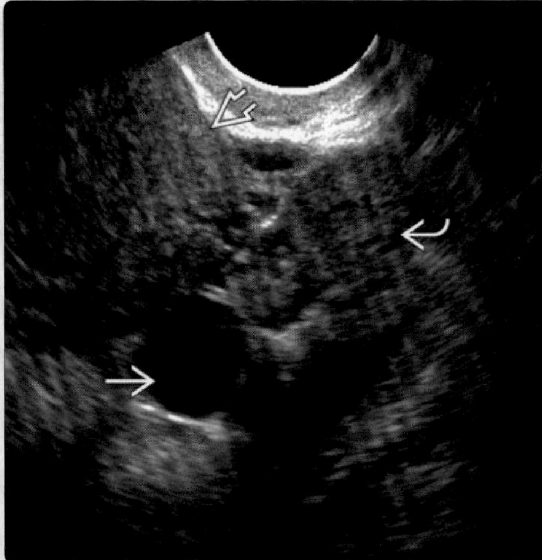

(Left) *Longitudinal transvaginal ultrasound of the adnexa shows a small, simple paraovarian cyst ➡ next to a normal ovary ➡. They were separable with probe pressure.* **(Right)** *Coronal transvaginal ultrasound of the left adnexa shows a small, simple paraovarian cyst ➡, next to a normal ovary ➡. They were separable from each other and from the uterus ➡ with probe pressure.*

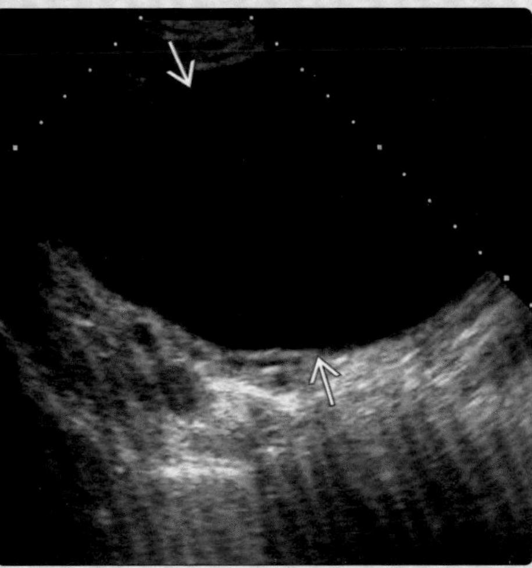

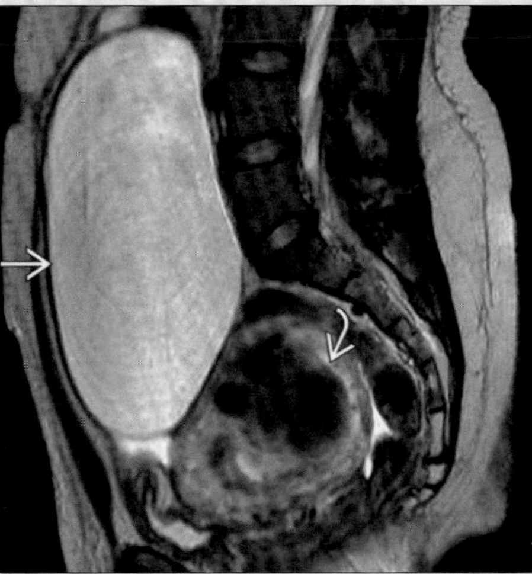

(Left) *Longitudinal transabdominal ultrasound of the pelvis shows a large unilocular cyst ➡ in the anterior pelvis. Neither ovary could be seen. MR was obtained for further evaluation.* **(Right)** *Sagittal T2 MR shows the large pelvic cyst ➡, anterior to a fibroid uterus ➡. Ovaries were normal, indicating that the cyst was a paraovarian cyst. Due to its size, surgery was performed.*

Peritoneal Inclusion Cyst

KEY FACTS

TERMINOLOGY

- Synonyms: Peritoneal pseudocyst, benign cystic mesothelioma
- Not true cyst but peritoneal or ovarian fluid trapped by peritoneal adhesions

IMAGING

- Unilocular or multilocular pelvic cystic lesion
- Boundaries defined by pelvic structures and walls
- Unilateral in 65%, bilateral in 35%, midline if large
- Normal ovary surrounded or displaced by fluid and septations; entrapped ovary: Spider in web appearance
- Fine septations most common
- Thick septations with nodules possible
- Blood flow can be seen in septations, especially if thick
- Transvaginal ultrasound 1st-line to localize ovary and exclude signs of malignancy

TOP DIFFERENTIAL DIAGNOSES

- Ovarian cystic neoplasm
- Hydrosalpinx
- Paraovarian cyst
- Lymphangioma/mesenteric cyst

PATHOLOGY

- Requires functioning ovary and peritoneal adhesions

CLINICAL ISSUES

- Almost exclusively premenopausal women
- Pelvic pain, palpable mass, abdominal distension, or pressure symptoms or incidentally noted on imaging
- Indolent course: May grow, remain stable, or regress
- Tend to recur after drainage

SCANNING TIPS

- Look for solid components and normal ovary using transabdominal and transvaginal probes

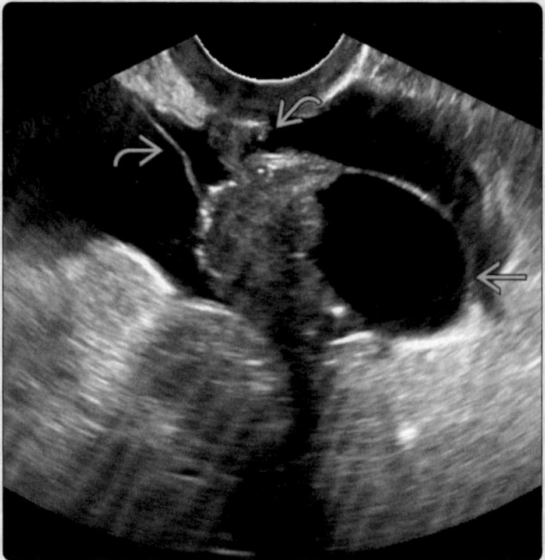

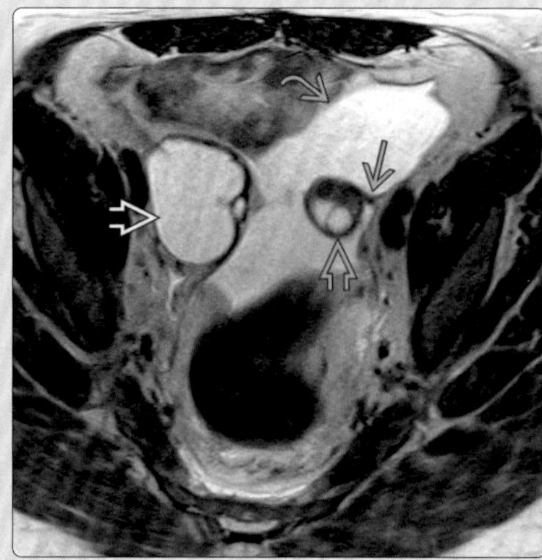

(Left) *Coronal transvaginal ultrasound shows a peritoneal inclusion cyst post hysterectomy. The cyst surrounds the left ovary, which contains a dominant follicle ➡, and consists of simple fluid with thin septa ➡.* **(Right)** *Axial T2 FSE MR of the same patient at a later time shows the fluid conforming to the peritoneal cavity ➡. A thin adhesion is present ➡. The left ovarian follicle ➡ is smaller; the right ovary has developed a larger cyst ➡.*

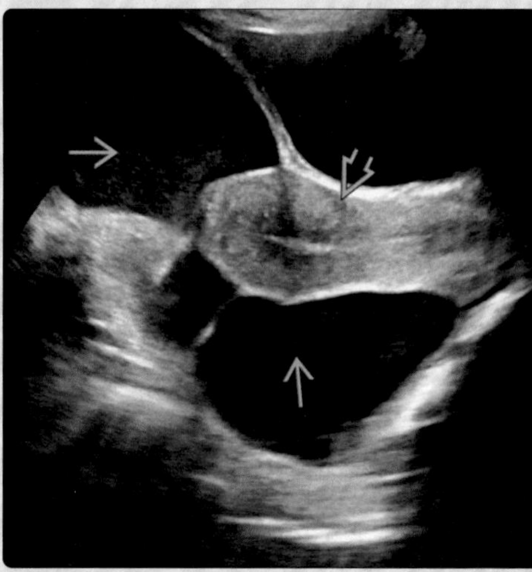

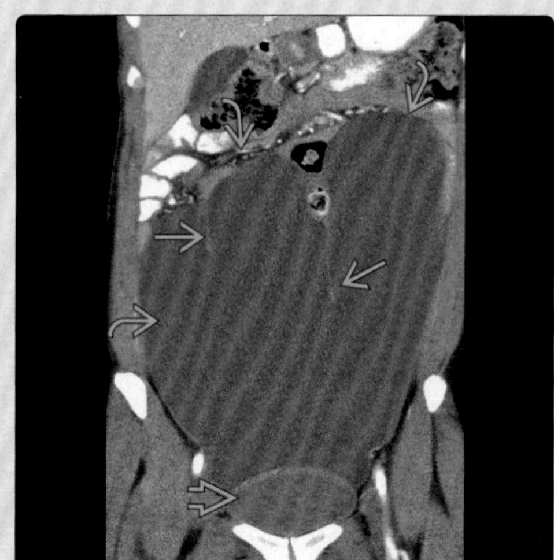

(Left) *Sagittal transabdominal ultrasound shows a peritoneal inclusion cyst ➡ superior and posterior to the uterus ➡. Internal echoes were from hemorrhage, confirmed at surgery.* **(Right)** *Coronal CECT of the same patient shows the extent of the huge peritoneal inclusion cyst ➡, displacing bowel. Thin septa ➡ are present. The bladder was normal ➡.*

Bartholin Cyst

KEY FACTS

TERMINOLOGY

- Bartholin glands (or greater vestibular glands) are mucus-secreting glands located in vulvar vestibule, just lateral and inferior to vaginal introitus
- Occlusion of Bartholin glands resulting in cyst formation

IMAGING

- Cystic structure on posterolateral distal vaginal wall, medial to labia minora, and at level of introitus
- Anechoic when simple
- Mixed echogenicity if complicated by hemorrhage or infection; → septations and thick wall
- Size ranges 1-4 cm
- No internal vascularity, may see reactive hyperemia around Bartholin abscess

TOP DIFFERENTIAL DIAGNOSES

- Sebaceous cyst
- Thrombophlebitis/other infections/varices
- Hematoma, endometrioma
- Skene gland cyst

PATHOLOGY

- Most common vulvar cystic mass; ~ 2% of women
- Usually asymptomatic
    - Superimposed infection can develop
        - Increase in size or preexisting cyst; local pain, dyspareunia
- Malignancy very rare
    - Squamous and adenocarcinoma most common types

CLINICAL ISSUES

- Usually found incidentally
- Palpable and sometimes visible mass
- Perineal pain, tender labial mass when infected (Bartholin abscess)

SCANNING TIPS

- Use higher frequency transducer for transperineal scanning

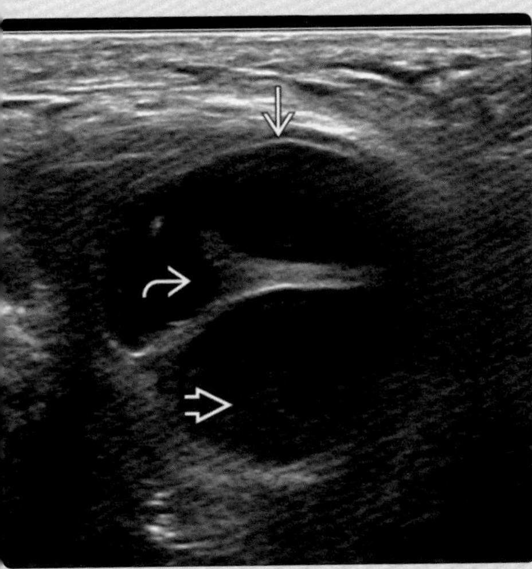

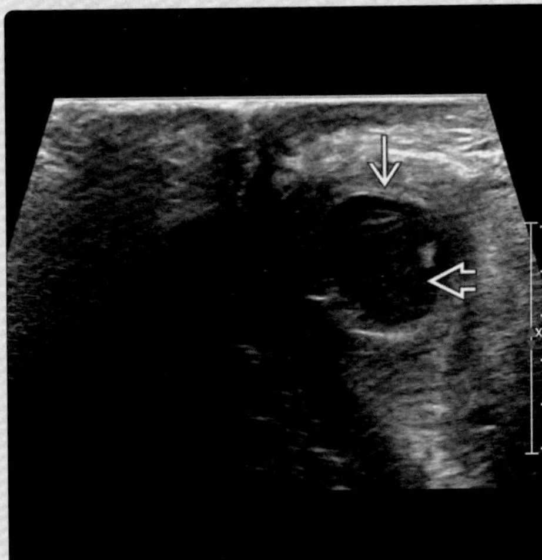

(Left) *Transverse ultrasound of the left labia shows a Bartholin abscess ➔, which is multiloculated with thick septa ↪ and internal debris ⇨. The patient had a history of recurrent abscesses.* **(Right)** *Transverse ultrasound of both labia shows a left Bartholin abscess ➔ with internal debris ⇨.*

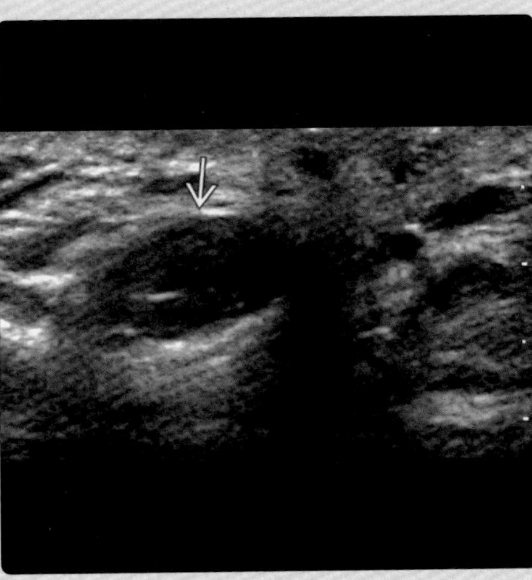

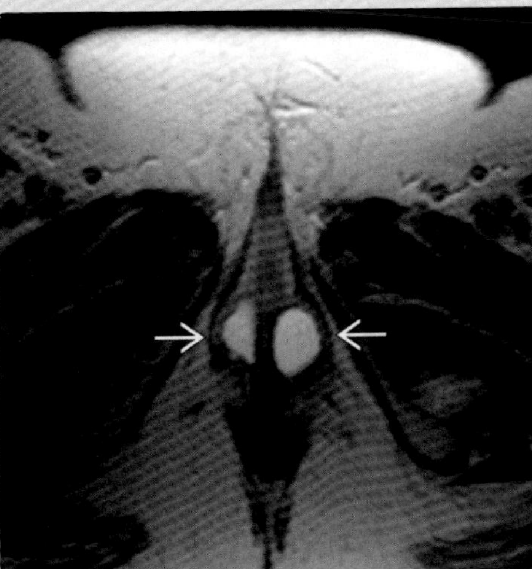

(Left) *Transverse ultrasound shows a hemorrhagic right Bartholin cyst ➔ in a patient who presented with acute pain but no signs of infection.* **(Right)** *T2 MR shows the typical location of Bartholin cysts ➔, which are often an incidental finding. Note the high T2 signal from internal fluid.*

KEY FACTS

TERMINOLOGY

- Gartner duct cyst: Embryonic remnant of wolffian (mesonephric) duct, lined with nonmucinous columnar cells
  - Associated with renal/ureteral/müllerian anomalies

IMAGING

- Ultrasound is modality of choice
- Well-defined cyst with thin walls, may contain septa
- Anechoic to hypoechoic with increased through transmission
- Separate from cervix, in anterolateral vaginal wall
- Infection or hemorrhage → increased echogenicity of fluid
- Rarely, large enough to cause urethral obstruction
- Cyst may be seen posterior to bladder or protrude into bladder, mimicking ureterocele or urethral diverticulum
- No internal flow on Doppler

TOP DIFFERENTIAL DIAGNOSES

- Nabothian cysts
- Vaginal inclusion cysts
- Urethral diverticulum
- Ectopic ureterocele
- Endometriosis
- If solid-appearing, consider vaginal tumors or cervical/vaginal polyp

CLINICAL ISSUES

- Occurs in 1-2% of women; usually asymptomatic
- Incidental finding on imaging or pelvic examination
- Symptomatic if large: Pelvic pressure symptoms, dyspareunia, obstructed labor
- Infection/hemorrhage may cause acute pain
- May present with urologic symptoms

SCANNING TIPS

- Partial withdrawal of transvaginal probe or light pressure helpful to minimize cyst compression
- Transperineal sonography can be alternative

(Left) *Longitudinal transabdominal ultrasound shows an ovoid cyst ➡ inferior to the cervix ➡. The endometrium ➡ is normal in this retroverted uterus.* **(Right)** *Coronal transvaginal ultrasound in the same patient shows 2 ovoid cysts ➡ in the upper vagina, consistent with Gartner duct cysts.*

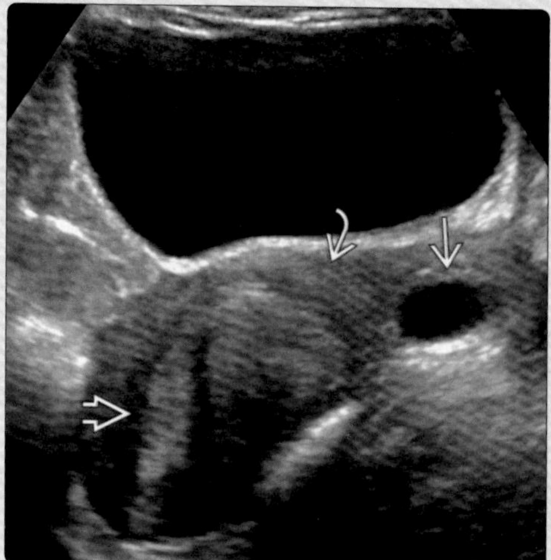

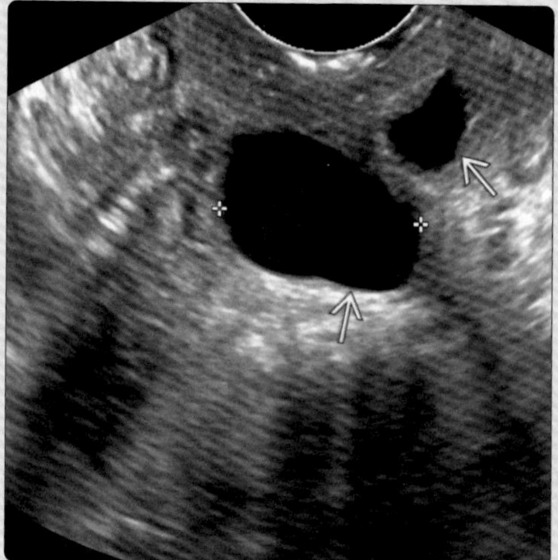

(Left) *Sagittal T2 FSE MR in the same patient confirms the location of the Gartner duct cysts ➡, inferior to the cervix ➡, which contains a nabothian follicle ➡.* **(Right)** *Transverse transabdominal ultrasound shows an incidental ovoid cyst ➡ posterior to the bladder ➡ and lateral to the cervix ➡, consistent with a Gartner duct cyst.*

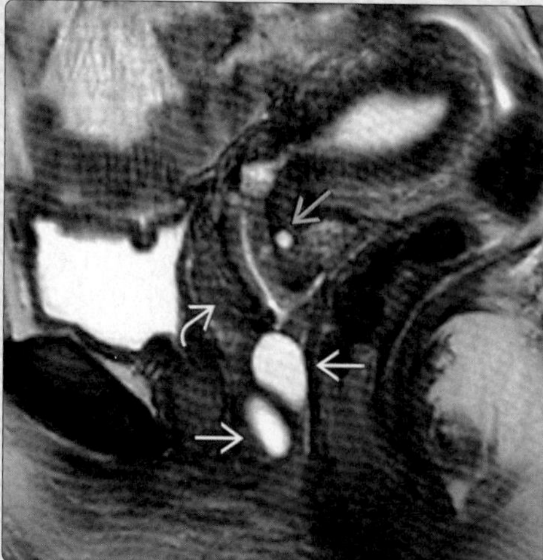

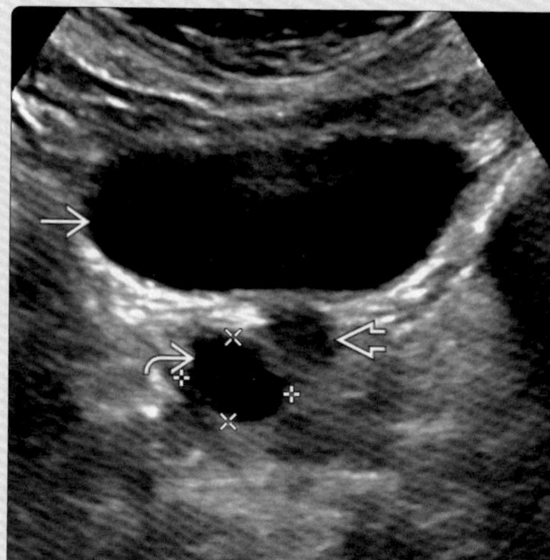

KEY FACTS

TERMINOLOGY

- Group of ovarian tumors arising from either embryonic sex cords or mesenchyme
  - Fibroma, thecoma, fibrothecoma
  - Granulosa cell tumor
  - Sertoli-Leydig tumor (androblastoma)
  - Sclerosing stromal tumor, steroid cell tumors, gynandroblastoma, and sex cord tumor with annular tubules

IMAGING

- Ultrasound findings of sex cord-stromal tumors are diverse and nonspecific
- Range from small, solid tumors to large, multicystic masses
- Sex cord-stromal tumors are generally solid or have significant solid components
- Hormonally active tumors may be small and difficult to find
- **Granulosa cell tumors**
  - More often contain cysts with sponge-like appearance
  - Cysts may be complex and contain hemorrhagic fluid
- **Fibrothecomas**
  - Hypoechoic with posterior acoustic attenuation
  - May have appearance similar to uterine leiomyoma

TOP DIFFERENTIAL DIAGNOSES

- Ovarian carcinoma
- Germ cell tumors

CLINICAL ISSUES

- Symptoms related to hormone production
- Some are estrogen-producing tumors: Bleeding in postmenopausal patient
- May be associated with Meigs syndrome (triad of ovarian fibroma, ascites, pleural effusion)

SCANNING TIPS

- May mimic pedunculated fibroid; use color Doppler to look for "bridging vessels" between uterus and mass, which would suggest pedunculated fibroid over ovarian tumor

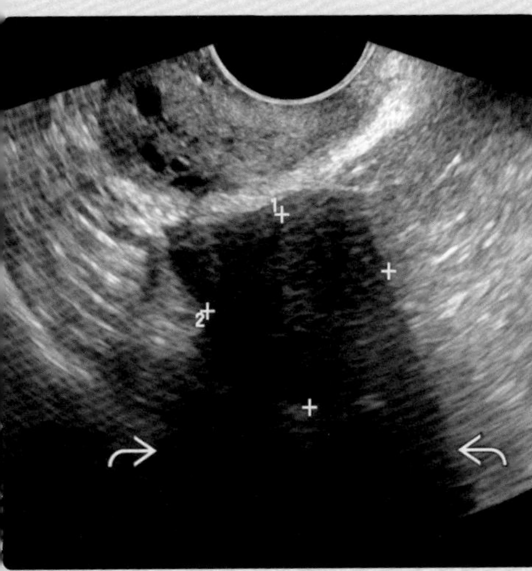

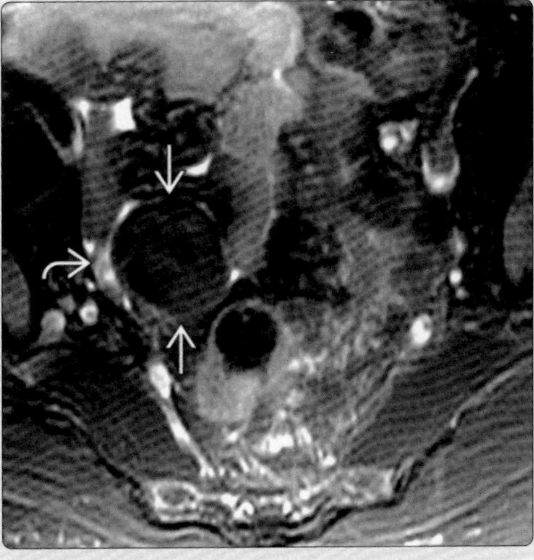

(Left) *Endovaginal US shows a right adnexal hypoechoic solid mass (calipers) with a dense posterior acoustic shadow ➔, > expected given the hypoechoic appearance of the mass. The ovary is not identified separately, and the imaging appearance is most consistent with an ovarian fibroma.* **(Right)** *Axial T2 FS MR in the same patient shows the mass ➔ is homogeneously T2 dark and associated with a small claw of normal ovarian tissue ➔, consistent with an ovarian fibroma.*

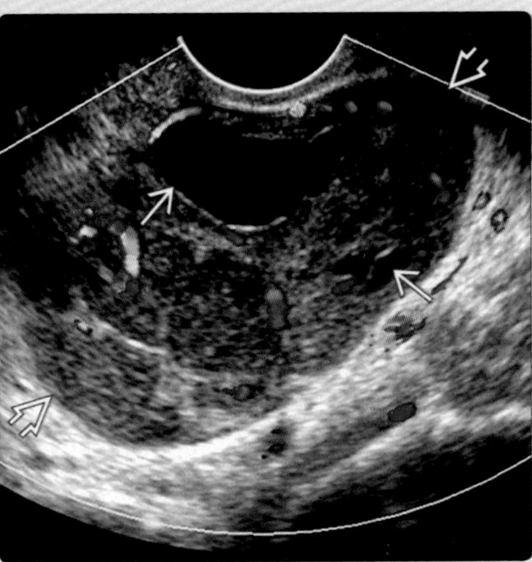

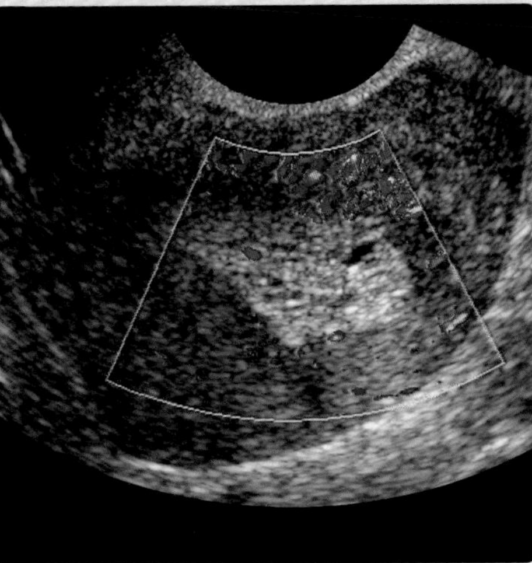

(Left) *Color Doppler endovaginal US in a perimenopausal woman with heavy vaginal bleeding shows a heterogeneous left adnexal mass ➔, which is predominately solid and vascular but also contains small cystic foci ➔. This was confirmed to be a granulosa cell tumor at pathology.* **(Right)** *Color Doppler endovaginal US in the same patient shows a thickened endometrium with multiple cysts, consistent with hyperplasia from estrogen stimulation in the setting of a granulosa cell tumor.*

Adnexal/Ovarian Torsion

KEY FACTS

TERMINOLOGY

- Adnexal torsion is more accurate term than ovarian torsion, as torsion usually also includes fallopian tube

IMAGING

- Ovary > 4 cm long or > 20 cm^3 in volume
- Enlarged, heterogeneously echogenic ovarian stroma
- Multiple small, fluid-filled follicles displaced peripherally due to edematous stroma &/or mass
  - May see follicular ring sign: Thin echogenic rim around follicles in early torsion
- Whirlpool sign: Coiled, twisted pedicle
- Flow pattern depends on degree of vascular obstruction and chronicity of torsion
- Venous flow affected 1st
- Due to dual arterial blood supply to ovary, arterial flow may be preserved

TOP DIFFERENTIAL DIAGNOSES

- Hemorrhagic corpus luteum
- Pelvic inflammatory disease
- Ectopic pregnancy

PATHOLOGY

- In adults, 50-90% have associated ovarian mass that serves as lead point
  - Large physiologic follicular cyst or corpus luteum cyst most common, followed by dermoid
- Presence of venous flow suggests viable ovary

SCANNING TIPS

- Compare with asymptomatic contralateral side
- Presence of normal blood flow does **not** exclude torsion
- Ovaries are highly mobile and when torsed, may be located in unusual locations
- When ovaries are deep in location, it may be difficult to detect color Doppler flow even in normal ovaries

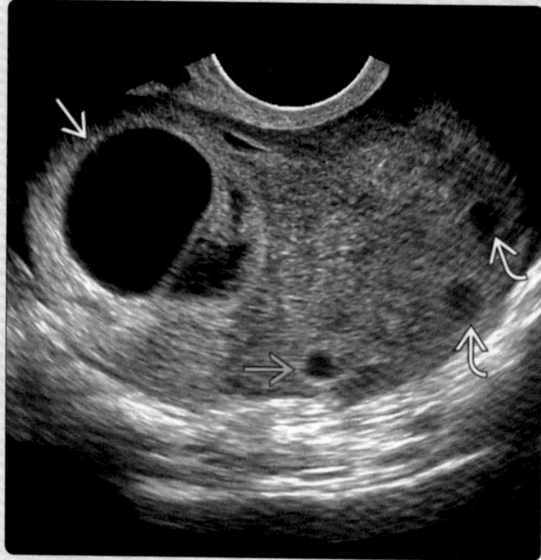

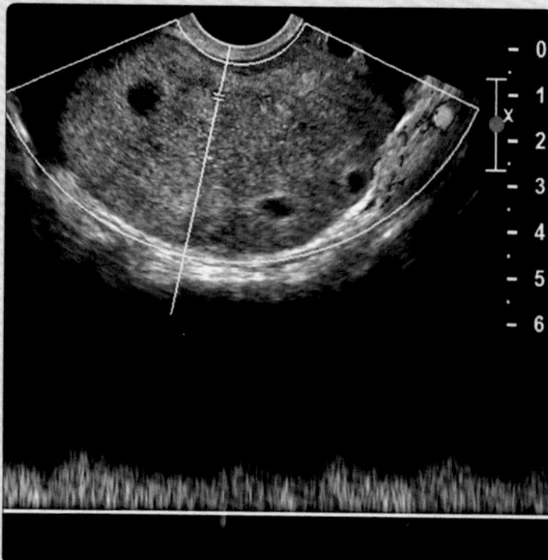

(Left) *Longitudinal endovaginal ultrasound with adnexal torsion shows an enlarged, 6-cm ovary ➔ containing a hemorrhagic cyst with multiple peripheral follicles ➔. One of the follicles demonstrates the follicular ring sign ➔.* **(Right)** *Endovaginal pulse wave Doppler ultrasound in the same patient with adnexal torsion shows low-resistance arterial flow in the ovary. It is important to remember that the presence of blood flow does not exclude ovarian torsion.*

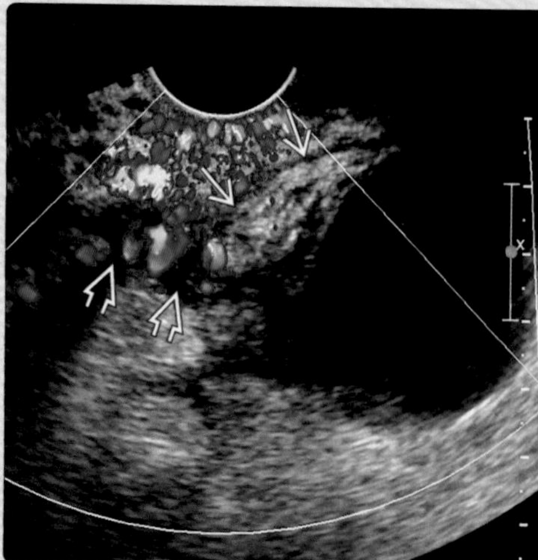

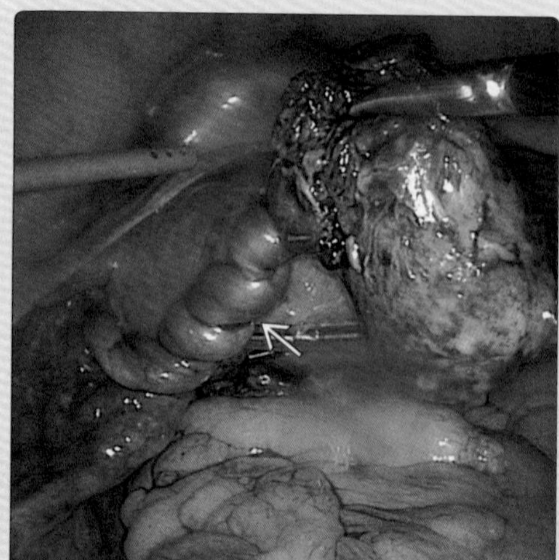

(Left) *Endovaginal ultrasound in a woman with acute pelvic pain shows a large cyst in the ovary with adjacent edematous parenchyma ➔ with no color Doppler signal. Alternating red and blue color signal ➔ represents a twisted vascular pedicle, which is best seen during real time.* **(Right)** *Intraoperative photo in the same patient looking caudally confirms torsion and shows dusky infarcted right ovary (grasped) and twisted vascular pedicle ➔.*

KEY FACTS

TERMINOLOGY

- Secondary (metastatic) neoplasms to ovary
- Krukenberg tumor: Subtype of metastatic tumors containing > 10% mucin-filled signet cells in cellular stroma
- High-stage mucinous tumors involving ovary frequently represent metastases from extraovarian primary sites and are often misdiagnosed as primary ovarian mucinous tumors

IMAGING

- Bilateral ovarian masses in patients with known primary carcinoma
- Metastases to ovary are usually solid masses
- Often large
- Lobulated masses with smooth external contour
- US
  - Solid or cystic and solid
  - Solid components demonstrate vascularity on Doppler evaluation
  - Typically heterogeneous
  - May be complicated by hemorrhage
- MR
  - T2WI: Solid components demonstrate heterogeneous signal intensity
  - T1WI C+: Solid components show marked heterogeneous enhancement

TOP DIFFERENTIAL DIAGNOSES

- Primary ovarian cancer
- Ovarian lymphoma

SCANNING TIPS

- Look for ascites, which is often seen in the setting of Krukenberg tumor

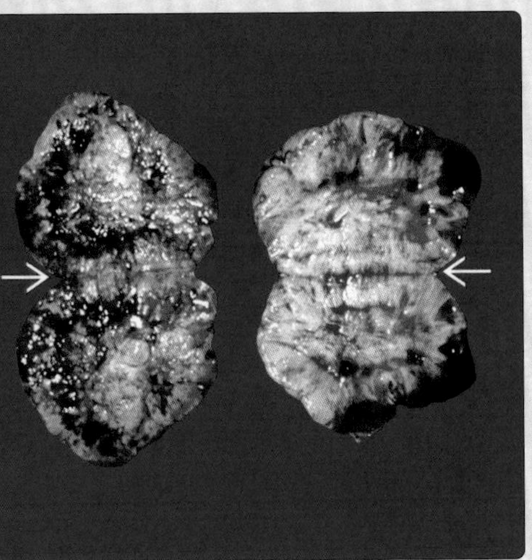

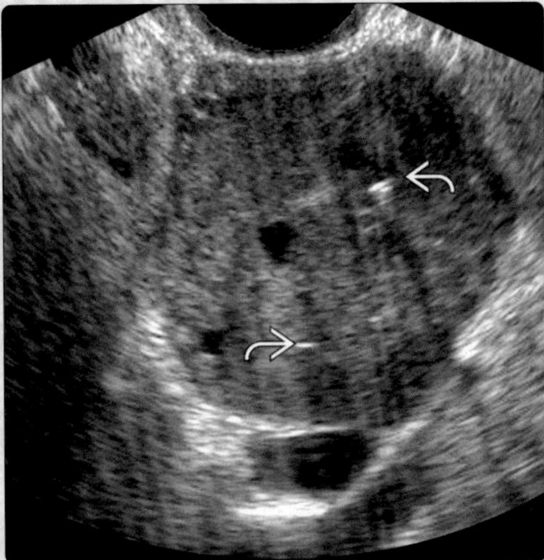

(Left) *Gross pathology specimen shows ovarian metastasis from gastric cancer (Krukenberg tumor). Bilateral, solid ovarian masses* ➡ *are depicted.* **(Right)** *Longitudinal endovaginal US shows a large, solid adnexal mass in a patient with gastric cancer. Note the small foci of calcification* ➦*, which can rarely be seen in mucinous gastric adenocarcinomas.*

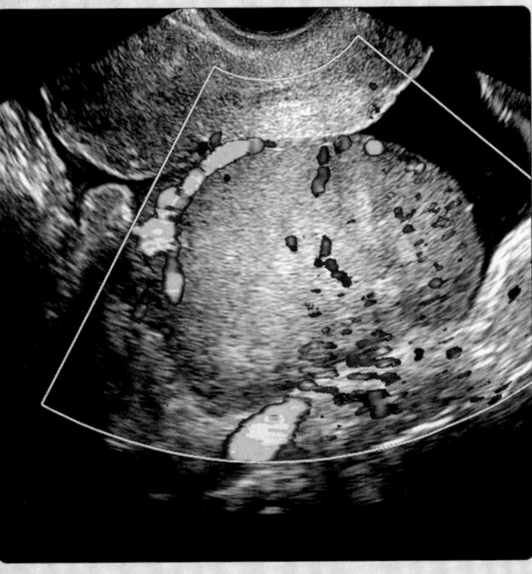

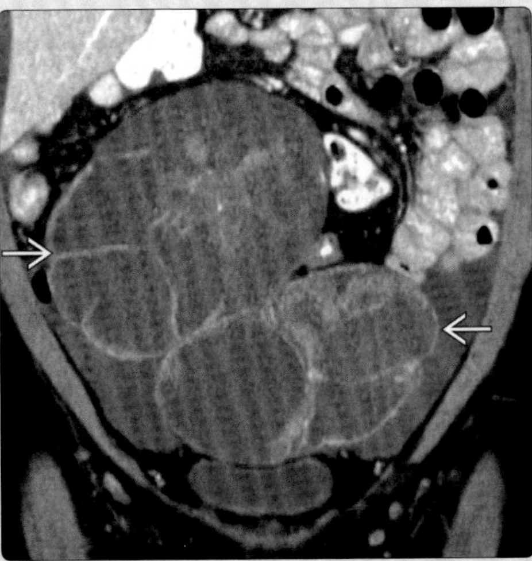

(Left) *Longitudinal color Doppler US shows flow within a solid, large right adnexal mass in a patient with metastatic melanoma to the ovary. Note the free fluid in the cul-de-sac.* **(Right)** *Coronal CECT in a 45-year-old woman shows large, bilateral, complex cystic and solid adnexal masses* ➡*. The patient had a recent history of colon cancer, and these were confirmed metastases at oophorectomy.*

Part III
SECTION 1
Anatomy and Approach

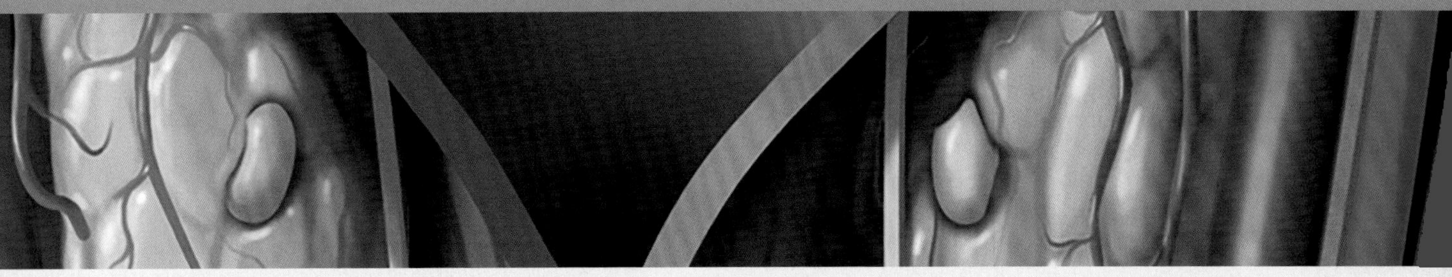

GROSS ANATOMY

Thyroid Gland

- **H- or U-shaped gland** in anterior cervical neck formed from 2 elongated lateral lobes with superior and inferior poles connected by median isthmus
- Thyroid gland lies anterior and lateral to trachea in visceral space of infrahyoid neck
  - Extends from level of 5th cervical vertebra to 1st thoracic vertebra
  - Posteromedially are **tracheoesophageal grooves**
    - Contains paratracheal lymph nodes, recurrent laryngeal nerve, parathyroid glands
  - Posterolaterally are **carotid spaces**
    - Contains common carotid artery, internal jugular vein, vagus nerve
  - Anteriorly are infrahyoid **strap muscles**
  - Anterolaterally are **sternocleidomastoid muscles**
- Thyroid gland
  - **2 lateral lobes** (i.e., right and left lobes)
    - Measure ~ 4 cm in height
    - Each lobe has upper and lower poles
    - Lateral lobes are commonly asymmetric in size
  - Lateral lobes are joined by **midline isthmus**
  - **Pyramidal lobe** present in 30-50% of cases
    - Extends superiorly from isthmus toward hyoid bone
    - More common on left
- Superior thyroid arteries
  - 1st anterior branch of external carotid artery
- Inferior thyroid arteries
  - Arise from thyrocervical trunk, branch of subclavian artery
- Thyroidea ima occasionally present (3%)
  - Single vessel originating from aortic arch or brachiocephalic artery
  - Enters thyroid gland at inferior border of isthmus
- **Lymphatic drainage**
  - Lymphatic drainage is extensive and multidirectional
  - Initial lymphatic drainage courses to periglandular nodes
    - Prelaryngeal, pretracheal, and paratracheal nodes along recurrent laryngeal nerve
    - Paratracheal nodes drain into mediastinum
    - Regional drainage occurs laterally into internal jugular chain (levels 2-4) and spinal accessory chain (level 5)
- Embryology
  - Thyroid gland forms near base of tongue (foramen cecum) and descends into neck along thyroglossal duct
    - **Ectopic thyroid** gland can be seen from base of tongue into superior mediastinum
      - Most common location is just deep to foramen cecum at tongue base (i.e., lingual thyroid)
    - **Thyroglossal duct cyst** results from failure of complete involution of thyroglossal duct

Parathyroid Glands

- Small lentiform glands posterior to thyroid gland
  - Extracapsular in most cases but can be located within thyroid gland
- Located in region of tracheoesophageal groove
- Normal measurements
  - ~ 6 mm in length, 3- to 4-mm transverse, and 1-2 mm in anteroposterior diameter
- Variable number, but typically 4
  - 2 superior and 2 inferior
- **Superior parathyroid glands**
  - More constant in position as compared with lower glands
  - Lie on posterior border of middle 1/3 of thyroid in 75%
- **Inferior parathyroid glands**
  - More variable in location
  - 50% of inferior glands lie lateral to lower pole of thyroid gland
  - 15% lie within 1 cm of inferior thyroid poles
  - 35% position is variable, residing anywhere from angle of mandible to lower anterior mediastinum

ANATOMY IMAGING ISSUES

Thyroid Gland

- Use high-resolution linear array transducer (10-15 MHz)
- Normal thyroid parenchyma has fine, uniform echoes and is hyperechoic compared to adjacent muscles
- Echogenic **thyroid capsule** is clearly visualized and helps to differentiate thyroid lesions from extrathyroidal masses
- Both longitudinal and transverse scans are required for comprehensive ultrasound assessment of thyroid gland
  - Measurements taken in all 3 planes
- Midline transverse view for isthmus
- **Document size of all nodules** with particular attention to **sonographic characteristics** (all features are listed from least concerning to most concerning for malignancy)
  - **Composition**: Cystic, spongiform, mixed cystic and solid, solid, or predominantly solid
  - **Echogenicity**: Anechoic, hyperechoic, isoechoic, hypoechoic, very hypoechoic
  - **Shape**: Wider than tall, taller than wide
  - **Margin**: Smooth, ill-defined, lobulated or irregular, extrathyroid extension
  - **Echogenic foci**: Comet-tail artifacts, macrocalcifications, peripheral (rim) calcifications, punctate echogenic foci
- Assess adjacent structures (including trachea, esophagus, strap muscles, carotid artery, and internal jugular vein) and cervical lymph nodes

Parathyroid Glands

- Normal glands often not seen
  - **Look carefully in tracheoesophageal groove** behind mid- to lower thyroid
  - Small, well-circumscribed, hypoechoic nodules posterior to thyroid gland separated by echogenic thyroid capsule
- Best 1st examination for localizing parathyroid adenoma
  - May be in ectopic location so start above thyroid at angle of mandible and move downward, scanning through thyroid to level of clavicle
  - Hypoechoic on grayscale with hypervascularity on color flow imaging
    - Color flow imaging best done in longitudinal plane
- Easy to confuse with other structures, especially cervical lymph nodes
  - Look for echogenic hilum and classic central hilar vessel in lymph node

THYROID AND PARATHYROID GLANDS

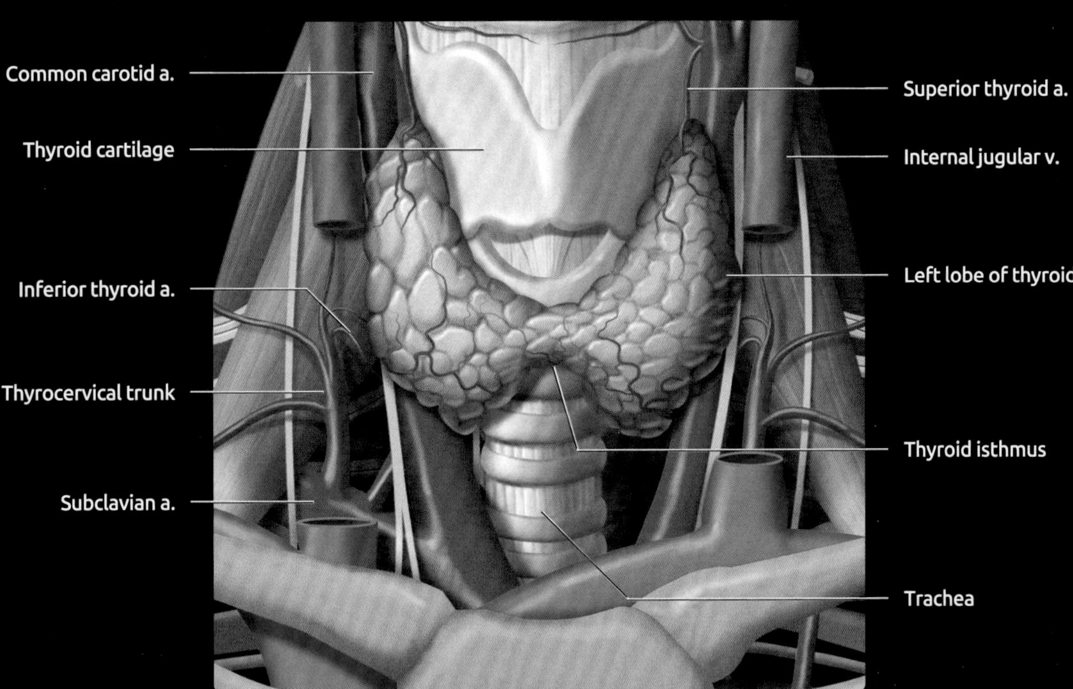

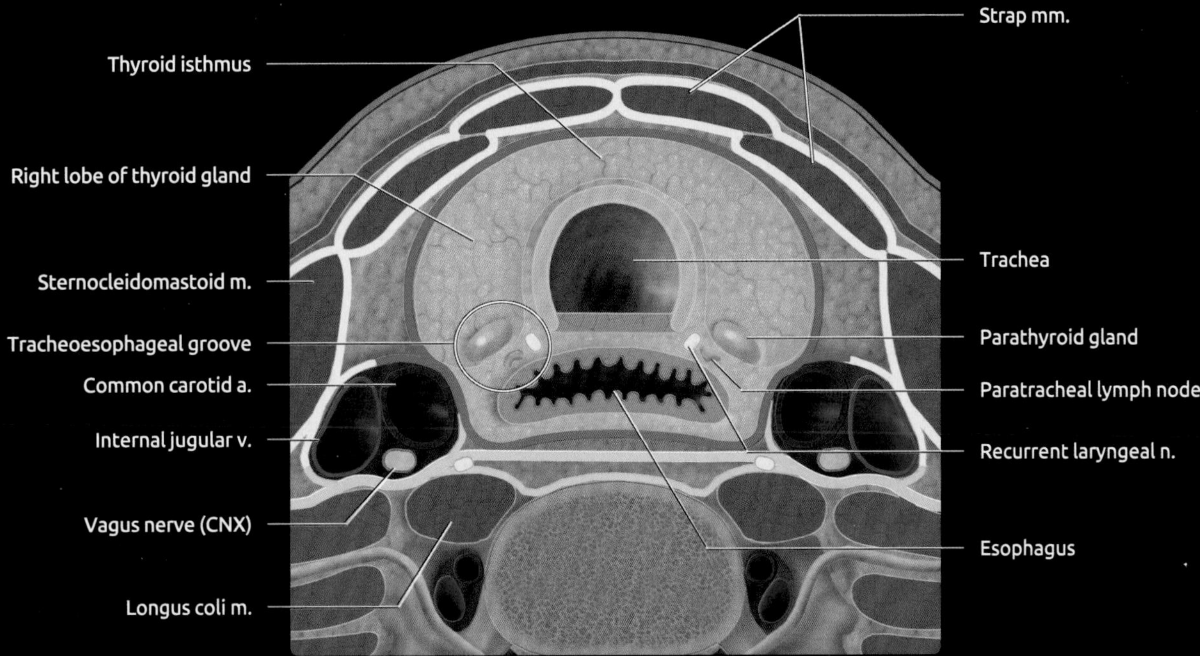

(Top) *The thyroid is located in an anatomically complex area. It has a H or U shape and drapes over the trachea with the lobes adjacent to a rich network of nerves and vessels.* **(Bottom)** *Axial graphic at the thyroid level depicts the superior parathyroid glands just posterior to the thyroid gland. Note that there are 3 key structures found in the area of the tracheoesophageal groove: The recurrent laryngeal nerve, paratracheal lymph node chain, and parathyroid glands. Lateral to this is the carotid space with the common carotid artery, internal jugular vein, and vagus nerve. The surrounding muscles include the strap muscles anteriorly, the sternocleidomastoid muscles laterally, and longus coli muscles posteriorly.*

THYROID AND PARATHYROID GLANDS

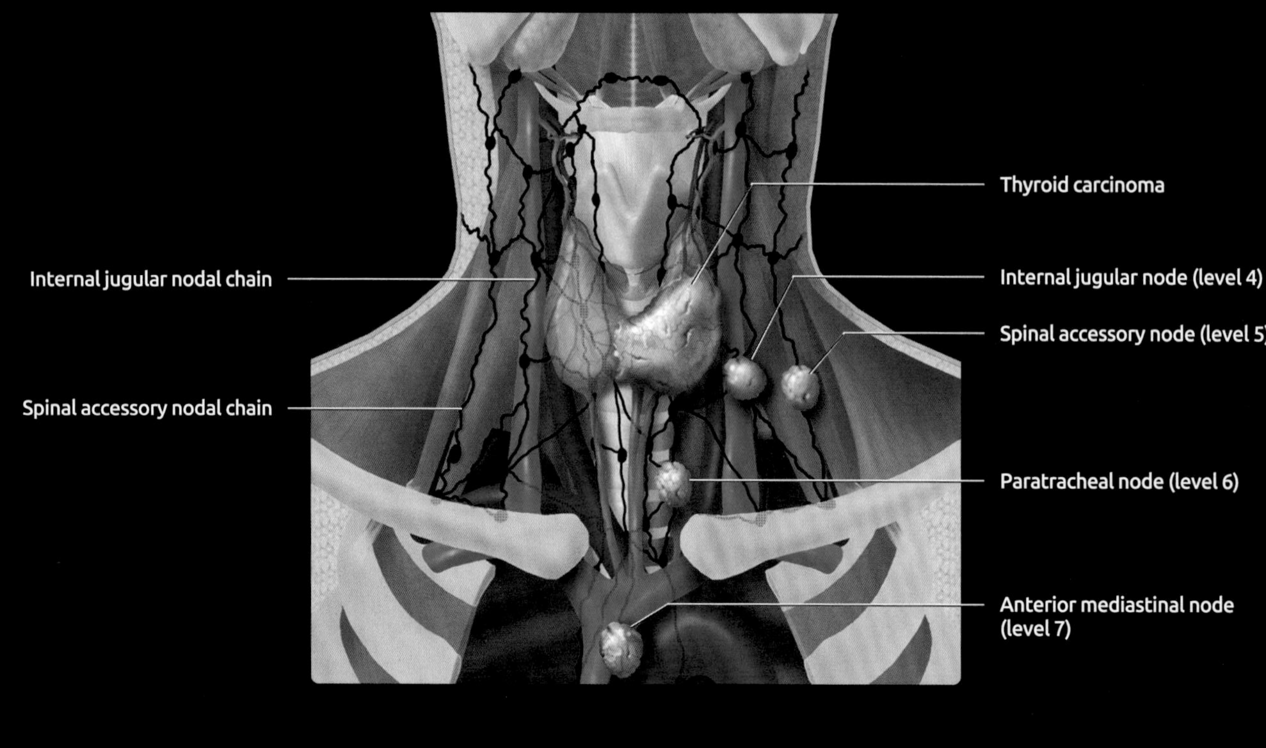

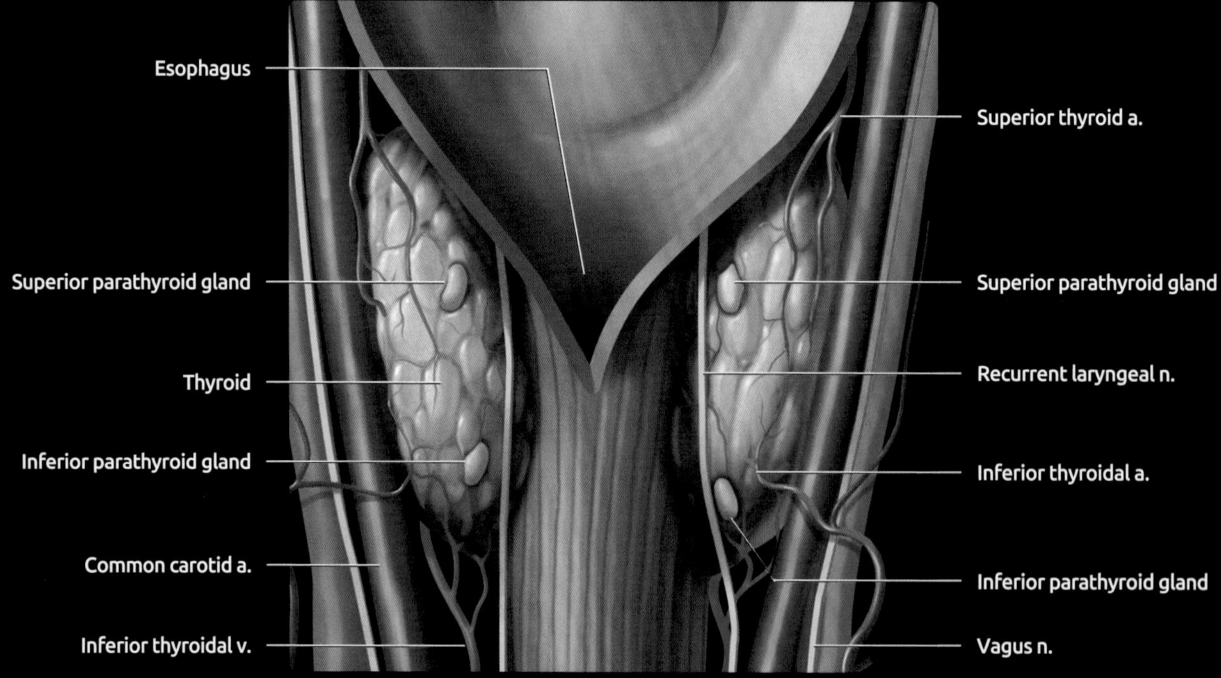

(Top) *Graphic shows a tumor within the thyroid gland with metastases to surrounding lymph nodes. There is a very rich surrounding lymphatic network within the neck, which extends down into the superior mediastinum. Lymphatic drainage is extensive and multidirectional, so it is important to perform complete sweeps through the lymph node chains when performing a neck ultrasound. Although limited in the chest by air within the lungs, an angled scan at the suprasternal notch may detect a superior mediastinal node.* **(Bottom)** *Coronal graphic illustrates the esophagus, parathyroid glands, and thyroid gland from behind. The drawing depicts the typical anatomic relationships of the paired superior and inferior parathyroid glands. Note the arterial supply to superior and inferior parathyroid glands is from the superior and inferior thyroid arteries, respectively.*

THYROID GLAND

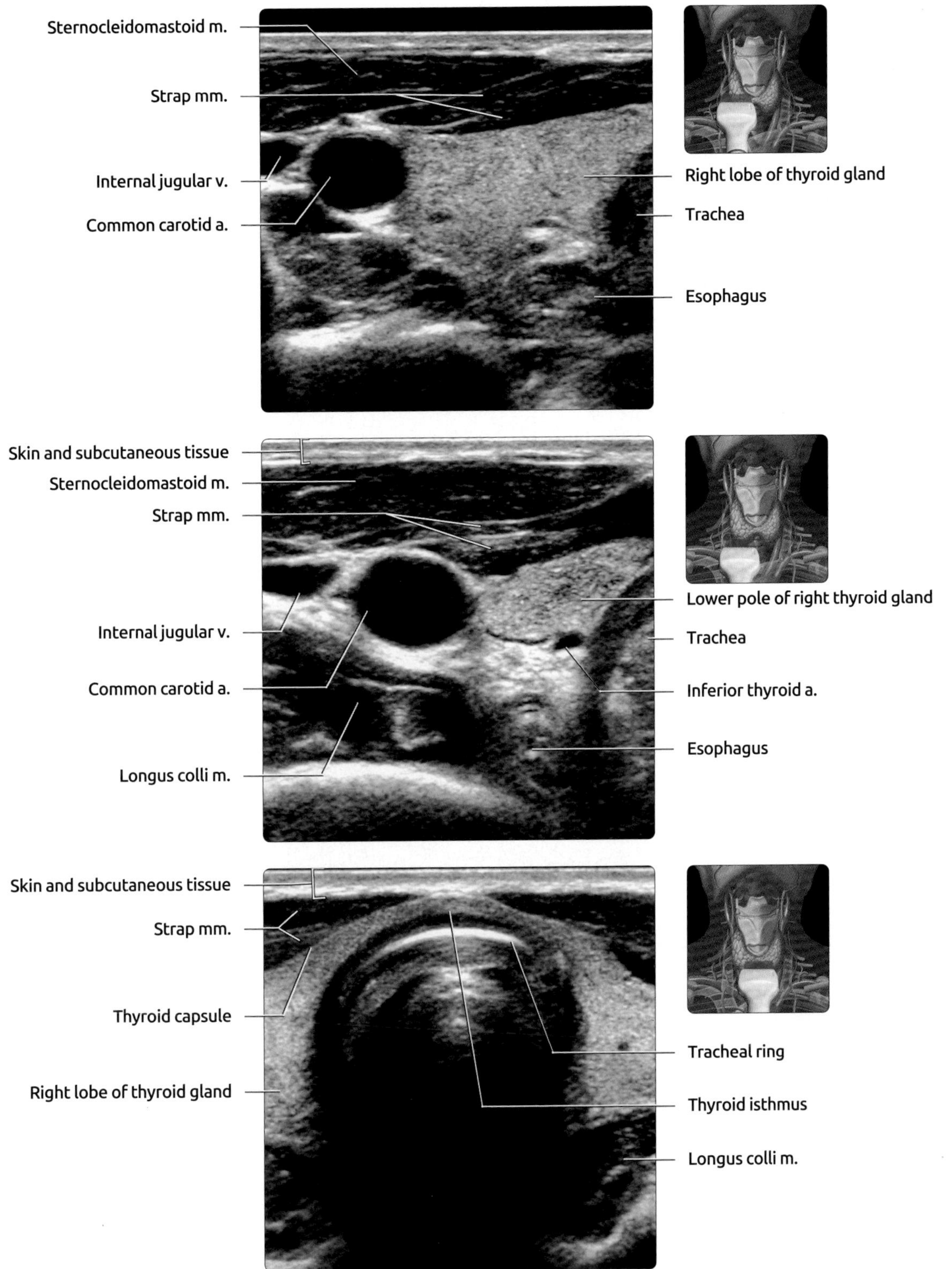

(Top) *Transverse grayscale ultrasound of the right lobe of the thyroid gland shows the homogeneous, hyperechoic echo pattern of the glandular parenchyma. Note its close anatomical relationship with the major vessels (internal jugular vein and common carotid artery) laterally, the trachea medially, and the cervical esophagus posteromedially.* **(Middle)** *Transverse grayscale ultrasound shows the level of the inferior pole of the thyroid gland. The inferior thyroid artery is a consistent finding related to and supplying the inferior pole.* **(Bottom)** *Midline transverse grayscale ultrasound shows the thyroid isthmus connecting the 2 lobes. The isthmus lies on the anterior surface of the trachea. In view of the intimate anatomical relationship between the thyroid gland and the trachea, tumor invasion into the trachea from malignant thyroid carcinoma may occur, rendering surgical excision more extensive than total thyroidectomy.*

THYROID GLAND

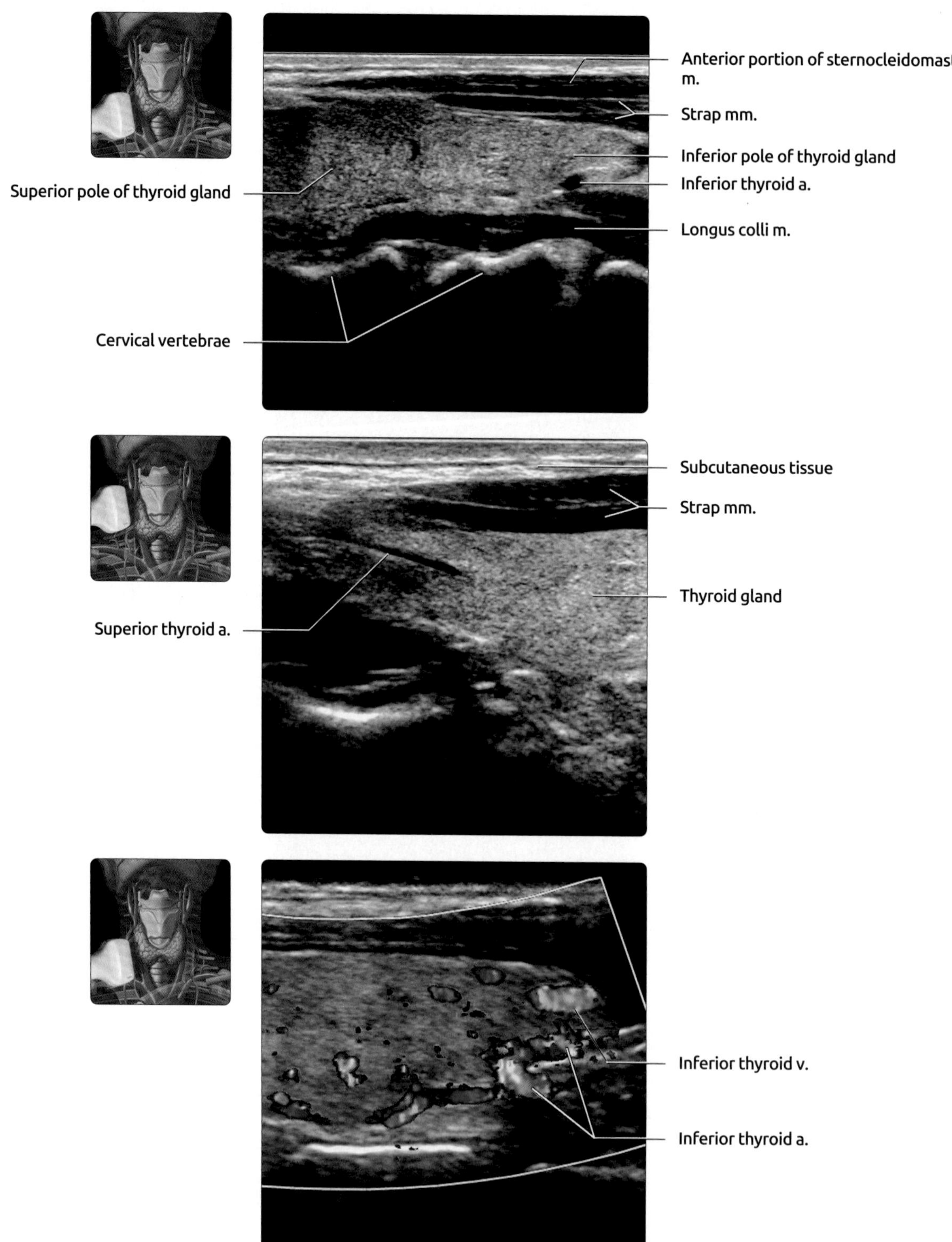

(Top) *Parasagittal longitudinal grayscale ultrasound shows the homogeneous, hyperechoic echo pattern the thyroid gland. Part of the tortuous course of the inferior thyroid artery is seen in relation to the lower pole.* **(Middle)** *Parasagittal longitudinal grayscale ultrasound shows the superior thyroid artery, the 1st anterior branch of the external carotid artery, running inferiorly within and supplying the upper pole of the thyroid gland. Longitudinal scans best evaluate the glandular parenchyma and vascularity.* **(Bottom)** *Longitudinal color Doppler ultrasound shows both the inferior thyroid artery and vein. The thyroid gland is a very vascular organ.*

PYRAMIDAL LOBE

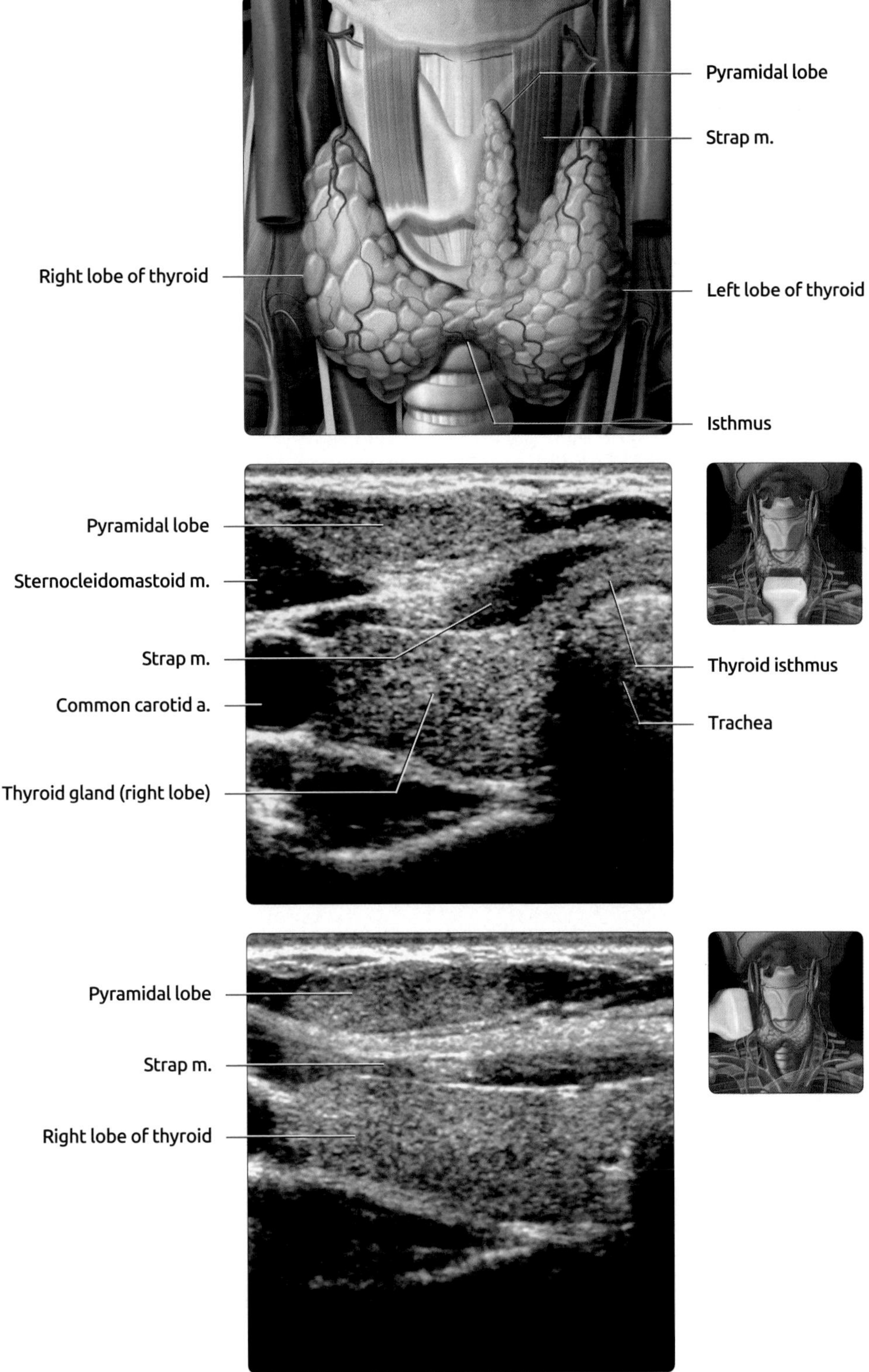

(Top) *There are many variants in the size and shape of the thyroid gland. This graphic shows the most common, a pyramidal lobe, which formed along the thyroglossal duct, and is present to some degree in 30-50% of the population. They more commonly project to the left but can be in the midline or to the right. Note that it is anterior to the strap muscles, while the main thyroid lobe is posterior.* **(Middle)** *Transverse grayscale ultrasound shows the pyramidal lobe of the thyroid gland. The echo pattern is identical to the normal right thyroid lobe (i.e., homogeneous, hyperechoic). It is located anterior to the anterior strap muscle. This should not be mistaken for a mass. Careful scanning will show it connects to the isthmus of the thyroid.* **(Bottom)** *Longitudinal ultrasound in the same patient shows the pyramidal lobe anterior to the strap muscle.*

PARATHYROID GLANDS

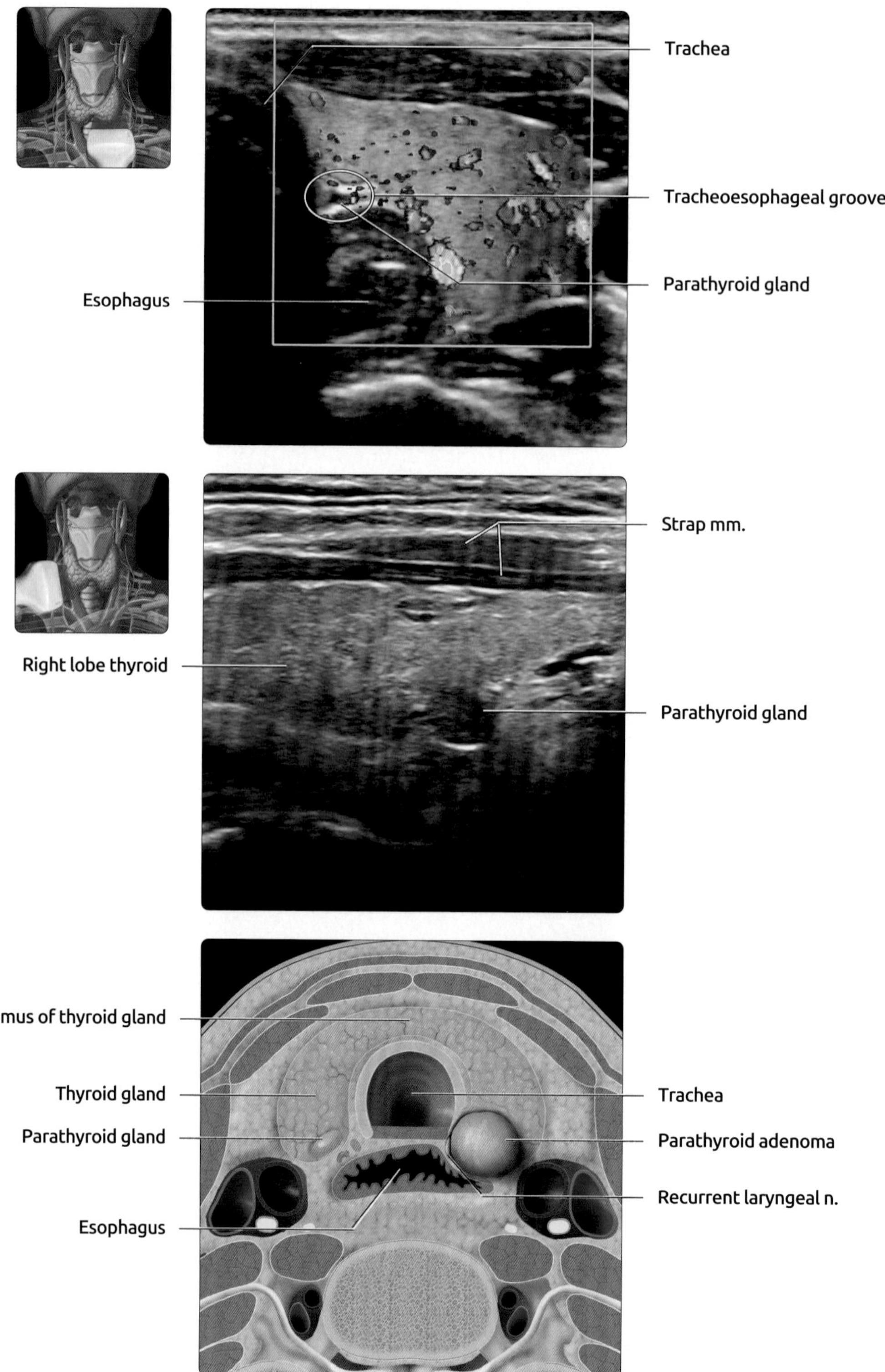

(Top) *Transverse color Doppler ultrasound at the level of the midthyroid shows a small, ovoid, hypoechoic area of soft tissue in the tracheoesophageal groove. Although it is difficult to tell with certainty, this is likely a normal parathyroid gland. Normal parathyroid glands are often difficult to identify.* **(Middle)** *Longitudinal scan of the right thyroid shows a larger, hypoechoic nodule in the expected location of the parathyroid gland, posterior to the middle 1/3 of the thyroid gland. This is the typical location of the superior parathyroid glands. Careful analysis during a real-time scan should be done to prove they are outside the thyroid capsule and not a thyroid nodule. A parathyroid gland may also sometimes be confused with a small lymph node, but a normal lymph node should have an echogenic hilum.* **(Bottom)** *Axial graphic shows a well-circumscribed mass in the left tracheoesophageal groove causing mass effect on the recurrent laryngeal nerve, esophagus, trachea, and left thyroid lobe. This is typical of a parathyroid adenoma, but a recurrent laryngeal nerve schwannoma or nodal disease in the paratracheal nodal chain could also cause such an appearance.*

PARATHYROID GLANDS

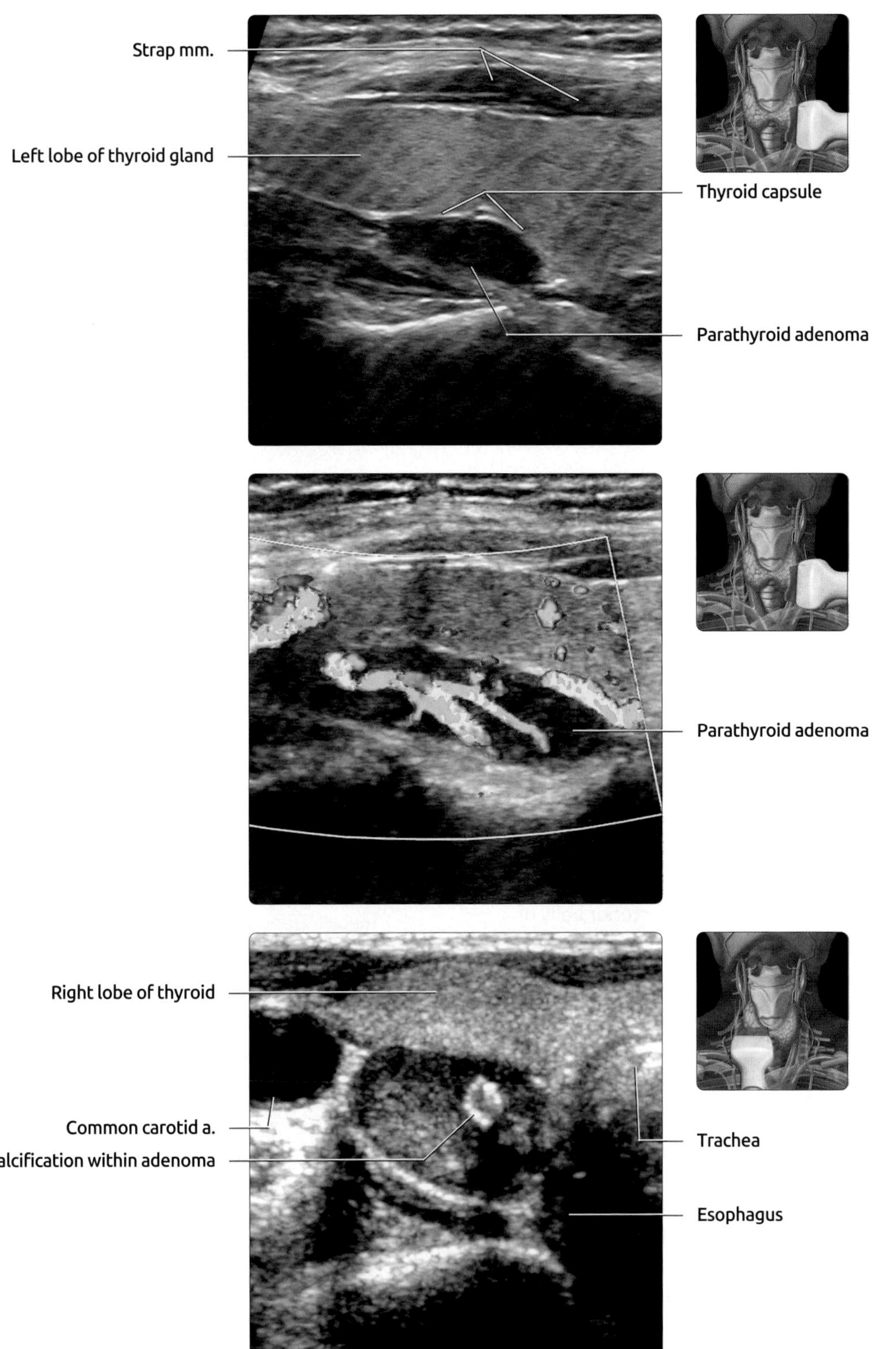

(Top) *Longitudinal ultrasound of the left lobe of the thyroid in a patient with hypercalcemia shows a well-defined, ovoid, hypoechoic mass. Note the distinct thyroid capsule, confirming this is posterior to the thyroid and therefore likely a parathyroid gland rather than a thyroid nodule.* **(Middle)** *Color Doppler ultrasound in the same patient shows increased vascularity, typical of a parathyroid adenoma.* **(Bottom)** *Transverse grayscale ultrasound shows a well-circumscribed, solid, round, hypoechoic parathyroid adenoma posterior to the right thyroid lobe in the region of the tracheoesophageal groove. This patient had biochemical evidence of primary hyperparathyroidism. Note that the presence of calcification within an adenoma is uncommon; it is more commonly seen with carcinoma.*

TERMINOLOGY

Synonyms

- Internal jugular chain (IJC): Deep cervical chain
- Spinal accessory chain (SAC): Posterior triangle chain
- Transverse cervical chain: Supraclavicular chain
- Anterior cervical chain: Prelaryngeal, pretracheal, paratracheal nodes
- Paratracheal node: Recurrent laryngeal node

Definitions

- Jugulodigastric node: "Sentinel" (highest) node, found at apex of IJC at angle of mandible
- Virchow node: "Signal" node, lowest node of deep cervical chain
- Troisier node: Most medial node of transverse cervical chain
- Omohyoid node: Deep cervical chain node superior to omohyoid as it crosses jugular vein
- Delphian node: Pretracheal node

IMAGING ANATOMY

Overview

- In normal adult neck, may be up to 300 lymph nodes
  - Internal structures: Capsule, cortex, medulla, hilum
- US appearances of normal cervical lymph node
  - Small, oval/reniform shape with well-defined margin
  - Homogeneous, hypoechoic cortex with echogenic fatty hilum
  - Hilar vascularity on color/power Doppler examination
- Imaging-based nodal classification
  - **Level I: Submental and submandibular nodes**
    - Level IA: Submental nodes: Found between anterior bellies of digastric muscles
    - Level IB: Submandibular nodes: Found around submandibular glands in submandibular space
  - **Level II: Upper IJC nodes: From posterior belly of digastric muscle to hyoid bone**
    - Level IIA: Level II node anterior, medial, lateral, or posterior to IJV; if posterior to IJV, node must be inseparable from IJV; contains jugulodigastric nodal group
    - Level IIB: Level II node posterior to IJV with fat plane visible between node and IJV
  - **Level III: Mid IJC nodes**
    - From hyoid bone to inferior margin of cricoid cartilage
  - **Level IV: Lower IJC nodes**
    - From inferior cricoid margin to clavicle
  - **Level V: Nodes of posterior cervical space/spinal accessory chain**
    - SAC nodes lie posterior to back margin of sternocleidomastoid muscle
    - Level VA: Upper SAC nodes from skull base to bottom of cricoid cartilage
    - Level VB: Lower SAC nodes from cricoid to clavicle
  - **Level VI: Nodes of visceral space**
    - Found from hyoid bone above to top of manubrium below
    - Midline group of cervical lymph nodes
    - Includes prelaryngeal, pretracheal, and paratracheal subgroups
  - **Level VII: Superior mediastinal nodes**
    - Between carotid arteries from top of manubrium above to innominate vein below
- Other nodal groups not included in standard imaging-based nodal classification
  - Parotid nodal group: Intraglandular or extraglandular
  - Retropharyngeal (RPS) nodal group: Medial RPS nodes and lateral RPS nodes (Rouvière node)
  - Facial nodal group

ANATOMY IMAGING ISSUES

Imaging Approaches

- Nodal metastases from primary tumors are site specific; therefore, it is critical to understand usual patterns of lymphatic spread
- Equivocal nodes outside usual pattern less suspicious
- Likely location of primary tumor can be suspected in patients presenting with nodal mass
- Nodal disease outside usual pattern may suggest aggressive tumor or prompt search for 2nd primary

Imaging Pitfalls

- RPS nodes and superior mediastinal nodes cannot be assessed by US

Key Concepts

- Useful US features suspicious of malignancy
  - Shape: Round, long:short axis ratio < 2
  - Loss of echogenic hilum
  - Presence of intranodal necrosis (cystic/coagulation)
  - Presence of extracapsular spread: Ill-defined margin
  - Peripheral/subcapsular flow on color/power Doppler ultrasound
  - Increased intranodal intravascular resistance: Resistive index (RI) > 0.8, pulsatility index (PI) > 1.6
  - Internal architecture: Punctate calcifications in metastatic node from papillary thyroid carcinoma, reticulated/pseudocystic appearance of lymphomatous node
- No single finding sensitive or specific enough; these signs should be used in combination
- Fine-needle aspiration biopsy helps to improve diagnostic accuracy
- Tuberculous nodes mimic metastatic nodes
  - Differentiating features: Intranodal necrosis, nodal matting, soft tissue edema and displaced hilar vascularity/avascularity, calcification (post treatment)

CLINICAL IMPLICATIONS

Clinical Importance

- Presence of malignant SCCa nodes on staging associated with 50% ↓ in long-term survival
  - If extranodal spread present, further 50% ↓
- Location of metastatic nodes in neck may help predict site of primary tumor
  - RPS and posterior triangle nodes seen in nasopharyngeal carcinoma, and lower cervical nodes in lung cancer
  - When Virchow node found on imaging without upper neck nodes, primary not in neck, and whole-body imaging warranted

LYMPH NODE GROUPS

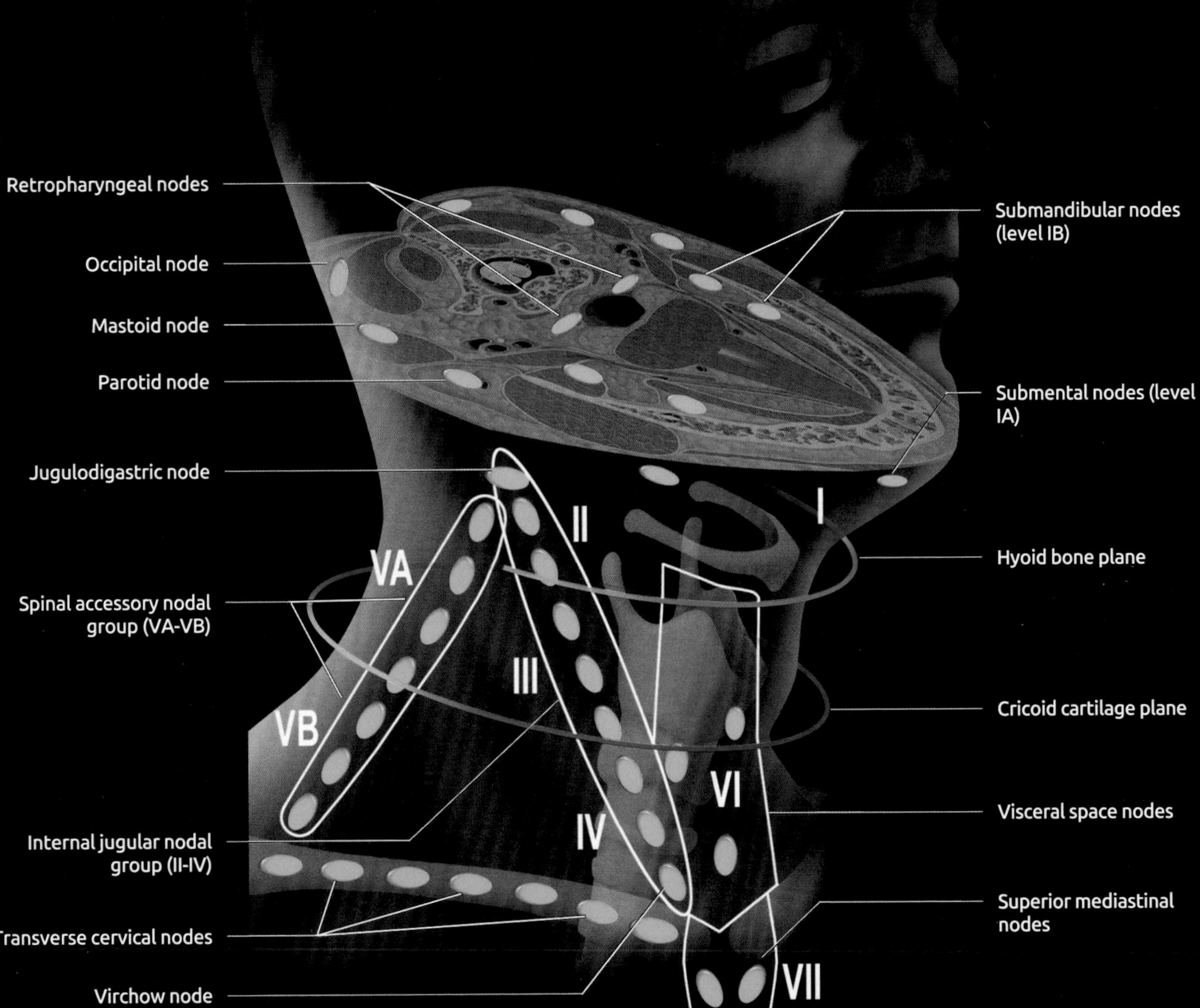

Lateral oblique graphic of the cervical neck depicts an axial slice through the suprahyoid neck. The retropharyngeal nodes behind the pharynx are often clinically occult. The hyoid bone (blue arc) and cricoid cartilage (orange circle) planes are highlighted, as they serve to subdivide the internal jugular and spinal accessory nodal group levels. Regional lymph nodes are staged the same way for almost all head and neck tumors, largely based on size, bilaterality, and number of nodes involved. N stages for most pharyngeal and oral cavity tumors are determined by this generic head and neck nodal classification. Tumors of the nasopharynx, however, have a unique N classification scheme.

FACE AND NECK LYMPH NODES

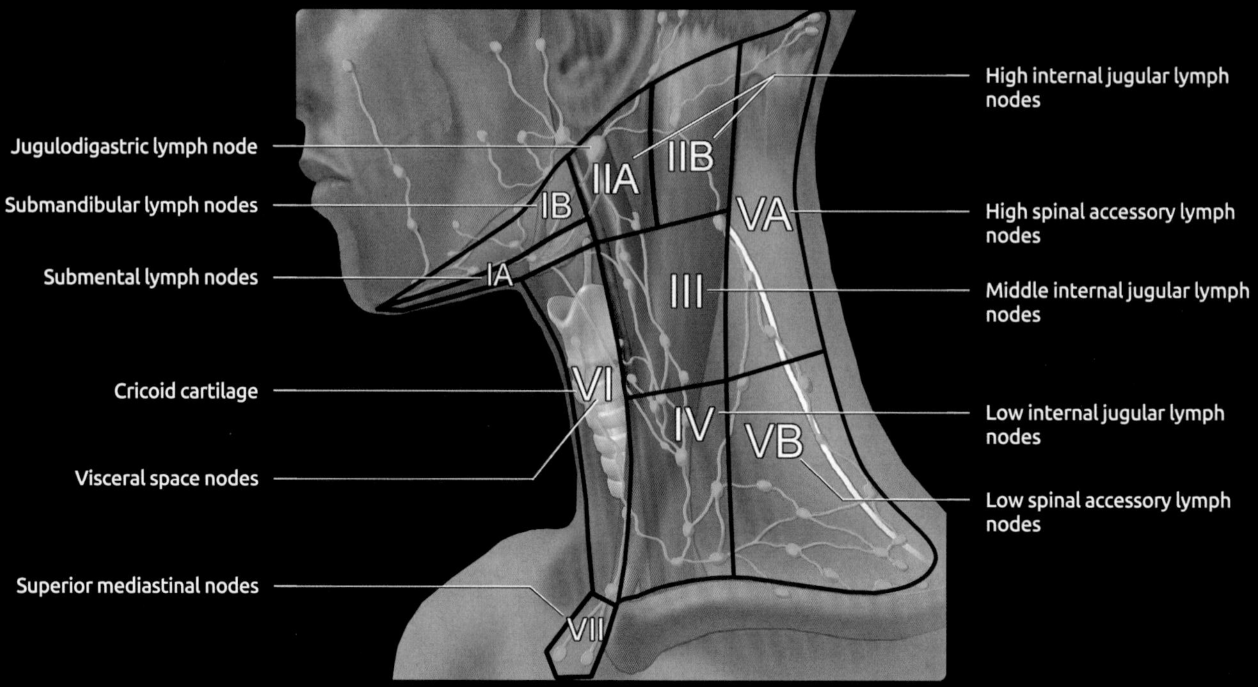

Jugulodigastric lymph node
Submandibular lymph nodes
Submental lymph nodes
Cricoid cartilage
Visceral space nodes
Superior mediastinal nodes
IIA
IIB
IB
IA
VA
III
VI
IV
VB
VII
High internal jugular lymph nodes
High spinal accessory lymph nodes
Middle internal jugular lymph nodes
Low internal jugular lymph nodes
Low spinal accessory lymph nodes

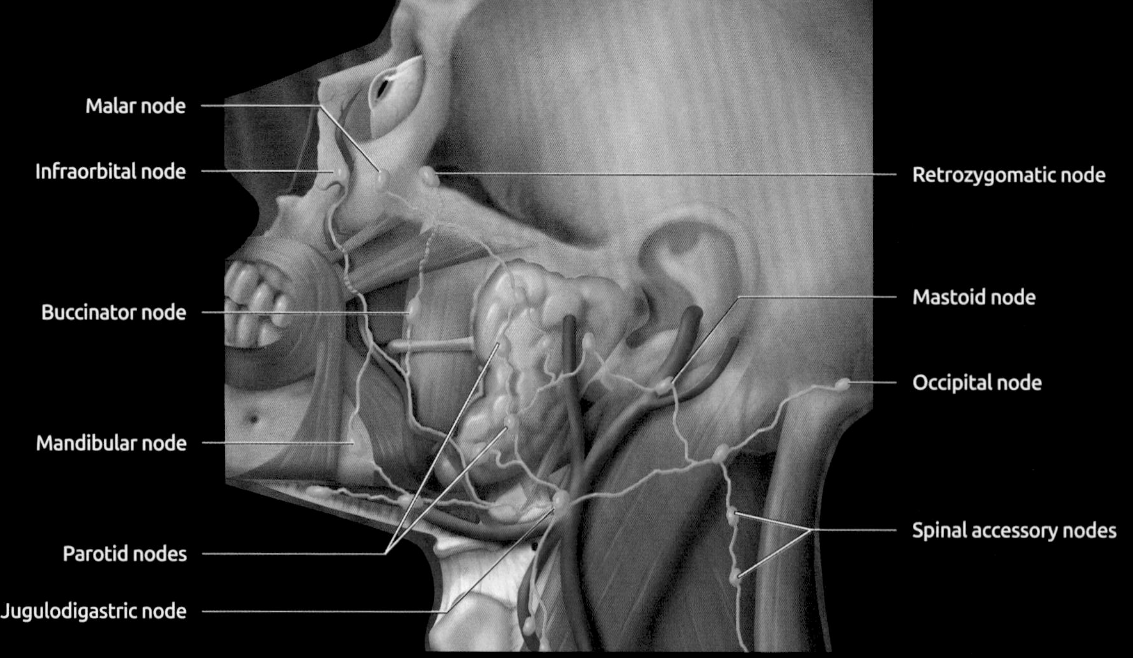

(Top) *Lateral oblique graphic of the neck shows the anatomic locations for the major nodal groups of the neck. Division of the internal jugular nodal chain into high, middle, and low regions is defined by the level of the hyoid bone and cricoid cartilage. Similarly, the spinal accessory nodal chain is divided into high and low regions by the level of the cricoid cartilage.* **(Bottom)** *Lateral view shows facial nodes plus parotid nodes. None of these nodes bear level numbers but instead must be described by their anatomic location. Note that the internal jugular chain is the final common pathway for all lymphatics of the upper aerodigestive tract and neck.*

NORMAL LYMPH NODES

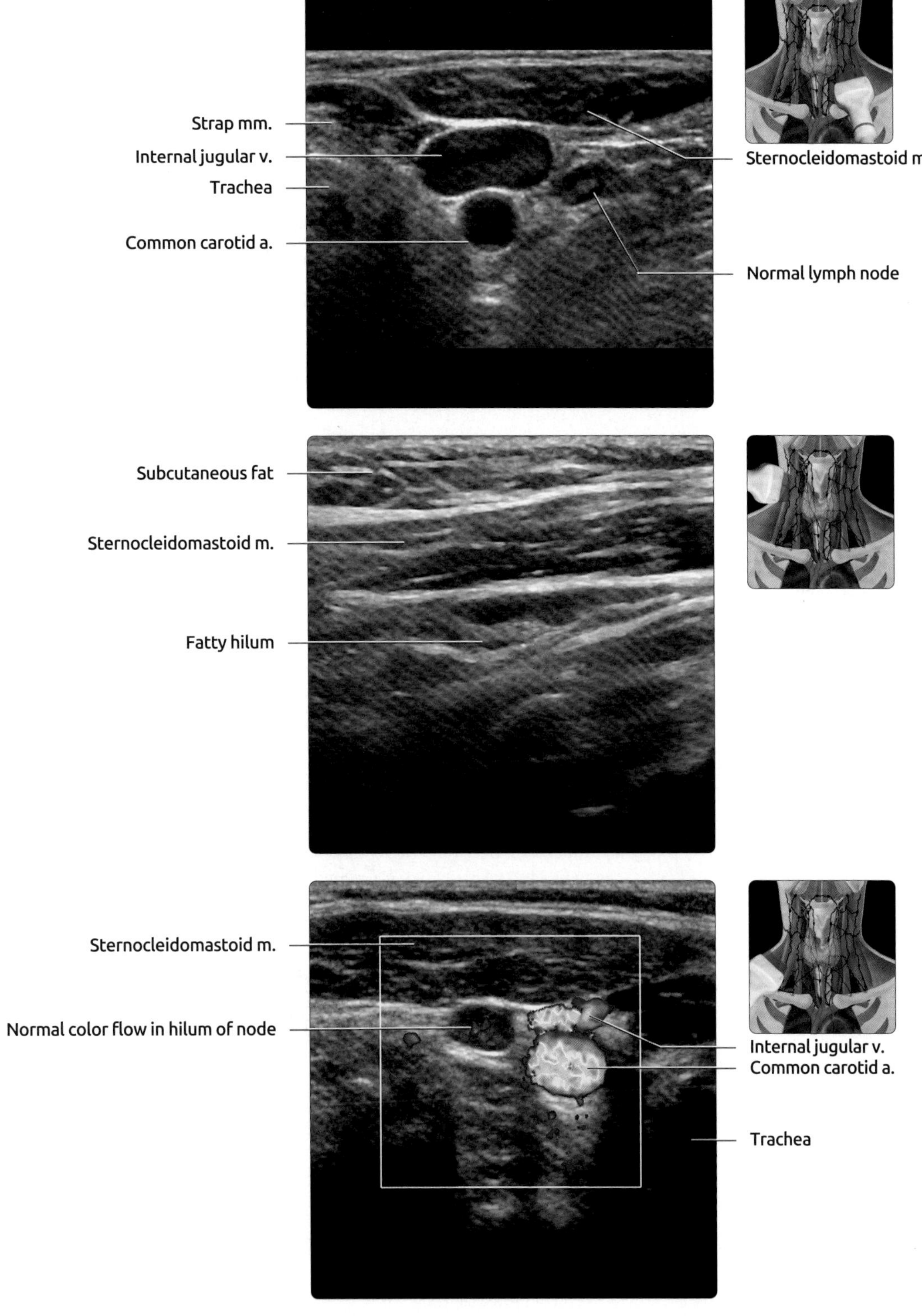

(Top) *Transverse ultrasound of the left upper neck post thyroidectomy shows a small lymph node at level III. There is a central fatty hilum.* **(Middle)** *Longitudinal ultrasound of the neck at level IV shows an elliptical lymph node with a normal central fatty hilum.* **(Bottom)** *Transverse color Doppler ultrasound of the neck at level III for neck surveillance post thyroidectomy is shown. There is a small lymph node with color flow in the hilum. The node was elliptical in the longitudinal axis.*

BENIGN LYMPH NODES

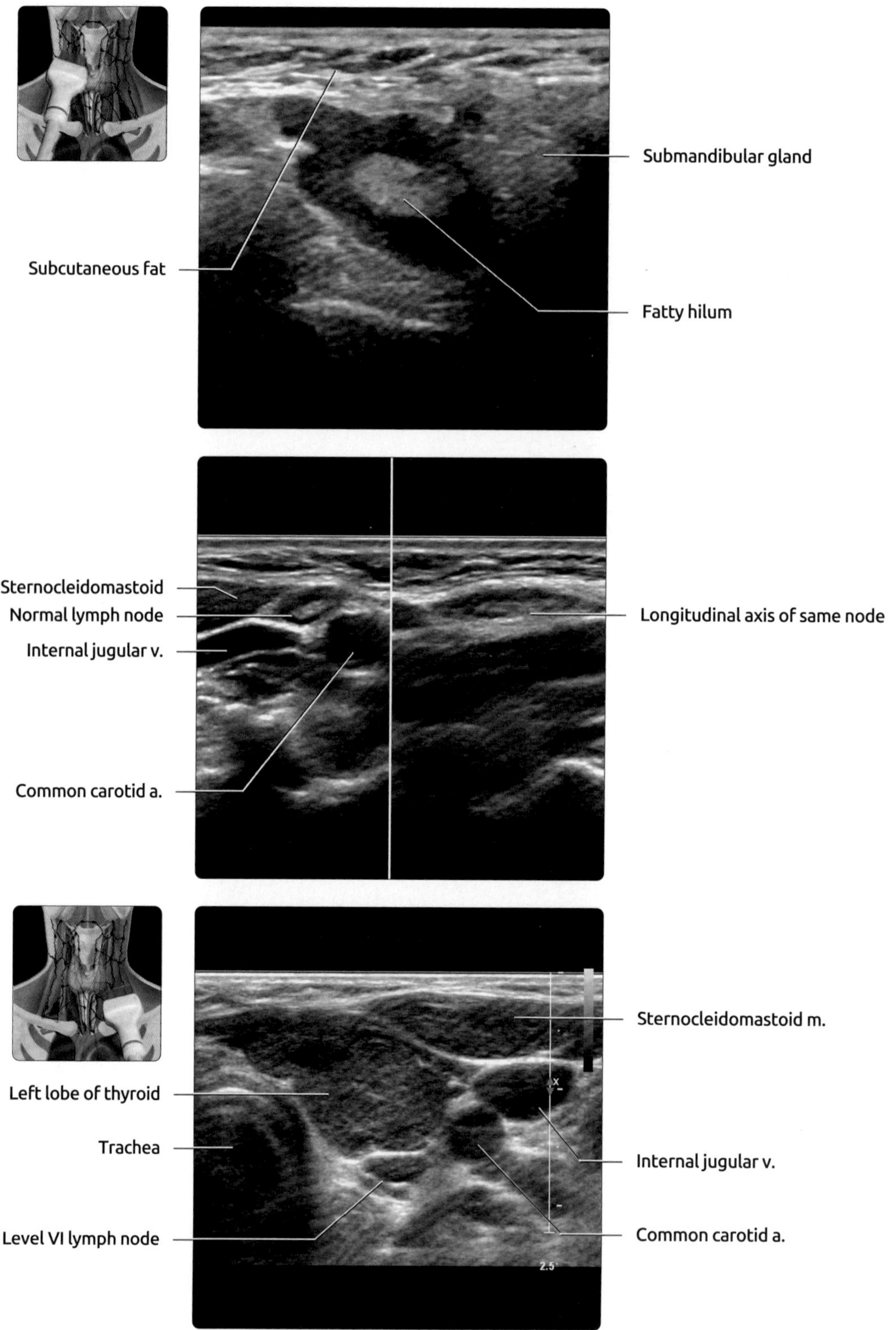

(Top) *Transverse ultrasound of the submandibular region shows a more rounded benign lymph node with a fatty hilum. Reactive nodes are common in this region.* **(Middle)** *Split screen ultrasound (transverse on left, longitudinal on the right) of a normal upper cervical lymph node is shown. The node is elliptical with a fatty hilum.* **(Bottom)** *Transverse ultrasound of the left neck at the level of the thyroid in a patient with Hashimoto thyroiditis is shown. There were multiple reactive nodes in the neck. Note the characteristic changes of Hashimoto in the left lobe of thyroid.*

ABNORMAL LYMPH NODES

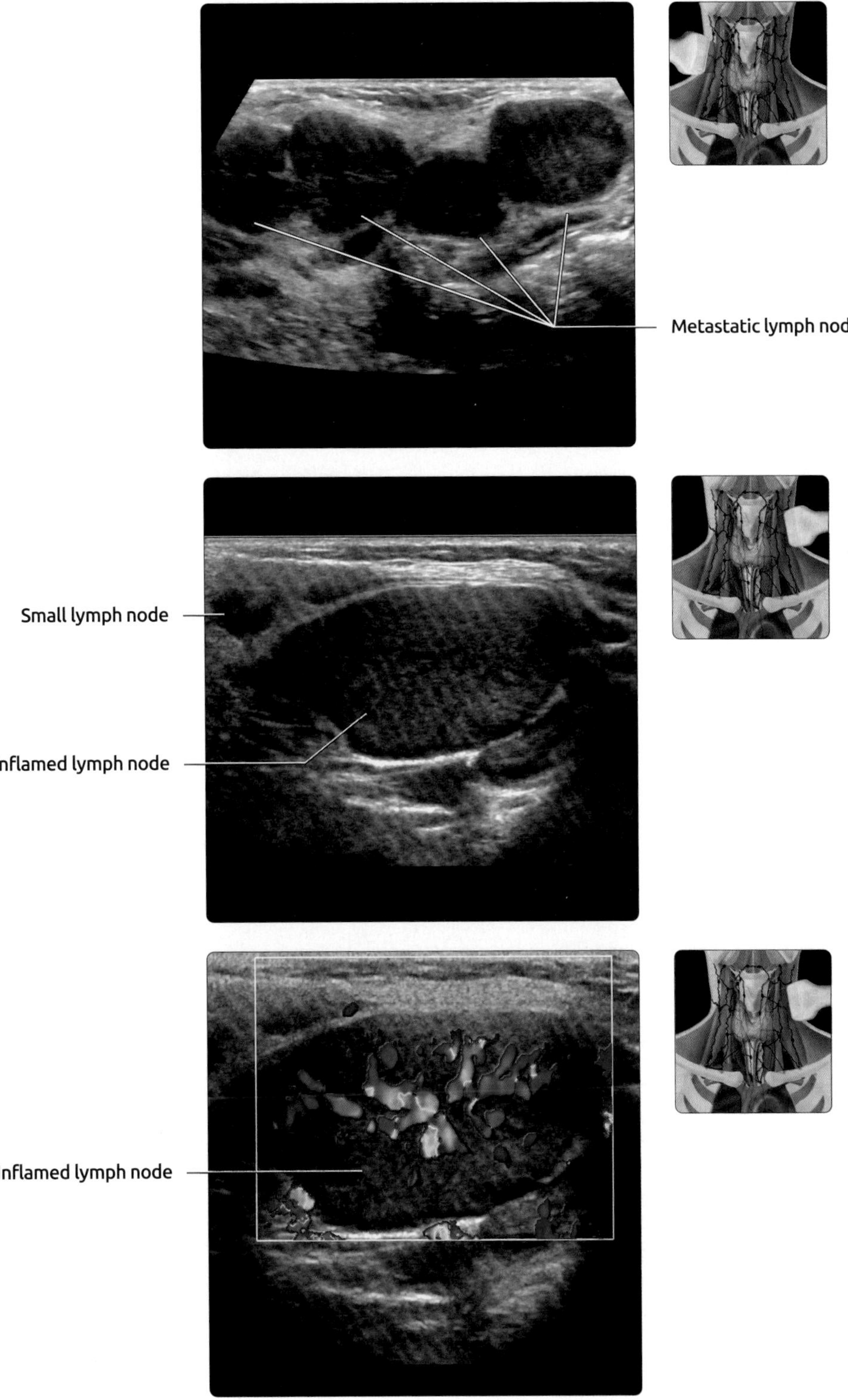

(Top) *Longitudinal ultrasound of the right upper neck in a patient with laryngeal cancer and a palpable mass is shown. There are multiple round nodes with no fatty hila.* **(Middle)** *Longitudinal ultrasound of the left upper neck in a patient with a palpable mass is shown. There are multiple small surrounding lymph nodes.* **(Bottom)** *Longitudinal color Doppler ultrasound of the left upper neck in the same patient shows prominent central color flow in an inflammatory lymph node.*

METASTATIC LYMPH NODES

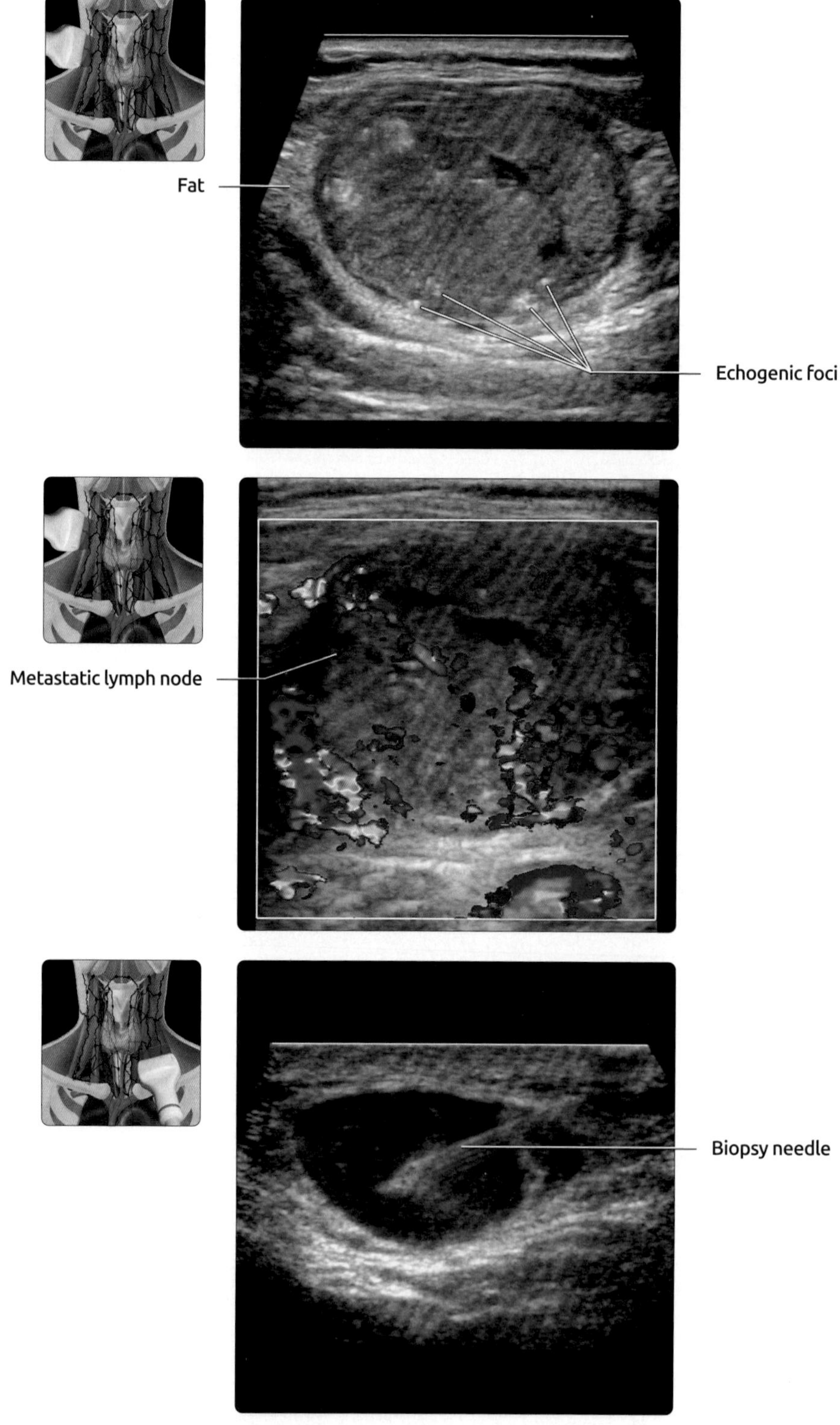

(Top) *Longitudinal ultrasound of the lower neck shows a 4-cm abnormal lymph node proven to be metastatic papillary thyroid carcinoma. The node is ovoid with increased short to long axis ratio. It contains small echogenic foci, which are highly suggestive of papillary thyroid carcinoma.* **(Middle)** *Longitudinal color Doppler ultrasound of metastatic papillary carcinoma in a lymph node shows disorganized internal color flow.* **(Bottom)** *Transverse ultrasound obtained during fine-needle aspiration of an abnormal cervical lymph node that lacked a fatty hilum is shown. Pathology was metastatic melanoma.*

METASTATIC LYMPH NODES

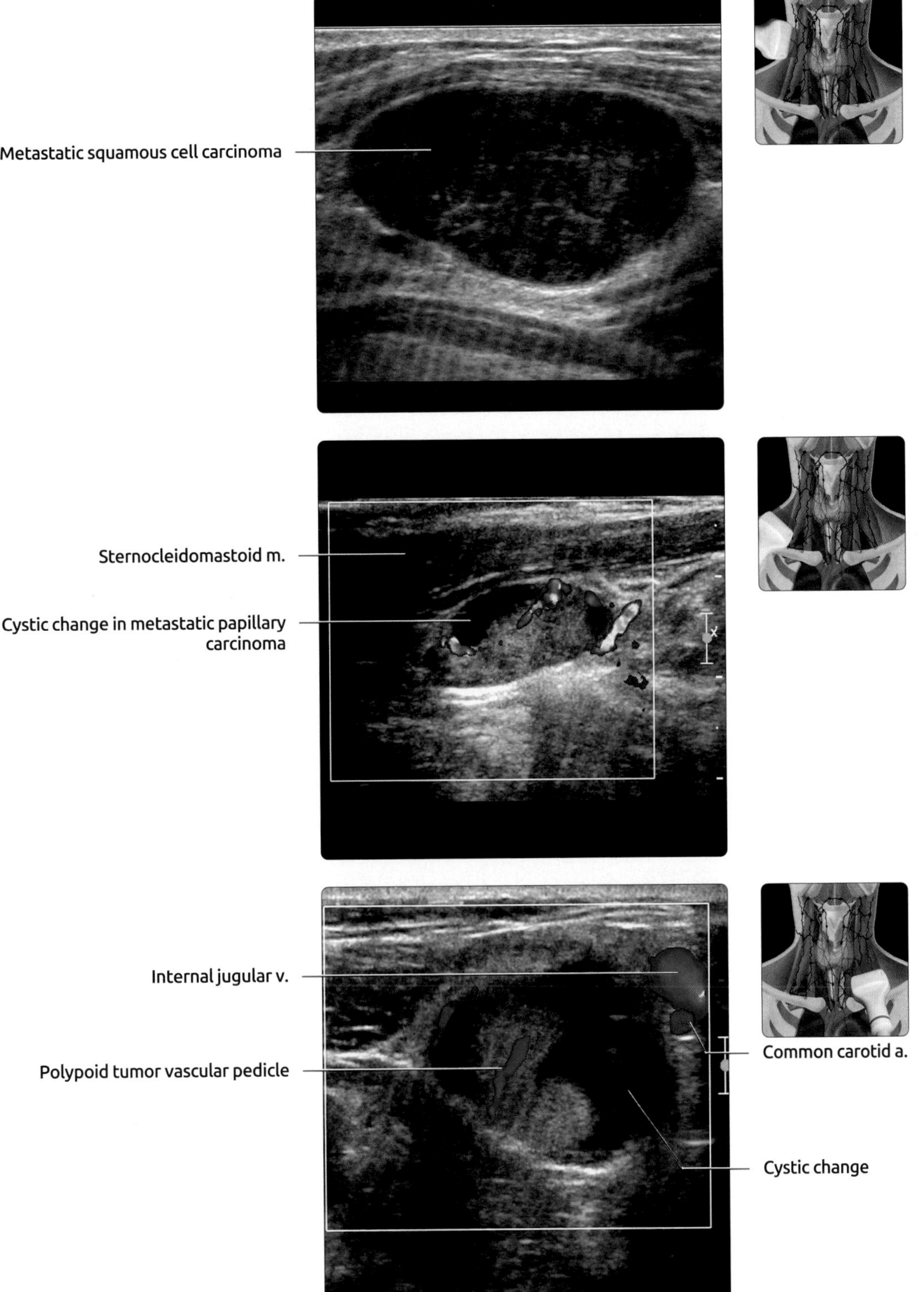

(Top) *Longitudinal ultrasound of the upper neck in a patient with oropharyngeal squamous cell carcinoma is shown. The lymph node is enlarged, ovoid, and solid with no echogenic hilum.* **(Middle)** *Longitudinal color Doppler ultrasound of the lower neck in a patient who had a thyroidectomy for papillary thyroid carcinoma is shown. There is an elliptical lymph node with eccentric cystic change. Despite preservation of the elliptical shape, the morphology of this node is abnormal.* **(Bottom)** *Transverse ultrasound of the left lower neck shows a mixed cystic and solid lymph node from metastatic papillary thyroid carcinoma. There is a papillary solid nodule with a vascular pedicle surrounded by cystic change.*

PART III
SECTION 2
Neck Lesions

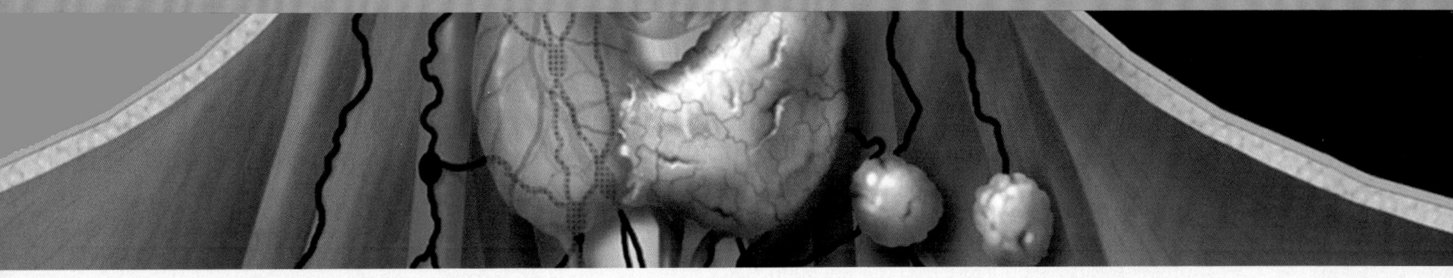

Differentiated Thyroid Carcinoma

KEY FACTS

TERMINOLOGY

- Well-defined histology: Papillary and follicular carcinoma

IMAGING

- **Papillary carcinoma (~ 80% of thyroid cancer)**
  - Majority are ill-defined with irregular outlines
  - 10-20% multifocal, 70% solid; 77-90% hypoechoic
  - Calcifications: Punctate small echogenic foci highly specific; larger calcifications also concerning
  - Cystic variant: Rare, eccentric polypoid solid vascular nodule within cyst ± microcalcifications
  - Nodes predominantly hyperechoic (80%) compared to muscles; 50% with punctate microcalcification; cystic change in 25%
- **Follicular carcinoma (~ 10% of thyroid cancer)**
  - Ill-defined solid tumor; hypoechoic, heterogeneous
- Large tumors invade strap muscles, esophagus, trachea, recurrent laryngeal nerve, neck vessels
- Color Doppler: Profuse chaotic vascularity within nodule or in wall, and septa of partially cystic tumors

TOP DIFFERENTIAL DIAGNOSES

- Multinodular goiter
- Thyroid adenoma
- Aggressive thyroid carcinomas and metastases

CLINICAL ISSUES

- Painless, palpable thyroid nodule or incidental finding on imaging
- Rapid growth of thyroid mass, extrathyroidal hard nodes, hoarseness; history of radiation exposure
- Low mortality from malignancy; 20-year survival rate: 90% papillary, 75% follicular
- Peak incidence in 3rd and 4th decade; F:M = 3:1

SCANNING TIPS

- Look for extrathyroidal extension by evaluating capsule and mobility during swallowing; evaluate nodal chains

(Left) *Transverse ultrasound of a left lobe papillary thyroid carcinoma shows that the tumor ⇨ is taller than it is wide, with lobulated margins, and hypoechoic relative to normal thyroid ➡.* **(Right)** *Transverse color Doppler ultrasound of the same left lobe papillary thyroid carcinoma ⇨ shows color flow in the center of the tumor.*

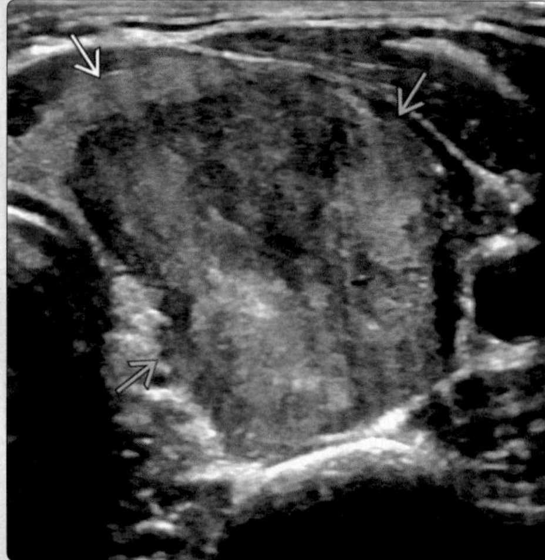

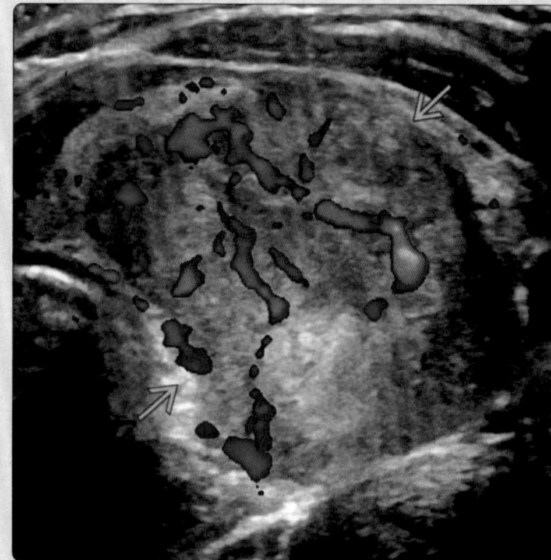

(Left) *Longitudinal ultrasound of papillary thyroid carcinoma shows the tumor ⇨ is markedly hypoechoic relative to normal thyroid ➡.* **(Right)** *Longitudinal ultrasound of classic papillary thyroid carcinoma shows the tumor ➡ is poorly marginated and is hypoechoic in comparison to the thyroid with multiple echogenic foci.*

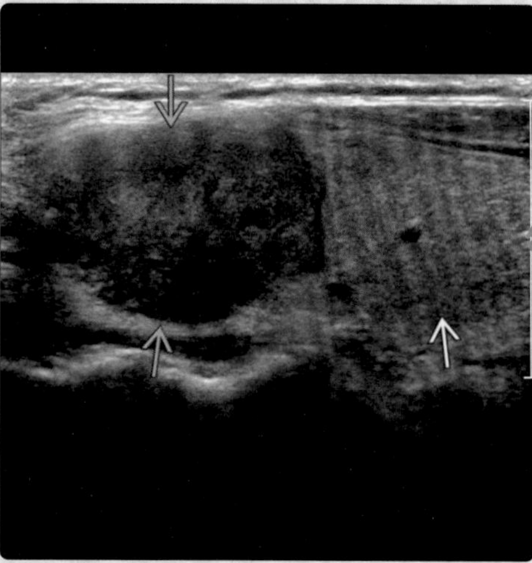

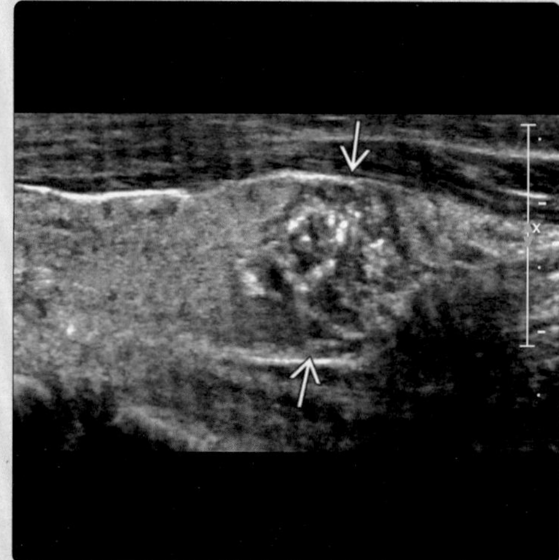

Anaplastic Thyroid Carcinoma

KEY FACTS

MAGING

- Ill-defined, hypoechoic tumor diffusely involving entire lobe or gland, often invading adjacent structures
- Background of multinodular goiter or differentiated thyroid cancer
- Typically > 5 cm at presentation
- Necrosis (78%), dense amorphous calcification (58%)
- Extracapsular spread with infiltration of trachea, esophagus, & perithyroid soft tissues & nerves
- May see thrombus in internal jugular vein & carotid artery, causing expansion & occlusion of vessels
- Color Doppler shows prominent, small, chaotic intratumoral vessels
- Nodal or distant metastases in 80% of patients
  - Abnormal vascularity seen within metastatic nodes

OP DIFFERENTIAL DIAGNOSES

- Differentiated thyroid carcinoma
- Non-Hodgkin lymphoma
- Thyroid metastases

CLINICAL ISSUES

- Rapidly growing, large, painful neck mass, 1-2% of thyroid malignancy
- Presents at later age than other thyroid malignancies, most typically 6th or 7th decade
- 50% have associated symptoms from local invasion: Dyspnea, hoarseness, or dysphagia
- Rapidly fatal, mean survival of 6 months after diagnosis

SCANNING TIPS

- Rapidly enlarging, infiltrative thyroid mass suggests anaplastic carcinoma or thyroid non-Hodgkin lymphoma; biopsy essential for diagnosis
- Use curvilinear transducer to encompass entire tumor when large
- Ultrasound may be unable to completely evaluate infiltration into trachea, larynx, adjacent soft tissues, & mediastinal spread; CECT or MR may be necessary

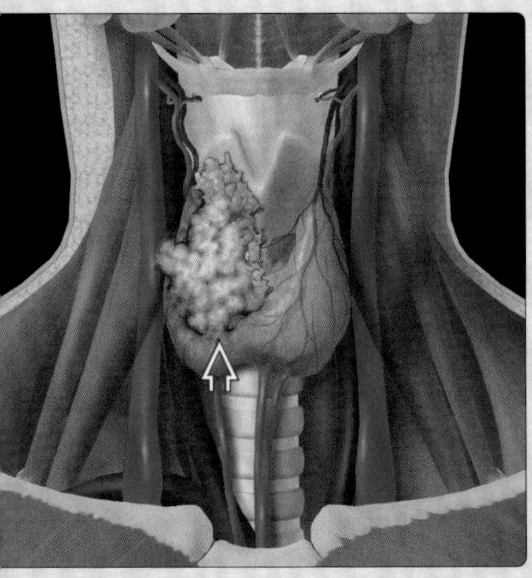

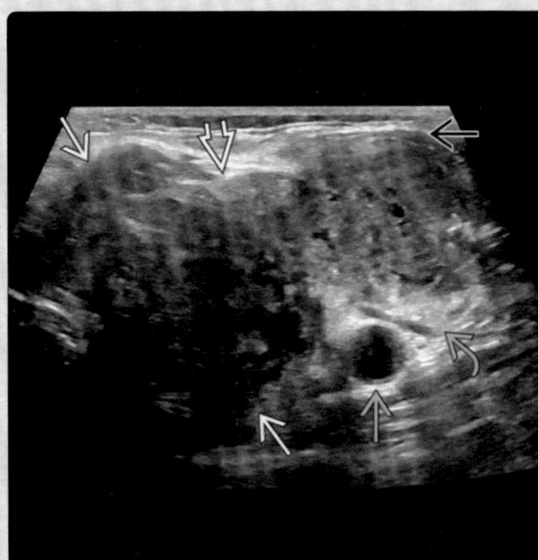

(Left) *Coronal graphic shows a thyroid tumor [T4a (stage IVa) disease].* **(Right)** *Transverse ultrasound of a rapidly growing neck mass is shown. There is a heterogenous mass infiltrating the left lobe of thyroid and extending anterolaterally. There is invasion of the sternocleidomastoid muscle and compression of the internal jugular vein. The common carotid artery was normal.*

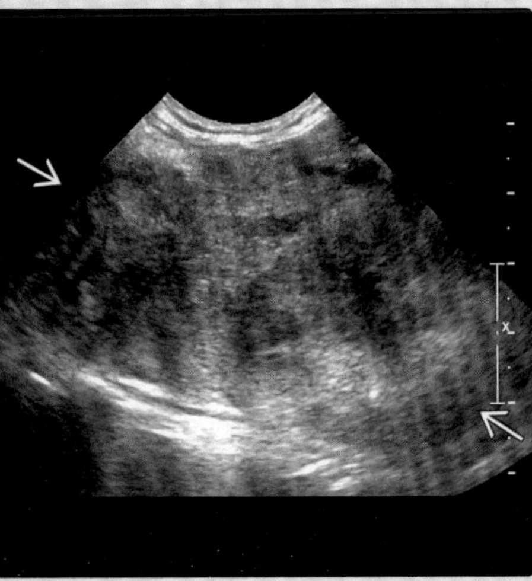

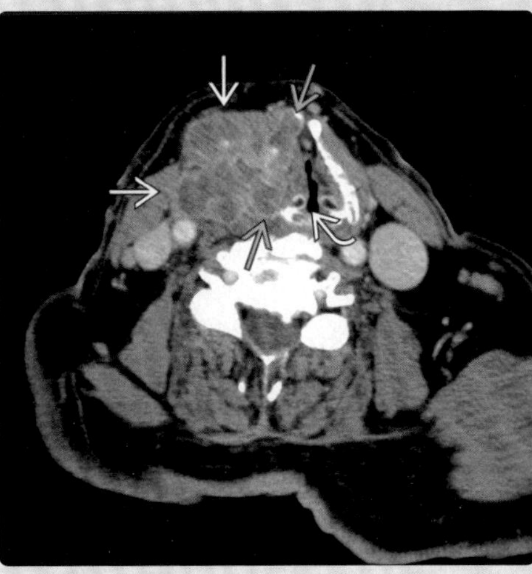

(Left) *Longitudinal ultrasound of a large anaplastic carcinoma is shown. A curved transducer was required to include the entire mass. The mass is heterogeneous in echotexture.* **(Right)** *Axial CECT of the same patient shows a large heterogenous mass that is destroying the right thyroid cartilage and displacing and narrowing the airway.*

Thyroid Non-Hodgkin Lymphoma

KEY FACTS

IMAGING

- Thyroid mass in patient with history of Hashimoto thyroiditis (in 40-80%)
- Focal lymphomatous mass/nodule
  - Well defined, solid, hypoechoic, heterogeneous, noncalcified, solitary/multiple, unilateral/bilateral
- Diffuse involvement
  - Hypoechoic, heterogeneous, rounded gland
  - Simple thyroid enlargement, minimal change in echo pattern (often missed); adjacent lymphadenopathy and background Hashimoto may be only clue
- Evidence of background Hashimoto thyroiditis: Echogenic fibrous bands in lobulated, hypoechoic gland
- Lymphadenopathy: Multiple ± bilateral
  - Reticulated or pseudocystic pattern, but nodes are solid with no necrosis
- Color Doppler: Thyroid nodules are nonspecific: Hypovascular or chaotic intranodular vessels
  - Lymph nodes: Central > peripheral vascularity

TOP DIFFERENTIAL DIAGNOSES

- Anaplastic thyroid carcinoma, differentiated thyroid carcinoma, metastases to thyroid, multinodular goiter

CLINICAL ISSUES

- 2-5% of all thyroid malignancies
- Rapidly enlarging thyroid mass, frequently with associated neck adenopathy
- Compression of surrounding tissues may cause dysphagia, dyspnea, or pressure symptoms
- Older females, known Hashimoto thyroiditis
- Pathologic diagnosis may require core needle biopsy in addition to fine-needle biopsy

SCANNING TIPS

- Rapidly enlarging thyroid mass in elderly patient is usually due to thyroid non-Hodgkin lymphoma or anaplastic carcinoma; lack of calcification, invasion, and necrosis favors non-Hodgkin lymphoma

(Left) *Longitudinal ultrasound shows a lobulated, hypoechoic, noncalcified tumor ➡ with a small amount of residual normal thyroid ➡ posteriorly. This was a B-cell lymphoma.* **(Right)** *Longitudinal color Doppler ultrasound of the same patient shows color flow ➡ in the lymphomatous infiltration.*

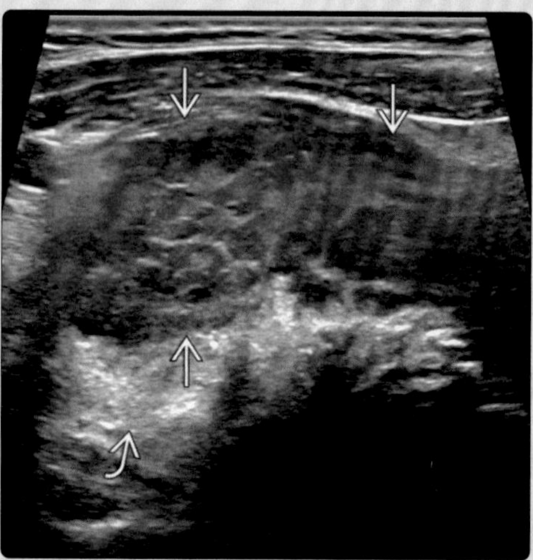

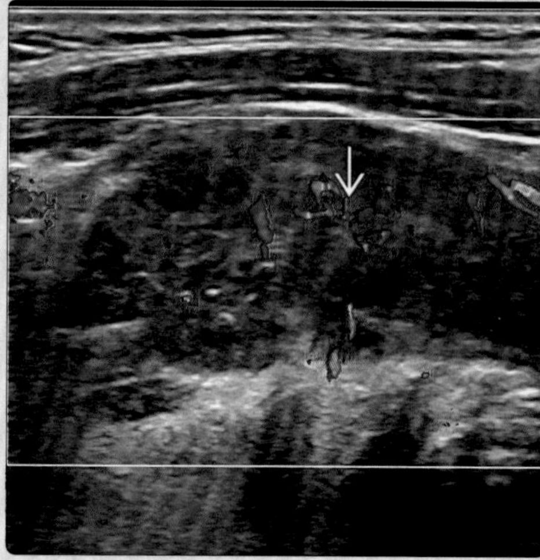

(Left) *Transverse ultrasound in a patient with Hashimoto thyroiditis and a previously atrophic thyroid shows a lobulated hypoechoic, noncalcified tumor ➡, biopsy proven to be lymphoma.* **(Right)** *Axial CECT through the thyroid gland in the same patient shows asymmetric enlargement of the right thyroid with hypodense tumor ➡ extending into the isthmus. Note the small left lobe ➡ from Hashimoto thyroiditis and enlarged lymph nodes ➡. The right internal jugular vein is occluded.*

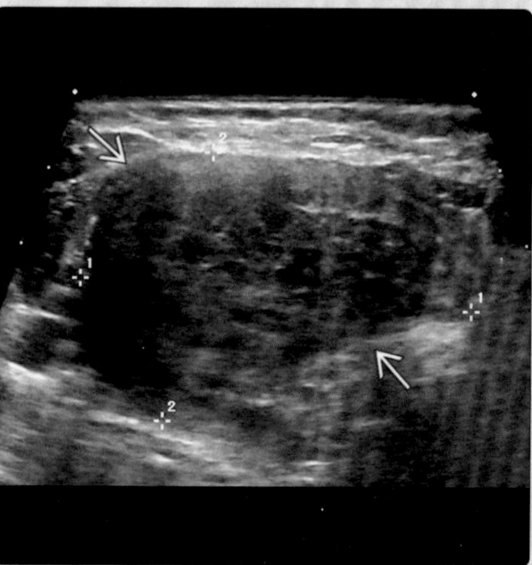

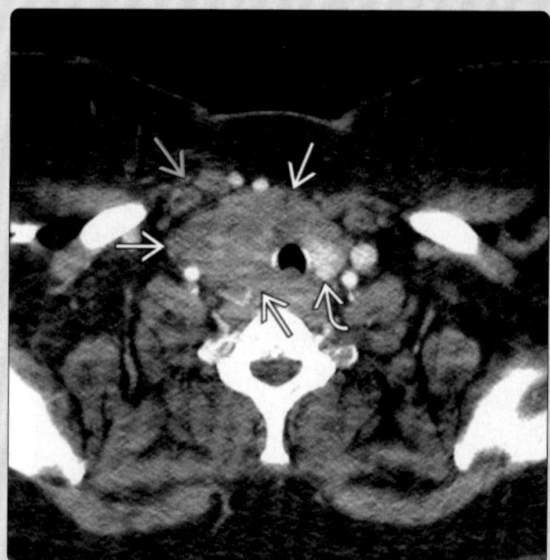

Multinodular Goiter

KEY FACTS

IMAGING

- Multiple nodules with bilateral diffuse involvement
- Solid nodules most often isoechoic; 5% hypoechoic
- Nodules are sharply defined with haloes but may conglomerate
- Heterogeneous internal echo pattern: Solid/cystic portions, internal debris, septa, "spongiform" nodules
  - Cystic component due to degeneration, hemorrhage, or colloid within nodule
- Dense shadowing calcification (curvilinear, dysmorphic, coarse)
- Nodules with comet-tail artifact; highly suggestive of colloid nodule (may mimic microcalcification)
- Background thyroid may be heterogeneous
- Color Doppler: Peripheral > intranodular vascularity
  - Septa and intranodular solid portions are avascular (organizing blood, clot)

TOP DIFFERENTIAL DIAGNOSES

- Papillary and follicular carcinoma
- Anaplastic and medullary thyroid carcinoma

CLINICAL ISSUES

- Incidence of sporadic multinodular goiter (MNG): ~ 5% in US
- Sporadic goiter has no specific age incidence, F:M = 2-4:1
- Most asymptomatic and euthyroid
- Can become hyperthyroid or hypothyroid
- Symptoms related to mass effect: Airway compression, hoarseness, dysphagia, and superior vena cava syndrome

SCANNING TIPS

- Change transducer frequency to evaluate colloid, calcification and cystic components
- Use curvilinear transducer if thyroid is too large for linear transducer
- Look for suspicious nodules

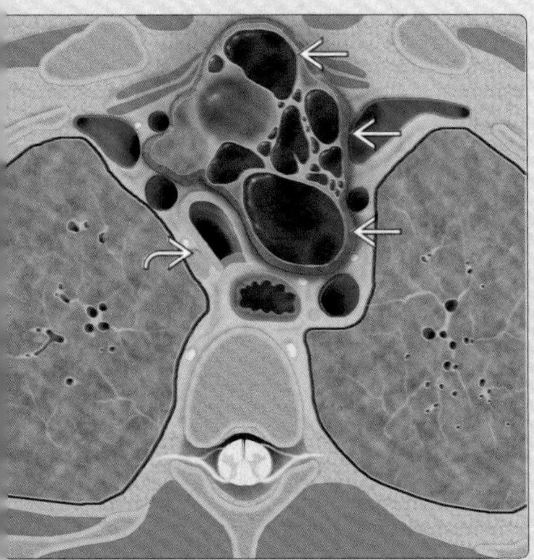

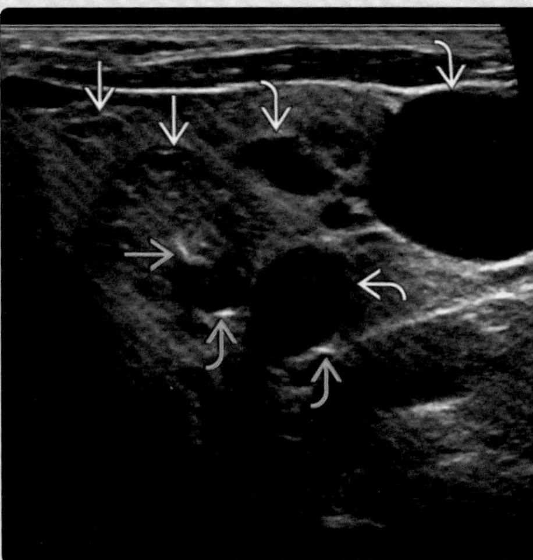

(Left) *Graphic shows an enlarged, lobulated thyroid gland with multiple cystic nodules ➡. The trachea ➡ is displaced to the right.* **(Right)** *Transverse ultrasound of a patient with asymptomatic neck swelling is shown. There are multiple nodules in this multinodular goiter, including mixed solid and cystic ➡ and entirely cystic ➡ nodules. Coarse calcification ➡ was present in one nodule and colloid ➡ in others.*

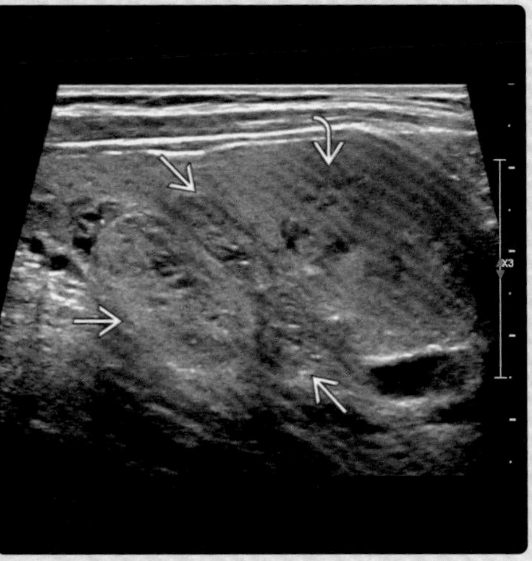

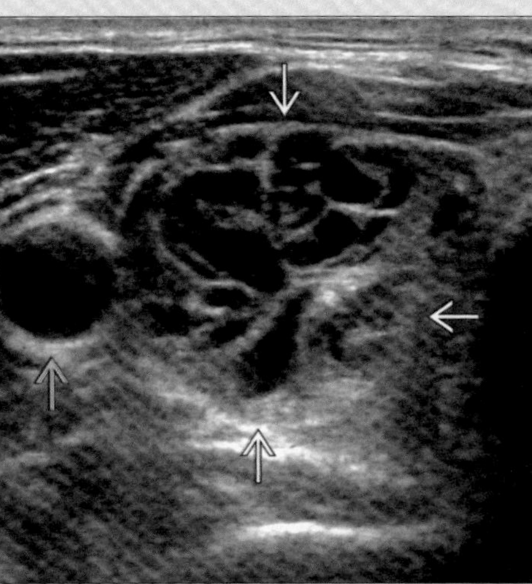

(Left) *Longitudinal ultrasound of a multinodular goiter shows multiple well-marginated isoechoic nodules ➡ with internal cystic changes. There is also cystic change ➡ without a discrete nodule.* **(Right)** *Transverse ultrasound of a spongiform nodule ➡ entirely composed of multiple cystic spaces with intervening septa. The common carotid artery ➡ was normal.*

Colloid Cyst of Thyroid

KEY FACTS

IMAGING

- Typically, unilocular, thin-walled cyst
- Anechoic content with posterior acoustic enhancement
- Echogenic foci with comet-tail artifacts are characteristic
    - Represent suspended colloid aggregates
- Hemorrhage into cyst results in thick wall with debris, septa, or fluid level
- Colloid cyst can arise in hyperplastic nodule
    - Background solid, isoechoic nodule with colloid aggregates in cystic spaces of variable sizes; no punctate calcification
- Ultrasound-guided fine-needle aspiration is not necessary for diagnosis

TOP DIFFERENTIAL DIAGNOSES

- Thyroid adenoma
- Simple thyroid cyst
- Differentiated thyroid carcinoma
- Thyroglossal duct cyst

PATHOLOGY

- Benign lesion without malignant potential

CLINICAL ISSUES

- Common (15-25% of thyroid nodules)
- Most are incidentally detected on ultrasound
- May present as palpable nodule when large or as rapidly enlarging nodule if bleeding occurs into cyst

SCANNING TIPS

- Colloid crystals may mimic echogenic foci from punctate calcification seen in papillary thyroid carcinoma
- Compound imaging may show comet-tail artifacts behind punctate echogenic focus
    - Scanning in fundamental mode helps to distinguish comet tail from posterior shadowing
- Beware of cystic malignancy if cystic lesion contains eccentric solid nodule with color flow or if there are pathologic lymph nodes

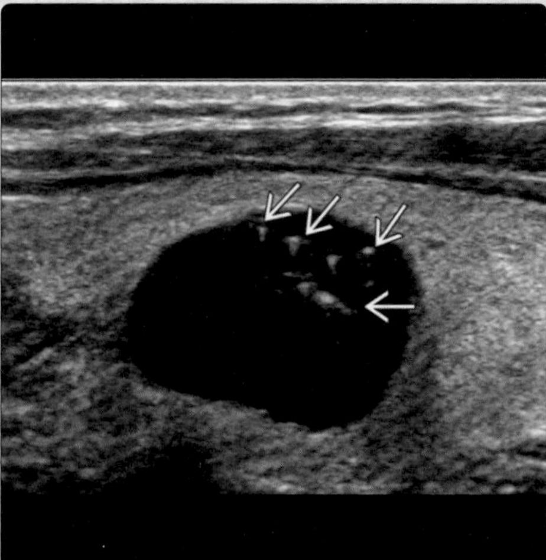

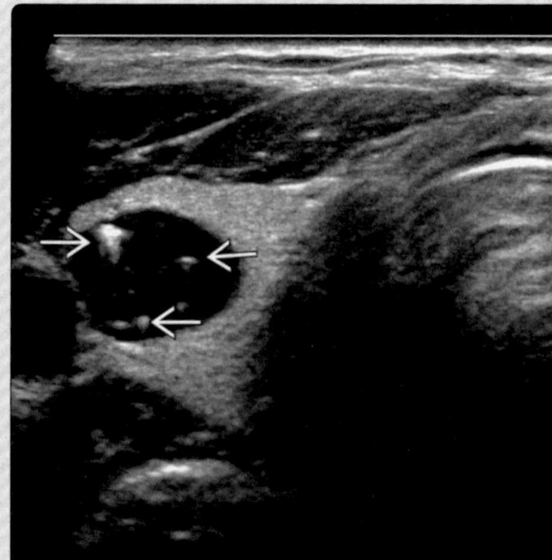

(Left) *Longitudinal grayscale ultrasound shows a typical colloid nodule with multiple echogenic foci and comet-tail artifacts suspended in the cyst* ➡*. These represent colloid aggregates in viscous fluid containing thyroglobulin.* **(Right)** *Transverse ultrasound shows a typical colloid nodule in the right lobe. There are multiple echogenic foci and comet-tail artifacts suspended in the cyst* ➡*.*

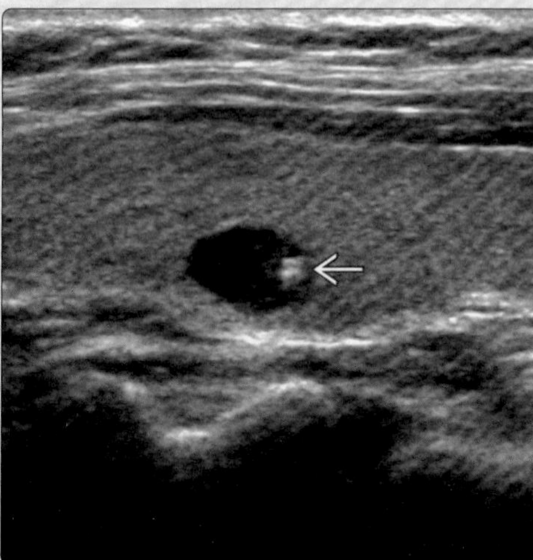

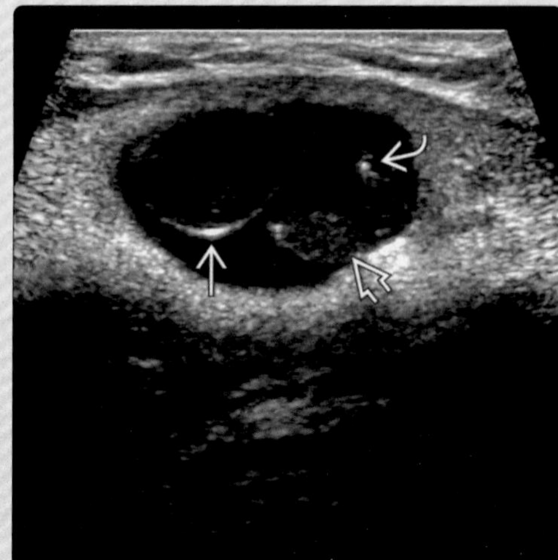

(Left) *Longitudinal ultrasound shows a small unilocular cystic nodule with colloid* ➡*. The comet-tail artifact is not V-shaped.* **(Right)** *Longitudinal high-frequency ultrasound of a more complex-appearing colloid cyst is shown. There is a thin internal septum* ➡ *and avascular debris* ➡ *with little colloid* ➡*.*

KEY FACTS

TERMINOLOGY

- Chronic, autoimmune-mediated lymphocytic inflammation of thyroid gland

IMAGING

- Features vary with stages of disease (acute, chronic, end stage) and extent of involvement (diffuse or focal)
- Acute diffuse: Enlarged heterogeneous hypoechoic thyroid with lobulated contour; multiple hypoechoic micronodules throughout with intervening echogenic septa
- Acute focal: Discrete, hypoechoic or hyperechoic nodules against normal or altered background thyroid, ± calcifications, halo
- End stage: Small, hypoechoic gland with heterogeneous echo pattern
- Color Doppler: Vascularity depends on stage and type of involvement
  - Acute focal/diffuse: Variable vascularity, focal nodule may mimic benign/malignant thyroid nodule
- Enlarged nodes are common, especially in central neck

TOP DIFFERENTIAL DIAGNOSES

- Thyroid Non-Hodgkin lymphoma
- Graves disease
- de Quervain thyroiditis
- Riedel thyroiditis (invasive fibrosing thyroiditis)

CLINICAL ISSUES

- Most common cause of hypothyroidism in USA
- Gradual, painless enlargement of thyroid with later atrophy
- ↑ thyroid peroxidase and antithyroglobulin antibodies
- ↑ risk of non-Hodgkin lymphoma and papillary carcinoma

SCANNING TIPS

- Be on lookout for developing cancer: Look for nodules that are different from others and for those that are enlarging or contain microcalcifications

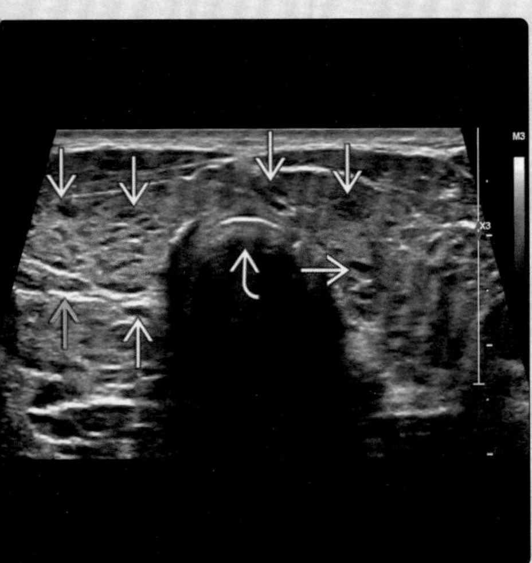

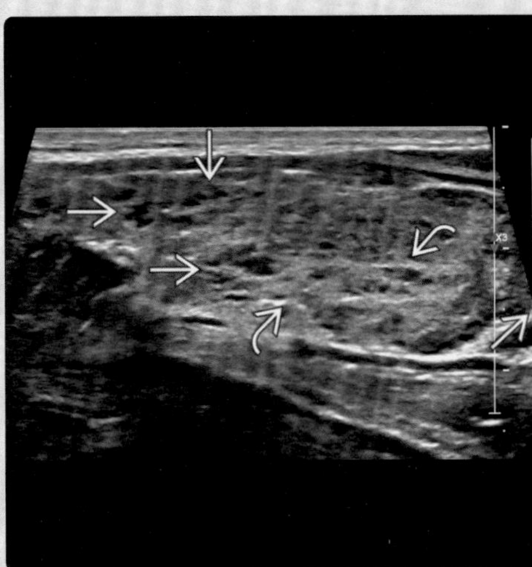

(Left) *Transverse grayscale ultrasound shows both thyroid lobes and the trachea ➡ in a patient with diffuse Hashimoto thyroiditis. In addition to numerous tiny hypoechoic nodules ➡, there are echogenic septa ➡.* **(Right)** *Longitudinal ultrasound of Hashimoto thyroiditis shows diffuse heterogeneity with hypoechoic nodules of varying sizes ➡ and echogenic septa ➡.*

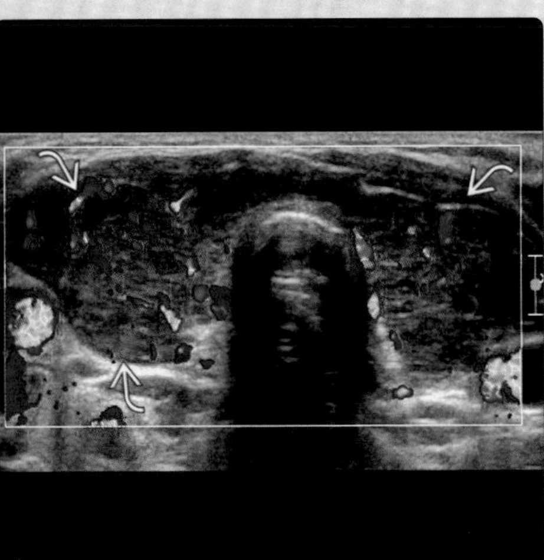

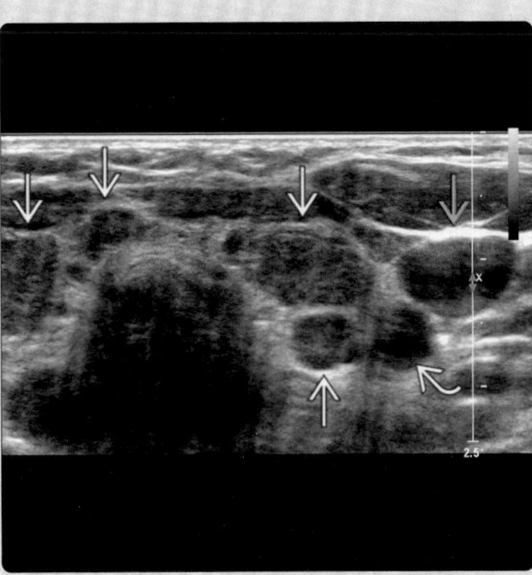

(Left) *Transverse color Doppler ultrasound shows the heterogeneous texture and lobulated contour of both thyroid lobes ➡ representing acute Hashimoto thyroiditis in a teenager.* **(Right)** *Transverse ultrasound of the same patient shows multiple enlarged lymph nodes ➡ in the central neck, below the thyroid. Note the common carotid artery ➡ and internal jugular vein ➡.*

Graves Disease

KEY FACTS

TERMINOLOGY

- Autoimmune disorder with long-acting, thyroid-stimulating antibodies producing hyperplasia and hypertrophy of thyroid

IMAGING

- Mild/moderate diffuse, symmetric enlargement of thyroid gland, including isthmus
- Hypoechoic, heterogeneous, spotty parenchymal echo pattern
- Marked increase in parenchymal vascularity (turbulent flow with AV shunts): "Thyroid inferno"
- Increased vascularity does not correlate with thyroid function but reflects inflammatory activity
- Spectral Doppler: Increase in peak flow velocity (≤ 120 cm/s) as measured in inferior thyroid artery
- ↑ vascularity tends to ↓ in response to treatment
- Diagnosis based on clinical signs and symptoms and laboratory findings, ultrasound is not needed

TOP DIFFERENTIAL DIAGNOSES

- Hashimoto thyroiditis
- de Quervain thyroiditis
- Nodular goiter

CLINICAL ISSUES

- 3rd-4th decade; M:F = 1:7
- Palpitations, loss of weight despite increased appetite, sweating, and wet palms
- Hyperdynamic circulatory state, muscle weakness, fatigue
- Thyroid-associated ophthalmopathy: Periorbital edema, lid retraction, ophthalmoplegia, proptosis, malignant exophthalmos
- Elevated T_3 + T_4 levels and depressed TSH level
- Strong family history of autoimmune disorders

SCANNING TIPS

- US may be used to establish thyroid volume prior to radioactive iodine treatment

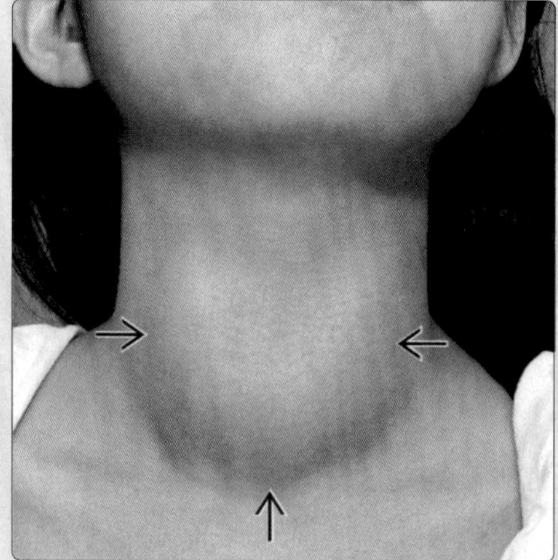

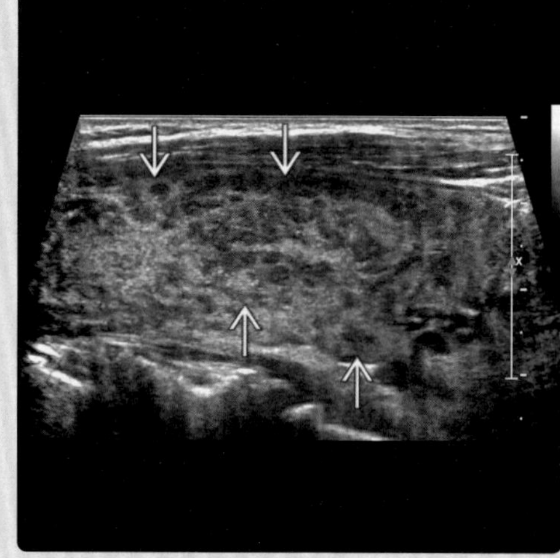

(Left) *Clinical photograph shows diffuse thyroid enlargement ➡ in a patient with Graves disease (GD). Diagnosis of GD is based on clinical features and laboratory tests. Ultrasound is usually not indicated for patient management.* **(Right)** *Longitudinal ultrasound of a patient with GD shows a mildly enlarged heterogeneous thyroid with multiple small hypoechoic nodules ➡. This appearance overlaps with Hashimoto thyroiditis, but the clinical picture is different.*

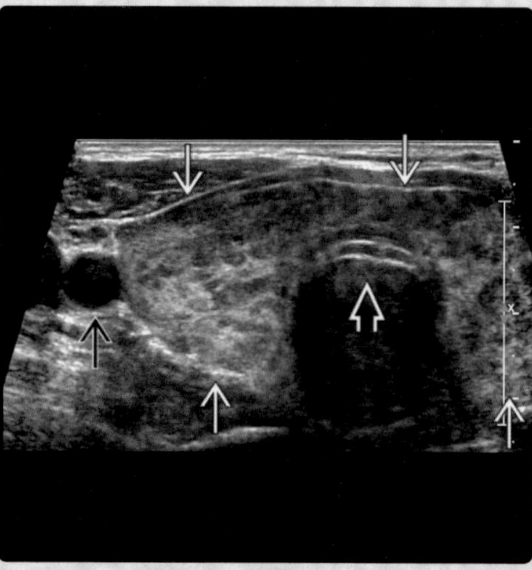

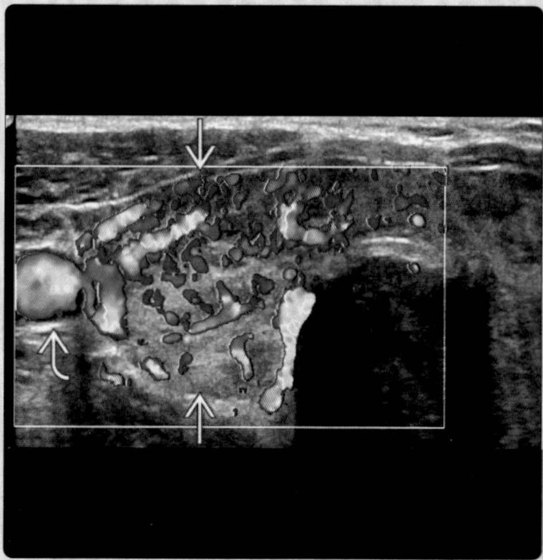

(Left) *Transverse ultrasound shows an enlarged thyroid ➡ with rounded contour and hypoechoic, heterogeneous thyroid parenchymal echo pattern. Note the right CCA ➡ and trachea ➡.* **(Right)** *Transverse color Doppler ultrasound of the same patient shows marked hypervascularity in the right thyroid lobe ➡. Note the right CCA ➡.*

Parathyroid Adenoma

KEY FACTS

IMAGING

- Round or oval, well-circumscribed, solid mass
- Typically 1-3 cm in size
- Most are hypoechoic to thyroid and homogeneous
- Some show cystic degeneration
- Calcification is rare; more common in carcinoma or hyperplasia due to hyperparathyroidism
- Location
  - Upper glands: Posterior to upper or mid pole of thyroid
  - Lower glands: 65% inferior, lateral to lower pole of thyroid
  - ≤ 20% in ectopic location: Tracheoesophageal groove, thymus, carotid sheath, superior mediastinum, intrathyroid (~ 6%)
- Color Doppler: Adenomas are hypervascular; vessels enter at poles, unlike lymph nodes

TOP DIFFERENTIAL DIAGNOSES

- Exophytic thyroid nodule
- Paratracheal lymph node
- Parathyroid carcinoma

CLINICAL ISSUES

- Asymptomatic hypercalcemia, kidney stones, low bone density
- Single adenoma responsible for 75-85% of primary hyperparathyroidism: ↑ serum calcium and PTH
- Secondary hyperparathyroidism in chronic kidney disease: Usually 4 enlarged parathyroid glands

SCANNING TIPS

- Scan with patient supine and neck hyperextended, ask patient to turn neck or swallow if adenoma is not found
- Look deep to thyroid (and in mediastinum with lower frequency transducer)
- Use color Doppler to find vascular supply from inferior thyroid artery
- US may be limited in obese patients with short necks, postoperative necks, or ectopic parathyroid adenomas

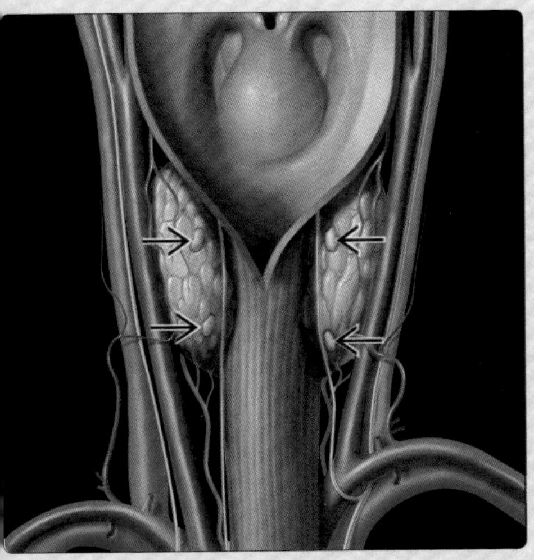

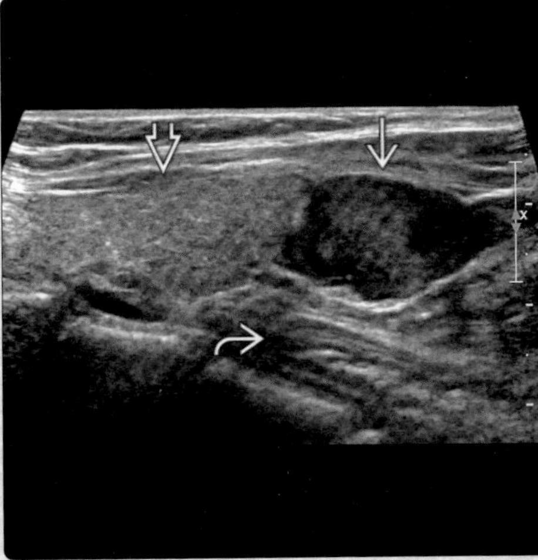

(Left) *Graphic shows the normal location of the parathyroid glands and their relationship to the thyroid gland. Ultrasound is sensitive for the detection of adenomas in these locations.* **(Right)** *Longitudinal ultrasound shows an inferior parathyroid adenoma. The adenoma is lobulated and homogeneously hypoechoic. It is separate from the thyroid and lies anterior to the esophagus.*

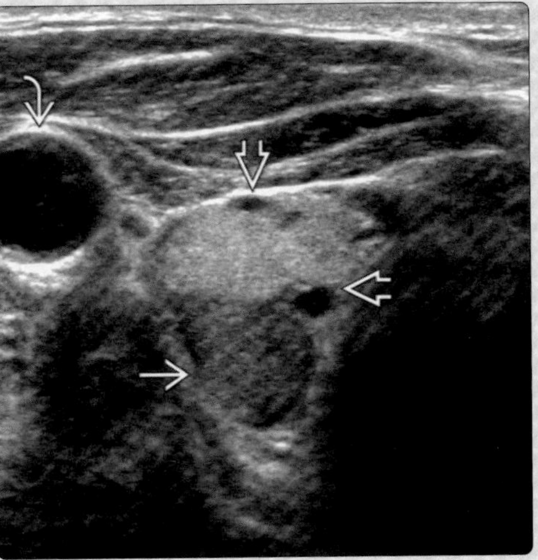

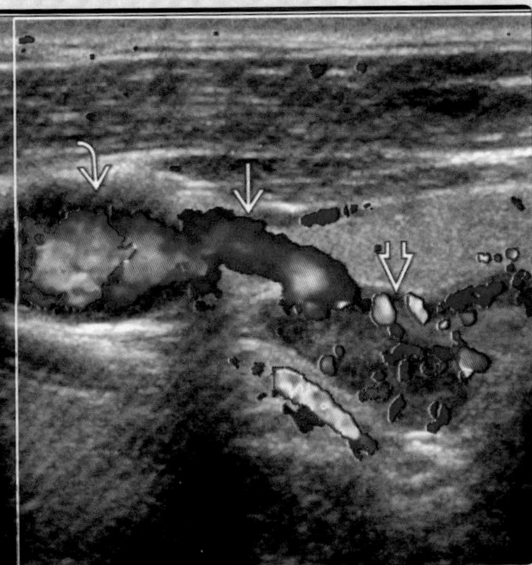

(Left) *Transverse ultrasound shows an inferior right parathyroid adenoma, hypoechoic to thyroid. Incidental colloid cysts are noted in the thyroid. Note the common carotid artery.* **(Right)** *Transverse color Doppler ultrasound shows a large feeding artery arising from the common carotid artery to supply an inferior parathyroid adenoma.*

Reactive Adenopathy

KEY FACTS

IMAGING

- US is ideal imaging modality for initial assessment of enlarged lymph nodes
- Unilateral or bilateral
- Reactive adenopathy: Absence of intranodal necrosis
  - Hypoechoic cortex compared with adjacent muscle ± cortical hypertrophy
  - Preserved hilar architecture usually
  - Oval in shape
  - Color Doppler: Hilar vascularity
- Suppurative adenopathy: Loss of fatty hilum and cortical hypertrophy
  - Central fluid; surrounding inflammation resulting in blurring of margins
  - Complicated by nodal matting and abscess
  - Color Doppler: Peripheral increase in vascularity

TOP DIFFERENTIAL DIAGNOSES

- Metastatic node
- Tuberculosis
- Non-Hodgkin lymphoma

CLINICAL ISSUES

- Reactive adenopathy: Any age, most common in pediatric age group
  - Firm, sometimes fluctuant, freely mobile subcutaneous nodal masses, associated with viral infection
- Suppurative adenopathy: Any age, upper respiratory tract/odontogenic/salivary gland bacterial infections
  - Tender, warm neck mass, fever, ↑ white blood cells
  - Pus on aspiration

SCANNING TIPS

- Map out cervical nodes by level
- Rule out abnormal morphology, such as necrosis or microcalcification
- Look for surrounding cellulitis or abscess

(Left) *Transverse ultrasound of multiple palpable reactive submental lymph nodes is shown. These nodes are round and lack fatty hila* ➡. **(Right)** *Transverse color Doppler ultrasound of multiple palpable reactive submental lymph nodes is shown. There is a normal color flow in the center of the node* ➡.

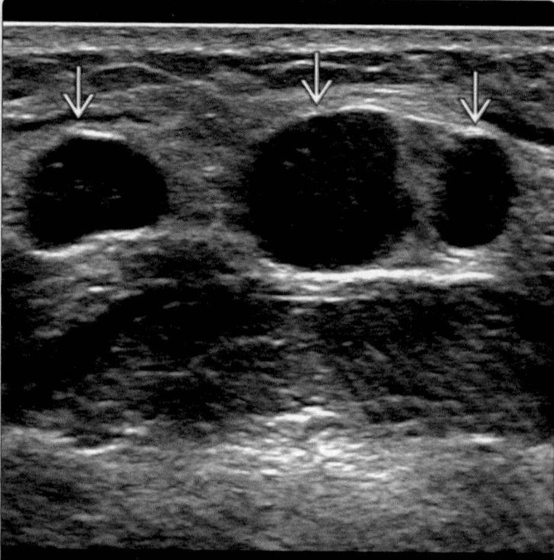

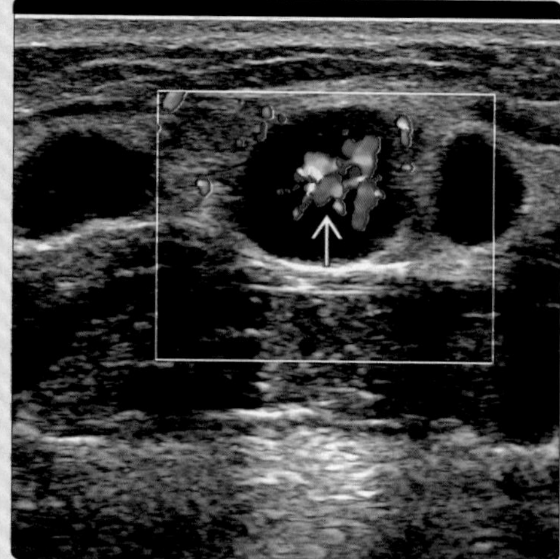

(Left) *Transverse ultrasound of suppurative lymphadenitis in the left submandibular region is shown. The center is liquefied* ➡*, representing pus. There is surrounding inflammation* ➡. **(Right)** *Longitudinal ultrasound of suppurative lymphadenitis in the left submandibular region is shown. There is a multilocular purulent center* ➡. *Inflammation has spread beyond* ➡ *the nodal conglomerate.*

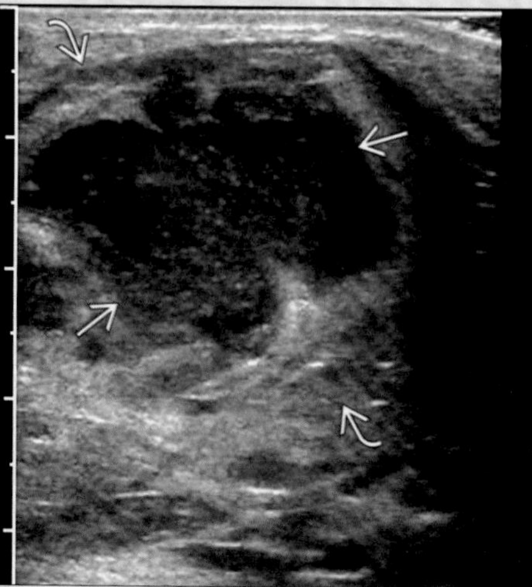

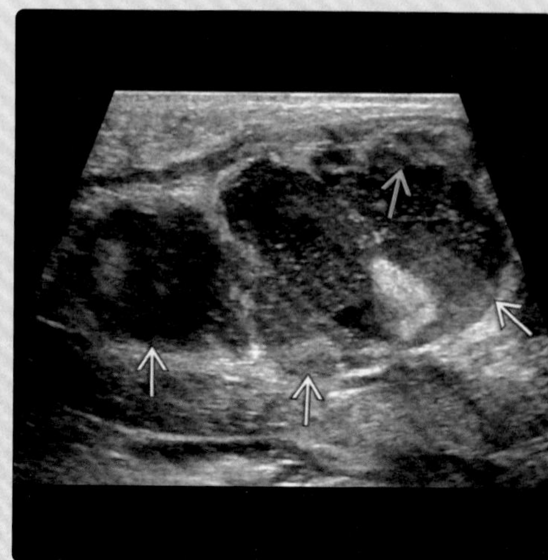

KEY FACTS

IMAGING

- Location: Levels I-VI
- Head and neck squamous cell cancers: Most common in upper neck, at level II
- Thyroid cancers: Most common at levels VI, III, and IV
- Supraclavicular nodes are usually from distant primary tumor (e.g., lung, gastrointestinal tract, breast)
- Size less important than morphology
- Malignant nodes are round with sharp borders, (long = short axis < 2)
- Irregular borders suggest extracapsular extension; ± invasion of adjacent structures (e.g., vessels, muscles)
- Loss of fatty hilum
- Eccentric cortical thickening
- Most hypoechoic but can be hyperechoic in papillary thyroid cancer
- Cystic component: Consider necrosis in squamous cell carcinoma or cystic metastasis from papillary thyroid cancer
- Punctate calcifications: Consider papillary thyroid cancer or medullary thyroid carcinoma
- Color Doppler: Chaotic/disorganized intranodal vascularity, peripheral vascularity

TOP DIFFERENTIAL DIAGNOSES

- Reactive lymphadenopathy
- Non-Hodgkin lymphoma
- Tuberculosis

CLINICAL ISSUES

- Patients may present with painless, firm neck mass
  - Nodes may be asymptomatic and found during staging
- Nodes more likely with larger primary, initially ipsilateral then contralateral to primary tumor
- Even when nodes are sonographically suspicious, fine-needle aspiration may be required to confirm tumor involvement

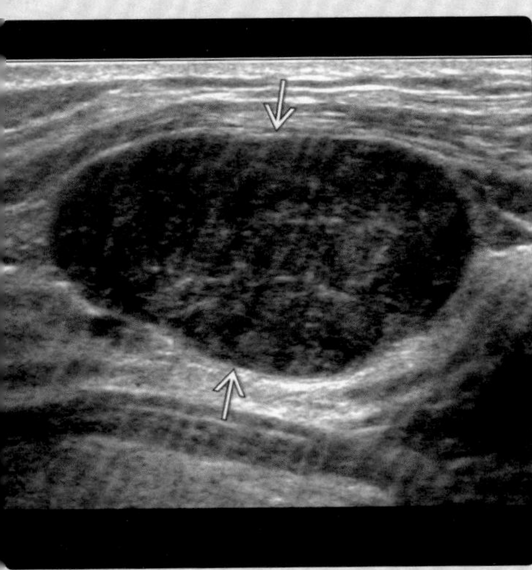

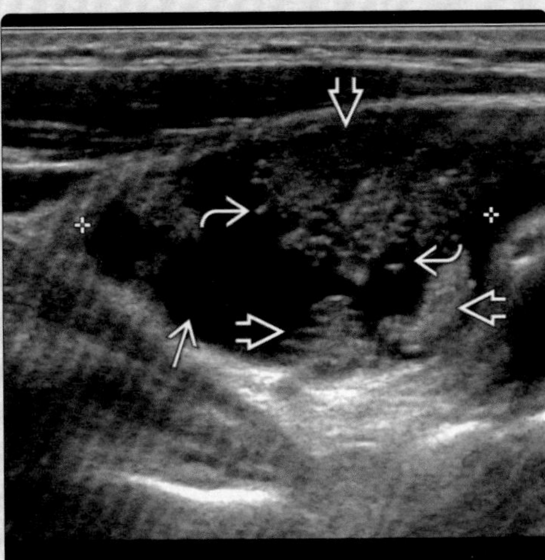

(Left) *Longitudinal ultrasound of a hypoechoic, enlarged (in short axis) lymph node ➡, lacking a fatty hilum, is shown. This was confirmed to be metastatic squamous cell carcinoma by fine-needle aspiration.* **(Right)** *Longitudinal ultrasound of a lymph node with characteristic findings of metastatic cystic papillary cancer is shown. The node is enlarged (3.5 cm in length) and cystic ➡. There are internal papillary soft tissue nodules ➡ with echogenic foci ➡.*

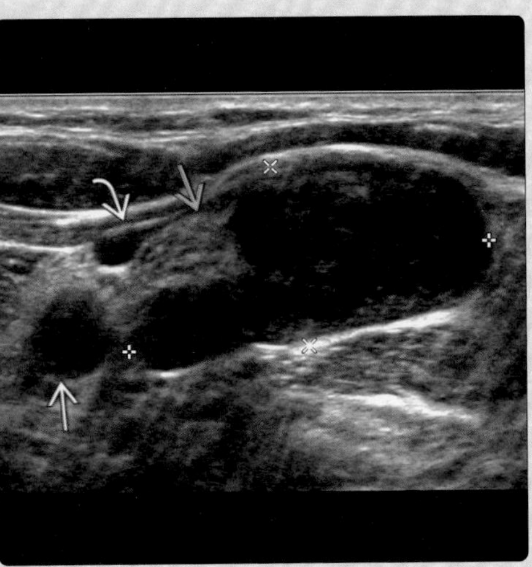

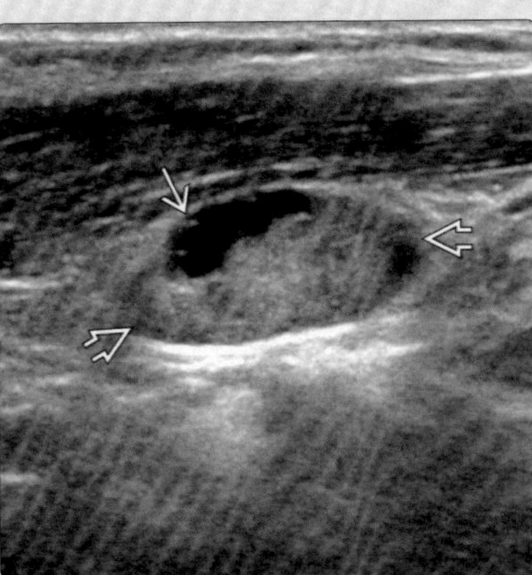

(Left) *Transverse ultrasound of the left neck at level IV in a patient with a history of cervical cancer shows there is an abnormal, enlarged lymph node with a displaced fatty hilum ➡ compressing the internal jugular vein ➡. Fine-needle aspiration showed metastatic cervical cancer. The common carotid artery ➡ was normal.* **(Right)** *Longitudinal ultrasound of a predominantly hyperechoic ➡ lymph node in metastatic papillary thyroid cancer is shown. An eccentric cystic component ➡ with a few echogenic foci is noted.*

Parotid Tumors

KEY FACTS

IMAGING

- Pleomorphic adenoma
  - Most common parotid space tumor (80%)
  - Well defined, lobulated, solid, hypoechoic
  - Homogeneous internal echoes with posterior enhancement
  - Large tumors more heterogeneous from hemorrhage and necrosis
  - Intratumoral calcification may occur if longstanding
  - Malignant transformation if untreated
- Warthin tumor
  - Arises in intraparotid lymphoid tissue, 2nd most common benign parotid tumor
  - Well defined, heterogeneous, hypoechoic
  - Cystic change, posterior acoustic enhancement
  - Multiseptated when large
  - Multicentric in 20%, unilateral or bilateral, malignant change in 1%
- Malignant parotid tumors
  - Include mucoepidermoid carcinoma, adenoid cystic and acinic cell carcinoma, and adenocarcinoma
  - Ill-defined, irregular border, hypoechoic, necrosis, local invasion, and adenopathy
  - Internal vascularity
  - Low-grade tumors may mimic benign tumors

TOP DIFFERENTIAL DIAGNOSES

- Non-Hodgkin lymphoma
- Parotid nodal metastasis

CLINICAL ISSUES

- Painless or painful cheek mass
- Facial nerve paralysis

SCANNING TIPS

- Evaluate for signs of invasion and regional lymphadenopathy

(Left) *Longitudinal ultrasound of a parotid pleomorphic adenoma ➡ is shown. The tumor is hypoechoic to normal parotid ➡ with posterior acoustic enhancement ➡.* **(Right)** *Longitudinal color Doppler ultrasound of a parotid pleomorphic adenoma ➡ is shown. There is both peripheral and central color flow, confirming that the tumor is solid despite posterior acoustic enhancement ➡.*

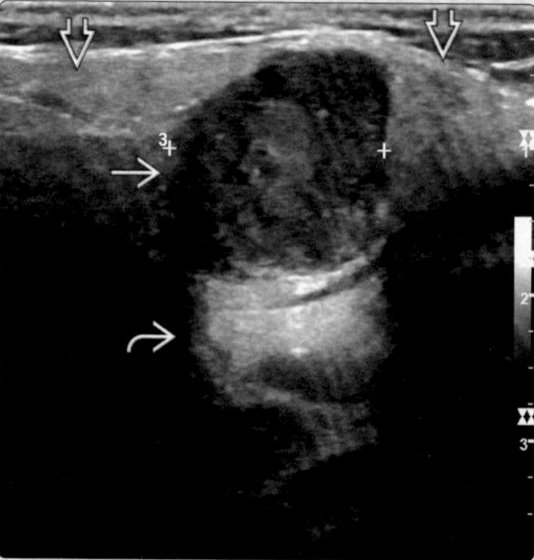

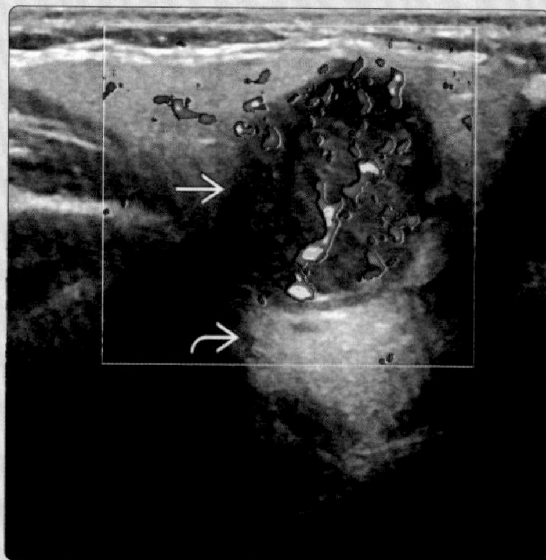

(Left) *Longitudinal color Doppler ultrasound of a parotid Warthin tumor is shown. The tumor is well marginated and has both solid, vascularized components ➡ and a cystic component ➡.* **(Right)** *Longitudinal ultrasound of a parotid adenoid cystic carcinoma is shown. The tumor is poorly marginated, infiltrating, and hypoechoic ➡. The deeper margin is hard to define, but it abuts the mandible ➡ and the masseter muscle ➡.*

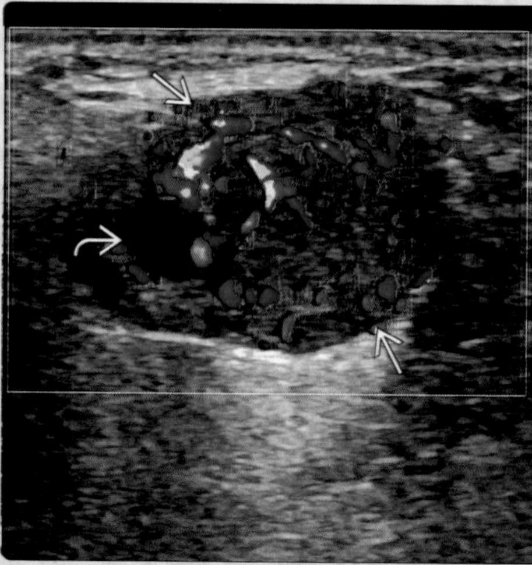

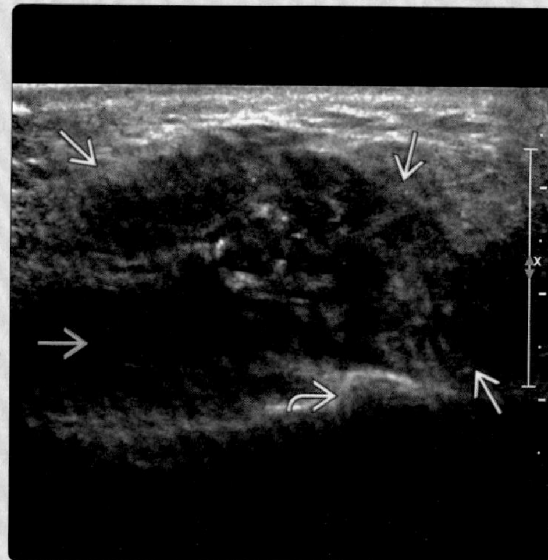

KEY FACTS

IMAGING

- Acute sialadenitis, calculous
  - Unilateral, enlarged, hypoechoic, heterogeneous submandibular gland (SMG)
  - Intra-/extraglandular duct dilatation and calculus
  - Tender on transducer pressure ± ↑ in vascularity
- Acute sialadenitis, acalculous
  - Unilateral, enlarged hypoechoic gland
  - No duct dilatation or calculi
  - Tender on transducer pressure, ↑ vascularity
- Salivary gland abscess
  - Liquefied component with mobile internal debris and thick walls, surrounding soft tissue edema
  - Enlarged, reactive-type regional lymph nodes
- Chronic sclerosing sialadenitis
  - Hypoechoic, heterogeneous nodules/cirrhotic appearance, bilateral involvement

TOP DIFFERENTIAL DIAGNOSES

- Enlarged submandibular (SM) lymph node
- Benign mixed tumor, SMG
- SMG carcinoma

CLINICAL ISSUES

- Unilateral, painful SMG swelling associated with eating or psychological gustatory stimulation (salivary colic)
- 80% of cases presenting with painful SMG swelling are secondary to calculus disease
- If SMG affected without ductal pathology, consider Sjögren, AIDS, or primary SMG infection

SCANNING TIPS

- Look for dilated SM duct and follow to point of transition/calculus/stenosis
- Compare to other side
- Evaluate for complications, such as abscess formation and for reactive lymph nodes

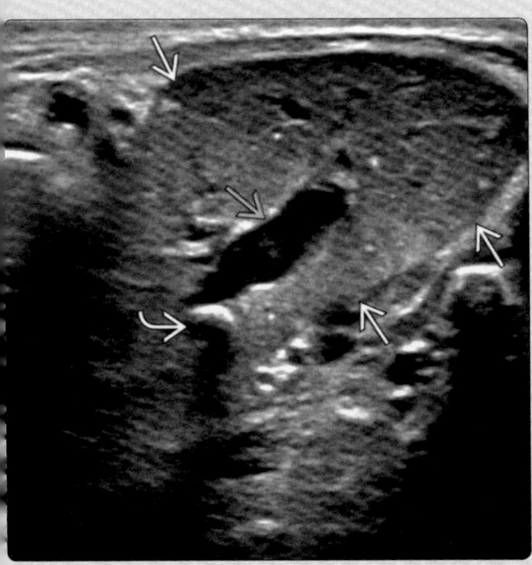

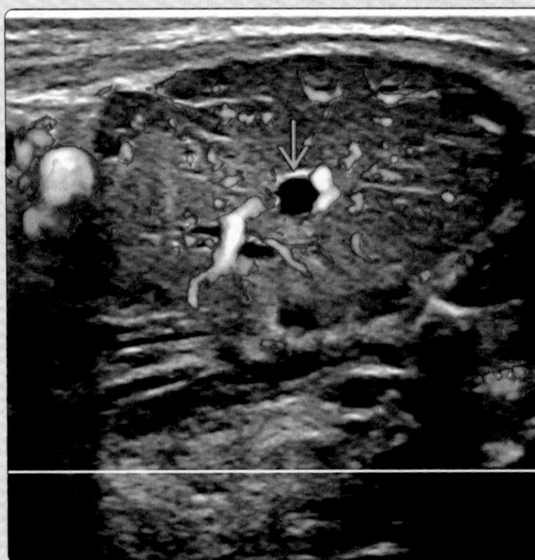

(Left) *Transverse ultrasound of acute calculous submandibular sialadenitis is shown. The submandibular gland ➡ is swollen, and the duct ⇨ is dilated secondary to a shadowing stone ➡.* **(Right)** *Transverse power Doppler ultrasound of acute calculous submandibular sialadenitis is shown. The main submandibular duct ⇨ is dilated, and there is increased color flow in the gland.*

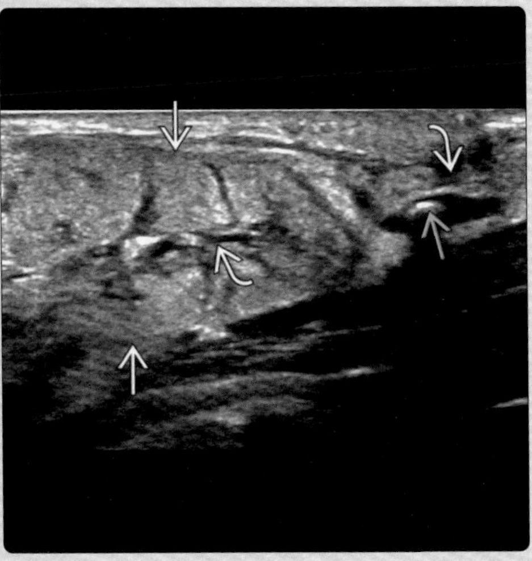

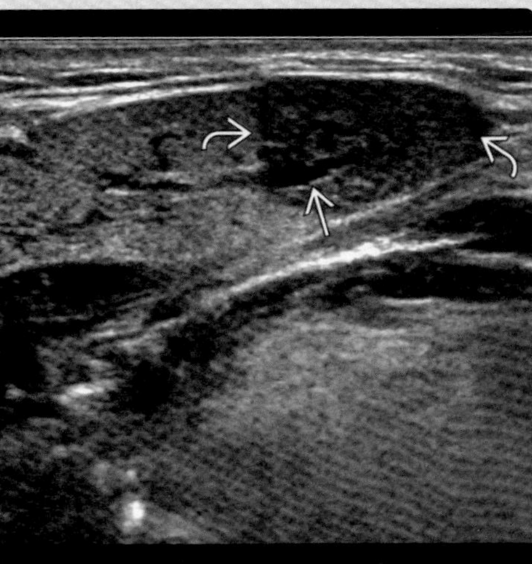

(Left) *Longitudinal ultrasound of acute submandibular sialadenitis is shown. There is ductal dilation ➡ and a small stone ⇨ within the duct. The submandibular gland ➡ is swollen.* **(Right)** *Longitudinal ultrasound of the right submandibular gland is shown. A well-marginated zone of decreased echogenicity ➡ with ductal dilation ➡ was noted. There was no mass effect on vessels. This was pathologically proven to be chronic fibrosing sialadenitis.*

PART IV
SECTION 1

Anatomy and Approach

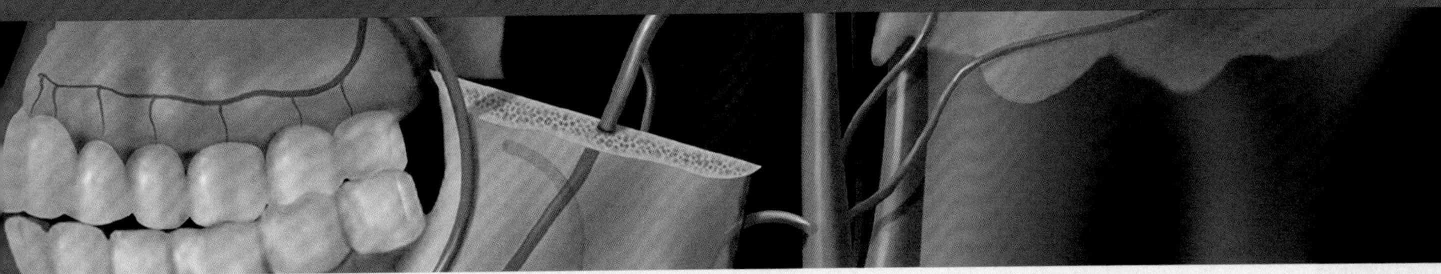

TERMINOLOGY

Abbreviations

- Common (CCA), internal (ICA), and external (ECA) carotid arteries; vertebral artery (VA)

GROSS ANATOMY

Overview

- CCA terminates by dividing into ECA and ICA
- ECA is smaller of 2 terminal branches
  - Supplies most of head and neck (except eye, brain)
  - Has numerous anastomoses with ICA and VA (may become important source of collateral blood flow)
- ICA has no normal extracranial branches

IMAGING ANATOMY

Overview

- CCA
  - Right CCA originates from brachiocephalic trunk; left CCA originates from aortic arch
  - Courses superiorly in carotid space, anteromedial to internal jugular vein
  - Divides into ECA and ICA at ~ C3-C4 level
- Cervical ICA
  - 90% are posterolateral to ECA
  - Carotid bulb
    - Focal dilatation of ICA at its origin from CCA
    - Flow reversal occurs in carotid bulb
  - Ascending cervical segment
    - Courses superiorly within carotid space
    - Enters carotid canal (petrous temporal bone)
    - No named branch in neck
- ECA
  - Smaller and medial compared with ICA
  - Has 8 major branches in neck
  - Superior thyroid artery
    - 1st ECA branch (may arise from CCA bifurcation)
    - Arises anteriorly, courses inferiorly to apex of thyroid
    - Supplies superior thyroid and larynx
    - Anastomoses with inferior thyroid artery (branch of thyrocervical trunk)
  - Ascending pharyngeal artery
    - Arises from posterior ECA (or CCA bifurcation)
    - Courses superiorly between ECA and ICA
    - Visceral branches, muscular branches, and neuromeningeal branches
  - Lingual artery
    - 2nd anterior ECA branch
    - Loops anteroinferiorly, then superiorly, to tongue
    - Major vascular supply to tongue, oral cavity, and submandibular gland
  - Facial artery
    - Originates just above lingual artery
    - Curves around mandible, then passes anterosuperiorly across cheek and is closely related to submandibular gland
    - Supplies face, palate, lip, and cheek
  - Occipital artery
    - Originates from posterior aspect of ECA
    - Courses posterosuperiorly between occiput and C1
    - Supplies scalp, upper cervical musculature, and posterior fossa meninges
  - Posterior auricular artery
    - Arises from posterior ECA above occipital artery
    - Courses superiorly to supply pinna, scalp, external auditory canal, and chorda tympani
  - Superficial temporal artery
    - Smaller of 2 terminal ECA branches
    - Runs superiorly behind mandibular condyle, across zygoma
    - Supplies scalp and gives off transverse facial artery
  - Internal maxillary artery
    - Larger of 2 terminal ECA branches
    - Arises within parotid gland, behind mandibular neck
    - Gives off middle meningeal artery (supplies cranial meninges)

ANATOMY IMAGING ISSUES

Imaging Recommendations

- Normal ultrasonography appearances of carotid arteries
  - CCA diameter: 6.3 ± 0.9 mm, smooth and thin intima, antegrade low-resistance arterial flow
  - ICA diameter: 4.8 ± 0.7 mm, smooth and thin intima, antegrade low-resistance flow
  - ECA diameter: 4.1 ± 0.6 mm, smooth and thin intima, antegrade high-resistance flow
- In assessing carotid arteries on ultrasonography, the following parameters should be examined
  - Intimal-medial thickness
    - Distance between leading edges of lumen-intima interface and media-adventitia interface at far edge
    - 0.5-1.0 mm in healthy adults
  - Presence of atherosclerotic plaques
    - Eccentric/concentric, noncircumferential/circumferential
    - Calcified plaque/soft plaque
  - Luminal diameter/area reduction
    - Should be measured on true cross-sectional view of affected artery
    - Color flow helps to detect residual lumen in tight stenosis or in assessing indeterminate total occlusion
  - Spectral Doppler analysis
    - Arterial flow pattern: Low-resistance/high-resistance flow, antegrade/retrograde flow, special waveform (e.g., damped waveform, preocclusive "thump")
    - Peak systolic velocity measurement
    - Systolic velocity ratio measurement

Imaging Pitfalls

- Scanning technique must be meticulous to produce reliable Doppler ultrasound results
- Obliquity of imaging plane in relation to cross section of artery may wrongly estimate degree of stenosis

CLINICAL IMPLICATIONS

Clinical Importance

- Consider acute idiopathic carotidynia: Tender mass around distal carotid, near bifurcation

GRAPHIC & DIGITAL SUBTRACTION ANGIOGRAM

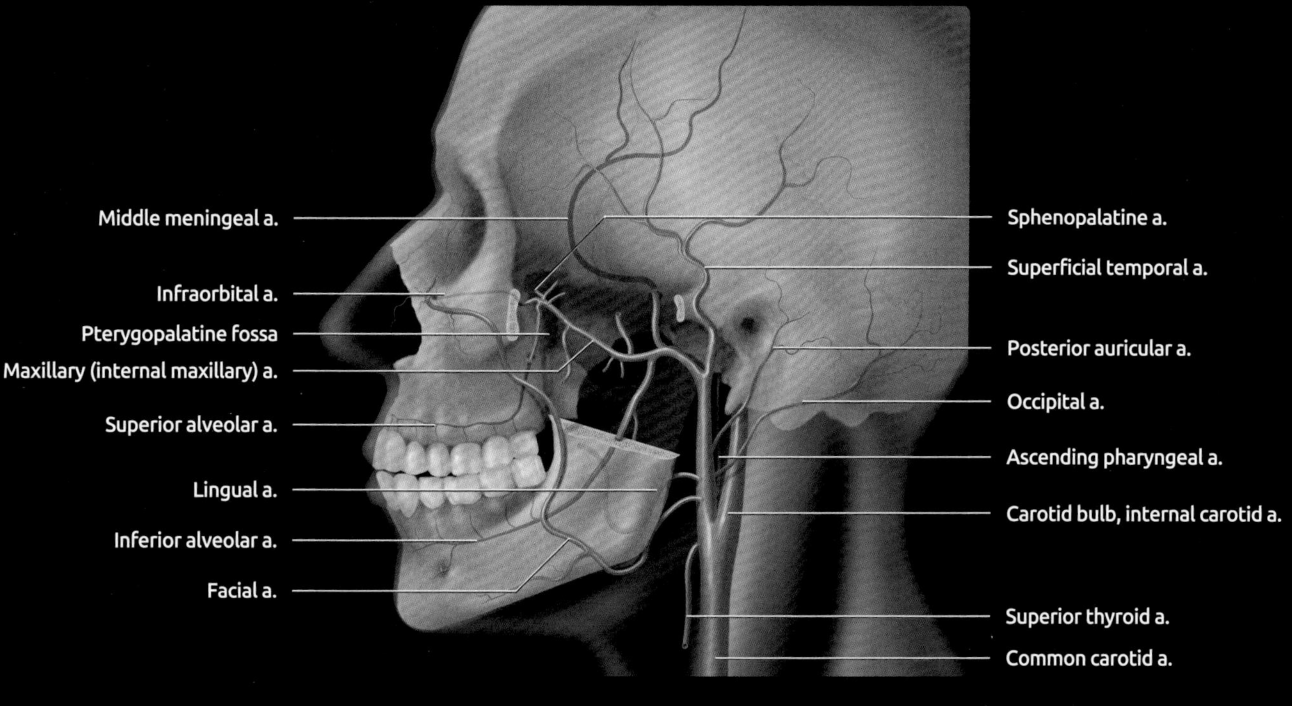

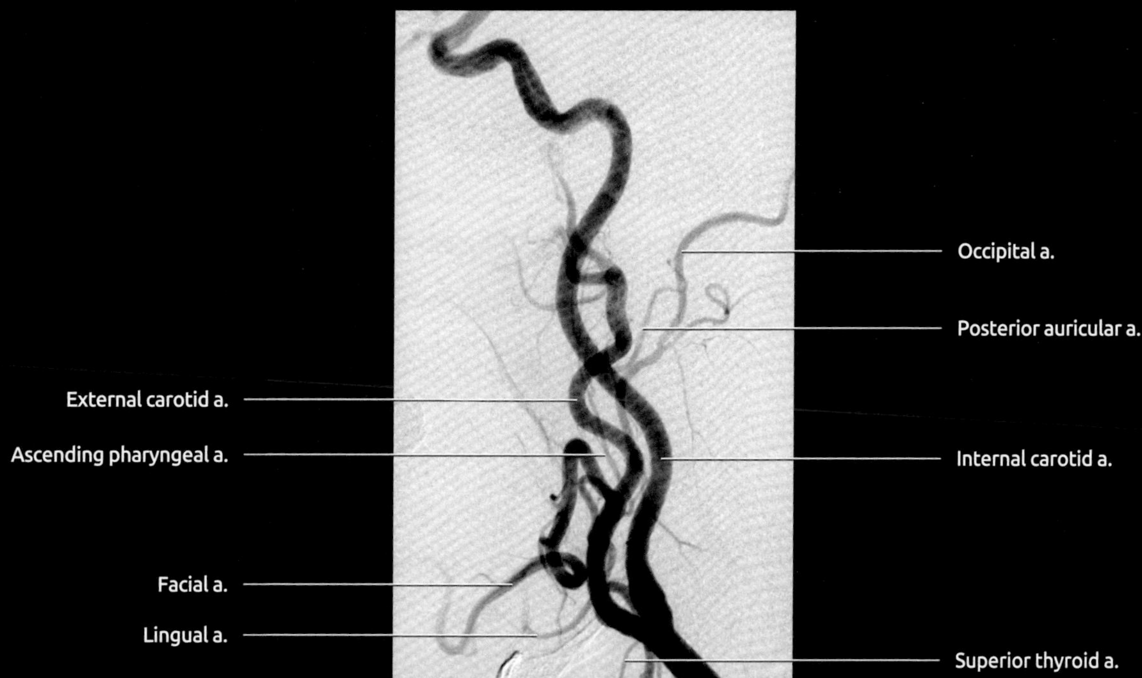

(Top) *Lateral graphic depicts the common carotid artery (CCA) and its 2 terminal branches, the external (ECA) and internal (ICA) carotid arteries. The scalp and the superficial facial structures are removed to show the deep ECA branches. The ECA terminates by dividing into the superficial temporal and internal maxillary arteries (IMA). Within the pterygopalatine fossa, the IMA divides into numerous deep branches. Its distal termination is the sphenopalatine artery, which passes medially into the nasal cavity. Numerous anastomoses between the ECA branches (e.g., between the facial and maxillary arteries) and between the ECA and the orbital and cavernous branches of the ICA provide potential sources for collateral blood flow.* **(Bottom)** *The early arterial phase of CCA angiogram is shown with bony structures subtracted. The major ECA branches are opacified.*

COMMON CAROTID ARTERY

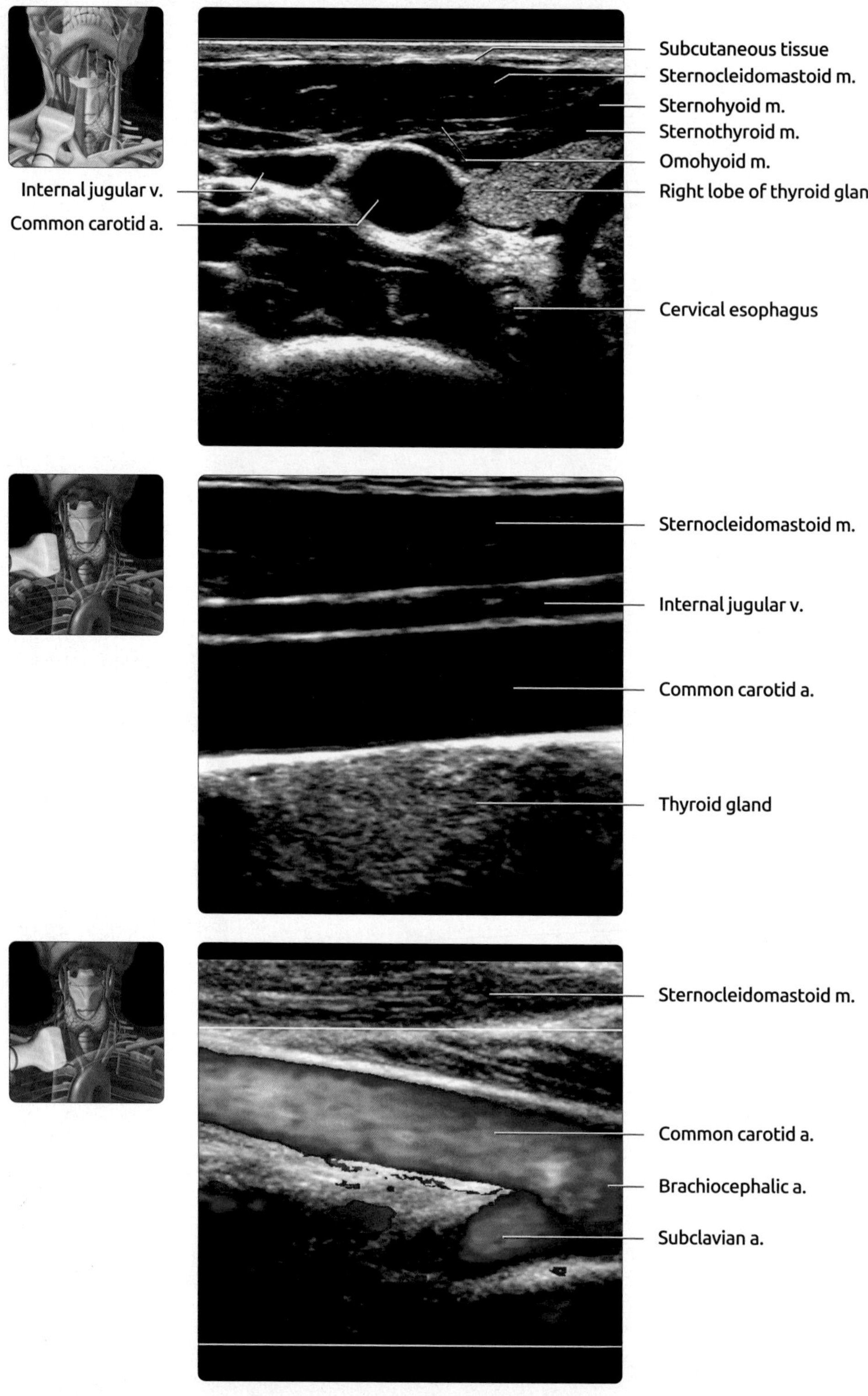

(Top) *Transverse grayscale ultrasound shows the distal CCA at the level of the upper pole of the thyroid gland. Note that the wall in a normal individual is smooth with no intimal thickening or atherosclerotic plaque. The lumen is circular in cross section. There is no major named branch in the neck apart from the termination into the ECA and ICA at the level of the hyoid bone.* **(Middle)** *Longitudinal grayscale ultrasound of the CCA shows the smooth outline of the intimal layer.* **(Bottom)** *Color Doppler ultrasound of the proximal CCA at the root of the neck in the longitudinal plane demonstrates the normal antegrade arterial flow in the cranial direction. Its origin along with the subclavian artery from the brachiocephalic artery is also well demonstrated.*

COMMON CAROTID ARTERY

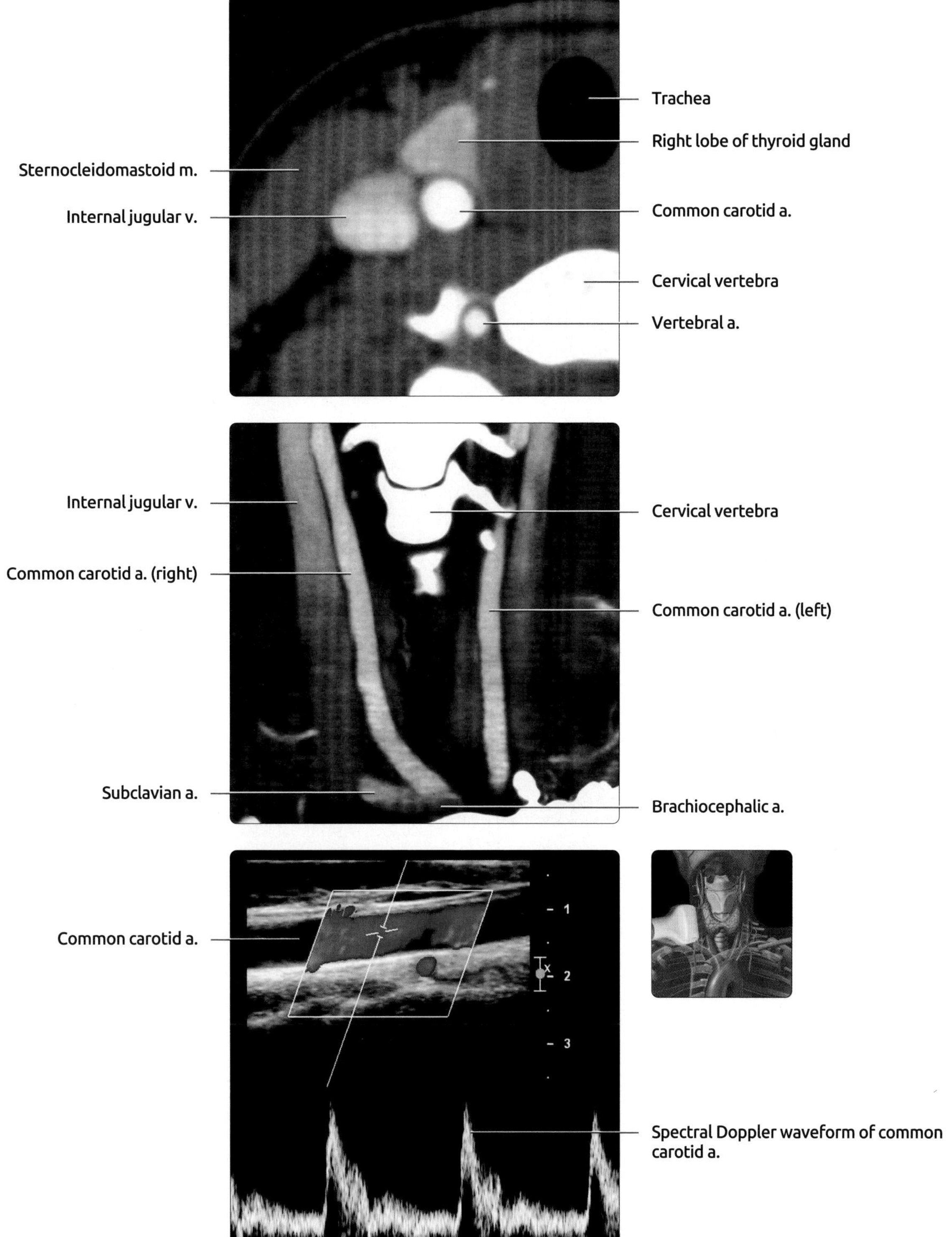

(Top) *Axial CECT of the lower neck shows contrast-filled CCA related anteriorly and medially to the right lobe of the thyroid gland and laterally to the internal jugular vein.* **(Middle)** *Coronal reformatted CECT shows the normal contour and vertical course of the CCA. It originates from the brachiocephalic artery on the right at the root of the neck with the right subclavian artery.* **(Bottom)** *Spectral Doppler ultrasound of the CCA shows low-resistance arterial flow with a forward diastolic component. The scanning technique must be meticulous to produce a reliable Doppler assessment.*

CAROTID BIFURCATION

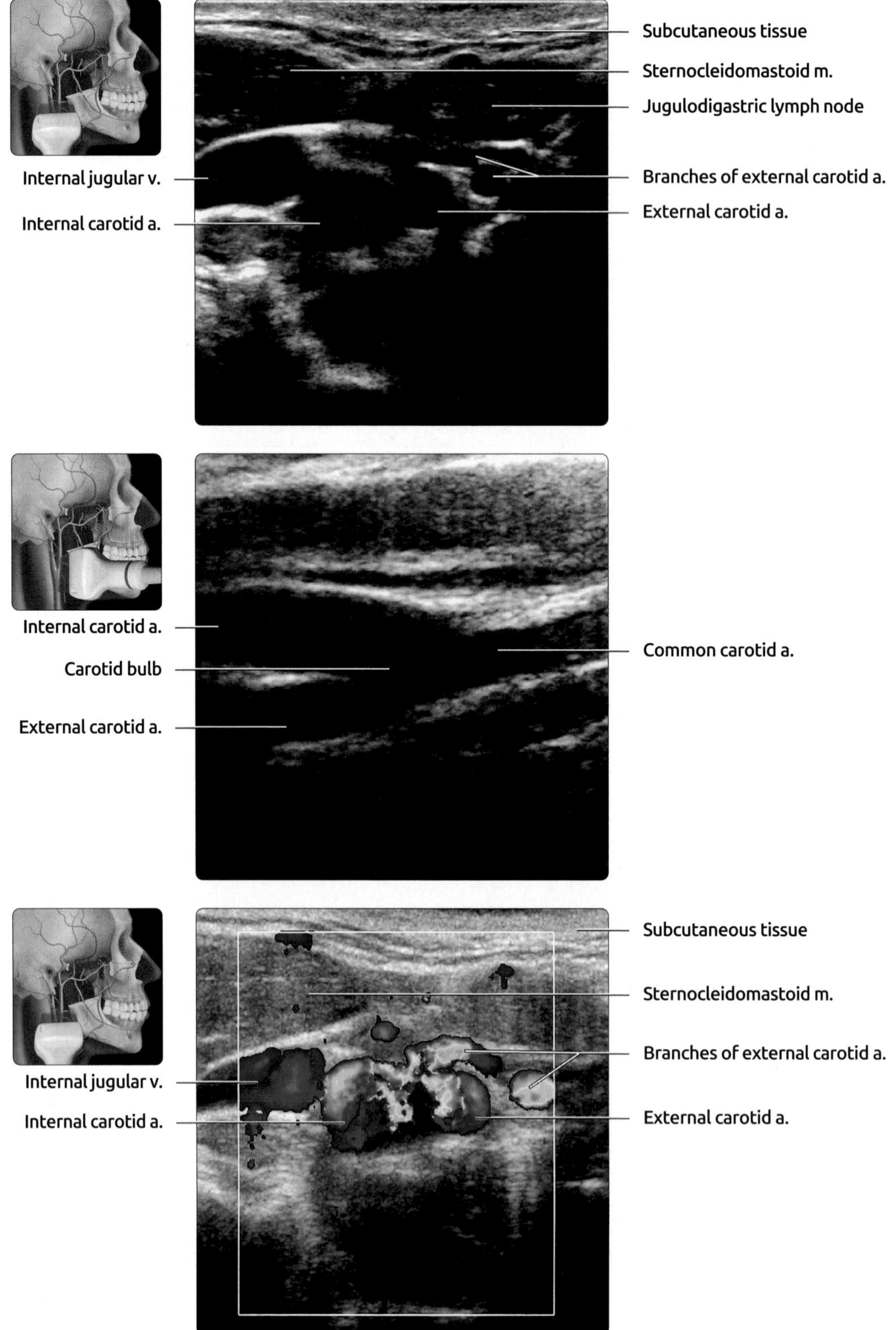

(Top) *Transverse grayscale ultrasound shows the upper cervical level at the carotid bifurcation. The CCA bifurcates into the ICA and ECA. The former is usually of larger caliber, laterally located, and has no branches in the neck.* **(Middle)** *Longitudinal grayscale ultrasound in coronal orientation demonstrates the carotid bifurcation. The proximal portion of the ICA is usually mildly dilated and is termed carotid bulb. At this site, the color/spectral Doppler study is more complex due to a disturbance of laminar flow and should not be misinterpreted as an abnormality.* **(Bottom)** *Color Doppler ultrasound of carotid bifurcation in a transverse plane demonstrates turbulent flow in the carotid bulb. Branches of ECA are easier to depict than on grayscale examination.*

CAROTID BIFURCATION

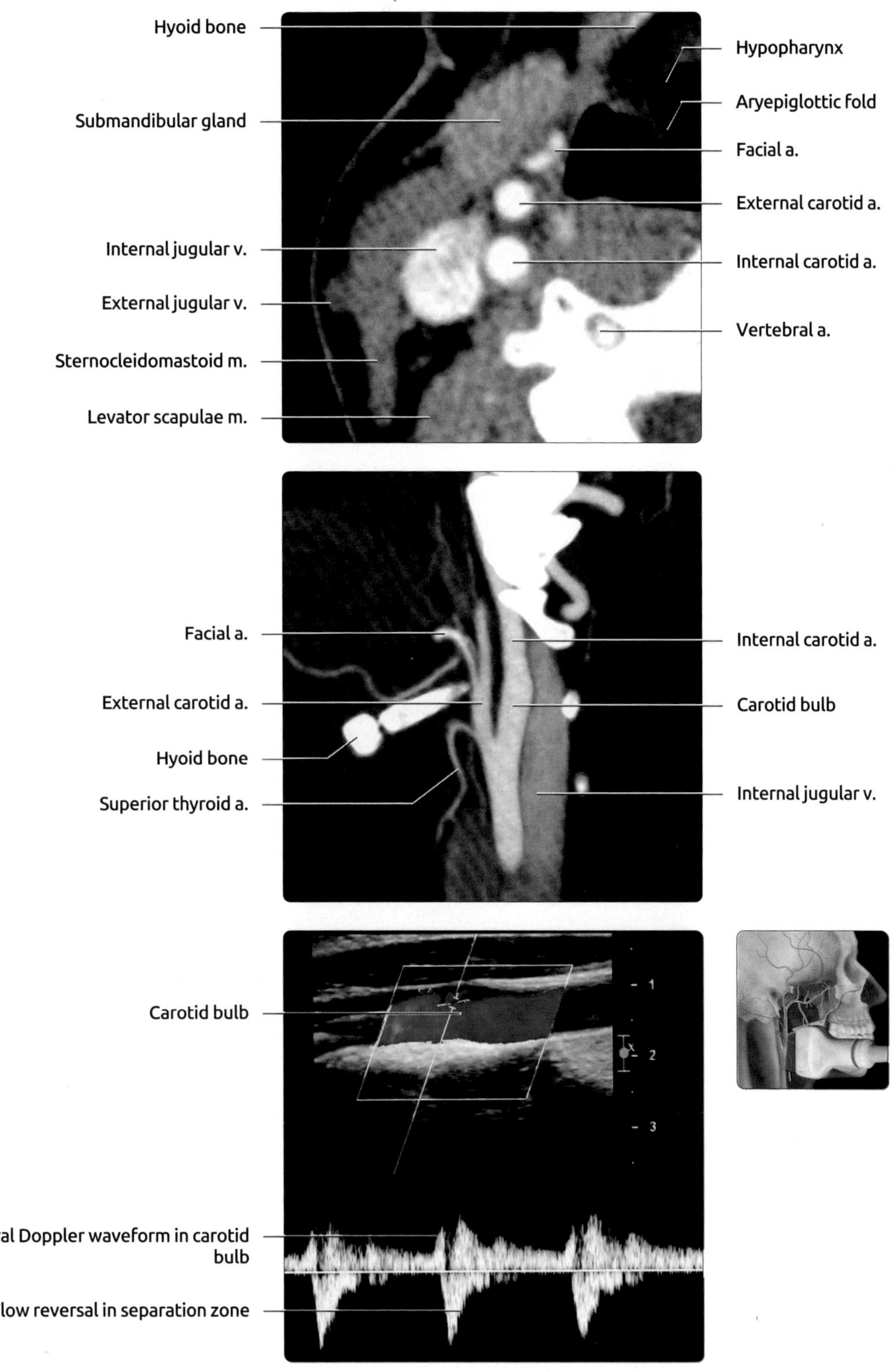

(Top) *Axial CECT shows the upper neck just beyond the carotid bifurcation. The ICA is larger and more posterolateral in position than the ECA.* **(Middle)** *Maximum-intensity projection in the sagittal plane demonstrates carotid bifurcation into the ECA and ICA at the level of the hyoid bone. Note the branching nature of the ECA in contrast to the ICA.* **(Bottom)** *Spectral Doppler ultrasound shows the carotid bulb, which has a different flow pattern than the rest of the ICA. In early systole, blood flow is accelerated in a forward direction. As the peak systole is approached, a large separation zone with flow reversal develops. Flow separation should be seen in normal individuals, and its absence should raise the suspicion of plaque formation.*

INTERNAL CAROTID ARTERY

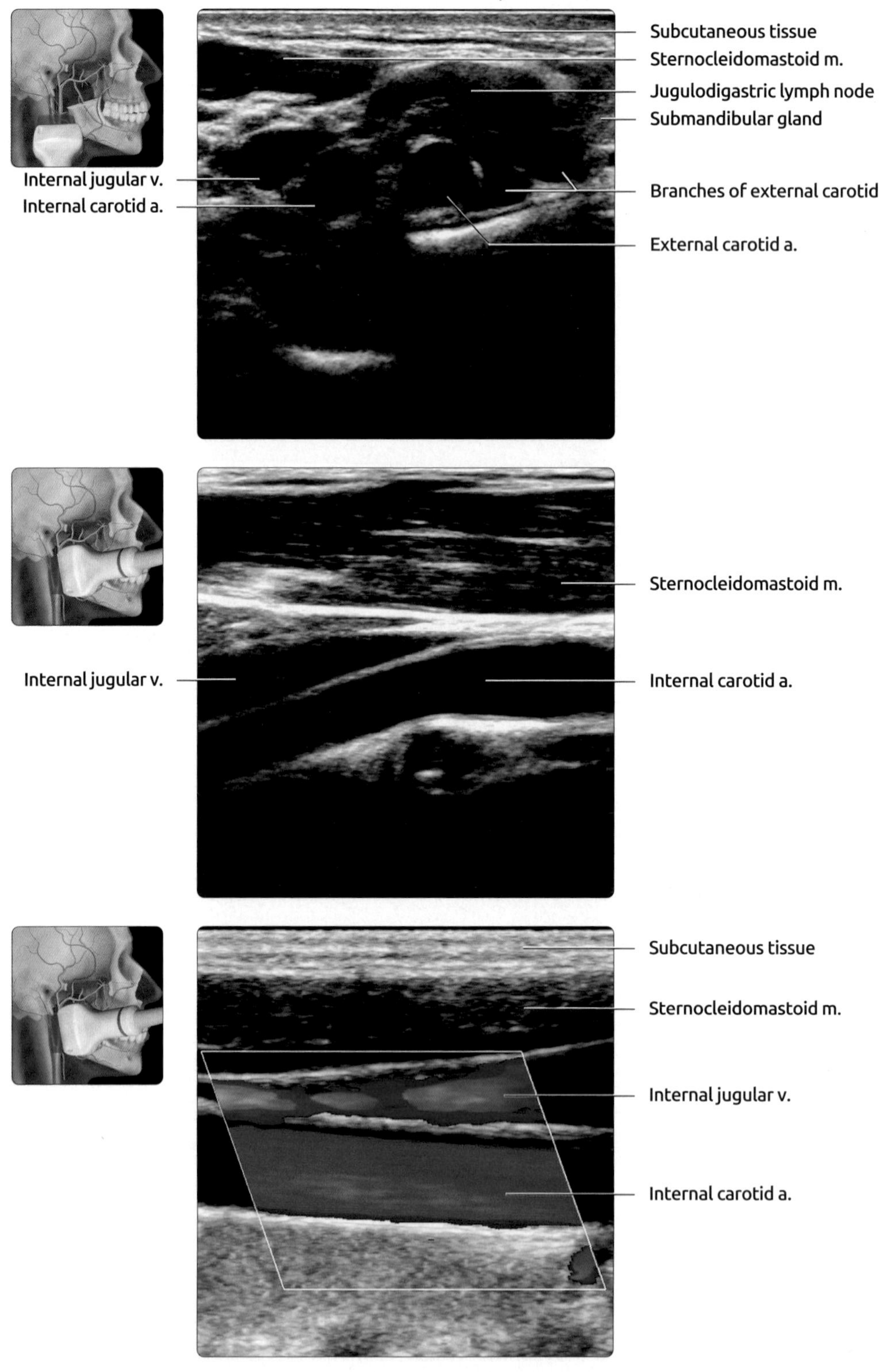

(Top) *Transverse grayscale ultrasound of the upper neck, just beyond the carotid bifurcation, shows the close anatomical relationship of the upper neck with the internal jugular vein, ECA, and jugulodigastric lymph node.* **(Middle)** *Longitudinal grayscale ultrasound shows the ICA. Note its smooth wall with no intimal thickening; it is free of atherosclerotic plaque in a normal individual. No branch is seen in the cervical region.* **(Bottom)** *Color Doppler ultrasound shows the ICA and the internal jugular vein in the longitudinal plane. Note that the normal antegrade flow is toward the cranial direction of the ICA and opposite the caudal direction of flow in the adjacent internal jugular vein.*

INTERNAL CAROTID ARTERY

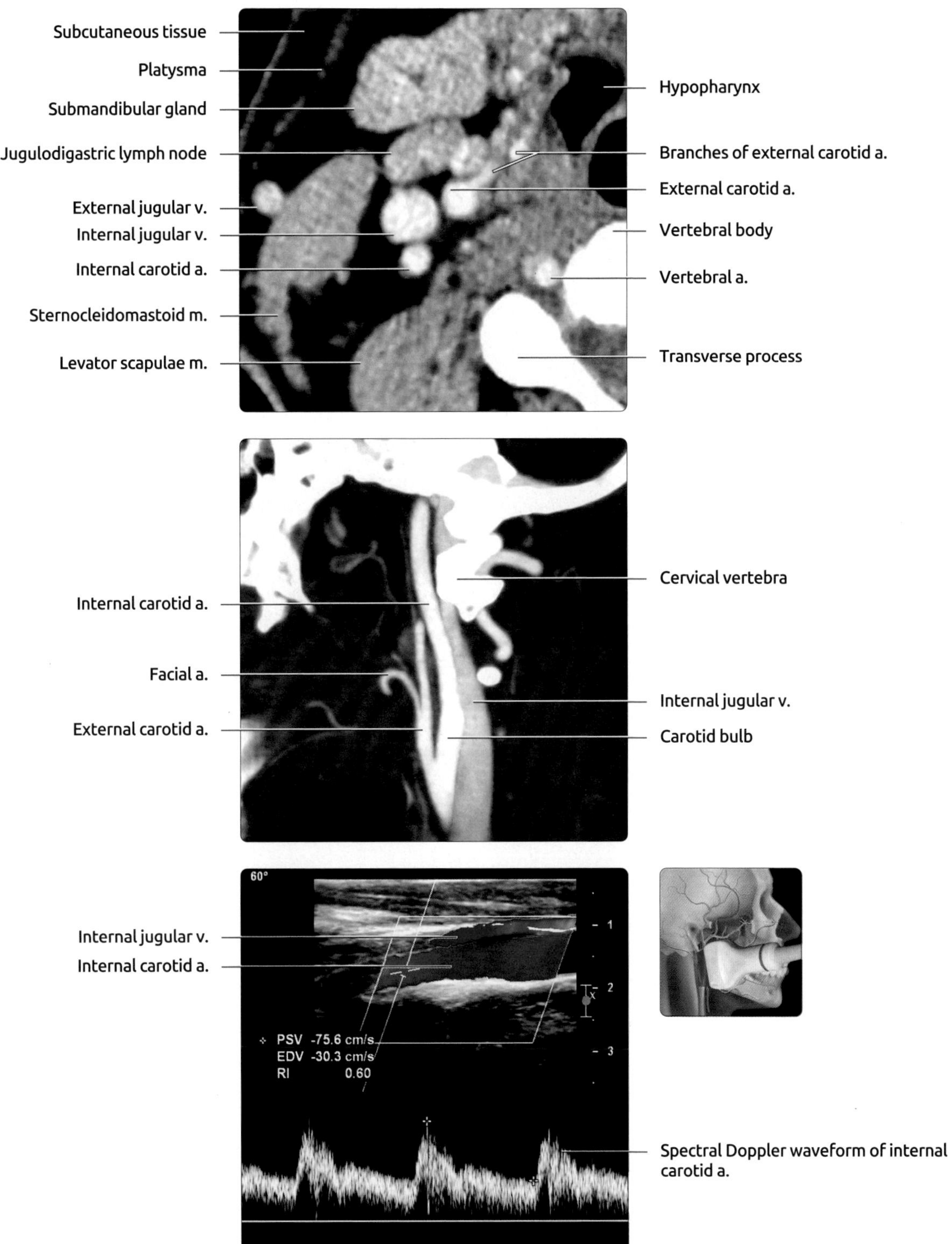

(Top) *Axial CECT of the upper neck shows the anatomical relation of the ICA with the internal jugular vein and branches of the ECA.* **(Middle)** *Maximum-intensity projection CECT in the sagittal plane shows the normal configuration and contour of the cervical portion of the ICA. Note the lack of an arterial branch from the cervical ICA in the neck in contrast to the ECA. Note the mild dilatation of the ICA at its origin (carotid bulb).* **(Bottom)** *Spectral Doppler ultrasound in the longitudinal plane shows the cervical portion of the ICA, which has a low-resistance flow pattern with antegrade flow in the diastolic phase. The waveform is different from that of the carotid bulb.*

EXTERNAL CAROTID ARTERY

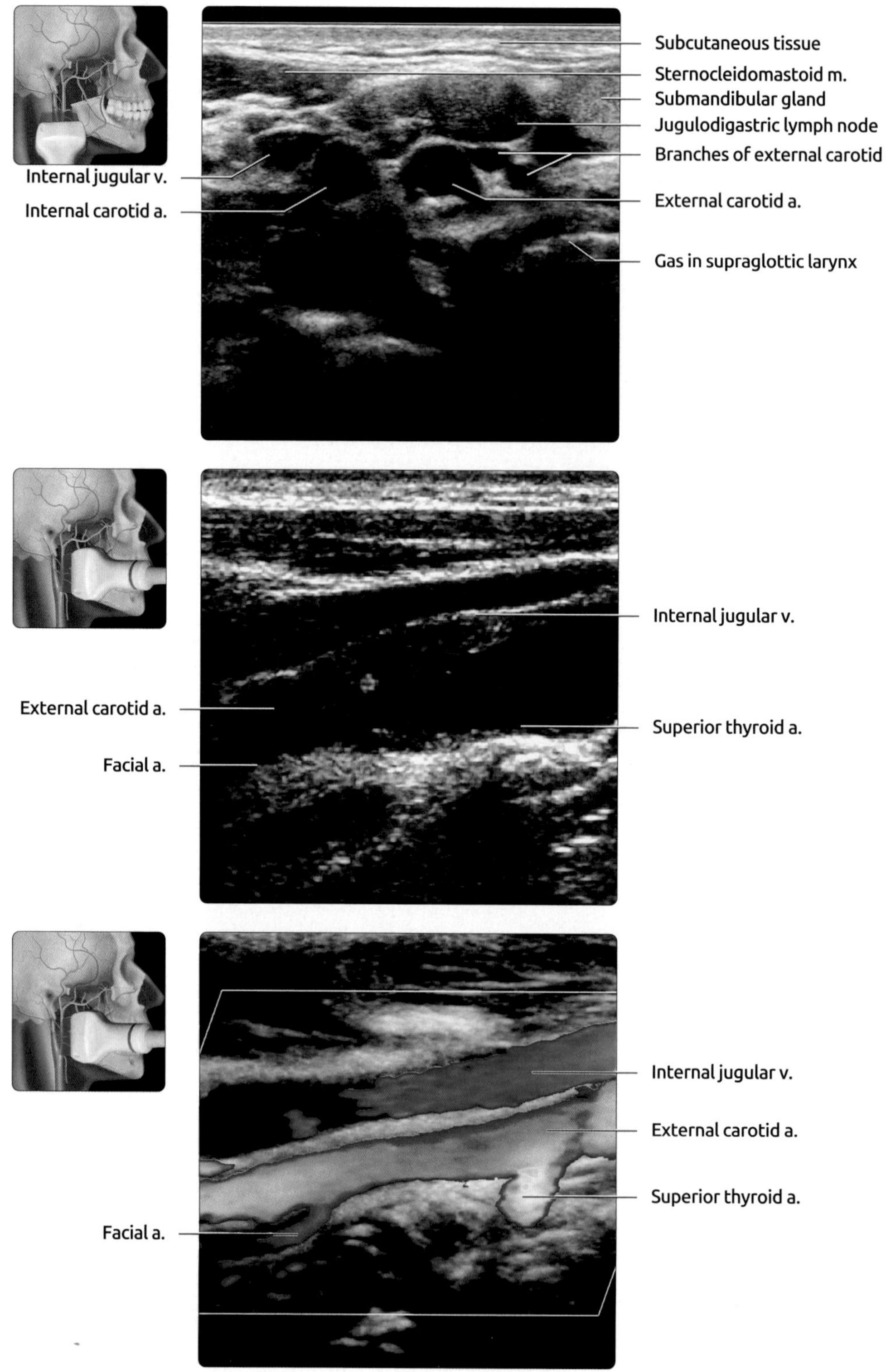

(Top) *Transverse grayscale ultrasound shows the upper neck above the carotid bifurcation. The position of the ECA medial to the ICA and internal jugular vein, posterior to the jugulodigastric lymph node, is well demonstrated.* **(Middle)** *Longitudinal grayscale ultrasound shows the ECA. Two anterior branches, the superior thyroid artery and the facial artery, are seen arising from the proximal portion of the ECA. They course inferiorly to the upper pole of the thyroid and superiorly to the facial region.* **(Bottom)** *Color Doppler ultrasound shows the ECA in the longitudinal plane. The antegrade flow in the cranial direction of the ECA is demonstrated. Note the opposite flow direction of the adjacent internal jugular vein.*

EXTERNAL CAROTID ARTERY

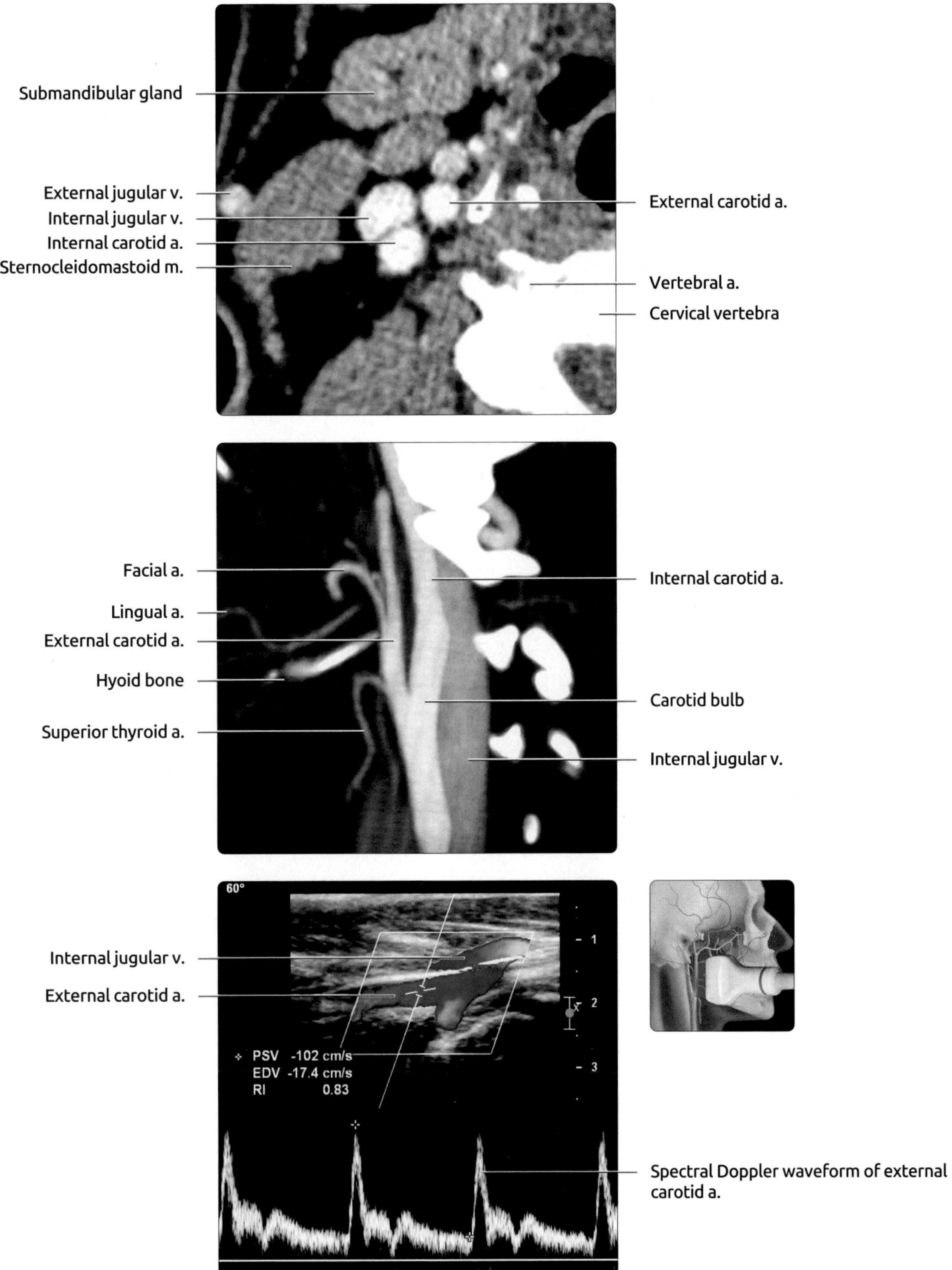

(Top) *Axial CECT of the upper neck at the hyoid bone level shows the relationship of the ECA with the adjacent ICA and the internal jugular vein.* **(Middle)** *Maximum-intensity projection CECT in the sagittal plane shows the normal contour and configuration of the ECA. Note some of its major branches, including the superior thyroid artery, lingual artery, and facial artery, in its proximal portion.* **(Bottom)** *Spectral Doppler ultrasound of the ECA in longitudinal plane shows a high-resistance flow pattern with a low diastolic component. Contrarily, the CCA and ICA are of a low-resistance pattern with a high diastolic component.*

GRAYSCALE AND DOPPLER ULTRASOUND

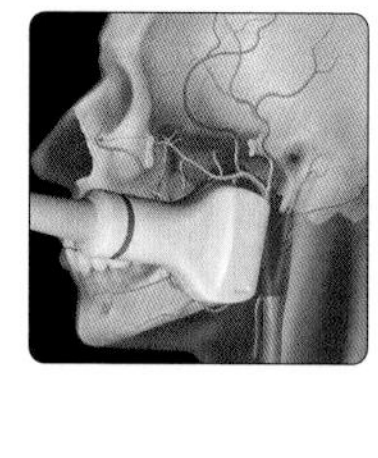

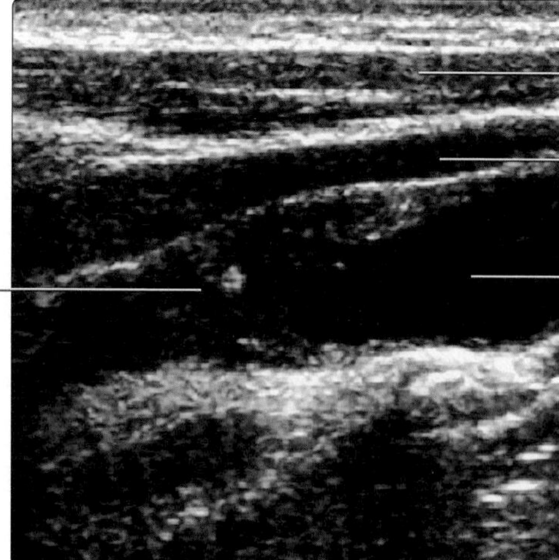

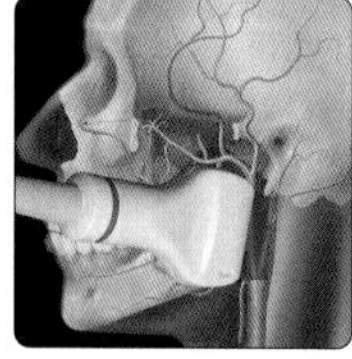

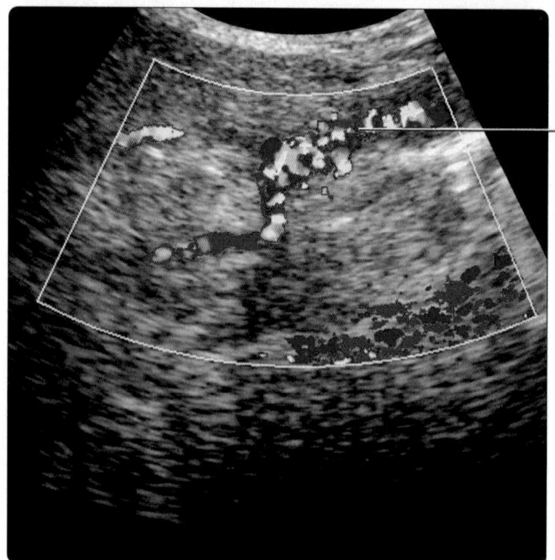

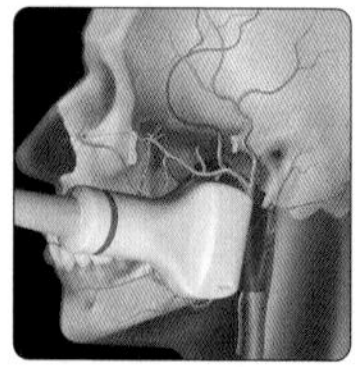

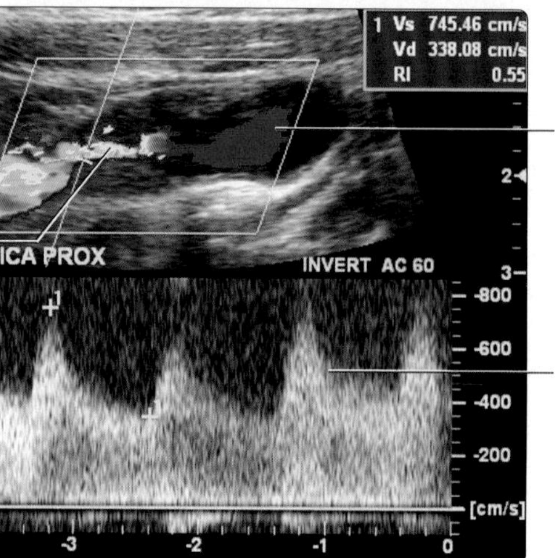

(Top) *Longitudinal grayscale ultrasound of the cervical portion of the ICA shows hypoechoic atherosclerotic plaque with marked luminal narrowing.* **(Middle)** *Longitudinal color Doppler ultrasound in the same patient helps to demonstrate the turbulent arterial flow through the severe stenotic segment in the proximal ICA. Color flow imaging is a useful tool to distinguish severe stenosis from complete occlusion.* **(Bottom)** *Spectral Doppler ultrasound of the proximal ICA demonstrates markedly elevated peak systolic and peak diastolic velocity, indicating severe stenosis.*

GRAYSCALE AND DOPPLER ULTRASOUND

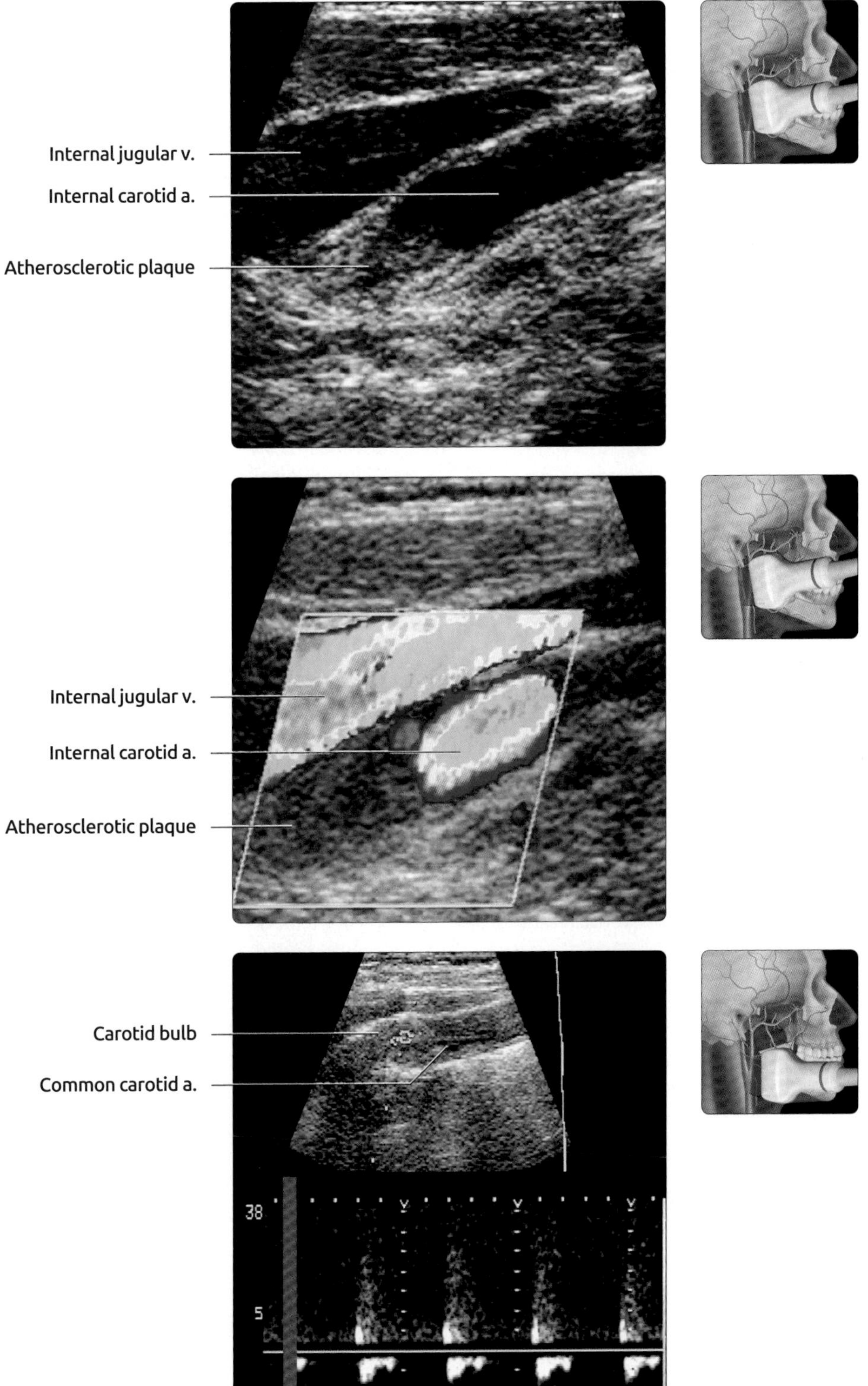

(Top) *Longitudinal grayscale ultrasound of the cervical portion of the ICA shows a slightly hyperechoic atherosclerotic plaque causing complete arterial occlusion.* **(Middle)** *Color Doppler ultrasound in the same patient reveals an absence of arterial flow in the occluded segment of the ICA.* **(Bottom)** *Spectral Doppler ultrasound at the carotid bifurcation shows no detectable signal within the occluded segment and preocclusive "thump" proximal to the occluded segment. The carotid bulb was occluded on grayscale imaging (not shown).*

IMAGING ANATOMY

Overview

- Vertebral artery (VA): 4 segments
  - V1 segment (extraosseous segment)
    - Arises from 1st part of subclavian artery
    - Courses posterosuperiorly to enter C6 transverse foramen
    - Branches: Segmental cervical muscular, spinal branches
  - V2 segment (foraminal segment)
    - Ascends through C6-C3 transverse foramina
    - Turns superolaterally through inverted L-shaped transverse foramen of axis (C2)
    - Courses short distance superiorly through C1 transverse foramen
    - Branches: Anterior meningeal artery, unnamed muscular/spinal branches
  - V3 segment (extraspinal segment)
    - Exits top of atlas (C1) transverse foramen
    - Lies on top of C1 ring, curving posteromedially around atlantooccipital joint
    - As it passes around back of atlantooccipital joint, turns sharply anterosuperiorly to pierce dura at foramen magnum
    - Branches: Posterior meningeal artery
  - V4 segment (intradural/intracranial segment)
    - After VA enters skull through foramen magnum, courses superomedially behind clivus
    - Unites with contralateral VA at or near pontomedullary junction to form basilar artery (BA)
    - Branches: Anterior, posterior spinal arteries (ASA, PSA), perforating branches to medulla, posterior inferior cerebellar artery (PICA)
    - Arises from distal VA, curves around/over tonsil, gives off perforating medullary, choroid, tonsillar, cerebellar branches
- BA
  - Courses superiorly in prepontine cistern (in front of pons, behind clivus)
  - Bifurcates into its terminal branches, posterior cerebral arteries (PCAs), in interpeduncular or suprasellar cistern at or slightly above dorsum sellae
  - Branches: Pontine, midbrain perforating branches (numerous), anterior ICA (AICA), superior cerebellar arteries (SCAs), PCAs (terminal branches)

Vascular Territory

- VA
  - ASA: Upper cervical spinal cord, inferior medulla
  - PSA: Dorsal spinal cord to conus medullaris
  - Penetrating branches: Olives, inferior cerebellar peduncle, part of medulla
  - PICA: Lateral medulla, choroid plexus of 4th ventricle, tonsil, inferior vermis/cerebellum
- BA
  - Pontine perforating branches: Central medulla, pons, midbrain
  - AICA: Internal auditory canal, CNVII, and CNVIII, anterolateral cerebellum
  - SCA: Superior vermis, superior cerebellar peduncle, dentate nucleus, brachium pontis, superomedial surface of cerebellum, upper vermis

Normal Variants, Anomalies

- Normal variants
  - VA: Variation in size from right to left, dominance common; origin from aortic arch in 5%
- Anomalies
  - VA/BA may be fenestrated or duplicated (may have increased prevalence of aneurysms)
  - Embryonic carotid-basilar anastomoses (e.g., persistent trigeminal artery)

ANATOMY IMAGING ISSUES

Imaging Recommendations

- V1 and V2 segments are amenable to US examination
- Examination usually starts in V2 segment and proceeds downward to V1 segment, then to its origin
- Examination of V2 segment
  - Transducer oriented longitudinally in midcervical region between trachea and sternocleidomastoid muscle
  - Angle transducer laterally from common carotid artery (CCA) and locate V2 segment posterior to acoustic shadowing of transverse processes
- Examination of V1 segment
  - Trace caudally from V2 to its origin
  - Left VA more difficult to visualize than right VA
  - Do not confuse with vertebral vein lying adjacent to VA, which can appear pulsatile
    - Color flow imaging helps to differentiate
- Normal waveform of VA on spectral Doppler analysis
  - Low-resistance flow
  - Similar to that of CCA but with lower amplitude
  - PSV: 59 ± 17 cm/s; EVD: 19 ± 8 cm/s
  - Flow velocity asymmetry is common and related to caliber of VA

Imaging Pitfalls

- VA distal to V2 cannot be properly assessed by US
  - Abnormalities in spectral Doppler waveform of VA at V1/V2 segment provide clue for disease beyond V2

EMBRYOLOGY

Embryologic Events

- Plexiform longitudinal anastomoses between cervical intersegmental arteries → VA precursors
- Paired plexiform dorsal longitudinal neural arteries (LNAs) develop, form precursors of BA
- Transient anastomoses between dorsal LNAs develop, and ICAs appear (primitive trigeminal/hypoglossal arteries, etc.)
- Definitive VAs arise from 7th cervical intersegmental arteries, anastomose with LNAs
- LNAs fuse as temporary connections with ICAs regress → definitive BA, vertebrobasilar circulation formed

GRAPHICS AND VOLUME-RENDERED CTA

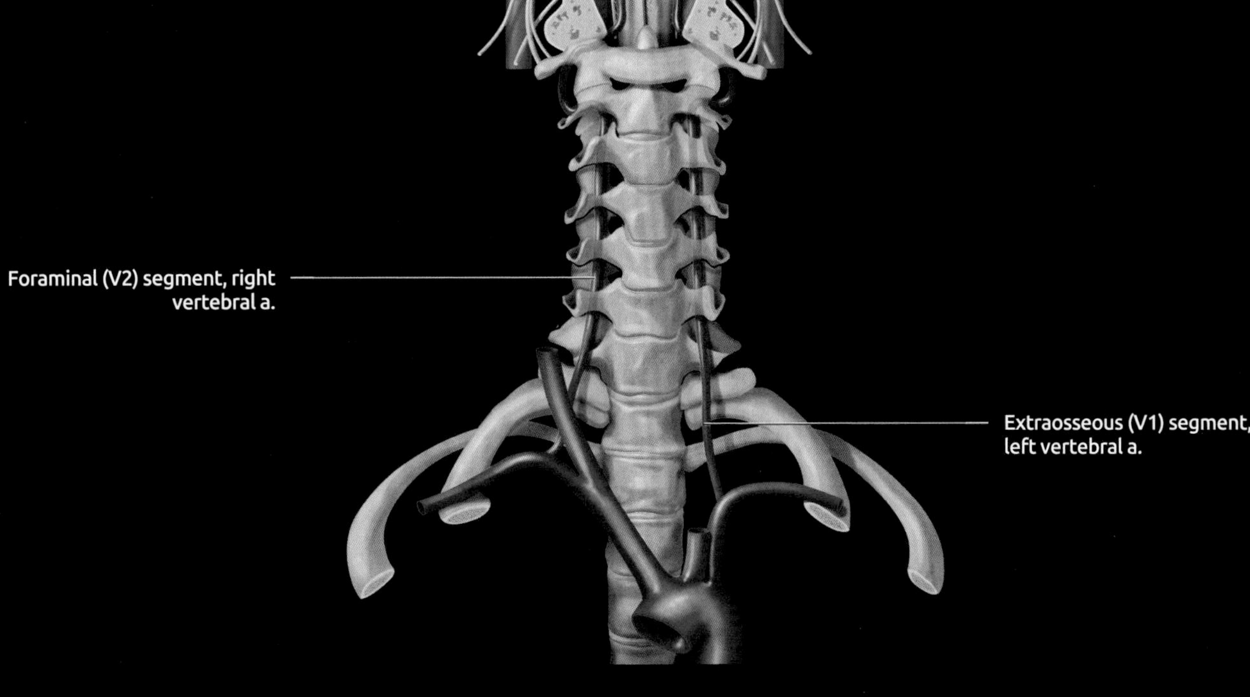

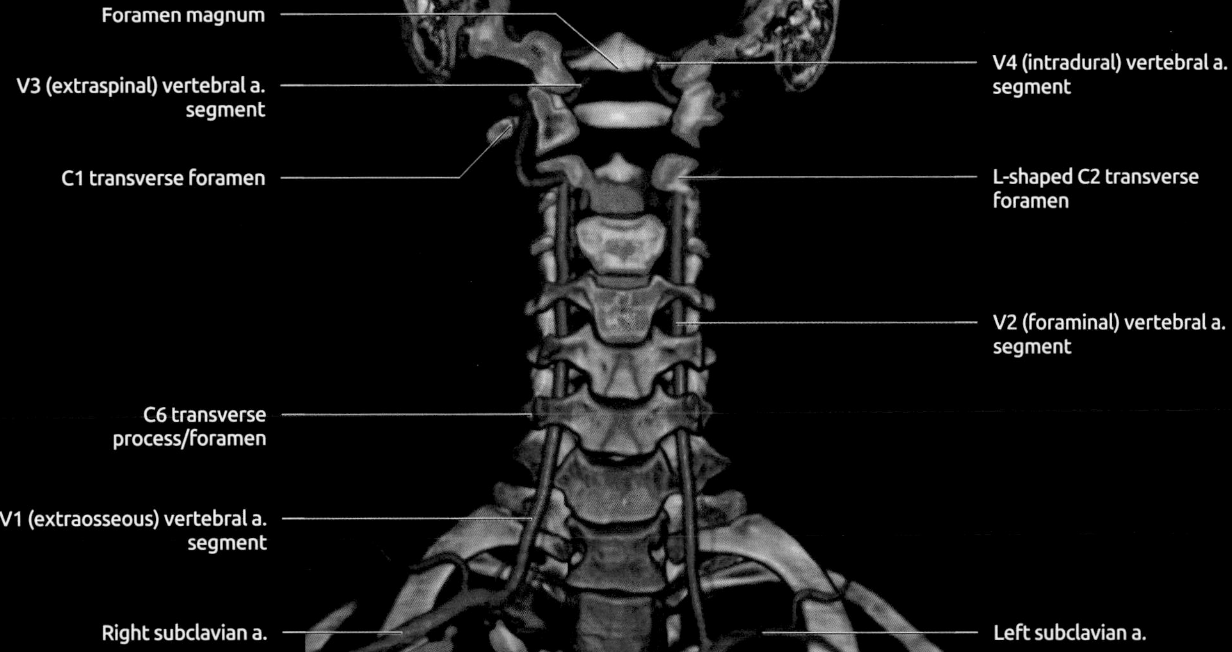

(Top) *AP graphic shows 2 of the 3 extracranial segments of the vertebral arteries and their relationship to the cervical spine. The extraosseous (V1) vertebral artery segments extend from the superior aspect of the subclavian arteries to the C6 transverse foramina. The V2 (foraminal) segment extends from C6 to the vertebral artery exit from the C1 transverse foramina.* **(Bottom)** *3D-VRT CTA shows the extracranial vertebral arteries, which originate from the superior aspect of the subclavian arteries. The vertebral arteries typically enter the transverse foramina of C6 and ascend almost vertically to C2, where they make a 90° turn laterally in the L-shaped C2 transverse foramina before ascending vertically again to C1.*

TRANSVERSE, LONGITUDINAL GRAYSCALE AND COLOR DOPPLER ULTRASOUND

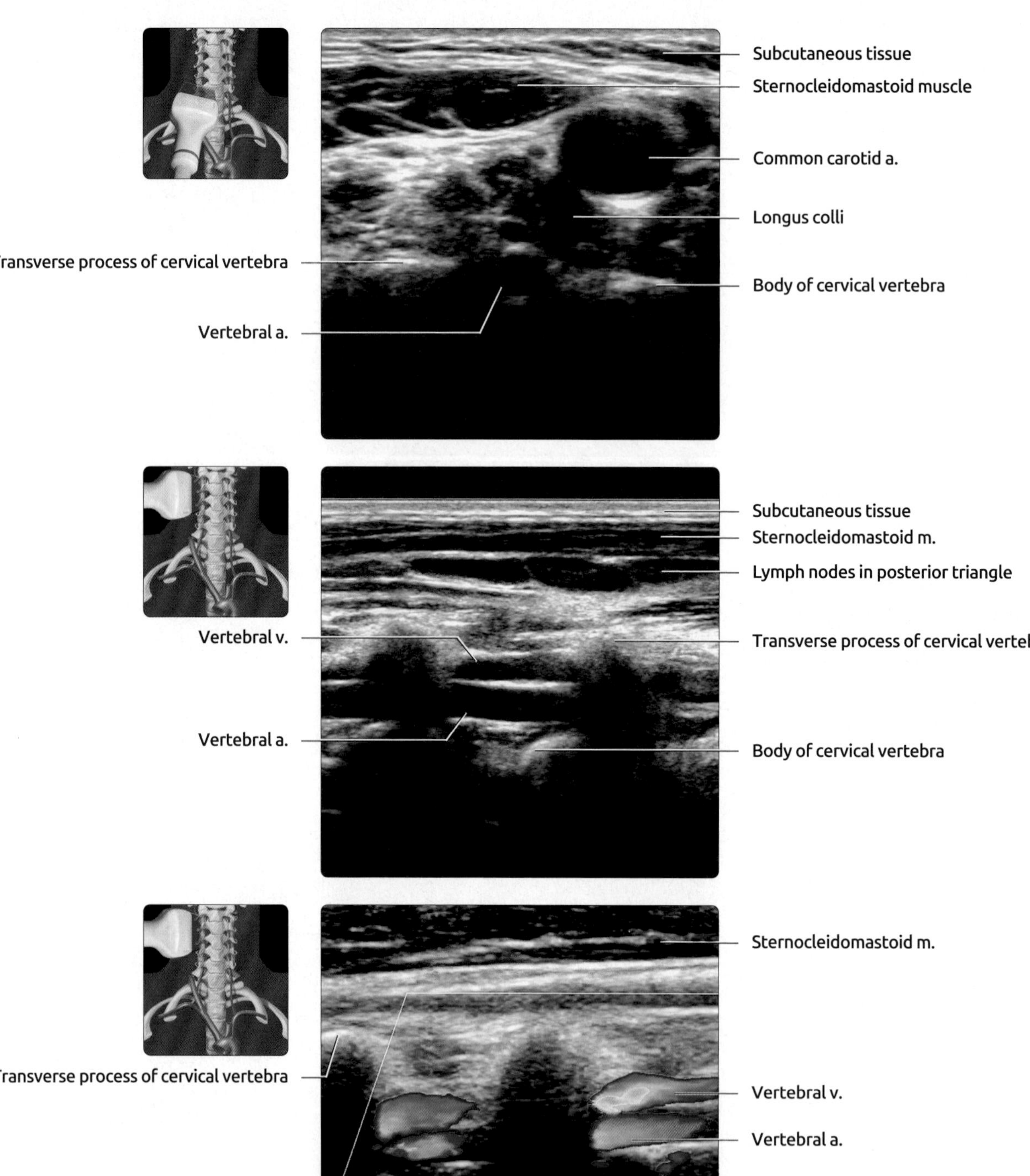

(Top) *Transverse grayscale ultrasound of the lower neck shows the proximal V1 segment of the vertebral artery, which arises from the 1st part of the subclavian artery and courses superiorly to enter the transverse foramina of the lower cervical vertebra. Note its posterior relationship to the longus colli at this level.* **(Middle)** *Longitudinal grayscale ultrasound of the posterior neck demonstrates the V2 segment of the vertebral artery within the transverse foramina of the cervical vertebrae. Note the presence of dense posterior acoustic shadowing from the transverse processes, obscuring a clear view of the underlying vertebral vessels.* **(Bottom)** *Color Doppler ultrasound shows the V2 segment of the vertebral artery in the longitudinal plane. Note the opposite flow direction of the vertebral vein (i.e., craniocaudal direction) as compared with that of the vertebral artery (caudocranial direction).*

AXIAL AND CORONAL CECT, SPECTRAL DOPPLER ULTRASOUND

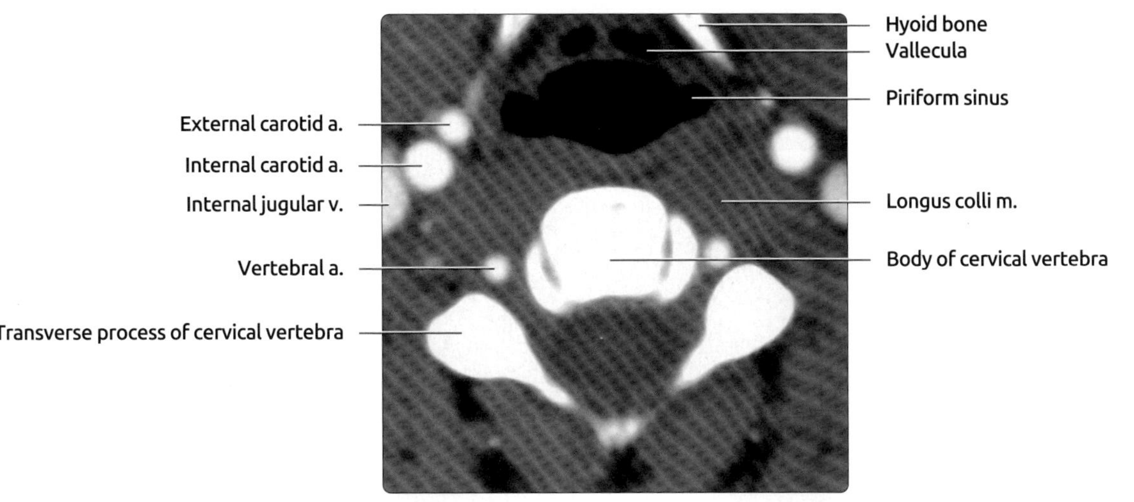

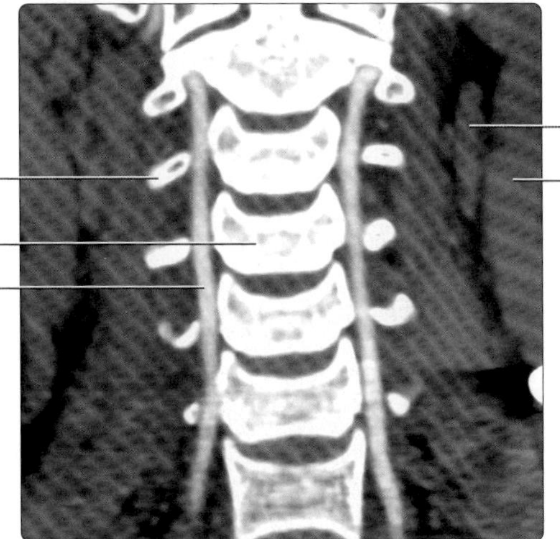

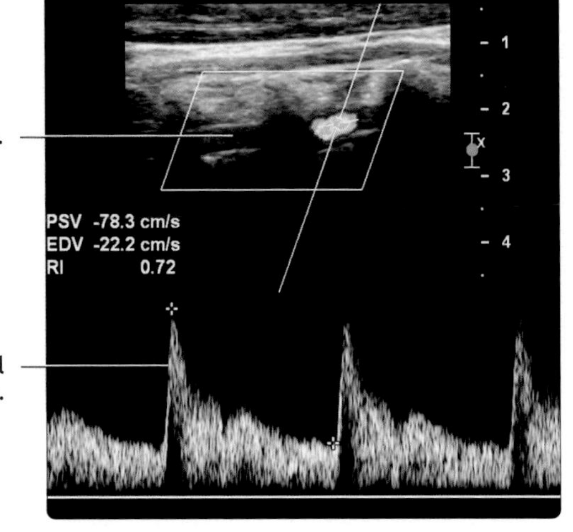

(Top) *Axial CECT of the neck at the level of the hyoid bone shows the vertebral artery running in a caudocranial direction within the foramen transversarium of the cervical vertebrae. This portion is amenable for ultrasound examination.* **(Middle)** *Coronal reformatted CECT of the neck shows the vertical course of the vertebral arteries through the transverse foramina of C6-C2 vertebrae. Note its close anatomical relationship with the transverse processes and bodies of the cervical vertebrae.* **(Bottom)** *Spectral Doppler ultrasound of the V2 segment of the vertebral artery is of low resistance, similar to that of the common carotid artery, but with lower amplitude. Spectral analysis of the V2 segment provides a clue to stenosis/occlusion proximally and distally. For example, a high-resistance flow pattern without a diastolic flow component is often associated with a distal flow obstruction.*

GRAYSCALE AND DOPPLER ULTRASOUND

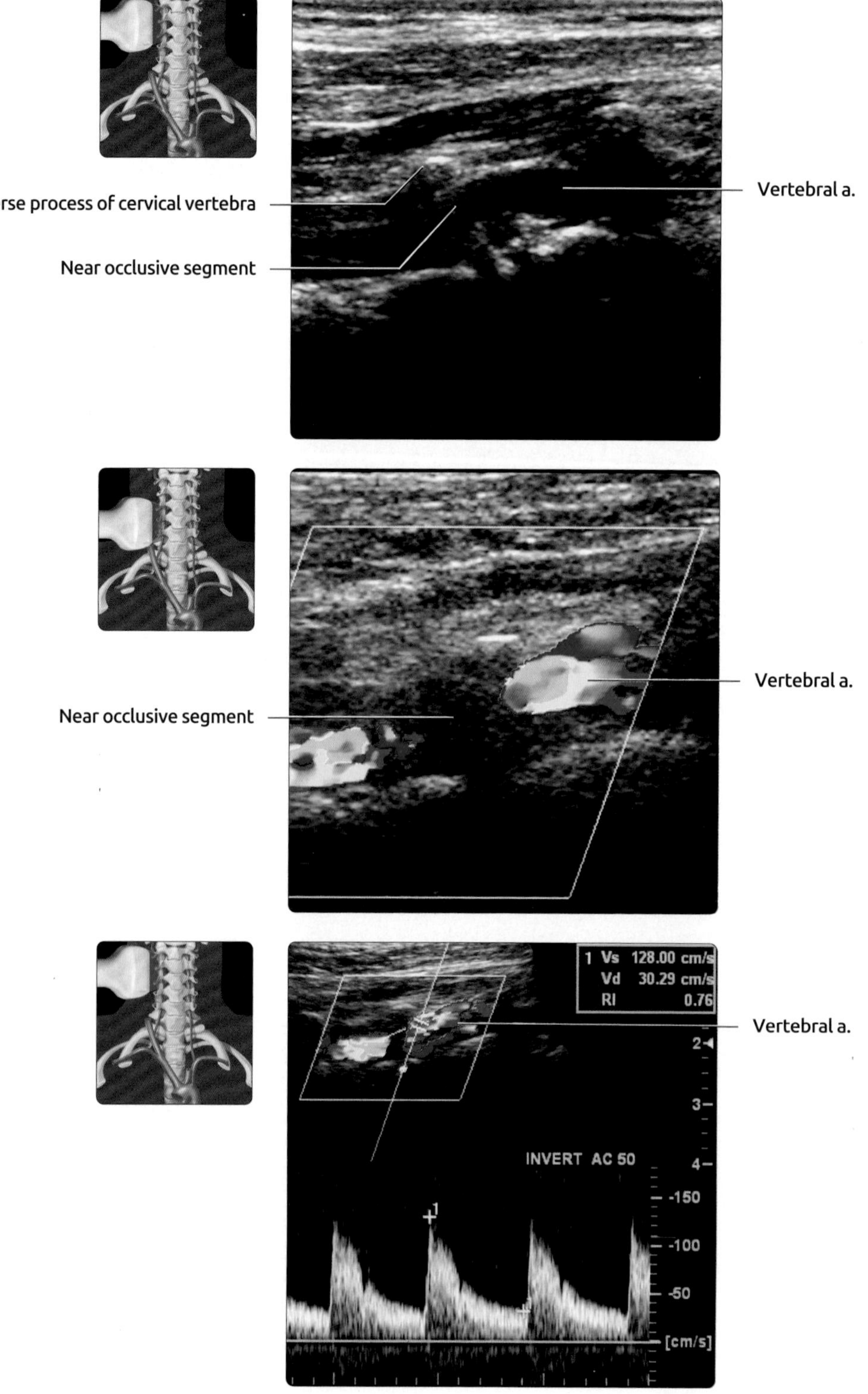

(Top) *Longitudinal grayscale ultrasound of the V2 segment of the vertebral artery shows the presence of hypoechoic atherosclerotic plaque, causing near-complete occlusion.* **(Middle)** *Color Doppler ultrasound of the vertebral artery in the same patient shows a lack of arterial color flow within the nearly occluded segment.* **(Bottom)** *Spectral Doppler ultrasound in the same patient shows a high-resistance flow pattern with elevated peak systolic and diastolic velocities.*

GRAYSCALE AND DOPPLER ULTRASOUND

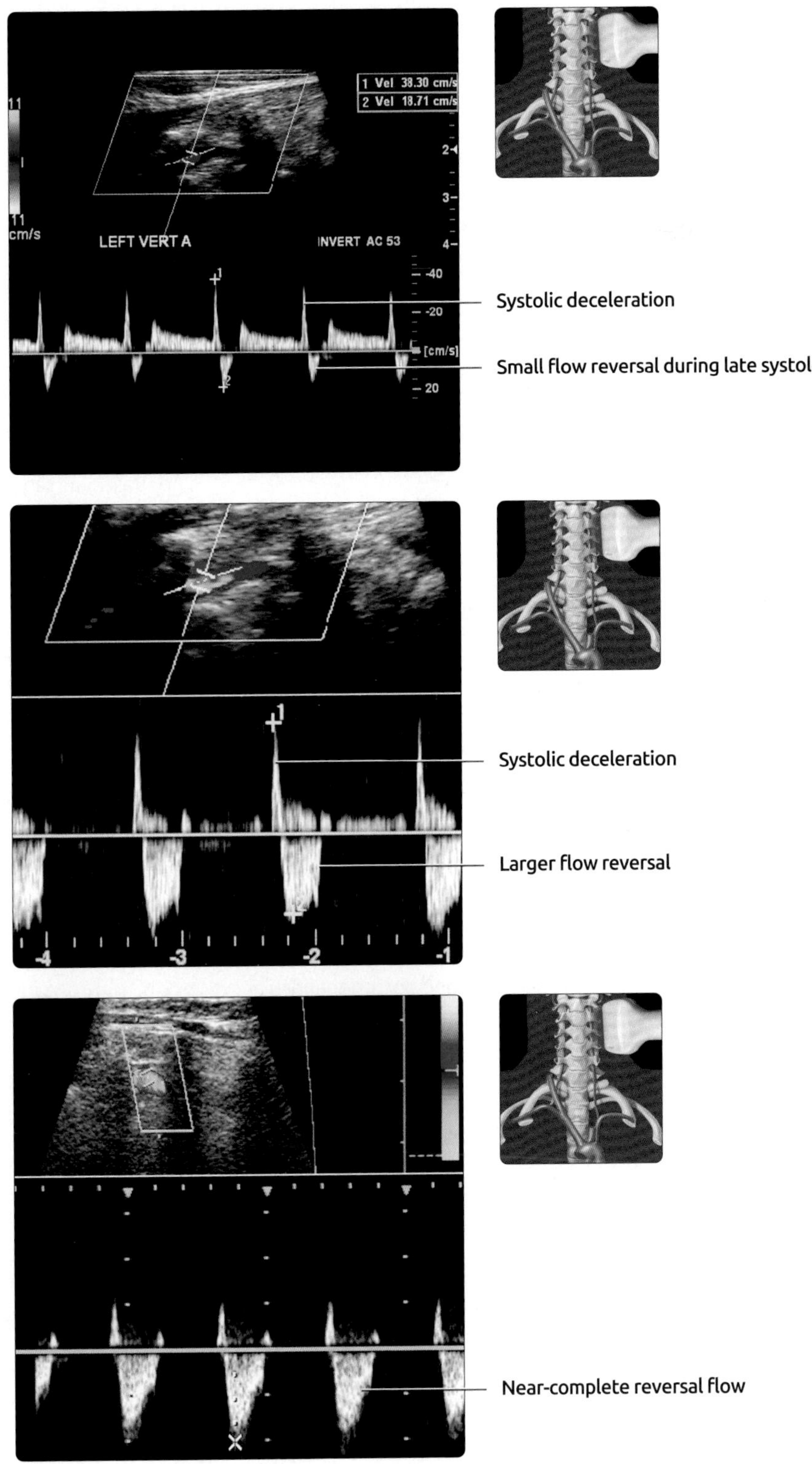

(Top) *Spectral Doppler ultrasound shows a mild degree of subclavian steal syndrome. There is systolic deceleration of the vertebral flow in an antegrade direction with small flow reversal during late systole.* **(Middle)** *Spectral Doppler ultrasound shows a moderate degree of subclavian steal syndrome. The degree of systolic deceleration and flow reversal is more pronounced with alternating vertebral flow demonstrated.* **(Bottom)** *Spectral Doppler ultrasound shows severe subclavian steal syndrome. There is near-complete reversal of flow in the vertebral artery with relative absent antegrade flow. This pattern is commonly associated with the occurrence of vertebrobasilar symptoms.*

TERMINOLOGY

Abbreviations

- Internal jugular vein (IJV)
- External jugular vein (EJV)
- Retromandibular vein (RMV)

GROSS ANATOMY

Overview

- Major extracranial venous system composed of facial veins, neck veins, scalp, skull (diploic), and orbital veins
- Facial veins
  - Facial vein
    - Begins at angle between eye, nose
    - Descends across masseter, curves around mandible
    - Joins IJV at hyoid level
    - Tributaries from orbit (supraorbital, superior ophthalmic veins), lips, jaw, facial muscles
  - Deep facial vein
    - Receives tributaries from deep face, connects facial vein with pterygoid plexus
  - Pterygoid plexus
    - Network of vascular channels in masticator space between temporalis/lateral pterygoid muscles
    - Connects cavernous sinuses and clival venous plexus to face/orbit tributaries
    - Drains into maxillary vein
  - RMV
    - Formed from union of maxillary and superficial temporal veins
    - Lies within parotid space
    - Passes between external carotid artery (ECA) and CNVII to empty into IJV
- Neck veins
  - EJV
    - From union of retromandibular and posterior auricular veins
    - Courses inferiorly on surface of sternocleidomastoid muscle
    - Drains into subclavian vein in supraclavicular fossa
    - Receives tributaries from scalp, ear, and face
    - Size, extent highly variable
  - IJV
    - Caudal continuation of sigmoid sinus from jugular foramen at skull base
    - Jugular bulb = dilatation at origin
    - Courses inferiorly in carotid space posterolateral to internal/common carotid arteries underneath sternocleidomastoid muscle
    - Unites with subclavian vein to form brachiocephalic vein
    - Size highly variable; significant side-to-side asymmetry common; right usually larger than left
  - Subclavian vein
    - Proximal continuation of axillary vein in thoracic inlet
    - EJV drains into subclavian vein
    - Subclavian vein joins IJV to form brachiocephalic vein
  - Vertebral venous plexus
    - Suboccipital venous plexus
    - Tributaries from basilar plexus, cervical musculature
    - Interconnects with sigmoid sinuses, cervical epidural venous plexus
    - Terminates in brachiocephalic vein

IMAGING ANATOMY

Overview

- Low pressure inside; easily compressible
  - Light probe pressure with good surface contact between transducer and skin to ensure optimal visualization
  - Valsalva maneuver helps to distend major neck veins
- IJV
  - Largest vein of neck
  - Deep cervical chain lymph nodes commonly found along its course
  - Beware of thrombosis in patients with previous central venous catheterization or adjacent tumors
  - Always check for compressibility and phasicity on respiration
  - Vascularity in IJV thrombosis usually seen with tumor thrombus rather than bland venous thrombus
- Subclavian vein
  - Accessible on US by inferior tilting of transducer in supraclavicular fossa
  - Venous valves present in most patients
  - Thrombosis/stenosis commonly seen in patients on chronic hemodialysis or with previous subclavian venous catheterization
- RMV
  - Serves as landmark on US to infer position of intraparotid portion of facial nerve
  - Anterior division of RMV sandwiched between submandibular gland anteriorly and parotid tail posteriorly
    - Its displacement helps to determine origin of mass in posterior submandibular region

ANATOMY IMAGING ISSUES

Imaging Pitfalls

- Neck veins often overlooked as most sonologists pay more attention to arteries than veins in neck
- Not all neck veins readily assessed by US
  - Only large and superficial veins clearly seen
- Asymmetric IJVs common; 1 IJV may be many times the size of contralateral IJV
  - IJV venous varix: Extreme dilatation of IJV upon Valsalva maneuver with clinically palpable neck lump
- Slow flow within IJV may appear as low-level, hyperechoic intraluminal "mass"
  - May mimic IJV thrombus
  - Moving nature of echoes on real-time US and sharp linear near-field interface help to distinguish artifacts from slow flow and IJV thrombus

CLINICAL IMPLICATIONS

Clinical Importance

- US safely guides needle for venous access
- Absence of respiratory phasicity is strong indicator of abnormality

GRAPHIC

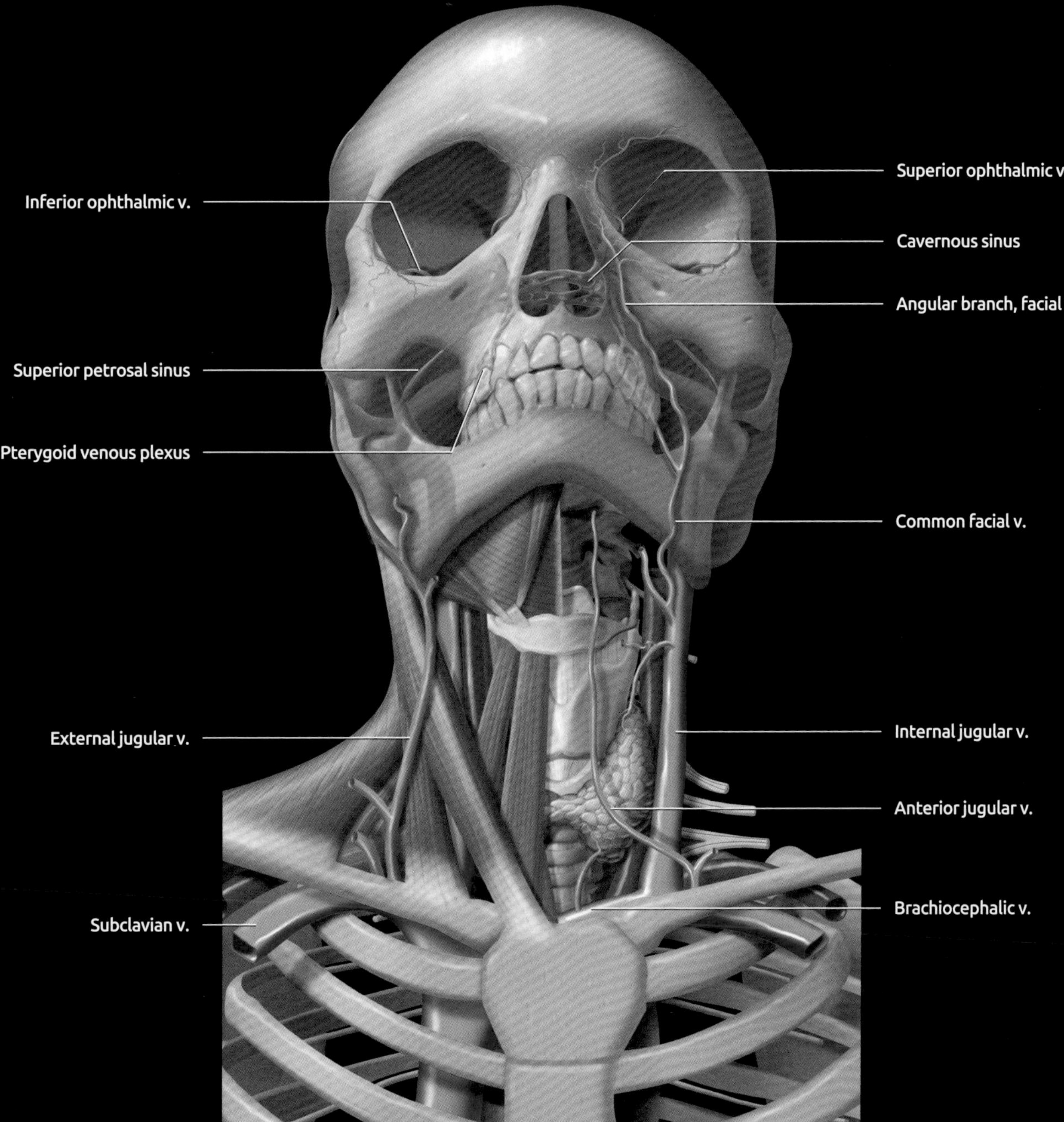

Anteroposterior view of the extracranial venous system depicts the major neck veins, their drainage into the mediastinum, and their numerous interconnections with the intracranial venous system. The pterygoid venous plexus receives tributaries from the cavernous sinus and provides an important potential source of collateral venous drainage if the transverse or sigmoid sinuses become occluded.

GRAYSCALE AND COLOR DOPPLER ULTRASOUND INTERNAL JUGULAR VEIN

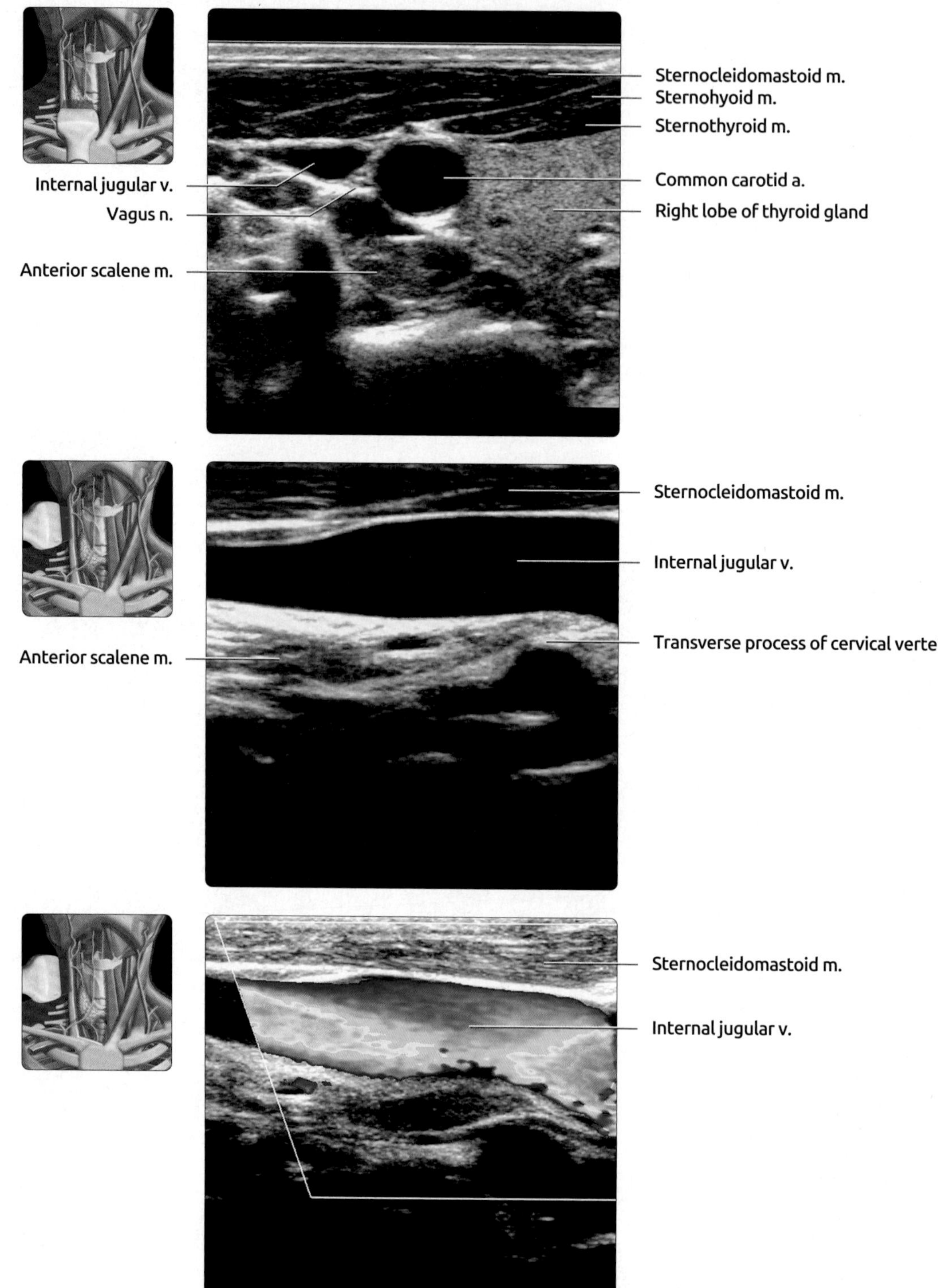

(Top) *Transverse grayscale ultrasound of the lower cervical level shows the normal anatomical relationship between the internal jugular vein and the adjacent structures. It is underneath the sternocleidomastoid muscle and lateral to the common carotid artery and vagus nerve within the carotid sheath.* **(Middle)** *Longitudinal grayscale ultrasound shows the internal jugular vein in the midcervical level. The internal jugular vein appears as a tubular anechoic structure coursing in a vertical direction. It should be examined with light probe pressure and with compression to exclude a venous thrombosis.* **(Bottom)** *Corresponding color Doppler ultrasound in the longitudinal plane shows color flow filling the entire lumen of the internal jugular vein. The use of color Doppler helps to identify and evaluate the presence and nature of an internal jugular vein thrombus.*

CECT AND SPECTRAL DOPPLER ULTRASOUND INTERNAL JUGULAR VEIN

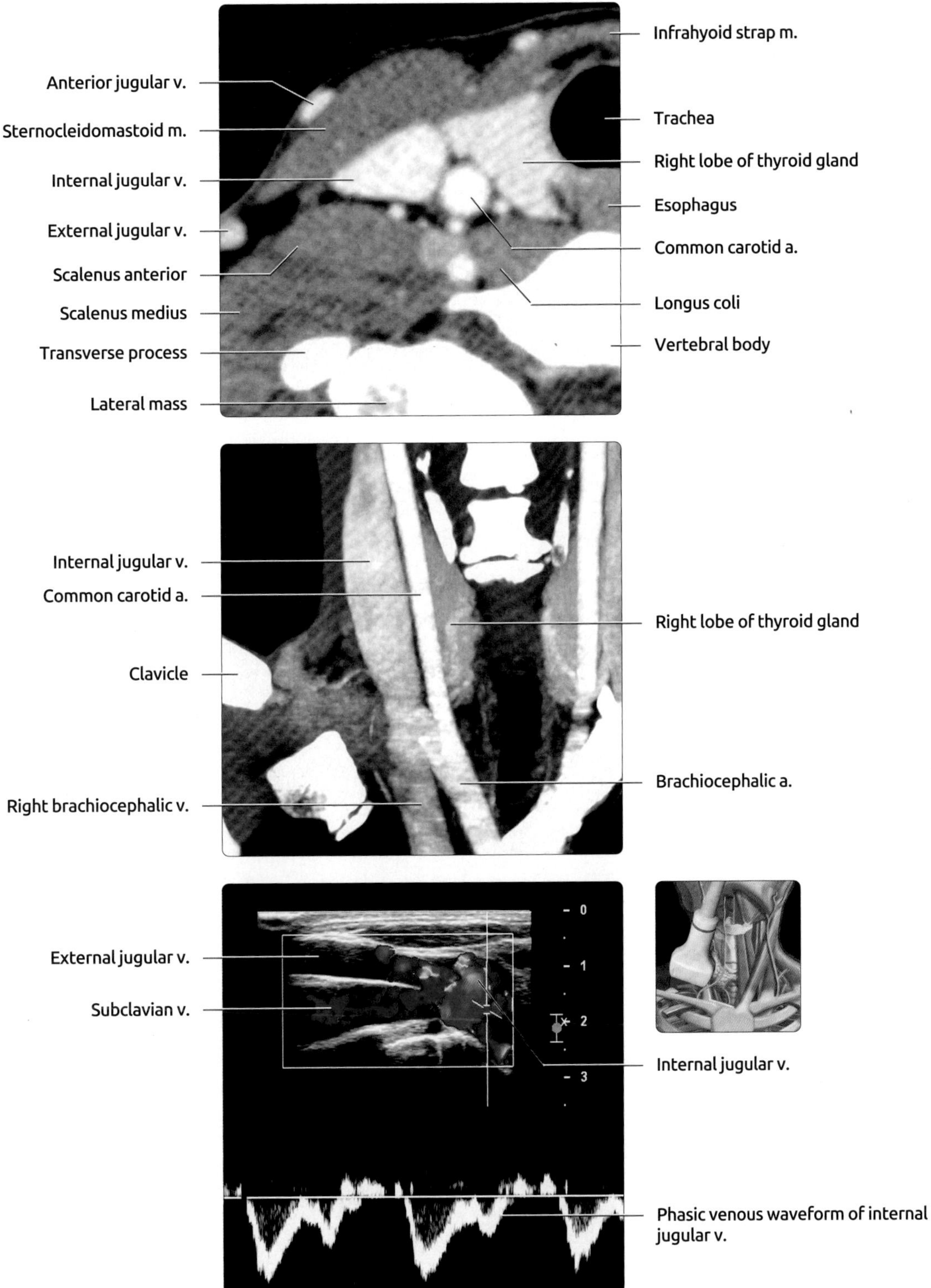

(Top) *Axial CECT of the lower neck shows the internal jugular vein, which is usually larger than and lateral to the common carotid artery. The external jugular vein is in a subcutaneous location.* **(Middle)** *Coronal reformatted CECT of the lower neck shows the close anatomical relationship of the internal jugular vein and common carotid artery within the carotid sheath. The internal jugular vein continues inferiorly below the clavicle to join the subclavian vein to form the brachiocephalic vein.* **(Bottom)** *Transverse spectral Doppler ultrasound shows the internal jugular vein at the level of the supraclavicular fossa at the junction with the subclavian vein. The normal triphasic venous waveform, which varies with respiratory motion, can be easily demonstrated and helps to exclude the presence of obstructing venous thrombus.*

GRAYSCALE AND COLOR DOPPLER ULTRASOUND EXTERNAL JUGULAR VEIN

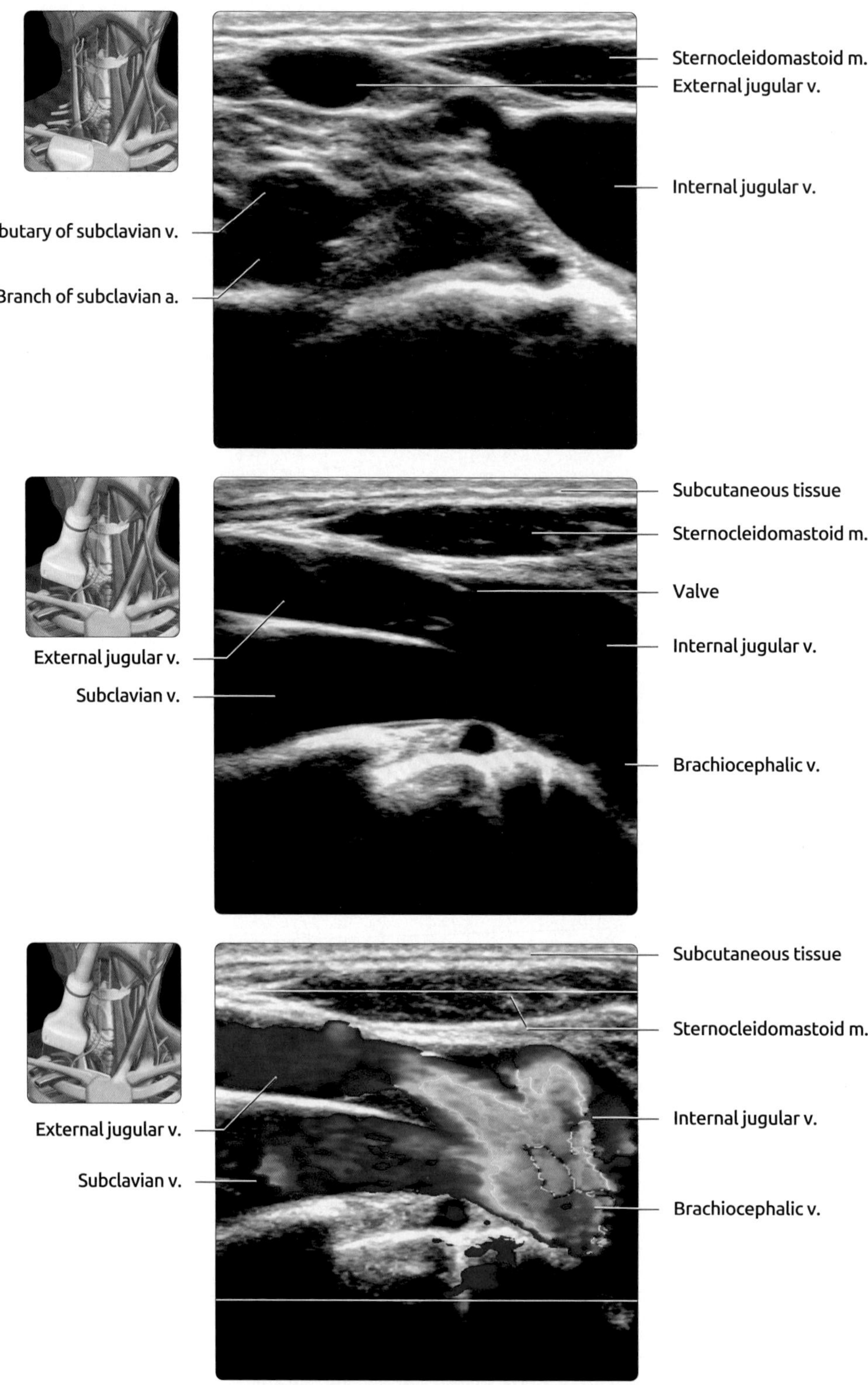

(Top) *Transverse grayscale ultrasound of the right lower neck shows the location of the external jugular vein in relation to the sternocleidomastoid muscle. It appears as a distended, round, anechoic structure on Valsalva maneuver using light transducer pressure.* **(Middle)** *Transverse grayscale ultrasound shows the external jugular vein at the supraclavicular level, at the site of union with the subclavian vein, close to the terminal portion of the internal jugular vein. Valve leaflets are commonly seen within the major veins at the thoracic inlet level.* **(Bottom)** *Corresponding transverse color Doppler ultrasound at the supraclavicular level helps to depict the venous drainage of the external jugular vein to the subclavian vein. Note that the subclavian vein joins the internal jugular vein to form the brachiocephalic vein.*

CECT AND SPECTRAL DOPPLER ULTRASOUND EXTERNAL JUGULAR VEIN

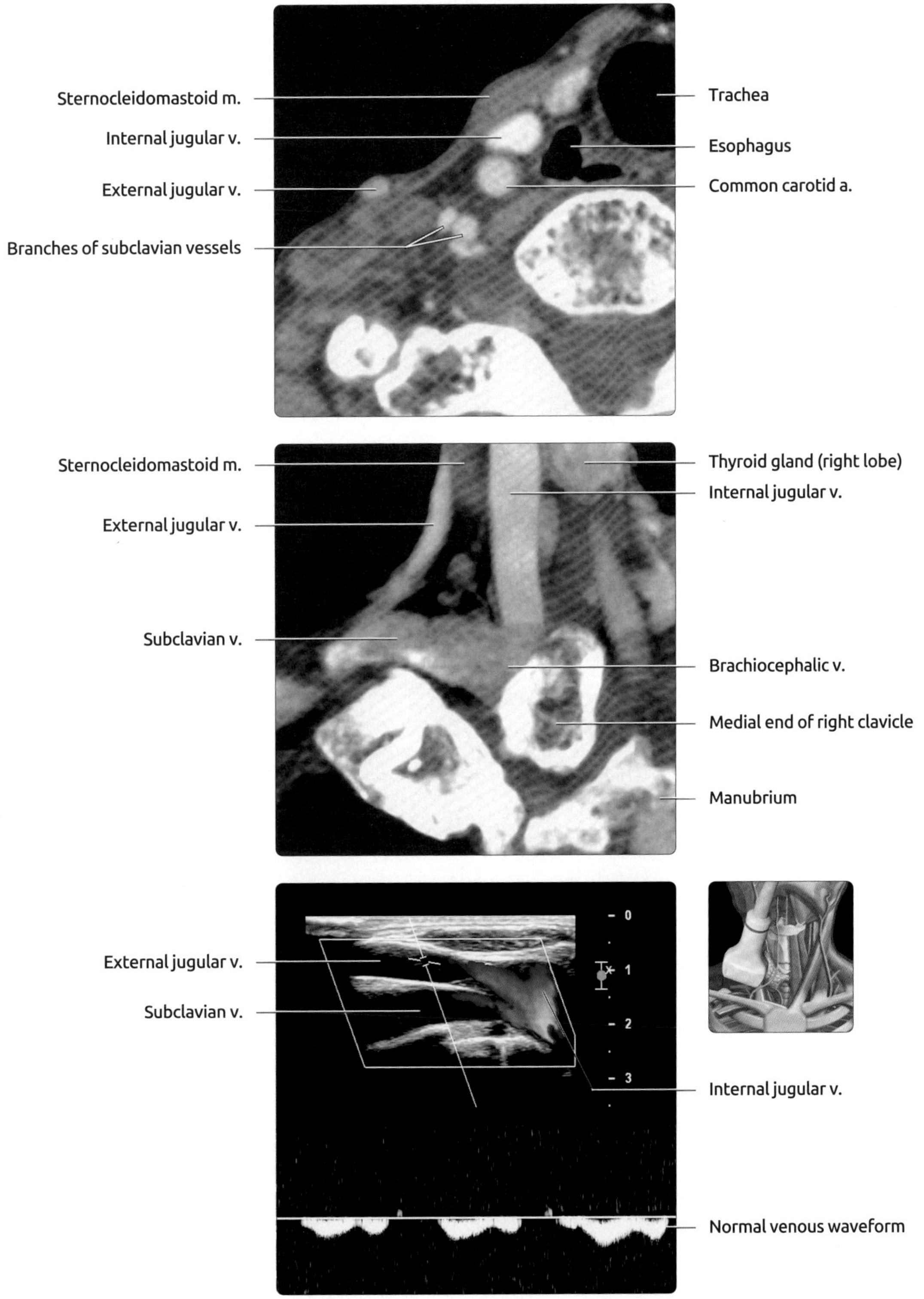

(Top) *Axial CECT shows the right lower neck. Note the superficial anatomical location of the external jugular vein. Thus, light probe pressure is necessary for the assessment of the external jugular vein on ultrasound, because with increasing pressure, the vein will be compressed.* **(Middle)** *Coronal reformatted CECT shows the right lower neck. Note the drainage of the external jugular vein to the subclavian vein, which joins the internal jugular vein to form the brachiocephalic vein at the thoracic inlet level.* **(Bottom)** *Spectral Doppler ultrasound interrogating the terminal portion of the external jugular vein shows a normal, phasic, low-pressure venous waveform, which helps to confirm its patency.*

LONGITUDINAL AND TRANSVERSE ULTRASOUND

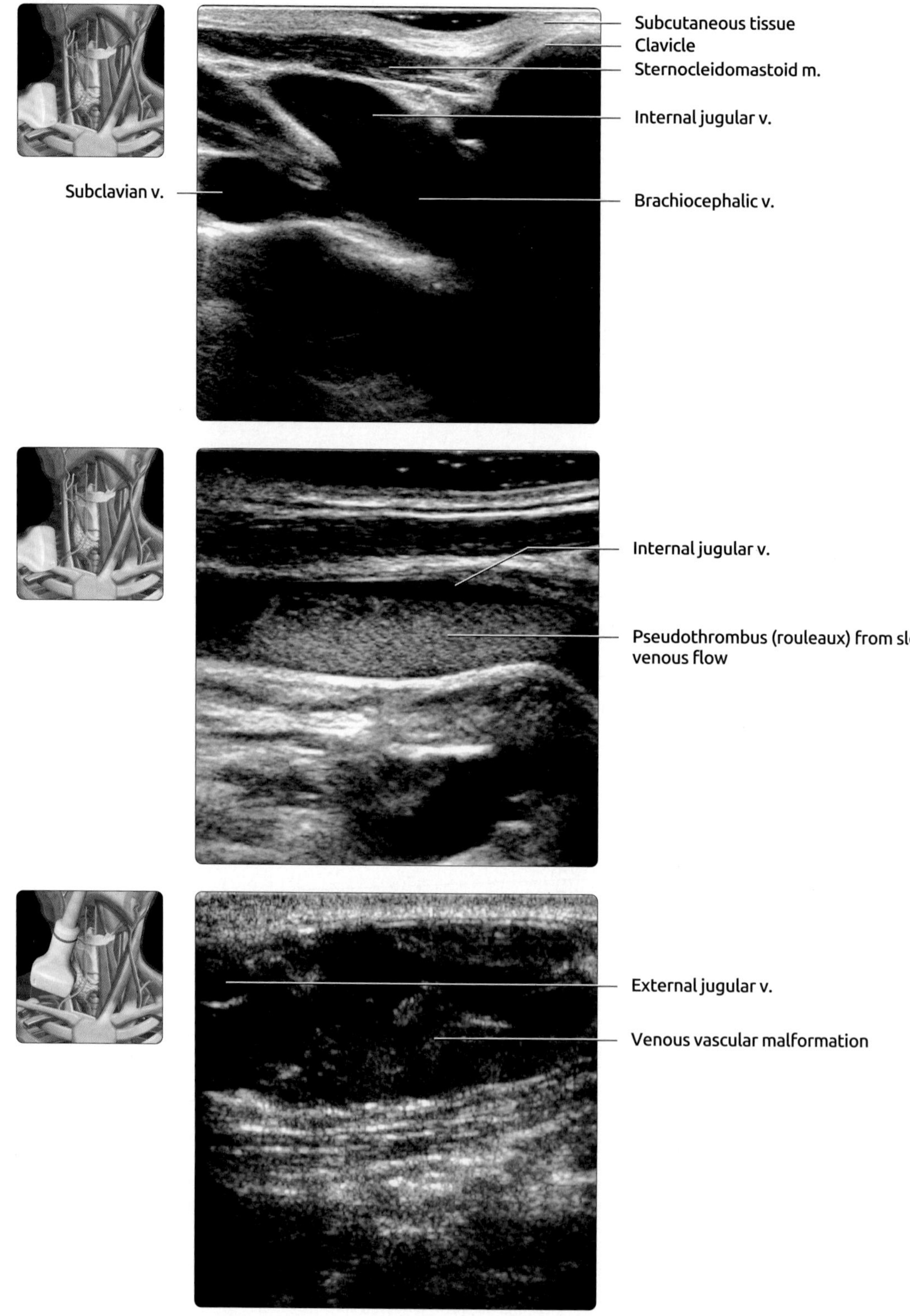

(Top) *Longitudinal grayscale ultrasound at the supraclavicular level shows the union of the internal jugular vein and subclavian vein to form the brachiocephalic vein. The more distal portion of the brachiocephalic vein is obscured by the overlying clavicle and is therefore not assessed by ultrasound.* **(Middle)** *Longitudinal grayscale ultrasound of the right internal jugular vein shows a pseudothrombus (rouleaux) phenomenon due to slow venous flow within the internal jugular vein. Note the layering with a sharp linear border in the internal jugular vein lumen in the near field, which is the clue to distinguish it from venous thrombus.* **(Bottom)** *Transverse grayscale ultrasound of the right posterior triangle shows a well-defined, hypoechoic mass with multiple internal sinusoidal spaces. The lesion is inseparable from the external jugular vein. Surgery confirmed a venous vascular malformation arising from the external jugular vein.*

CECT, COLOR AND POWER DOPPLER ULTRASOUND

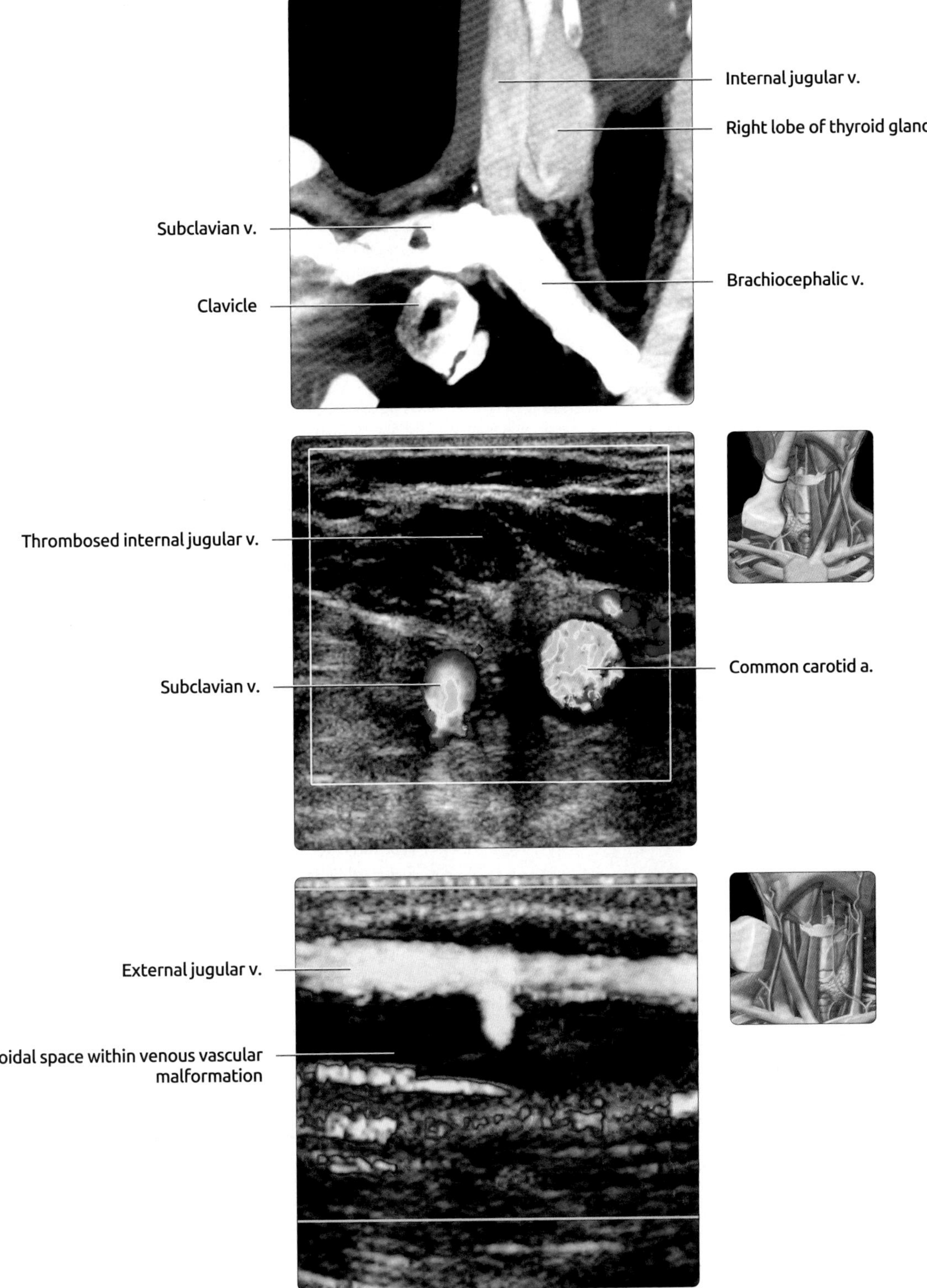

(Top) *Coronal reformatted CECT of the right supraclavicular fossa shows the formation of the brachiocephalic vein by union of the subclavian vein (dense contrast filling due to injection in ipsilateral antecubital fossa) and internal jugular vein. The brachiocephalic vein can be fully assessed on CECT as compared with ultrasound.* **(Middle)** *Transverse color Doppler ultrasound of the right supraclavicular level reveals intraluminal, hypoechoic, avascular echoes causing occlusion of the internal jugular vein. The appearances are of a bland venous thrombus due to prolonged central venous catheterization.* **(Bottom)** *Longitudinal power Doppler ultrasound shows the external jugular vein venous vascular malformation. Note the intimate relationship of the venous vascular malformation and the external jugular vein. Sinusoidal spaces are usually not color filled due to very slow flow within.*

TERMINOLOGY

Abbreviations

- Inferior vena cava (IVC)

Definitions

- "Proximal" and "distal" in arterial and venous systems apply to position of arterial and venous segment in relation to heart (rather than direction of flow)
- Aneurysm: Focal increase in caliber of artery with diameter of dilated segment measuring at least 1.5x > adjacent unaffected segments

GROSS ANATOMY

Overview

- Abdominal aorta
  - Enters abdomen at T12 level, bifurcates at L4
  - Level of origins of major branches: Celiac axis (T12), superior mesenteric artery (SMA) (L1), renal arteries (L1/2), IMA (L3), common iliac arteries (L4)
- IVC
  - Blood from alimentary tract passes through portal venous system before entering IVC through hepatic veins
  - Begins at L5 level with union of common iliac veins
  - Leaves abdomen via IVC hiatus in diaphragm at T8 level
  - IVC tributaries correspond to paired visceral and parietal branches of aorta
  - IVC development has complex embryology
    - Various anomalies common (up to 10% of population), especially at and below level of renal veins
    - All are variations of persistence/regression of embryologic sub- and supracardinal veins

IMAGING ANATOMY

Overview

- Not all branches of abdominal aorta and tributaries of IVC can be well seen on ultrasound examination
- Major arterial branches of abdominal aorta seen on ultrasound
  - Celiac artery, common hepatic artery, splenic artery, SMA, inferior mesenteric artery (IMA), renal arteries, common iliac arteries
- Major venous tributaries draining into IVC
  - Common iliac veins, renal veins, hepatic veins

Internal Contents

- Abdominal aorta
  - Normal peak systolic velocity (PSV): 60-110 cm/s
  - Spectral Doppler waveform
    - Upper: Narrow, well-defined systolic complex with forward flow during diastole
    - Mid: Reduced diastolic flow
    - Distal: Absent diastolic flow, similar to lower limb arteries
  - Normal caliber: 15-25 mm
    - Upper: 22 mm above renal arteries
    - Middle: 18 mm below renal arteries
    - Lower: 15 mm above bifurcation
  - Best imaging plane: Both transverse and longitudinal
- Celiac axis
  - Normal PSV: 98-105 cm/s
  - Spectral Doppler demonstrates low-resistance flow with high end-diastolic velocities
  - Flow velocity not dependent on food intake
  - Normal caliber: 6-10 mm
  - Best imaging plane: Transverse plane to show typical T-shaped bifurcation
- Common hepatic artery
  - Normal PSV: 70-120 cm/s
  - Spectral Doppler shows low-resistance flow characteristics with large amount of continuous flow in diastole
  - Normal caliber: 4-10 mm
  - Best imaging plane
    - Start transverse midline to follow common hepatic artery to right of T-shaped bifurcation from celiac axis
    - Gastroduodenal artery may be seen to arise from common hepatic artery along anterosuperior aspect of pancreas; thereafter, common hepatic artery becomes proper hepatic artery
      - Proper hepatic artery normal PSV: 60-100 cm/s
- Splenic artery
  - Normal PSV: 70-110 cm/s
  - Spectral Doppler shows typically turbulent flow due to tortuosity of vessel
  - Normal diameter: 4-8 mm
  - Best imaging plane
    - Transverse midline approach shows proximal portion of artery wall
    - Intercostal through spleen, using it as acoustic window; useful for showing distal splenic artery around hilum
- SMA
  - Normal PSV: 97-142 cm/s
  - Spectral Doppler demonstrates high impedance flow with low diastolic velocities during fasting due to relative vasoconstriction
  - End-diastolic velocity increases typically 30-90 minutes after meals due to vasodilation of mesenteric branches
  - Normal caliber: 5-8 mm
  - Best imaging plane
    - Longitudinal midline approach best for evaluation of SMA blood flow
    - Transverse plane useful for identifying short anteriorly directed stump; shows dot-like appearance, surrounded by distinctive triangular mantle of fat
- IMA
  - Normal PSV: 93-189 cm/s
  - Spectral Doppler demonstrates high impedance flow with low diastolic velocities during fasting due to relative vasoconstriction
  - End-diastolic velocity increases after meal due to vasodilation of mesenteric branches
  - Normal caliber: 1-5 mm
  - Best imaging plane: Transverse plane following line of aorta; origin of IMA arises from below origins of renal arteries and may be anterior or slightly to left of midline
- Renal arteries
  - Normal PSV: 60-140 cm/s, not > 180 cm/s

  - Spectral Doppler demonstrates open systolic window, rapid systolic upstroke occasionally followed by secondary slower rise to peak systole with subsequent gradual diastolic delay but with persistent forward flow in diastole
  - Normal caliber: 5-8 mm
  - Best imaging plane
    - Transverse anterior midline approach best for identification of origins of renal arteries
    - Posterolateral approach using kidneys as acoustic window useful for visualization of distal portions of renal arteries
- Common iliac arteries
  - Normal spectral Doppler shows characteristic triphasic waveform
    - Initial high-velocity peak forward-flow phase resulting from cardiac systole
    - Brief phase of reverse flow in early diastole
    - Low-velocity forward flow in diastole
  - Normal caliber: 8-12 mm
  - Best imaging plane: Transverse anterior approach and oblique anterior approach along long axis of iliac arteries
  - Stenosis causing 1-19% diameter reduction
    - Triphasic waveform with minimal spectral waveform broadening
    - PSV increase < 30% relative to adjacent proximal segment; proximal and distal waveform remain normal
  - Stenosis causing 20-49% diameter reduction
    - Triphasic waveform usually maintained, though reverse flow component may be diminished
    - Spectral broadening prominent with filling in of area under systolic peak
    - PSV increase 30-100% relative to adjacent proximal segment; proximal and distal segment remain normal
  - Stenosis causing 50-99% diameter reduction
    - Monophasic waveform with loss of reverse flow component, forward flow throughout cardiac cycle
    - Extensive spectral broadening
    - PSV increase > 100% relative to adjacent proximal segment
    - Distal waveform monophasic with reduced systolic velocity
  - Occlusion
    - No flow, preocclusive thump may be heard proximal to site of obstruction
    - Distal waveforms are monophasic with reduced systolic velocities
- IVC
  - Normal PSV: 44-118 cm/s
  - Spectral Doppler shows slow flow that varies with respiration and cardiac pulsation
  - Normal caliber: 5-29 mm during quiet inspiration
  - Best imaging plane: Both transverse and longitudinal
- Common iliac veins
  - Spectral Doppler shows 5 normal characteristics
    - Spontaneous flow, phasic flow, flow ceases with Valsalva maneuver, flow augmentation with distal compression, unidirectional flow toward heart
  - Best imaging plane: Transverse anterior approach and oblique anterior approach along long axis of iliac veins
- Renal veins
  - Normal PSV: 18-33 cm/s
  - Right renal vein relatively short and drains directly into IVC
  - Left renal vein runs a slightly longer course; receives left gonadal vein, usually courses anterior to aorta before joining IVC
  - Spectral Doppler of right renal vein mirrors pulsatility of IVC
  - Spectral Doppler of left renal vein may show only slight variability of flow velocities consequent upon cardiac and respiratory activity
  - Normal caliber: 4-9 mm
  - Best imaging plane: Transverse anterior approach
- Hepatic veins
  - Normal PSV: 16-40 cm/s
  - Spectral Doppler shows triphasic waveform due to transmitted cardiac activity
  - Best imaging plane: Transverse/oblique subcostal approach with cranial angulation

ANATOMY IMAGING ISSUES

Imaging Recommendations

- Use 2- to 5-MHz transducer
- Fasting for 12 hours recommended to reduce interference by bowel gas; satisfactory Doppler signal for aorta and IVC can be obtained in up to 90% of patients
- Imaging patient in morning after overnight fast most convenient protocol
- Lateral decubitus position and graded compression to displace intervening bowel gas may be useful
- Angle correction crucial in spectral Doppler assessment
- Detailed delineation of branches of aorta and IVC better assessed on CTA or MRA
- Digital subtractive angiography usually reserved for when intervention may be required (e.g., embolization of mesenteric artery branches in gastrointestinal bleed, renal artery stenting, etc.)

Imaging Approaches

- **Proximal aorta** can be scanned either from an anterior epigastric approach or right coronal approach
- **Midaorta** can be scanned either from a midanterior abdominal approach or by placing the patient in the left lateral decubitus or the right lateral decubitus position, which will allow partial visualization of aorta in the region of the kidney
- **Distal aorta** can be scanned from inferior anterior abdominal window or a coronal approach
  - A coronal approach allows visualization of the distal aorta and both common iliac arteries simultaneously
- Because there is usually no gap between the spine and aorta, when measuring the longitudinal aorta in anterior-posterior dimension, ensure that the spine is not included in the measurement; the aorta wall and spine are both very echogenic and may be difficult to delineate

Imaging Pitfalls

- Bowel gas, patient body habitus, and operator dependence are main factors contributing to suboptimal ultrasound examination of aorta and IVC

AORTA AND INFERIOR VENA CAVA

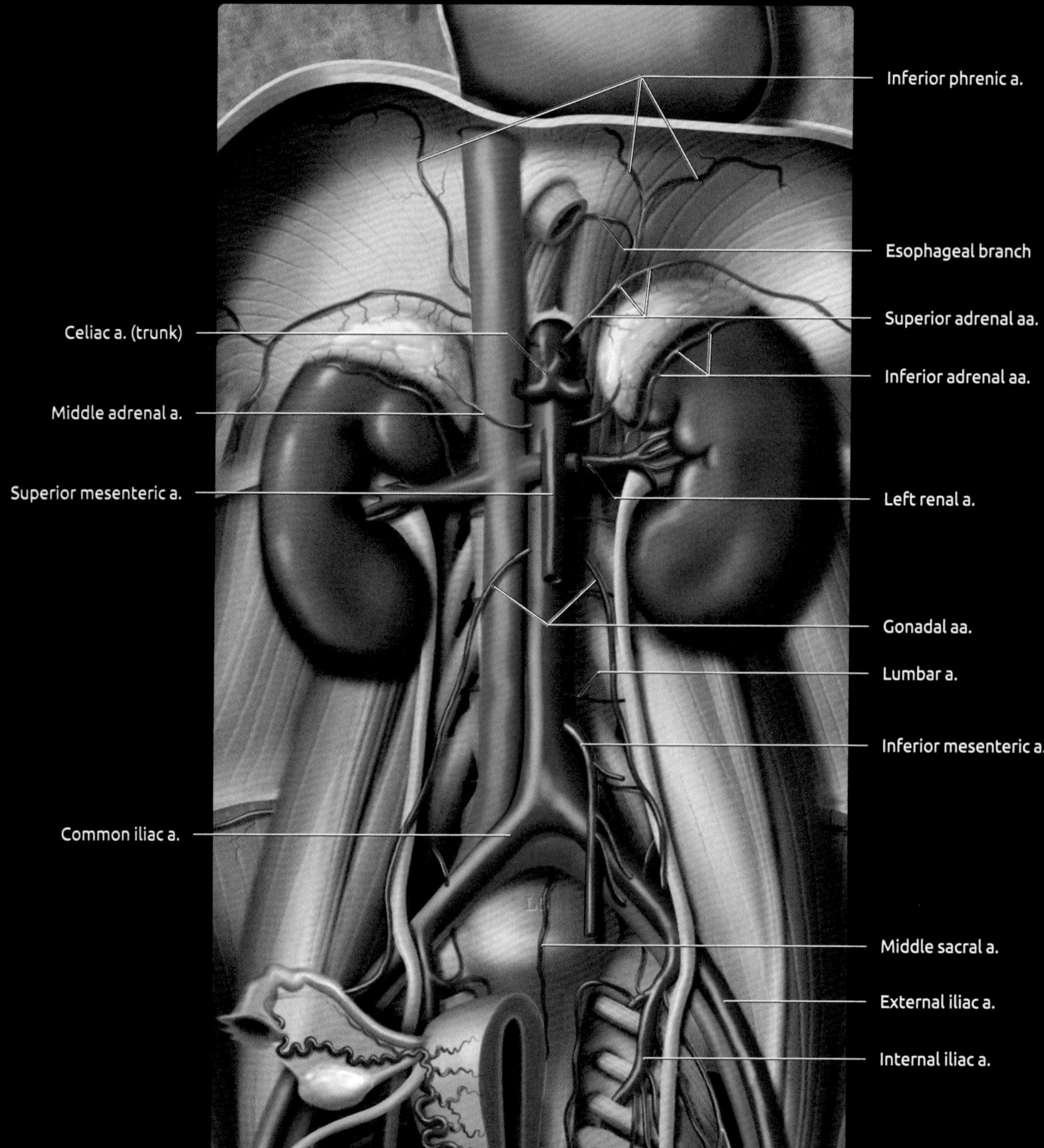

Graphic shows the major arteries to the gastrointestinal tract arise as unpaired vessels from the aortic midline plane and include the celiac, superior, and inferior mesenteric arteries. Branches to the urogenital and endocrine organs arise as paired vessels in the lateral plane and include the renal, adrenal, and gonadal (testicular or ovarian) arteries. The diaphragm and posterior abdominal wall are supplied by paired branches in the posterolateral plane, including the inferior phrenic and lumbar arteries (4 pairs, only 1 of which is labeled here). The anterior abdominal wall is supplied by the inferior epigastric and deep circumflex iliac arteries, both branches of the external iliac artery. The inferior epigastric artery turns superiorly to run in the rectus sheath, where it anastomoses with the superior epigastric artery, a terminal branch of the internal mammary (thoracic) artery.

COMMON VARIATIONS OF INFERIOR VENA CAVA

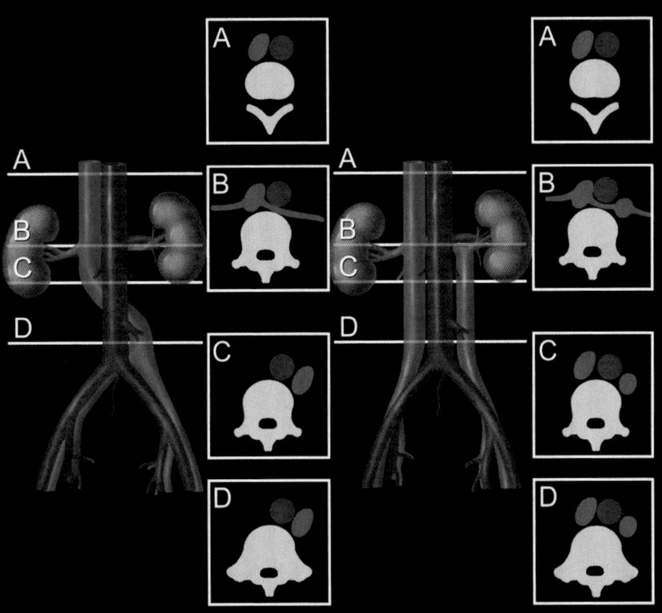

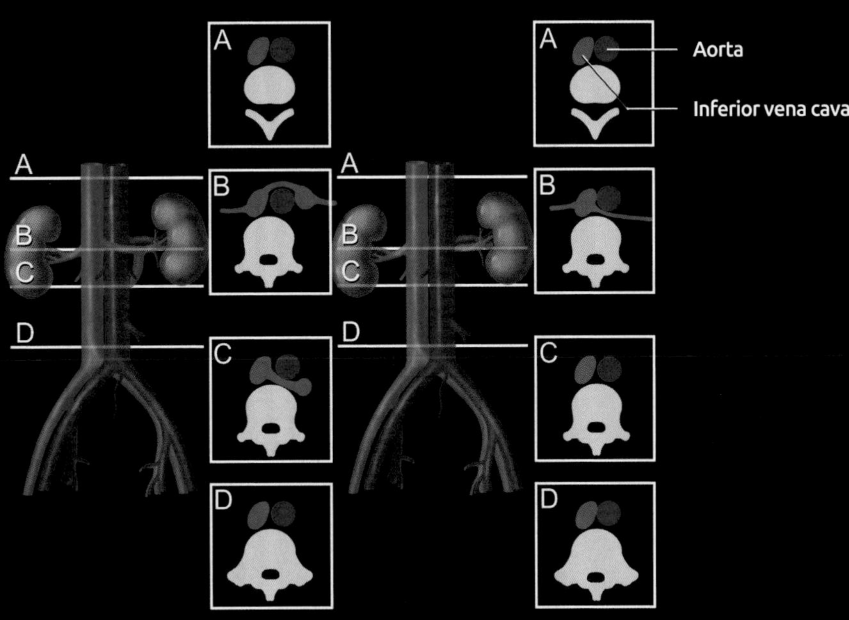

(Top) *First 2 of 4 graphics illustrating common variations of the inferior vena cava (IVC) are shown. The labeled lines on the frontal graphics correspond to the levels of the axial sections. The left graphic shows transposition of the IVC in which the infrarenal portion of the IVC lies predominantly to the left side of the aorta. A more common anomaly is shown on the right graphic, a "duplication" of the IVC in which the left common iliac vein continues in a cephalad direction without crossing over to join the right iliac vein. Instead, it joins the left renal vein and then crosses over to the right. The suprarenal IVC has a conventional course and appearance.* **(Bottom)** *The left graphic shows a circumaortic left renal vein with the smaller, more cephalic vein passing in front of the aorta and the larger vein passing behind and caudal. The right graphic shows a completely retroaortic renal vein.*

PROXIMAL AORTA, SAGITTAL VIEW

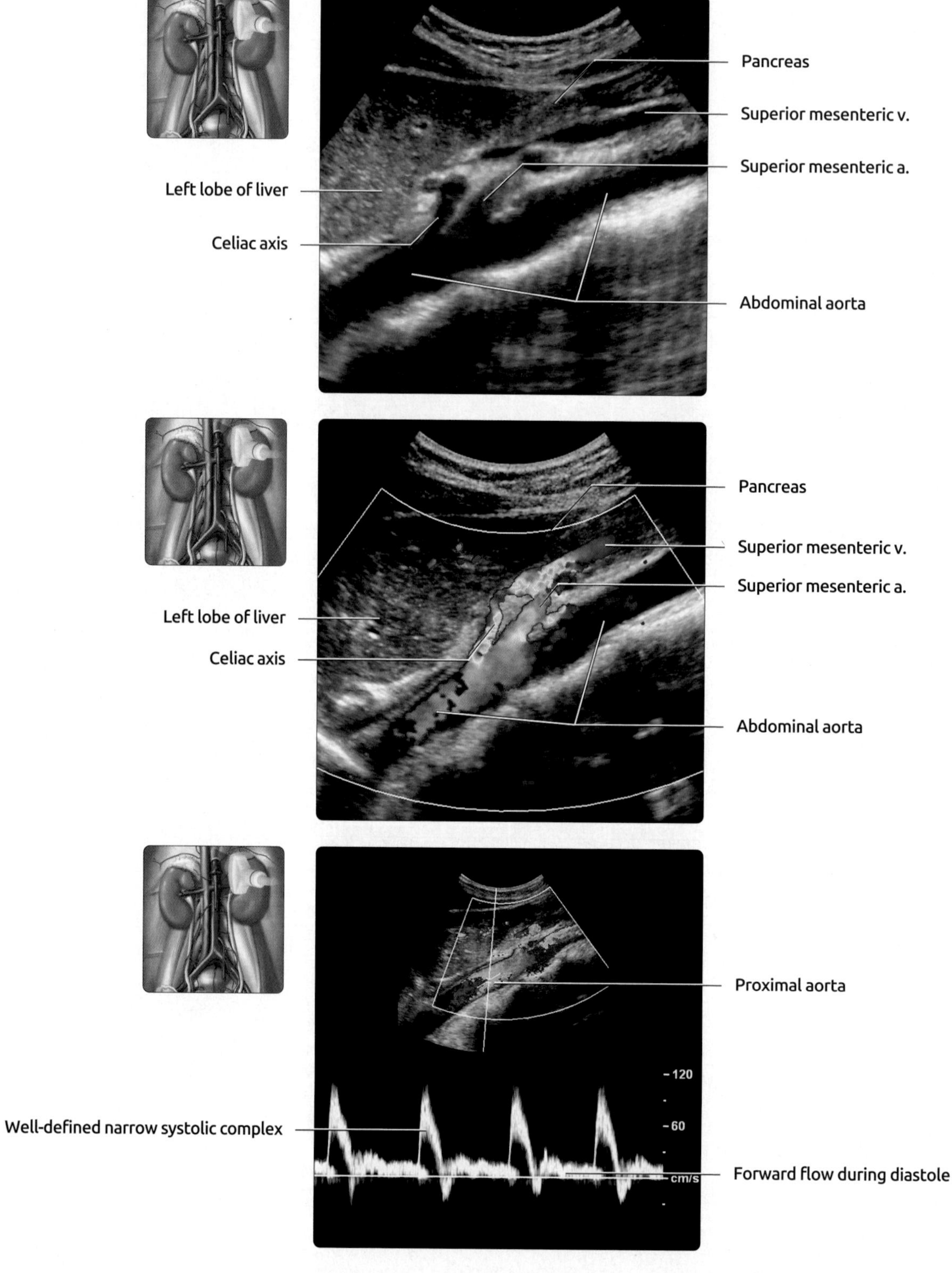

(Top) *Longitudinal grayscale US of the proximal abdominal aorta shows the origins of the celiac axis and superior mesenteric artery (SMA). The origin of the celiac axis is usually seen at T12, whereas the origin of the SMA is usually seen at L1, immediately below the origin of the celiac axis on this view. The normal diameter of the abdominal aorta is 15-25 mm, and the average diameter of the proximal abdominal aorta above the renal arteries is around 22 mm.* **(Middle)** *Longitudinal color Doppler US of the proximal abdominal aorta shows the origins of the celiac axis and SMA. Apart from assessment of flow through the aorta, this is also a useful view for assessment of flow in the SMA.* **(Bottom)** *Spectral Doppler US of the proximal aorta shows a narrow, well-defined systolic complex with forward flow during diastole.*

MIDDLE AND DISTAL AORTA, SAGITTAL VIEW

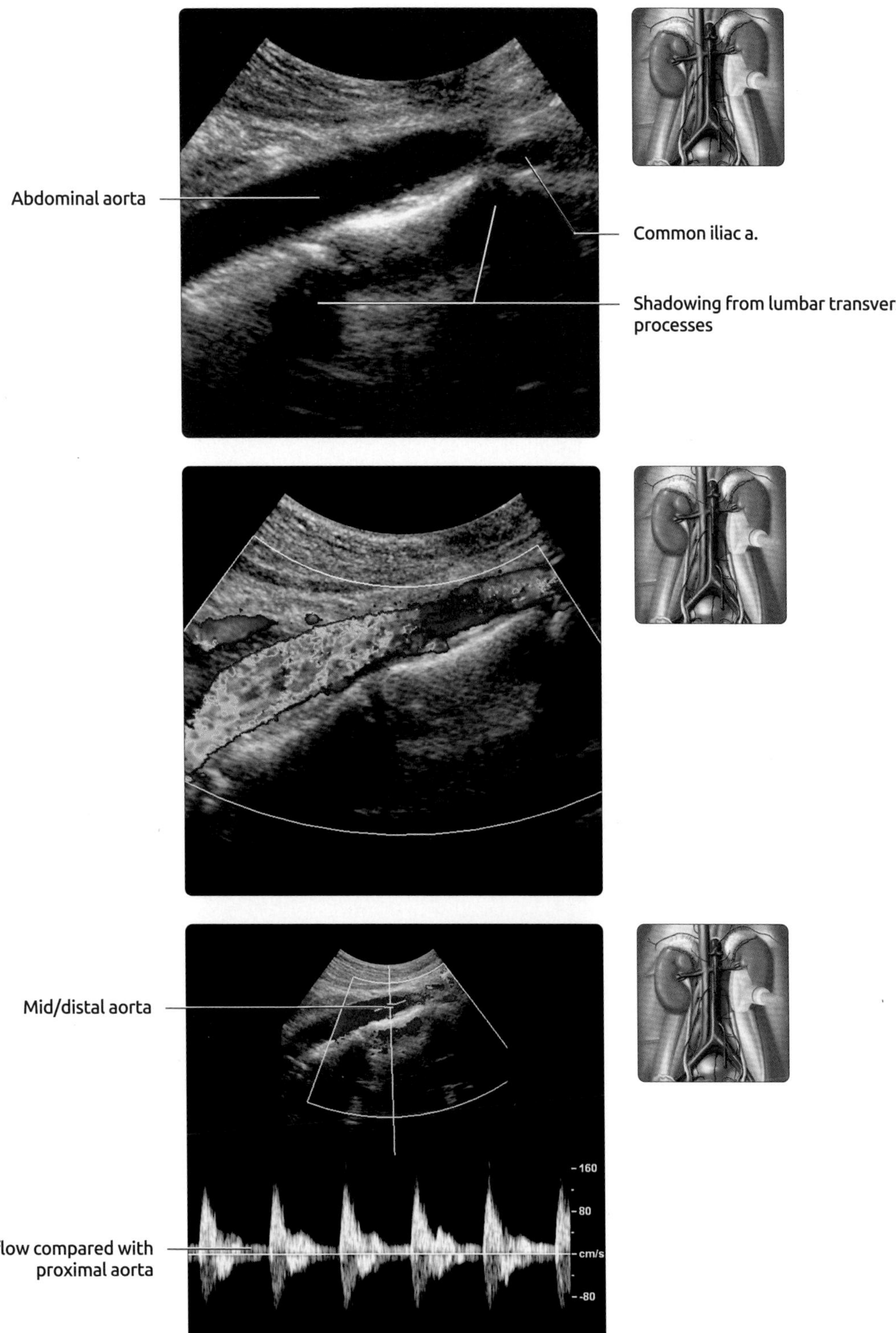

(Top) *Longitudinal grayscale US of the mid/distal abdominal aorta shows 1 of the common iliac arteries coming off the aortic bifurcation. The aortic bifurcation is usually seen at the L4 level. The average diameter of the midportion of the abdominal aorta is ~ 18 mm below the renal arteries and 15 mm above the aortic bifurcation.* **(Middle)** *Color Doppler US of the mid/distal abdominal aorta shows one of the common iliac arteries coming off the aortic bifurcation.* **(Bottom)** *Spectral Doppler US of the mid/distal abdominal aorta shows reduced diastolic flow compared with the proximal aorta. The spectral Doppler waveform to be expected in the distal abdominal aorta usually shows absent diastolic flow, similar to that seen in the lower limb arteries.*

CELIAC AXIS

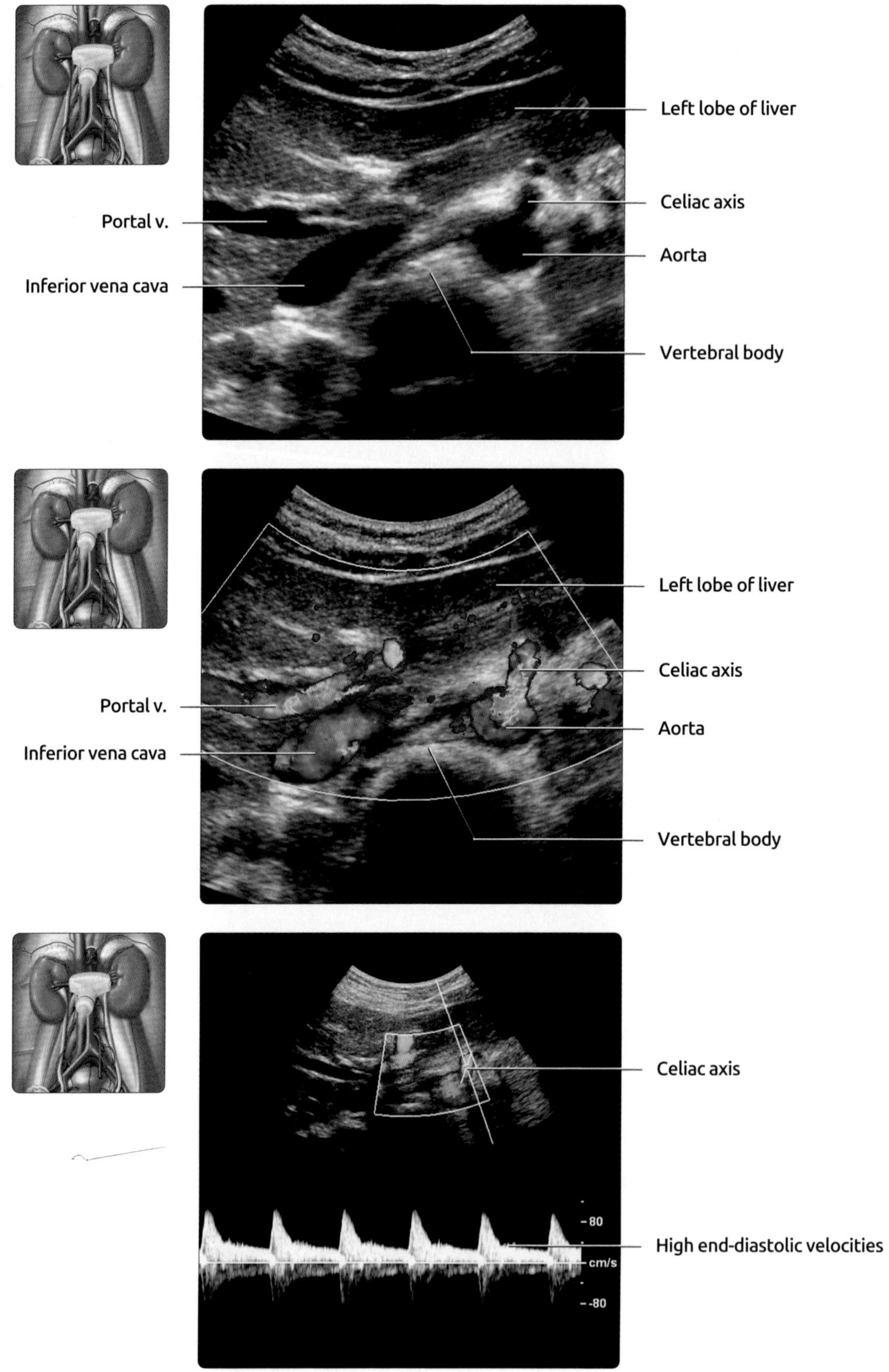

(Top) *Transverse grayscale US shows the abdominal aorta at the level of the celiac axis via a midline approach. The celiac axis is the 1st branch of the abdominal aorta seen arising anteriorly, usually at the level of T12. The normal caliber of the celiac axis is between 6-10 mm. Note the normal position of the IVC to the right of the abdominal aorta.* **(Middle)** *Transverse color Doppler US shows the abdominal aorta at the level of the celiac axis via a midline approach. As the celiac axis is perpendicular to the transducer, a small amount of cranial angulation was used to improve the color Doppler signal obtained.* **(Bottom)** *Spectral Doppler US of the celiac axis shows low-resistance flow with high end-diastolic velocities. Flow velocity in the celiac axis is not dependent on food intake, and the normal peak systolic velocity (PSV) ranges from 98-105 cm/s.*

SPLENIC ARTERY

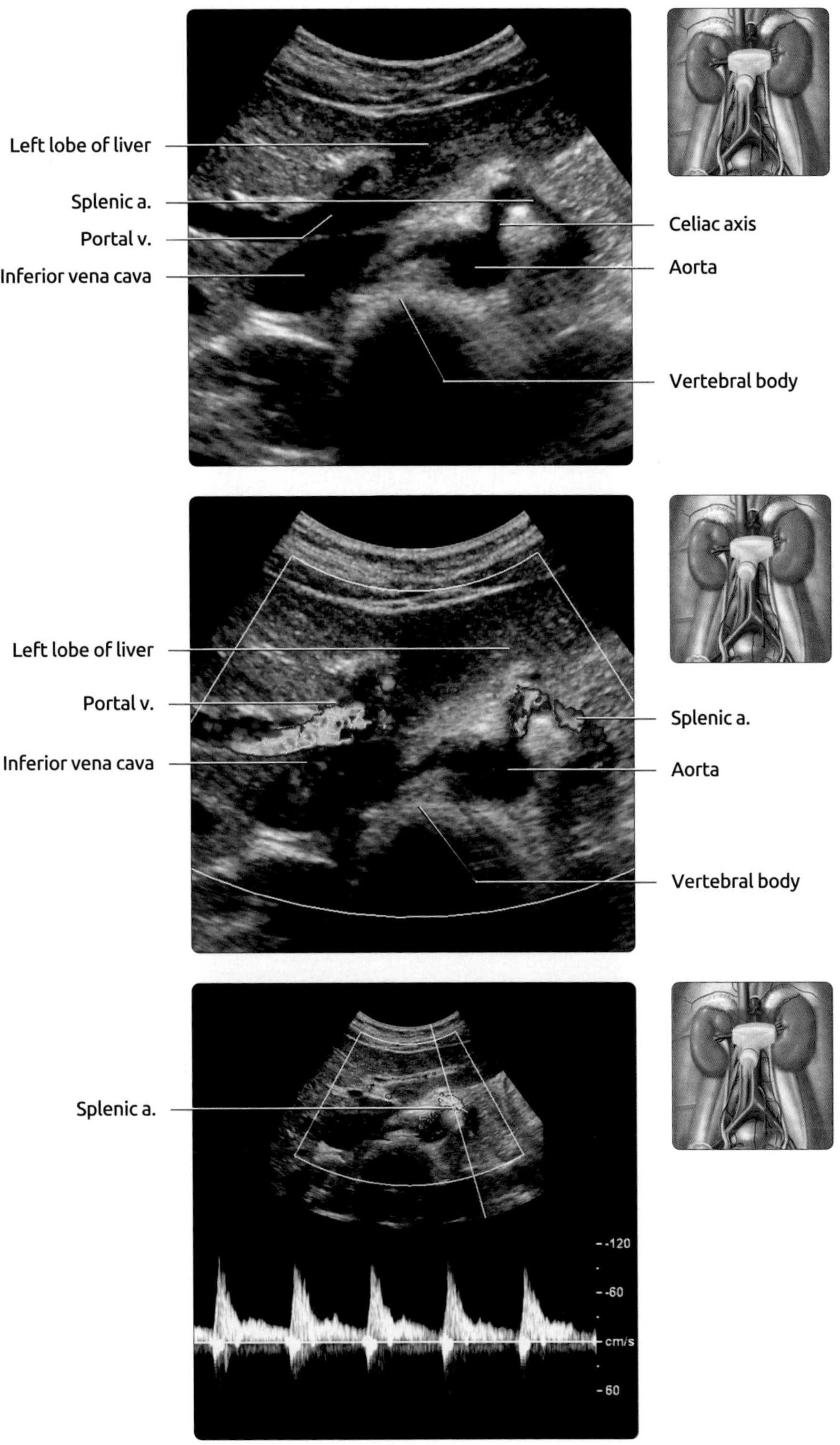

(Top) *Transverse grayscale US via a midline approach shows the origin of the splenic artery as it branches from the celiac axis and hooks to the left. This is usually the best view for visualizing the proximal portion of the splenic artery. The more distal splenic artery is tortuous in its course. An intercostal approach using the spleen as an acoustic window may be useful for showing the distal splenic artery around the hilum. The normal caliber of the splenic artery ranges from 4-8 mm.* **(Middle)** *Transverse color Doppler US via a midline approach shows flow within the proximal splenic artery.* **(Bottom)** *Spectral Doppler US of the proximal splenic artery shows typically turbulent flow due to tortuosity of the vessel. The normal PSV in the splenic artery ranges from 70-110 cm/s.*

COMMON HEPATIC ARTERY

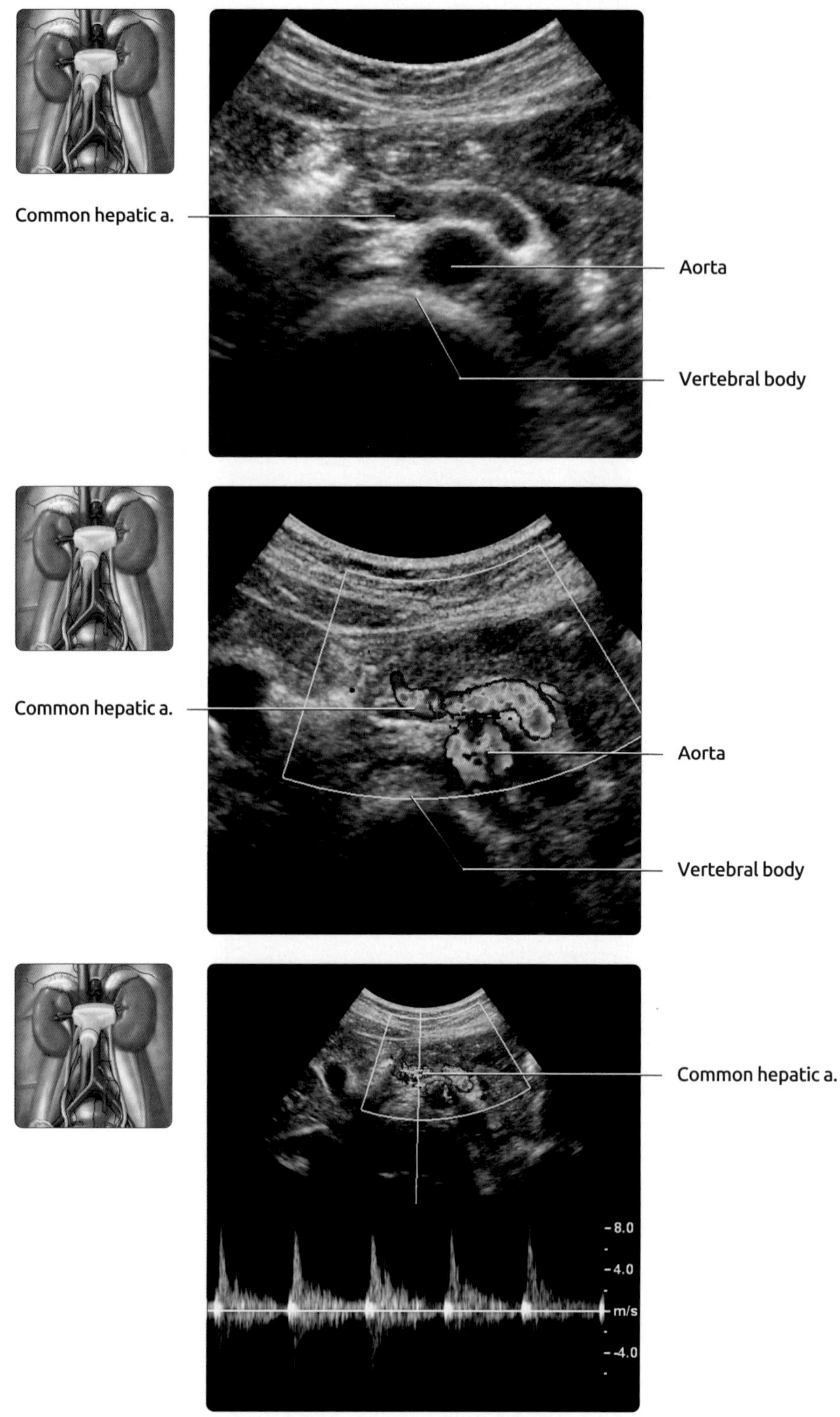

(Top) *Transverse grayscale US via a midline approach shows the proximal portion of the common hepatic artery as it branches to the right, off the T-shaped bifurcation of the celiac axis (not imaged). The normal diameter of the common hepatic artery ranges from 4-10 mm.* **(Middle)** *Color Doppler US shows flow within the proximal portion of the common hepatic artery. The gastroduodenal artery may be seen to arise from the common hepatic artery along the anterosuperior aspect of the pancreas; thereafter, the common hepatic artery becomes the proper hepatic artery.* **(Bottom)** *Spectral Doppler US of the common hepatic artery shows low-resistance flow characteristics with large amount of continuous flow in diastole. The normal PSV for the common hepatic artery ranges from 70-120 cm/s.*

SUPERIOR MESENTERIC ARTERY

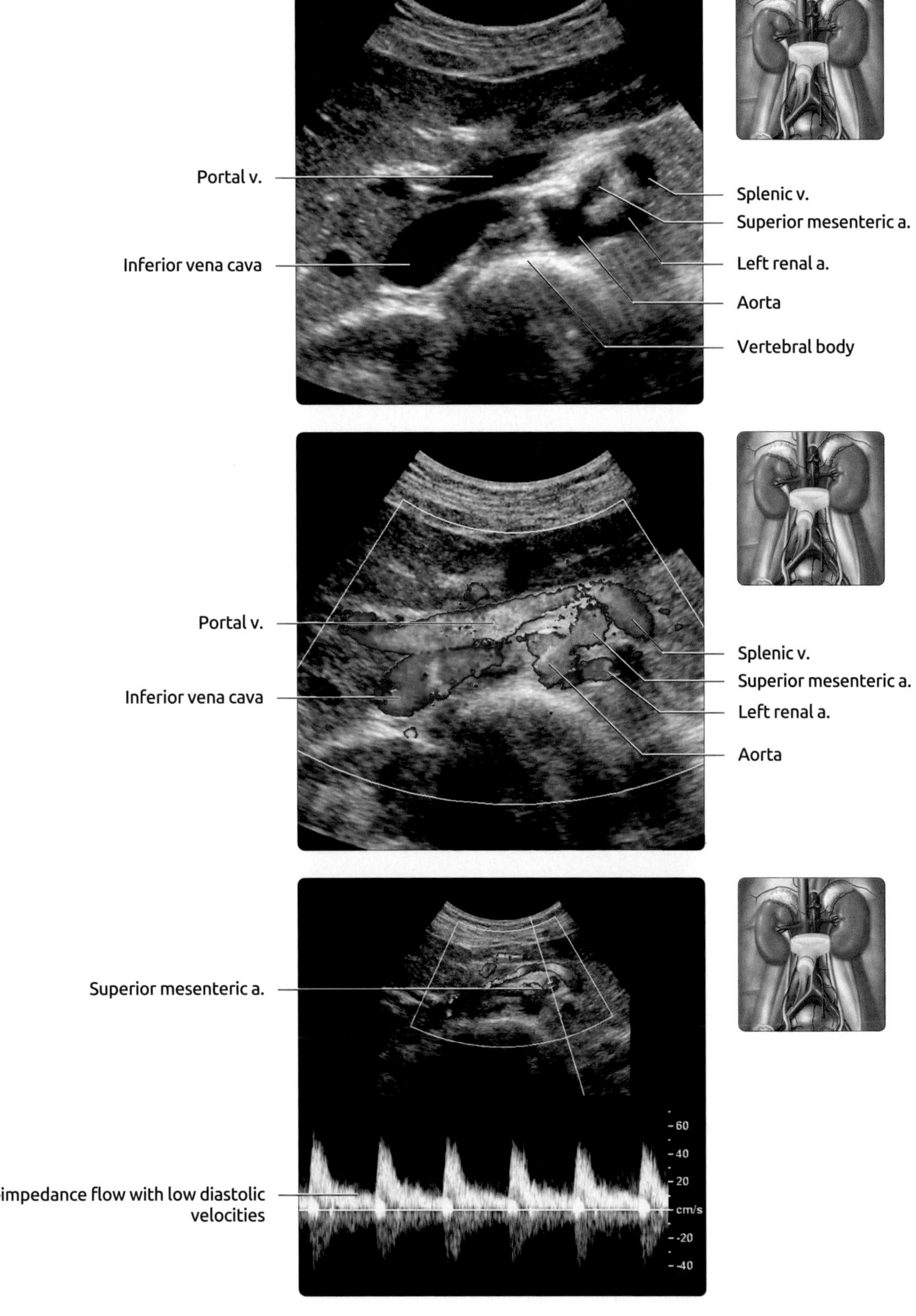

(Top) *Transverse grayscale US shows the origin of the SMA arising anteriorly from the aorta. The origin of the SMA is usually seen at L1 between the celiac axis (T12) and the renal arteries (L1/2). The normal caliber of the SMA ranges from 5-8 mm.* **(Middle)** *Transverse color Doppler US shows the proximal SMA. The transducer has been angled slightly cranially with the arterial blood coming toward the transducer, shown in red, and the venous blood going away from the transducer, shown in blue.* **(Bottom)** *Spectral Doppler US shows the proximal portion of the SMA. High-impedance flow with low diastolic velocities is observed during fasting due to relative vasoconstriction. End-diastolic velocity increases after meals due to vasodilation of the mesenteric branches, typically 30-90 minutes after meals.*

RIGHT RENAL ARTERY

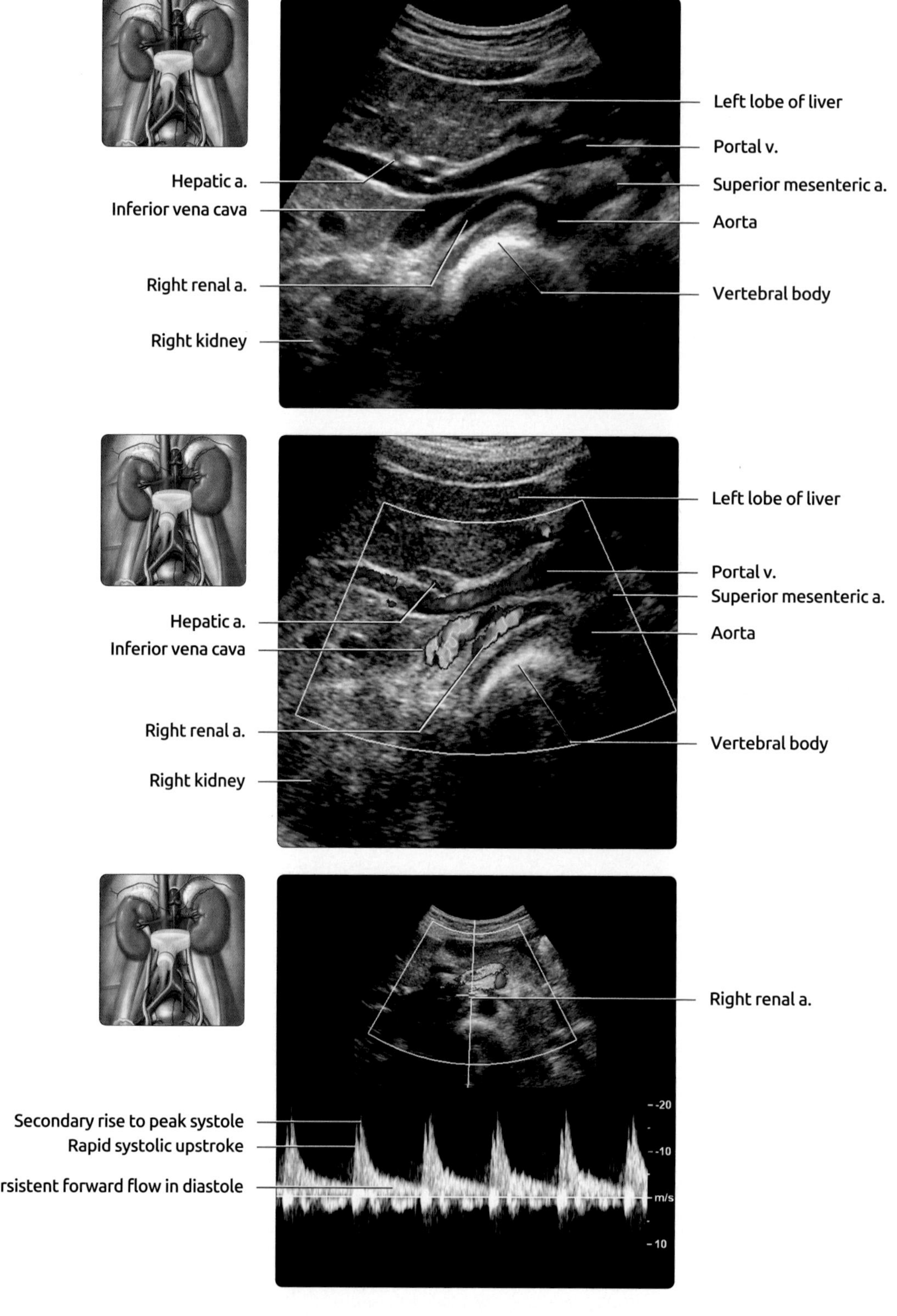

(Top) *Transverse grayscale US shows the proximal right renal artery as it branches from the aorta and courses behind the IVC. This midline anterior approach is usually the best for evaluating the origin of the renal arteries. The normal diameter of the renal arteries ranges from 5-8 mm. The renal arteries arise around the L1/2 level at or below the level of the SMA.* **(Middle)** *Transverse color Doppler US of the abdominal aorta shows the proximal right renal artery as it branches from the aorta and courses behind the IVC.* **(Bottom)** *Spectral Doppler US of the right renal artery shows open systolic window, rapid systolic upstroke followed by a secondary slower rise to peak systole with subsequent gradual diastolic delay but with persistent forward flow in diastole. The normal PSV ranges from 60-140 cm/s, but not > 180 cm/s.*

LEFT RENAL ARTERY

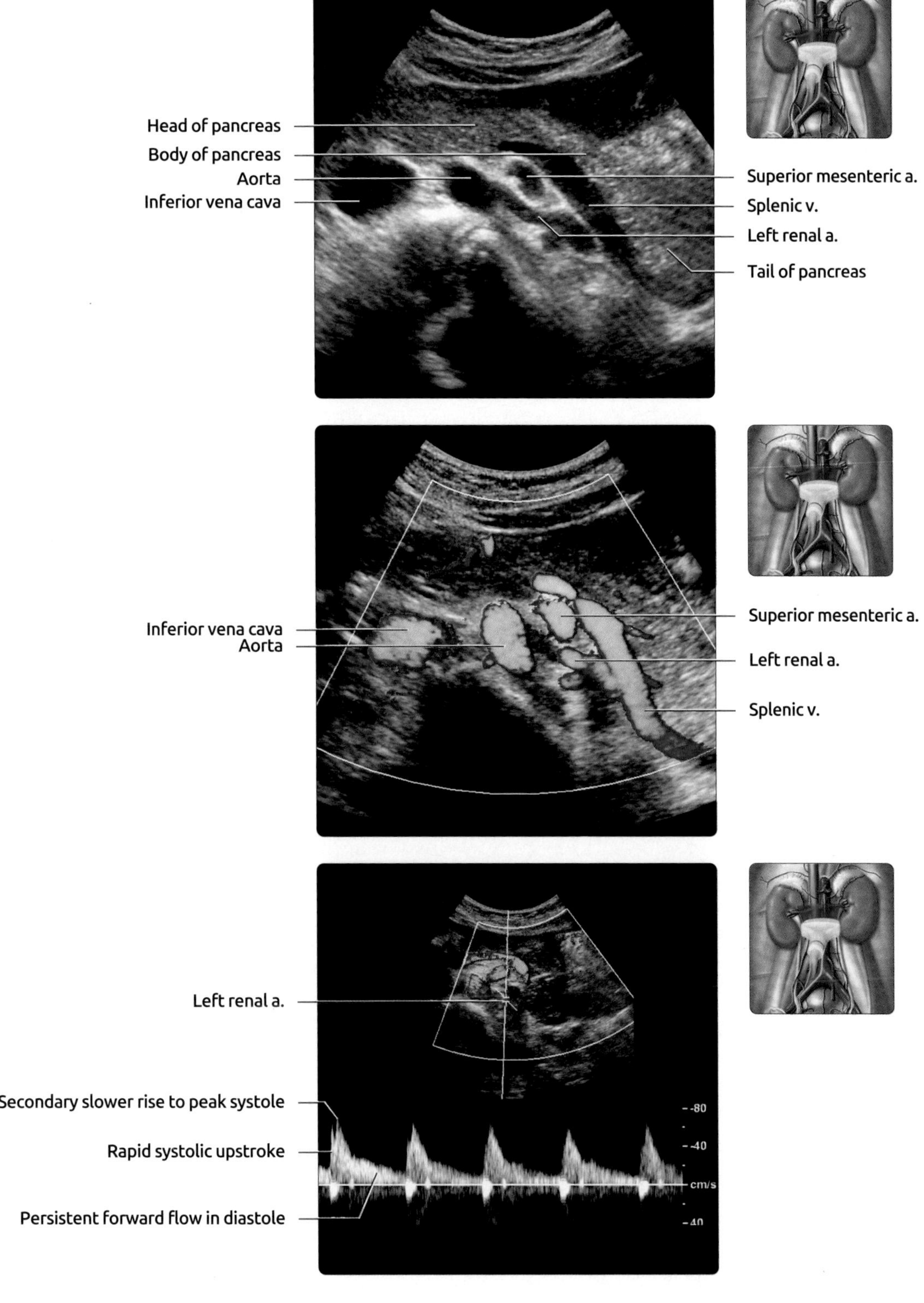

(Top) *Transverse grayscale US shows the proximal left renal artery as it branches from the aorta and courses posterior to the SMA and splenic vein. This midline anterior approach is usually the best for evaluating the origin of the renal arteries. The normal diameter of the renal arteries ranges from 5-8 mm. The renal arteries arise around the L1/2 level.* **(Middle)** *Power Doppler US shows flow in the proximal left renal artery as it branches from the aorta and courses posterior to the SMA and splenic vein.* **(Bottom)** *Spectral Doppler US of the left renal artery shows open systolic window, rapid systolic upstroke followed by a secondary slower rise to peak systole with subsequent gradual diastolic delay but with persistent forward flow in diastole. The normal PSV ranges from 60-140 cm/s but not > 180 cm/s.*

INFERIOR MESENTERIC ARTERY

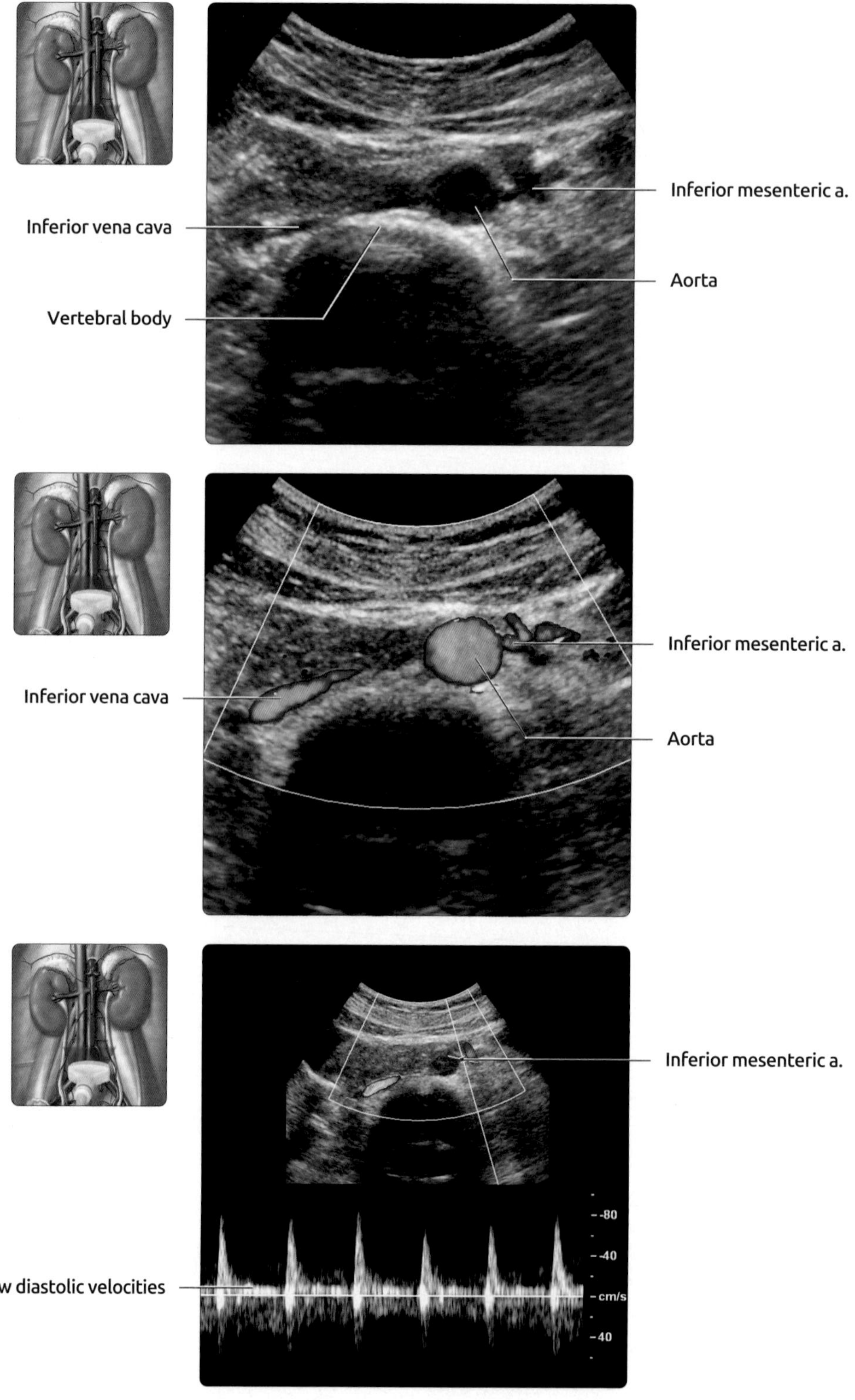

(Top) *Transverse grayscale US shows the distal abdominal aorta at the level of the origin of the inferior mesenteric artery (IMA). The IMA arises from the anterior or left anterolateral aspect of the abdominal aorta at the L3 level. The transverse plane following the line of the aorta is the best imaging plane for identification of the origin of the IMA. The normal caliber of the IMA ranges from 1-4 mm.* **(Middle)** *Transverse power Doppler US shows flow in the proximal IMA.* **(Bottom)** *Spectral Doppler US of the IMA shows high-impedance flow with low diastolic velocities during fasting due to relative vasoconstriction. End-diastolic velocity increases after a meal due to vasodilation of the mesenteric branches. Normal PSV ranges from 93-189 cm/s.*

AORTIC BIFURCATION

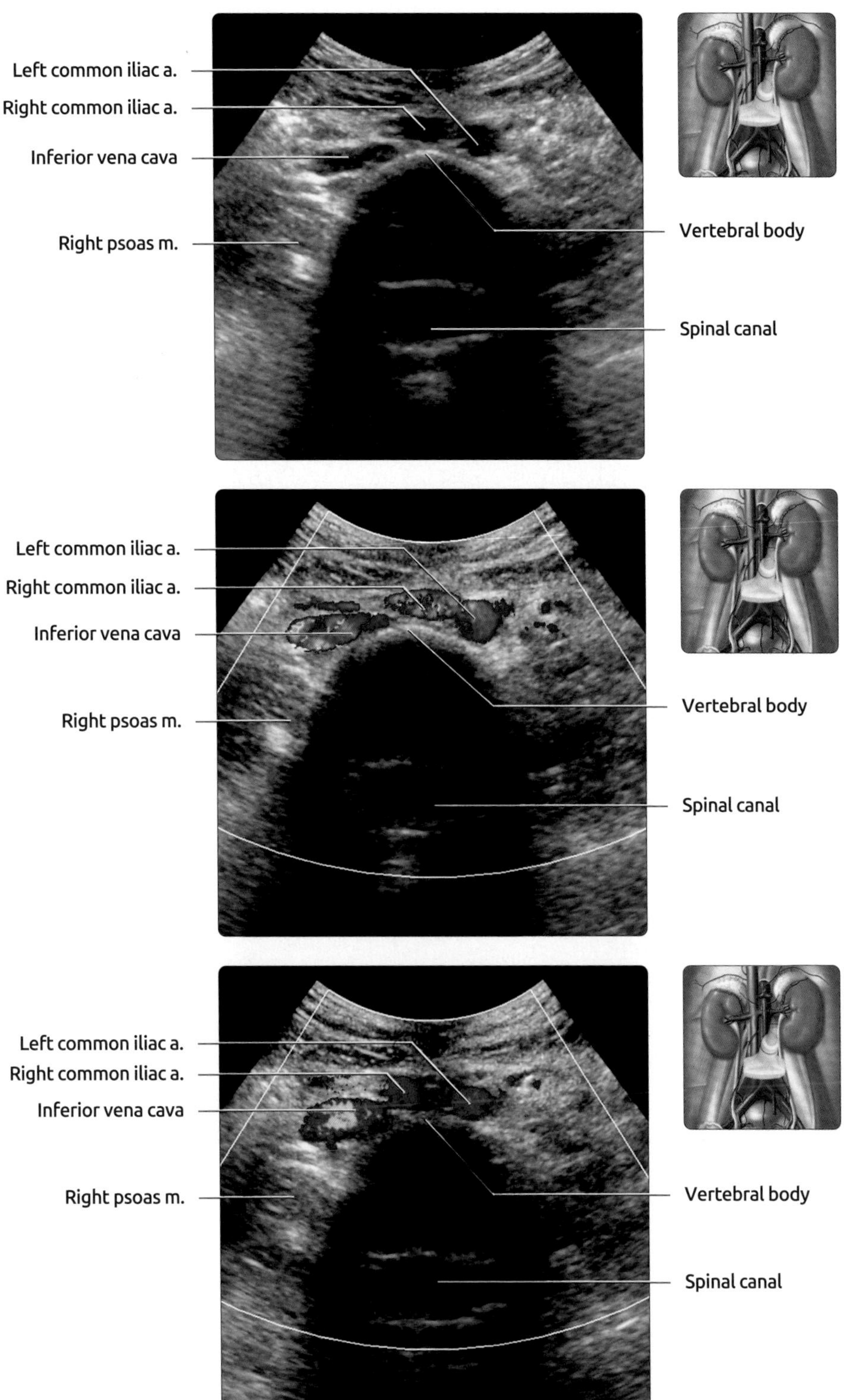

(Top) *Transverse grayscale US of the aortic bifurcation shows the origins of the right and left common iliac arteries. The aortic bifurcation is usually seen at the L4 level.* **(Middle)** *Transverse color Doppler US shows flow in the origins of the right and left common iliac arteries.* **(Bottom)** *Transverse power Doppler US shows flow in the origins of the right and left common iliac arteries. Power Doppler is less angle dependent and demonstrates flow more readily, particularly in vascular structures that are close to a right angle with the transducer.*

RIGHT COMMON ILIAC ARTERY

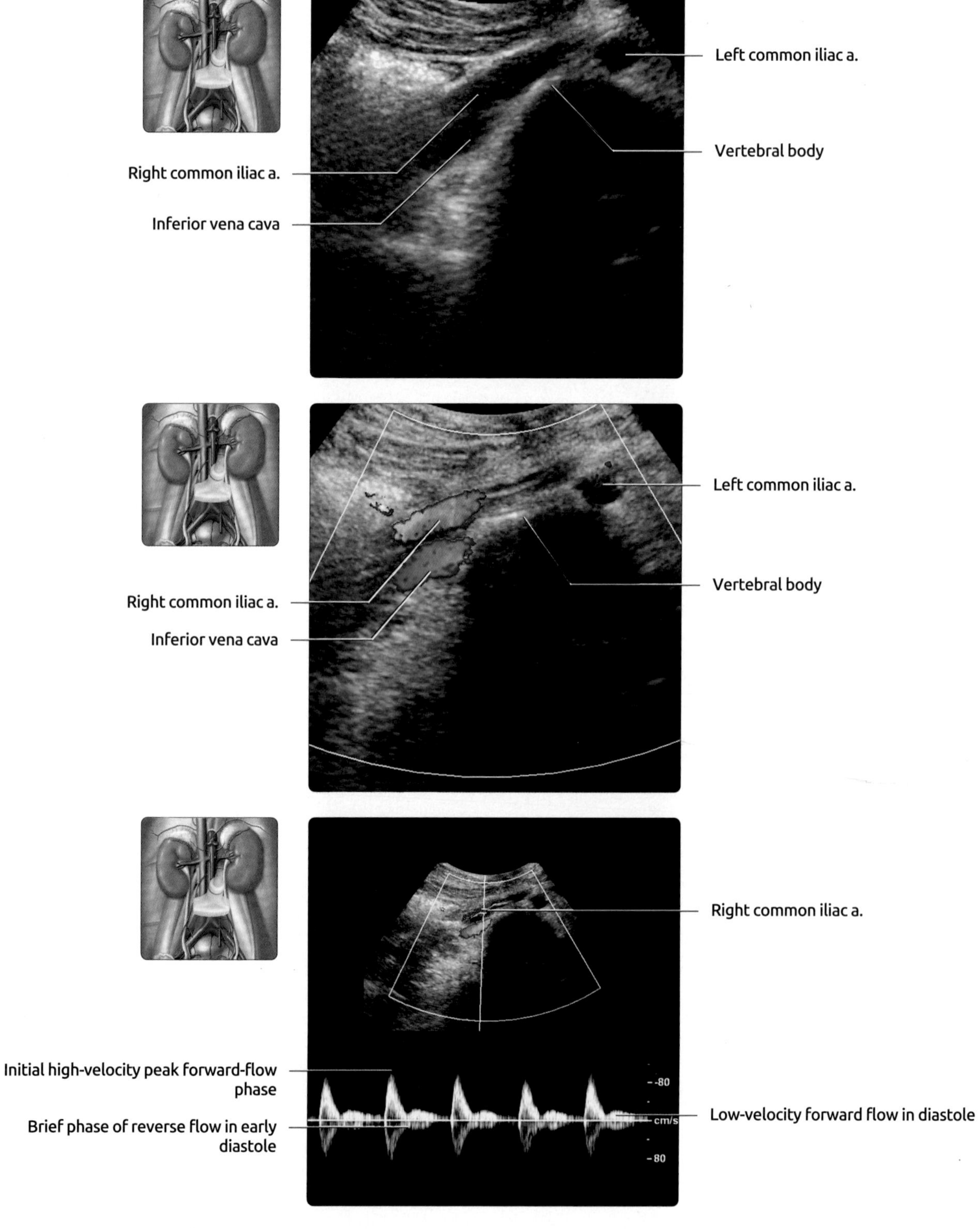

(Top) *Oblique grayscale US shows the course of the right common iliac artery as it branches off the aortic bifurcation. The proximal common iliac artery is first identified on the transverse plane, and the transducer is then angulated along the long axis of the right common iliac artery. The normal diameter of the common iliac arteries ranges from 8-12 mm.* **(Middle)** *Oblique color Doppler US shows flow in the proximal right common iliac artery.* **(Bottom)** *Spectral Doppler US of the right common iliac artery shows triphasic waveform. Initial high-velocity peak forward-flow phase results from cardiac systole, brief phase of reverse flow in early diastole, and low-velocity forward flow in diastole.*

LEFT COMMON ILIAC ARTERY

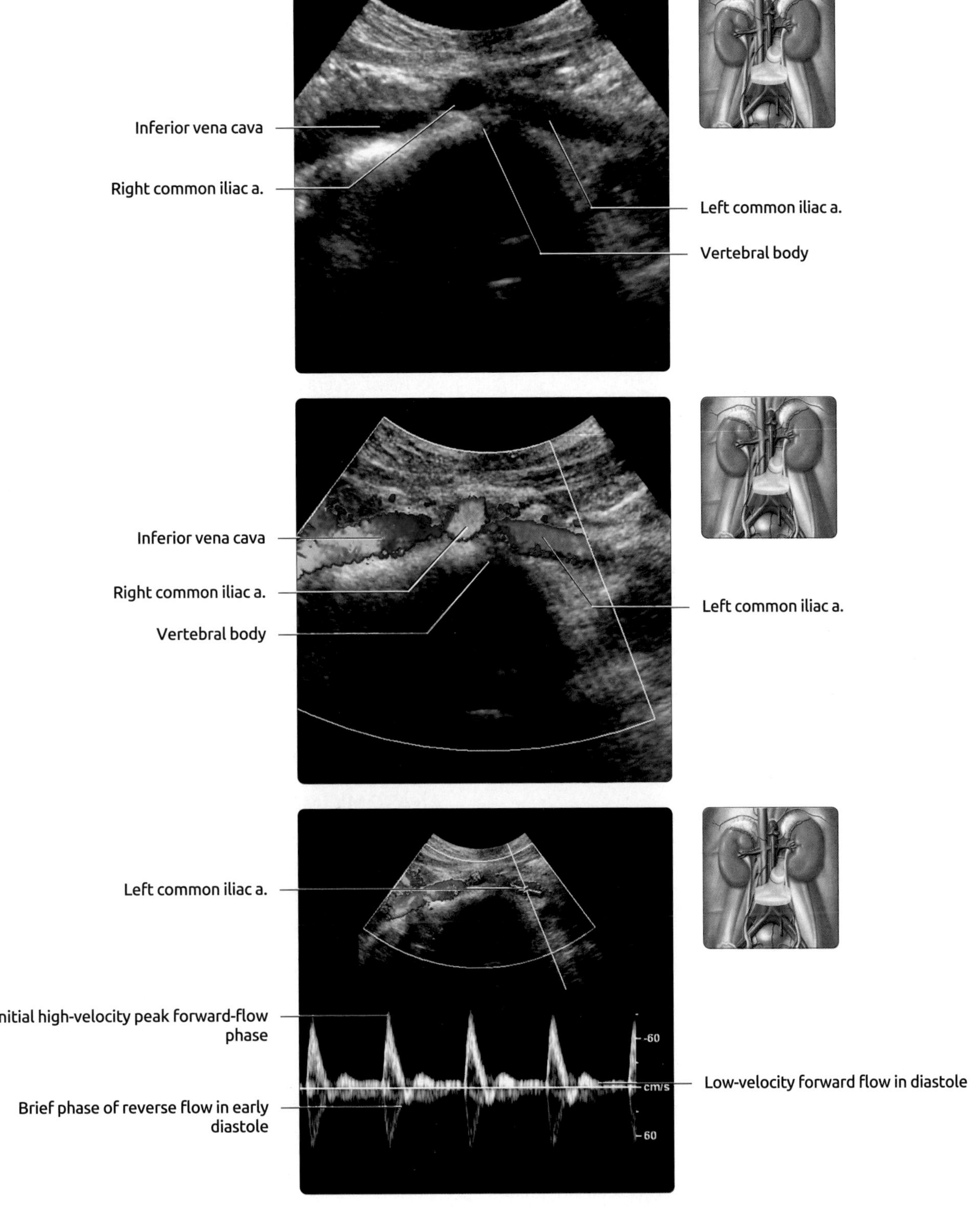

(Top) *Oblique grayscale US shows the course of the left common iliac artery as it branches off the aortic bifurcation. The proximal common iliac artery is first identified on the transverse plane, and the transducer is then angulated along the long axis of the left common iliac artery. The normal diameter of the common iliac arteries ranges from 8-12 mm.* **(Middle)** *Oblique color Doppler US shows flow in the proximal left common iliac artery.* **(Bottom)** *Spectral Doppler US of the left common iliac artery shows characteristic triphasic waveform. Initial high-velocity peak forward-flow phase results from cardiac systole, brief phase of reverse flow in early diastole, and low-velocity forward flow in diastole.*

GROSS ANATOMY

Arteries

- Abdominal aorta
  - Testicular and ovarian arteries originate below renal arteries
  - Median (middle) sacral artery is small, unpaired branch from posterior aspect of distal aorta
  - Divides into common iliac arteries at L4-5
- Common iliac arteries
  - Run anterior to iliac veins and inferior vena cava
  - Usually no major branches
    - Rarely, gives off aberrant iliolumbar or accessory renal arteries
  - ~ 4 cm long
- External iliac artery
  - No major branches
  - Exits pelvis beneath inguinal ligament
  - Larger than internal iliac artery
  - Inferior epigastric (medial) and deep iliac circumflex (lateral) arteries demarcate junction between external iliac and common femoral arteries
- Internal iliac (hypogastric) artery
  - Principal vascular supply of pelvic organs
  - Divides into anterior and posterior trunk
    - Anterior trunk to pelvic viscera
    - Posterior trunk to pelvic musculature
- Anterior trunk of internal iliac artery
  - Branching pattern quite variable
  - Umbilical artery
    - Only pelvic segment remains patent after birth
    - Remainder becomes fibrous medial umbilical ligament
  - Obturator artery
    - Exits pelvis through obturator canal to supply medial thigh muscles
  - Superior vesicle artery
    - Supplies bladder and distal ureter
    - Gives off branch to ductus deferens in males
  - Inferior vesicle artery (male)
    - May arise from middle rectal artery
    - Supplies prostate, seminal vesicles and lower ureters
  - Uterine artery (female)
    - Passes over ureter at level of cervix ("water under the bridge")
    - Anastomoses with vaginal and ovarian arteries
  - Vaginal artery (female)
  - Middle rectal artery runs above pelvic floor and anastomoses with superior and inferior rectal arteries to supply rectum
    - Also anastomoses with inferior vesicle artery
  - Internal pudendal artery
    - Supplies external genitalia (penis, clitoris) and rectum
  - Inferior gluteal (sciatic) artery
    - Largest and terminal branch of anterior division of hypogastric artery
    - Supplies muscles of pelvic floor, thigh, buttocks and sciatic nerve
- Posterior division of internal iliac artery
  - Iliolumbar artery
    - Ascends laterally to supply iliacus, psoas, and quadratus lumborum muscles
  - Lateral sacral artery
    - Runs medially toward sacral foramina to anastomose with middle sacral artery
  - Superior gluteal artery
    - Largest and terminal branch of posterior division
    - Supplies piriformis and gluteal muscles

Veins

- External iliac vein
  - Upward continuation of femoral vein at level of inguinal ligament
  - Receives inferior epigastric, deep iliac circumflex, and pubic veins
- Internal iliac vein begins near upper part of greater sciatic foramen
  - Gluteal, internal pudendal and obturator veins have origins outside pelvis
  - Pelvic viscera drain into multiple, deep pelvic venous plexuses
    - These drain into veins, which roughly parallel pelvic arteries
- Right gonadal vein drains into IVC, left gonadal vein drains into left renal vein
- Common iliac vein formed by union of external and internal iliac veins
  - Unites with contralateral side to form IVC

IMAGING ANATOMY

Overview

- CT angiography (CTA) and MR angiography (MRA) are imaging modalities of choice to evaluate pelvic vessels
  - Ultrasound limited to demonstrating common iliac, external iliac, and proximal internal iliac vessels

ANATOMY IMAGING ISSUES

Imaging Recommendations

- Transducer: 2-5 MHz
- Patient examined in supine position
  - Place transducer lateral to rectus muscles, angulating medially
- Fasting for > 4 hours may help decrease overlying bowel gas

Imaging Pitfalls

- Pelvic vessels usually obscured by overlying bowel gas

CLINICAL IMPLICATIONS

Clinical Importance

- Abdominal aortic aneurysms may extend to involve iliac arteries
- Rich, complex collateral circulation helps ensure delivery of blood to pelvic organs and lower limbs in event of proximal obstruction
- Patients with deep venous thrombosis of lower limbs may have involvement of iliac veins

ILIAC ARTERIES AND VEINS IN SITU

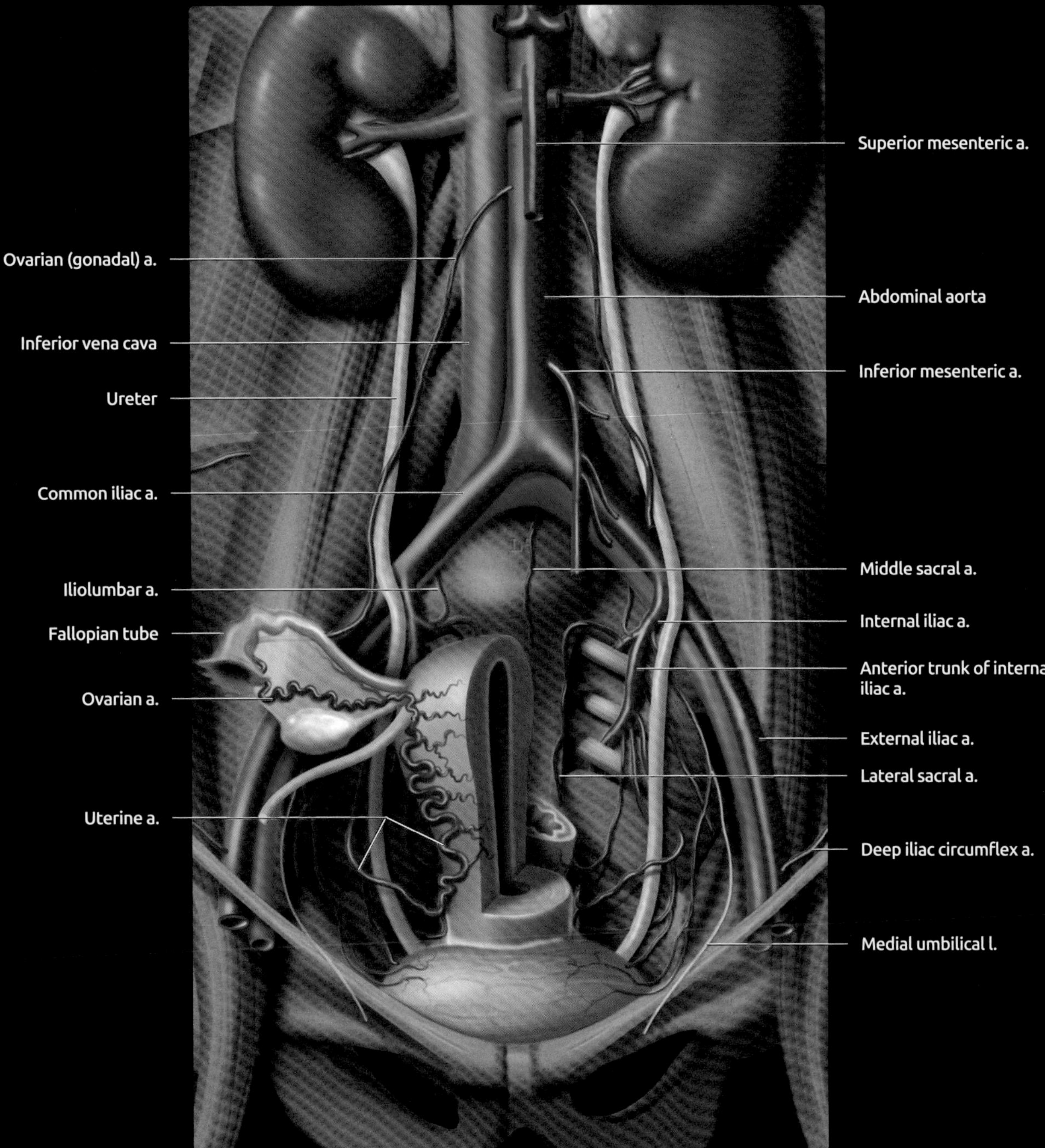

Frontal graphic shows the abdominal aorta, inferior vena cava, and iliac vessels in a female subject. The inferior mesenteric artery is the smallest of the anterior mesenteric branches of the aorta and continues in the pelvis as the superior rectal artery. The paired ovarian arteries arise from the aorta below the renal arteries and pass inferiorly on the posterior abdominal wall to enter the pelvis. The ureters cross anterior to the bifurcation of the common iliac arteries on their way to the urinary bladder. The common iliac artery divides into the external iliac artery, which supplies the lower extremity, and the internal iliac (hypogastric) artery, which supplies the pelvis. The internal iliac artery divides into an anterior trunk for the pelvic viscera and a posterior trunk for the muscles of the pelvis.

COMMON ILIAC ARTERY AND BRANCHES

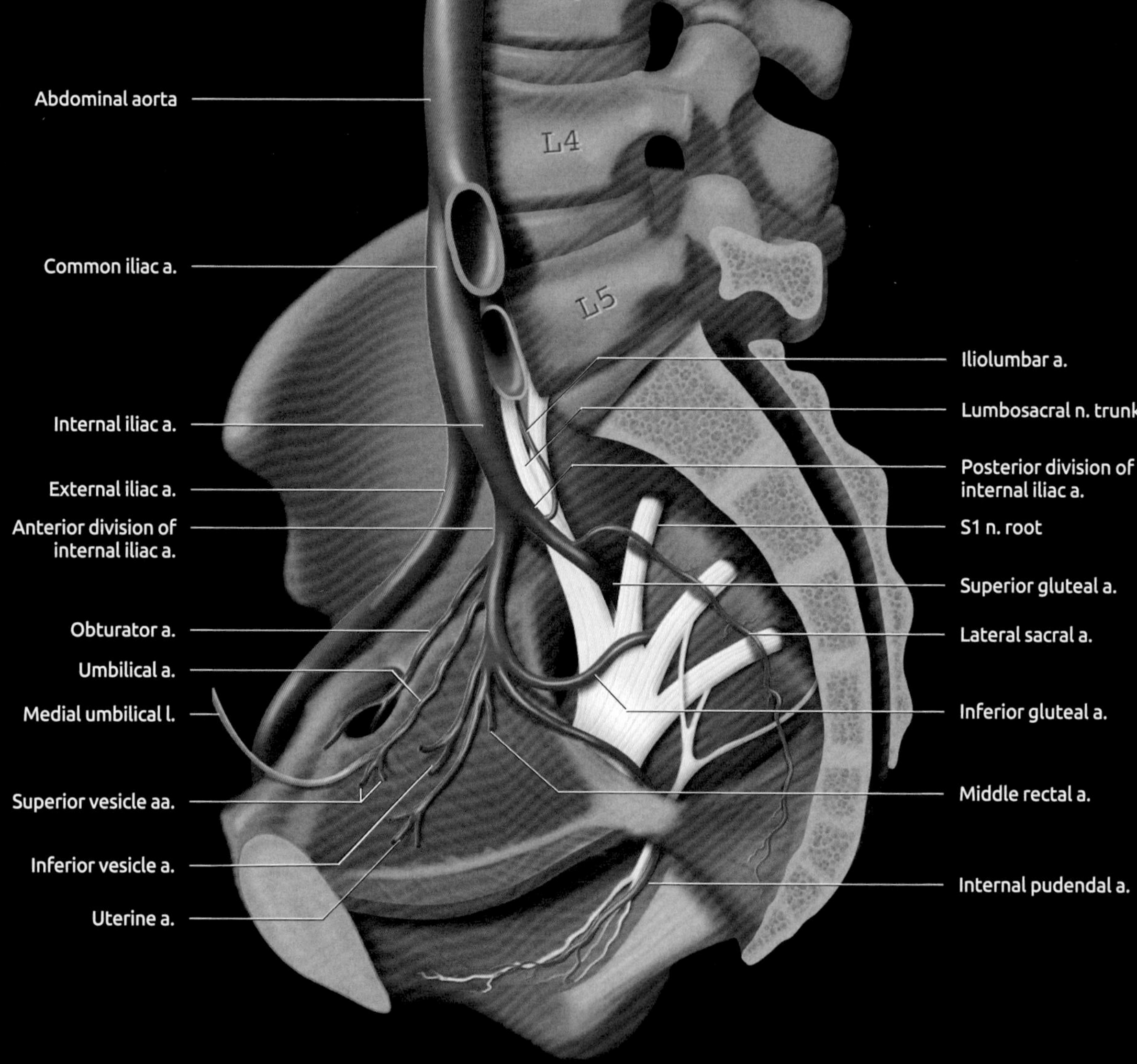

Graphic shows the pelvic arteries and their relation to the sacral nerves. The superior gluteal artery passes posteriorly and runs between the lumbosacral trunk and the anterior ramus of the S1 nerve, whereas the inferior gluteal artery usually runs between the S1-2 or S2-3 nerve roots to leave the pelvis through the inferior part of the greater sciatic foramen. Only the proximal portion of the umbilical arteries remains patent after birth, while the distal portion obliterates forming the medial umbilical ligaments. Arteries to the deep pelvic viscera include the superior and inferior vesicle, uterine, middle rectal and internal pudendal. The individual branching pattern is quite variable.

ILIAC VEINS IN SITU

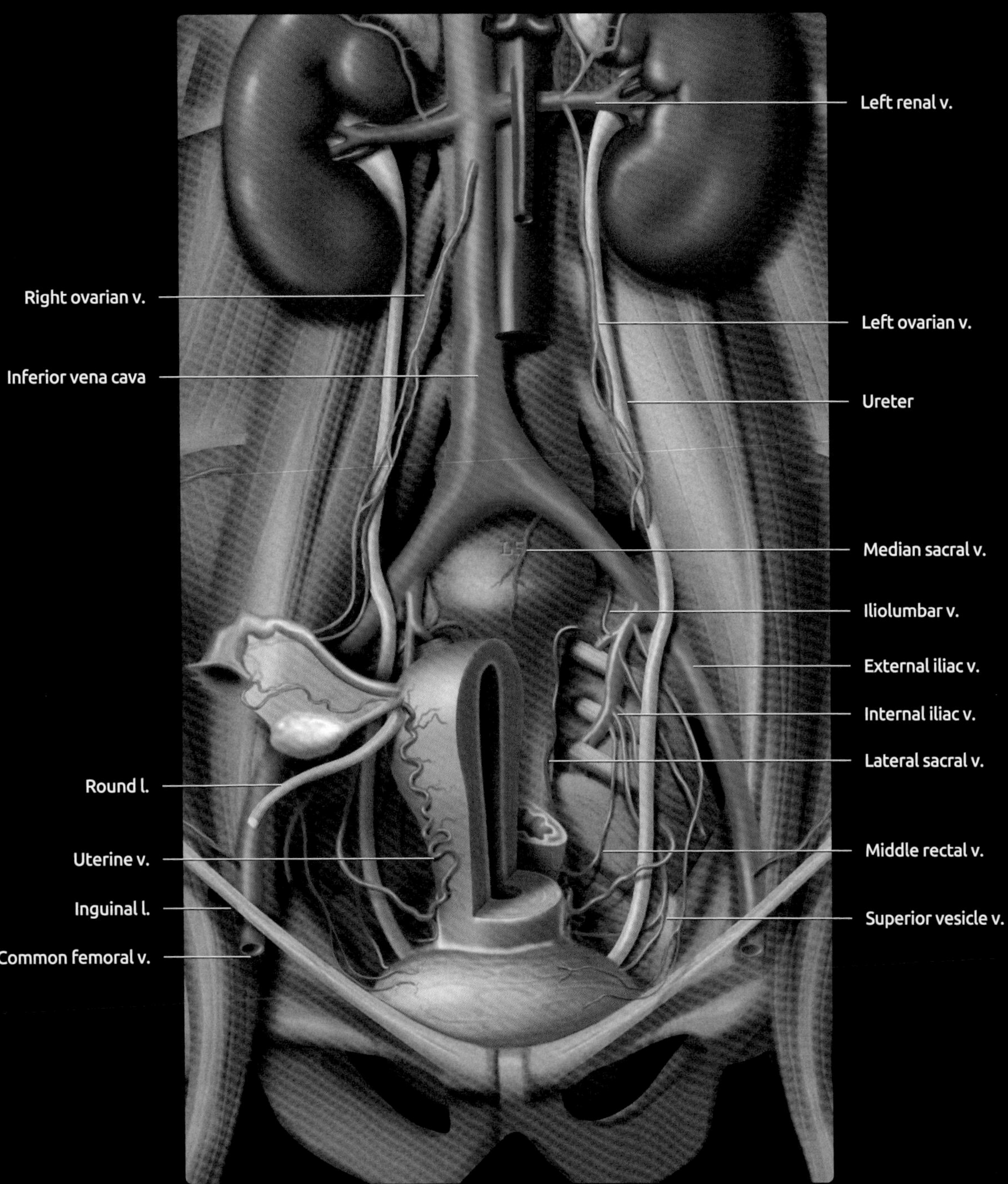

Graphic shows the veins of the pelvis. The left ovarian vein drains into the left renal vein, whereas the right ovarian vein drains directly into the inferior vena cava. Multiple intercommunicating pelvic venous plexuses (rectal, vesicle, prostatic, uterine, and vaginal) drain mainly to the internal iliac veins. There is a communication between the pelvic veins and the intraspinal epidural plexus of veins through the sacral venous plexus.

AORTIC BIFURCATION

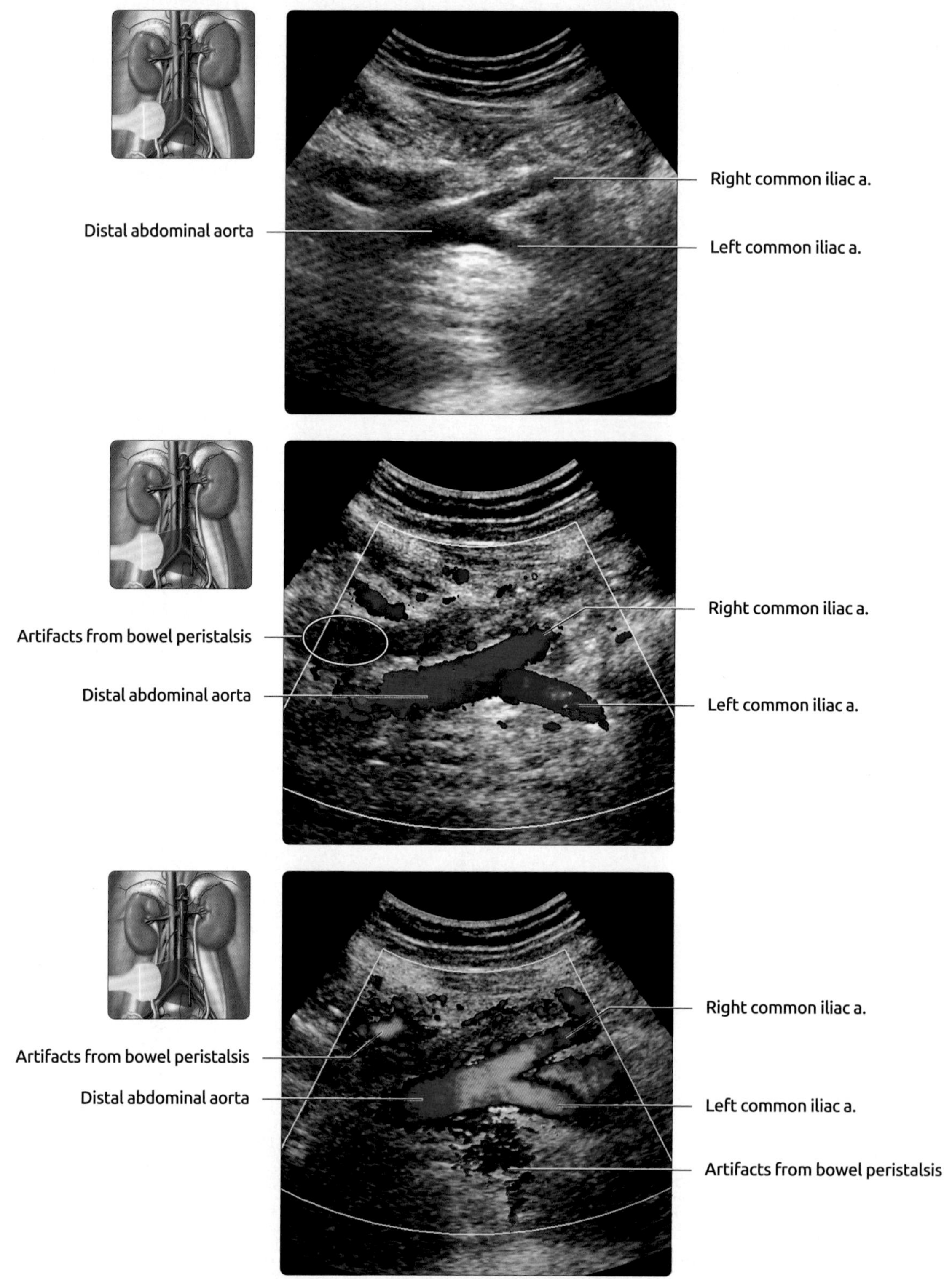

(Top) *Coronal grayscale ultrasound shows the bifurcation of the distal aorta into the common iliac arteries. This occurs at the level of L4 vertebra and corresponds to the umbilicus, serving as a useful landmark for transducer placement for common iliac artery insonation.* **(Middle)** *Coronal color Doppler ultrasound demonstrates color flow in the distal aorta and bifurcation. The left common iliac artery assumes a blue color (as opposed to the red color of the distal aorta and right common iliac artery) owing to its flow direction. Peristalsis of adjacent bowel segments also demonstrates color on color Doppler ultrasound, rendering artifacts.* **(Bottom)** *Coronal power Doppler is more sensitive than color Doppler ultrasound in demonstrating blood flow without providing information on flow direction. There is also significant increase in image artifacts from peristalsis.*

COMMON ILIAC ARTERY

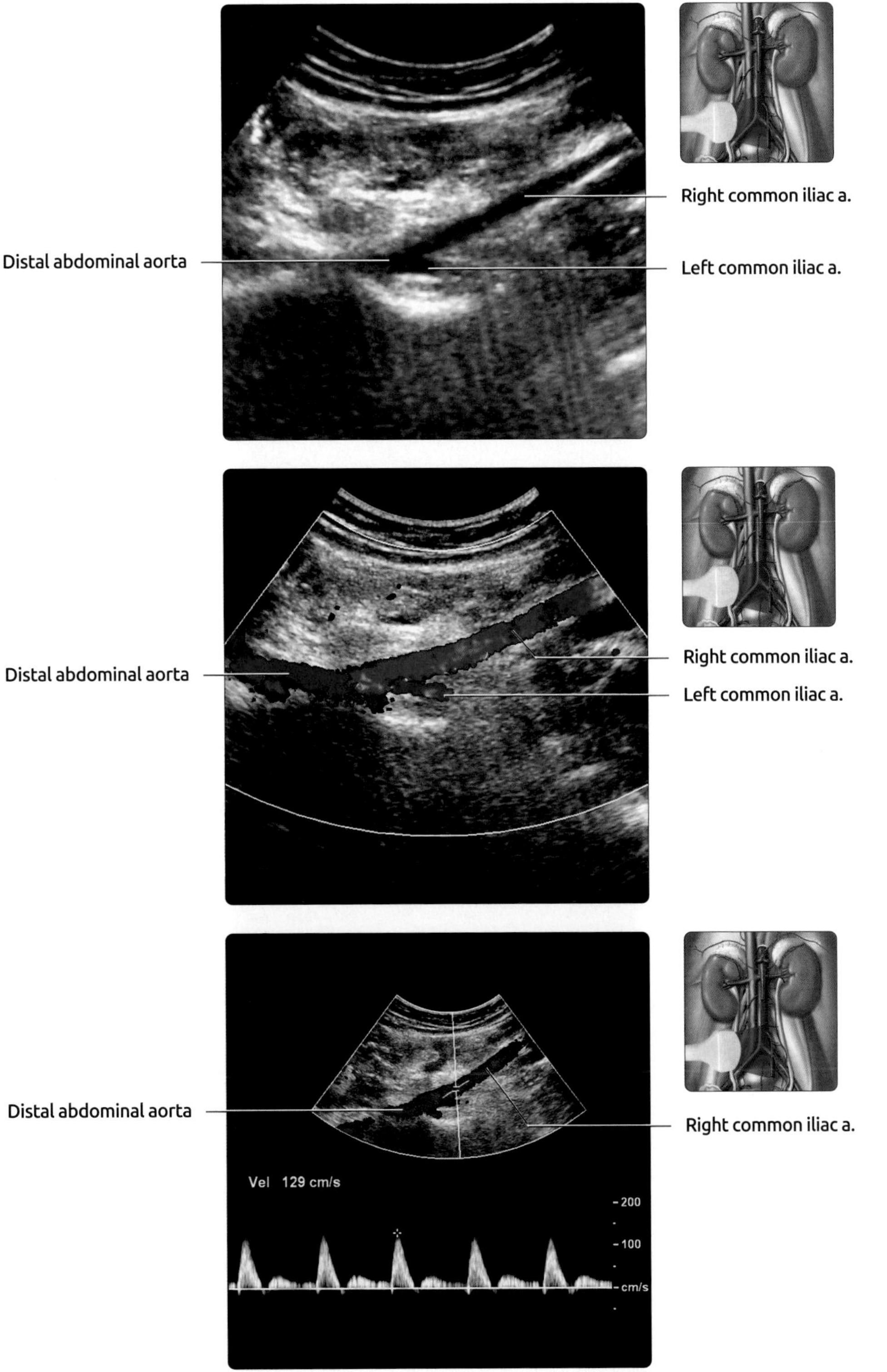

(Top) *Coronal transabdominal grayscale ultrasound, angulating the transducer to demonstrate the course of the right common iliac artery, is shown. The common iliac artery is about 5 cm long with diameters of 1.3 cm (females) and 1.5 cm (males).* **(Middle)** *Coronal transabdominal color Doppler ultrasound shows the right common iliac artery (shown in red) with consistent intense color indicating uniform mean flow velocity. This is a useful plane for examining abdominal aortic aneurysms when there is extension into the common iliac arteries.* **(Bottom)** *Transabdominal color pulsed Doppler ultrasound of the right common iliac artery shows peak systolic velocity of 129 cm/s, within the normal range of 80-187 cm/s. Note normal triphasic spectral waveform.*

INTERNAL ILIAC ARTERY

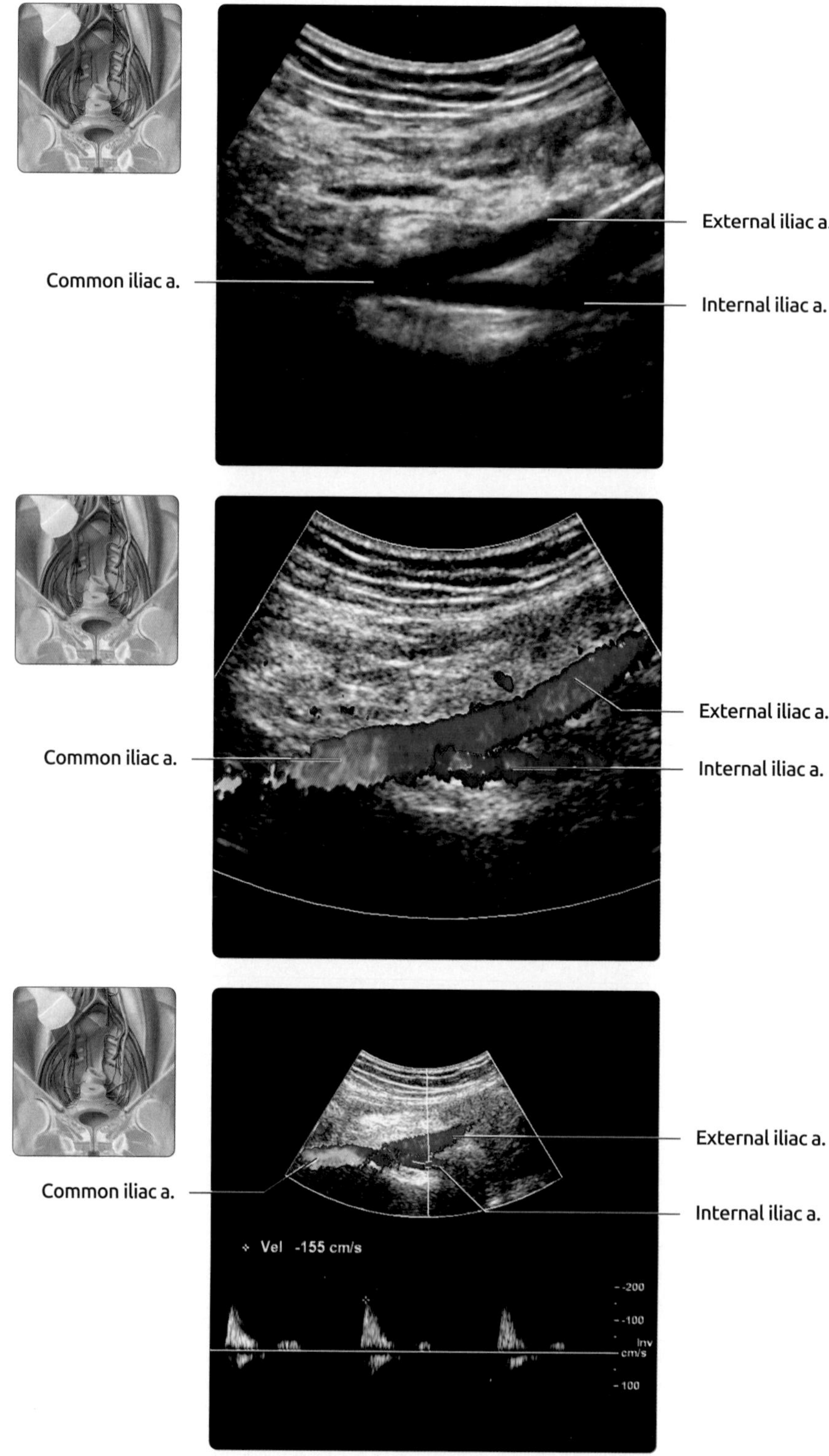

(Top) *Oblique transabdominal grayscale ultrasound of the distal common iliac artery demonstrates its bifurcation into the external iliac and internal iliac arteries. The internal iliac artery has a smaller caliber compared to the external iliac artery and courses more posteriorly. The internal iliac artery divides into 2 trunks, which are usually too deep to be demonstrated on ultrasound.* **(Middle)** *Longitudinal transabdominal color Doppler ultrasound shows intense color in the distal common iliac (shown in red) and external iliac (shown in red) arteries, suggesting uniform mean velocity in the arterial segments. The branches of the internal iliac artery (shown in blue) supply the wall and viscera of the pelvis, including the reproductive organs.* **(Bottom)** *Pulsed Doppler ultrasound shows the internal iliac artery, which is usually investigated in graft kidneys and some cases of erectile dysfunction.*

EXTERNAL ILIAC ARTERY

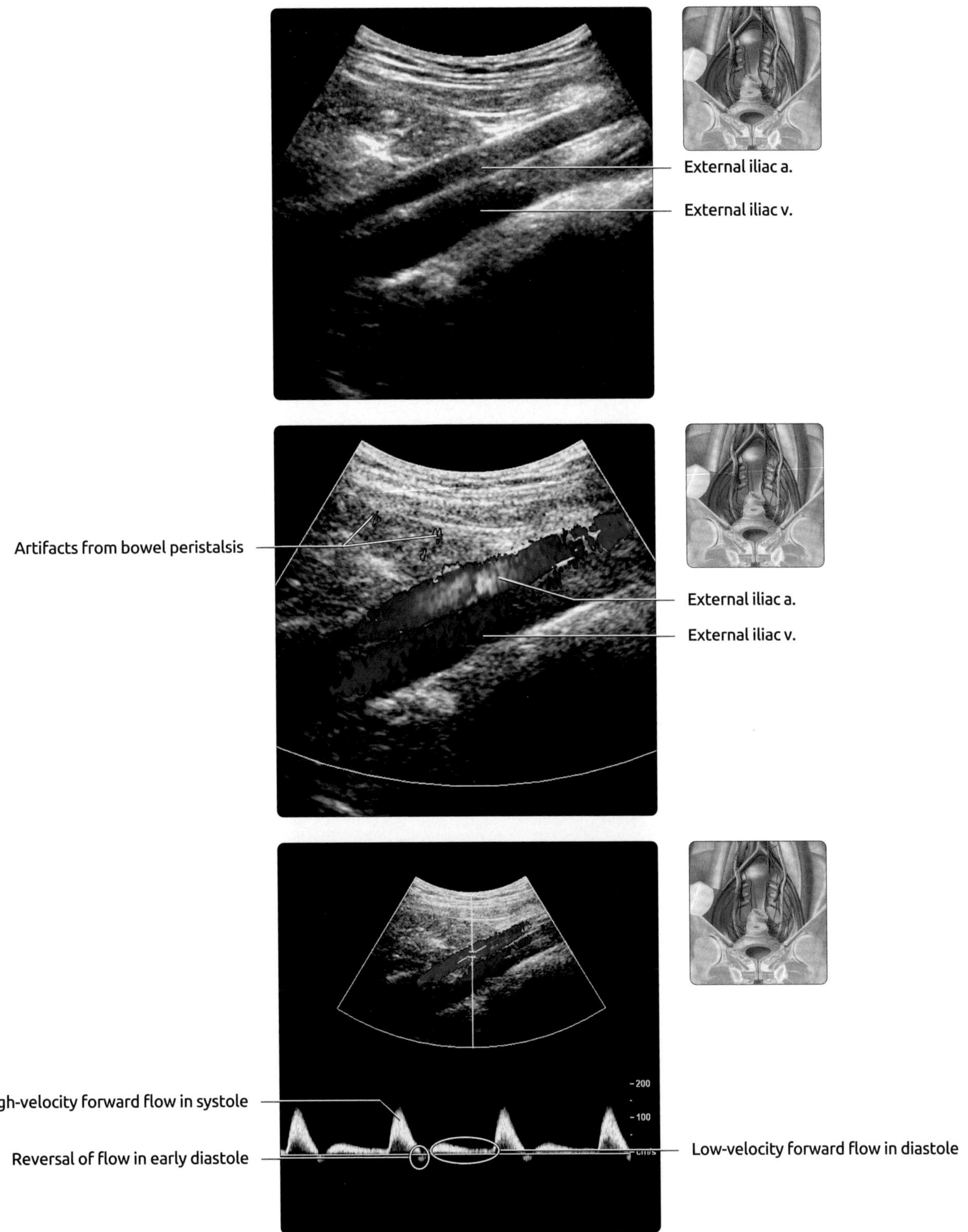

(Top) *Longitudinal transabdominal grayscale ultrasound shows the external iliac artery, usually easily demonstrated owing to its superficial location and absence of overlying bowel gas. Normal diameters are up to 11 mm in females and 12 mm in males.* **(Middle)** *Longitudinal transabdominal color Doppler ultrasound shows the relationship of the external iliac artery (shown in red) with the external iliac vein (shown in blue), which is located posteriorly. The two vessels run along the same course as they enter the thigh.* **(Bottom)** *Pulsed Doppler ultrasound shows the external iliac artery; the waveform resembles those from lower extremity arteries. Note high-velocity forward flow during systole and low-velocity forward flow during diastole. There is an intervening short reversal of flow in early diastole, due to peripheral resistance. Peak systolic velocity of 129 cm/s is within the normal range (< 140 cm/s).*

ILIAC VESSELS, TRANSVERSE US

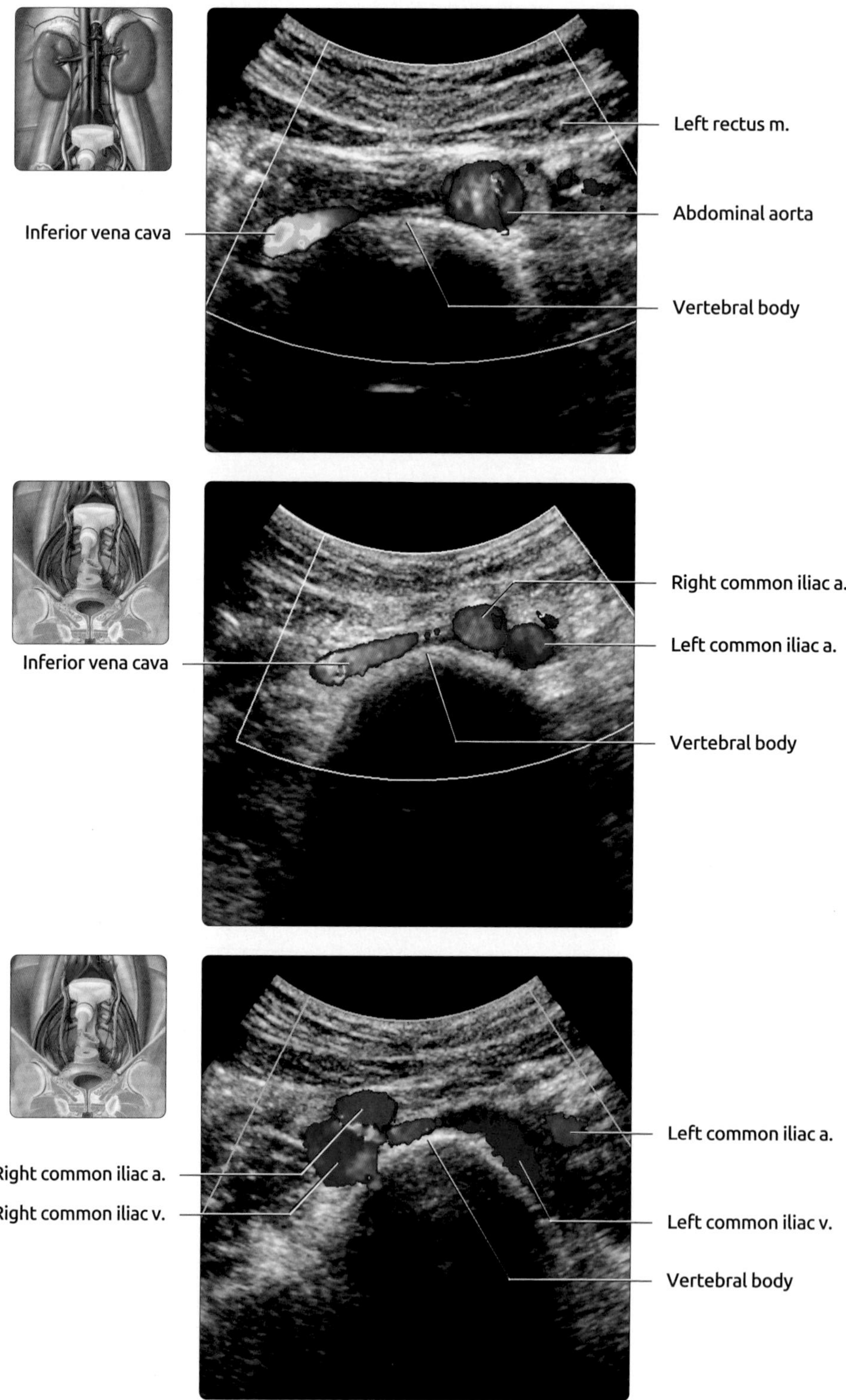

(Top) *Transverse transabdominal color Doppler ultrasound at the supraumbilical level shows the distal aorta (shown in red) and inferior vena cava (shown in blue), both of which have not yet bifurcated. The inferior vena cava is to the right of the abdominal aorta; a left-sided inferior vena cava is rarely encountered (0.2-0.5%) and may be associated with other vascular anomalies, such as circumaortic or retroaortic renal vein.* **(Middle)** *Transverse transabdominal color Doppler ultrasound at the infraumbilical level is shown. The distal aorta has bifurcated into the paired common iliac arteries at the level of L4, occurring more proximally than the formation of the inferior vena cava.* **(Bottom)** *Transverse transabdominal color Doppler ultrasound continued inferiorly in the same patient is shown. The paired common iliac veins (shown in blue) are now identified, which run posterior to their arterial counterparts (shown in red).*

ILIAC VESSELS, CT

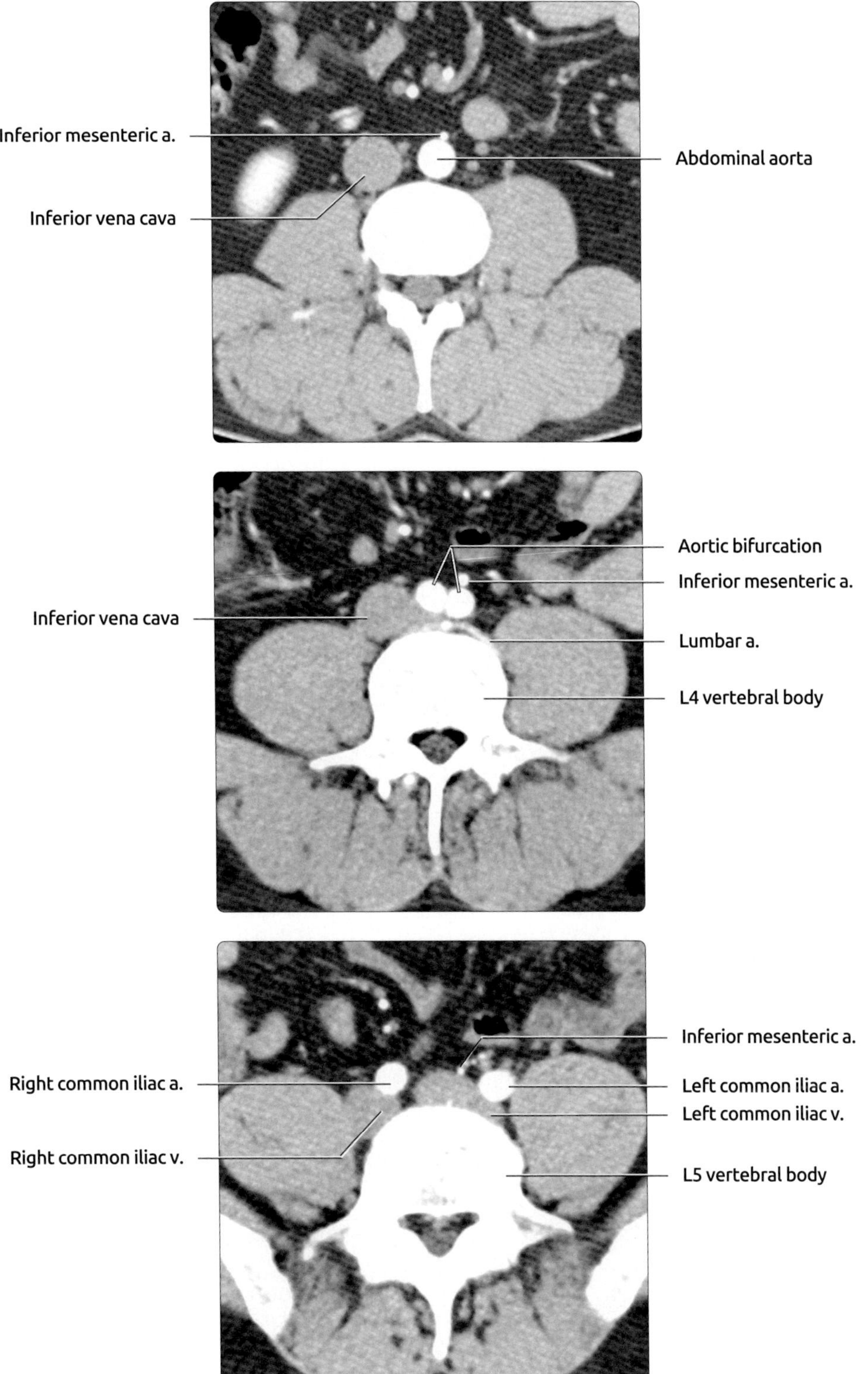

(Top) *First of 3 axial CECT images of the pelvic vessels is shown. The abdominal aorta rests on the vertebral body; its distal portion gives off the inferior mesenteric artery, the smallest of the mesenteric arteries. The inferior vena cava is identified to the right of the abdominal aorta and spine.* **(Middle)** *The aorta bifurcates at the level of L4 into the 2 common iliac arteries. Despite its diminutive caliber, the lumbar artery is identified on CT.* **(Bottom)** *The common iliac arteries usually give off no visceral branches. They may, however, give origin to accessory renal arteries. At this lower level, the termination of the common iliac veins are identified just before forming into the inferior vena cava. The left common iliac vein is longer than the right as it traverses the spine to form the IVC, which is located in the right paraspinal region.*

ILIAC VESSELS, TRANSVERSE US

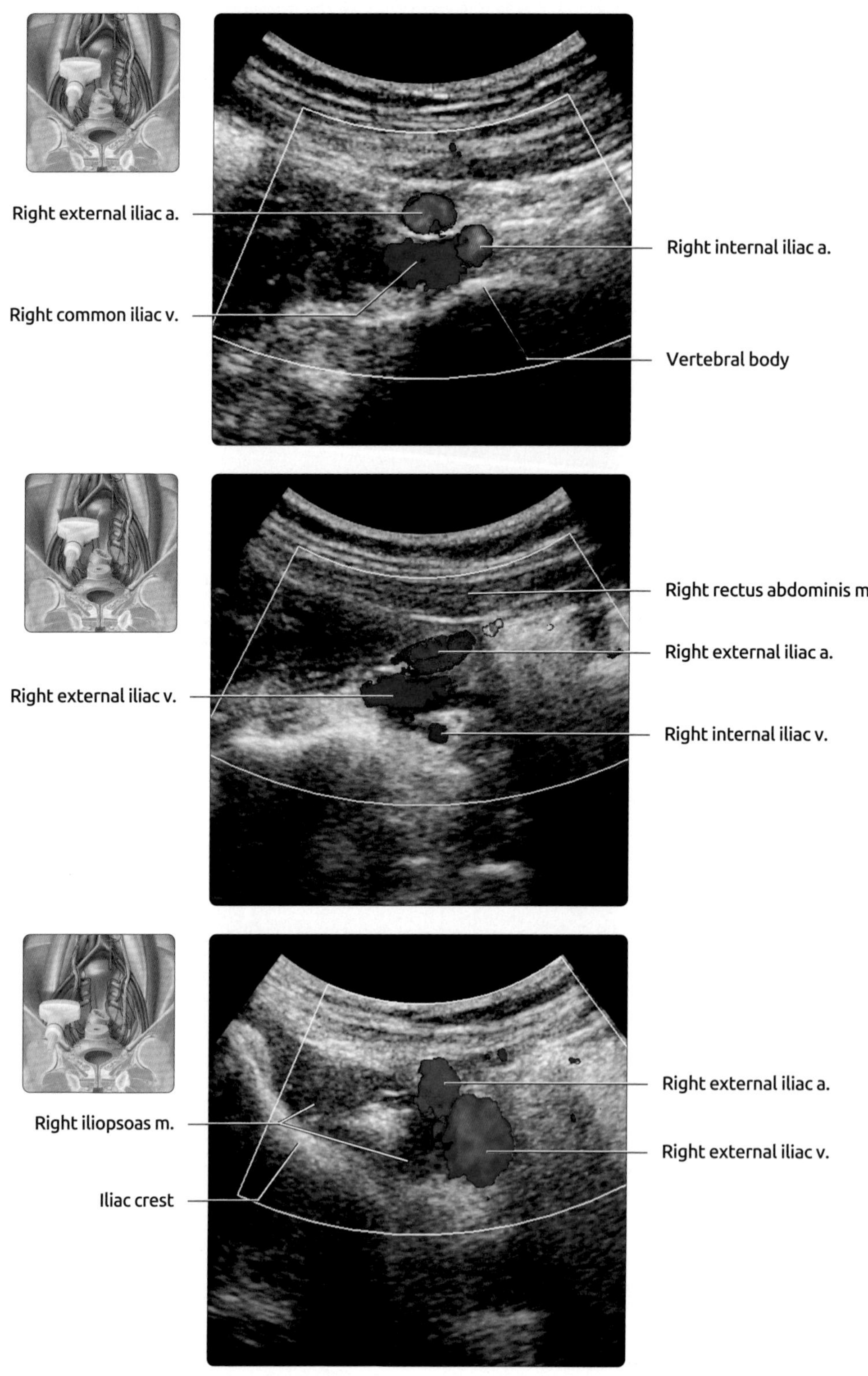

(Top) *Transverse transabdominal color Doppler ultrasound shows dichotomous branching of the right common iliac artery into the larger caliber external iliac artery (red) and smaller caliber internal iliac artery (red). The common iliac vein (blue) maintains its posterior location in relation to the 2 arteries.* **(Middle)** *Transverse transabdominal color Doppler ultrasound, continued more inferiorly in the same patient, demonstrates the right external iliac vein and smaller internal iliac vein (shown in blue). The right external iliac artery (shown in red) is identified anterior to its venous counterpart.* **(Bottom)** *Transverse color Doppler ultrasound at the right iliac fossa is shown. The right external iliac artery (shown in red) and vein (shown in blue) course medial to the psoas major/iliopsoas muscle and maintain their relationship until they exit the pelvis beneath the inguinal ligament. Note the larger diameter of the vein compared to the artery.*

ILIAC VESSELS, CT

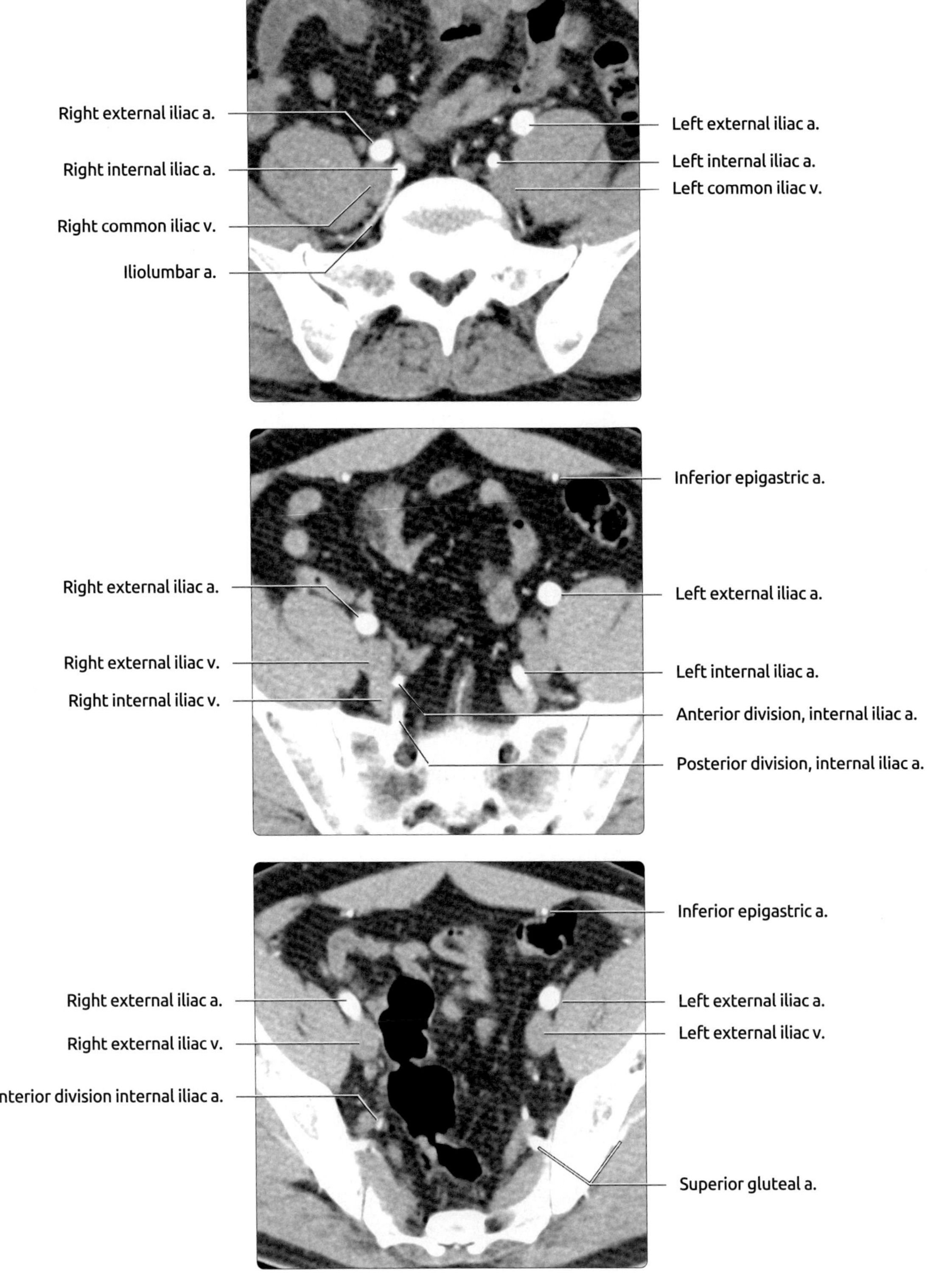

(Top) *First of 3 axial CECT images of the pelvic vessels is shown. The common iliac arteries bifurcate more proximal to the formation of the common iliac veins. The iliolumbar artery, usually a branch of the posterior trunk of the internal iliac artery, arises in this subject from the main internal iliac artery. CT is the imaging modality of choice in the examination of smaller pelvic vessels.* **(Middle)** *The internal iliac artery divides into an anterior and posterior trunk. The anterior trunk mainly supplies the pelvic viscera, whereas the posterior trunk supplies the pelvic musculature. Note their deep location relative to the external iliac vessels, which limits ultrasound examination of internal iliac vessel branches and tributaries.* **(Bottom)** *The external iliac artery and vein continue in an anterolateral direction as they course out of the pelvis and into the thigh.*

COMMON ILIAC VEIN

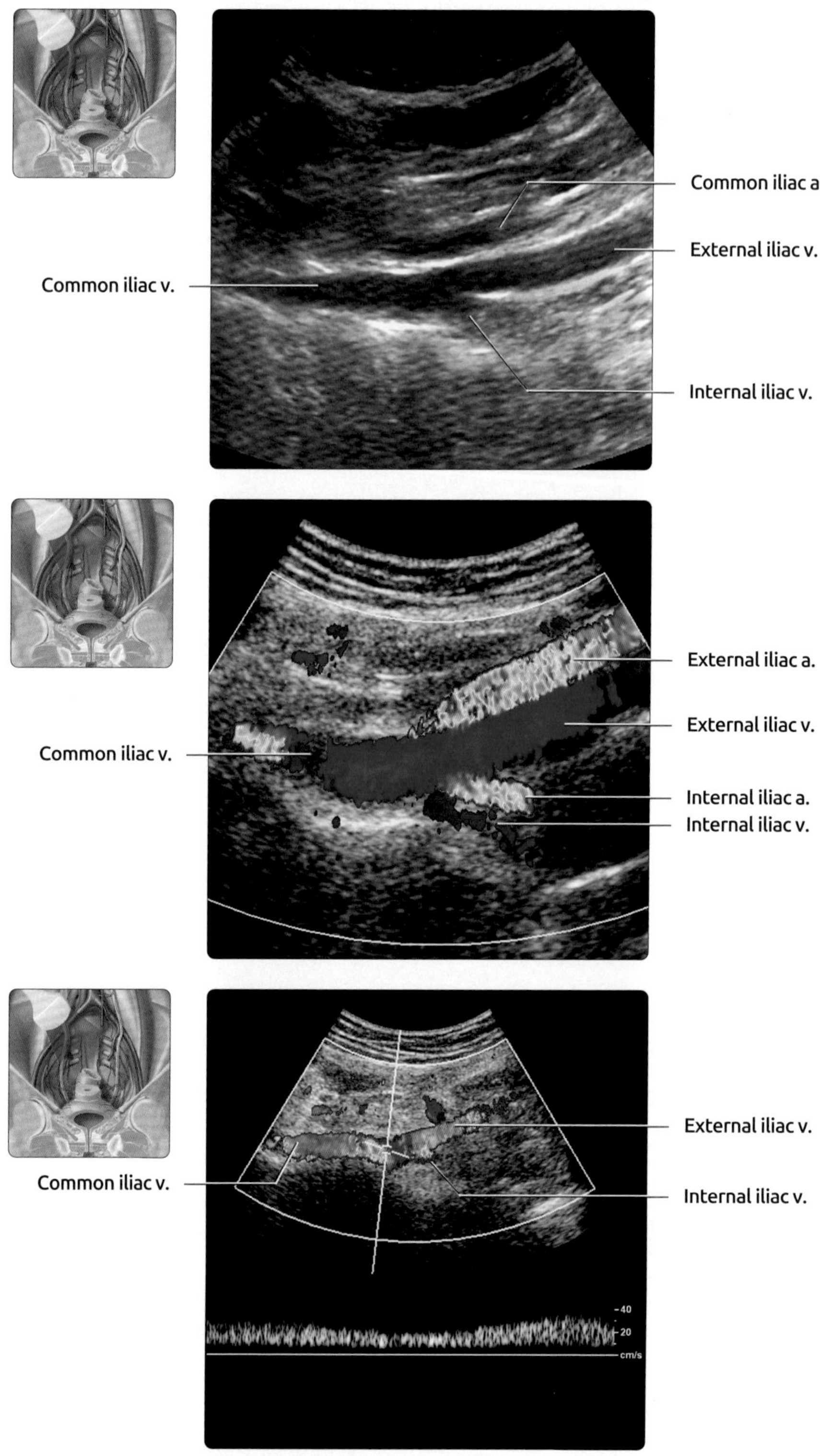

(Top) *Longitudinal transabdominal grayscale ultrasound shows the external and internal iliac veins converging to form the common iliac vein.* **(Middle)** *Longitudinal transabdominal color Doppler ultrasound provides information on the direction of blood flow in the pelvic vessels, facilitating identification and differentiation of the veins from arteries. The external iliac vein (shown in blue) is a large-caliber vessel seen posterior to its arterial counterpart (shown in multicolor). Note its uniform intensity in color flow. The internal iliac vein (shown in red) is smaller in diameter and directed inferomedially.* **(Bottom)** *Pulsed Doppler ultrasound of the common iliac vein shows uniform velocity with mild phasic changes associated with respiration.*

INTERNAL ILIAC VEIN

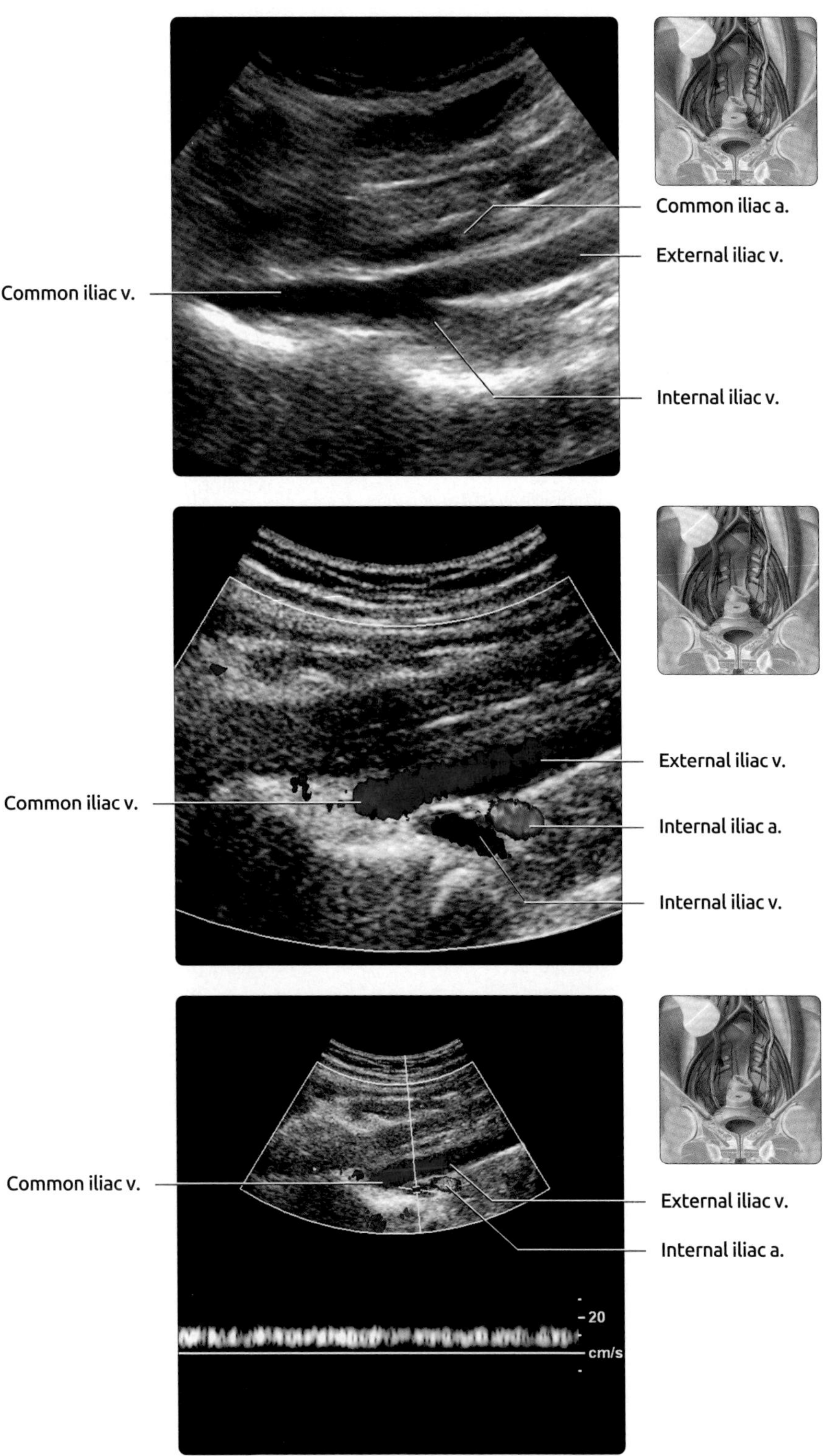

(Top) *Longitudinal transabdominal grayscale ultrasound shows the external and internal iliac veins converging to become the common iliac vein. The internal iliac vein drains various veins from outside the pelvis, the sacrum, and from the venous plexuses connected to pelvic viscera.* **(Middle)** *Longitudinal transabdominal color Doppler ultrasound shows a short segment of the internal iliac vein (shown in red) draining into the common iliac vein (shown in blue). Owing to its depth, the internal iliac vein cannot be identified on ultrasound in its entirety.* **(Bottom)** *Pulsed Doppler ultrasound of the internal iliac vein shows continuous venous flow and uniform velocity devoid of phasic changes and unaffected by respiration.*

GROSS ANATOMY

Vessels of Leg

- **Popliteal artery**
  - Begins as continuation of superficial femoral artery after it has passed through adductor hiatus (inferior end of adductor canal)
  - Runs through fat of popliteal fossa
  - Relationships
    - Deep to artery: Femoral shaft, knee joint capsule, popliteus fascia
    - Superficial to artery: Popliteal vein, semimembranosus muscle, and gastrocnemius muscle
  - Artery lies just deep to vein in 40%, deep and medial to vein in 43%, deep and lateral to vein in 9%, and just medial or lateral to vein in 8%
  - Ends at distal border of popliteus muscle dividing into 2 branches: Anterior tibial artery and tibioperoneal trunk
- **Anterior tibial artery**
  - Smaller of the 2 terminal branches of popliteal artery
  - Origin in back of leg, at distal border of popliteus muscle
  - Passes through upper part of interosseous membrane
  - Straight course down front of leg to become dorsalis pedis artery
  - Runs on anterior surface of interosseous membrane, deep to extensor muscles
  - Muscular branches along length
  - Malleolar branches ramify over malleoli; lateral branch anastomoses with perforating branch of peroneal artery
- **Posterior tibial artery**
  - Larger of 2 terminal branches of popliteal artery
  - Main blood supply to foot
  - Passes downward and slightly medially along with tibial nerve to end in space between medial malleolus and calcaneus
  - Within calf, artery runs just deep to transverse intermuscular septum
  - Divides into lateral and medial plantar arteries in tarsal tunnel behind medial malleolus
  - Branches
    - Circumflex fibular (may arise from anterior tibial), runs laterally around neck of fibula
    - Nutrient artery to tibia
    - Muscular branches
- **Peroneal artery**
  - Largest branch of posterior tibial artery
  - Runs obliquely downward and laterally beneath soleus to fibula
  - Descends deep to flexor hallucis longus
- **Popliteal vein**
  - Paired venae comitantes of anterior and posterior tibial arteries join to form popliteal vein
  - Also receives small saphenous vein in popliteal fossa
  - Usually begins at inferior border of popliteus muscle
  - Crosses from medial to lateral side of popliteal artery as it runs in popliteal fossa, aside from always being superficial to popliteal artery
  - Ends at adductor hiatus by becoming superficial femoral vein
- **Great saphenous vein**
  - Begins at medial border of foot
  - Ascends in front of medial malleolus
  - Passes obliquely upward and backward across medial surface of distal 1/3 of tibia
  - Passes vertically upward along medial border of tibia to posterior part of medial side of knee
- **Small saphenous vein**
  - Extends behind lateral malleolus, ascends lateral to Achilles tendon
  - At midline of calf in lower popliteal region, pierces popliteal fascia, and terminates in popliteal vein

ANATOMY IMAGING ISSUES

Imaging Recommendations

- Ultrasound
  - Examination of lower limb vessels requires use of morphological and functional techniques
    - Morphology: Documentation of areas of stenosis or occlusion, sites of venous valves, aberrant branches, aneurysm formation, etc.
    - Functional: Combination of color and spectral Doppler examination
  - Veins require use of dynamic maneuvers
    - Compression: To demonstrate absence of thrombus by using transducer pressure to cause complete luminal occlusion
    - Valsalva: To increase abdominal pressure and accentuate reverse flow and incompetent venous valves
    - Augmentation: To increase venous return (to demonstrate venous flow and patency) by manually squeezing calf or by gently moving toes
  - Arteries require use of spectral Doppler scanning to show their phasicity; normal scan is triphasic
    - Sharp forward flow upstroke (systolic phase)
    - Small reversed flow (early diastolic phase)
    - Final smaller forward flow (late diastolic phase)

Imaging Pitfalls

- Augmentation frequently required to demonstrate flow in deep calf veins (which normally show no color Doppler flow)

ANTERIOR AND POSTERIOR LEG VESSELS

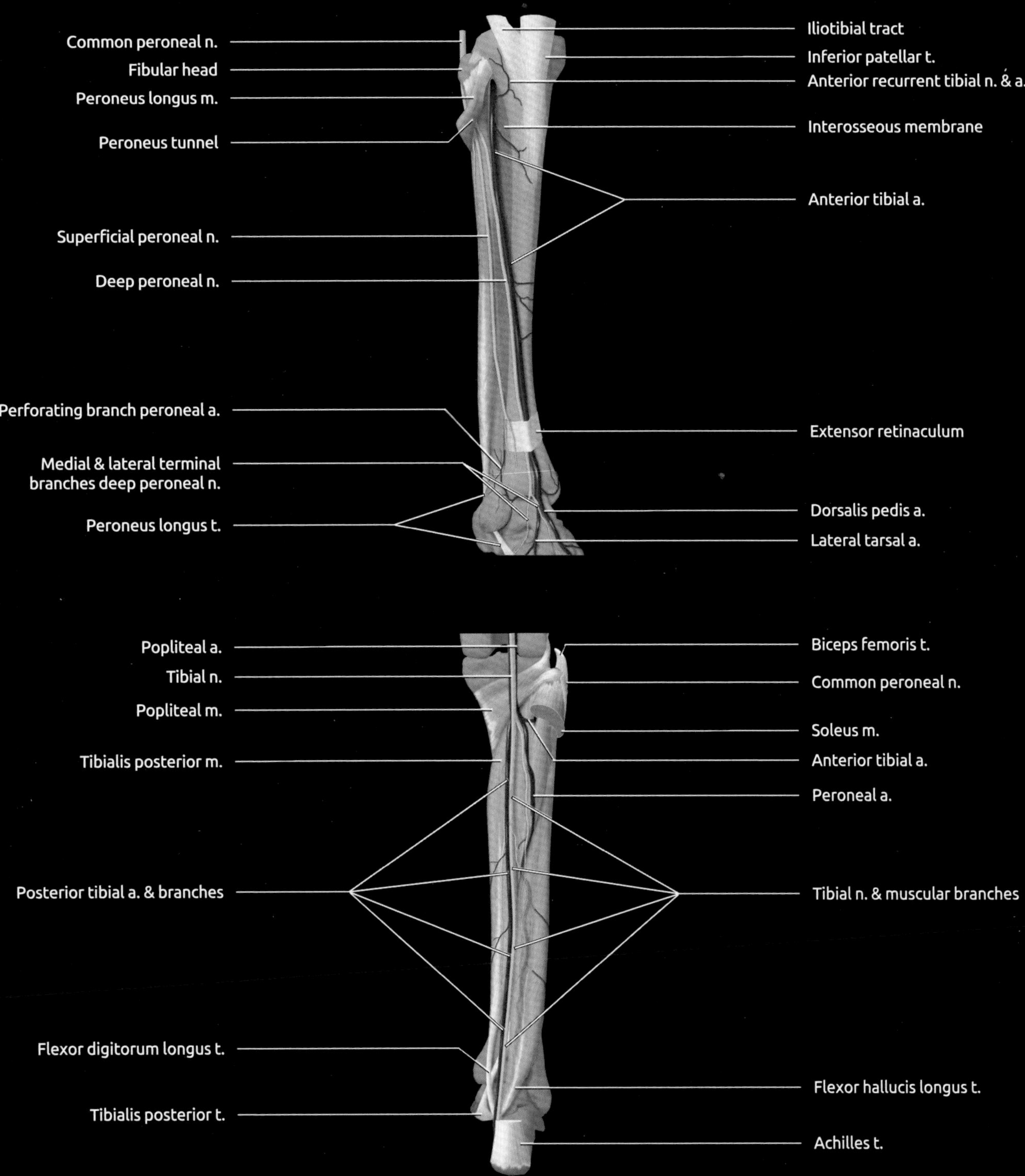

(Top) *Graphic of anterior leg shows the anterior tibial artery perforating the interosseous septum proximally and descending along this membrane down the front of leg to terminate as the dorsalis pedis. Distally, a perforating branch of the peroneal artery is seen, which in a variant situation may provide the major blood supply to the dorsum of the foot.* **(Bottom)** *The popliteal artery ends at the distal border of popliteus in 2 branches: (1) Anterior tibial artery passes through a slit in the tibialis posterior muscle and the interosseous membrane to the anterior compartment, and (2) the posterior tibial artery passes downward and slightly medially adjacent to the tibial nerve to end in the space between the medial malleolus and calcaneus. The largest branch of the posterior tibial artery is the peroneal artery, which runs obliquely downward and laterally beneath the soleus to the fibula.*

POPLITEAL VESSELS

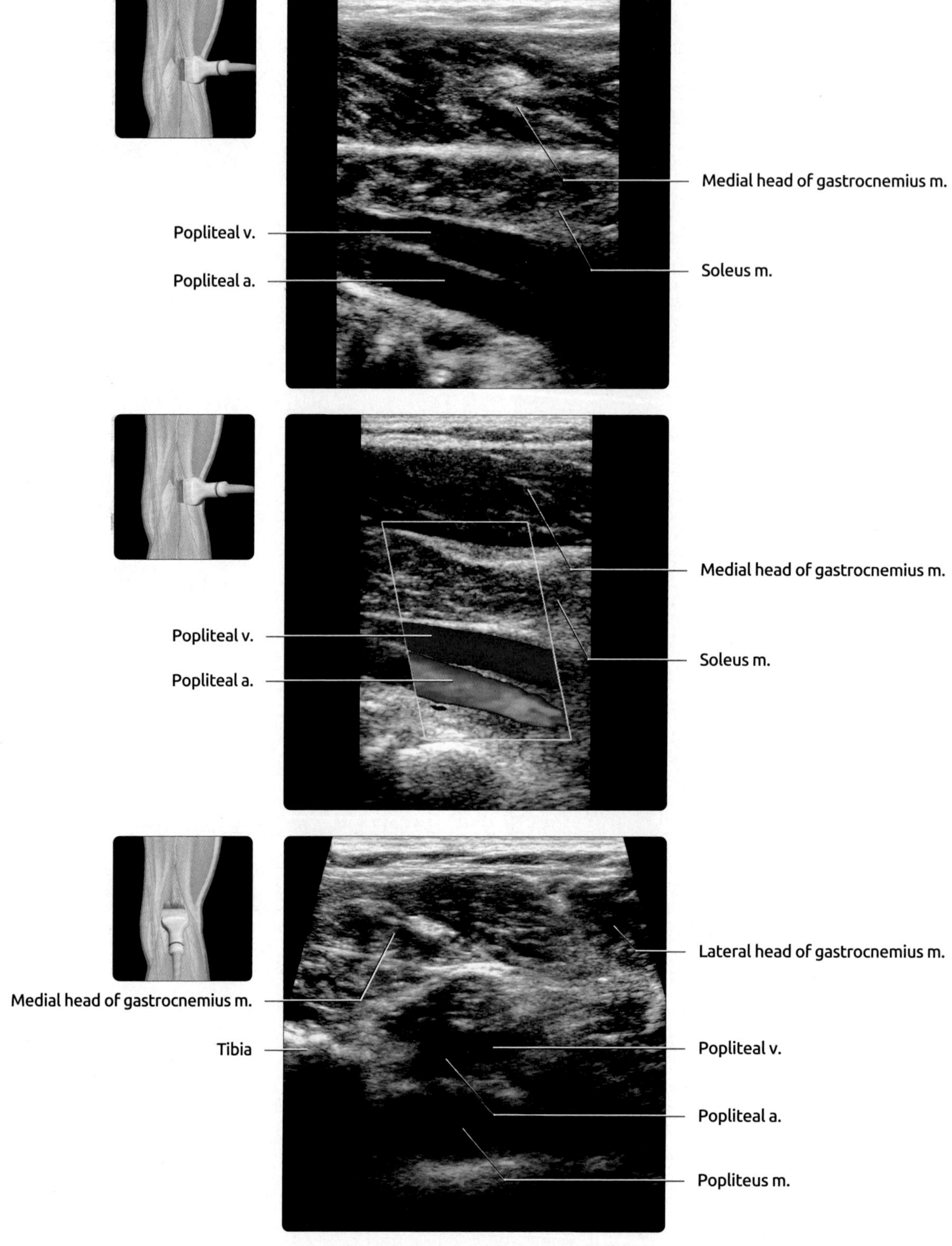

(Top) *Sagittal US shows the lower part of the popliteal vessels, which are continuations of the superficial femoral vessels after they have exited the adductor canal through the adductor hiatus. The popliteal vein lies superficial to the popliteal artery, a reverse of the relationship between the superficial femoral vein and artery. The popliteal vessels pass inferolaterally through the fat of the popliteal fossa.* **(Middle)** *Sagittal color Doppler US of the popliteal vessels shows complete color filling of the lumina (excluding luminal thrombus) and normal flow direction, toward the trunk (blue) for the vein and away from the trunk (red) for the artery.* **(Bottom)** *Transverse US shows the lower part of the popliteal vessels. The popliteal vein runs superficial to the popliteal artery and usually bifurcates at the inferior margin of the popliteus muscle.*

POPLITEAL VESSEL BIFURCATION

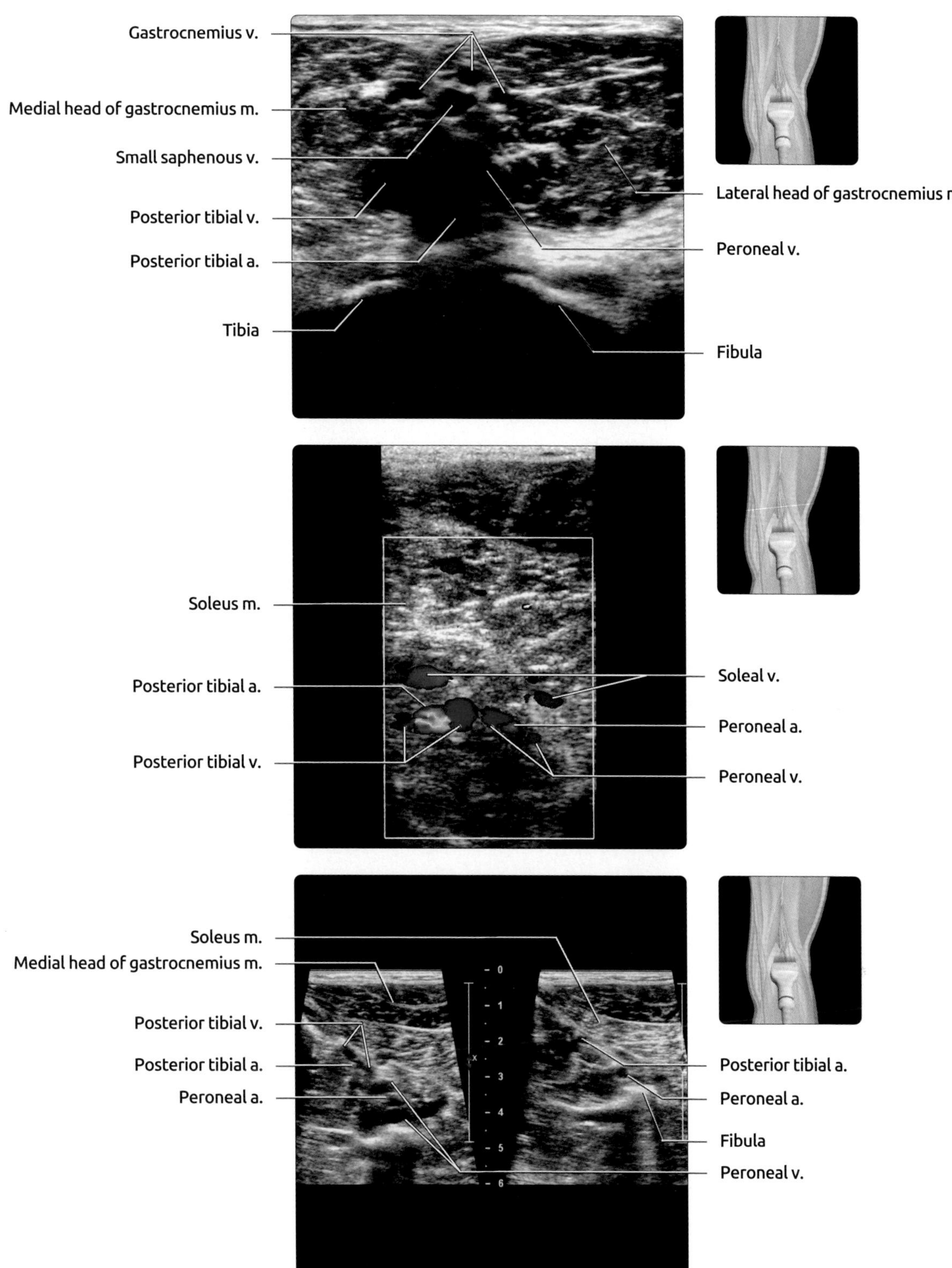

(Top) *Transverse US below the bifurcation of the popliteal artery is shown. The popliteal artery bifurcates into the anterior and posterior tibial arteries. The posterior tibial artery is the larger of the 2 terminal branches of the popliteal artery and passes inferiorly for a short distance before giving out its largest branch, the peroneal artery.* **(Middle)** *Transverse color Doppler US shows the posterior compartment vessels of the proximal calf. Color flow highlights the paired venae comitantes nature of the posterior tibial and peroneal veins, lying on both sides of the corresponding artery.* **(Bottom)** *Transverse US at the midproximal calf, scanning from the medial side is shown. The lumina of the peroneal and tibial veins can be compressed by firm transducer pressure (right side of image), indicating the lack of thrombus.*

TRANSVERSE POSTERIOR TIBIAL VESSELS

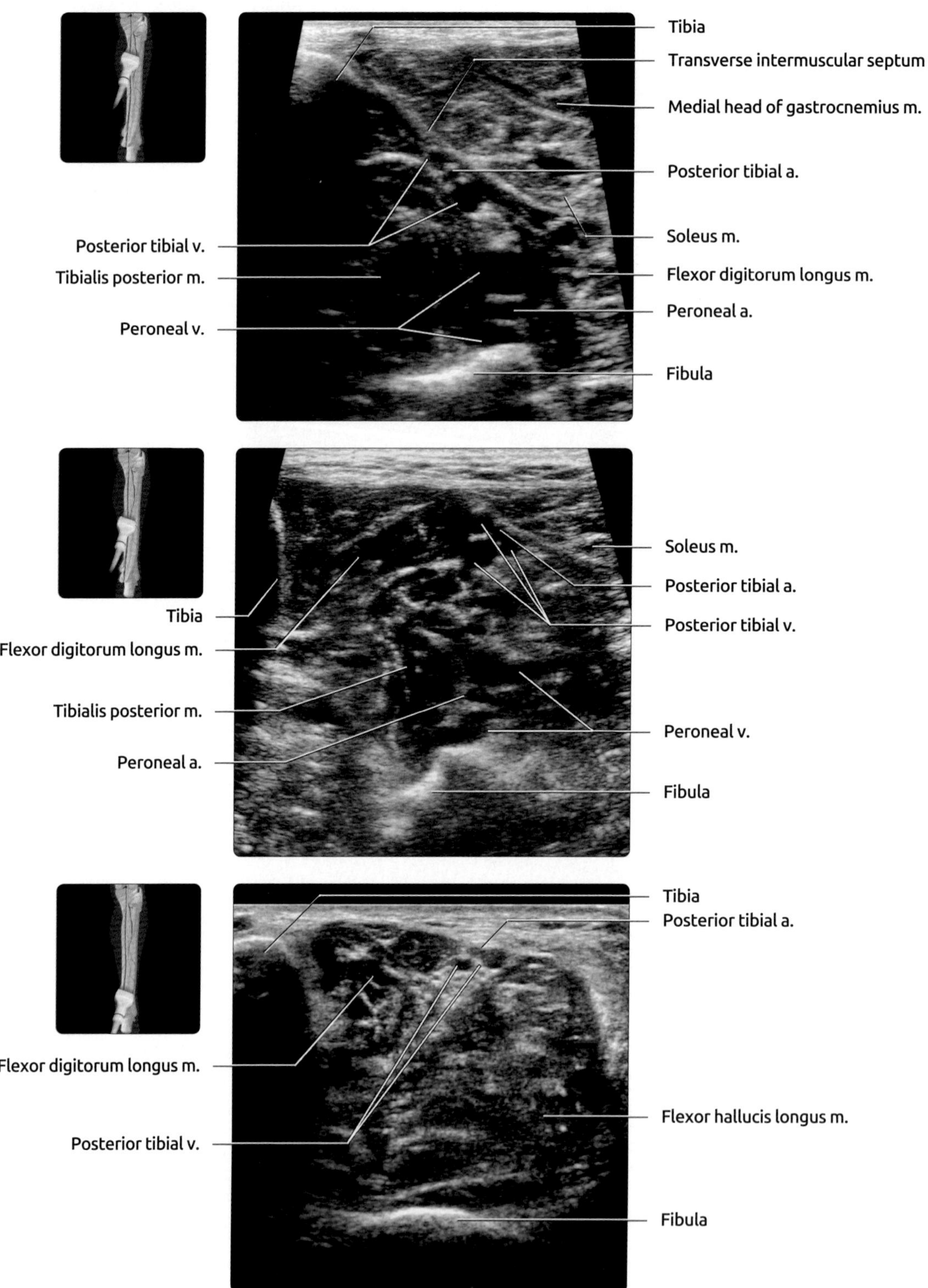

(Top) *Three transverse scans show the posterior tibial vessels using a medial approach. Superiorly, the posterior tibial vessels give off their main branches, the common peroneal vessels. The posterior tibial artery lies just deep to the transverse intermuscular septum while the peroneal arteries are deep to the flexor digitorum muscle.* **(Middle)** *At the midcalf level, the posterior tibial vessels no longer line up side by side (3 in a line). Anatomical variations occur, as seen here with 3 posterior tibial veins accompanying 1 artery. The peroneal vessels continue their deeper course, running on the surface of the tibialis posterior, which separates them from the anterior leg compartment.* **(Bottom)** *Further inferiorly, the posterior tibial vessels emerge superficially as they prepare to enter the tarsal tunnel behind the medial malleolus.*

LONGITUDINAL POSTERIOR TIBIAL VESSELS

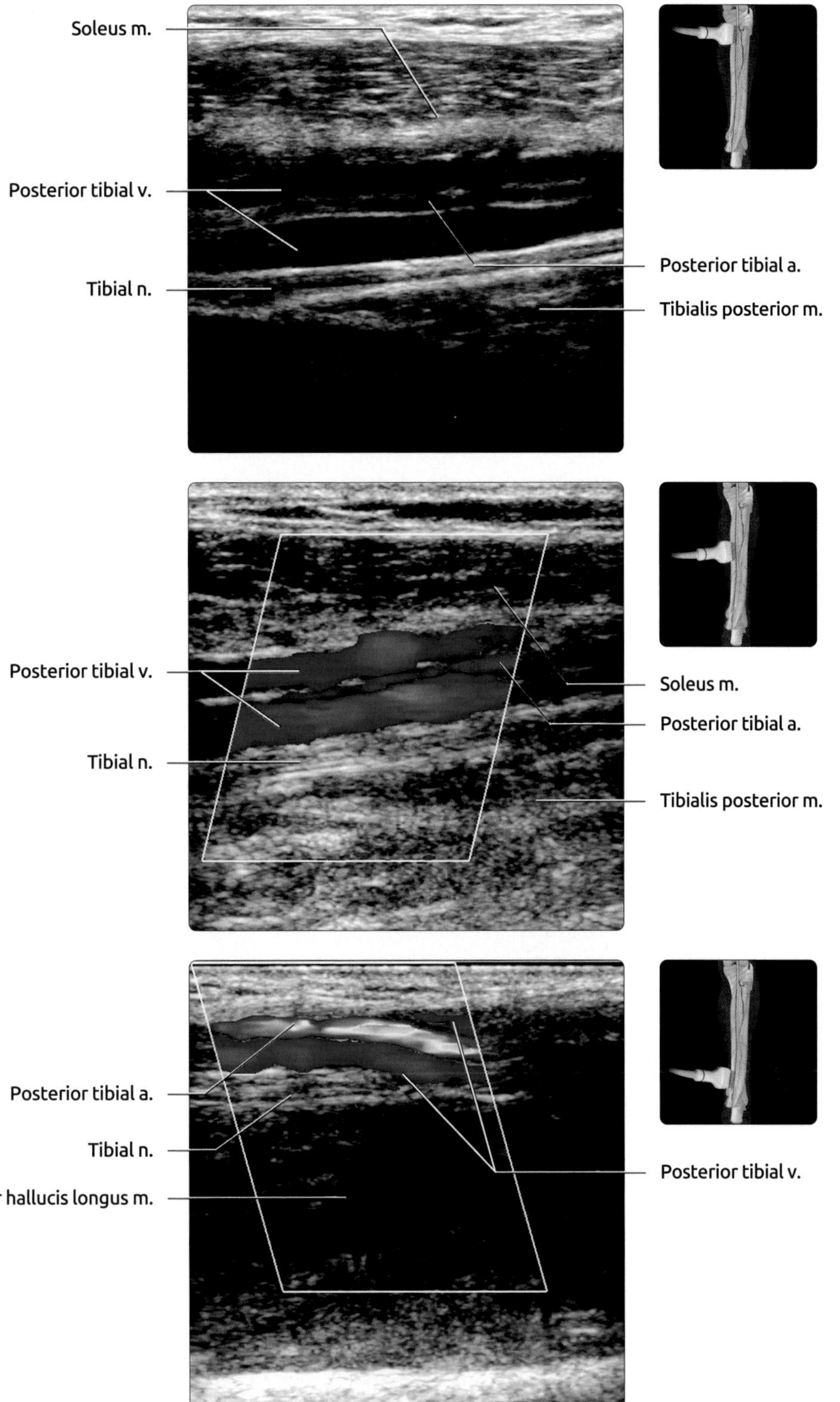

(Top) *Oblique coronal US shows the posterior tibial vessels using a medial approach. The posterior tibial artery is accompanied by paired venae comitantes (posterior tibial veins) and the tibial nerve. They run deep to the transverse intermuscular septum of the leg.* **(Middle)** *Color Doppler US shows the posterior tibial vessels. Notice the marked difference in caliber between the artery and the veins, all of which show normal, complete color filling and normal direction of flow.* **(Bottom)** *Further inferiorly, oblique coronal US of the lower calf shows the distal part of the posterior tibial vessels running superficial to the flexor hallucis muscle and getting ready to curve under the medial malleolus. The posterior tibial vessels and tibial nerve run in the tarsal tunnel together with the tendon flexors of the foot.*

TRANSVERSE PERONEAL VESSELS

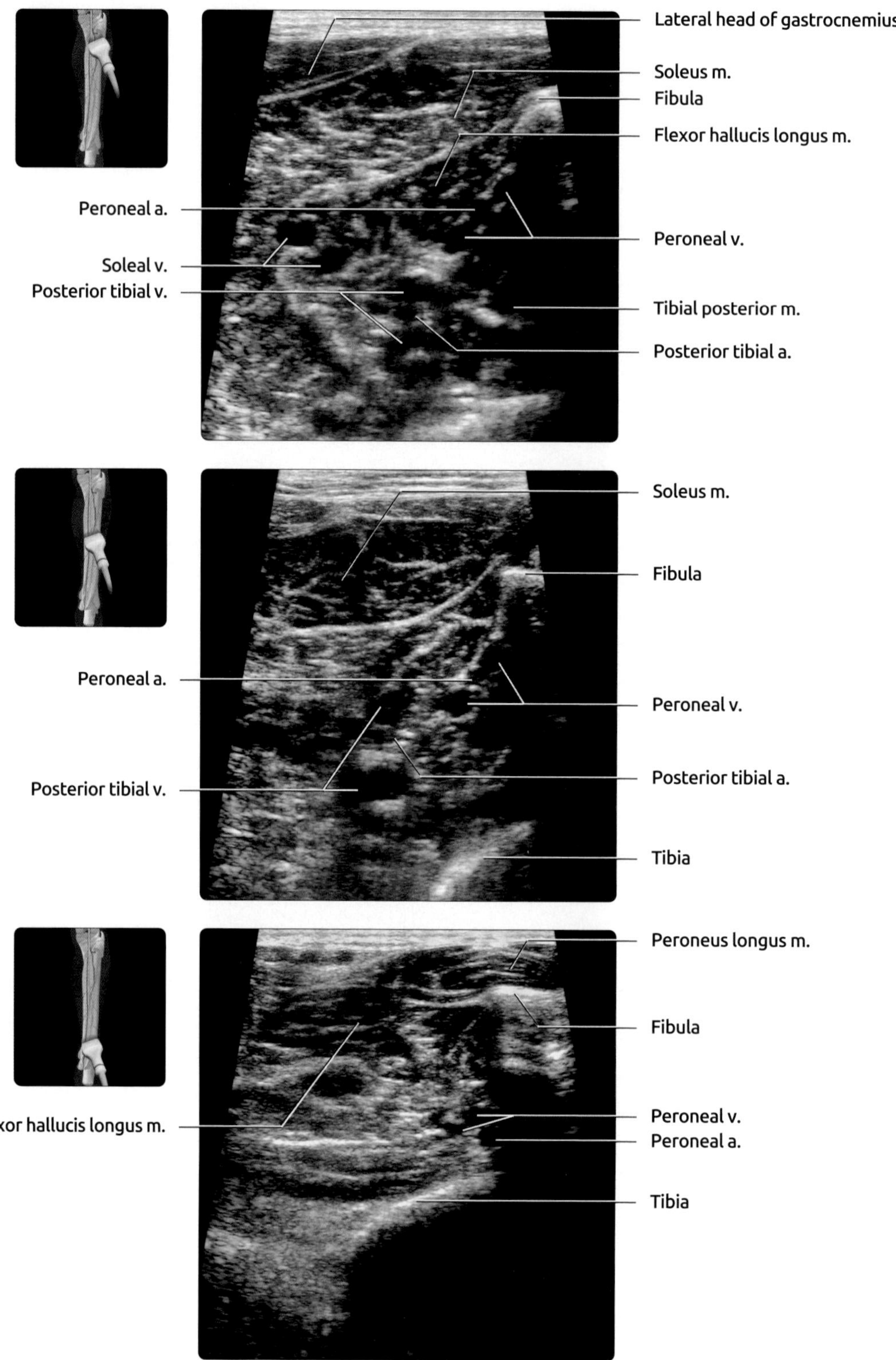

(Top) *Three transverse scans of the calf using a lateral approach are shown. The peroneal artery is a branch of the posterior tibial artery. It runs obliquely toward the fibula and then along the medial surface of the fibula distally, sandwiched between the flexor hallucis longus muscle and tibialis posterior muscle.* **(Middle)** *More distally, the relationship between the peroneal vessels and the fibula and flexor muscles remains the same. Nutrient vessels branch out to supply the fibula and the adjacent muscles.* **(Bottom)** *Most distally, the peroneal artery runs behind the tibiofibular syndesmosis before dividing into lateral calcaneal branches, which run over the lateral and posterior surfaces of the calcaneum.*

LONGITUDINAL PERONEAL VESSELS

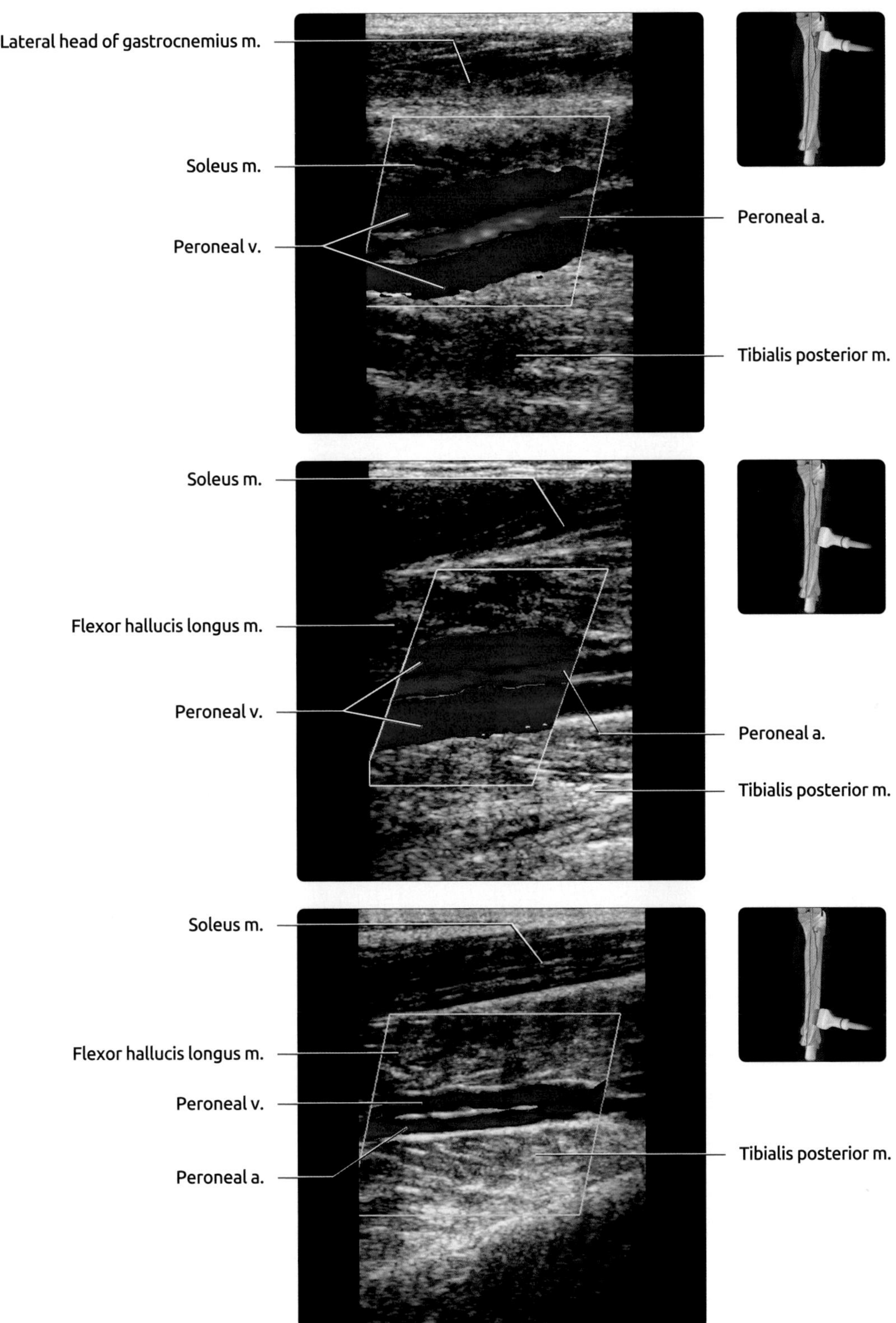

(Top) *Oblique coronal US shows the peroneal vessels using a lateral approach. The peroneal artery, like the posterior tibial, is also accompanied by venae comitantes (peroneal veins); the difference is that there is no peroneal nerve to accompany the vessels. The peroneal nerve runs in the lateral leg compartment after curving around the neck of the fibula.* **(Middle)** *More inferiorly, oblique coronal US shows the peroneus vessels lie deep to the flexor hallucis longus and soleus muscles while running superficial to the tibialis posterior muscle.* **(Bottom)** *Further inferiorly, the peroneal vessels are much smaller in caliber after giving out many branches, passing posterior to the tibiofibular syndesmosis.*

TRANSVERSE ANTERIOR TIBIAL VESSELS

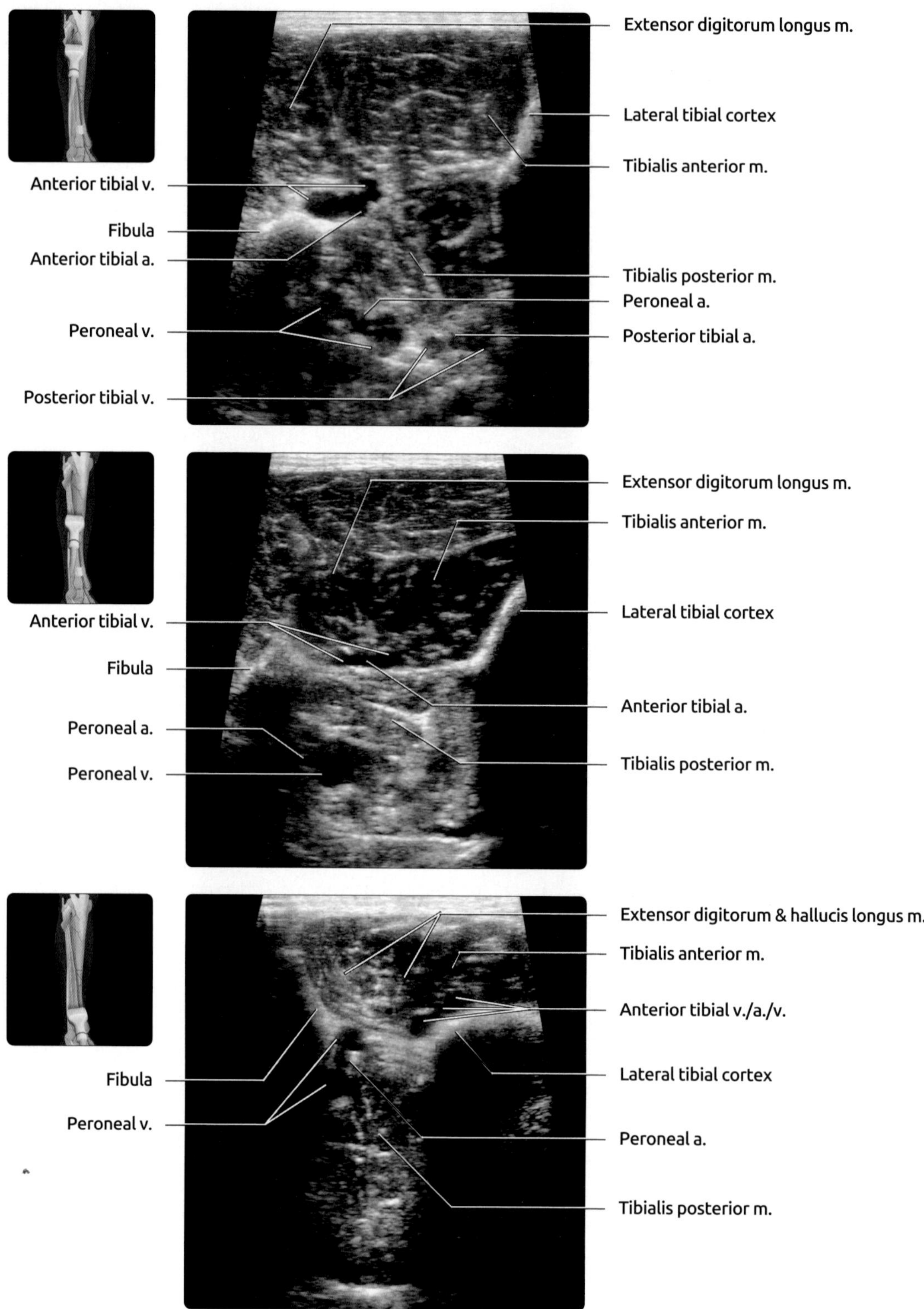

(Top) *Three transverse scans show the anterior tibial vessels using an anterior approach. The anterior tibial vessels are the smaller terminal branches of the popliteal vessels (smaller compared to the posterior tibial vessels at the bifurcation). After its origin, the anterior tibial vessels run anterior through the interosseous membrane and then pass inferiorly on the anterior surface of this membrane.* **(Middle)** *At midleg level, the anterior tibial vessels continue to run in a deep position on the surface of the interosseous membrane. Through the window between the tibia and fibula, the peroneal vessels and tibialis posterior muscle are seen.* **(Bottom)** *In the most distal part of the leg, the anterior tibial vessels move medially to lie on the surface of the tibia. At this level, the peroneal artery branches run anteriorly to penetrate the interosseous membrane.*

LONGITUDINAL ANTERIOR TIBIAL VESSELS

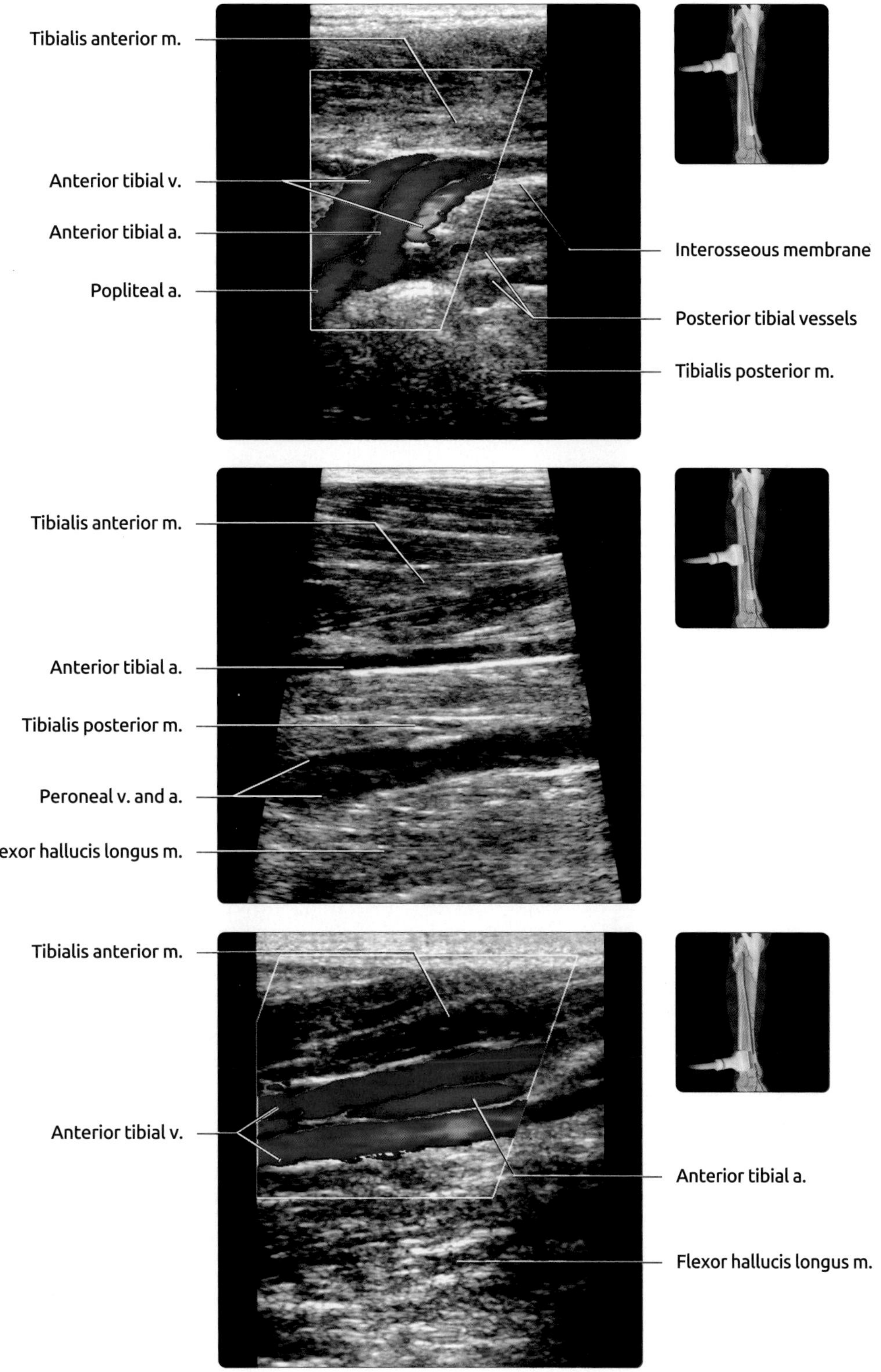

(Top) *Oblique sagittal color Doppler US shows the anterior tibial vessels as they bifurcate from the popliteal vessels. The anterior tibial vessels run anteriorly to penetrate the interosseous membrane into the anterior compartment.* **(Middle)** *Sagittal US shows the anterior tibial artery in the midleg level. The anterior tibial artery runs deep within the anterior compartment and on the surface of the interosseous membrane, being covered by the tibialis anterior muscle.* **(Bottom)** *Sagittal color Doppler US shows the lower aspect of the anterior tibial vessels. The vessels begin to run more superficially, and in the foot, the anterior tibial artery continues as the dorsalis pedis artery.*

SPECTRAL DOPPLER OF LEG ARTERIES

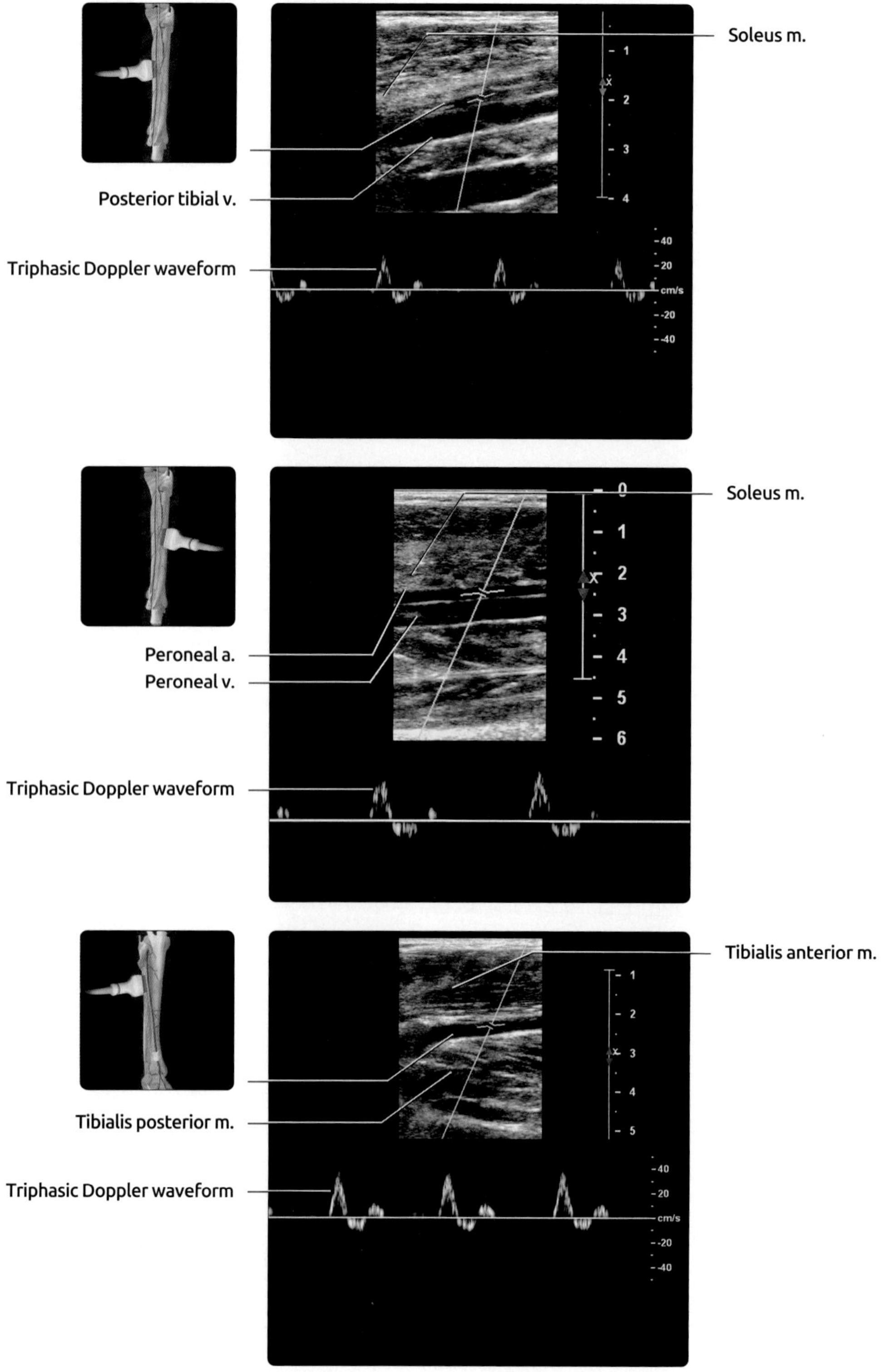

(Top) *Spectral Doppler US of the posterior tibial artery demonstrates the typical triphasic pattern seen in normal arteries. Loss of the reverse flow in the diastolic phase is termed a biphasic pattern and would suggest stenosis proximal to the point of interrogation. With proximal stenosis, the peak flow velocity would also be decreased.* **(Middle)** *Similarly, the peroneal artery shows a triphasic waveform on spectral Doppler US.* **(Bottom)** *Oblique coronal spectral Doppler US of the anterior tibial artery in the upper calf level also shows a normal triphasic pattern. Abnormal increase in reversed flow (negative flow in early diastolic phase) would suggest increased distal resistance from stenosis.*

SPECTRAL DOPPLER OF LEG VEINS

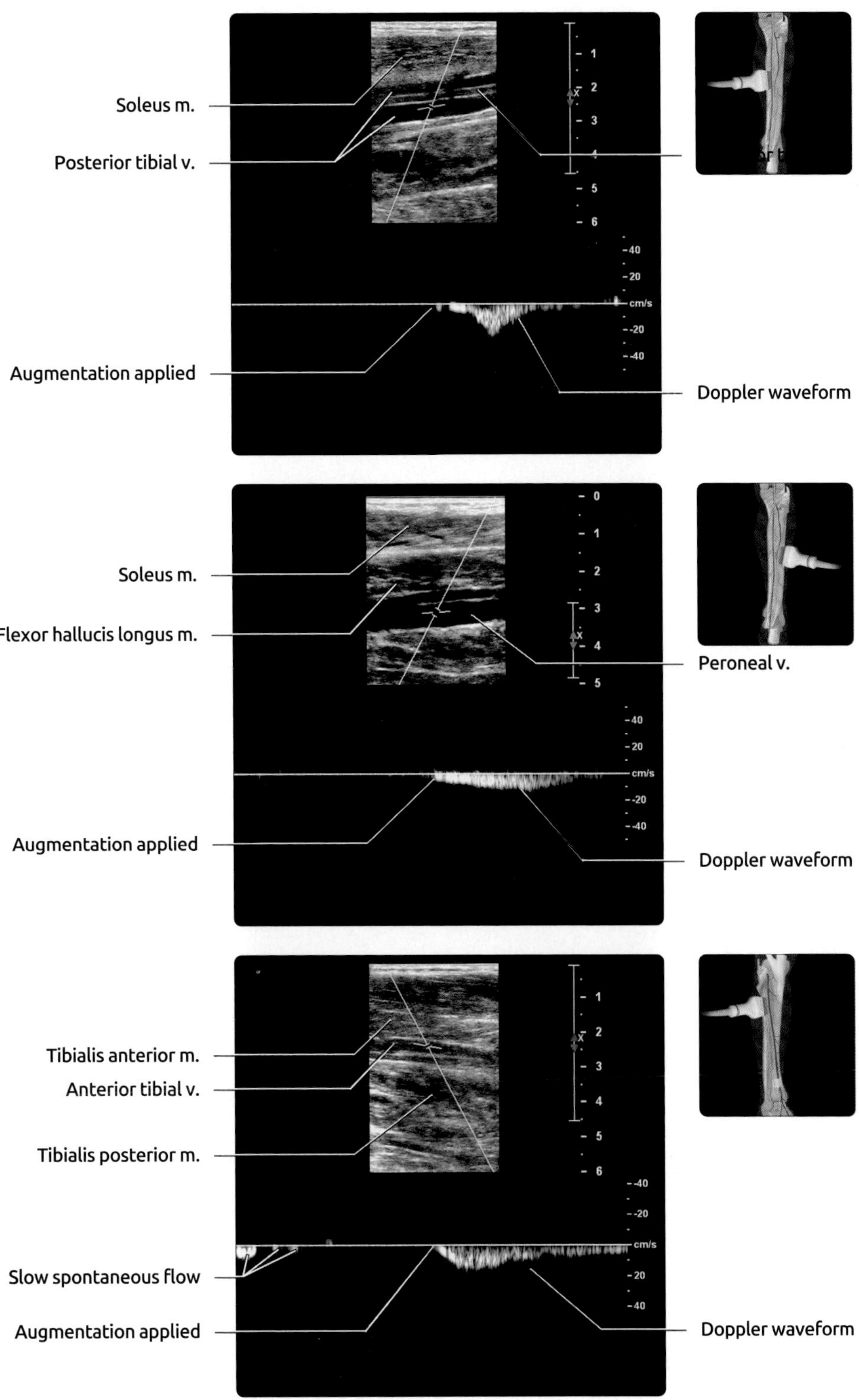

(Top) *Oblique coronal spectral Doppler US of the posterior tibial vein shows absence of spontaneous flow at rest (left 1/2 of the spectral trace). After augmentation (squeezing calf muscles distal to transducer), a surge of blood flow toward the trunk (negative values) can be demonstrated and indicates luminal patency.* **(Middle)** *Oblique coronal spectral Doppler US of the peroneal vein before and after augmentation shows a similar sudden surge of blood flow.* **(Bottom)** *Oblique coronal spectral Doppler US of the anterior tibial vein demonstrates slow spontaneous flow at rest. After augmentation, a sustained surge of flow is demonstrated.*

SOLEAL VEINS

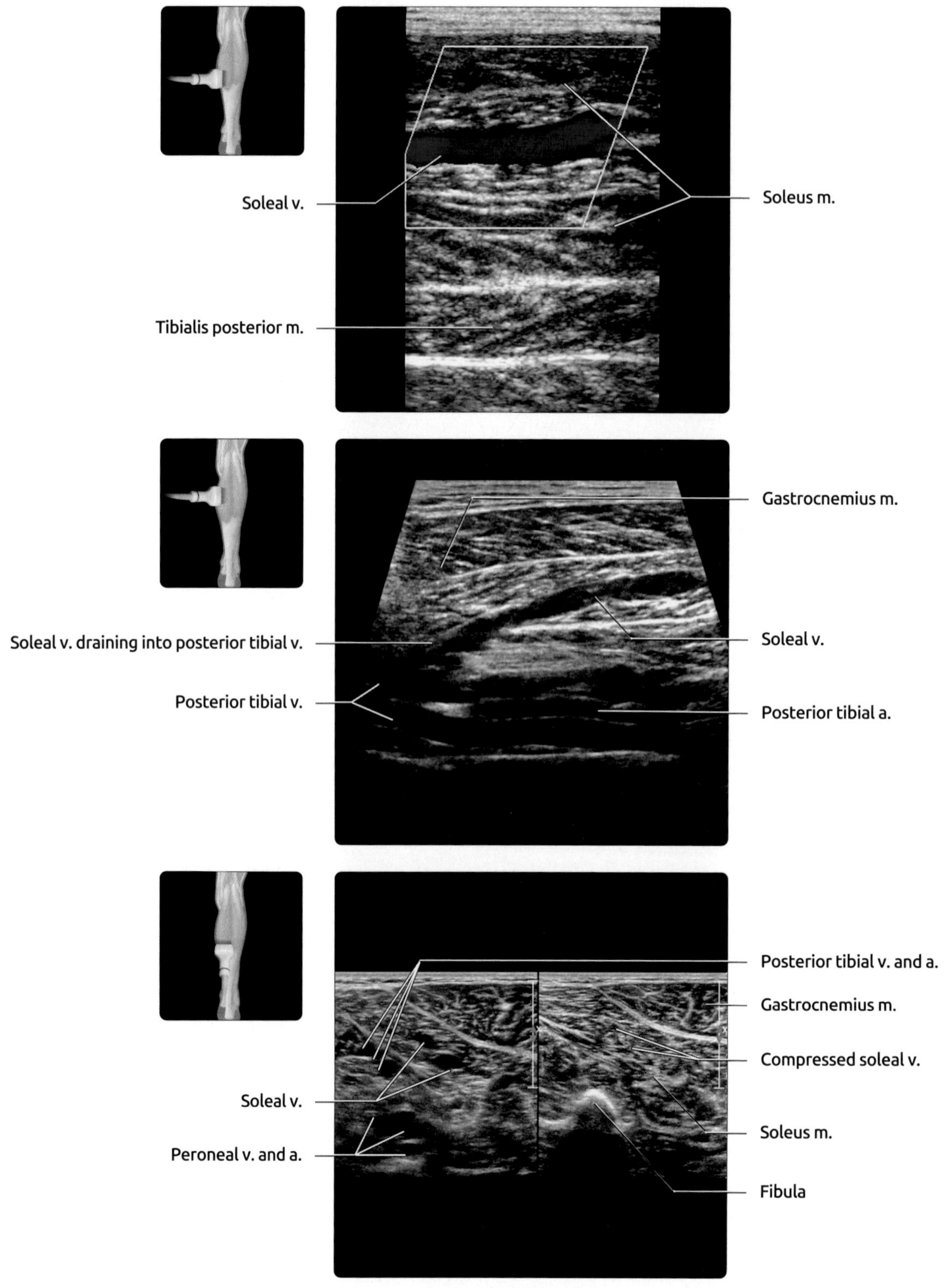

(Top) *Oblique sagittal color Doppler US shows the posterior compartment in the midcalf level. The soleal vein shows complete color filling of its lumen, indicating the absence of thrombus. Soleal veins are the most common veins to develop thrombosis and should be assessed when scanning for deep venous thrombosis.* **(Middle)** *Oblique sagittal US of the posterior compartment shows the soleal vein running proximally and joining the posterior tibial vein. This pathway allows a soleal vein thrombus to extend into the posterior tibial vein and propagate proximally.* **(Bottom)** *Dual transverse US shows the posterior compartment using a medial approach, before (left) and during (right) firm transducer compression. The soleal veins are completely compressed by transducer pressure, indicating an absence of thrombus.*

GASTROCNEMIUS VEINS

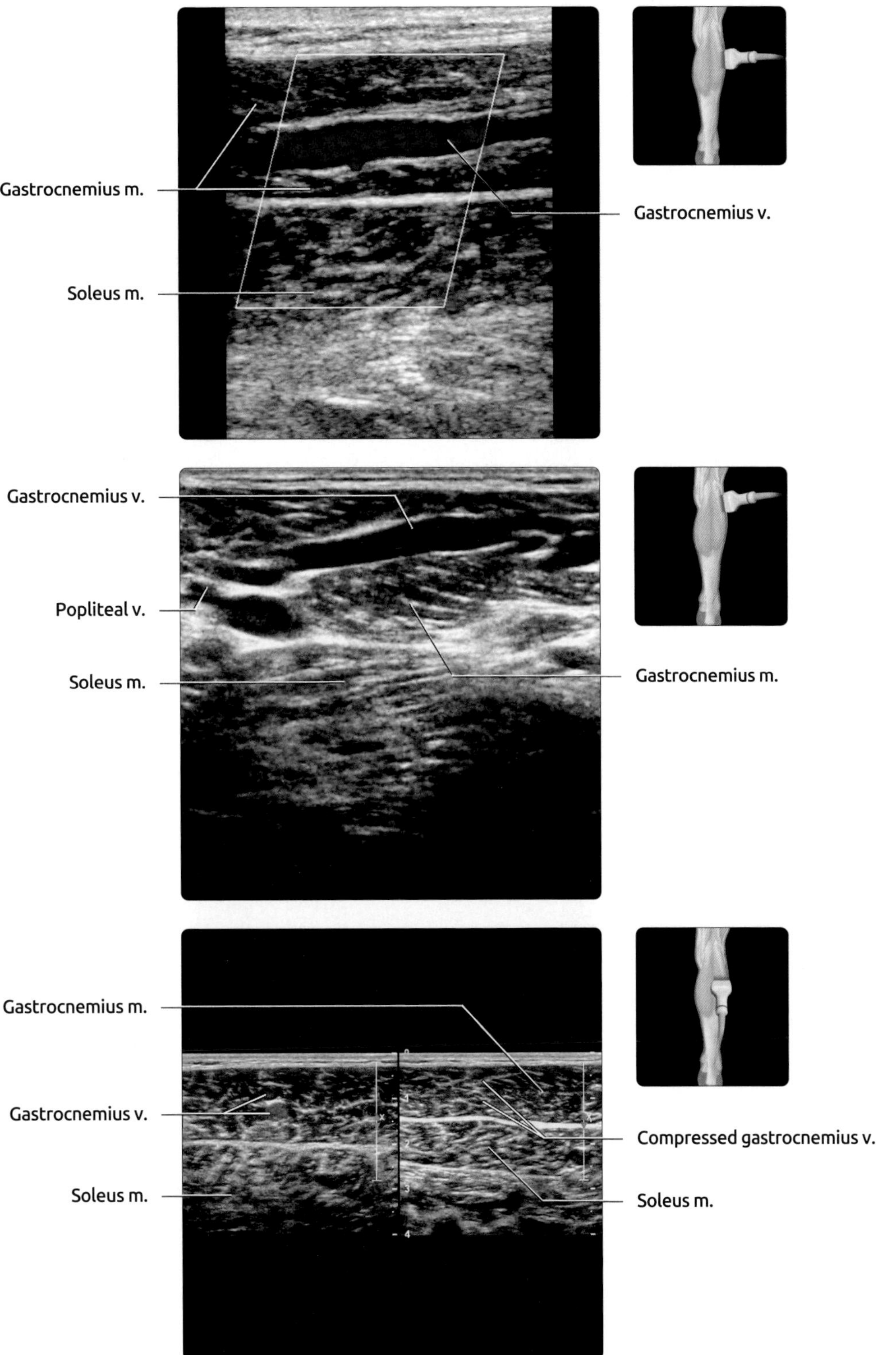

(Top) *Oblique sagittal color Doppler US shows the posterior leg compartment. The gastrocnemius vein shows complete color filling, indicating absence of thrombus. The gastrocnemius veins are the 2nd most common site for venous thrombosis.* **(Middle)** *Oblique sagittal US of the posterior compartment of the upper calf shows the gastrocnemius vein joining the popliteal vein, allowing a gastrocnemius vein thrombus to extend proximally to the popliteal vein.* **(Bottom)** *Dual transverse US shows gastrocnemius veins before (left) and during (right) compression. The gastrocnemius veins are completely compressed during compression, indicating an absence of thrombus. Compression is regarded as the most reliable technique to rule out venous thrombosis.*

SMALL SAPHENOUS VEIN

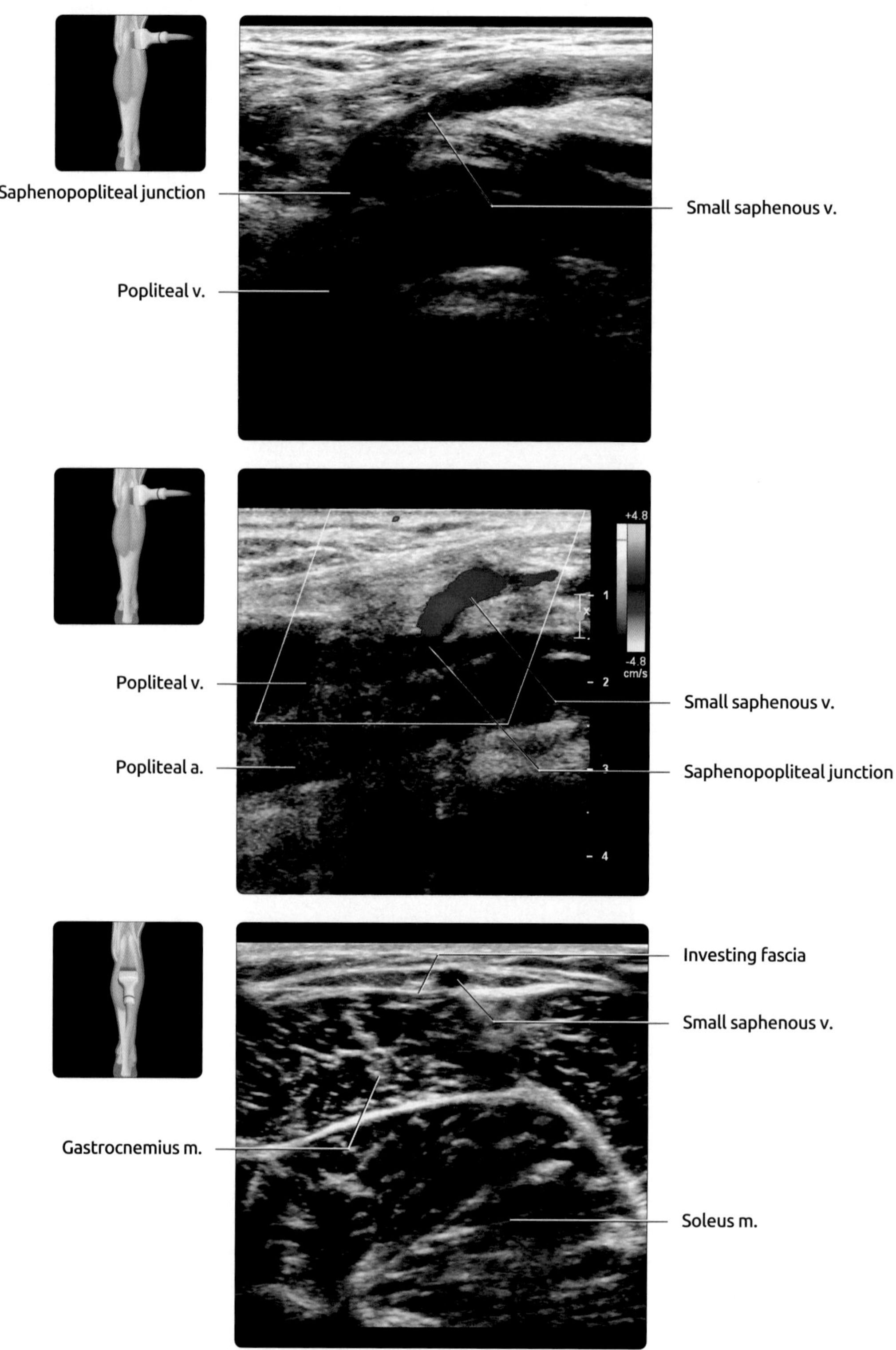

(Top) *Sagittal US shows central popliteal fossa. The small saphenous vein running from the lateral surface of the calf turns medially and penetrates the popliteal fascia to drain into the popliteal vein. Varicose veins arise as a result of reflux and stasis due to incompetent valves. Varicose veins on the lateral side of the calf would suggest an incompetent small saphenous system.* **(Middle)** *Sagittal color Doppler US shows the central popliteal fossa with augmentation. Flow toward the popliteal vein (red) is demonstrated at the saphenopopliteal junction. Reverse flow into the small saphenous vein would suggest valvular incompetence.* **(Bottom)** *Transverse US shows the posterior surface of the upper calf. The small saphenous vein is sandwiched between 2 layers of investing fascia. Minimal probe pressure is required to avoid inadvertent compression of the small saphenous vein.*

GREAT SAPHENOUS VEINS

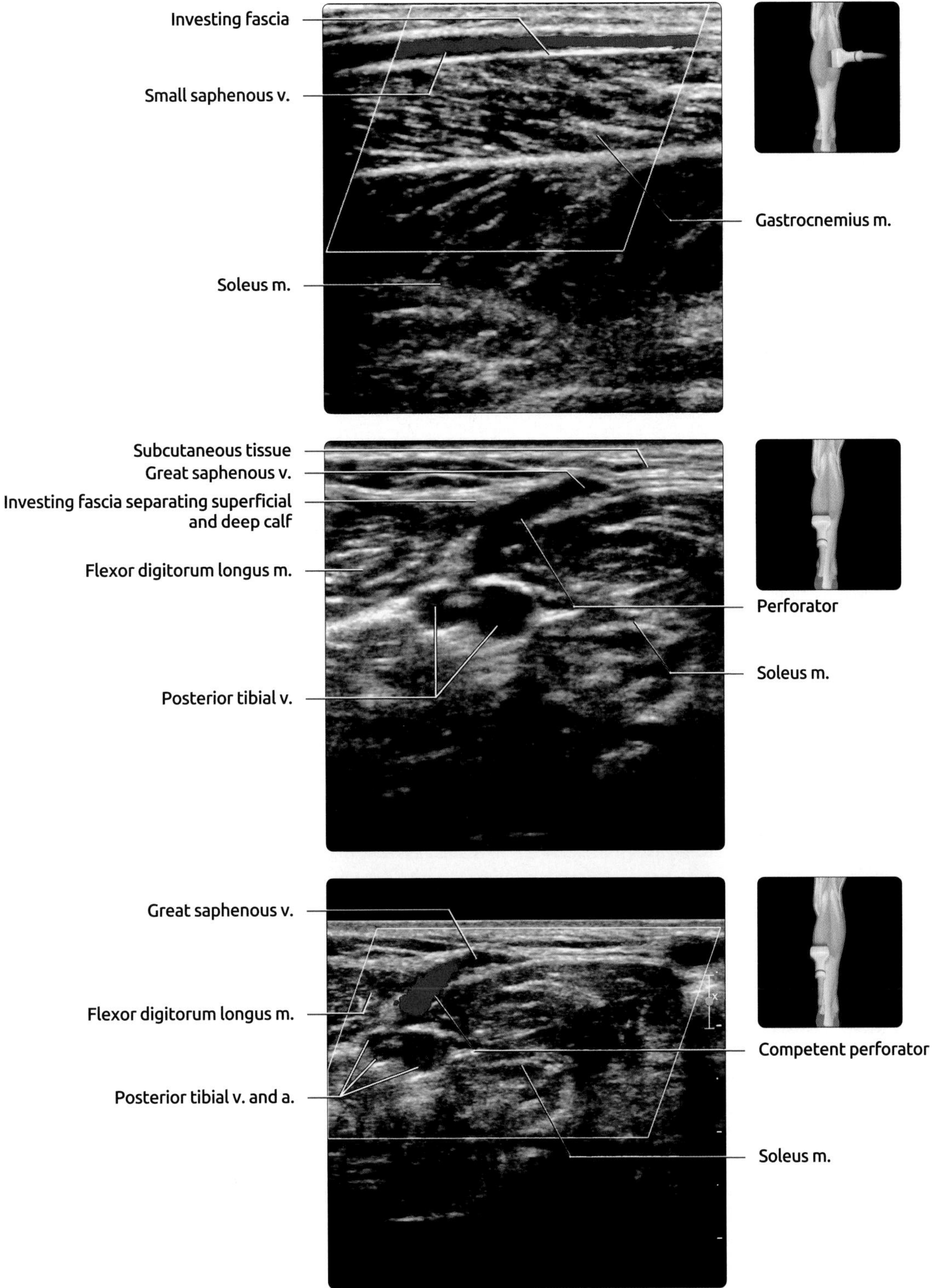

(Top) *Sagittal color Doppler US shows the upper midcalf with augmentation. The complete filling of the venous lumen of the small saphenous vein is demonstrated, indicating the absence of a superficial vein thrombus. If flow toward the trunk is demonstrated, valvular incompetence can be excluded.* **(Middle)** *Transverse US shows the medial aspect of the lower 1/3 of the calf. A perforator arising from the great saphenous vein is seen penetrating through the investing fascia to join the posterior tibial vein.* **(Bottom)** *Transverse color Doppler US shows the medial aspect of the lower 1/3 of the calf. With augmentation, color filling of the perforator lumen is demonstrated in the perforator between the great saphenous vein and the posterior tibial vein, indicating patency of vessel. If flow toward the posterior tibial vein can be documented on Doppler study, incompetence can be excluded.*

PART IV
SECTION 2
Vascular Lesions

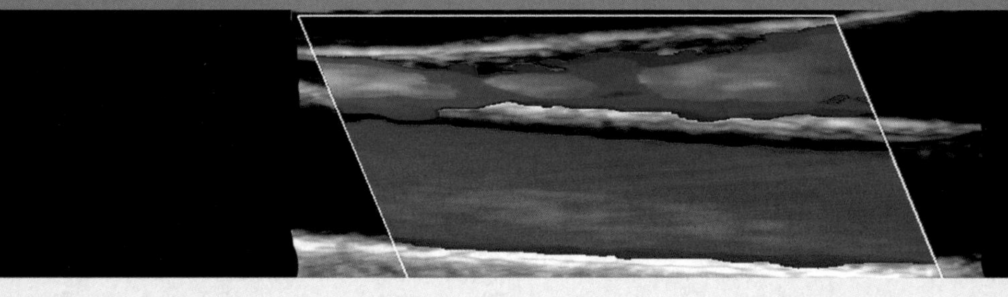

Jugular Vein Thrombosis

KEY FACTS

TERMINOLOGY

- Chronic internal jugular vein (IJV) thrombosis (> 10 days after acute event) where clot persists within lumen after soft tissue inflammation is gone
- JV thrombophlebitis: Acute-subacute thrombosis of IJV with associated adjacent tissue inflammation

IMAGING

- Acute thrombophlebitic phase
  - Loss of fascial planes between IJV & surrounding soft tissues + cellulitis
  - Echogenic intraluminal thrombus, distended, noncompressible IJV
  - Acute thrombus may be anechoic & difficult to distinguish from flowing blood; lack of compressibility & absent color or flow signal on Doppler may be only clues
  - Loss of venous pulsation & respiratory phasicity
  - No flow seen within echogenic venous thrombus
  - Tumor infiltration of IJV causes tumor thrombus with ↑ vascularity on Doppler US, most commonly from thyroid anaplastic carcinoma or follicular carcinoma
- Chronic phase
  - Collateral veins may be detected
  - Central liquefaction or heterogeneity of thrombus
  - Thrombus tends to be well organized & echogenic
  - May be difficult to separate from perivascular echogenic tissues
  - Absence of phasicity in jugular or subclavian veins may suggest more central nonocclusive thrombus

SCANNING TIPS

- Scan neck in neutral flat supine position; if head is elevated, cerebral venous drainage occurs mainly via vertebral vein & IJV will be collapsed
- Avoid over-rotation of head to contralateral side, as this may cause neck musculature to compress vein

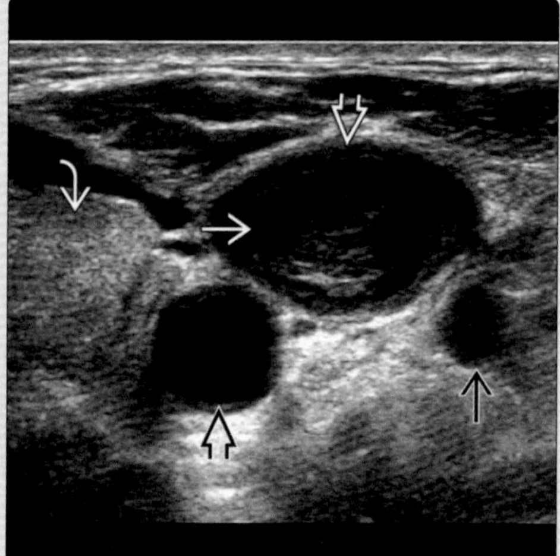

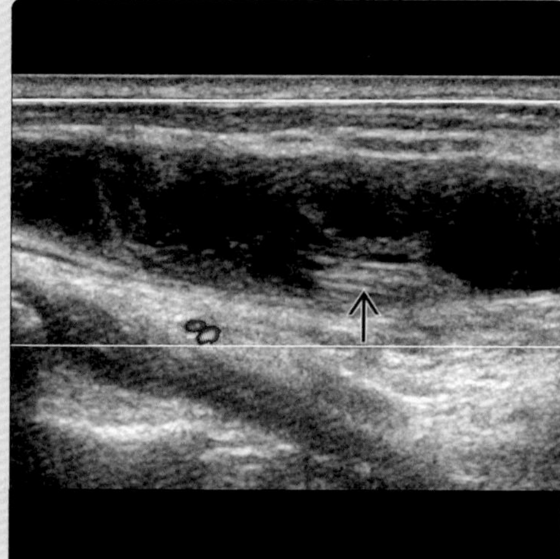

(Left) *Transverse grayscale US shows enlarged left internal jugular vein (IJV) ➡ filled with heterogeneous, laminated intraluminal thrombus ➡. This patient had known H&N squamous cell carcinoma, and thrombosed IJV could well be mistaken for metastatic node. Note the adjacent round, hypoechoic, metastatic node ⇨, CCA ⇨, and thyroid gland ➡.* **(Right)** *Corresponding power Doppler US shows the "lesion" to be in fact tubular, consistent with IJV thrombus ⇨. Note absence of flow signal within venous lumen & thrombus.*

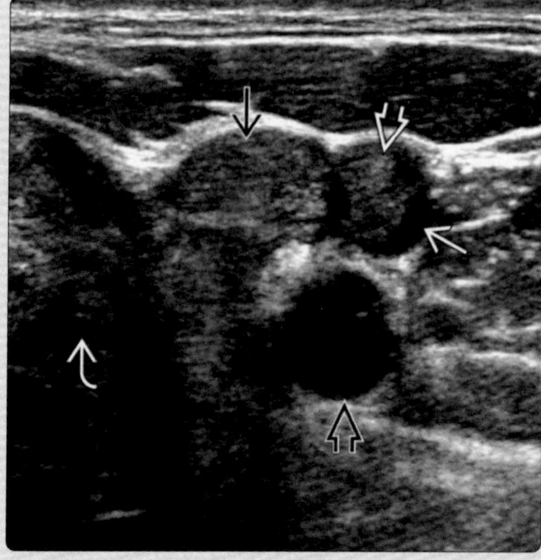

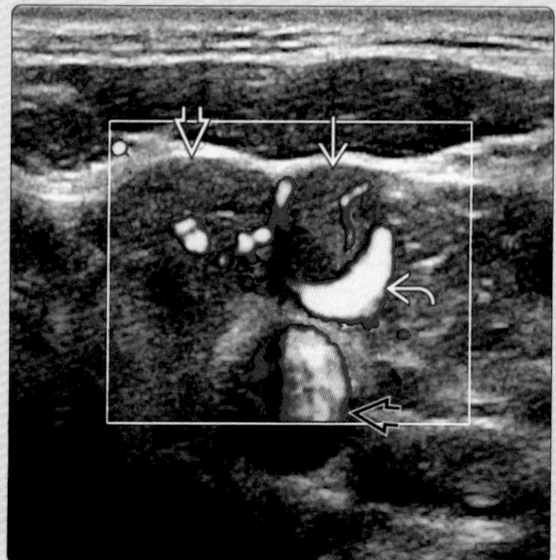

(Left) *Transverse grayscale US shows a tumor thrombus in the left IJV ➡, arising from a malignant thyroid mass ➡ and extending into the IJV via the middle thyroid vein ⇨ (also filled with thrombus & distended). Note remnant lumen of the vein ➡ and uninvolved CCA ⇨.* **(Right)** *Corresponding transverse power Doppler US shows vascularity within the IJV thrombus ➡ & in the middle thyroid vein thrombus ➡, suggesting these to be tumor thrombi. Note flow signal within remnant lumen of the IJV ➡ and uninvolved CCA ⇨.*

KEY FACTS

TERMINOLOGY

- Carotid artery dissection (CAD): Tear in carotid artery wall allows blood to enter and delaminate wall layers

IMAGING

- Extracranial internal CAD (ICAD) > > intracranial ICAD or CCAD
- 20% of ICADs bilateral or involve vertebral arteries
- Pathognomonic findings of dissection: Intimal flap or double lumen
- Turbulent flow caused by fluttering intimal flap
- Smooth tapering stenosis typical sonographic appearance of ICAD; often occurs in young patients with no visible atherosclerotic plaque
- High ICAD beyond reach of ultrasound may only manifest as ↑ flow resistance in Doppler waveform and ↓ flow velocity due to distal obstruction
- Flap may be obscured by color blooming artifact on color Doppler and better seen on grayscale
- False lumen commonly demonstrates low peak flow velocity and reversed diastolic flow direction
- "Slosh" phenomenon of systolic forward-and-backward flow proximal to dissection highly typical

CLINICAL ISSUES

- Ipsilateral pain in face, jaw, head, or neck
- Oculosympathetic palsy (miosis and ptosis, partial Horner syndrome), bruit (40%), pulsatile tinnitus
- Ischemic symptoms (cerebral or retinal TIA or stroke)
- Lower cranial nerve palsies (especially CNX)

SCANNING TIPS

- Beware of mirror image artifact in which IJ vein anterior to carotid is mirrored over carotid artery and can mimic dissection; rescan in different position
- B-flow technique may confirm flap more clearly due to lack of color blooming artifact
- In suspected dissection, reimage with higher frequency linear transducer (10-15 MHz) to help delineate flap

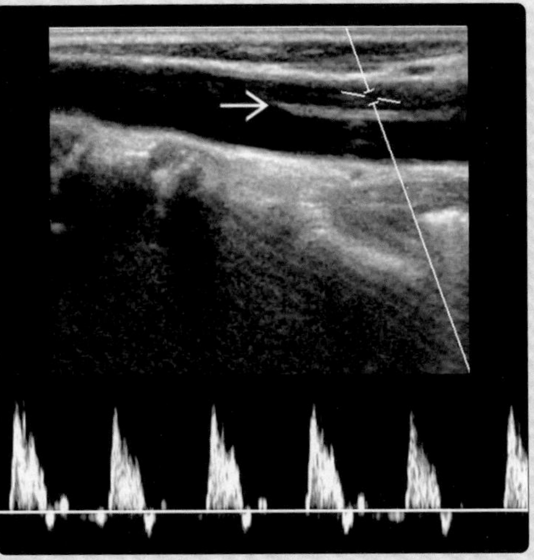

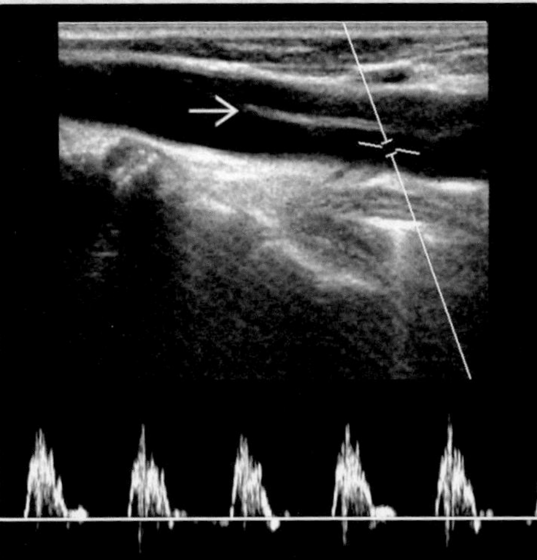

(Left) *Longitudinal pulsed Doppler ultrasound shows a common carotid artery dissection (CCAD) with 2 lumina separated by a thick dissection membrane ➡.* **(Right)** *Longitudinal pulsed Doppler ultrasound shows a CCAD with 2 lumina separated by a thick dissection membrane ➡. Doppler waveforms of these 2 lumina both show high-resistance flow with rapid systolic upstroke and minimal forward flow during diastole.*

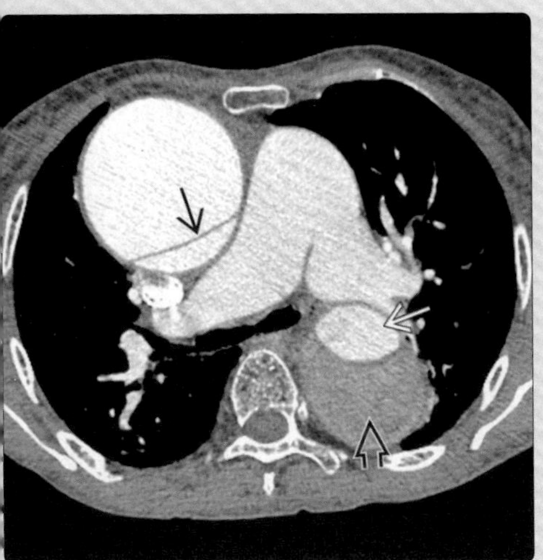

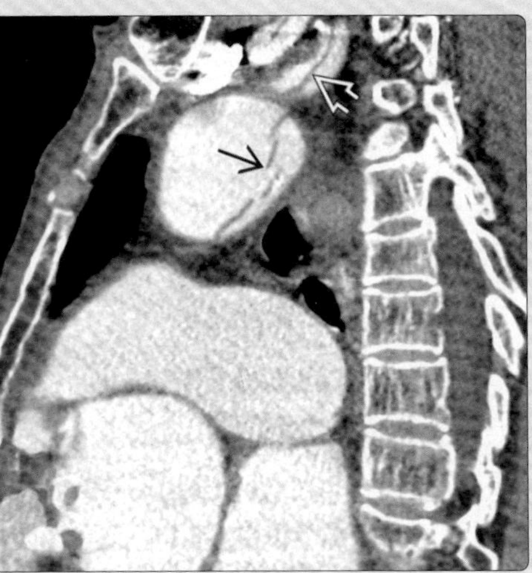

(Left) *Dissection commonly originates from the thoracic aorta and extends into the carotid arteries, as shown on this axial CECT. Note the dissection membrane ➡ and thrombosed false lumen ⇨. The larger thrombosed false lumen causes narrowing of the true lumen ➡.* **(Right)** *Corresponding sagittal CECT reconstruction (in the same patient) again demonstrates the intimal flap ➡. Note the extension of the dissection into the left CCA ➡.*

Carotid Stenosis/Occlusion

KEY FACTS

IMAGING

- Characterization of plaques
  - Uniformly echolucent or predominantly echolucent; fatty or fibrofatty; ↑ risk of embolization
  - Uniformly/mildly echogenic and predominantly echogenic; fibrous; ↓ risk of embolization
  - Highly echogenic with distal shadowing, focal/diffuse; calcified; ↓ risk of embolization
  - Ulcerated: Focal crypt in plaque with sharp or overhanging edges; ↑ risk of embolization
- Grading of internal carotid artery (ICA) stenosis
  - < 50% stenosis: Peak systolic velocity (PSV) < 125 cm/s; PSV ratio (PSVR) < 2.0
  - 50-69% stenosis: PSV 125-229 cm/s; PSVR 2.0-3.9
  - ≥ 70% stenosis: PSV ≥ 230 cm/s; PSVR ≥ 4.0
  - Near occlusion: High-/low-velocity (trickle) flow
  - Occlusion: Absent flow
- Common carotid artery and external carotid artery stenosis
  - No well-established Doppler criteria for grading stenosis
  - Measuring stenosis on color-coded images may underestimate degree of stenosis
- Diagnostic pitfalls
  - Trickle flow at near occlusion may be undetected
  - ICA stenosis may be underestimated due to poor cardiac function or tandem stenoses
  - Contralateral ICA stenosis may be overestimated due to crossover collateral flow
  - Moderate carotid stenosis may be underestimated due to normalization of flow at bulb

SCANNING TIPS

- Obtain color Doppler view of stenotic area during systole, because aliasing (indicative of stenosis) may not be seen during diastole
- Small parts/high-frequency probes (10-15MHz) can better delineate grayscale detail of ulcerated plaques, but color and power Doppler will have limited steering angles

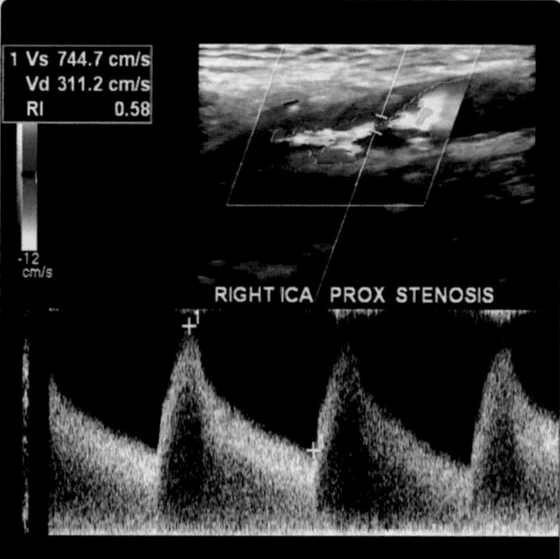

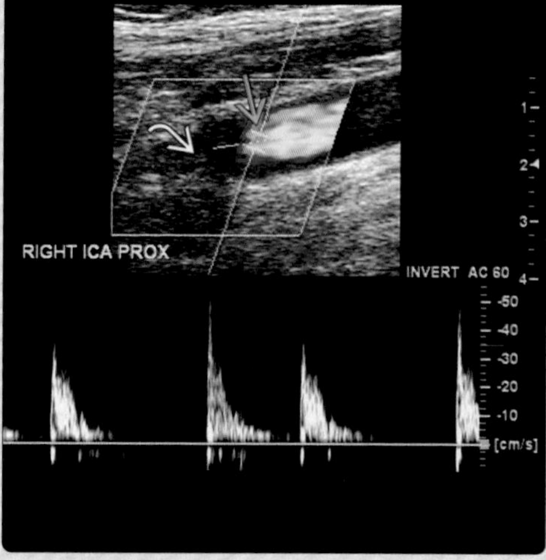

(Left) *Longitudinal spectral Doppler US shows a tight stenosis at the proximal internal carotid artery (ICA) causing significant focal increase in flow velocity (> 700 cm/s). Aliasing artifacts are depicted within the stenotic lumen. Findings are predictive of a > 70% stenosis.* **(Right)** *Longitudinal spectral Doppler US shows total ICA occlusion. The proximal ICA segment is devoid of any Doppler signals ➡, whereas high-resistance monophasic waveforms are detected in the preocclusive segment ➡.*

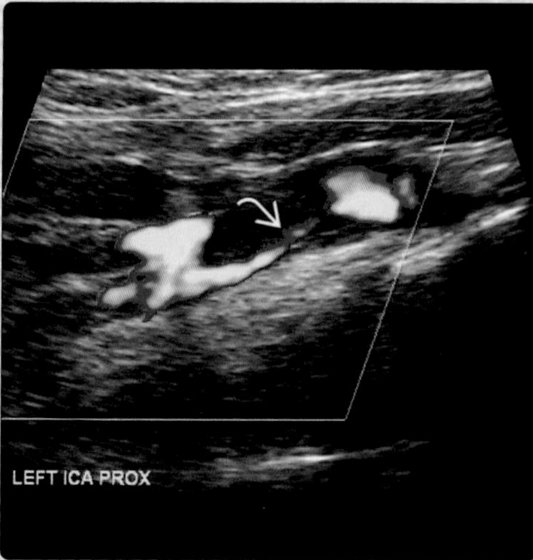

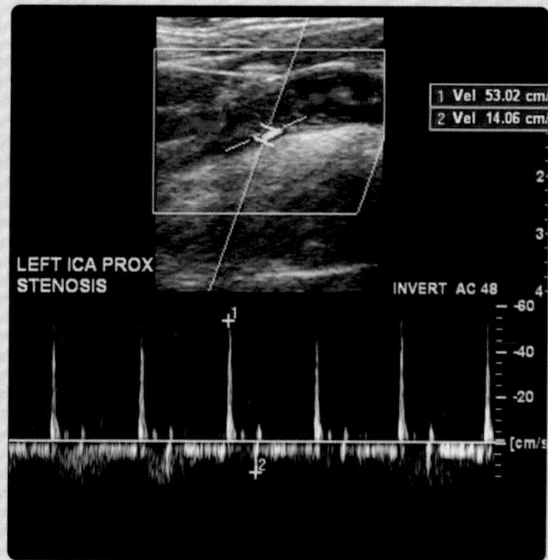

(Left) *Longitudinal power Doppler US shows near occlusion at the proximal ICA with a slender residual lumen ➡. Compared with color Doppler, power Doppler is more sensitive to delineating the residual lumen with low-velocity flow.* **(Right)** *Corresponding spectral Doppler US shows "to-and-fro" flow within the severely stenotic segment due to high-flow resistance. The findings are suggestive of near occlusion.*

Vertebral Stenosis/Occlusion

KEY FACTS

IMAGING

- Plaque formation: Proximal vertebral artery (VA) > distal VA
- Grayscale imaging
  - Chronic occlusion: Contracted vessel caliber; VA may be hard to demonstrate
- Spectral Doppler
  - Stenosis: Significant focal ↑ in peak systolic velocity (PSV) + poststenotic turbulence or dampened flow
  - Occlusion: Absent Doppler signals; vertebral venous signals may be prominent
  - Asymmetrical VA velocities may be due to difference in vessel caliber or unilateral occlusive disease
  - Mild subclavian steal (SS): Systolic deceleration
  - Moderate SS: Alternating flow
  - Complete SS: Flow reversal
  - Dynamic test with affected arm exercise is recommended to evaluate severity of SS
- Color Doppler
  - Stenosis: Aliasing or trickle flow at stenosis
  - Occlusion: Absent Doppler signals ± surrounding neck collaterals
  - Mild SS: Antegrade or minimal retrograde flow
  - Moderate SS: Bidirectional flow
  - Severe SS: Predominantly retrograde flow

DIAGNOSTIC CHECKLIST

- Check for presence of intraluminal plaque with abnormal ↑ or ↓ of PSV and neck arterial collaterals
- Consider alteration of VA flow velocity, flow asymmetry, and flow resistance as causes for stenosis/occlusion if it cannot be accounted for by VA size

SCANNING TIPS

- To avoid mistaking musculoskeletal branch of external carotid artery for VA, use transverse process as landmark for identification of VA
- Vertebral vein is always anterior to VA

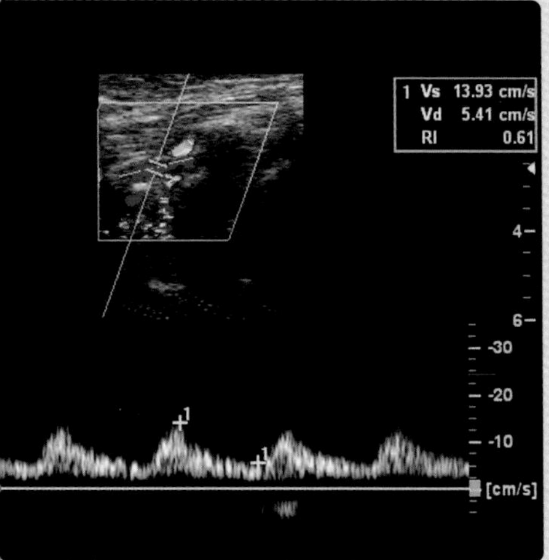

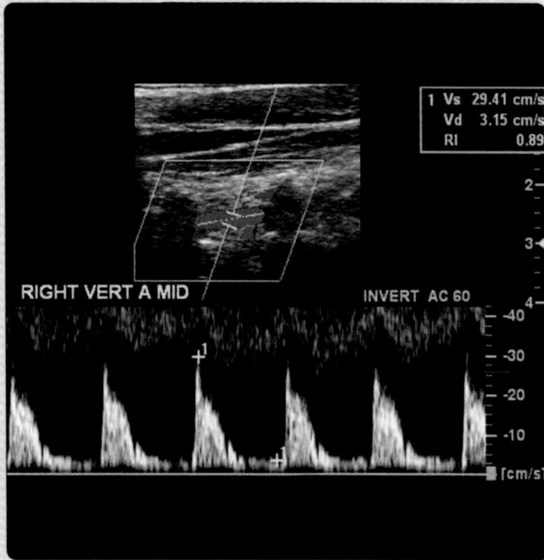

(Left) *Spectral Doppler US shows dampened waveforms of the V2 segment with delayed upstroke and reduced flow velocities. Findings are indicative of significant proximal arterial stenosis or occlusion.* **(Right)** *Spectral Doppler US shows high-resistance waveforms with sharp upstroke and low end-diastolic velocity of the normal-sized V2 segment. Findings may be due to significant distal stenosis. Note that flow resistance is usually higher than normal in hypoplastic vertebral artery (VA).*

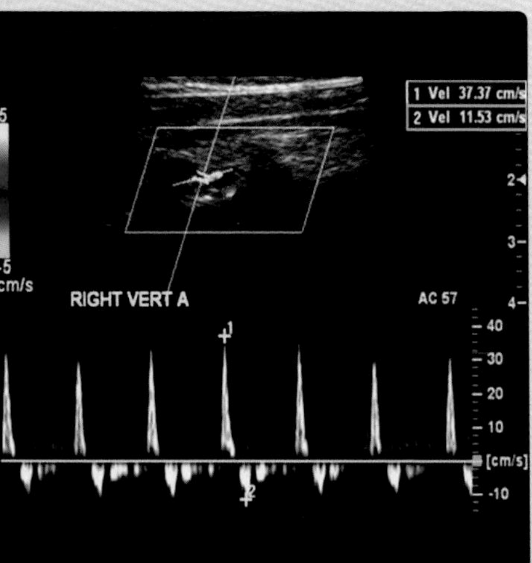

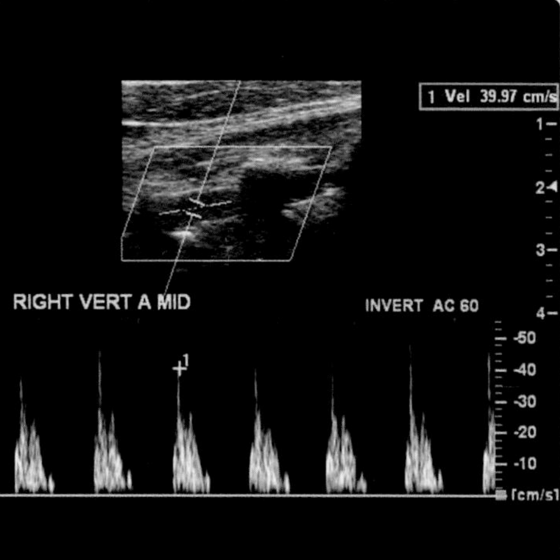

(Left) *Spectral Doppler US shows abnormal biphasic flow in a small VA. The finding is suspicious of near or total arterial occlusion in the distal segment.* **(Right)** *Spectral Doppler US shows monophasic waveforms with sharp upstroke and absent diastolic components of the V2 segment. The finding is typical in preocclusive arterial segment.*

Deep Vein Thrombosis

KEY FACTS

TERMINOLOGY

- Deep vein thrombosis (DVT): Thrombus forms within deep venous system, typically in lower limbs

IMAGING

- Complete compression ensures no thrombus is present
- Augmentation (↑ in flow velocity with distal compression)
  - Poor augmentation suggests downstream obstruction
- **Acute thrombosis (~ 14 days)**
  - Thrombus hypoechoic, may distend vein if occlusive
  - May see free-floating thrombus
  - Associated slow flow may be seen as visible mobile echoes moving back and forth in real time/cine clip
- **Subacute thrombosis (~ 2 weeks to 6 months)**
  - Thrombus becomes more echogenic, variable
  - Luminal flow may be restored or vein may stay occluded
  - Collateral venous channel continues to develop
- **Chronic phase (≥ 6 months)**
  - Postthrombotic scarring forms
  - Scarred veins are thick-walled with reduced diameter
  - Plaque-like fibrous scars, synechiae form along vein periphery and may occasionally calcify
  - Fibrous cord: In nonrecannalized vein, vein reduced to echogenic cord smaller than normal vein
  - Valve abnormalities

SCANNING TIPS

- Femoral vein (FV) and popliteal veins are often duplicated
- If 9 linear transducer is not able to penetrate to level of vein due to patient body habitus or limb swelling, try curvilinear probe
- Refractive edge shadow from fascial planes may obscure distal FV; slightly anterior/medial approach using vastus medialis muscle as acoustic window may help visualization
- Calcified arteries may obscure visualization of adjacent deep vein and create pseudo filling defect on color Doppler images; avoid using adjacent artery as acoustic window in these patients

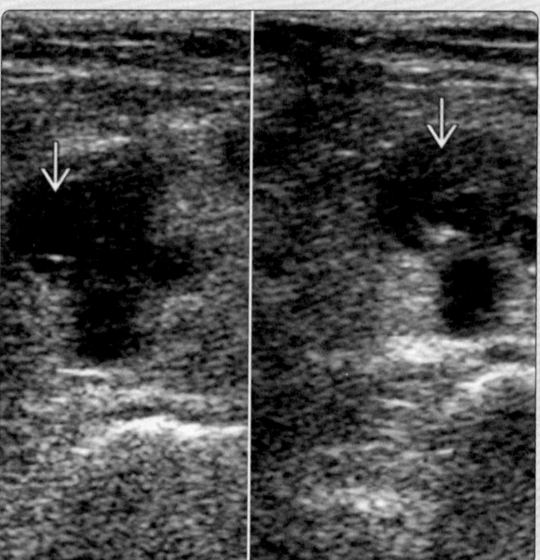

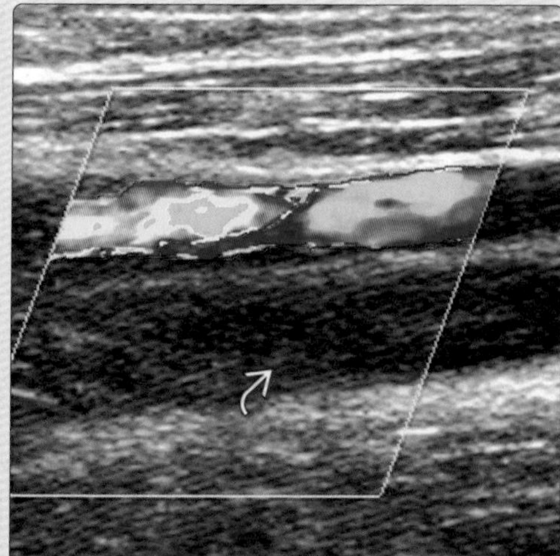

(Left) *Transverse ultrasound shows acute deep vein thrombosis (DVT) of the popliteal vein, filled with hypoechoic thrombus ➡ (right) and incompressible with transducer pressure (left).* **(Right)** *Longitudinal color Doppler ultrasound shows acute thrombosis of the femoral vein ➡. Of note, the term femoral vein is now used instead of superficial femoral vein per ACR recommendation.*

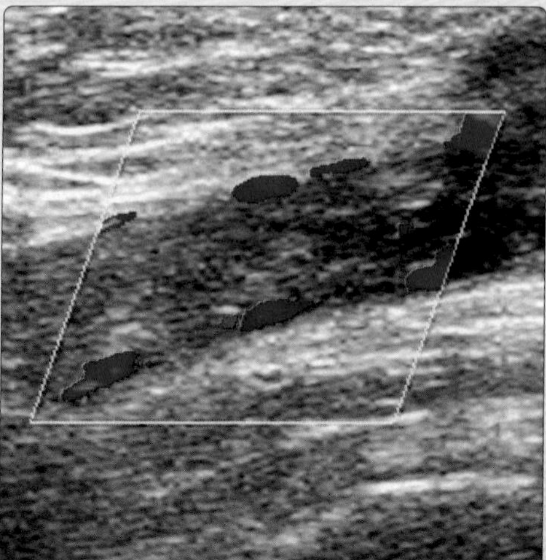

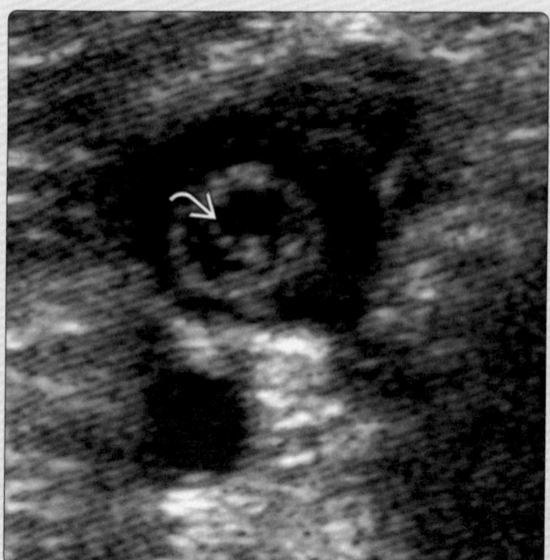

(Left) *Corresponding longitudinal color Doppler ultrasound shows DVT of common femoral vein with partial color filling.* **(Right)** *Transverse ultrasound shows chronic DVT with a contracted, echogenic, and probably calcified thrombus ➡.*

KEY FACTS

TERMINOLOGY

- Chronic venous insufficiency refers to venous valvular incompetence in superficial, deep, and perforating veins
- Venous reflux that persists for longer than 0.5 s at any level is considered clinically significant

IMAGING

- **Grayscale ultrasound**: Evaluate definition of vein lumen, vein valve leaflets, and wall morphology
  - Evaluate compressibility of vein and echogenicity of thrombus, which may indicate chronicity
- **Pulsed Doppler**: Differentiate venous from arterial flow
  - Assess duration of venous reflux
  - Assess augmentation with distal limb compression (use contralateral limb as reference)
  - Evaluate reflux in deep vs. superficial veins at saphenofemoral junction and saphenopopliteal junction
- **Color Doppler**: Differentiate partial thrombosis from complete venous occlusion
  - Distinguish reflux in deep veins from reflux in superficial system at saphenofemoral junction and saphenopopliteal junction
  - Identify incompetent perforating veins
  - Demonstrate recanalization of chronically thrombosed venous segment and collateralization around thrombosed veins
- **At each level, evaluate for the following**
  - Cephalad flow when limb compressed distally
  - No retrograde flow with release of distal compression with Valsalva maneuver or with limb compression proximal to probe

SCANNING TIPS

- Optimize color flow imaging parameters for detection of low-velocity flow
- When venous insufficiency suggested in recumbent ultrasound, confirm by moving patient to standing position

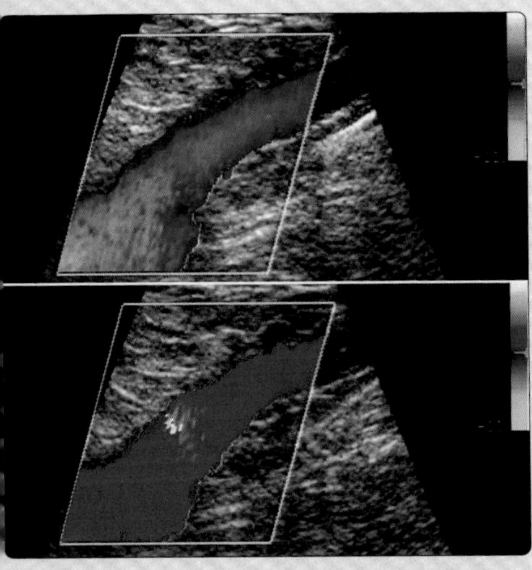

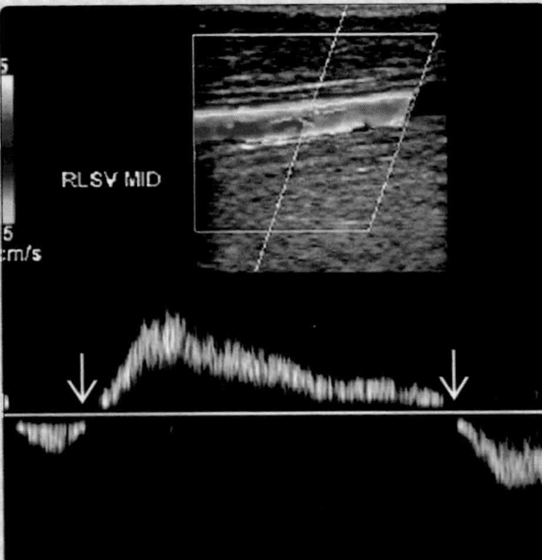

(Left) *Longitudinal color Doppler ultrasound shows reflux at the saphenofemoral junction. Note change in color code from blue to red demonstrating reversal of flow at the saphenofemoral junction during Valsalva maneuver.* **(Right)** *Longitudinal color Doppler ultrasound shows the incompetent great saphenous vein (formerly called long saphenous vein) with significant flow reflux > 2.0 s during Valsalva maneuver ➡.* *Findings are consistent with valvular incompetence.*

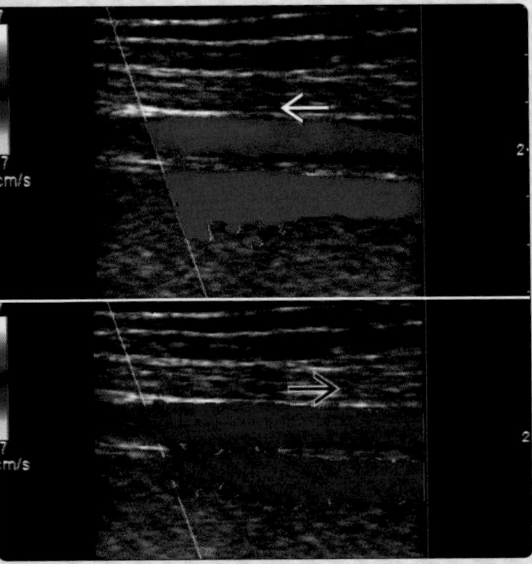

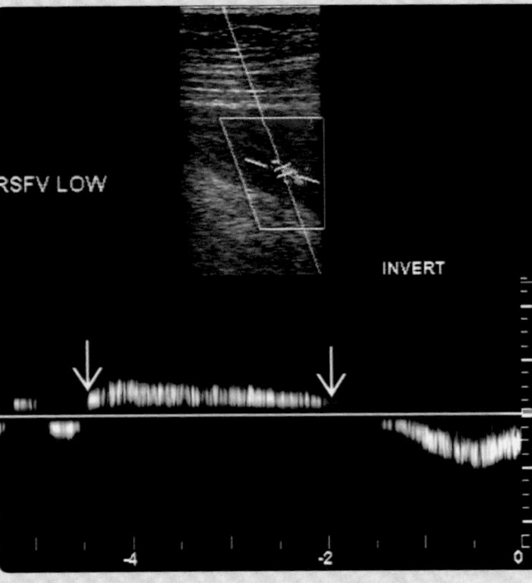

(Left) *Longitudinal color Doppler ultrasound shows a duplicated femoral vein with antegrade ➡ and retrograde ➡ flow during normal respiration (top) and Valsalva maneuver (bottom), respectively.* **(Right)** *Longitudinal color Doppler ultrasound shows the incompetent femoral vein (formerly called superficial femoral vein) with significant flow reflux ➡. Note abnormal reflux time is respectively taken as > 0.5 s and > 2.0 s with patient standing and supine.*

PART V
SECTION 1
Anatomy and Approach

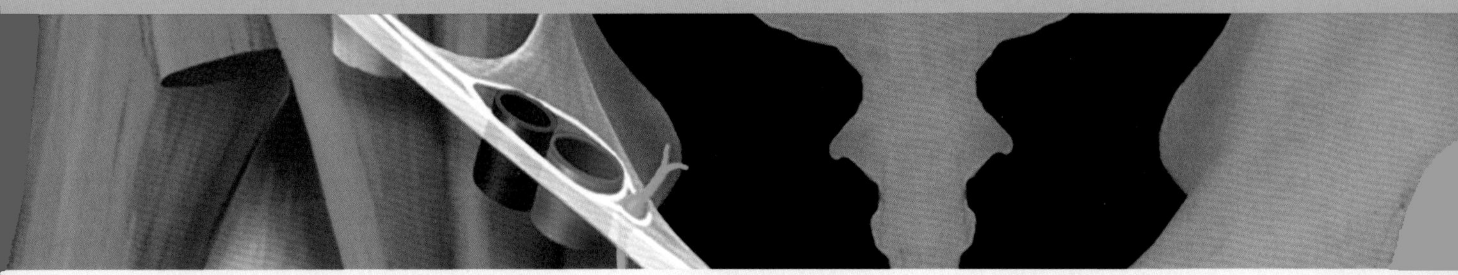

IMAGING ANATOMY

Overview

- **Rotator cuff**
  - Consists of supraspinatus, infraspinatus, teres minor, subscapularis muscles, and tendons
  - Cuff tendons blend with shoulder joint capsule
  - Supraspinatus and infraspinatus tendons are inseparable at insertion
  - Anterior 2.25 cm of tendon comprises supraspinatus tendon insertional area
- **Supraspinatus muscle**
  - Origin: Supraspinatus fossa of scapula
  - Insertion: Superior facet (horizontal orientation) and anterior portion of middle facet of greater tuberosity
    - Broad insertional area
  - Nerve supply: Suprascapular nerve
  - Blood supply: Suprascapular artery and circumflex scapular branches of subscapular artery
  - Action: Abduction of humerus
  - Muscle consists of 2 distinct portions
    - Anterior portion is larger, fusiform in shape, has dominant tendon, and is more likely to tear
    - Posterior portion is flat and has terminal tendon
  - Most commonly injured rotator cuff tendon
- **Infraspinatus muscle**
  - Origin: Infraspinatus fossa of scapula
  - Insertion: Mid to posterior aspects of middle facet of greater tuberosity; centrally positioned within tendon
  - Nerve supply: Suprascapular nerve, distal fibers
  - Blood supply: Suprascapular artery and circumflex scapular branches of subscapular artery
  - Action: External rotation of humerus and resists posterior subluxation
- **Teres minor muscle**
  - Origin: Lateral scapular border, middle 1/2
  - Insertion: Inferior facet (vertical orientation) of greater tuberosity
  - Nerve supply: Axillary nerve
  - Blood supply: Posterior circumflex humeral artery and circumflex scapular branches of subscapular artery
  - Action: External rotation of humerus
  - Least commonly injured rotator cuff tendon
- **Subscapularis muscle**
  - Origin: Subscapular fossa of scapula
  - Insertion: Lesser tuberosity and up to 40% may insert at surgical neck
  - Some fibers cross over to lateral lip of bicipital groove, reinforcing and blending with transverse ligament
  - Nerve supply: Subscapular nerve, upper and lower
  - Blood supply: Subscapularis artery
  - Action: Internal rotation of humerus, also adduction, extension, depression, and flexion
  - 4-6 tendon slips converge into main tendon; multipennate morphology increases strength
- **Rotator cuff tendon blood supply**
  - Derived from adjacent muscle, bone, and bursae
  - Normal hypovascular regions in tendons
    - Termed critical zone: ~ 1 cm proximal to insertion
    - Vulnerable to degeneration and calcific deposition
    - However, insertional area is more prone to tearing than critical zone
- **Biceps tendon, long head**
  - Origin: Superior glenoid labrum (biceps anchor)
    - Portions may attach to supraglenoid tubercle, anterosuperior labrum, posterosuperior labrum, and coracoid base
  - Runs along superior aspect of shoulder to bicipital groove
  - Action: Stabilizes and depresses humeral head
  - Anatomic variants: Anomalous intra- and extraarticular origins from rotator cuff and joint capsule
  - Tendon sheath communicates with glenohumeral joint and normally contains small amount of fluid
- **Subacromial-subdeltoid fat plane**
  - Subacromial and subdeltoid portions
    - ± subcoracoid extension in some patients
  - Fat plane is superficial to bursa
  - May be interrupted or absent in normal patients
  - Attached along free border of coracoacromial ligament, deep surface of deltoid muscle, and humeral neck
- **Rotator cuff interval**
  - Space between supraspinatus and subscapularis tendon through which biceps tendon passes
  - **Borders of rotator cuff interval**
    - Triangular-shaped space
    - Reflections of glenohumeral ligament and coracohumeral ligament form biceps reflection pulley
    - Biceps reflection pulley stabilizes biceps tendon within rotator cuff interval
    - Superior border: Leading edge of supraspinatus
    - Inferior border: Superior aspect of subscapularis tendon
    - Lateral border: Long head of biceps tendon and bicipital groove
    - Medial border: Base of coracoid process
  - **Contents of rotator interval**
    - Long head of biceps tendon; biceps reflection pulley
- **Coracoacromial ligament**
  - Forms coracoacromial arch along with acromion and coracoid process
    - Reinforces inferior aspect of acromioclavicular joint
  - Extends from distal coracoid to subacromial area
  - Broad insertion to undersurface acromion
    - Ligament is thicker at acromion (normal thickness < 2.5 mm) and may be associated with spurs
- **Glenoid labrum**
  - Triangular-shaped rim of fibrocartilage, which extends around periphery of glenoid

ANATOMY IMAGING ISSUES

Imaging Approaches

- Tendons best seen when on stretch
  - High-resolution linear transducer
  - Long-axis (longitudinal) & transverse view of each tendon
  - Each part of tendon needs to be examined; anisotropy prevents all parts of curved rotator cuff tendons from being seen at same time
  - Need to realign ("toggle") probe to see different parts of tendons

- Supraspinatus tendon
  - Arm extended and internally rotated behind lumbar region (Crass position)
    - If too painful, hand behind hip (back pocket) with elbow close to body (modified Crass position)
- Infraspinatus and teres minor tendons
  - Arm flexed and internally rotated with hand placed on contralateral shoulder
  - Teres minor tendon located posteroinferior to infraspinatus tendon
- Subscapularis tendon: Arm neutral and externally rotated
- Long head of biceps tendon
  - Arm neutral and externally rotated
  - Vary degree of external rotation for optimal view of biceps tendon
  - Check for tendon subluxation
- Subacromial-subdeltoid bursa
  - Stretching tendons may squeeze fluid from area of bursa under inspection
  - Examine in all positions and also in neutral position
  - Fluid collects preferentially just lateral to acromion and proximal humerus and near coracoacromial ligament
- Coracoid process and coracoacromial ligament
  - Neutral position
- Acromioclavicular joint
  - Neutral position
  - Can pull down on arm to assess joint laxity
- Glenohumeral joint
  - Neutral position
  - Best seen from posterior aspect of joint
  - Passive movement of arm during scanning can help in identifying posterior glenoid labrum
- Spinoglenoid notch
  - Neutral position just medial to glenohumeral joint
- Supraspinatus and infraspinatus muscles
  - Neutral position with hands resting on thigh
  - Examine thickest part of muscles from behind (in coronal and sagittal planes)
  - ↓ muscle bulk, ↑ echogenicity, and ↓ visibility of central tendon are signs of atrophy with fatty replacement
    - Compare muscle echogenicity to that of trapezius or deltoid muscle

Imaging Sweet Spots

- Look for tears particularly at anterior leading edge of supraspinatus tendon
  - Unexplained bursal fluid is good secondary sign of rotator cuff tear
- Bursal fluid is often best seen with arm in neutral position or ↓ internal rotation (hand in back pocket)

Imaging Pitfalls

- **Anisotropy**
  - Echoes are optimally reflected when transducer is parallel to tendon fibers
  - Rotator cuff tendons are prone to anisotropy due to curved course
  - If transducer is not at right angles to tendon, it will appear either isoechoic or hypoechoic to muscle
    - May simulate tendinosis or partial tear
- **Tendon edges**
  - Interfaces of tendons with adjacent structures may simulate tears
  - All pathology should be confirmed in 2 planes
- **Rotator cuff cable**
  - Thick band of fibers running perpendicular to supraspinatus tendon
  - Located on deeper aspect of tendon just proximal to insertional area
  - May reinforce critical zone supraspinatus fibers
  - Cable thicker in young subjects but more easily seen in elderly subjects due to supraspinatus tendinosis
  - Can simulate tendinosis or partial-thickness tear
- **Tendinous interspace at rotator cuff interval**
  - Interspace between leading (anterior) edge of supraspinatus and long head of biceps tendon may simulate tear
  - Overcome by recognizing ovoid or rounded shape of biceps tendon
  - Rotator cuff interval best seen with external rotation
- **Focal thinning at supraspinatus-infraspinatus junction**
  - Mild diffuse thinning of supraspinatus and infraspinatus tendon junction is normal finding
  - Should not be mistaken for tendon attenuation or partial-thickness tear
- **Musculotendinous junction**
  - Supraspinatus tendon
    - Hypoechoic muscle extending along superficial aspect of tendon may simulate subacromial-subdeltoid bursal distension
    - Interdigitating tendons of anterior and posterior portions may simulate tendinosis or tear
  - Infraspinatus tendon
    - Muscle fibers surrounding centrally positioned tendon may be confused with tear
  - Subscapularis tendon
    - 4-6 tendon slips converging into main tendon may simulate tendinosis
- **Fibrocartilaginous insertion**
  - Thin layer of fibrocartilage exists between tendon and bone at insertional area
  - Steeper tendon insertion = thicker fibrocartilaginous layer
  - This thin hypoechoic layer of fibrocartilage may simulate avulsive tear
- **Subacromial-subdeltoid fat plane**
  - Fat plane lies mainly superficial to bursa and deep to deltoid muscle
  - Normal bursa is very thin
  - Thickness of echogenic fat plane is variable among patients though usually similar from side to side
  - May be wrongly interpreted as bursal fluid
    - Look for intrabursal fluid ± hyperemia (latter is feature of inflammatory arthropathy)
- **Fluid in biceps tendon sheath**
  - Communicates with glenohumeral joint
  - Small amount of fluid is normal
    - Do not misinterpret as long head of biceps tenosynovitis
  - ↑ fluid in biceps tendon sheath usually reflects ↑ fluid in glenohumeral joint

MUSCLES AND LIGAMENTS

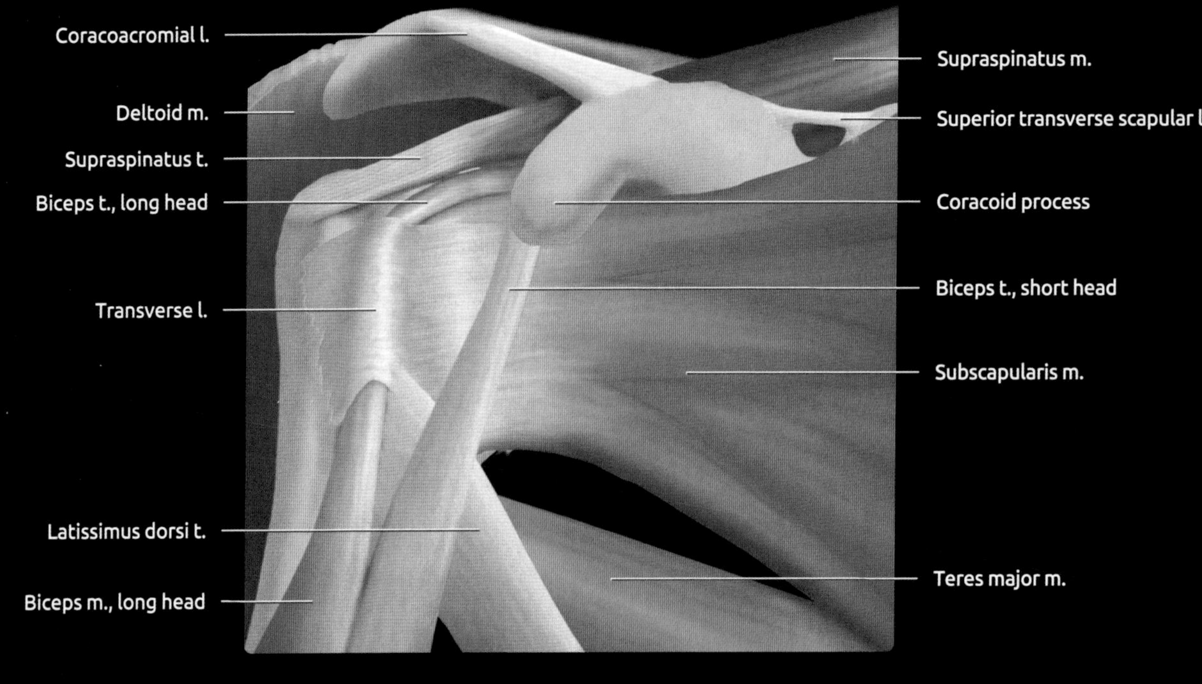

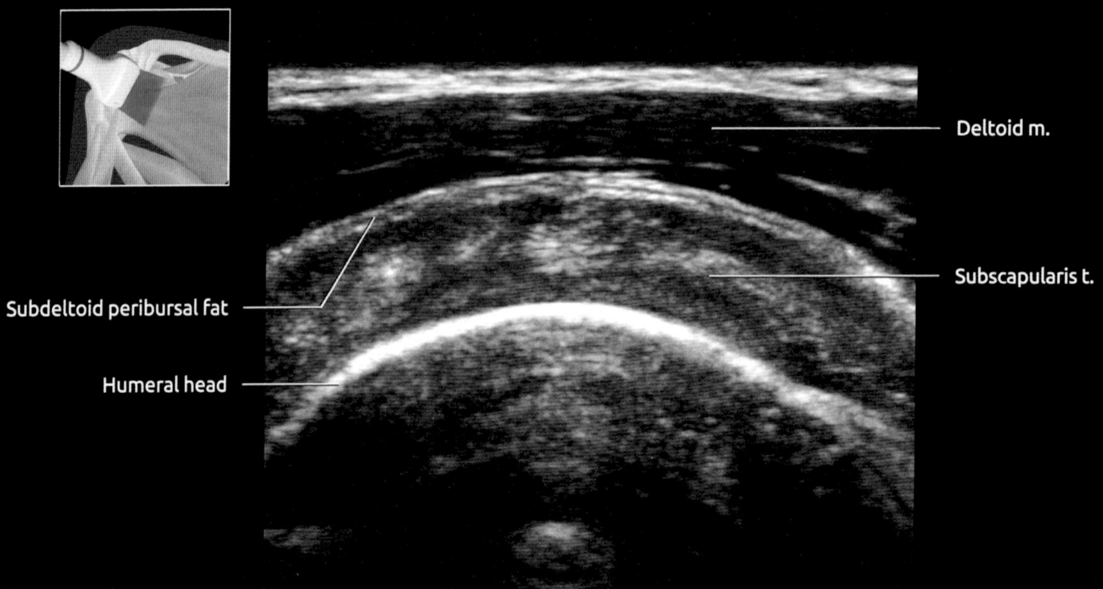

(Top) *Anterior graphic of the shoulder illustrates the rotator cuff and adjacent structures. The rotator cuff consists of supraspinatus, infraspinatus, teres minor, and subscapularis muscles and tendons. The biceps tendon courses the rotator cuff interval between the supraspinatus and subscapularis tendons, then descends along the bicipital groove, which is covered by the transverse ligament.* **(Bottom)** *Transverse grayscale US shows the subscapularis tendon midfibers. As they converge toward the insertion, fiber bundles of the multipennate subscapularis tendon give the tendon a mixed echogenic appearance. This is normal and should not be mistaken for tendinosis.*

BICEPS TENDON

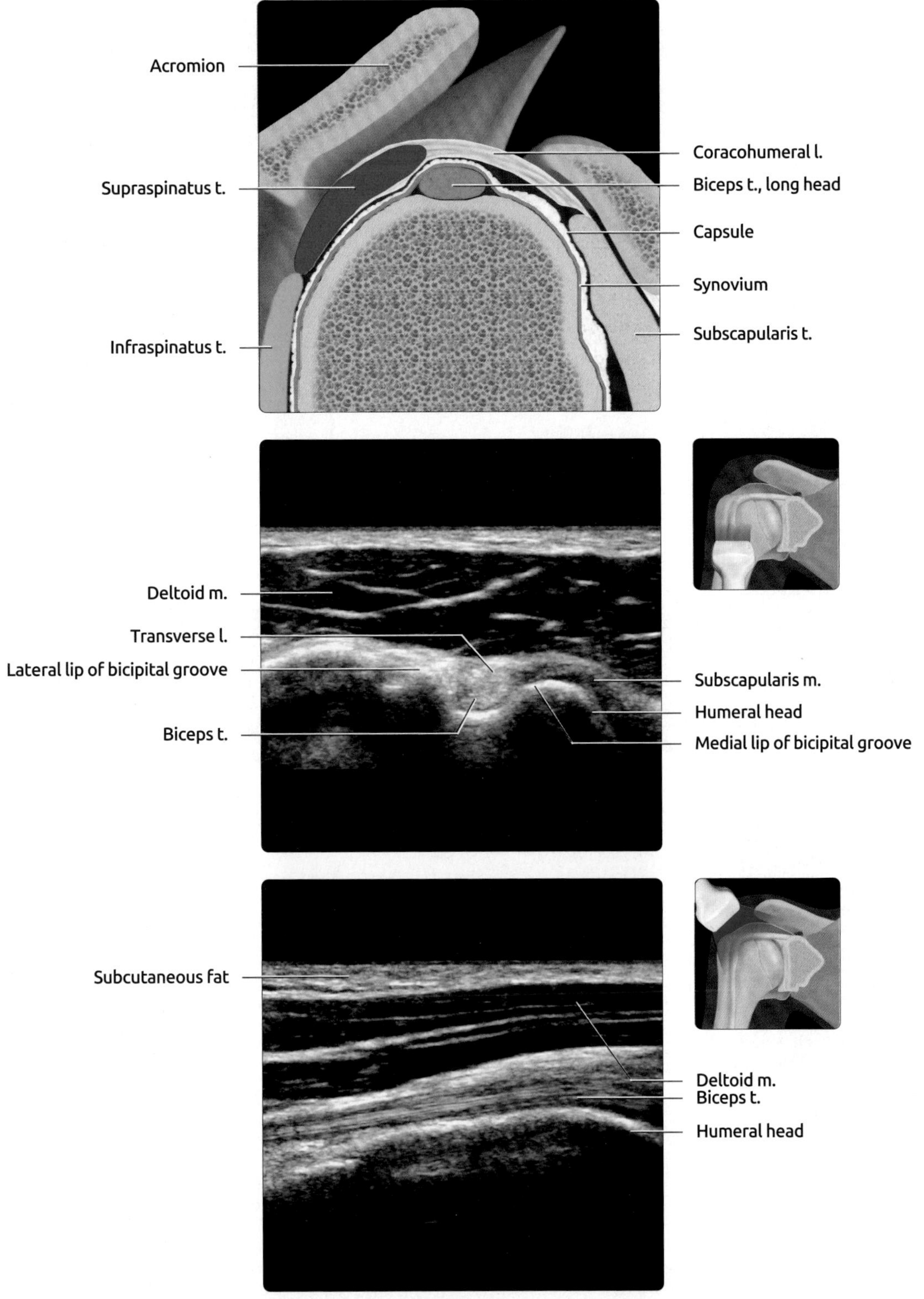

(Top) *Graphic shows the relationship of the coracohumeral ligament to the rotator cuff tendons. The coracohumeral ligament is not a true ligament but a folded portion of the glenohumeral capsule that extends from the coracoid process to the humerus. The undersurface is lined by synovium. Portions of the coracohumeral ligament pass superficial and deep to the supraspinatus tendon. The coracohumeral ligament attaches to the superior border of the subscapularis tendon as well as to the greater tuberosity.* **(Middle)** *Transverse grayscale US shows relations of the biceps tendon. The transverse ligament is not a distinct entity but consists of a fibrous expansion of both the pectoralis major tendon and subscapularis tendon inserting into the lateral lip of the bicipital groove.* **(Bottom)** *Longitudinal grayscale US shows the upper section of the biceps tendon. A small amount of fluid in the biceps tendon sheath, which is continuous with the glenohumeral joint, is normal and should not be mistaken for tenosynovitis. No fluid is depicted in this image.*

DEEP STRUCTURES

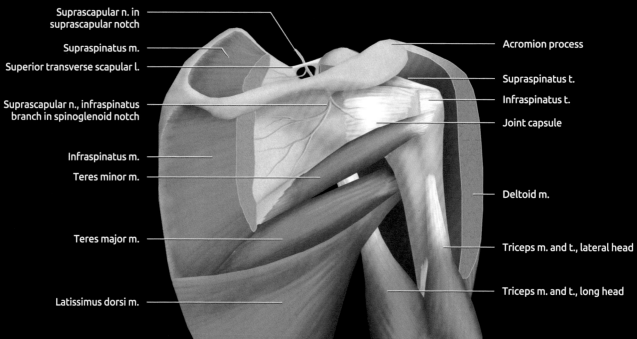

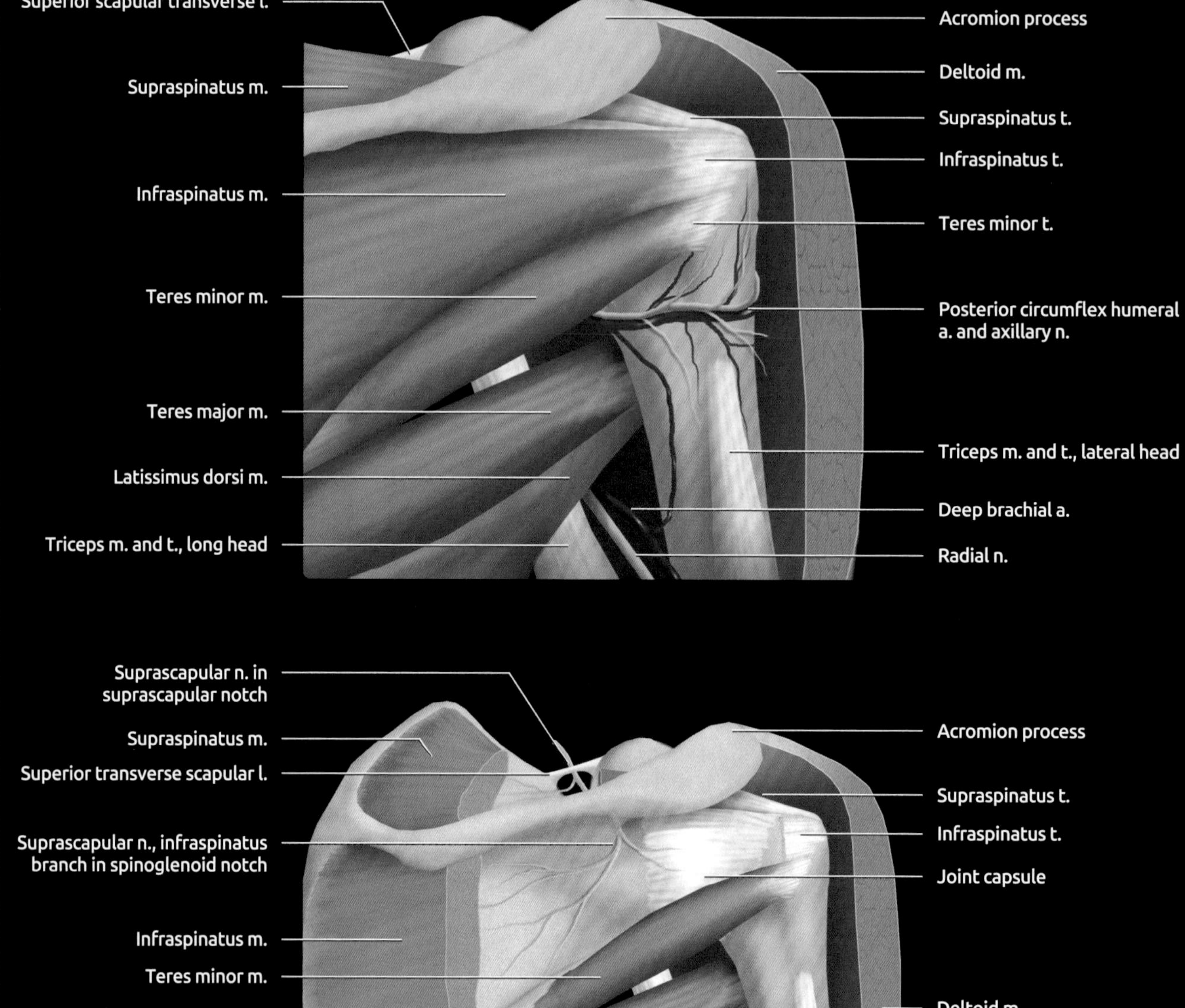

(Top) *Posterior graphic of the shoulder illustrates the rotator cuff and adjacent structures. The infraspinatus and teres muscles and tendons form the posterior wall of the rotator cuff. Inferior to the teres minor muscle and superior to the teres major is the axillary nerve and posterior circumflex humeral vessels running through the quadrilateral space.* **(Bottom)** *Deep scapulohumeral dissection shows the course of the suprascapular nerve. The nerve enters the supraspinous fossa through the suprascapular notch, below the superior transverse scapular ligament. The nerve then passes beneath the supraspinatus and curves around the lateral border of the spine of the scapula to enter the infraspinous fossa.*

LONGITUDINAL US, SUPRASPINATUS INSERTIONAL AREA

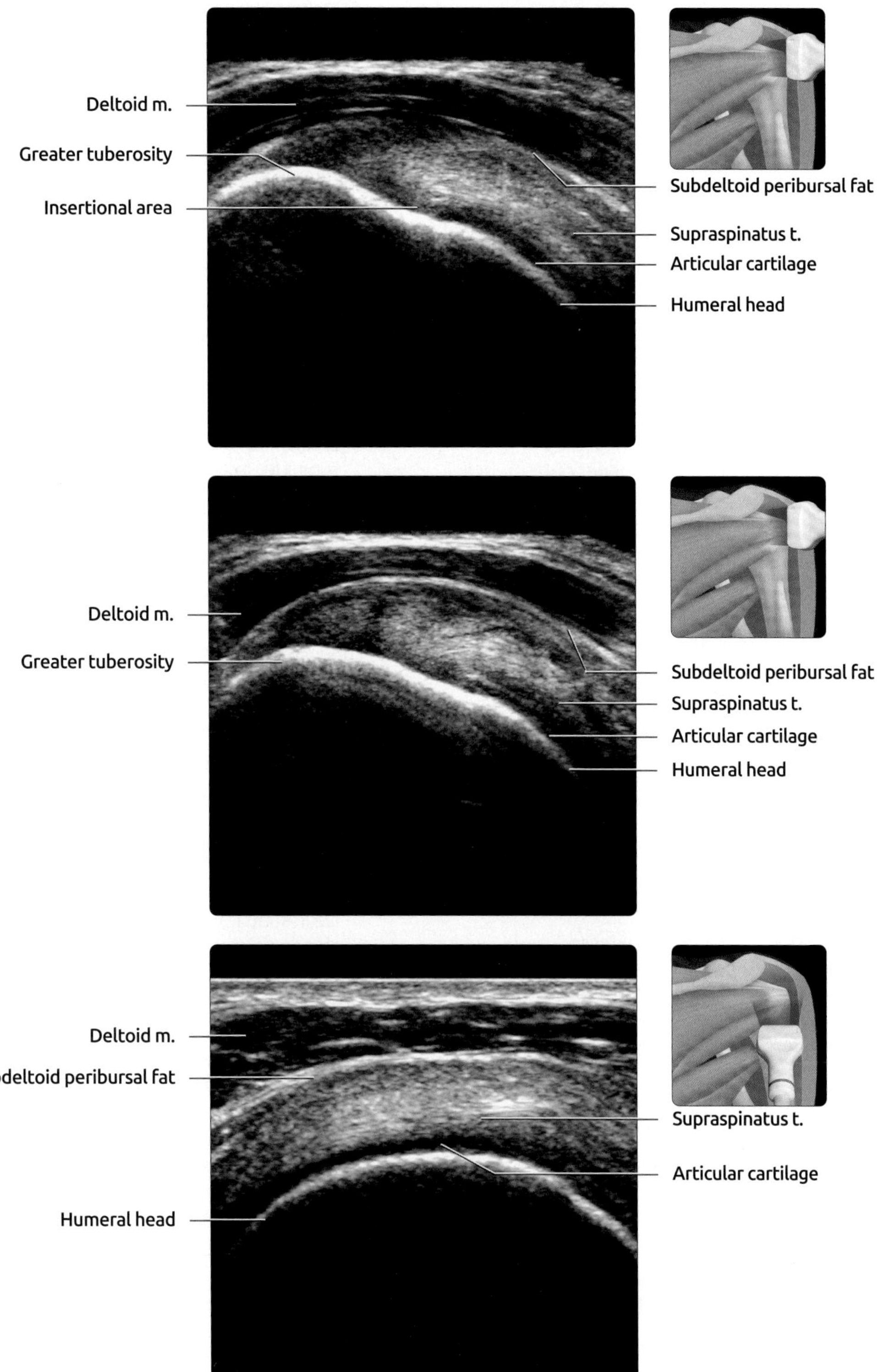

(Top) *Longitudinal grayscale US shows the anterior fibers of the supraspinatus tendon insertional area. The supraspinatus tendon inserts over a wide area (footprint) on the anterior aspect of the greater tuberosity. Many tears of the supraspinatus tendon involve avulsion of the tendon from its insertional site.* **(Middle)** *Longitudinal grayscale US shows the supraspinatus tendon midfibers. There is often a thin hypoechoic line at the insertional area. This represents Sharpey fibers and fibrocartilage.* **(Bottom)** *Transverse grayscale US shows the supraspinatus medial to the insertional area. The fibrillar pattern of the supraspinatus tendon is prone to anisotropy. With tendinosis, the fibrillar pattern is disrupted. The tendon becomes more hypoechoic and thickened.*

TERMINOLOGY

Abbreviations

- Origin (O), insertion (I)

Definitions

- Junctional region between thigh and trunk

IMAGING ANATOMY

Overview

- Incorporates lower abdominal wall, inguinal canal, femoral triangle, and femoral adductor muscles

Osseous Anatomy

- Pubic bone
  - **Pubic tubercle**: Small protuberance, lateral border pubic crest
    - Attachment: Inguinal ligament
  - **Superior and inferior rami**: Extend from pubis
  - **Pecten**: Ridge, posterior aspect superior pubis
    - O of pectineus muscle
    - I of conjoint tendon (internal oblique and transverse abdominis)
  - **Pubic crest**: Superior surface, anterior aspect pubic body
    - O of rectus abdominis muscle
    - I of transversus abdominis and external oblique muscles
  - **Pubic symphysis**: Cartilaginous joint between pubic bodies
  - **Superior pubic ligament**: Laterally extends to pubic tubercles

Anterior Abdominal Wall

- Abdominal wall muscles
  - **Rectus abdominis**: Paired midline muscles
    - O: Superior pubic ramus, pubic crest
    - I: Xiphoid process, costal cartilages 5-7
  - **Linea alba**: Aponeurotic junction of rectus femoris, transverse abdominis, and internal and external oblique muscles
  - **External oblique**: Most superficial
    - O: Ribs 5-12
    - I: Pubic crest, anterior iliac crest, linea alba
    - Lower border of aponeurosis contributes to inguinal ligament
  - **Internal oblique**: Between external oblique, transversus abdominis
    - O: Lateral inguinal ligament, iliac crest, thoracolumbar fascia
    - I: Pecten (conjoined tendon), pubic crest, inferior aspect of ribs 10-12, linea alba
    - O: Anterior to deep inguinal ring
    - I: Lateral to rectus abdominis muscle, posterior and medial to superficial inguinal ring
    - Arches over inguinal canal, forming roof
  - **Transversus abdominis**: Deepest
    - O: Iliac crest, posterior aspect of lateral inguinal ligament, thoracolumbar fascia
    - I: Pubic crest, pecten (conjoined tendon), linea alba
    - Remains posterior to inguinal canal

Inguinal Ligament

- Thickening inferior border of external oblique aponeurosis
- Attachments: Anterior superior iliac spine and pubic tubercle
- Separates lower extremity from pelvis
- Fascia lata attaches to inferior border
- **Subinguinal space**: Deep to inguinal ligament
  - Passageway for femoral vessels and nerve, iliopsoas muscle into femoral triangle
  - External iliac vessels become femoral vessels upon entering this space

Inguinal Canal

- Entrance: **Deep inguinal ring**
  - Located midinguinal ligament
  - Opening of evaginated transversalis fascia through which spermatic cord/round ligament pass
- Exit: **Superficial inguinal ring**
  - Division of external oblique aponeurosis lateral to pubic tubercle
- Contents: Ilioinguinal nerve; small arteries and veins; male: Spermatic cord; female: Round ligament
  - Covered by evaginated transversalis fascia

Adductor Musculature

- **Adductor longus muscle**: Thin tendon arises from medial superior pubic ramus
  - Overlies O of gracilis, adductor brevis, and magnus muscles
- **Gracilis muscle**: O from anterior aspect of symphysis pubis and medial aspect of inferior pubic ramus
  - O medial to adductor brevis muscle, deep to adductor longus muscle

Groin Lymph Nodes

- Superficial inguinal nodes
  - Lie in subcutaneous tissues below inguinal ligament and alongside great saphenous vein
  - Subdivided into 3 groups of lymph nodes
    - Inferior group are located distal to saphenous opening and receive drainage from lower limb
    - Superolateral group are located lateral to saphenous opening and receive drainage from lateral buttock and lower anterior abdominal wall regions
    - Superomedial group are located medial to saphenous opening and receive drainage from perineum and external genitalia
- Deep inguinal nodes
  - 3-5 nodes located in femoral triangle just medial to femoral vein
  - Cloquet node is most proximal of deep inguinal lymph nodes located just below inguinal ligament

ANATOMY IMAGING ISSUES

Imaging Recommendations

- Usual imaging pathway for assessing groin pathology includes radiography &/or ultrasound
- Use curvilinear abdominal transducer for deeper structures in addition to/or high-resolution linear transducers
- Dynamic imaging is important, particularly in assessment of hernias or other position dependent pathology

GROIN

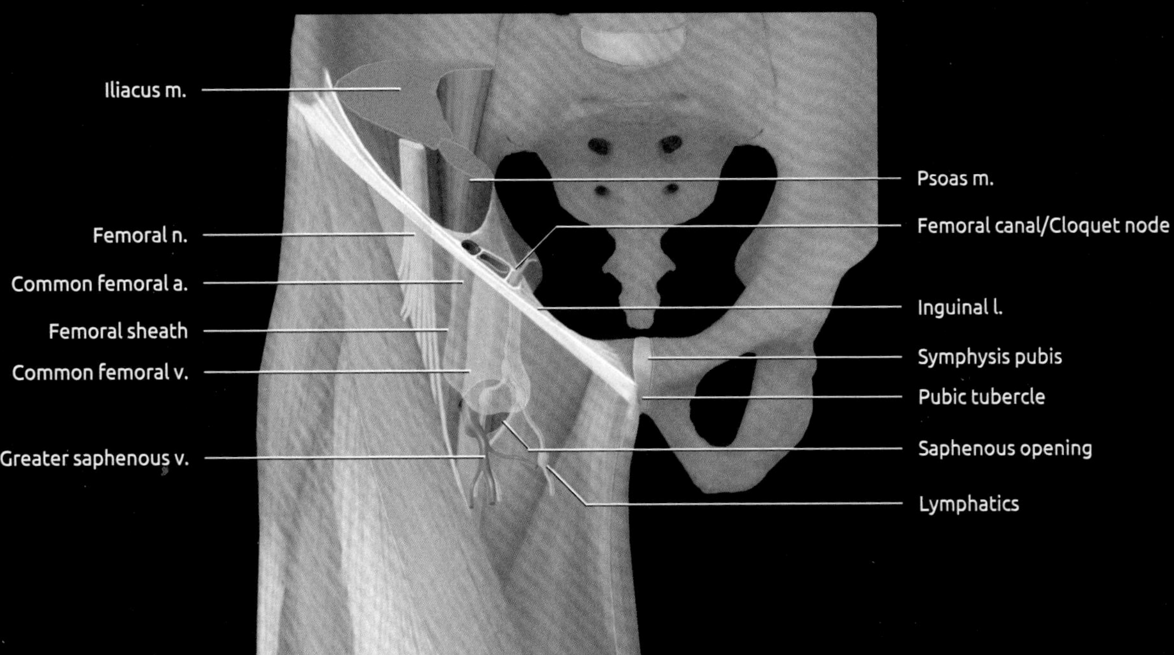

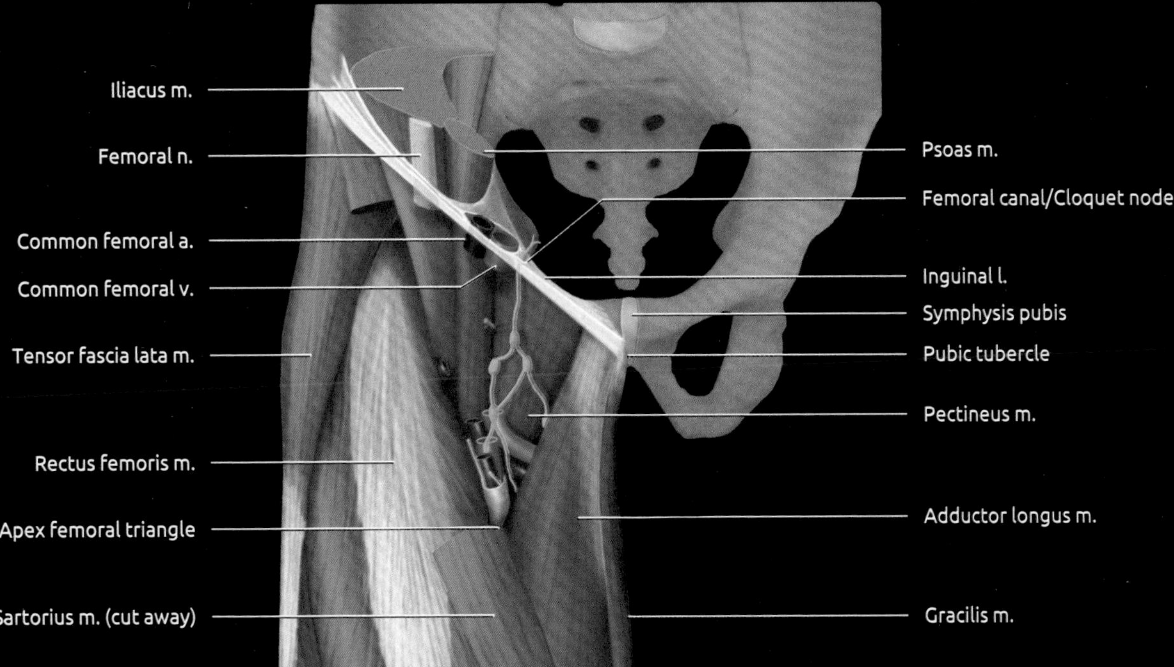

(Top) *The boundaries of the femoral triangle can be remembered by the mnemonic SAIL for sartorius, adductor longus, and inguinal ligament. The contents of the femoral triangle from lateral to medial (remembered by the mnemonic NAVeL) are the femoral nerve, femoral artery and vein, and lymphatics. The nerve lies superficial to the iliopsoas muscle. The fascia lata encases the structures of the thigh. The femoral sheath is the fascial covering over the proximal vessels. At the cut-away proximal boundary, note the septa dividing the sheath into compartments. The femoral canal is the medial compartment.* **(Bottom)** *Femoral triangle is shown after removal of the fascia lata, sartorius muscle, and the vessels. The apex of the triangle is at the crossing of the sartorius and adductor longus muscles. The pectineus, adductor longus, and iliopsoas muscles form the floor of the triangle.*

GROIN MUSCLES

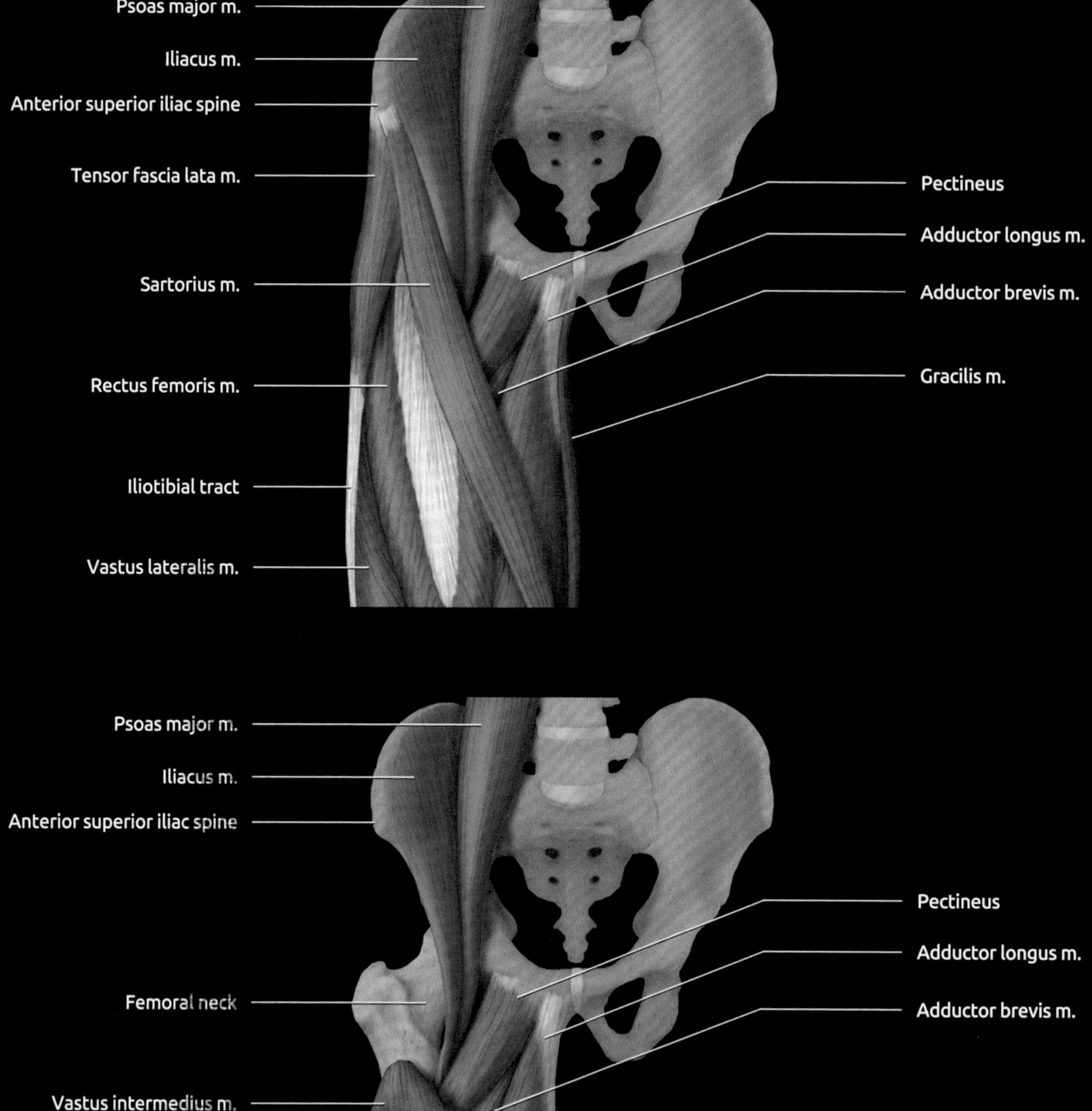

(Top) *Superficial muscles of the groin are shown. The most lateral muscle is the sartorius; its oblique course is easily appreciated. The psoas major and iliacus muscle exit from the pelvis toward the lesser trochanter. On the medial side, the most medial muscle is the gracilis. The adductor brevis muscle is deep to the adductor longus and pectineus muscles.* **(Bottom)** *After removing the superficial layer of muscles, the floor of the femoral triangle is better appreciated. The iliopsoas muscle dives deeply to its trochanteric insertion. The adductors fan out laterally from their pubic origin and constitute the major medial component at a midthigh level. The adductor magnus is in a deeper and more posterior position.*

GROIN OVERVIEW

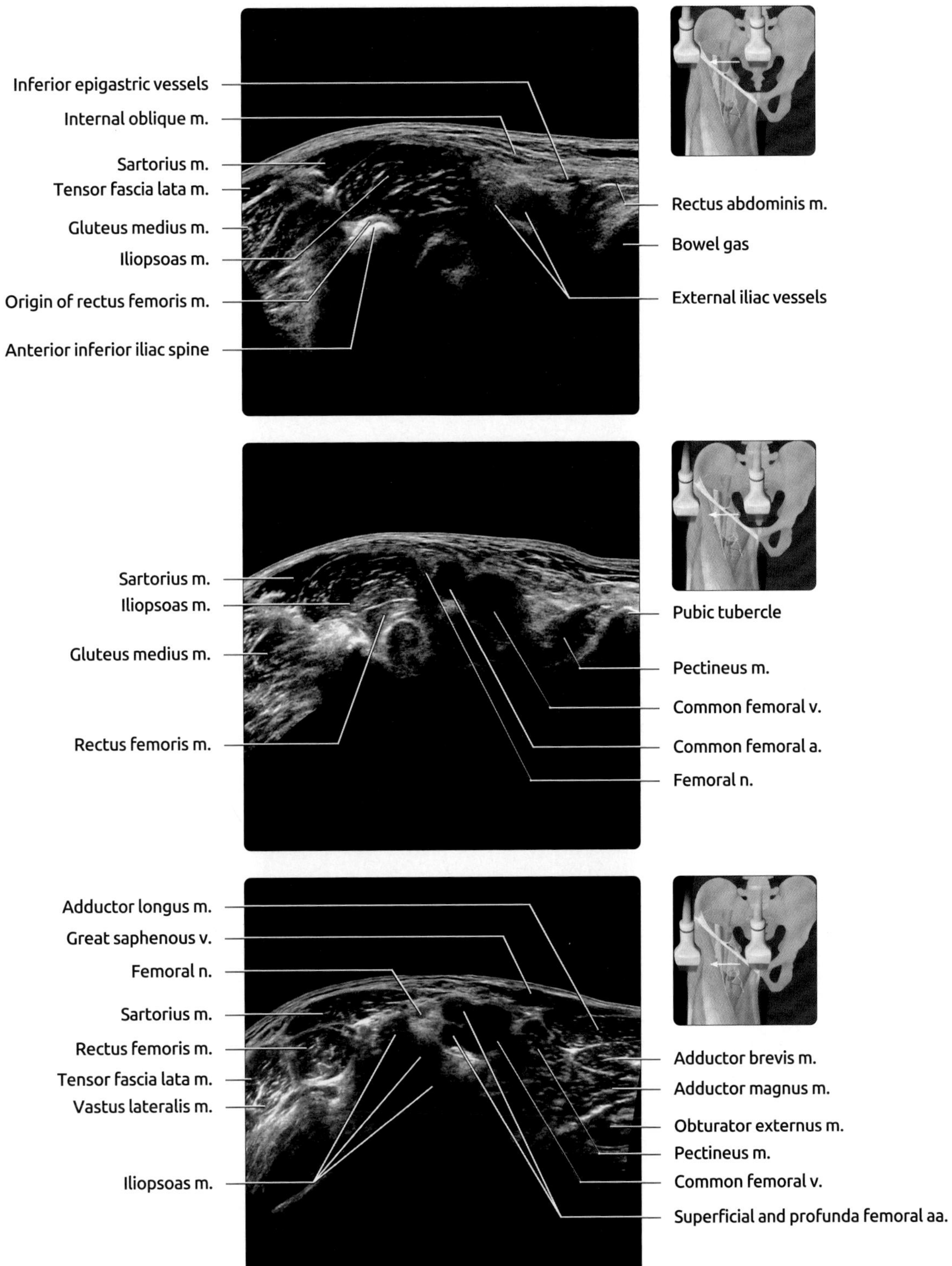

(Top) *Series of transverse panoramic scans show the groin. At this higher level, the lateral components of the groin include the sartorius and iliopsoas muscles and at the medial boundary, the rectus abdominis muscle. At this level, where most structures are above the inguinal ligament, there is bowel (containing gas, which produces shadowing artifact). At this level, vessels are named external iliac vessels.* **(Middle)** *At a lower level, through the pubic bone, the vessels have moved superficially after passing under the inguinal ligament and now become the common femoral vessels. Bowel is not normally present at this level; instead, the pectineus muscle and superior pubic ramus form the floor.* **(Bottom)** *Further inferiorly, the adductor muscles become the major medial component. Femoral vessels divide into superficial and profunda branches.*

MIDLINE GROIN

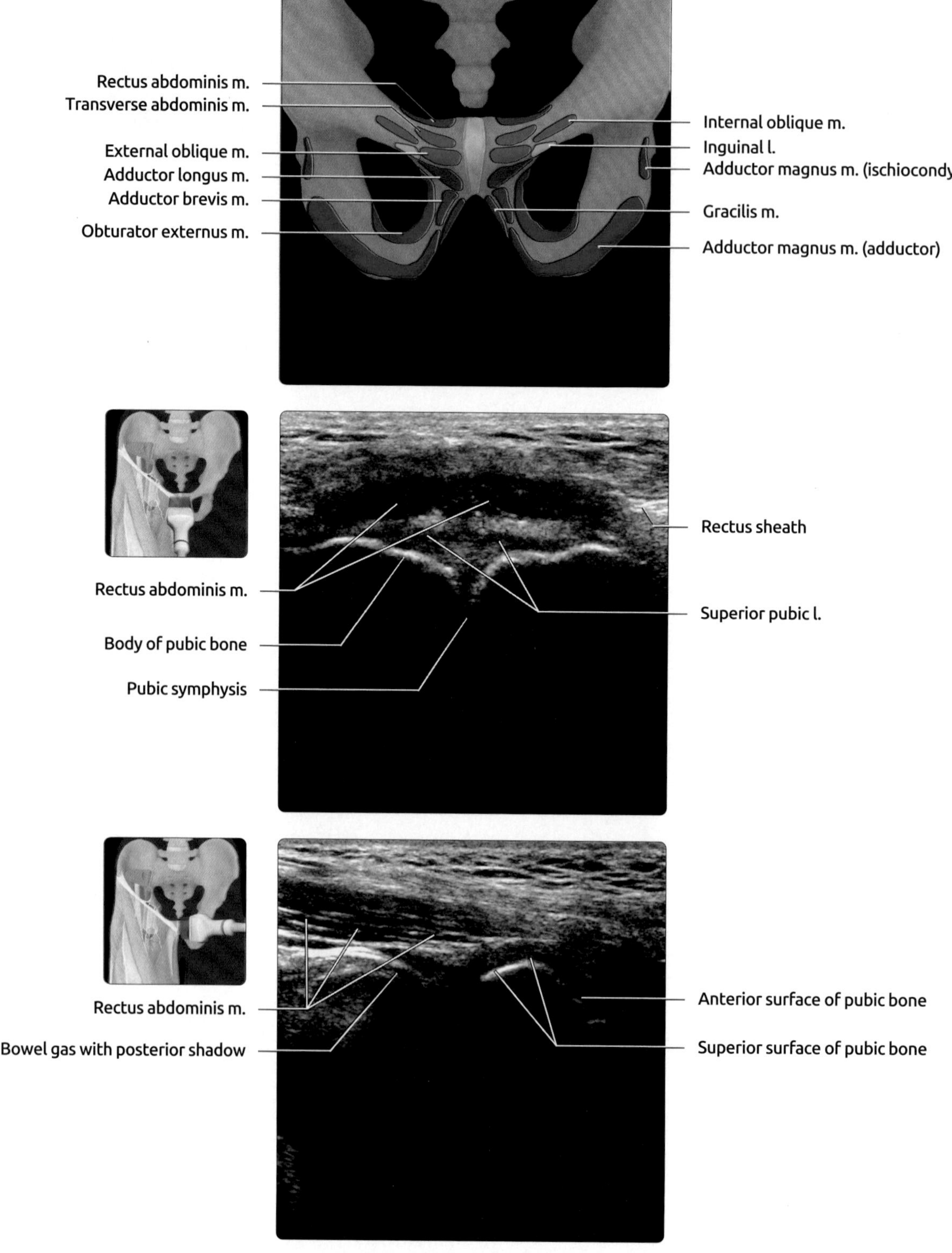

(Top) *Anterior view shows the anterior pelvis and the associated muscle attachments. A number of muscles take origin or insert onto the anterior aspect of the pelvis. These muscles aid in movement and stabilization of the trunk as well as movement and stabilization of the leg and form the medial components of the groin.* **(Middle)** *Transverse scan at the superior aspect shows pubic symphysis. The superior pubic ligament runs horizontally across the symphysis, deep to the rectus abdominis muscle origin.* **(Bottom)** *Sagittal image shows the lower rectus abdominis originating from the superior surface of the pubic bone (pubic crest). Deep to the rectus abdominis muscle is the peritoneal cavity and bowel. Bowel gas produces posterior shadowing artifact, which obscures deeper structures.*

MEDIAL GROIN

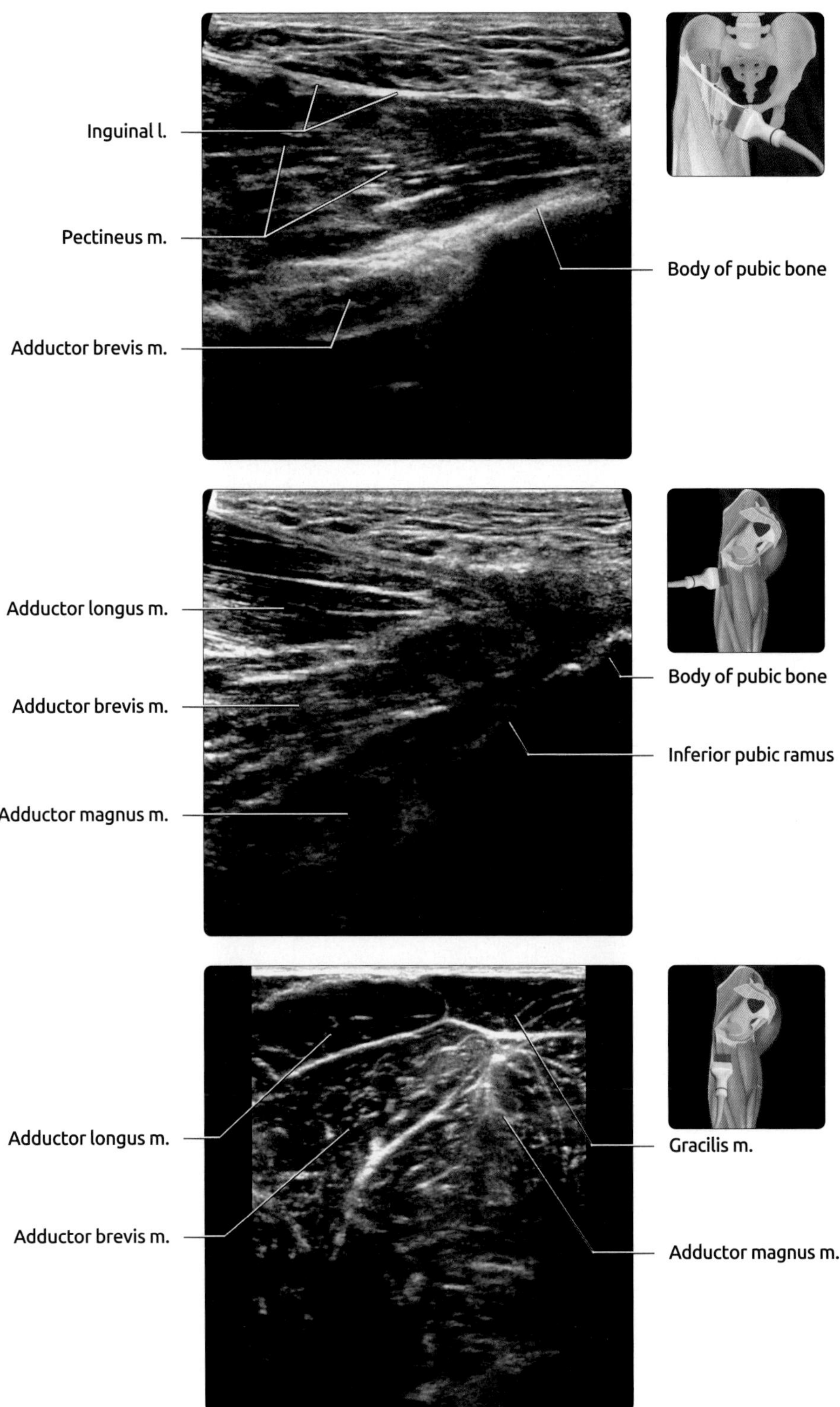

(Top) *First of a series of (oblique) transverse scans through the adductor muscles is shown. Superiorly, the pectineus muscle originates from the pectineal line (which is a ridge on the superior ramus of the pubic bone) and runs laterally to insert on the pectineal line of the proximal femur. The pectineal line of the proximal femur lies between the lesser trochanter and the linea aspera. The pectineus muscle runs lateral to the adductor longus muscle and superficial to the adductor brevis muscle.* **(Middle)** *Slightly inferiorly and scanning more obliquely, the adductor longus, brevis, and magnus can be seen originating from the pubic body and inferior ramus. Scanning this region requires thigh abduction and balancing the transducer head on the bony landmark. From here, individual muscles can be traced inferolaterally. Note that the scout image is a graphic in this sagittal plane.* **(Bottom)** *Oblique transverse scan of adductors using a medial approach is shown. Adductor longus and gracilis muscles form the superficial layer; adductor brevis and magnus muscles run deeper. All muscles run inferolaterally to their femoral insertions.*

CENTRAL GROIN, FEMORAL TRIANGLE

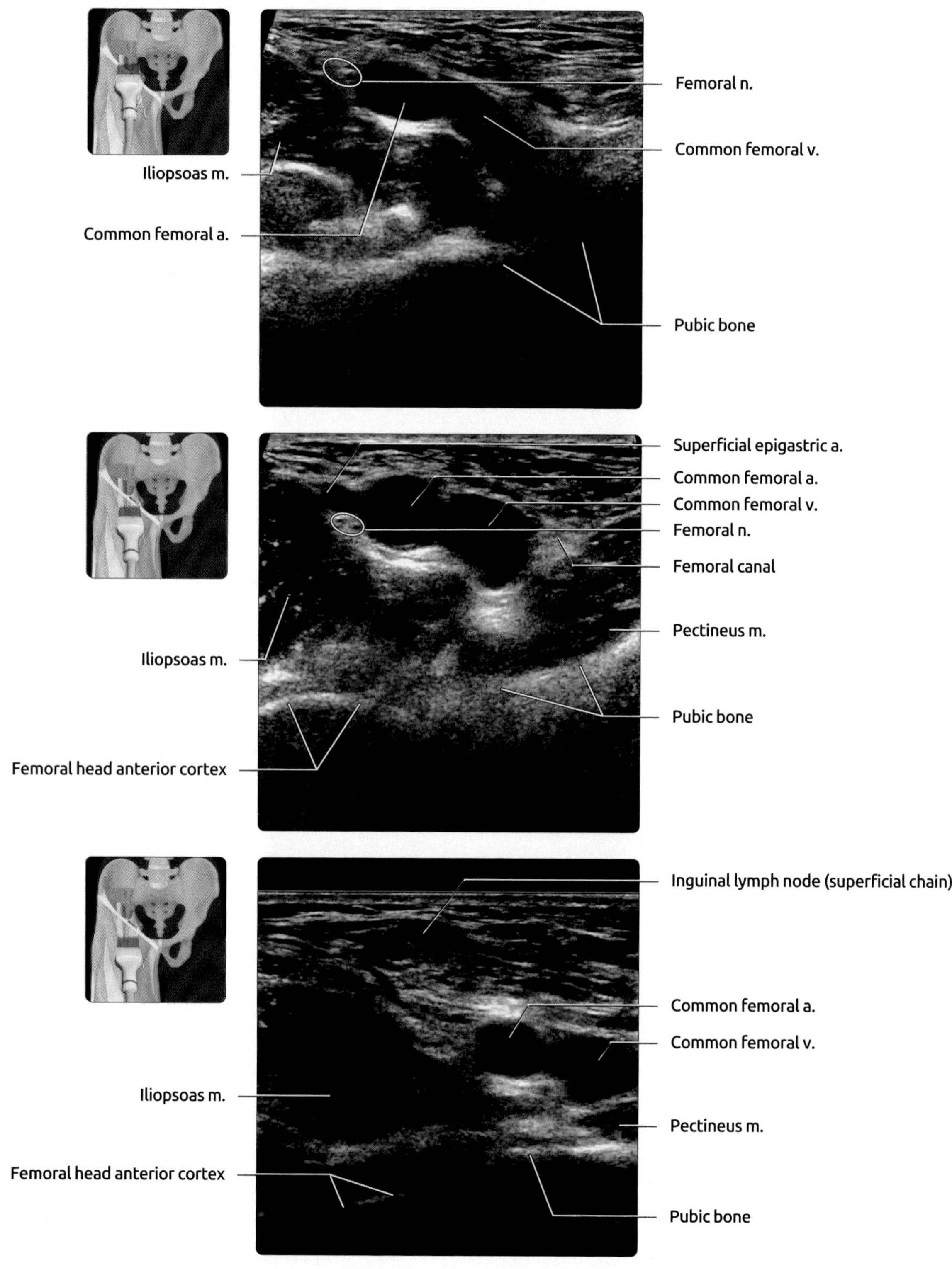

(Top) *Series of transverse scans through the femoral triangle is shown. Above the inguinal ligament, the femoral nerve, artery, and vein run medial to the iliopsoas tendon. The pubic bone acts as a hard support for the iliopsoas and pectineus muscular floor.* **(Middle)** *Slightly inferiorly, below the inguinal ligament, the femoral triangle commences. The mnemonic for the contents is NAVeL, standing for femoral nerve, common femoral artery, common femoral vein, and lymph nodes (within femoral canal). The pectineus muscle forms the floor of femoral triangle. This floor is supported by the pubic bone and hip joint.* **(Bottom)** *In addition to lymph nodes in the femoral canal, lymph nodes are frequently seen superficially (the superficial inguinal chain) in the subcutaneous tissue.*

CENTRAL GROIN, FEMORAL TRIANGLE

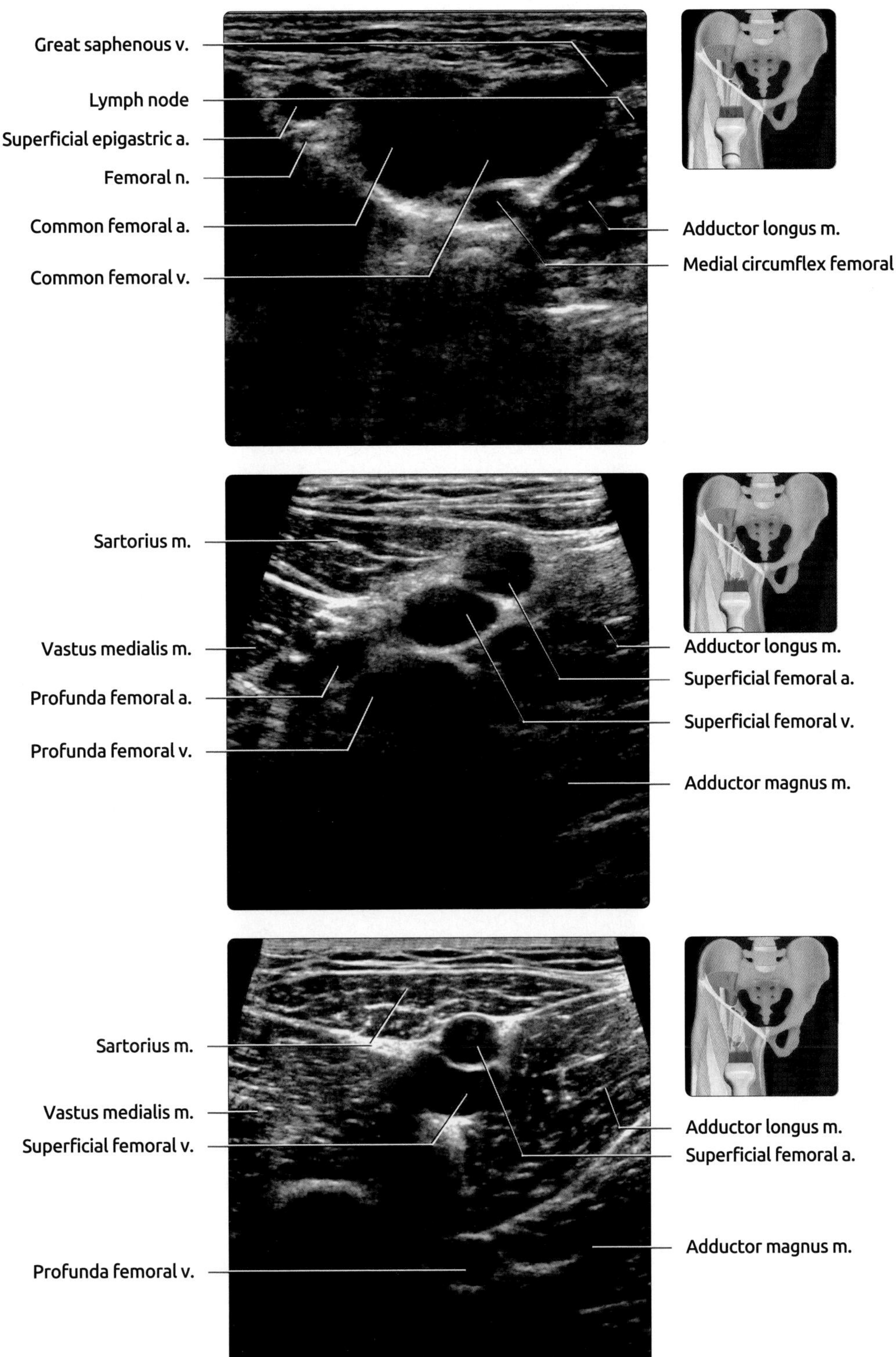

(Top) *Further inferiorly and still within the femoral triangle, the great saphenous vein perforates the anterior wall of the femoral sheath to enter the femoral vein. Also, the floor changes from the pectineus to adductor longus muscle with no bony support.* **(Middle)** *Transverse scan is shown at the apex of the femoral triangle, defined as where the sartorius muscle becomes the roof of the femoral triangle. Just before exiting the femoral triangle, the femoral vessels divide into superficial and profunda branches.* **(Bottom)** *Transverse scan shows the adductor canal. Distal to the femoral triangle, the superficial femoral vessels continue within a muscular conduit, the adductor canal. The groin muscles (the adductor longus and magnus muscles) form the medial wall and floor of this canal.*

LATERAL GROIN, ANTERIOR SUPERIOR ILIAC SPINE

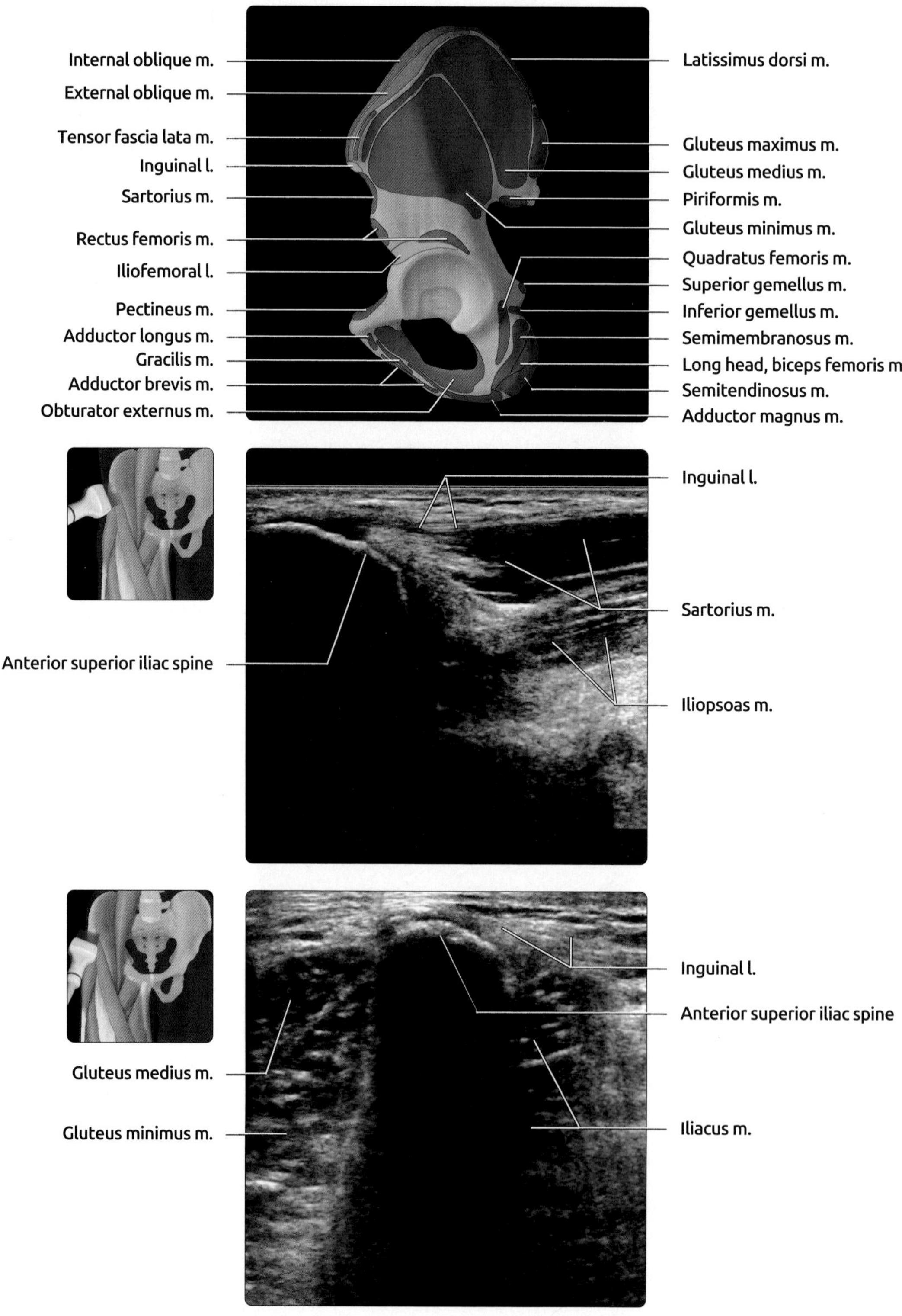

(Top) *Muscle and ligament attachments to the external surface of the pelvis are shown. Note the relatively small origin of the tendon of the adductor longus muscle. The adductor brevis muscle is just deep to the longus muscle. The origin of the gracilis muscle is lateral to the adductor brevis muscle. The adductor magnus muscle has a broad origin with its posterior fibers in close proximity to the hamstring tendon origins.* **(Middle)** *Oblique sagittal scan of the anterior superior iliac spine shows the origin of the sartorius muscle (longest muscle in the body). This slender muscle runs inferomedially over the iliopsoas muscle, covers the adductor canal, and inserts at the proximal tibia as part of the pes anserinus.* **(Bottom)** *Coronal scan of the anterior superior iliac spine shows division of muscle groups by this bone. Gluteal muscles lie lateral and hip flexors medial. The inguinal ligament originates here and runs inferomedially to the pubic tubercle.*

ACROSS GROIN, INGUINAL LIGAMENT

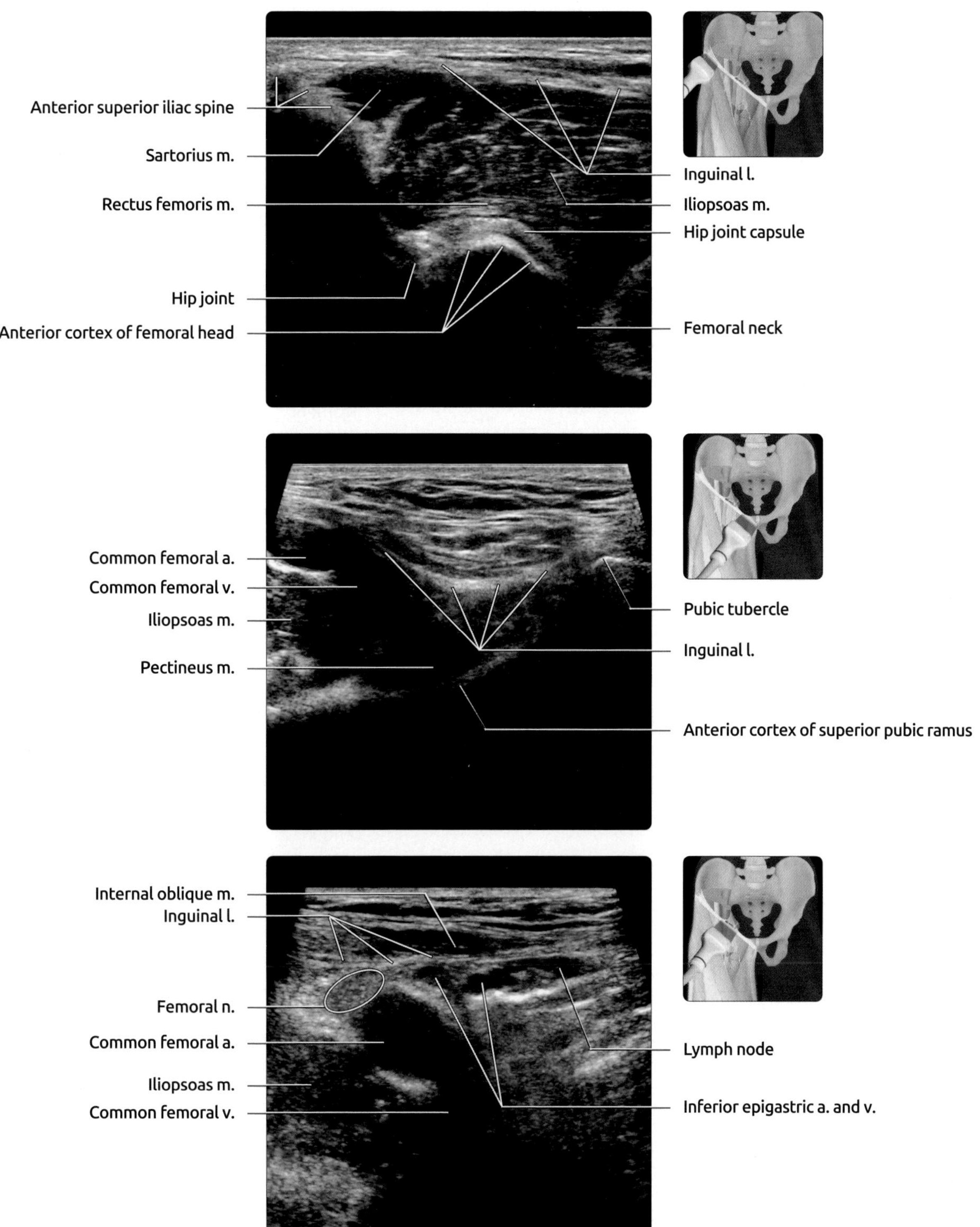

(Top) *Oblique transverse scan of the upper groin shows the inguinal ligament attachment on the anterior superior iliac spine with the sartorius muscle originating immediately inferior. The inguinal ligament runs inferomedially and covers the iliopsoas muscle.* **(Middle)** *Oblique transverse scan along the medial aspect of the inguinal ligament is shown. Medially, the inguinal ligament forms the roof of the femoral canal (covering the femoral vessels and nerve). It then runs over the pectineus muscle to insert on the pubic tubercle.* **(Bottom)** *Superficially focused oblique transverse scan over the upper femoral triangle shows the inguinal ligament forming its roof. Inferior epigastric vessels branch out from the femoral vessels and run superomedially. Clinically, the inferior epigastric vessels define the lateral boundary of direct inguinal hernias. Inguinal hernias that emerge lateral to the inferior epigastric vessels are considered indirect.*

TERMINOLOGY

Synonyms

- Lower leg; calf

GROSS ANATOMY

Osseous Anatomy

- **Tibia**
  - Proximal tibiofibular joint
    - Head of fibula and lateral condyle tibia joined by synovial-lined fibrous capsule
    - May communicate with knee joint (10%)
    - Posterolaterally located
    - Synovial joint, so can be affected by any synovial inflammatory process
  - Anterolateral tibia: Origin of anterior muscles of leg
  - Anterior border (shin): Sharp ridge running from tibial tuberosity proximally to anterior margin of medial malleolus
  - Medial tibial surface
    - Wide and flat
    - Proximally, covered by pes anserinus
    - Remainder is subcutaneous
  - Medial border of tibia: Saphenous nerve and great saphenous vein run along it
  - Posterior tibia: Origin of deep posterior muscles of leg
  - Lateral border of tibia: Ridge for attachment of interosseous membrane
  - Medial malleolus: 2 colliculi, anterior longer than posterior
  - Distal tibiofibular joint
    - Fibula articulates with tibia at fibular notch; joined by interosseous ligament
    - Strengthened by anterior and posterior tibiofibular ligaments
    - Posterolaterally located
- **Fibula**
  - Anterior fibula
    - Origin of lateral muscles of leg
  - Medial fibula
    - Origin of deep posterior muscles of leg
  - Posterolateral fibula
    - Origin of posterior muscles of leg
  - Lateral malleolus: 1 cm longer than medial malleolus

Interosseous Membrane

- Stretches across interval between tibia and fibula
- Greatly extends surface for origin of muscles
- Strong, oblique fibers run downward and laterally from tibia to fibula
- In upper part, below lateral condyle of tibia, there is opening for passage of anterior tibial vessels
- Distally, opening allows passage of perforating branch of peroneal artery
- Tibialis posterior and flexor hallucis longus take partial origin from back of membrane
- Tibialis anterior, long extensors of toes, and peroneus tertius take partial origin from front of membrane

Muscles of Leg

- Compartments separated by deep fascia, which give partial origin to several muscles
- **Posterior compartment: Superficial muscles**
  - **Gastrocnemius**
    - Origin: Medial from posterior femoral metaphysis; lateral from posterior edge of lateral epicondyle
    - Heads separated from posterior capsule by bursa
    - 2 heads unite to form main bulk of muscle
    - Join in thin aponeurotic tendon near midleg
    - Joins soleus aponeurosis to form Achilles tendon; concave in cross section; musculotendinous junction is 5 cm above calcaneal insertion
    - Nerve supply: Tibial nerve
    - Action: Plantar flexor of ankle and flexor of knee
  - **Plantaris**
    - Origin: Superior and medial to lateral head of gastrocnemius origin, as well as from oblique popliteal ligament
    - Continues deep to lateral head of gastrocnemius
    - Myotendinous junction at level of origin of soleus (muscle is 5-10 cm long)
    - Tendon then lies between medial head of gastrocnemius and soleus
    - Follows medial side of Achilles to insert either anteromedially on Achilles or on calcaneus
    - Plantaris absent in 7-10% of general population
    - Nerve supply: Tibial nerve
    - Action: Acts with gastrocnemius
  - **Soleus**
    - Origin: Extensive, from back of fibular head and upper 1/3 of posterior surface of shaft of fibula, from soleal line and middle 1/3 of medial border of tibia, and from tendinous arch joining these across popliteal vessels
    - Flat, thick, powerful muscle that ends in strong tendon
    - Joins with tendon of gastrocnemius to form Achilles tendon
    - Nerve supply: Tibial nerve
    - Action: Stabilizes ankle in standing, plantarflexes ankle
    - Accessory soleus: Rare variant, arises from anterior surface of soleus or from fibula and soleal line of tibia; inserts into Achilles or onto calcaneus anteromedially to Achilles; presents as mass
- **Posterior compartment: Deep muscles**
  - **Popliteus**
    - Origin: Tendon from popliteal groove of lateral femoral condyle
    - Passes through popliteal hiatus posteriorly and medially, pierces posterior capsule of knee
    - Muscle fibers directed medially and downward to insert on posterior surface of tibia above soleal line
    - Nerve supply: Tibial nerve
    - Action: Flexes knee and medially rotates tibia with respect to femur at onset of flexion (unlocking extension "screwing home" mechanism)
  - **Tibialis posterior**
    - Origin: Interosseous membrane and adjoining parts of posterior surfaces of tibia and fibula

- Superior end bifid; anterior tibial vessels pass forward between 2 attachments
- Distally, it inclines medially, under flexor digitorum longus
- Grooves and curves around medial malleolus
- Nerve supply: Tibial nerve
- Action: Plantarflexes and inverts foot

- **Flexor digitorum longus**
  - Origin: Posterior surface of tibia, below popliteus, and medial to vertical ridge
  - Crosses superficial to distal part of tibialis posterior
  - Tendon grooves lower end of tibia lateral to that of tibialis posterior, passes around medial malleolus to foot
  - Nerve supply: Tibial nerve
  - Action: Flexes interphalangeal and metatarsophalangeal joints of lateral 4 toes; plantarflexes and inverts foot
- **Flexor hallucis longus**
  - Origin: Posterior surface of fibula, below origin of soleus
  - Passes medially, descends down posterior to midtibia
  - Associated with os trigonum posterior to talus
  - Tendon occupies deep groove on posterior surface of talus, passes around medial malleolus, under sustentaculum tali, to great toe
  - Nerve supply: Tibial nerves
  - Action: Flexes interphalangeal and metatarsophalangeal joints of great toe; plantarflexes foot

- **Lateral compartment**
  - Peroneals separated from extensors by anterior intermuscular septum and from posterior muscles by posterior septum
  - **Peroneus longus**
    - Origin: Upper 2/3 lateral surface of fibula and intermuscular septa and adjacent muscular fascia
    - Becomes tendinous a few cm above lateral malleolus
    - Curves forward behind lateral malleolus, posterior to peroneus brevis
    - Nerve supply: Superficial peroneal
    - Action: Everts foot and secondarily plantarflexes foot
  - **Peroneus brevis**
    - Origin: Lower 2/3 lateral surface of fibula and intermuscular septa and adjacent muscular fascia
    - Muscle is medial to peroneus longus at origin but overlaps peroneus longus in middle 1/3
    - Tendon curves forward behind lateral malleolus, in front of peroneus longus tendon
    - Nerve supply: Superficial peroneal
    - Action: Everts foot and secondarily plantarflexes foot
  - Synovial sheath for peroneals begins 5 cm above tip of lateral malleolus and envelops both tendons; divides into 2 sheaths at the level of calcaneus
  - **Peroneus quartus**
    - Accessory muscle with prevalence of 10%
    - Originates from distal leg, frequently from peroneal muscles, with variable insertion sites at foot
    - At level of malleolus, located medial or posterior to both peroneal tendons
  - **Peroneus digiti minimi**
    - Accessory with prevalence of 15-36%
    - Extends from peroneus brevis muscle around medial malleolus to foot
    - Tiny tendinous slip
- **Anterior compartment**
  - **Tibialis anterior**
    - Origin: Upper 1/2 of lateral surface of tibia and interosseous membrane
    - Tendon originates in distal 1/3; passes deep to retinaculum
    - Nerve supply: Deep peroneal and recurrent genicular
    - Action: Dorsiflexor and invertor of foot
  - **Extensor digitorum longus**
    - Origin: From upper 3/4 of anterior surface fibula
    - Descends behind extensor retinacula to ankle
    - Nerve supply: Deep peroneal
    - Action: Extends interphalangeal and metatarsophalangeal joints of lateral 4 toes, dorsiflexes foot
  - **Peroneus tertius**
    - Small, not always present
    - Origin: Continuous with extensor digitorum longus, arising from distal 1/4 of anterior surface of fibula and interosseous membrane
    - Inserts into dorsal surface at base of 5th metatarsal
    - Nerve supply: Deep peroneal
    - Action: Dorsiflexes ankle and everts foot
  - **Extensor hallucis**
    - Thin muscle hidden between tibialis anterior and extensor digitorum longus
    - Origin: Middle 1/2 of anterior surface of fibula and interosseous membrane
    - Tendon passes deep to retinacula to great toe
    - Nerve supply: Deep peroneal
    - Action: Extends phalanges of great toe and dorsiflexes foot

ANATOMY IMAGING ISSUES

Imaging Recommendations

- Leg muscles and vessels are well demonstrated by ultrasound throughout their course and depth
- Start imaging at the ankle and move proximally to identify "hard to find" structures or ones that change course (i.e., plantaris)
- Gastrocnemius muscle tears at the myofascial junction and deep venous thrombosis in the leg are common

Imaging Pitfalls

- Deep structures of posterior compartment, such as peroneal vessels and tibialis posterior muscle, may be difficult to visualize in very muscular patients
  - Attempt scanning anteriorly through anterior compartment using the gap between the tibia and fibula as a window
- Intramuscular veins of the leg have variable anatomy
  - May be duplicated &/or asymmetric to the contralateral side
  - Any thrombus in a vein that is intramuscular (deep to a muscular fascia) is a deep venous thrombosis

ANTEROLATERAL LEG

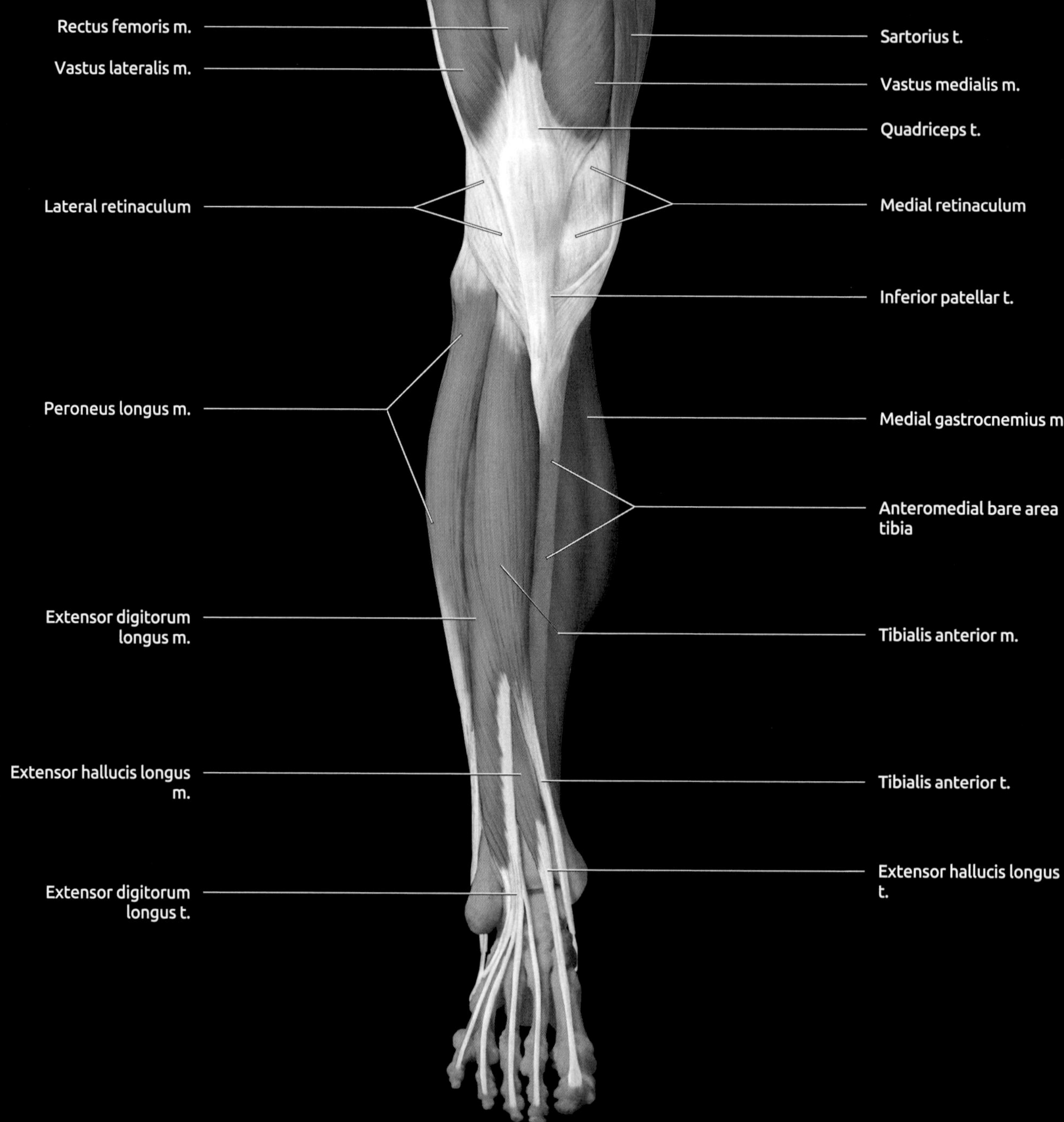

Graphic shows the anterior leg muscles. Note that nearly the entire anteromedial tibia is bare of muscle. Thus, it is poorly vascularized, resulting in slow fracture healing. The tibialis anterior has an extensive origin from both tibia and interosseous membrane and is the most substantial muscle of the anterior compartment. The extensor digitorum longus originates from the fibula. The extensor hallucis longus originates between the 2, from the fibula and the interosseous membrane. These 3 muscles retain the same orientation as they become tendinous anterior to the ankle. The mnemonic "Tom, Harry, & Dick" applies to the tendon order, from medial to lateral (tibialis anterior, extensor hallucis longus, extensor digitorum).

PANORAMIC ANTEROLATERAL LEG

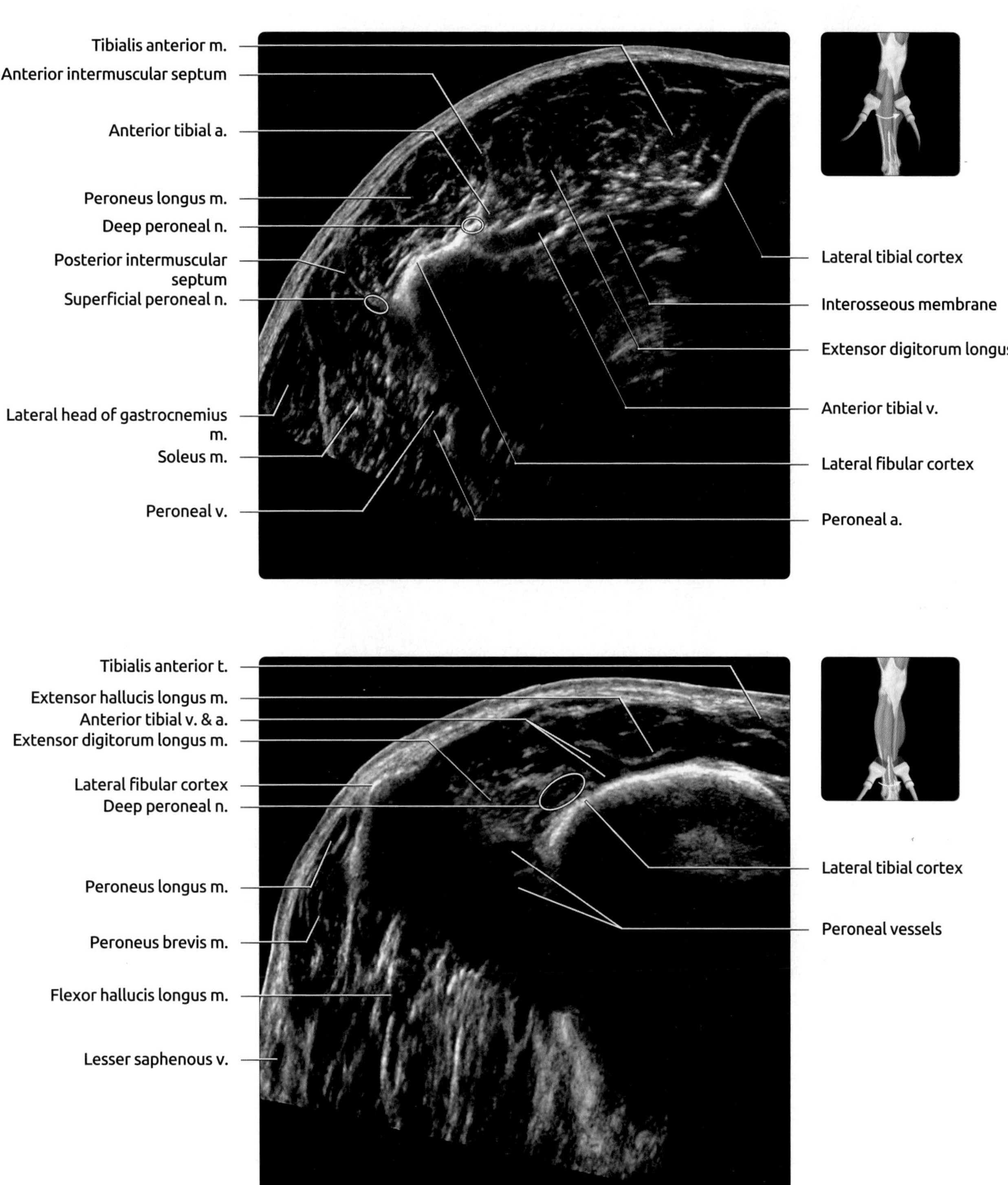

(Top) *Transverse panoramic view shows the anterior and lateral compartments of the upper leg. The crural compartments are divided by the tibia and the 2 intermuscular septa (anterior and posterior) into the anterior (extensor), lateral (peroneal), and posterior (flexor) compartments. The intermuscular septum separates the anterior from the posterior compartments.* **(Bottom)** *Transverse panoramic view shows the anterior and lateral compartments of the inferior leg. All muscles are smaller in caliber compared to those seen superiorly. An interosseous gap is still present between the tibia and fibula, but ultrasound interrogation through this gap is no longer possible and the interosseous membrane cannot be demonstrated.*

ANTERIOR COMPARTMENT

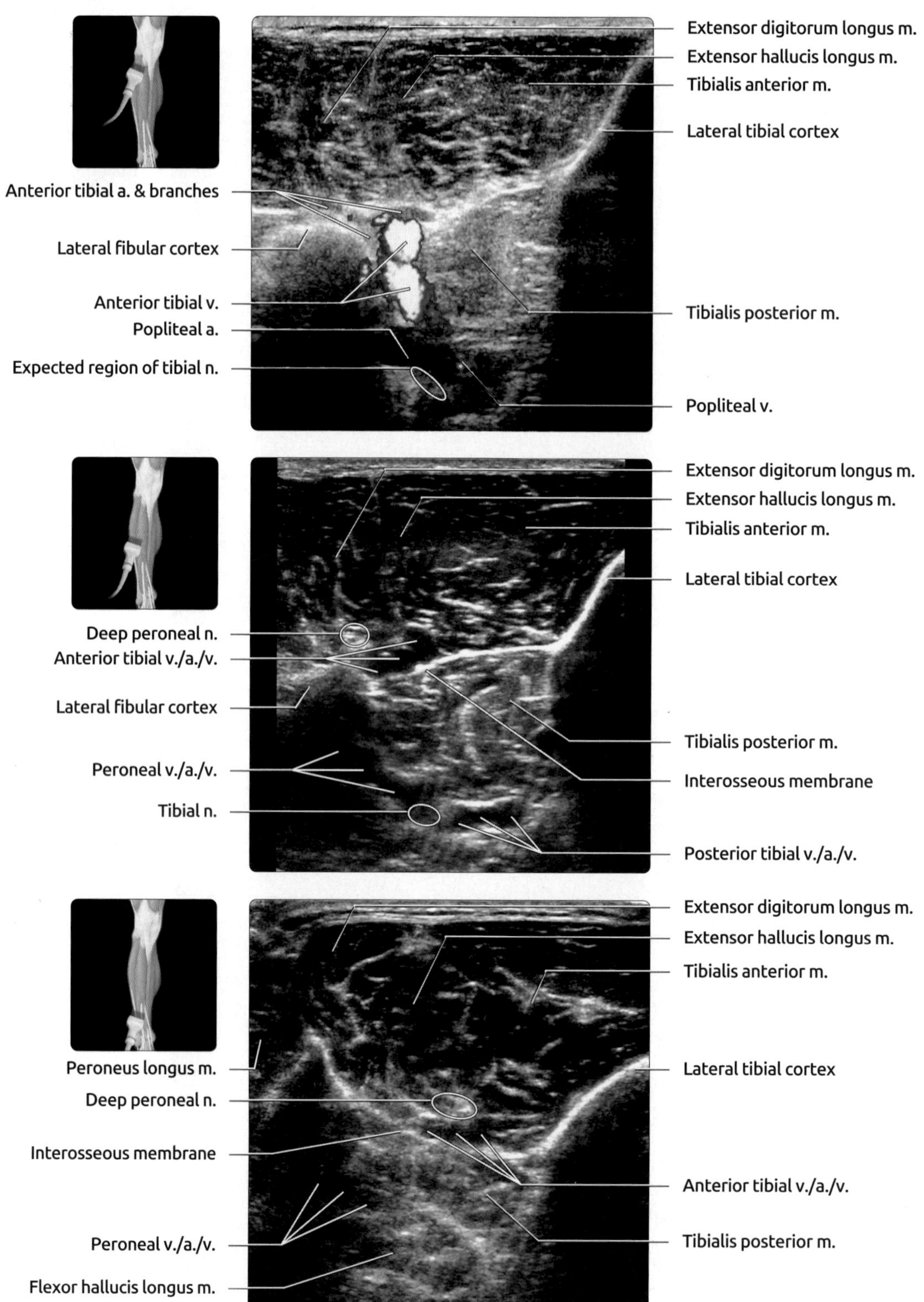

(Top) *Transverse color Doppler scan shows the anterior compartment at the upper leg level slightly below the proximal tibiofibular joint. At this level (above the superior margin of the interosseous membrane), the anterior tibial artery and vein (branches of the popliteal artery and vein) run anteriorly to supply the anterior compartment.* **(Middle)** *Transverse scan shows the anterior compartment at a slightly lower level. The tibialis anterior, extensor hallucis longus, and extensor digitorum longus muscles form the muscular component of this compartment. The deep peroneal nerve has penetrated laterally to supply this compartment. The anterior tibial vessels run on the surface of the interosseous membrane.* **(Bottom)** *Transverse scan more inferiorly shows a decrease in size of the extensor muscles and gradual migration of nerve and vessels more medially and superficially.*

ANTERIOR COMPARTMENT

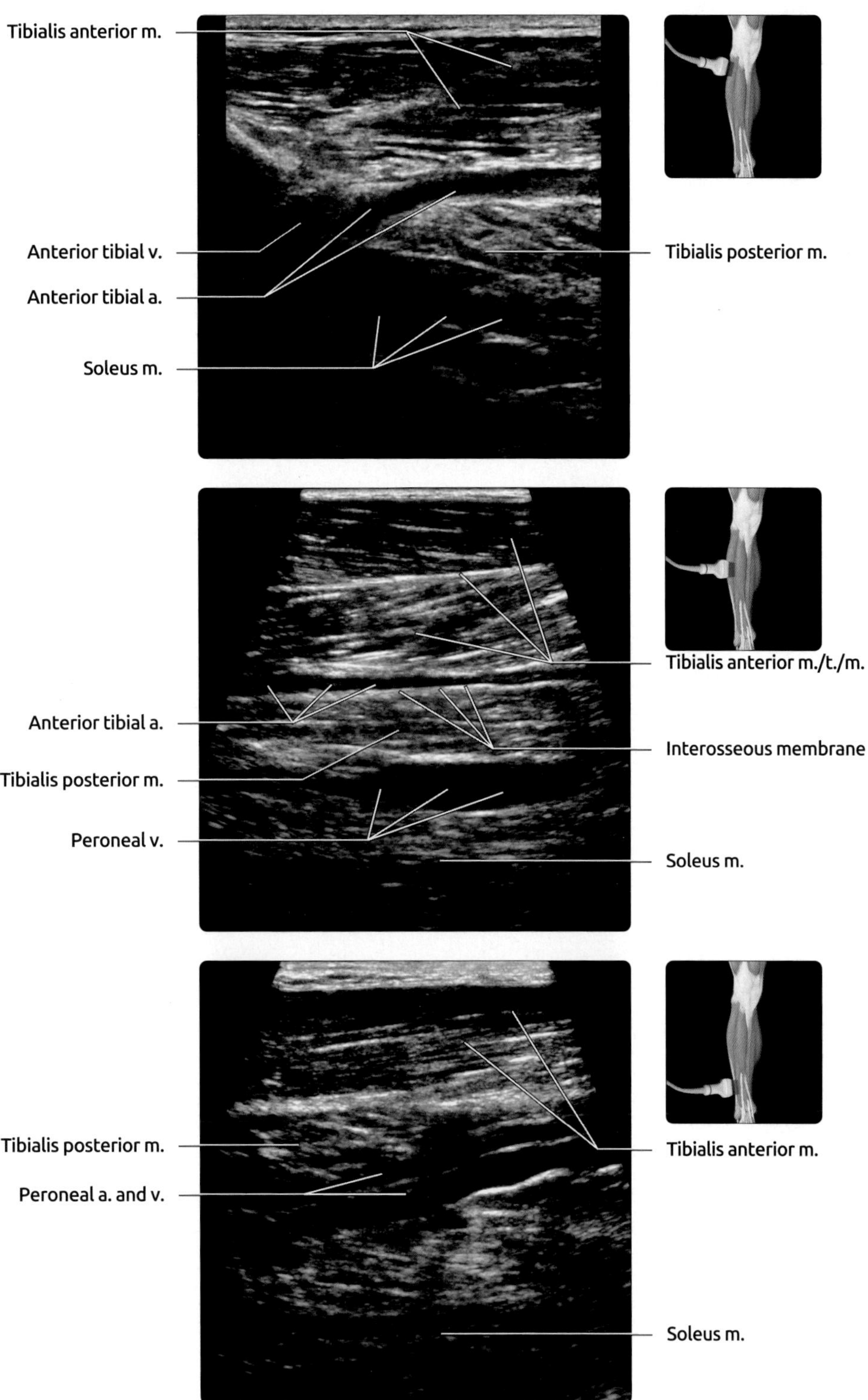

(Top) *Sagittal scan shows the anterior compartment at the upper leg level. The anterior tibial vessels pass above the superior margin of the interosseous membrane to enter the anterior compartment and supply the extensor muscles.* **(Middle)** *Sagittal scan of the anterior and posterior compartments at the midleg level shows that the interosseous gap between the tibia and fibula can be used as a window to interrogate the deep posterior structures.* **(Bottom)** *Sagittal scan shows the anterior compartment at a lower level. Within the posterior compartment, the peroneal vessels run anteriorly and just below the inferior margin of the interosseous membrane.*

LATERAL COMPARTMENT

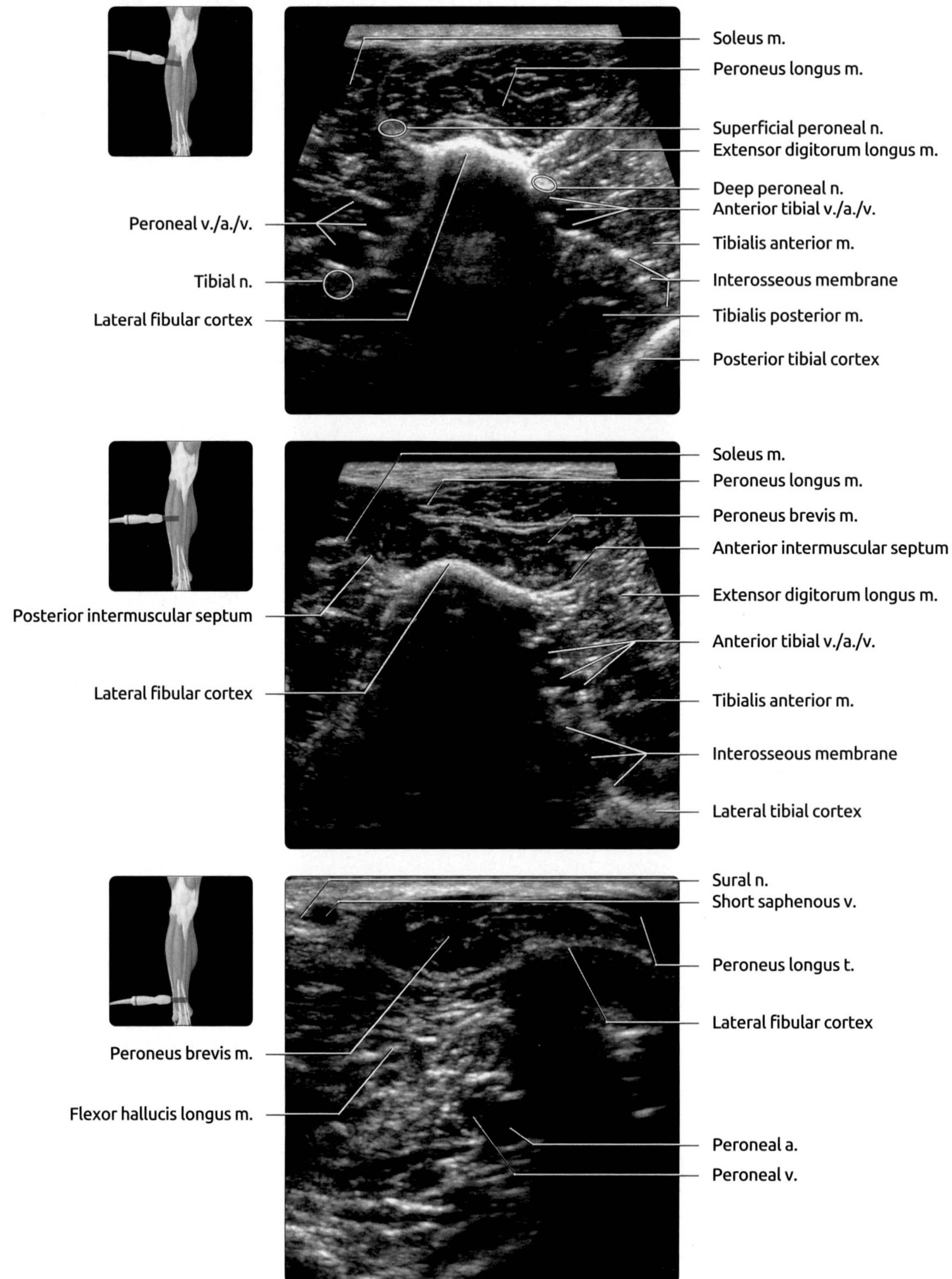

(Top) *Transverse scan shows the lateral compartment at a high level. At this level, only the peroneus longus muscle has originated and is the only muscle occupying this compartment. The superficial peroneal nerve lies on the posterior surface of the peroneus longus muscle. The deep peroneal nerve has already entered the anterior compartment after curving around the fibular neck (above this scan level).* **(Middle)** *Transverse scan at the midleg level shows that the peroneus brevis muscle has now originated and resides anterior and deep to the peroneus longus muscle. More inferiorly, the peroneus longus muscle will become smaller and turn into a tendon while the peroneus brevis will still have muscle fibers down to the level of the ankle joint.* **(Bottom)** *Transverse scan shows the level of the lateral malleolus. The peroneal tendons will run posterior to the lateral malleolus and curve around its tip to run toward the lateral foot.*

LATERAL COMPARTMENT

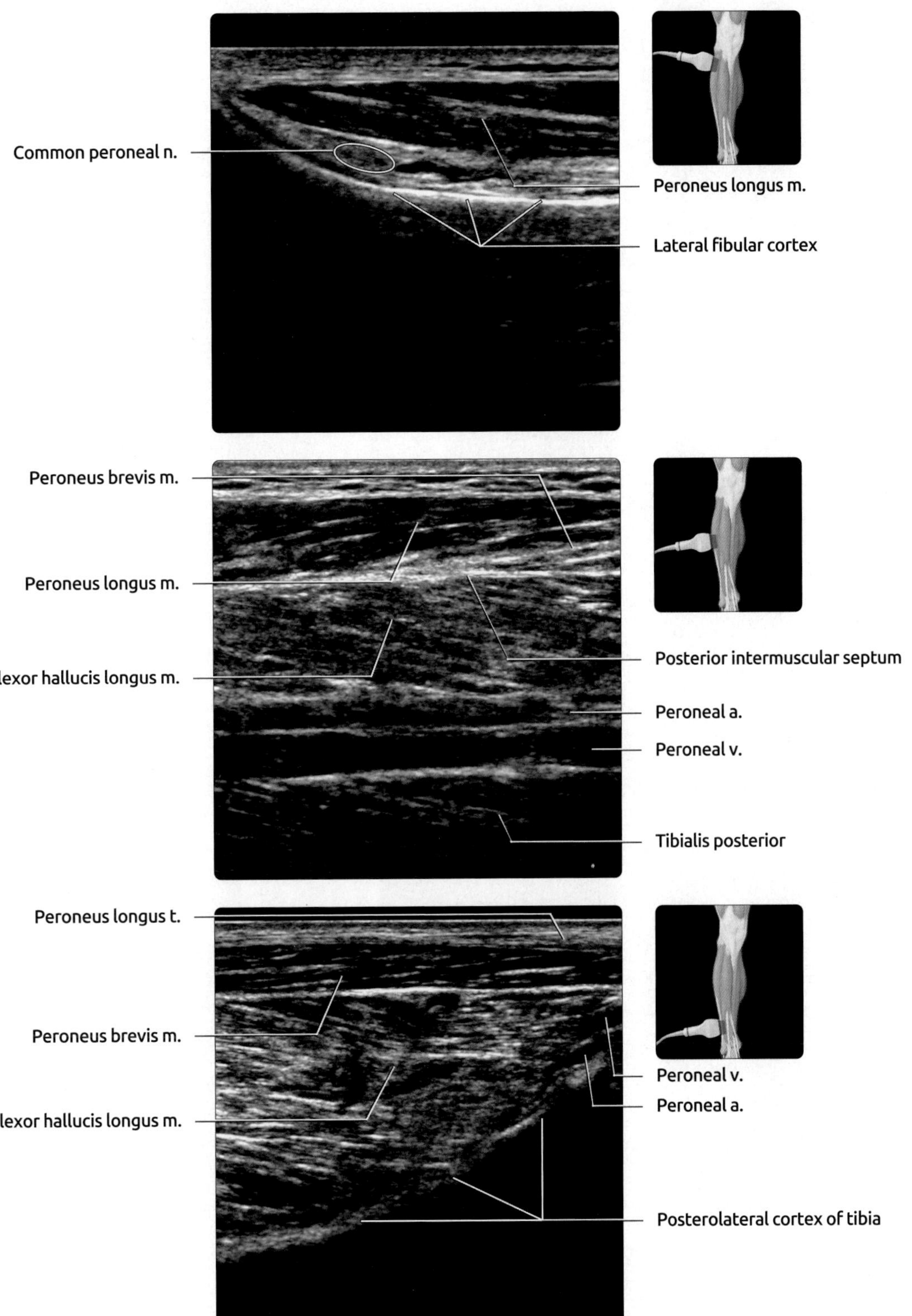

(Top) *Coronal scan shows the lateral compartment at the level of the fibular neck. The common peroneal nerve runs together with the biceps femoris tendon, then curves anteriorly around the neck of fibula to enter the lateral and then the anterior compartments.* **(Middle)** *Coronal scan of the lateral compartment at the midleg level shows the transition between the peroneus longus and peroneus brevis muscles. These are separated from the posterior compartment by the posterior intermuscular septum.* **(Bottom)** *Coronal scan further inferiorly shows that the peroneus longus muscle is now only a tendon, compared to the muscular peroneus brevis. Similarly, in the posterior compartment, the flexor hallucis longus muscle is the only muscle at this level, as the others have also become tendons.*

LATERAL LEG

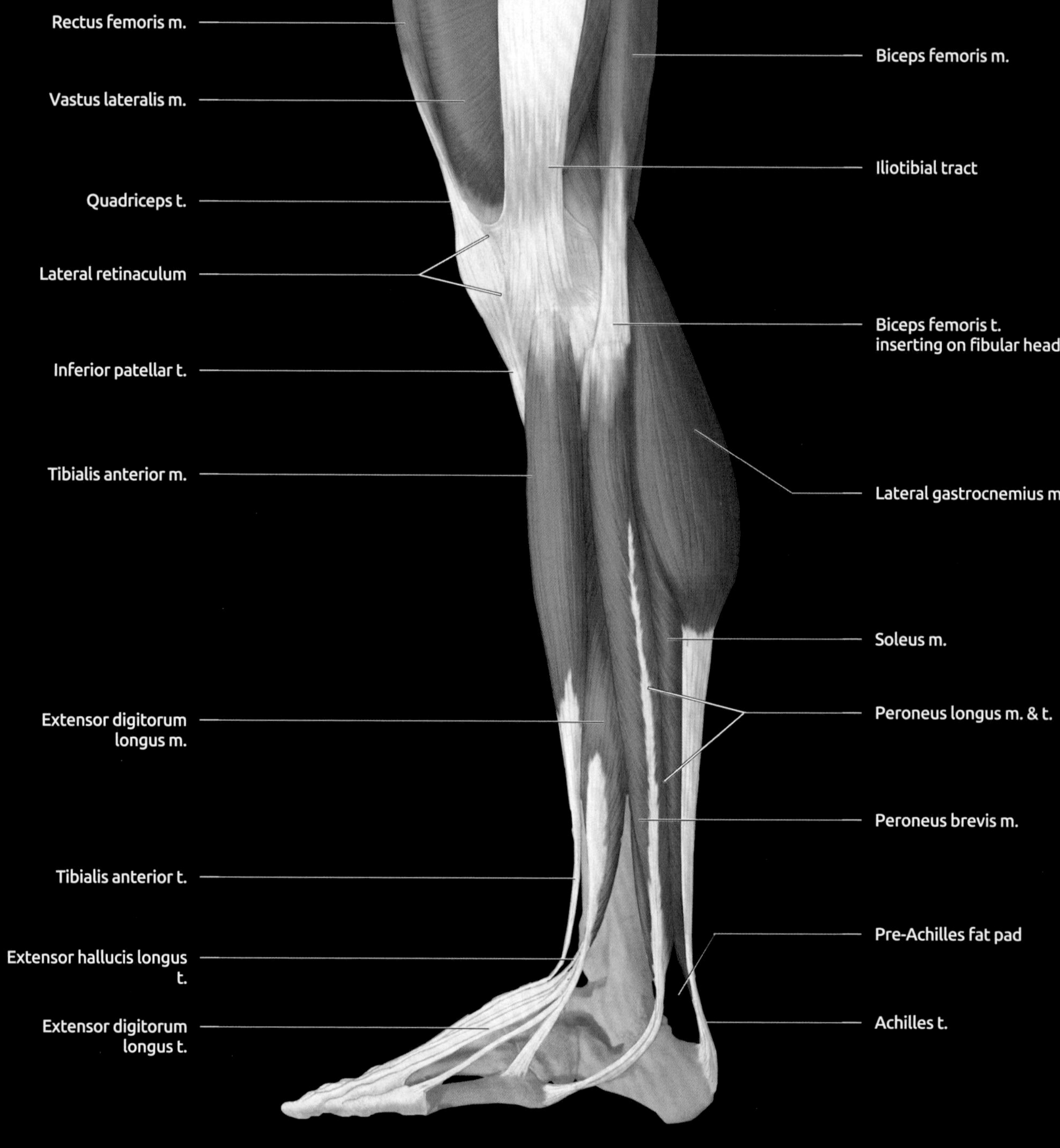

Graphic of the lateral leg shows the anterior compartment (extensors), lateral compartment (peroneals), and superficial muscles of the posterior compartment. Of the ankle tendons, tendinosis most commonly affects the Achilles tendon, the posterior tibialis tendon, and the peroneal tendons. The tibialis anterior tendon is also affected, though less commonly. As the peroneus brevis lies closest to the bone, it is more prone to trauma particularly in the retromalleolar region. Typically, this tear consists of a longitudinal split in which the overlying peroneus longus tendon pushes into the peroneus brevis tendon, splitting it into 2 sections. One may then see 3 rather than 2 tendons behind the lateral malleolus. Another reason to see 3 tendons behind the lateral malleolus is when there is a quartus tendon present.

POSTERIOR LEG

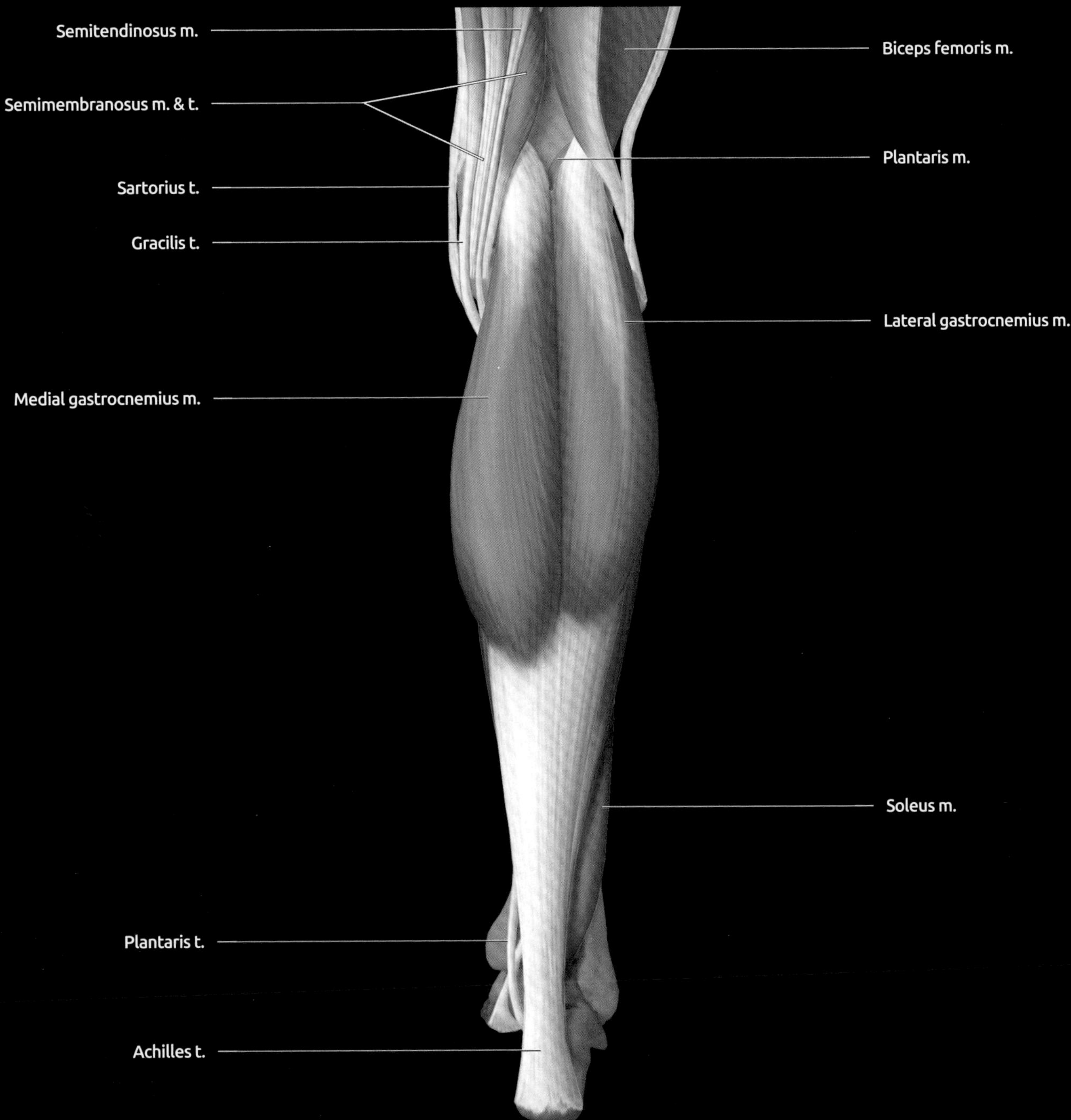

Posterior view shows superficial muscles and tendons of the leg. The gastrocnemius muscles are bulky in the proximal 1/2 of the leg and taper to an aponeurosis, which blends with the soleus more distally to become the Achilles tendon. The plantaris muscle is superficial only at its origin from the lateral femoral metaphysis, just medial to the origin of the lateral head of gastrocnemius. The muscle extends only a few centimeters before becoming tendinous, extending distally between the soleus and medial gastrocnemius. Eventually, the plantaris tendon merges with the medial side of the Achilles or inserts on the calcaneus, medial to the Achilles insertion.

PANORAMIC POSTERIOR LEG

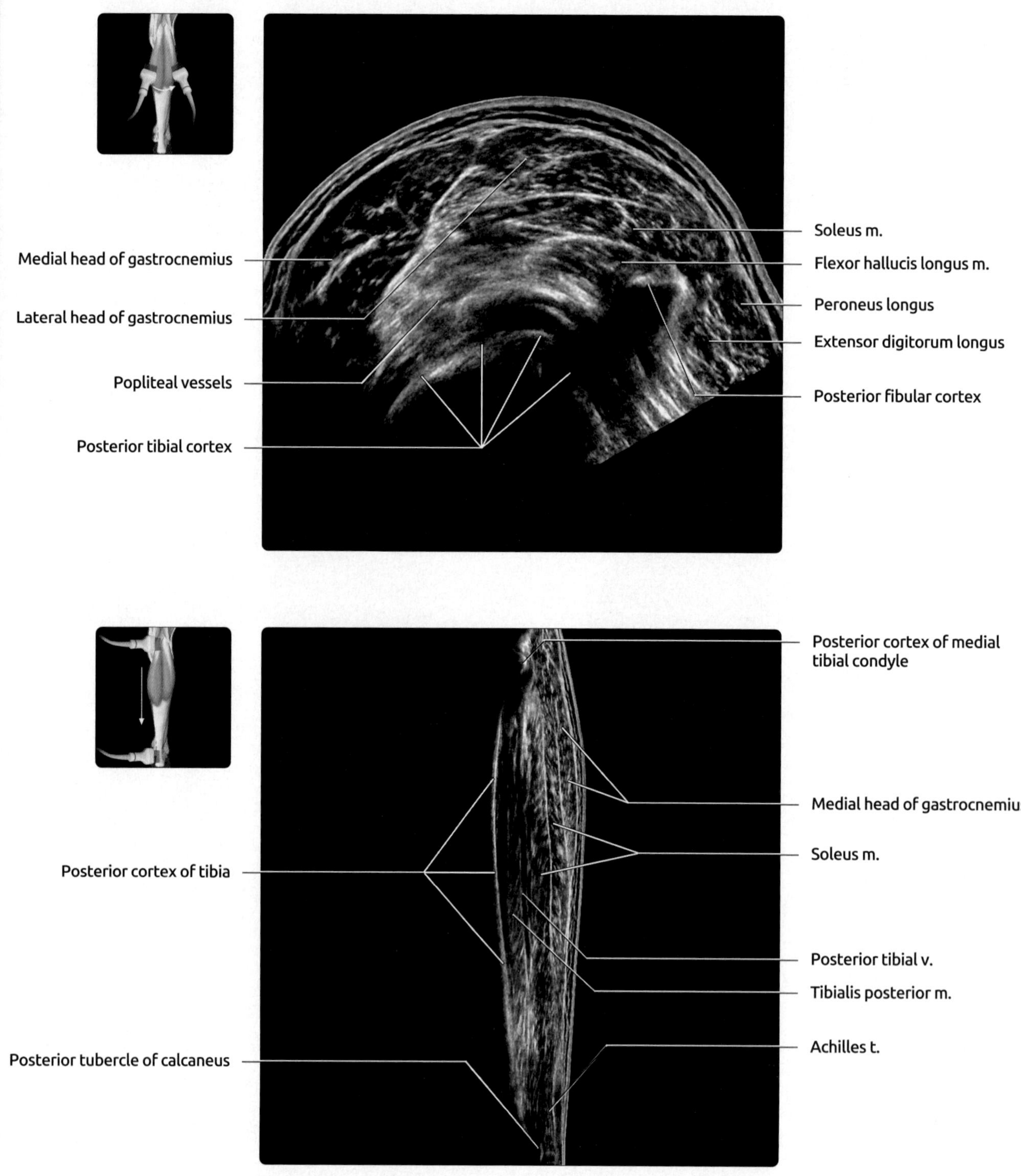

(Top) *Transverse panoramic scan shows the posterior compartment at the level of the midleg. The medial head of the gastrocnemius muscle is larger than the lateral head throughout its course. From this midcalf level downward, the soleus muscle will assume relatively more bulk as the gastrocnemius turns tendinous.* **(Bottom)** *Sagittal panoramic scan shows the posterior compartment. The gastrocnemius is muscular down to ~ the level of the midcalf. Below this level, it forms the Achilles tendon, receiving contributions from the soleus muscle. For the deep layer, the tibialis posterior muscle lies on the surface of the tibial shaft and interosseous membrane.*

TRANSVERSE POSTERIOR LEG

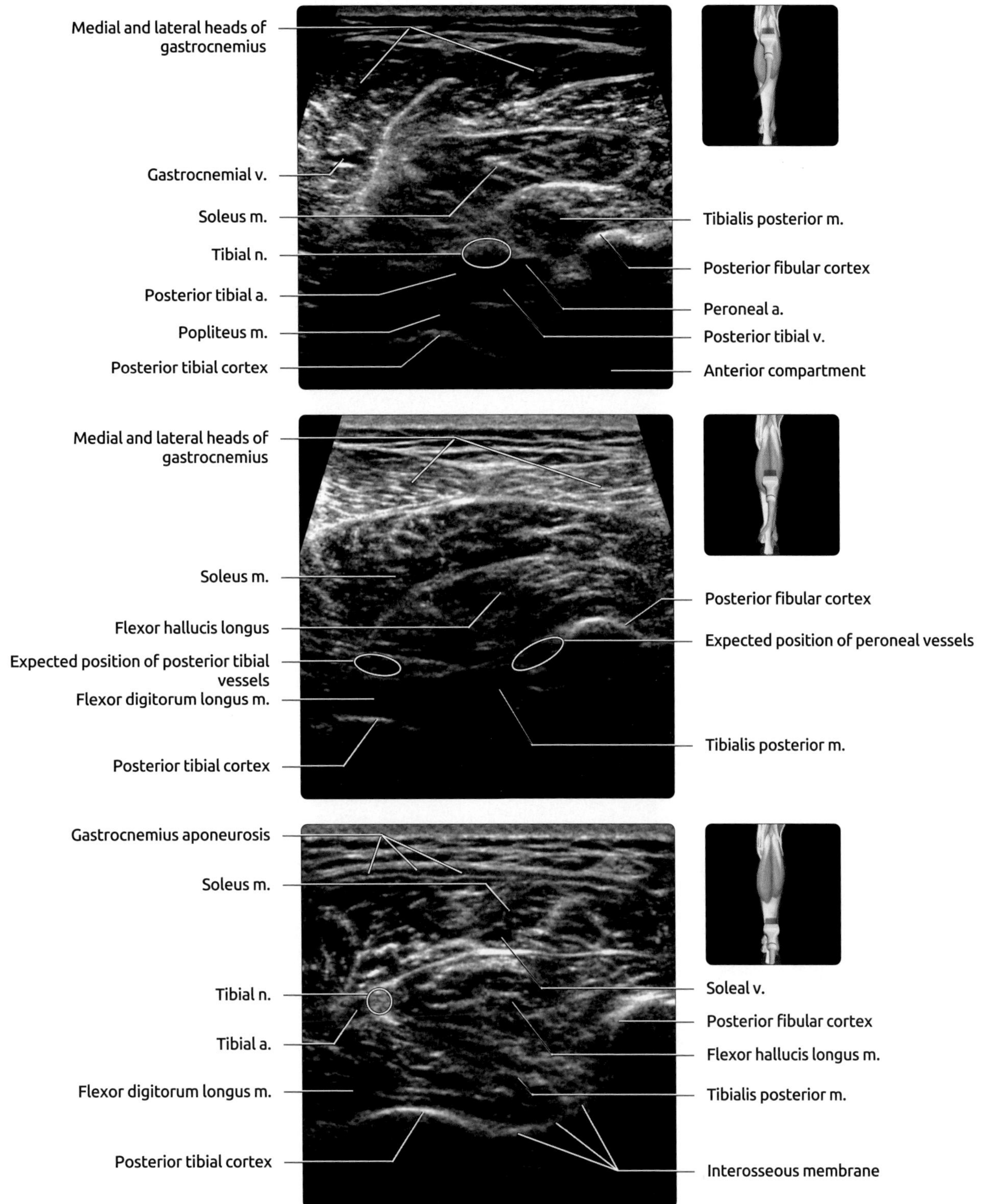

(Top) *Transverse scan is seen through the posterior compartment at the upper-calf level. For this compartment, the superficial layer consists of the gastrocnemius, plantaris, and soleus muscles. The deep layer consists of the popliteus, tibialis posterior, flexor digitorum longus, and flexor hallucis longus muscles.* **(Middle)** *Transverse scan shows the midcalf level. The tibial vessels have bifurcated into their peroneal and posterior tibial branches, which delineates a separation between the tibialis posterior and flexor digitorum longus from the rest of the calf muscles. Given the thickness of the gastrocnemius and soleus muscle, these deep muscles may be better seen using the anterior compartment as a window.* **(Bottom)** *Further inferiorly, the gastrocnemius has become a thin aponeurosis and, together with the tendon from the soleus muscle, will form the Achilles tendon.*

PART V
SECTION 2
Musculoskeletal Lesions

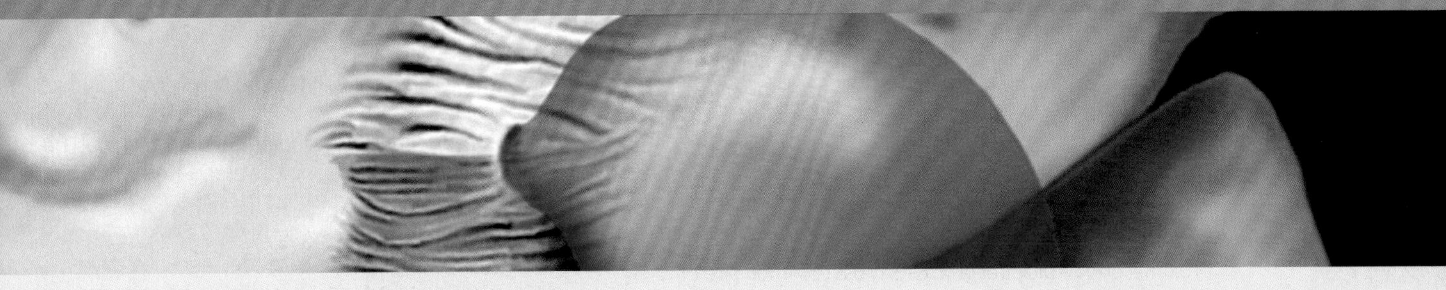

Rotator Cuff/Biceps Tendinosis

KEY FACTS

TERMINOLOGY

- Collagenous degeneration of rotator cuff ± biceps tendons with proteoglycan deposition

IMAGING

- Supraspinatus > infraspinatus > biceps > subscapularis
- Diffusely thickened tendon with diffuse hypoechogenicity and indistinct fibrillar pattern
  - Graded as mild, moderate, or severe
- Cortical irregularity of tendon insertional area
- Biceps tendinosis usually accompanies rotator cuff tendinosis
  - Proximal end of bicipital groove is most common site of biceps tendinosis
- Subclinical tendinosis of similar severity often present on opposite side
- Ultrasound is better than MR for assessing tendinosis as tendon detail, such as fibrillar pattern, is better appreciated
- Calcific tendinosis: Focal echogenic mass within rotator cuff tendon with acoustic shadowing

SCANNING TIPS

- Heel-toe ultrasound probe to remove anisotropy artifact and avoid mistaking for tendinosis
- Tendinosis is associated with tendon tears and should also be assessed
- Tears are more linear, hypoechoic, and sharper in outline than tendinosis; may or may not be associated with volume loss of tendon contour
- Suggested protocol
  - Supraspinatus: Crass (arm extended and internally rotated) or modified Crass position (hand in back pocket)
  - Infraspinatus and teres minor tendons: Arm abducted and internally rotated (hand on opposite shoulder)
  - Subscapularis and long head of biceps tendons: External rotation of arm with elbow flexed
  - Confirm all findings in 2 planes

(Left) *Oblique graphic shows a diffusely thickened supraspinatus tendon ➔ indicative of tendinosis. A normal subscapularis tendon ➔ and biceps tendon ➔ are also shown.* **(Right)** *Longitudinal ultrasound shows a diffusely thickened and hypoechoic infraspinatus tendon ➔. Multiple poorly demarcated, hypoechoic areas ➔ with loss of distinct fibrillary structure are present. Features are indicative of severe infraspinatus tendinosis.*

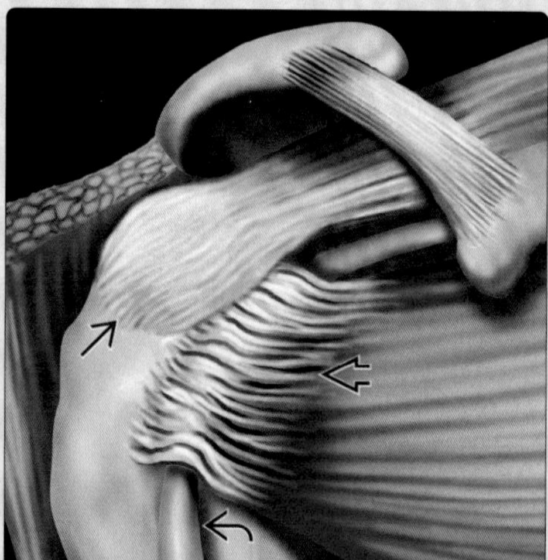

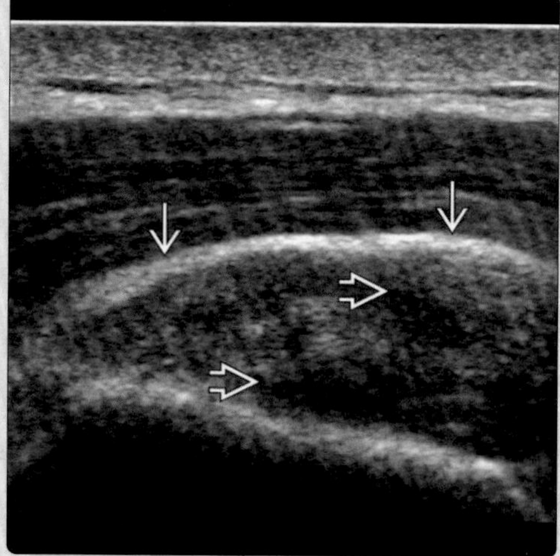

(Left) *Transverse ultrasound of the supraspinatus tendon shows several quite discrete areas of calcific deposition ➔ close to the tendon insertion. Moderate background tendinosis is present.* **(Right)** *Transverse ultrasound shows severe biceps tendinosis ➔. The tendon is enlarged and heterogeneous with loss of fibrillar pattern. Note the minimal degree of synovial sheath thickening and fluid ➔.*

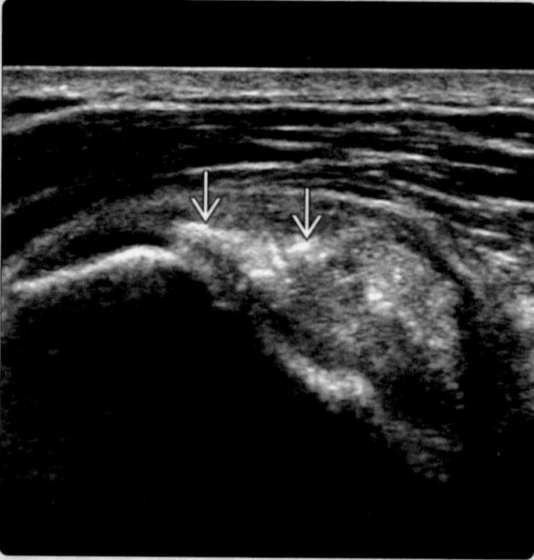

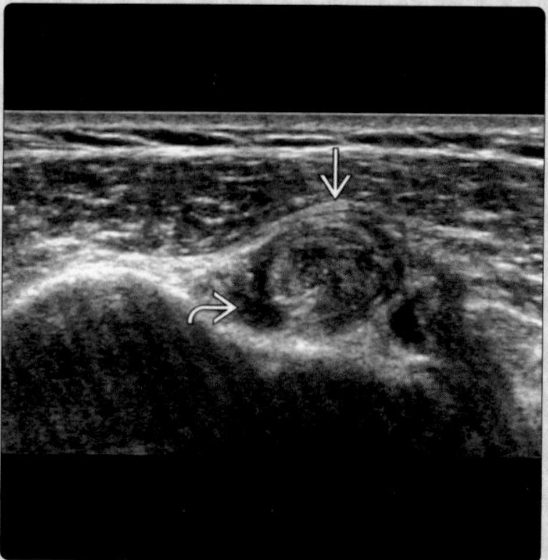

KEY FACTS

TERMINOLOGY

- Partial-thickness, full-thickness, or complete tear

IMAGING

- Supraspinatus tendon tears most common close to or at insertional area, especially anterior fibers
  - Most tears are avulsive type with retraction from insertional area; leading edge
  - Supraspinatus tears extending > 2.5 cm posterior to rotator cuff interval involve infraspinatus tendon
- Isolated tear of infraspinatus tendon is less common
- Underlying tendinosis is often present
- Partial tears of rotator cuff: Determine location and percentage of depth
  - Bursal sided: Tear abuts bursa surface; may see bursal fluid
  - Articular sided: Tear abuts hyaline cartilage
  - Intrasubstance: Tear is between tendon fibers and can extend to insertion
    - No contact with tendon surface; not visible at arthroscopy or bursoscopy
- Complete tear
  - Discontinuity of tendon filled with anechoic fluid
  - Focal flattening or concavity of bursal surface
  - With complete retraction, tendon may not be visualized; humeral head migrates superiorly

SCANNING TIPS

- Cortical irregularity is indirect sign of chronic rotator cuff tear
- Visualization of biceps tendon at rotator cuff interval ensures complete assessment of anterior supraspinatus where tears are most common
- With empty bicipital groove, ensure biceps is not dislocated or surgically relocated
  - Look for distal retracted tendon stump
- Assess for muscular atrophy, which affects prognosis
- Always confirm findings in 2 planes

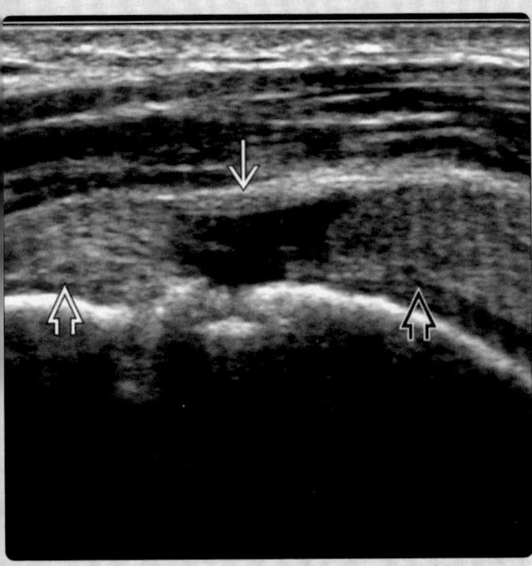

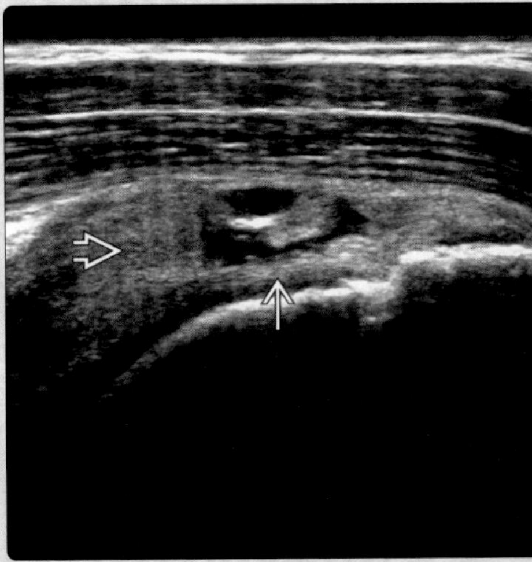

(Left) *Transverse ultrasound shows a full-thickness tear of supraspinatus tendon midfibers. Anterior fibers* ➡ *and posterior fibers* ⇨ *remain intact. Note the loss of volume with bursal surface contour depression* ➡. **(Right)** *Longitudinal ultrasound shows a near-full-thickness, partial tear of the supraspinatus tendon. The gap is filled with anechoic fluid. There are a few intact fibers close to the articular surface* ➡ *with moderate severity supraspinatus tendinosis* ➡.

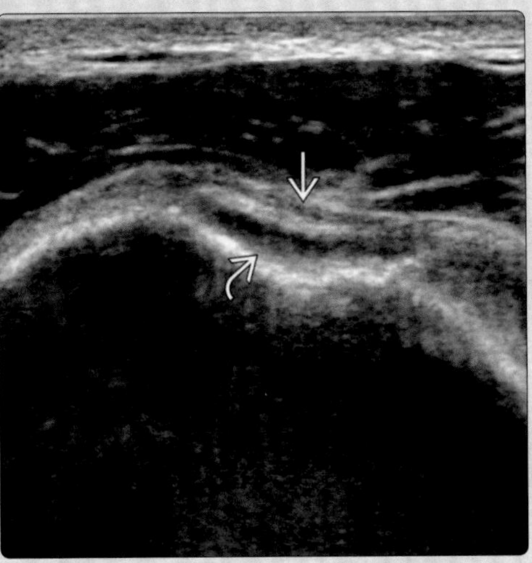

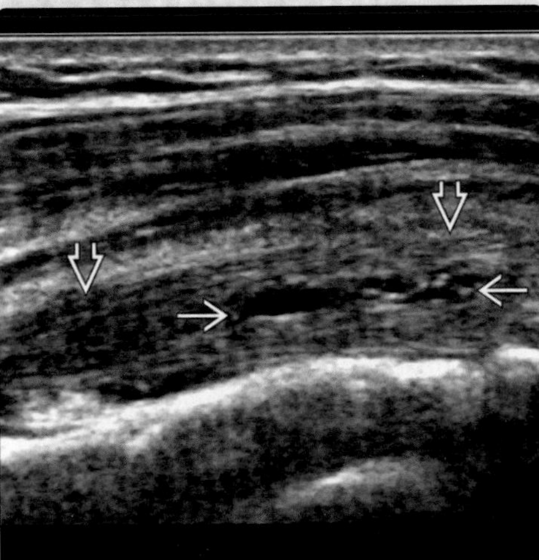

(Left) *Transverse ultrasound shows a complete rupture of the long head of the biceps tendon. There are no tendon fibers within the bicipital groove* ➡. *The transverse humeral ligament* ➡, *which attaches to the lateral lip of the bicipital groove, partially fills in the potential space of the groove.* **(Right)** *Longitudinal ultrasound shows moderate biceps tendinosis* ➡ *with an irregular, longitudinal, split-like, intrasubstance tear* ➡. *Intrasubstance tears of the rotator cuff have a similar appearance.*

Baker Cyst

KEY FACTS

TERMINOLOGY

- Synonym: Popliteal cyst

IMAGING

- Fluid distention of semimembranosus-medial gastrocnemius bursa
- C-shaped cyst usually anechoic, thin walled, and well defined
- Isoechoic or hyperechoic material within cyst can be complex fluid, hemorrhage, &/or synovitis
- Cysts with inflammation &/or intracystic hemorrhage can be thick walled, hyperemic, or septated
- Intraarticular bodies are common and appear hyperechoic with shadowing
- Inferior extension occurs superficial to medial gastrocnemius and can extend as far as ankle
- Free fluid tracking adjacent to cyst indicates recent leakage

CLINICAL ISSUES

- Intraarticular knee pathology is very frequently associated with Baker cysts in adults
- Cyst rupture can cause edema &/or reactive cellulitis
- Chronic Baker cyst rupture can be confused with soft tissue mass
- Can aspirate &/or inject steroid percutaneously, if not too viscous, but high rate of recurrence

SCANNING TIPS

- Examine with patient prone, knees extended
- Follow medial belly of gastrocnemius proximally and locate interspace between medial gastrocnemius head and semimembranosus tendon
- Look for characteristic "talk-bubble" configuration of cyst on transverse imaging
- Scan inferiorly to find cyst margin and assess for rupture
- Routinely scan contralateral side; subclinical Baker cysts are common

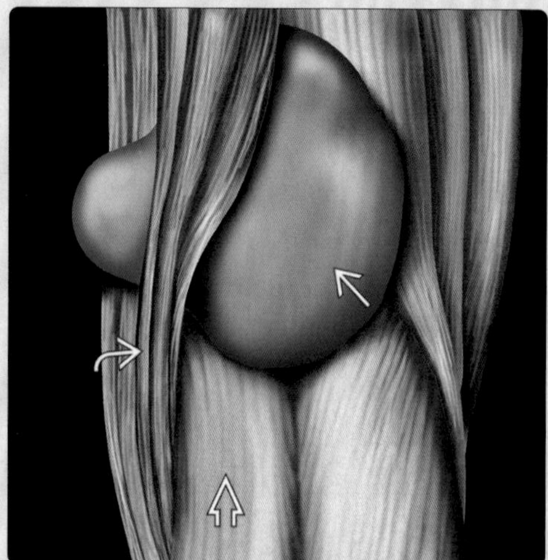

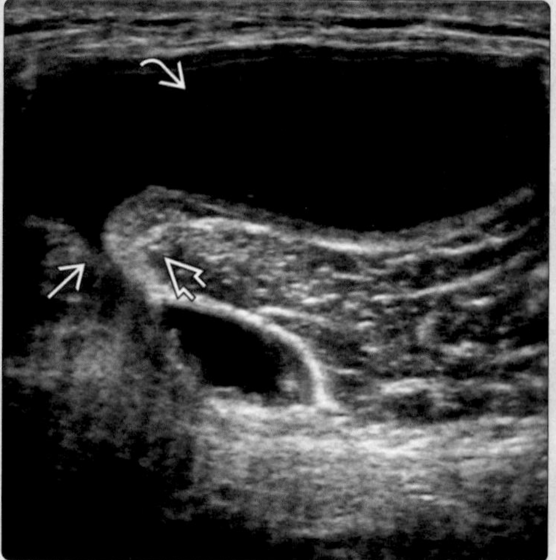

(Left) *Longitudinal graphic shows a Baker cyst ➡ located between the semimembranosus tendon ➡ and the medial belly of the gastrocnemius muscle ➡.* **(Right)** *Transverse ultrasound shows a typical Baker cyst ➡ with a "talk-bubble" configuration. The neck extends between the semimembranosus tendon ➡ and the medial belly of the gastrocnemius muscle ➡.*

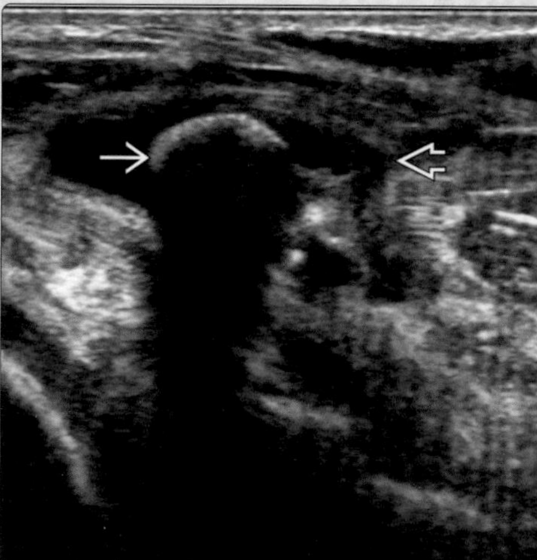

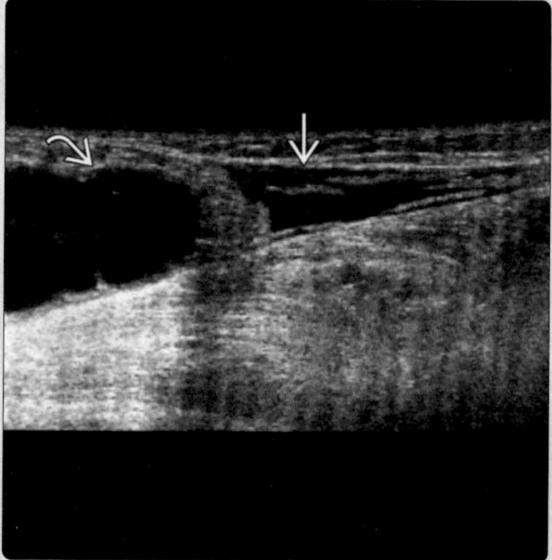

(Left) *Transverse ultrasound shows a calcified fragment ➡ within part of the Baker cyst ➡. Osseous fragments within the knee joint can extend into a Baker cyst. Osseous fragments may also enlarge within Baker cysts.* **(Right)** *Longitudinal ultrasound with extended field of view shows a complex cyst with fluid leakage ➡ tracking over the gastrocnemius muscle distal to the contained Baker cyst ➡. Note the lack of a wall around the free fluid.*

Lipoma

KEY FACTS

TERMINOLOGY

- Lipoma: Benign soft tissue tumor composed of mature adipose tissue

IMAGING

- Subcutaneous location more common than subfascial (intra- or intermuscular)
- Well-defined, oblong-shaped, encapsulated mass
- Fine linear striations parallel to long axis of tumor
- Hyper- or isoechoic to adjacent fat with absent or minimal color Doppler flow
- Compressible similar to adjacent fat

CLINICAL ISSUES

- Most common soft tissue tumor
- Soft, well-defined, painless mass enlarging over months, often during period of weight gain
- Classic appearance can be diagnosed definitively with ultrasound
- Atypical appearance needs evaluation with MR or biopsy
  - Large size, deep location, heterogeneity, vascularity, crossing fascial planes, rapid growth
- MR is better than ultrasound in differentiation of benign or malignant lipoma and in assessing deep masses

SCANNING TIPS

- Scan in area directed by patient in position they report is most exacerbating
- Use compression to demonstrate soft character of mass
- Use extended field of view to capture larger masses
- Use light pressure when assessing for color Doppler flow to avoid false absence from compression
- Look for "neck" as fat-containing ventral and lumbar hernias can mimic lipomas

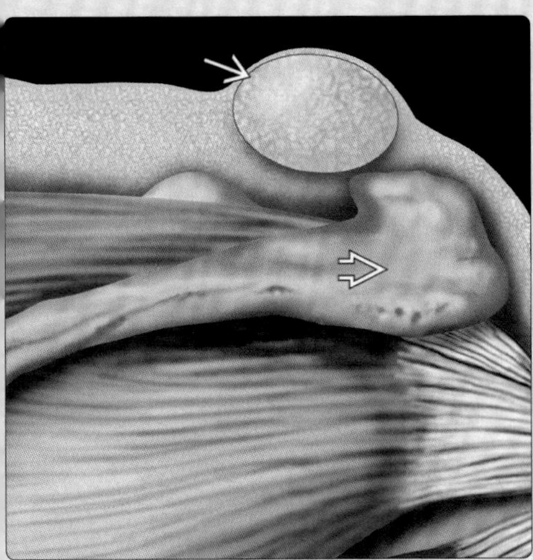

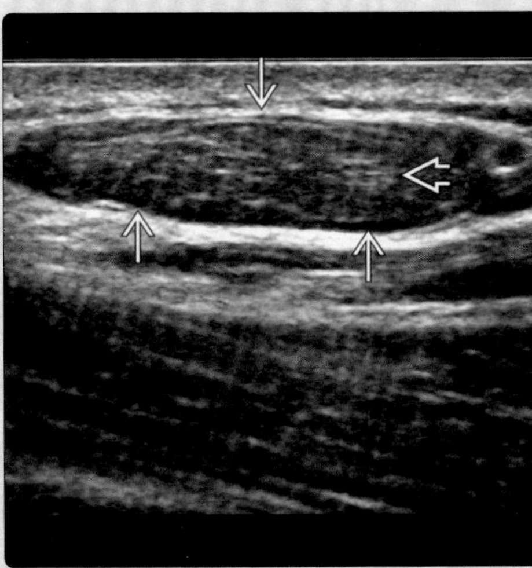

(Left) *Graphic shows a well-defined lipoma* ➡ *located in the subcutaneous tissue overlying the acromion* ➡. **(Right)** *Longitudinal ultrasound shows an encapsulated* ➡ *subcutaneous mass hypoechoic to adjacent subcutaneous fat and fine internal echogenic striations* ➡ *parallel to the long axis of the mass. These appearances are characteristic of lipoma.*

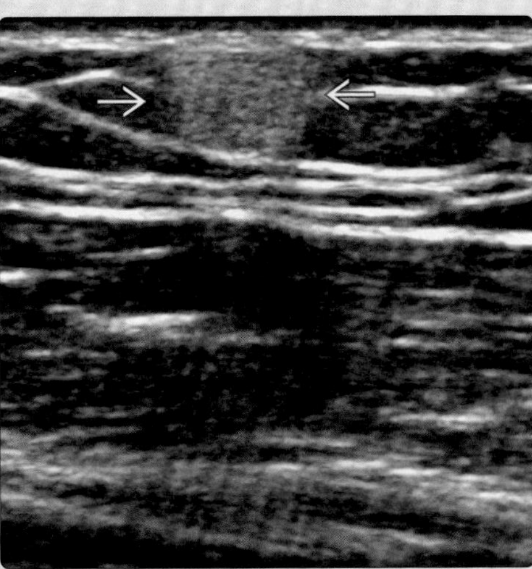

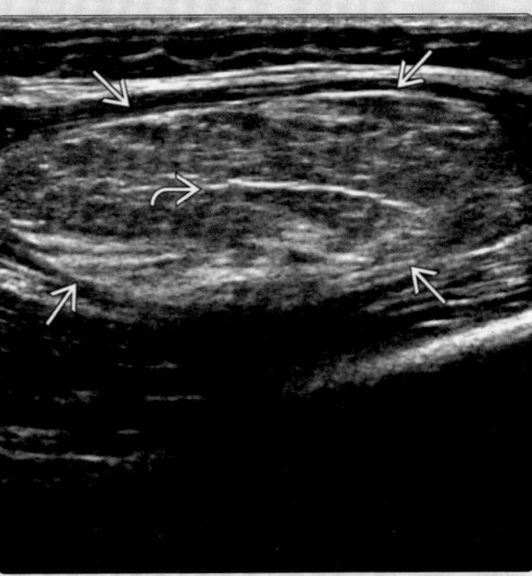

(Left) *Longitudinal ultrasound shows a small, well-defined homogeneously hyperechoic subcutaneous lipoma* ➡. *The fine striations are barely perceivable, though these appearances are still characteristic of a lipoma. Such lipomas are often multiple and tend to be located more centrally than peripherally.* **(Right)** *Longitudinal ultrasound shows an intramuscular hyperechoic lipoma within the vastus lateralis muscle. Note the well-defined hyperechoic capsule* ➡ *and the fine linear horizontal striations* ➡.

Epidermoid Cyst

KEY FACTS

TERMINOLOGY

- Slow-growing subdermal cyst that contains keratin and is lined by stratified squamous epithelium
  - Does not contain dermal elements (dermoid cyst)

IMAGING

- Ultrasound appearances depend on maturation of cyst and amount and compactness of keratin
  - Most epidermoids are avascular with thin, hypoechoic walls and posterior acoustic enhancement
  - Most are heterogeneous and mildly hyperechoic
  - Can appear homogeneous ("pseudotestis")
  - Well-circumscribed, ovoid (80%), lobulated (19%), or tubular (1%) configuration
  - Linear, hyperreflective, disc-like areas represent layered keratin aggregates ± cholesterol deposition
  - Hypoechoic tract extending from superficial wall to dermis (10%) (punctum)
  - Hypoechoic, small, cyst-like spaces
- Contained rupture → lobulated configuration of cyst

TOP DIFFERENTIAL DIAGNOSES

- Nerve sheath tumor, soft tissue abscess, lipoma

CLINICAL ISSUES

- Occur on face, scalp, neck, trunk, back
- Incidental or firm, nontender mass
- Complications include superinfection or rupture
- Can be electively surgically removed

SCANNING TIPS

- Internal debris, when present, is mobile and "swirls" with compression
- Assess periphery for vascularity indicating cyst rupture
- Ill-defined margin and irregular shape can also indicate rupture
- Look for layering hypoechoic and hyperechoic rings
- Look for cutaneous punctum (tract)

(Left) *Clinical photo shows 2 closely related superficial nodules ➡ associated with localized cutaneous erythema in the natal cleft region. Note the single small, whitish spot due to a punctum ↩.* **(Right)** *Longitudinal ultrasound shows a well-circumscribed, hypoechoic epidermoid cyst with dermal attachment ➡, multiple internal filiform anechoic areas ↩, linear hyperreflective strands ⇨, and posterior acoustic enhancement.*

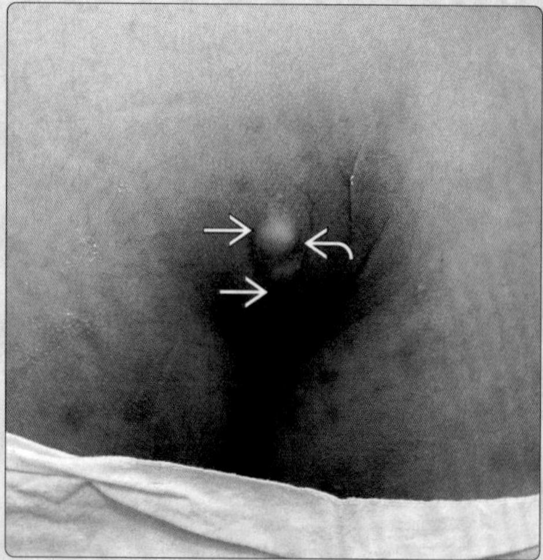

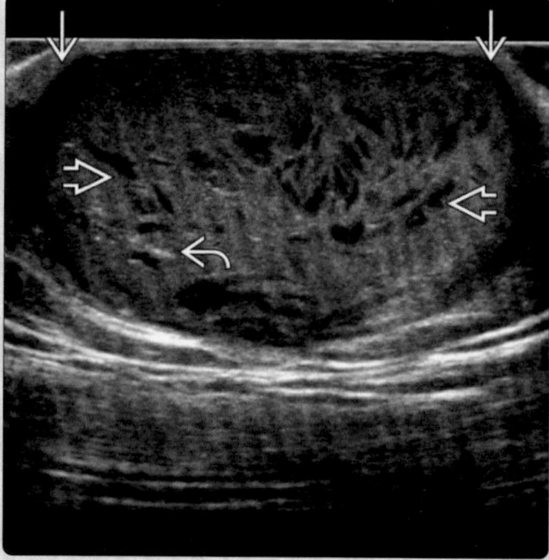

(Left) *Longitudinal ultrasound shows typical appearance of epidermoid cyst with a well-circumscribed, ovoid, heterogeneous nodule with dermal attachment, internal floating hyperreflective strands ➡, small hypoechoic areas ⇨, and a hypoechoic tract ↩ extending to a cutaneous punctum.* **(Right)** *Transverse color Doppler ultrasound shows moderate pericystic soft tissue hyperemia representing inflammation secondary to leakage of cyst contents.*

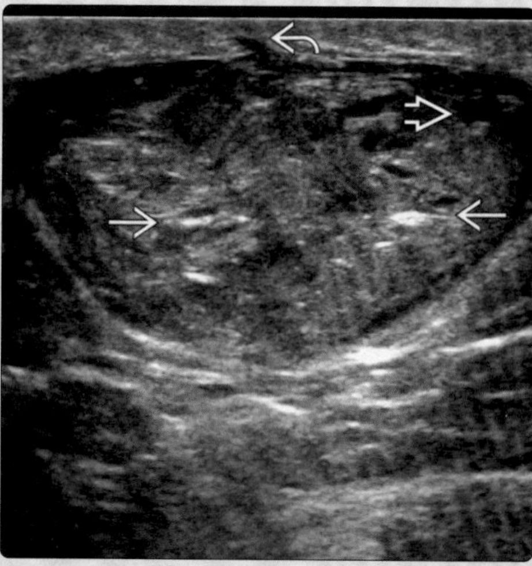

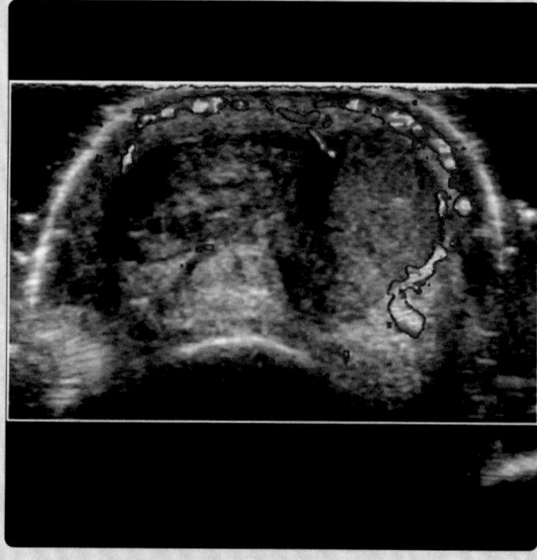

KEY FACTS

TERMINOLOGY

- Hematoma: Localized collection of blood outside of blood vessel
- Seroma: Serous fluid collection within soft tissues (plasma exudate from small blood vessels)
- Lymphocele: Collection of lymphatic fluid due to leakage/damage to lymphatics

IMAGING

- **Hematoma**
  - Acute
    - Heterogeneous pseudosolid appearance and can be echogenic or isoechoic
    - Underlying cause of hematoma such as muscle tear or vascular malformation may be apparent
    - No internal blood flow unless active bleeding
    - Surrounding edema
  - Subacute/chronic
    - Mild peripheral hyperemia
    - Decrease in size and become more echogenic around periphery over time
    - Layered appearance of fluid and solid debris from separation of cellular elements and serum
    - Solid matter retracts and remaining portion "liquefies" seen as cystic spaces or hypoechoic fluid
  - Organizing hematoma
    - Encapsulated with fibrous wall preventing reabsorption and allows for rebleeding
    - Mimics soft tissue mass
- **Seroma**
  - Echo-poor or anechoic with strong posterior acoustic enhancement
  - Absent or barely discernible wall depending on chronicity
  - Often near site of surgery (chest wall, abdomen, groin)
- **Lymphocele**
  - Unilocular and thin walled; indistinguishable sonographically from seroma
  - Occurs post surgery and is common after lymphadenectomy

CLINICAL ISSUES

- Hematoma can occur from minor trauma or spontaneously in patients on anticoagulation or with coagulopathy
- Unexplained, unusual, or nonresolving hematoma should raise concern for soft tissue mass
- Serial follow-up is helpful to confirm hematoma and to check for underlying cause
- Hematoma can be distinguished from seroma/lymphocele with ultrasound; seroma and lymphocele are differentiated by fluid analysis
- Seroma/lymphocele may need treatment with aspiration &/or pressure bandaging

SCANNING TIPS

- Always assess suspected fluid collection with color Doppler to avoid missing mass or vessel
- Use color and spectral Doppler around periphery of hyperacute hematoma to assess for active bleeding
- Seroma can have thin septa and jiggles like bowl of Jell-O with agitation
- Assess for mass effect on adjacent structures (i.e., hydronephrosis in transplant kidney)

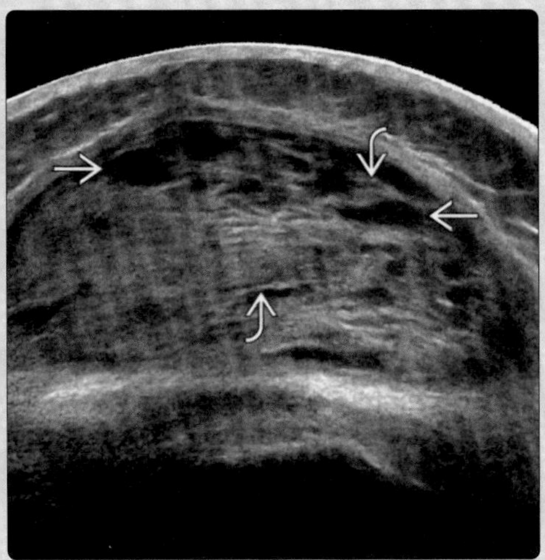

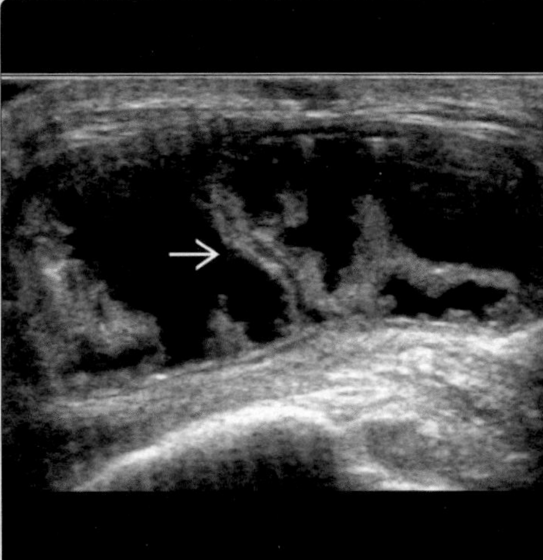

(Left) *Longitudinal ultrasound of the proximal thigh after total hip arthroplasty shows a well-defined mass with layering, anechoic liquefied areas ➡, and internal septations ⮫. Features are consistent with a resolving large hematoma.* **(Right)** *Transverse ultrasound 1 month later shows increased liquefaction of the hematoma with a greater cystic component, septa ➡, and fibrin clots. Features are consistent with liquefying hematoma.*

KEY FACTS

TERMINOLOGY

- Microbial infection of subcutaneous tissue (cellulitis), muscle (myositis), tendon (tenosynovitis), or fascia (fasciitis)
- Abscess is focal fluid collection containing suppurative inflammatory material

IMAGING

- **Cellulitis**
  - Edematous, hyperechoic, hyperemic subcutaneous fat with thickened interlobular septa
- **Infectious tenosynovitis**
  - Synovial tendon sheath is thickened, hyperemic, and contains fluid surrounding tendon
- **Infectious myositis**
  - Hyperechoic, hyperemic, and indistinct, ± abscess
- **Necrotizing fasciitis**
  - Spreads rapidly between tissue planes
  - Thickened, irregular fascia with perifascial fluid
  - Gas is highly specific but not always present
- **Abscess**
  - Variable echogenicity, peripheral hyperemia, ± septation/gas

CLINICAL ISSUES

- Route of spread can be direct (skin), postsurgical, or hematogenous
- Deep soft tissue infection may require hospitalization, IV antibiotics, &/or surgery
- Necrotizing fascitis is life threatening and early diagnosis decreases morbidity

SCANNING TIPS

- Use wide field of view and increase depth to ensure entire area of abnormal tissue is imaged
- Diagnose abscess by demonstrating fluctuance and lack of color Doppler flow
- Note and report visible skin changes, breeches, or crepitus
- Assess nearby joints for effusion (septic arthritis) and adjacent bone for cortical irregularity (osteomyelitis)

(Left) *Cellulitis is demonstrated on a transverse US of the ankle region showing severe subcutaneous tissue thickening and edema. There is fluid leading to thickened interlobular septa ➡ with intervening hyperechoic fat lobules ➡.* **(Right)** *Infectious tenosynovitis in an intravenous drug user. Longitudinal color Doppler US of the 3rd extensor digitorum tendon ➡ shows marked expansion of the tendon sheath ➡ with complex fluid ➡ as well as marked subcutaneous edema and hyperemia.*

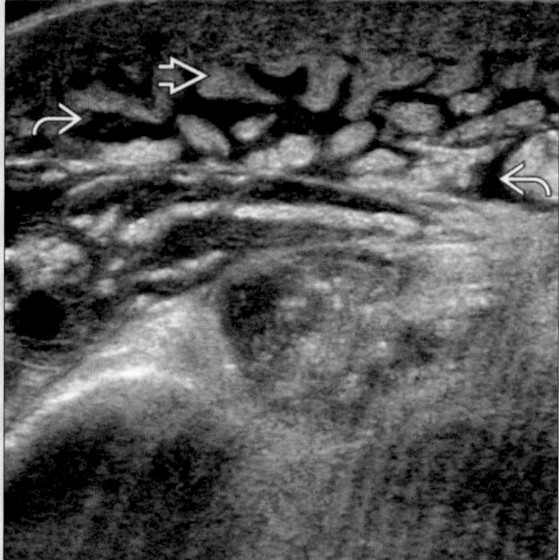

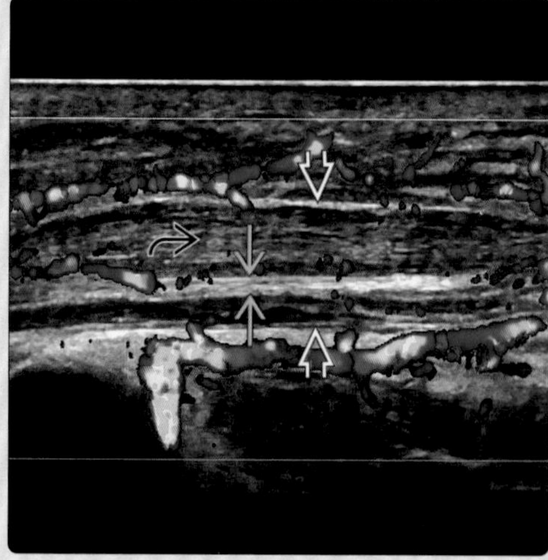

(Left) *Longitudinal color Doppler US along the anterior thigh shows hyperemia within the vastus medialis muscle ➡ with an intramuscular abscess ➡ containing layering debris.* **(Right)** *Fasciitis is shown on a longitudinal US of the calf region. There is severe thickening and edema of the investing fascia ➡ overlying gastrocnemius muscle associated with perifascial fluid ➡ as well as moderate subcutaneous and muscle edema ➡.*

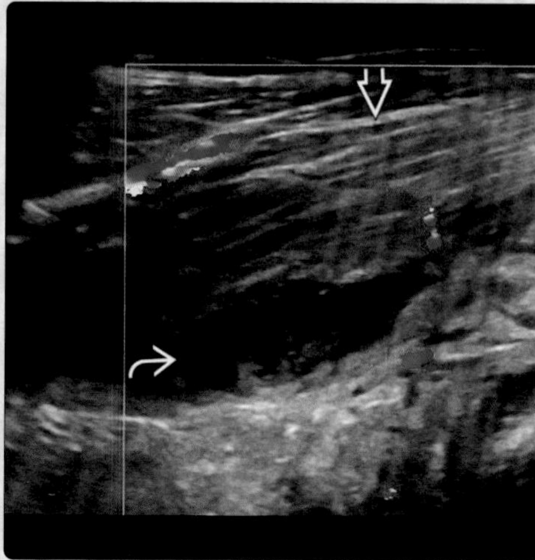

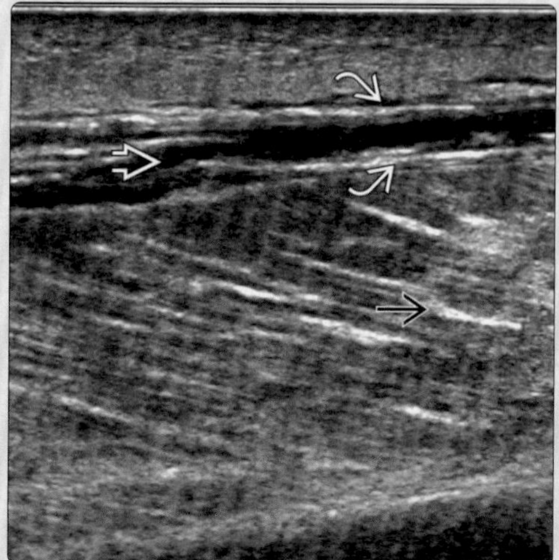

KEY FACTS

TERMINOLOGY

- Ganglion cyst: Myxoid tissue encased in fibroblastic collagenous wall with no synovial lining

IMAGING

- Fluid-filled mass with stalk emanating from joint
- Common in wrist but can occur in other joints, including fingers, ankle, knee, hip, and shoulder
- Readily diagnosed with ultrasound by characteristic features
- Contains hypoechoic fluid
  - ± septations
  - ± comet-tail artifacts (due to colloid aggregates)
- Very firm, not compressible
- Recent leakage can cause hyperemia and edema of surrounding tissues from inflammatory response

CLINICAL ISSUES

- Up to 50% of cysts in adults and > 90% in children; wrist ganglia will resolve without treatment
- Treated with ultrasound-guided aspiration or surgical excision
- Ultrasound-guided aspiration
  - Fluid is viscous, larger gauge needle is often required
  - Higher success rate alongside flexor tendon sheath, (> 70% vs. 50%)
  - Ganglia may become smaller/less symptomatic (partial response)

SCANNING TIPS

- Locate tell-tale stalk of cyst and trace it back toward joint of origin
- Note important relationships of cyst (i.e., to tendons and neurovascular bundle)
- Use color Doppler to differentiate from vascular anomaly or nerve sheath tumor, which also appears hypoechoic

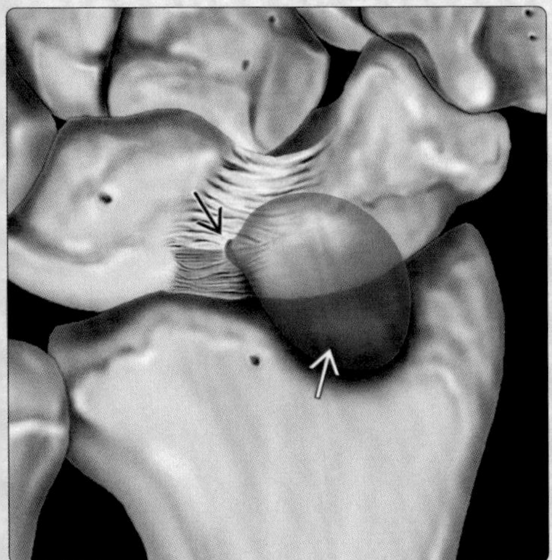

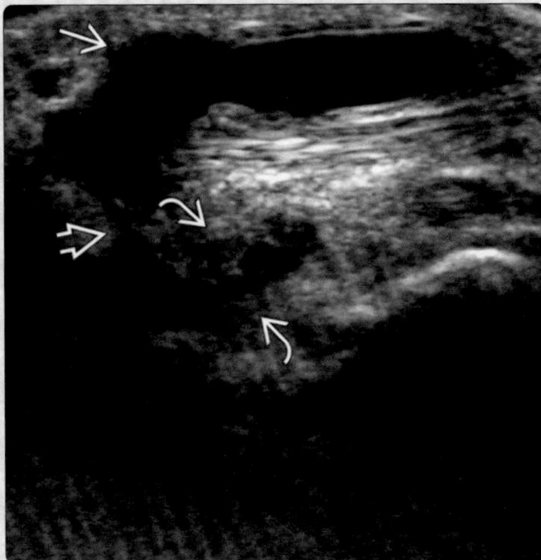

(Left) *Graphic shows the typical location of a dorsal wrist ganglion cyst ➡ arising from a defect in the dorsal capsule of the scapholunate ligament ➡. The ligament remains functionally intact.* **(Right)** *Longitudinal ultrasound shows an elongated ganglion ➡ on the radiovolar aspect of the wrist. The stalk ➡ of the ganglion extends deeply to lie between the radioscaphocapitate and radiolunotriquetral ligaments ➡.*

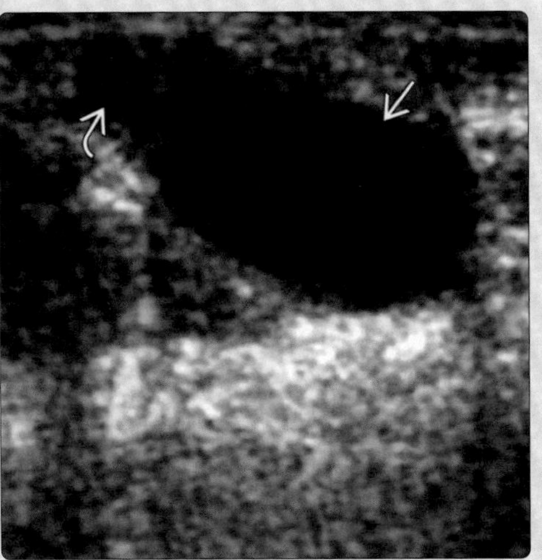

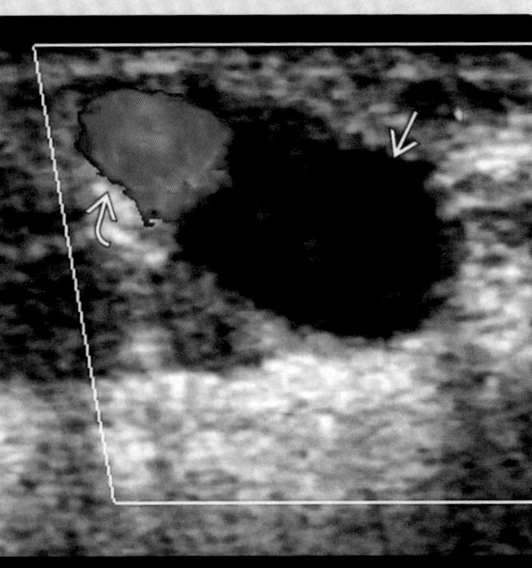

(Left) *Transverse ultrasound shows a volar wrist ganglion cyst ➡ located just proximal to the wrist crease. The radial artery ➡ is inseparable from the ganglion cyst.* **(Right)** *Transverse color Doppler ultrasound at the same location clearly shows the radial artery ➡ located at the edge of the ganglion cyst ➡ demonstrating the importance of color Doppler.*

KEY FACTS

TERMINOLOGY

- **Mechanisms of injury**
  - Overuse: Strenuous exercise results in diffuse muscular edema
  - Stretch: Causes torn muscle fibers + hematoma
  - Direct: Usually blunt trauma causes contusion, ± hematoma, ± tear

IMAGING

- **Delayed-onset muscle soreness**
  - Overuse leads to diffuse muscular edema
  - Muscle may appear normal or diffusely hyperechoic
- **Muscle contusion/hematoma**
  - Contusion: Ill-defined echogenic muscle; dispersed form of hematoma
  - Hematoma: Focal hemorrhage often associated with tear
- **Muscle or myofascial tear**
  - Usually partial at/near myofascial junction
  - Discontinuity ± retraction of fibers filled with hematoma (hematoma can obscure)
- **Muscle hernia**
  - Focal protrusion of fibers through investing fascia
  - Accentuated by contraction or standing

CLINICAL ISSUES

- Tears occur at common locations from common mechanisms
- Most injuries improve with conservative treatment and do not require follow-up ultrasound
- Clinical symptoms overlap with other diagnoses seen with ultrasound (deep vein thrombosis, tendinosis)

SCANNING TIPS

- Use contralateral side for comparison; even if bilateral, abnormalities often appear asymmetric
- Carefully assess distal medial gastrocnemius for small tears
- Use active contraction/passive joint movement to show retraction of fibers

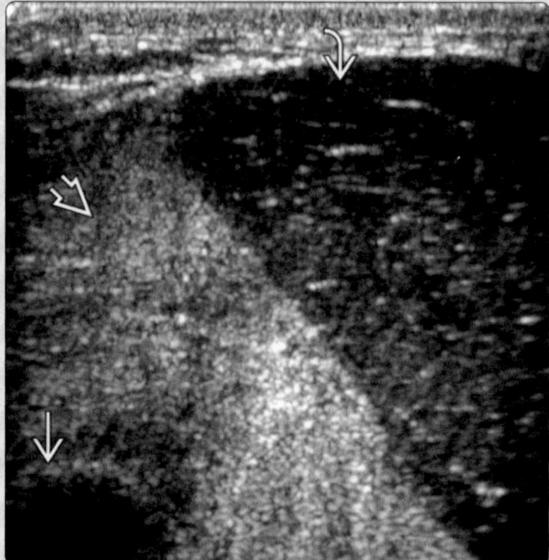

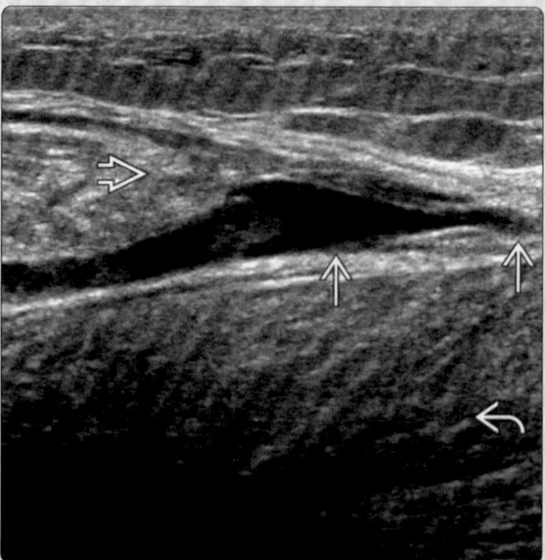

(Left) *Transverse ultrasound in a patient with unaccustomed overuse rowing injury and pain onset 1 day later shows severe edema of the brachialis muscle ➡ consistent with delayed-onset muscle soreness. The overlying biceps muscle ➡ and humeral shaft ➡ are normal.* **(Right)** *Longitudinal ultrasound shows a typical myofascial tear ("tennis leg") with stripping of the medial head of the gastrocnemius ➡ at the myofascial junction ➡ with the soleus muscle ➡. The retraction gap is filled with blood.*

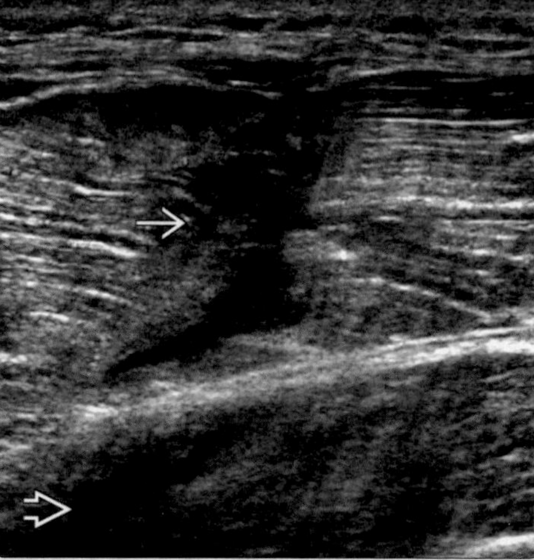

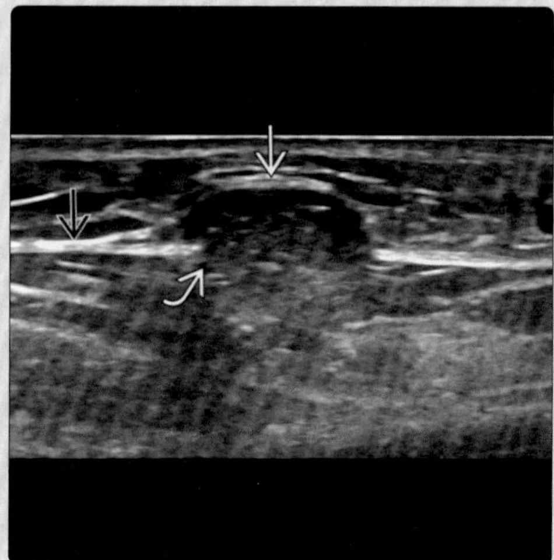

(Left) *Longitudinal ultrasound of the thigh in a patient recently kicked by a horse shows a full-thickness tear ➡ in the distal vastus lateralis muscle. The tear was associated with a surrounding hematoma (not shown). The adjacent vastus intermedius muscle ➡ is normal.* **(Right)** *High-resolution longitudinal ultrasound of the anterior tibialis muscle (most common location) shows focal herniation of the muscle ➡ through a defect ➡ in the muscular fascia ➡. This image was captured during muscular contraction.*

KEY FACTS

TERMINOLOGY

- Ligament: Fibrous band that connects 2 bones and helps stabilize intervening joint

IMAGING

- Ligament tears can be partial or complete and have same appearance irrespective of ligament location
- Acute stage
  - Diffuse or localized ligament swelling
  - Ligament fiber discontinuity with hypoechoic gap at site of tear
  - Surrounding soft tissue subcutaneous edema, hemorrhage, and hyperemia
- Chronic stage: 4 possible sequelae of ligament tear exist
  - Diffusely thickened, continuous ligament
  - Diffusely thickened, discontinuous ligament
  - Diffusely attenuated ligament
  - Absent ligament

CLINICAL ISSUES

- Most frequent musculoskeletal injury
- Leads to instability, impingement, dystrophic calcification, or contracture
- Often associated with other osseous or ligamentous injuries
- Healed ligament tissue post injury remains inferior to normal ligament
- Prior injury can confound clinical and imaging assessment

SCANNING TIPS

- Align transducer along long axis of ligament
- Adjust transducer alignment to minimize anisotropy
- Surrounding edema/fluid and hyperemia on color Doppler are clues to which ligament(s) could be injured
- Dynamically stretch ligament to maximize visibility of tear and determine joint laxity
- Examine contralateral, noninjured side for comparison

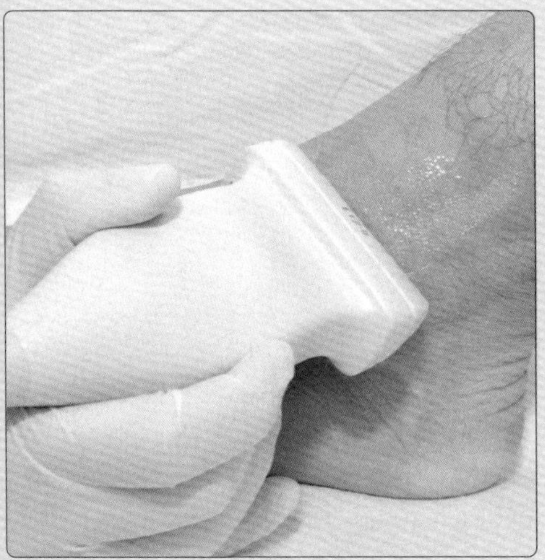

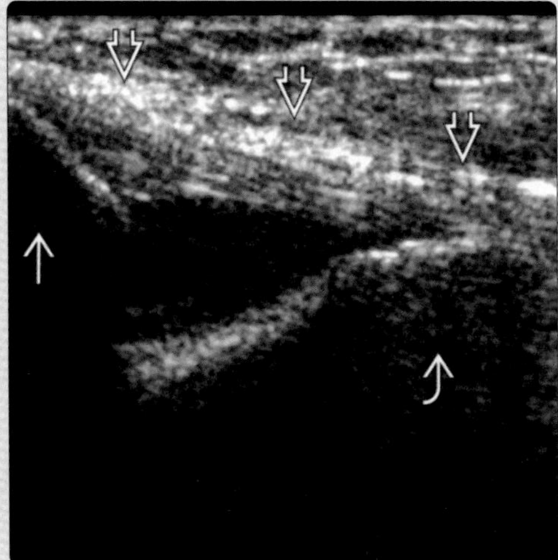

(Left) *Clinical photograph shows probe orientation for examining the anterior talofibular ligament (ATFL), the most commonly injured ligament. The ankle is slightly plantar flexed and the probe orientation is transverse.* **(Right)** *Transverse ultrasound of the anterolateral ankle in the same patient shows normal intact ATFL ➡ coursing between the fibula ➡ and talus ➡. Note how the ligament is echogenic and taut with continuity of fibers.*

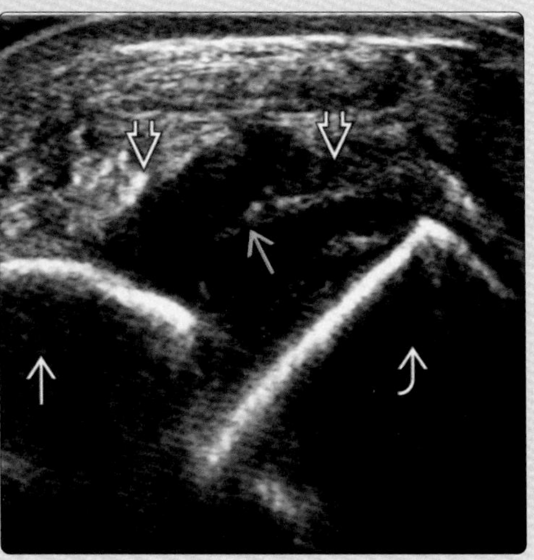

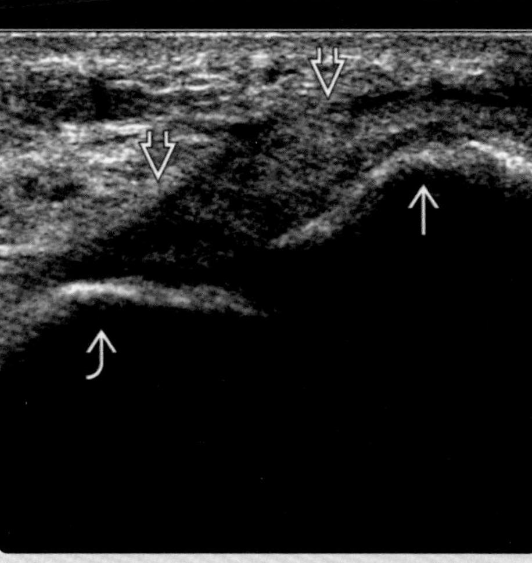

(Left) *Transverse ultrasound of the lateral ankle region shows an acute complete (grade 3) tear of the ATFL with loss of fibers in between the talus ➡ and the fibula ➡. Hematoma ➡ fills up the gap, and detached ligament fibers ➡ are seen.* **(Right)** *Longitudinal ultrasound of the lateral ankle region 4 weeks after inversion injury shows a severely thickened, hypoechoic ATFL ➡ with loss of normal fibrillar pattern between the distal fibula ➡ and talus ➡, compatible with a healing tear.*

PART VI
SECTION 1
First Trimester

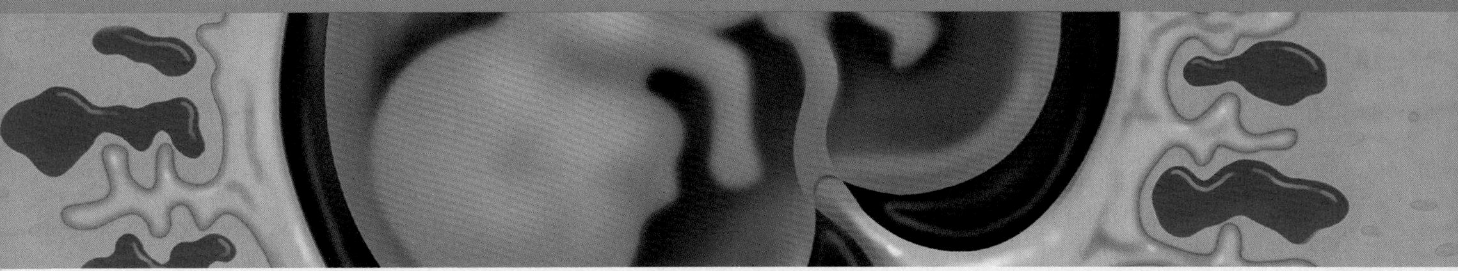

Anatomy and Approach

Abnormal Intrauterine Gestation

Ectopic Gestation

EMBRYOLOGY AND ANATOMY

Key Embryological Events

- Multiple events occur in 1st trimester
  - Ovulation with resultant corpus luteum in ovary
  - Fertilization of ovum → zygote
  - Zygote cleavage → blastocyst → embryoblast + trophoblast
  - Implantation → intrauterine sac-like structure
  - Embryonic development, organogenesis
  - Development of placenta, umbilical cord
- **Embryoblast cells form embryo and amnion**
  - Bilaminar embryonic disc forms when embryoblast splits into epiblast and hypoblast
  - Trilaminar disc develops by process of gastrulation, which moves cells to different locations
    - Creates 3 primary germ layers of ectoderm, mesoderm, endoderm
    - Determines axes of body
- **Embryonic disc lies between amnion and yolk sac**
  - Disc folds on itself to form a tube surrounded by amnion
    - Yolk sac is pinched off as embryonic disc sides come together to form tube
  - Series of tubes within tubes elongate, bud, rotate, and form all major organs by end of 13th week
- Trophoblast cells give rise to membranes and placenta, not embryo proper
- Gestational sac initially covered in chorionic villi, atrophy of those adjacent to uterine cavity → chorion laeve
- Chorionic villi adjacent to implantation site develop into mature tertiary villi
  - Tertiary villi contain fully differentiated blood vessels for gas exchange
  - This part of chorion increases in thickness and echogenicity → chorion frondosum
- Maternal endometrial cells differentiate into decidual cells
- Chorion frondosum + maternal decidua basalis = **placenta**
- Embryonic disc lies between amnion and yolk sac
  - Embryo initially connected to chorion by connecting stalk
  - **Umbilical cord** forms from incorporation of connecting stalk, allantois, vitelline duct

Anatomy

- Earliest visible structure is an **intrauterine sac-like structure**
  - Measure internal diameter (i.e., fluid component only, not echogenic wall)
    - Average of 3 orthogonal planes = mean sac diameter (MSD)
  - Sac-like structure is chorion; commonly referred to as gestational sac (GS)
  - Next visible structure is **yolk sac** (YS) inside GS
    - Round, distinct wall, normal size ≤ 6 mm
  - Next visible structure is **embryo**
    - 1st visible as thickening of YS wall
    - As amnion expands double bleb sign seen with embryo inside amnion, YS attached to embryo
    - Abdominal wall closure → YS separation from embryo
      - **Embryo inside amnion, YS outside amnion**
    - Embryo elongates, develops clear cranial (crown) vs. pelvic (rump) polarity, limb buds appear
    - At 10 weeks gestation, embryo → fetus
    - Organogenesis complete by 13 weeks
  - Measure crown rump length (CRL) as longest axis of embryo; do not include YS

SCANNING APPROACH AND IMAGING ISSUES

Where Is the Pregnancy?

- **Pregnancy of unknown location (PUL)**
  - Positive pregnancy test with no evidence of either intrauterine pregnancy (IUP) or ectopic pregnancy by transvaginal ultrasound (TVUS)
    - ~ 50% will resolve without definite diagnosis of IUP or ectopic
    - ~ 35% will have IUP
    - 10-20% will have ectopic pregnancy
- **Probable IUP**
  - Intrauterine sac-like structure without YS or embryo
    - If echogenic with round or oval shape, statistically highly likely to represent IUP
    - Positive pregnancy test, smooth-walled anechoic intrauterine sac-like structure, **no adnexal mass**
      - 99.98% probability of IUP
      - 0.02% probability of ectopic pregnancy
    - If sac-like structure has pointed edges, more likely to be intracavitary blood products or abnormal GS
- **Definite IUP**
  - Intrauterine sac-like structure with YS or embryo (regardless of cardiac activity)
- **Definite ectopic pregnancy**
  - Extrauterine GS with YS ± embryo (regardless of cardiac activity)
- **Probable ectopic pregnancy**
  - Inhomogeneous adnexal mass (described as blob sign)
  - Extrauterine sac-like structure (described as bagel sign)
  - Modern equipment resolution is so good that blob and bagel signs are often considered diagnostic of ectopic pregnancy

How Many Gestational Sacs Are There?

- In multiple pregnancies, prognosis depends on chorionicity, which is best determined in 1st trimester
  - 2 GS = dichorionic twins, 1 GS = monochorionic twins
    - Monochorionic twins can be diamniotic, monoamniotic, or conjoined
- Scan entire uterus
  - Müllerian duct anomalies may result in widely separated uterine horns
    - Multiple pregnancies may occur with implantation in 1 or both horns
    - Potential to miss an IUP in 1 horn if incomplete study performed
  - Heterotopic pregnancy occurs when there is an IUP and an ectopic pregnancy
    - Scan entire pelvis to evaluate adnexal structures
    - Commonest heterotopic pregnancy is IUP + tubal ectopic
      - Incidence in assisted reproduction patients can be as high as 1:60-100
    - **Pitfall**: Corpus luteum (CL) may look like extrauterine GS

- CL is intraovarian
- With transducer pressure, CL moves with ovary, tubal ectopic will separate from ovary
- Color Doppler does not differentiate CL from tubal ectopic; both may show ring of fire appearance of prominent peripheral flow

– **Pitfall**: Some ectopics may appear intrauterine
  - Cervical, interstitial, cesarean scar pregnancies

What is the Gestational Age?

- Gestational age assessment is most accurate in 1st trimester
  - GS usually visible by 4.0-4.5 weeks from last menstrual period (LMP)
  - YS usually visible by 5.0-5.5 weeks from LMP
  - Distinct embryo with cardiac activity usually visible by 6.0-6.5 weeks from LMP
- American College of Obstetric and Gynecology guidelines on redating recommend use of sonographic dates depending on menstrual age and number of days discrepancy between sonographic and menstrual dates
  - At ≤ 8 6/7 weeks, redate if > 5 days discrepancy
  - At 9 0/7 weeks to 15 6/7 weeks, redate if > 7 days discrepancy
  - At 16 0/7 weeks to 21 6/7 weeks, redate if > 10 days discrepancy
  - At 22 0/7 weeks to 27 6/7 weeks, redate if > 14 days discrepancy
  - At 28 0/7 weeks onward, redate if > 21 days discrepancy

Is the Pregnancy Viable?

- Viable pregnancy defined as one that **may potentially** result in liveborn baby
  - Embryo must be visible if MSD > 25 mm by TVUS
  - Embryo of > 7 mm CRL on TVUS must have cardiac activity
  - Embryo of > 15 mm CRL on abdominal scan must have cardiac activity
- Nonviable pregnancy defined as one that **cannot possibly** result in liveborn baby
  - Ectopic pregnancy, failed IUP
- Follow-up recommendations to prove viability in probable IUP or definite IUP without embryo
  - Lack of live embryo **≥ 14 days** from visualization of **sac without YS** (probable IUP) is diagnostic of failed pregnancy
  - Lack of live embryo **≥ 11 days** from visualization of **sac with YS** (definite IUP) is diagnostic of failed pregnancy
- IUP of uncertain viability
  - Mean sac diameter < 25 mm without embryo
  - Embryo < 7 mm without cardiac activity

Is There Evidence of Increased Risk for Aneuploidy?

- From 11-13 weeks, certain findings can be used to identify higher risk for aneuploidy
  - Increased nuchal translucency
  - Ductus venosus waveform
  - Nasal bone assessment
  - Facial angle
  - Tricuspid regurgitation
- Cell-free DNA testing in which maternal blood is analyzed for fragments of fetal DNA to detect aneuploidy has decreased emphasis on structural findings for risk stratification

Is the Fetal Anatomy Normal?

- Structural malformations may be visible even in absence of markers for aneuploidy
  - Abdominal wall defect
  - Limb reduction abnormalities
  - Alobar holoprosencephaly
  - Neural tube defect
  - Congenital heart disease

Is There Anything Else Noteworthy in Uterus or Adnexa?

- Chorionic bump
  - Focal protrusion of chorion often containing low-level swirling echoes
  - Thought to be arterial bleed within chorion
  - Associated with pregnancy failure if enlarges or if multiple
    – Strong association with partial mole
- Perigestational hemorrhage (PGH)
  - Hematoma in subchorionic space adjacent to GS
  - Use large field-of-view sweeps to assess size of bleed compared to sac size
  - Large PGH associated with increased risk of pregnancy loss, particularly if no living embryo
  - Early PGH (< 7 weeks) associated with higher risk of loss than later bleed
- Look at uterine contour for possible müllerian duct anomaly
  - Associated with recurrent pregnancy loss, fewer successful outcomes with assisted reproduction
  - IUP may be missed if only 1 horn of bicornuate uterus is scanned
  - Increased risk of preterm birth
- Document fibroid size and location
- Document nabothian or Gartner duct cysts
  - Potential cause of confusion during cervical evaluation later in gestation

Key Points

- 1st trimester is time of complex cell multiplication and differentiation with great potential for error if normal processes are not clearly understood
- Negative cell-free DNA screen does not change need for attention to detail as significant birth defects may occur without chromosomal abnormality
- Always use TVUS in early 1st-trimester scans for highest resolution
- In stable patient with IUP of uncertain viability, wait and see; avoid premature interruption of potentially viable pregnancy
- In PUL, close surveillance is mandatory with serial beta hCG measurement; repeat TVUS if levels rise
  - 10-20% risk of ectopic, in which case, methotrexate administration is appropriate
  - ~ 35% will have IUP, in which case, methotrexate administration is catastrophic as it is a potent teratogen

INTRAUTERINE SAC-LIKE STRUCTURE, PROBABLE INTRAUTERINE PREGNANCY

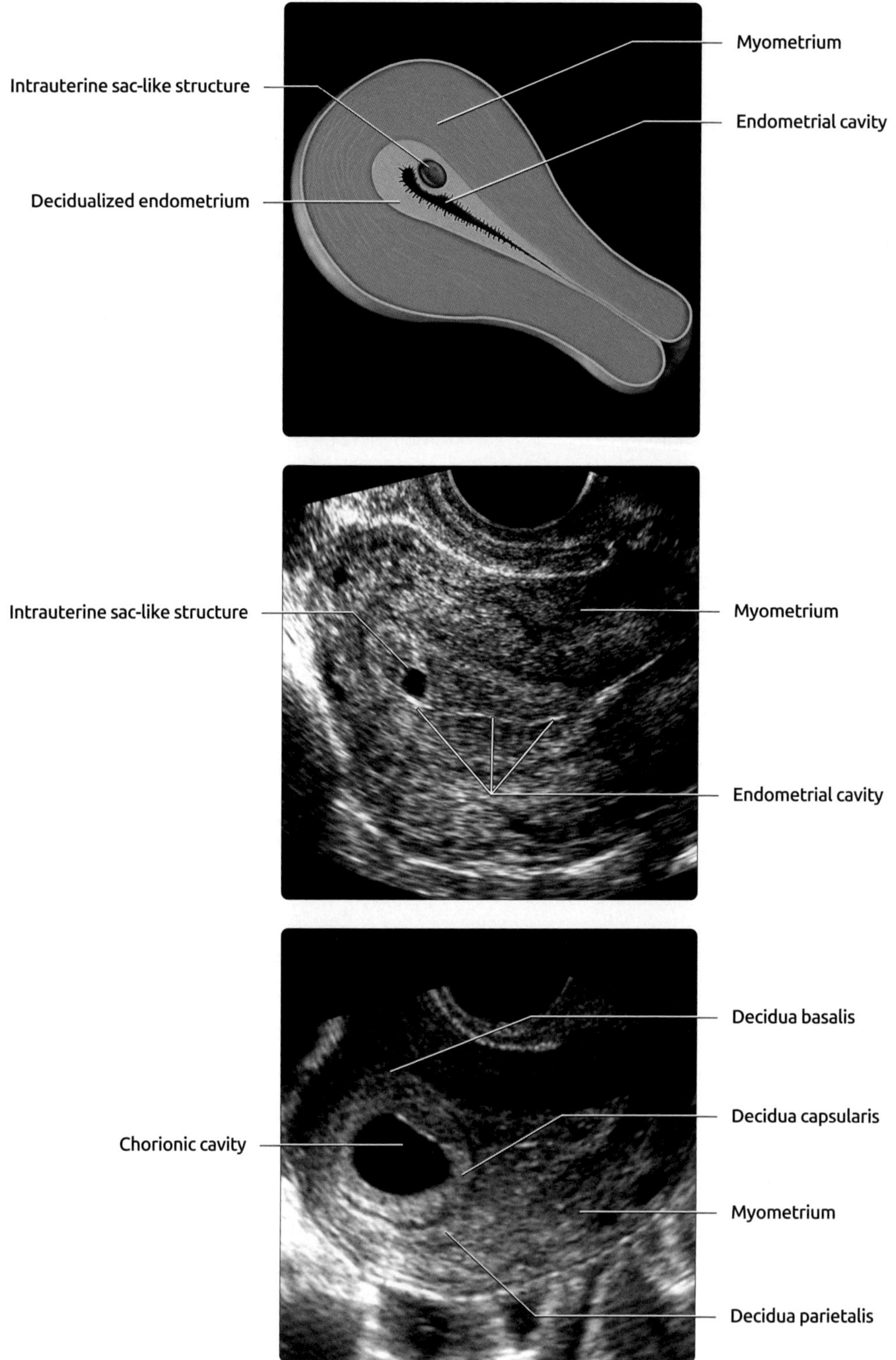

(Top) *The graphic illustrates the earliest sonographic manifestation of an intrauterine pregnancy (IUP). The gestational sac has burrowed into the decidualized endometrium, creating an asymmetrically placed, echogenic ring with a lucent center. This was initially described as the intradecidual sac sign. The sign is not always visible in early pregnancy, and it is subject to considerable interobserver variability; therefore, recommended terminology is now intrauterine sac-like structure.* **(Middle)** *An intrauterine sac-like structure is the earliest visible evidence of an IUP. In this example, the gestational sac is seen as an echogenic ring eccentric to the line created by apposition of the endometrial surfaces (i.e., implantation of the pregnancy has occurred). Currently, recommended terms for such an observation are intrauterine sac-like structure or probable IUP.* **(Bottom)** *As the pregnancy progresses, the gestational sac (i.e., the chorionic sac) enlarges. The concentric rings created by the decidua capsularis and parietalis were described as the double decidual sac sign of an IUP. Currently, this observation is also described as an intrauterine sac-like structure or probable IUP.*

INTRAUTERINE SAC-LIKE STRUCTURE, DEFINITE INTRAUTERINE PREGNANCY

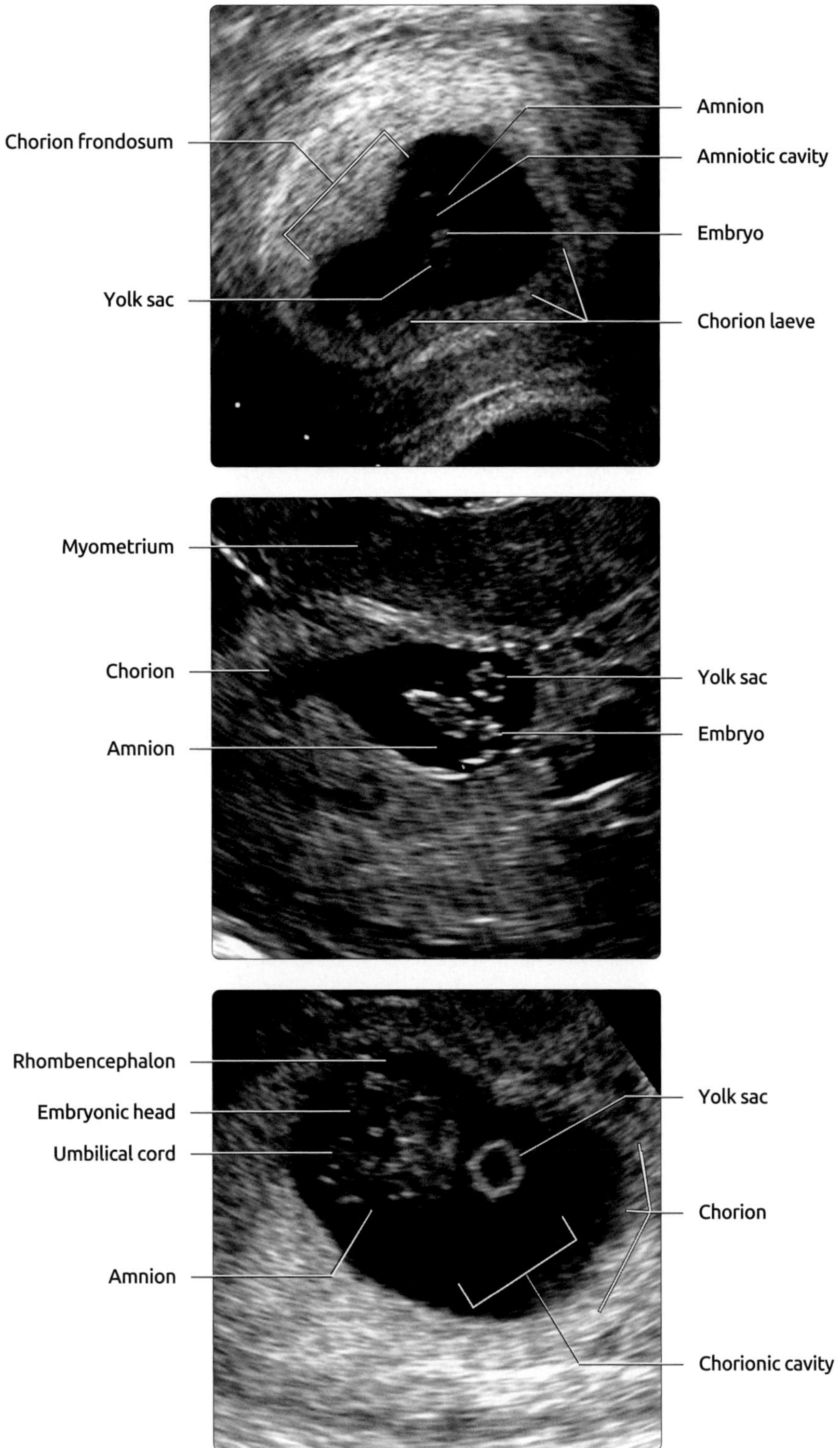

(Top) *Later in gestation, the yolk sac becomes visible followed by the embryo and the amnion. On this TVUS, the embryo is visible inside the amniotic cavity, but it is still intimately associated with the yolk sac, which is in continuity with the embryonic midgut at this stage. This has been described as the double bleb sign of an IUP. Approved current terminology is definite IUP when the gestational sac contains a yolk sac or an embryo, regardless of whether or not there is cardiac activity.* **(Middle)** *TVUS at 7 weeks, 4 days from last menstrual period shows that the yolk sac is now separate from the embryo, as at this stage, the abdominal wall has closed. It lies outside the amnion, which is visible as it surrounds the embryo. Remember that the yolk sac will always be outside the amnion; the embryo lies inside the amniotic sac.* **(Bottom)** *As further growth occurs, the embryo develops a clear, larger, cranial end in which the rhombencephalon may be seen from ~ 8 weeks. The rhombencephalon is 1 of the primary brain vesicles and is a precursor of the posterior fossa structures. It is a normal structure and should not be confused with an intracranial cystic mass. The umbilical cord has formed but is still short; it elongates as the embryo grows and starts to move independently.*

NORMAL EMBRYO

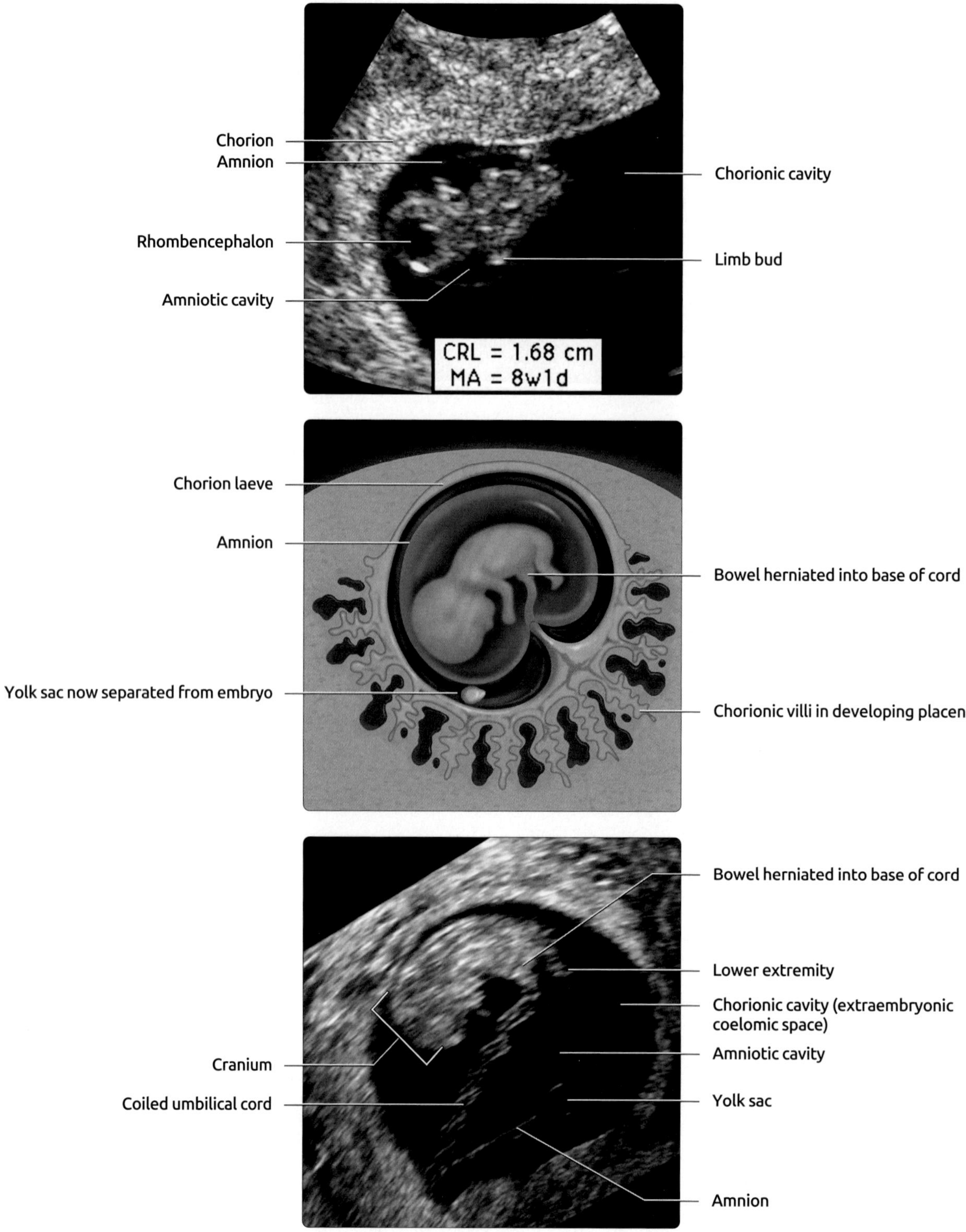

(Top) *Transvaginal scan at 8 weeks shows the rhombencephalic vesicle at the "crown" end of the embryo. The embryo is within the amniotic cavity. Limb buds are just becoming visible.* **(Middle)** *The embryo continues to grow and become increasingly human in appearance. At the same time, the chorionic villi in the chorion frondosum develop an increasingly complex branching pattern, leading to eventual development of the placenta. By the end of the 1st trimester, the amnion fills the chorionic cavity. The membranes do not "fuse" until 14-16 weeks.* **(Bottom)** *At 10 weeks, there is some residual herniation of bowel into the base of the cord. The embryo is freely suspended within the amniotic sac by the cord, which already shows evidence of coiling. The yolk sac will be obliterated as the amnion apposes to the chorion. Limb development continues with elongation of the limb buds.*

NORMAL FETUS

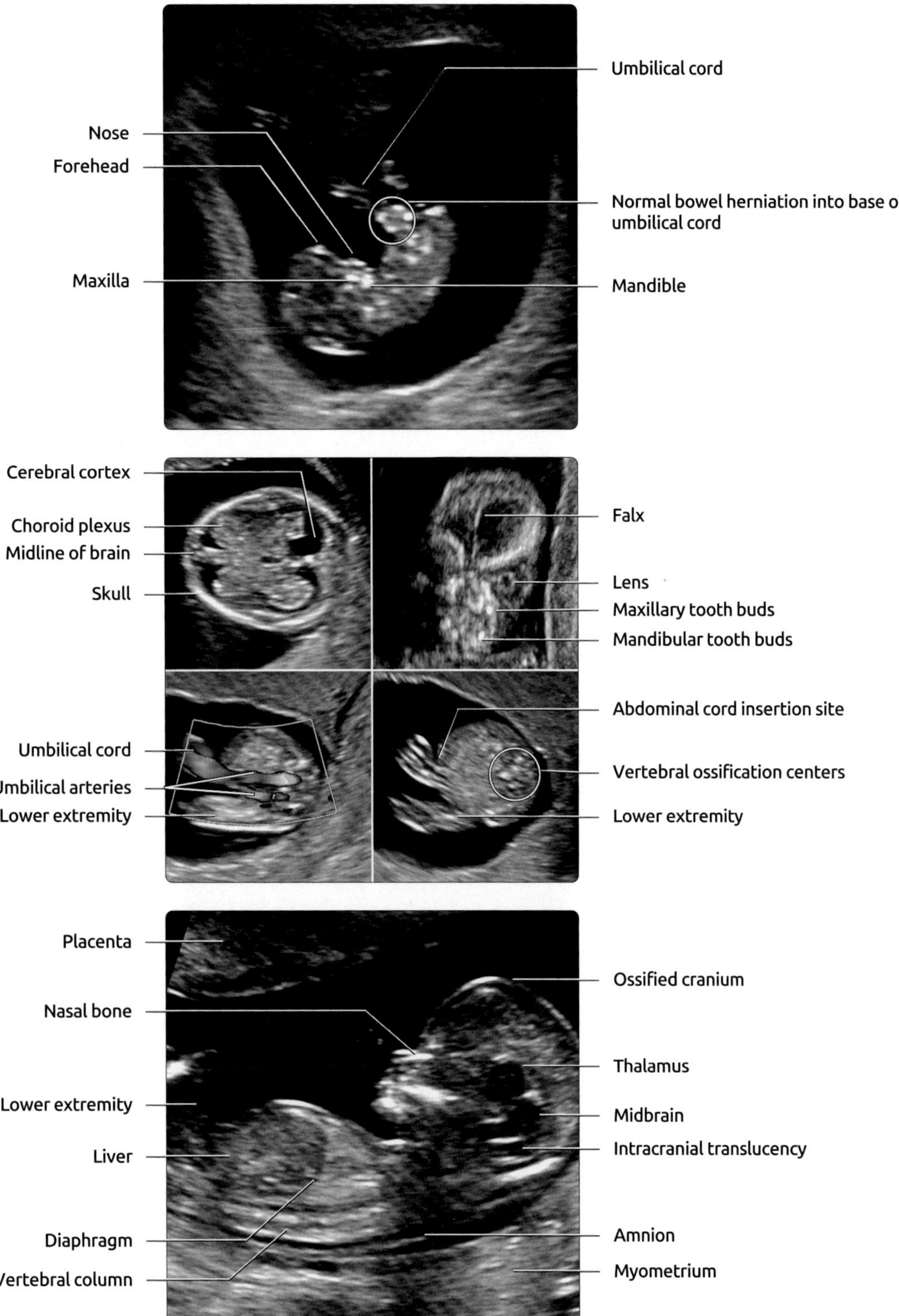

(Top) *Abdominal scan at 10 weeks, 1 day from last menstrual period shows a recognizable facial profile. Note the echogenic bowel loops herniated into the base of the umbilical cord. This is normal and should not be confused with an omphalocele.* **(Middle)** *Composite image shows normal structures seen on vaginal US at 12 weeks, 1 day. There are 2 visible cerebral hemispheres, recognizable facial structures including the lens of the eye, recognizable ossification centers of vertebral bodies, and a normal 3-vessel cord. Note that the cord insertion site is normal; all bowel has returned to the peritoneal cavity at this gestational age. The stomach and bladder are often visible as fluid-filled structures at this stage.* **(Bottom)** *Sagittal transabdominal ultrasound at 12 weeks, 6 days from last menstrual period shows recognizable anatomic features. Organogenesis is completed by the end of the 13th week. Growth and maturation of the various organ systems occurs during the remainder of gestation. The intracranial translucency is a precursor to the 4th ventricle. When seen, an open neural tube defect is highly unlikely.*

ABNORMAL FETUS

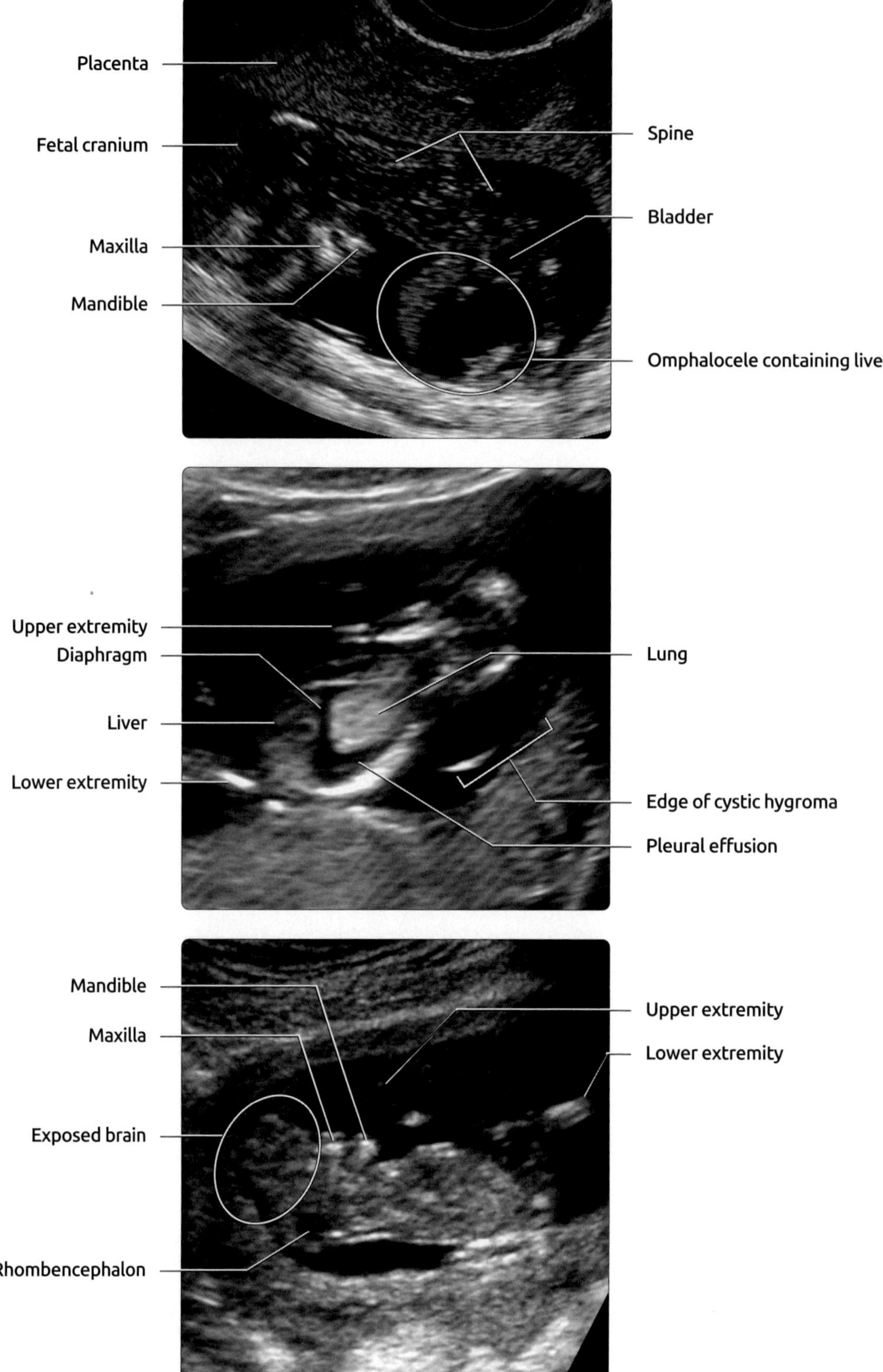

(Top) *This is an example of a major structural defect that can be diagnosed in the 1st trimester. This 12-week fetus has a large, liver-containing omphalocele. The family elected to terminate the pregnancy. Chromosomes were normal. This case serves as a reminder that not all birth defects are associated with aneuploidy.* **(Middle)** *This is a 12-week fetus with structural abnormalities. There is a pleural effusion, and there was also a large cystic hygroma. Intrauterine demise occurred within a week of this scan. The final diagnosis was Turner syndrome.* **(Bottom)** *In this fetus at 12 weeks gestation, the maxilla and mandible are clearly ossified but there are no cranial bones. The brain is unprotected, has an irregular contour, and "flops" forward over the forehead. This is exencephaly, a lethal anomaly that is not associated with aneuploidy.*

PITFALLS IN EARLY PREGNANCY

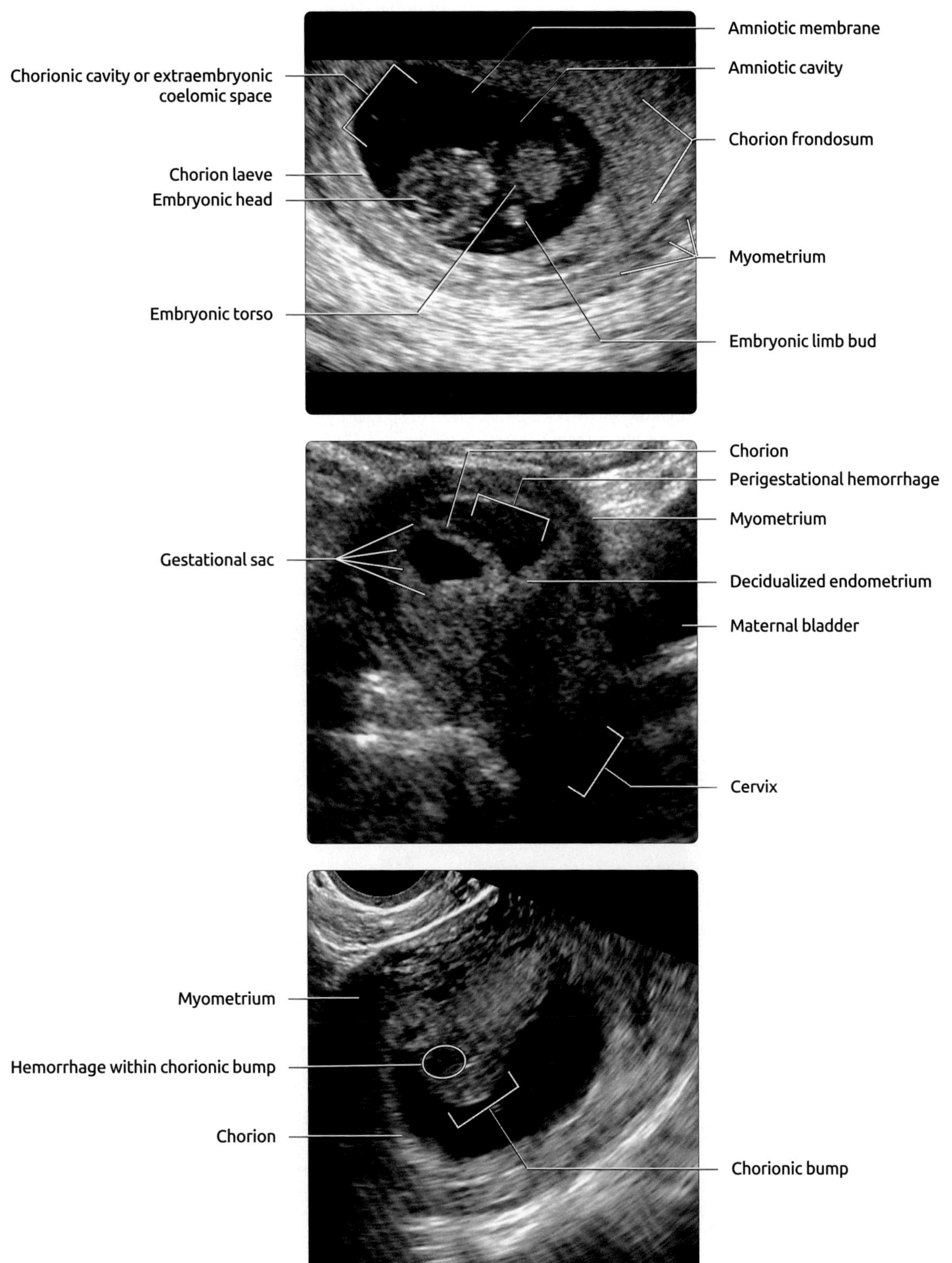

(Top) *As the pregnancy progresses, the amnion expands around the embryo. This 9-week TAUS shows the anechoic amniotic fluid surrounded by the echogenic, proteinaceous material in the chorionic cavity. This is normal and should not be confused with a perigestational hemorrhage, which is outside the gestational sac, between the chorion and the myometrium.* **(Middle)** *This TAUS shows the location of a perigestational hemorrhage, which is subchorionic (i.e., between the chorion and the myometrium). Do not confuse this with a twin pregnancy; the shape is crescentic rather than round, there are internal echoes of blood, and neither a yolk sac, amnion, nor embryo.* **(Bottom)** *This TVUS shows the typical appearance of a chorionic bump, which is a focal protuberance of the chorion and, as such, forms part of the wall of the gestational sac. Do not confuse this for an embryo, which should lie within the amnion, inside the chorionic cavity. An embryo should not be flush with the wall of the gestational sac. There is a strong association with partial mole.*

Abnormal and Failed First-Trimester Pregnancy

KEY FACTS

TERMINOLOGY

- **Viable** pregnancy defined as one with potential for live birth
- **Nonviable** pregnancy is one that will not result in live birth
- **Probable intrauterine pregnancy (IUP)**
  - Intrauterine sac-like structure without yolk sac (YS) or embryo
- **Definite IUP**
  - Intrauterine sac-like structure with YS or embryo (± cardiac activity)
- **Intrauterine pregnancy of uncertain viability**
  - Definite IUP that does not meet criteria to be called nonviable

IMAGING

- **Criteria for nonviable pregnancy on vaginal US**
  - Mean sac diameter > 25 mm without embryo
  - Crown rump length ≥ 7 mm without cardiac activity
  - Cessation of previously documented cardiac activity
- **Time follow-up intervals to allow for definitive diagnosis of nonviable pregnancy**
  - Lack of live embryo 11 days after demonstration of gestational sac **with** YS is diagnostic
  - Lack of live embryo 14 days after demonstration of gestational sac **without** YS is diagnostic

SCANNING TIPS

- Use vaginal US for highest resolution images
- With positive pregnancy test
  - Intrauterine sac-like structure with **rounded edges** is statistically IUP
  - Intrauterine sac-like structure with **pointed edges** concerning for nonviable IUP or blood products in setting of ectopic
  - Empty uterus + normal adnexa → **pregnancy of unknown location**
    - Must follow these patients with serial β-hCG as 10-20% have ectopic pregnancy

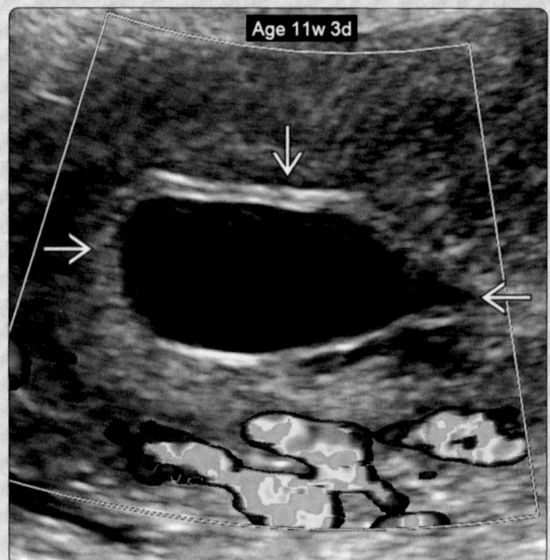

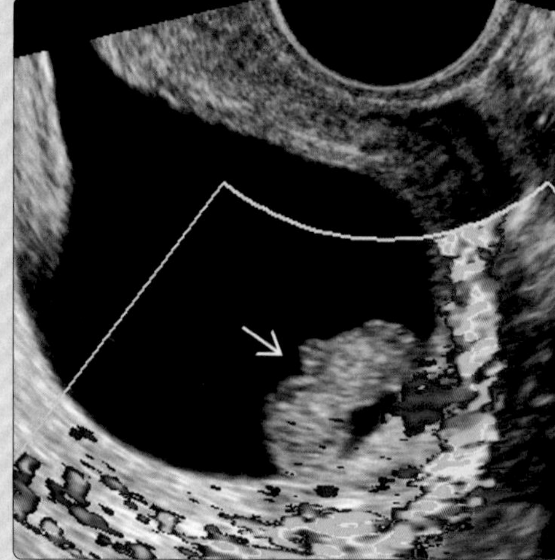

(Left) *Color Doppler US shows very little flow in the gestational sac wall ➡. The MSD was 27 mm, which was less than expected for dates. Lack of a live embryo with an MSD > 25 mm on vaginal US is definitive for nonviable pregnancy.* **(Right)** *Transvaginal color Doppler US confirms lack of cardiac motion in this 24-mm embryo ➡. An embryo > 7 mm should have demonstrable cardiac activity on vaginal sonography. Color Doppler or video clips may be used to confirm lack of cardiac activity on M-mode scans.*

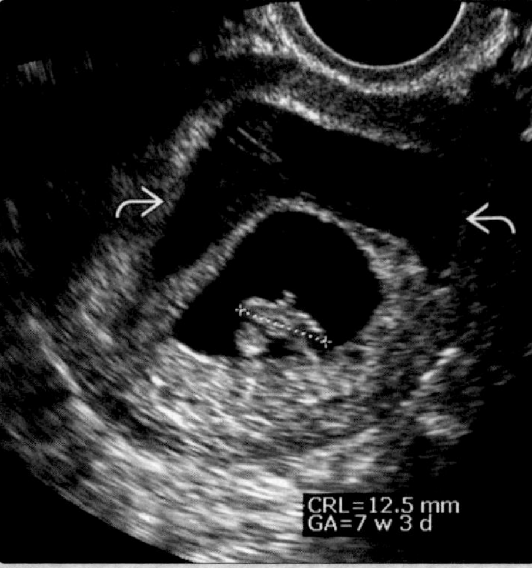

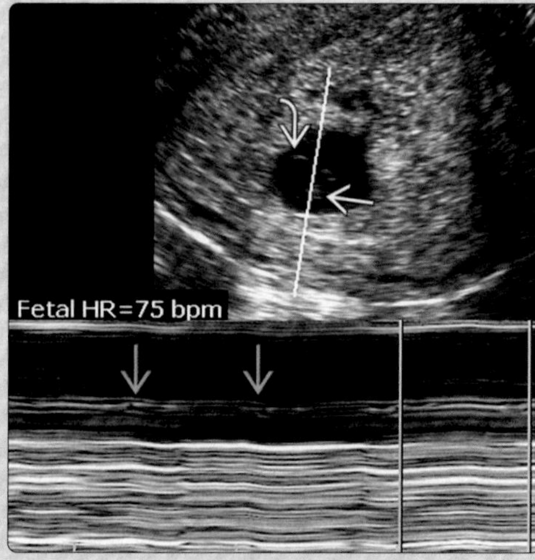

(Left) *TVUS shows a 12.5-mm embryo (calipers) without heart motion, confirming embryonic demise. Note the large subchorionic hemorrhage ➡.* **(Right)** *M-mode US shows bradycardia ➡ in a tiny embryo ➡ adjacent to the yolk sac ➡. Cardiac activity is often visible before the CRL can be measured accurately. Embryonic bradycardia indicates poor prognosis. One week later, this embryo was dead. Cessation of previously documented cardiac activity is diagnostic of nonviable pregnancy, regardless of CRL.*

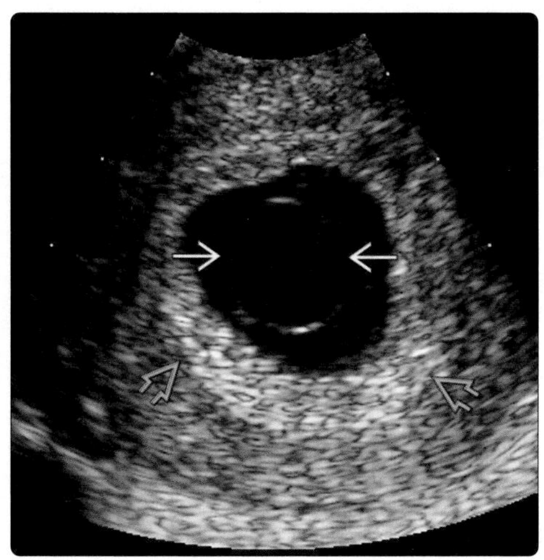

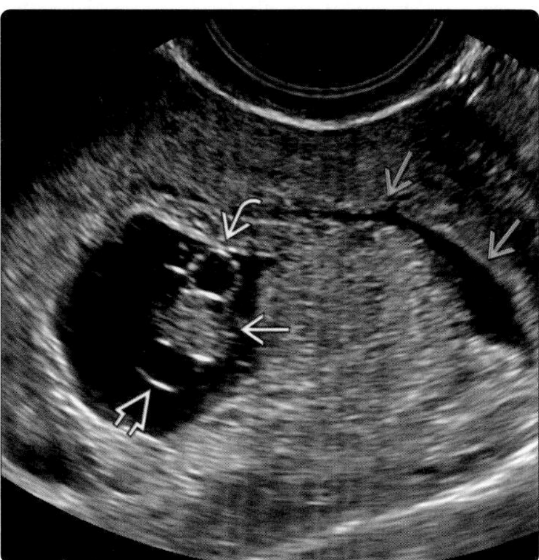

(Left) *TVUS shows an example of the empty amnion sign in which the amnion* ➡ *is visible inside the gestational sac* ➡*, but no embryo is present. Do not confuse this sign with the finding of a sac with a yolk sac.* **(Right)** *TVUS shows the expanded amnion sign in which an embryo* ➡ *is surrounded by a visible amnion* ➡*. The amnion forms before the embryo. Cardiac activity should be present in any embryo sufficiently developed to have a visible, separate amnion. The yolk sac* ➡ *is separate, and there is a subchorionic hemorrhage* ➡*.*

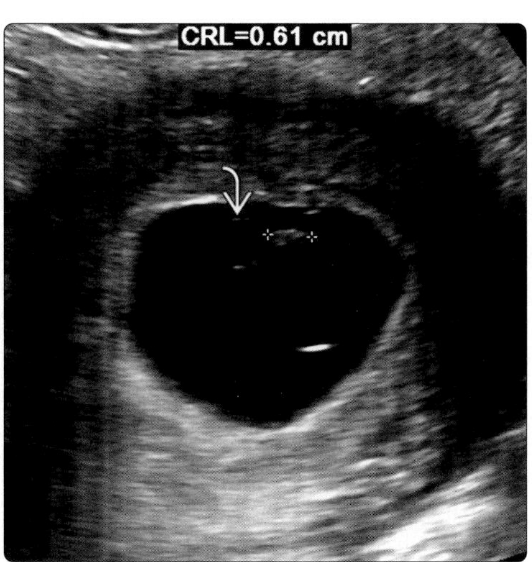

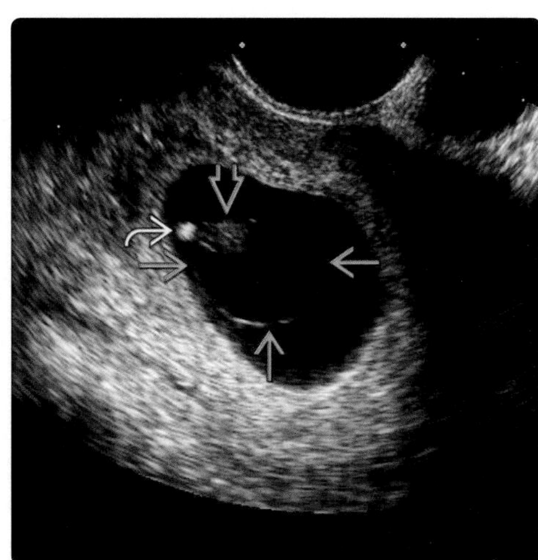

(Left) *TVUS shows a 6-mm embryo without cardiac activity. Per 2013 consensus guidelines, this is a pregnancy of uncertain viability. The yolk sac* ➡ *has separated (i.e., the embryological step of gastrulation has occurred), and there should be cardiac activity. This is known as the yolk stalk sign of embryonic demise.* **(Right)** *TVUS shows a calcified yolk sac* ➡*, dead embryo* ➡*, and expanded amnion* ➡*. Per consensus guidelines, an expanded amnion is suspicious for, but not diagnostic of, nonviable pregnancy.*

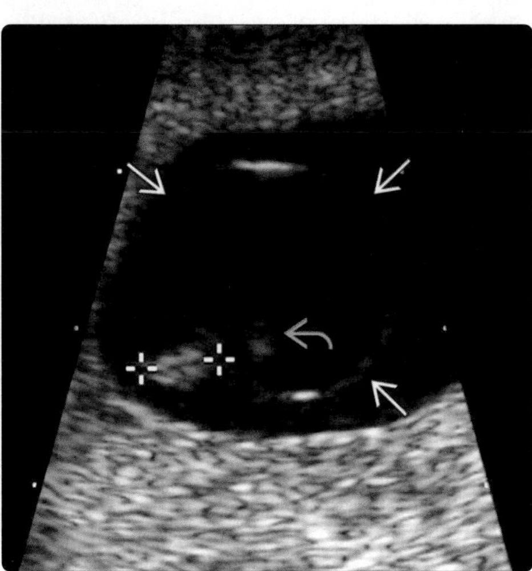

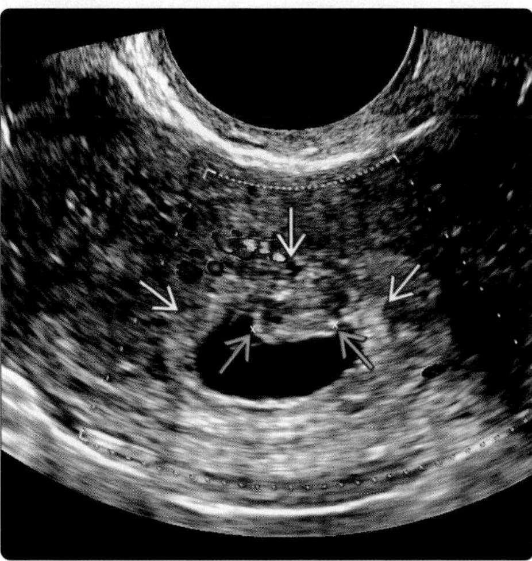

(Left) *TVUS shows the expanded amnion sign* ➡ *with a 3-mm embryo* ➡ *and a collapsed yolk sac (calipers), which was incorrectly measured as the embryo. This is an important pitfall that can be avoided if one remembers that the embryo is inside the amnion and the yolk sac is outside.* **(Right)** *TVUS shows a chorionic bump* ➡ *(focal hemorrhage within chorionic tissue), which was mistakenly measured (calipers) as an embryo. It is flush with the wall of the gestational sac* ➡*. An embryo should be free floating within the sac.*

KEY FACTS

TERMINOLOGY

- Perigestational hemorrhage (PGH): Hematoma in subchorionic space adjacent to gestational sac (GS)
- Subchorionic hematoma is synonymous with PGH

IMAGING

- Hematoma appearance depends on age of blood
  - Acute hematoma is echogenic
  - Subacute hematoma is complex, more hypoechoic
  - Old hematoma approaches sonolucent
- PGH has no blood flow on color Doppler
- Estimate PGH size compared with GS size (subjectively)
  - ≤ 10% vs. 11-25% vs. 26-50% vs. > 50%
  - Other measurement criteria shown to be less accurate (including amount of detachment of early placenta)

TOP DIFFERENTIAL DIAGNOSES

- Early twin gestation (PGH mimics 2nd sac)
- Chorioamniotic separation in late 1st trimester

CLINICAL ISSUES

- Large PGH associated with ↑ risk for pregnancy loss
  - PGH > 50% of GS (with living embryo) = 23% loss rate
  - PGH ≤ 10% of GS (with living embryo) = 6% loss rate
  - Loss rates higher if no living embryo at time of diagnosis
- Early PGH associated with ↑ risk of pregnancy loss
  - 20% loss rate if ≤ 7 weeks vs. 4% if > 8 weeks
- PGH is common (symptomatic or asymptomatic)
  - 2% of all 1st-trimester patients have PGH
  - 20% of patients with vaginal bleeding have PGH
- Guarded prognosis if embryonic bradycardia
- Guarded prognosis if cervix distended with blood

SCANNING TIPS

- Take large field of view or cine sweeps to show PGH size compared to GS size
- Zoom into GS to look for yolk sac, embryo (transvaginal scan often necessary)
- Document embryo heart rate with M-mode in every case

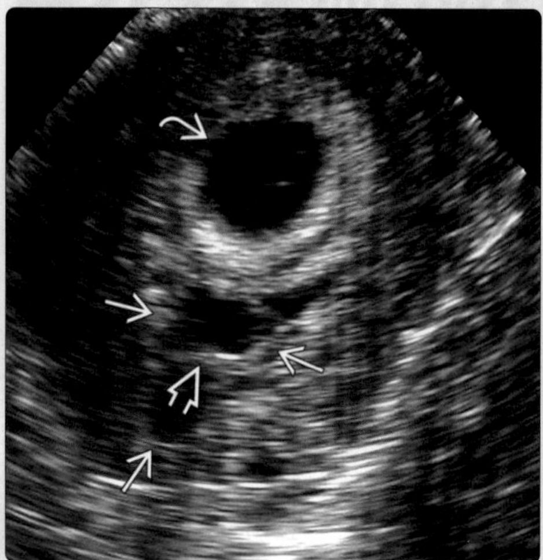

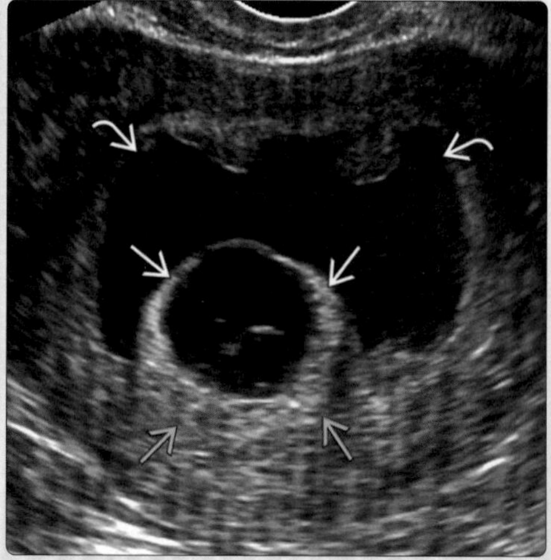

(Left) *Typical appearance of small perigestational hemorrhage (PGH) ➡ next to an early gestational sac (GS) ➡ is shown. The internal echogenicity in the subchorionic hematoma can mimic a yolk sac ➡ from a dichorionic twin. Sometimes follow-up is necessary to differentiate between the 2 diagnoses.* **(Right)** *A large PGH ➡ surrounds an early GS ➡. The sac is attached posteriorly ➡ but the PGH size is clearly > 50% of the GS size and the pregnancy is at a higher risk for failure.*

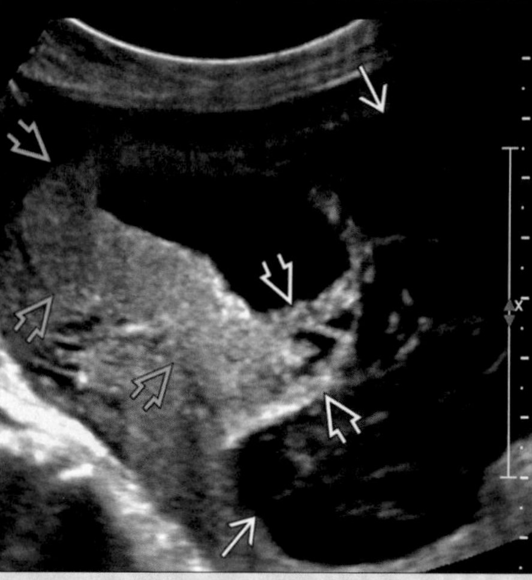

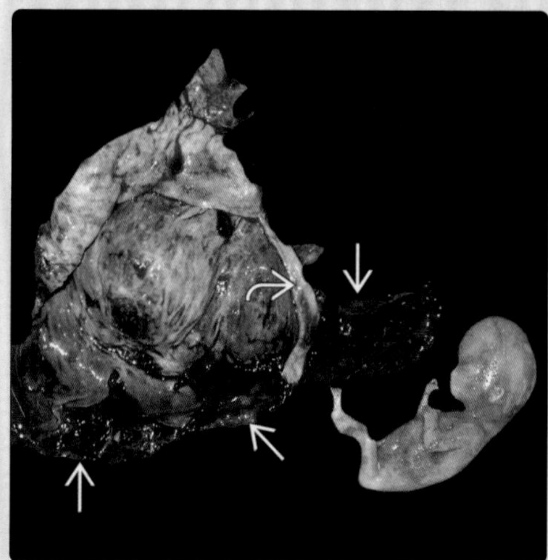

(Left) *In this 12-week pregnant patient, a large PGH ➡ with complex echogenicity lifts the inferior edge of the chorionic frondosum (CF), or early placenta ➡. The majority of the CF is otherwise well attached ➡, and the fetus survived to term in this case.* **(Right)** *In a case of an 11-week pregnancy loss from large PGH, gross pathology shows a large subchorionic hemorrhage ➡ that extends from behind the membranes ➡ and placenta.*

Complete Hydatidiform Mole

KEY FACTS

MAGING

- **Classic 2nd-trimester findings** described as "Swiss cheese" or "cluster of grapes" endometrium
  - No fetus or embryo
  - Increased vascularity on color Doppler
  - Areas of hemorrhage common
- **1st-trimester appearance** very different than seen later
  - Thickened, irregular endometrium
  - Appearance may mimic retained products of conception or anembryonic pregnancy
- Ovarian theca lutein cysts in 50% of cases
  - Result from ovarian hyperstimulation due to ↑ hCG
  - Rare < 13 weeks
- Invasive mole in 12-15%; choriocarcinoma in 5-8%

TOP DIFFERENTIAL DIAGNOSES

- Placental hydropic degeneration
  - Hydropic change of developing placenta after pregnancy failure
  - hCG will be low rather than elevated
- Triploidy (partial mole)
  - 3 complete sets of chromosomes
  - Placenta is cystic when extra set is from father
  - Fetus is present but abnormal; severe growth restriction

SCANNING TIPS

- Always evaluate with color Doppler, but be aware absence of flow **does not** mean it is not molar pregnancy
- Evaluate interface with myometrium carefully looking for invasion
- Must distinguish twin pregnancy with coexistent mole from triploidy
  - This will be dizygotic twin pregnancy with 1 normal fetus and 1 complete hydatidiform mole
  - Look for thick separating membrane (dichorionic)
- Evaluate ovarian size and appearance
  - Theca lutein cysts may cause massive ovarian enlargement

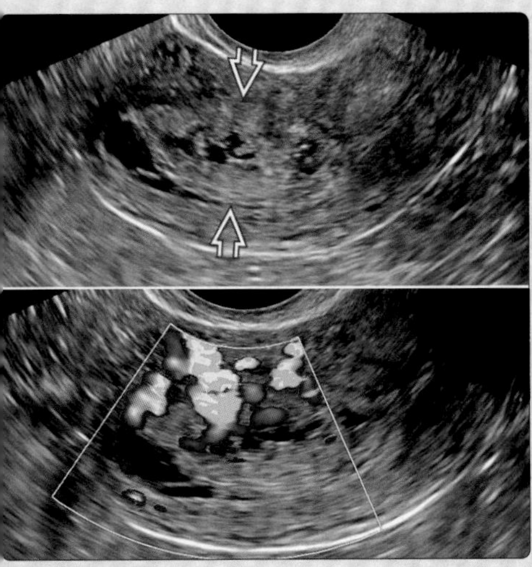

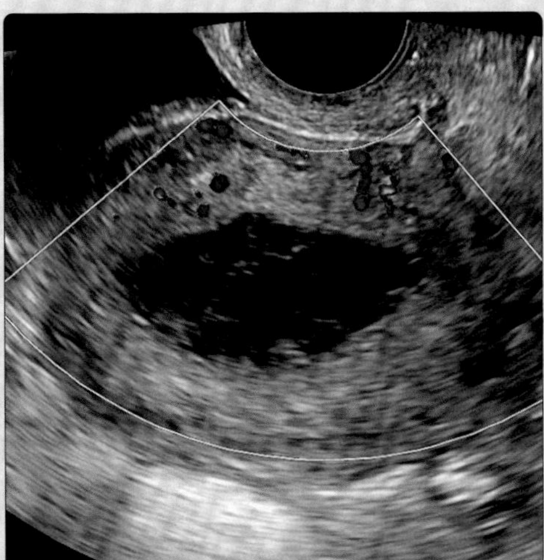

(Left) *Do not expect the classic bunch of grapes appearance of a complete hydatidiform mole (CHM) in the 1st trimester. It often appears as a thickened endometrium & can mimic retained products of conception or an anembryonic pregnancy. In this case, the endometrium is thickened ➡ with a few scattered lucencies and significant flow on color Doppler.* **(Right)** *This is another CHM in the 1st trimester that is hypovascular. The 1st-trimester appearance is quite variable, and it is essential to compare with the hCG levels.*

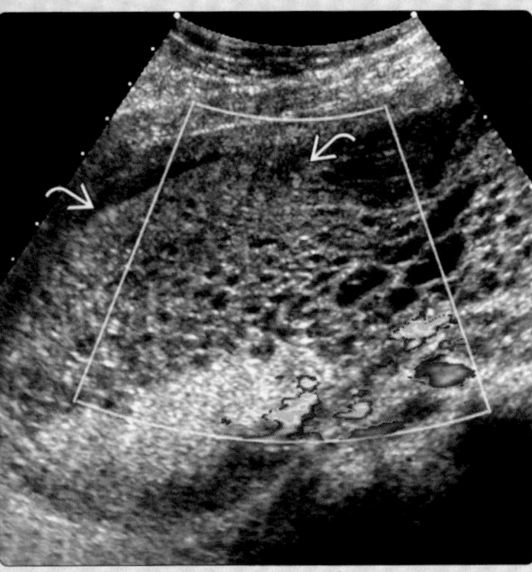

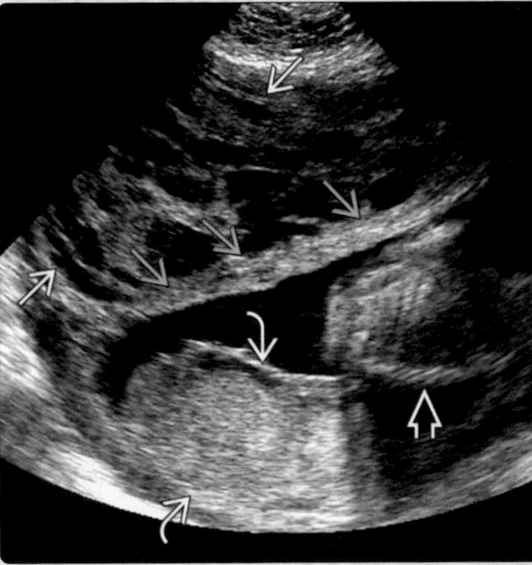

(Left) *By the 2nd trimester, a CHM will have a more classic Swiss cheese appearance. This longitudinal transabdominal ultrasound shows a large, cystic endometrial mass ➡ with multiple small, cystic areas representing the hydropic villi.* **(Right)** *Axial ultrasound in a 39-year-old woman shows a normal fetus with coexistent mole. This is the result of a dizygotic pregnancy. The normal twin ➡ and placenta ➡ are seen adjacent to a CHM ➡. A thick membrane ➡ separates the 2.*

KEY FACTS

IMAGING

- Classic findings of tubal ectopic pregnancy (EP)
  - No intrauterine pregnancy (IUP)
  - Tubal mass
  - Echogenic fluid in cul-de-sac (peritoneal blood)
- Nonspecific adnexal mass is most common finding
  - Tube dilated with blood
  - Ruptured tube causing adnexal hematoma
- Specific findings of tubal EP
  - Adnexal echogenic gestational sac ± yolk sac ± embryo (± heart beat)
  - Adnexal EP is vascular: "Ring of fire" with color Doppler
- Uterus may contain blood or decidual cysts: Can mimic IUP
- Peritoneal blood is important sign: Most often in cul-de-sac

CLINICAL ISSUES

- 90% of all EPs are tubal
- Treatment based on ultrasound findings and patient stability: Nonsurgical treatment preferred
  - Medical treatment with 1 or multiple doses of methotrexate if EP < 3-4 cm, patient stable, and no significant hemoperitoneum
    - Living embryo is not contraindication
  - Surgical treatment
    - Salpingostomy (spares tube): Tube incised and EP removed (for nonruptured cases)
    - Salpingectomy: Tube removed (for ruptured cases)

SCANNING TIPS

- Sagittal cul-de-sac view for abnormal fluid is part of every 1st-trimester protocol
  - Look in abdomen if a lot of blood seen in pelvis
- Corpus luteum (CL) can mimic tubal EP
  - Use endovaginal probe and hand on patient abdomen to move structures
    - EP slides independent of ovary, CL moves with ovary
  - CL also has "ring of fire" with color Doppler, showing it is **in** ovary, not next to ovary

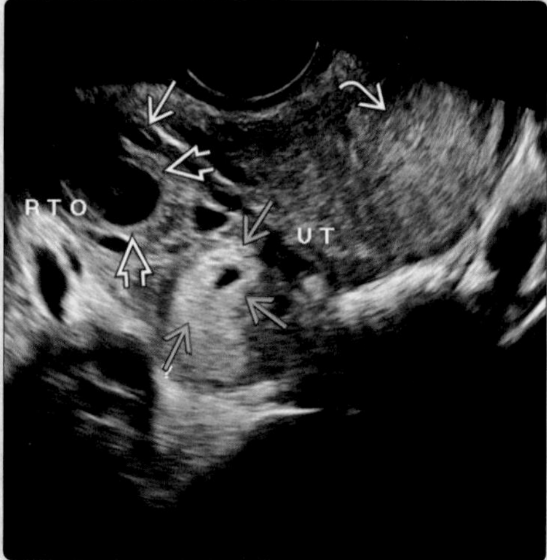

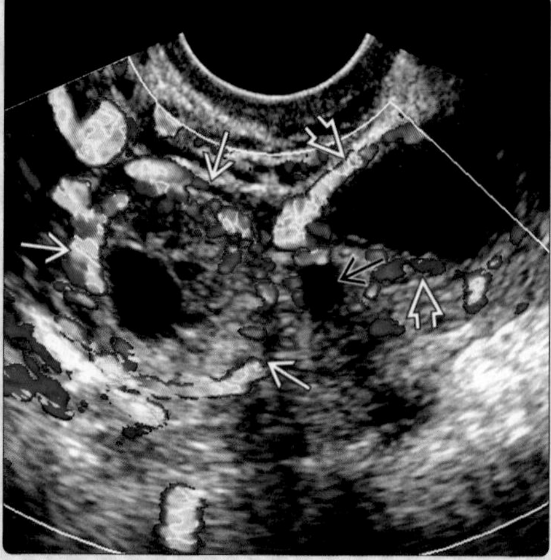

(Left) *Transvaginal US of a right tubal ectopic pregnancy (EP) shows an echogenic gestational sac (GS) ➔ adjacent to but separate from the right ovary ➔, which contains a corpus luteum (CL) ➔. Note that the uterus is empty ➔. Most tubal EPs occur on the same side as the ovarian CL.* **(Right)** *Color Doppler US of the adnexa shows the "ring of fire" of the left EP ➔ and the adjacent left ovarian CL ➔. The difference is that the CL is in the ovary (note follicle ➔), whereas the tubal EP is not.*

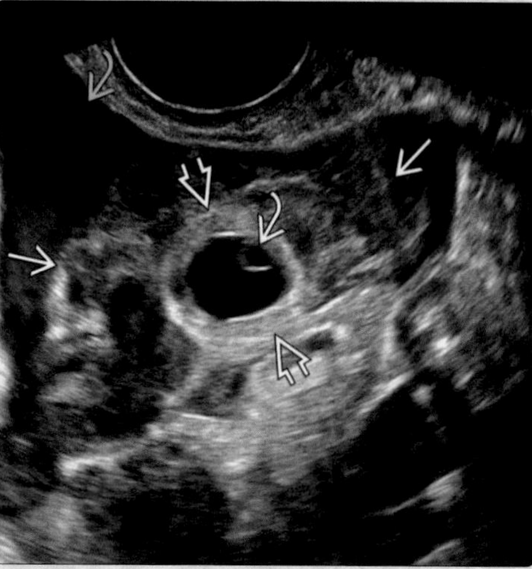

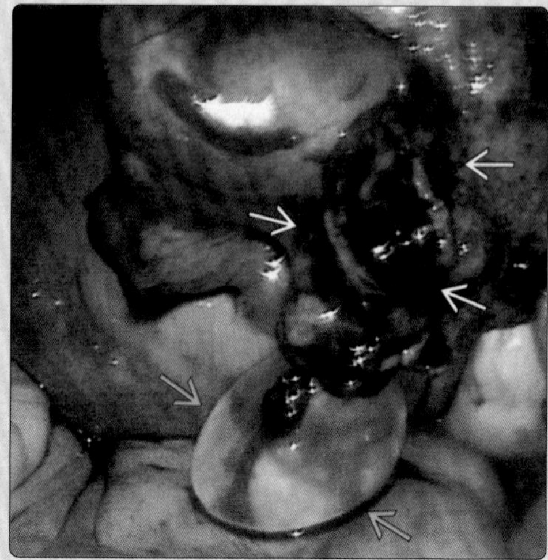

(Left) *Transvaginal US of a ruptured tubal EP shows an ectopic GS ➔ that contains a yolk sac ➔ and is surrounded by echogenic blood clot ➔. In addition, there is a moderate amount of free fluid with echoes in the pelvis ➔.* **(Right)** *Intraoperative photograph shows a ruptured fallopian tube ➔ with adherent blood clot. The intact amniotic sac ➔ lies in the cul-de-sac. Ruptured EPs are most often treated surgically. A large amount of intraperitoneal blood may be present with these cases.*

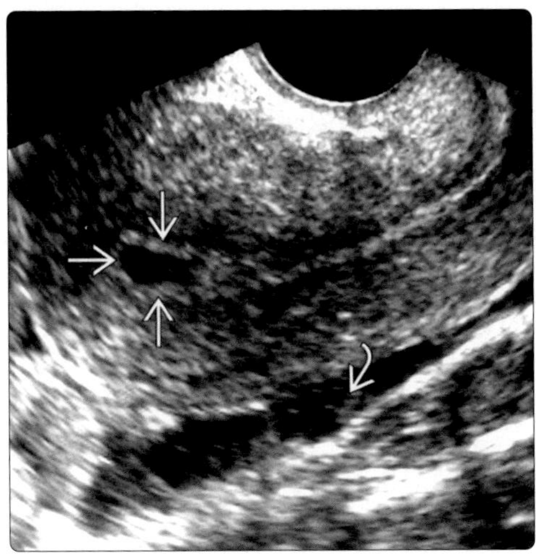

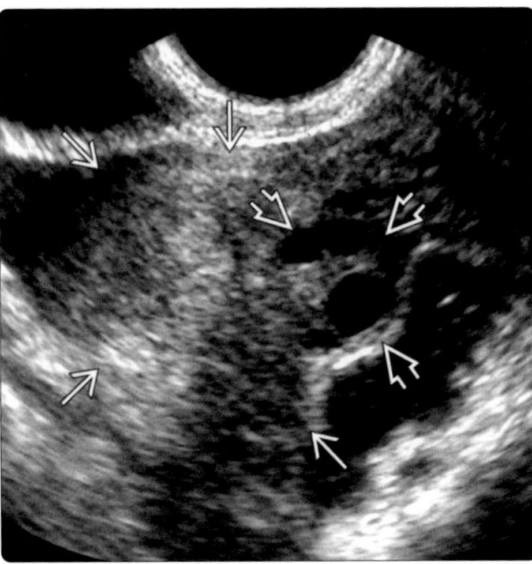

(Left) *Sagittal transvaginal US shows an intrauterine fluid collection ➡, which mimics an IUP. However, note that the fluid is oblong and centrally located in the uterine cavity instead of round and eccentric (as would be expected for an IUP). In addition, complex cul-de-sac fluid ➡ is also seen, raising suspicion for blood in the pelvis.* **(Right)** *Transvaginal US of the right adnexa in the same patient shows a heterogeneous adnexal mass ➡ adjacent to the ovary ➡. Nonspecific adnexal mass is a common finding with tubal EP.*

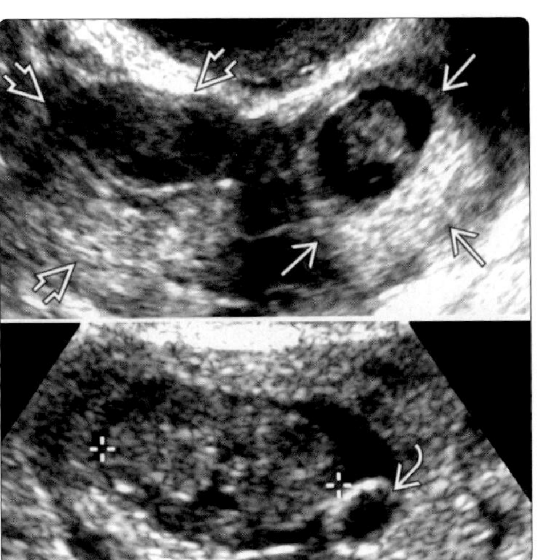

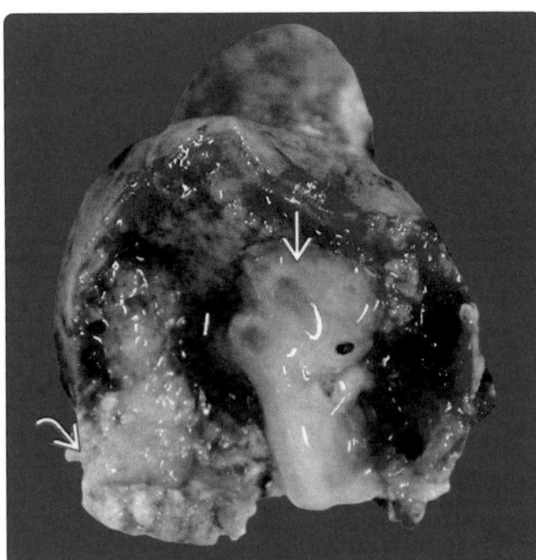

(Left) *Transvaginal US of a living embryo in a tubal ectopic reveals that the tubal ring ➡ is adjacent to the ovary ➡ and contains a distinguishable embryo (calipers) and yolk sac ➡. M-mode US confirmed cardiac activity.* **(Right)** *Gross pathology from the same patient shows a well-formed embryo ➡ within the tubal GS. Note the presence of extensive trophoblastic tissue ➡. It is unusual for an embryo to develop this fully in a fallopian tube without tubal rupture.*

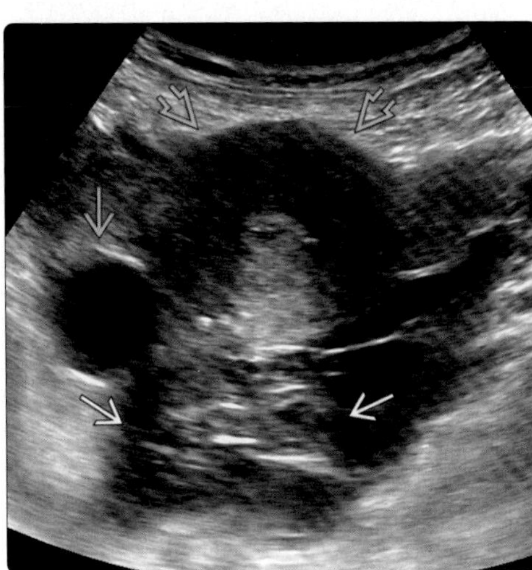

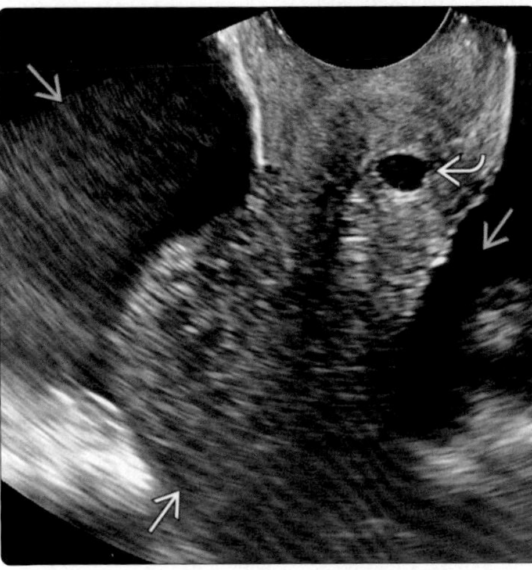

(Left) *In this case of ruptured tubal EP, echogenic clot is seen in the cul-de-sac ➡. The uterus ➡ is empty and a right ovarian CL cyst ➡ is seen. The findings are highly suspicious for ruptured EP, although a ruptured hemorrhagic CL can have similar findings. The biggest clue for EP is the lack of IUP.* **(Right)** *In a case of ruptured EP, the empty uterus ➡ is surrounded by nonclotted blood ➡. The incidental nabothian cyst ➡ should not be confused with an IUP. Patients can become unstable rapidly when there is significant hemoperitoneum.*

KEY FACTS

IMAGING

- **Interstitial ectopic**: Implantation in portion of tube crossing myometrium at cornua of uterus
  - Eccentrically located with respect to endometrial cavity
  - Bulges cornua of uterus
  - < 5 mm of surrounding myometrium very suggestive
  - Interstitial line sign: Echogenic line from endometrium to ectopic sac
  - 3D ultrasound shown to improve diagnosis and should be performed in every suspected case
  - Covered by myometrium so can grow to larger size than tubal ectopic; catastrophic bleeding if ruptures
- **Cervical ectopic**
  - Within cervical stroma separate from endocervical canal
  - Hourglass-shaped uterus: Cervical distention from pregnancy, with "waist" due to closed internal os
  - Primary differential is spontaneous abortion
    - Irregular, deformed, flattened sac in cervical canal
- **Cesarean scar ectopic**
  - Sac will be below midpoint of uterus within anterior myometrium at site of C-section scar
  - Must evaluate overlying myometrium
    - Deep implantation into defect, risk of impending rupture and life-threatening bleeding
    - Sac protruding into uterine cavity can lead to live birth but all will have placenta accreta
- **Abdominal ectopic**
  - Most often implants on uterus or in posterior cul-de-sac
  - May present quite late as not in contained space (e.g., fallopian tube), which would rupture
  - Membranes form sac around embryo/fetus and may be mistaken for myometrium
- **Ovarian ectopic**
  - Vascular echogenic ring in ovary far more likely to be corpus luteum cyst
  - More echogenic and rounder than typical corpus luteum
  - Location on/near surface of ovary

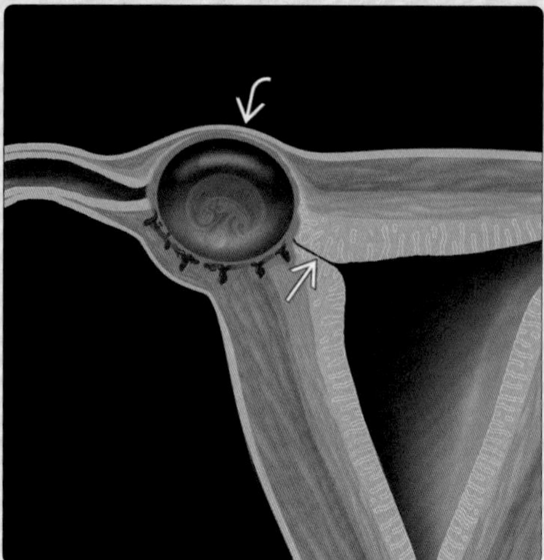

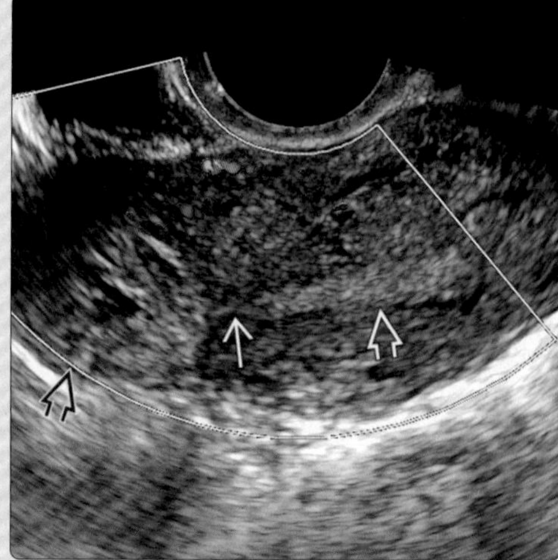

(Left) *Coronal graphic shows an interstitial ectopic pregnancy with bulging and thinning of the overlying myometrium ➡. The coapted margins of the interstitial portion of the tube create the interstitial line sign ➡. Cornual pregnancy is often used interchangeably, but there are inconsistent definitions, and this term should be dropped.* **(Right)** *TVUS shows an interstitial ectopic pregnancy ➡ with no clear myometrial covering. An interstitial line sign ➡ connects empty endometrial cavity ➡ to sac.*

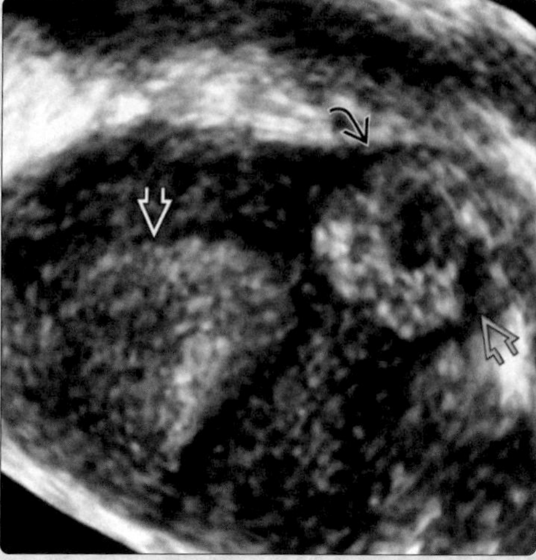

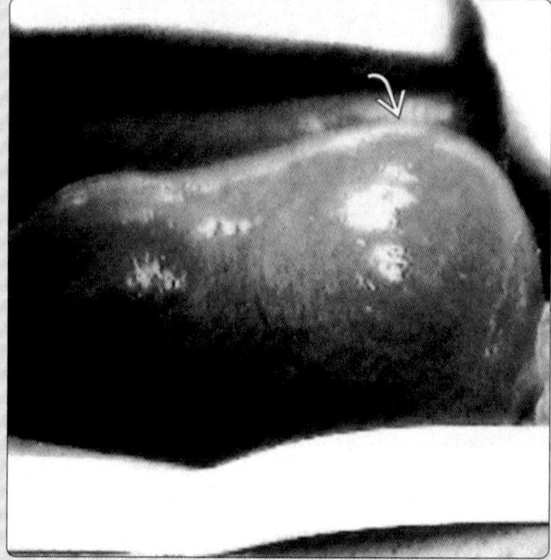

(Left) *3D US shows an interstitial ectopic pregnancy ➡ clearly separate from the endometrial cavity ➡. 3D US is the best way to make this diagnosis and should be performed in all suspected cases. Note the claw of myometrium ➡, which becomes imperceptibly thin along the fundal border of the sac. Rupture can lead to catastrophic bleeding.* **(Right)** *Intraoperative photograph shows the bulging, thinned myometrium at the site of the interstitial ectopic ➡.*

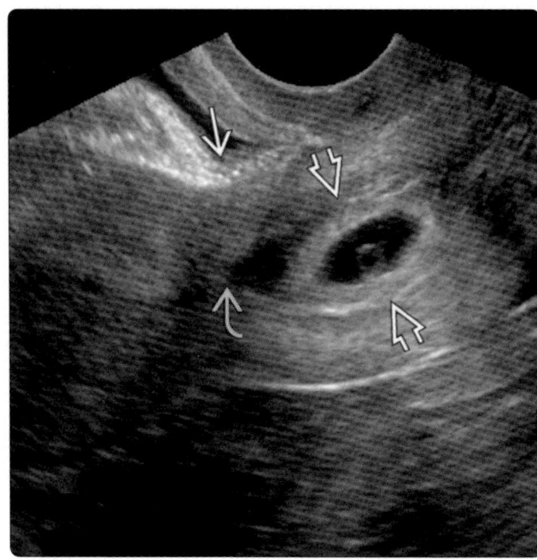

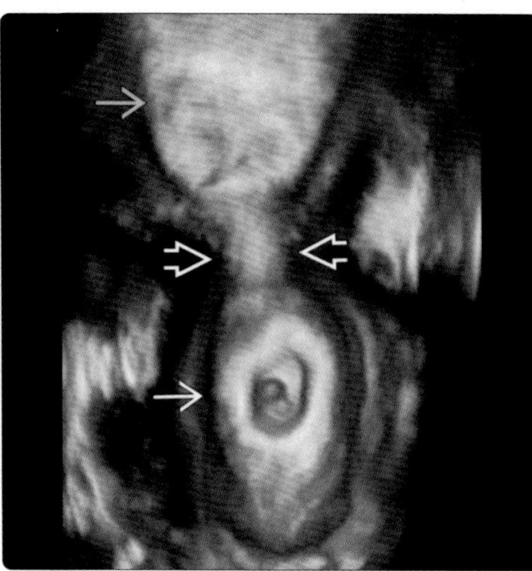

(Left) *Transvaginal US shows several classic features of a cervical ectopic pregnancy. The internal os ➔ is closed. The bladder neck ➔ is a landmark for the level of the internal os. The oval gestational sac ➔, which contains a yolk sac, is clearly implanted in the cervix, not the uterine cavity.* **(Right)** *3D reconstructions can help to visualize the hourglass shape typically seen with cervical ectopic pregnancy. The uterine cavity ➔ is empty and the gestational sac expands the cervix ➔. The waist ➔ is the closed internal os.*

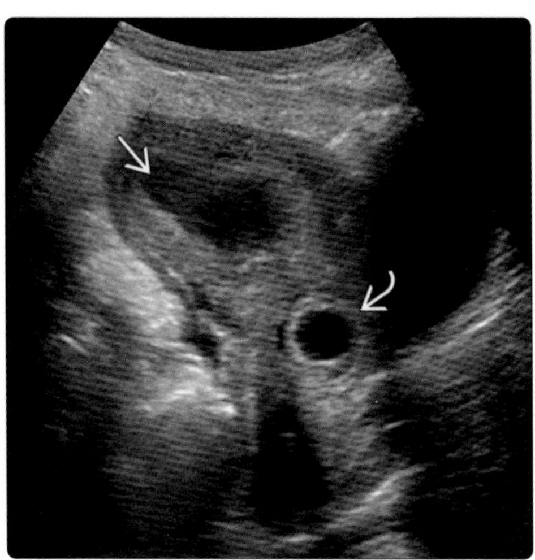

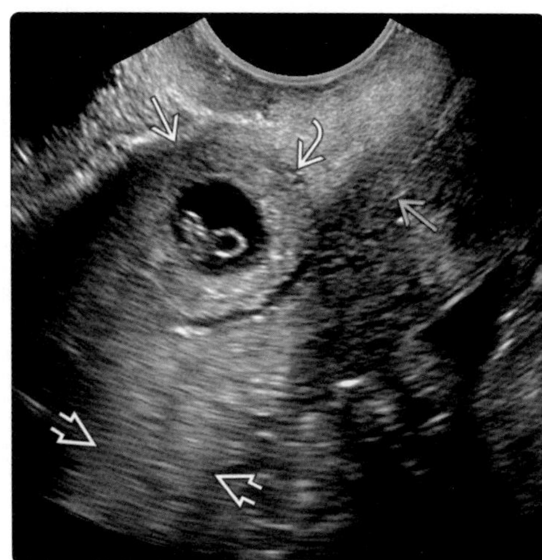

(Left) *Transabdominal US shows a gestational sac ➔ in the low anterior myometrium in a patient with a prior C-section. Also note the fluid ➔ in the endometrial cavity.* **(Right)** *Closer evaluation with transvaginal US shows the gestational sac ➔ eccentrically located in the C-section scar, with no clear covering of myometrium ➔. Decidualized endometrium is present in the uterine cavity ➔. The sac is implanted above the internal os ➔, differentiating it from a cervical ectopic.*

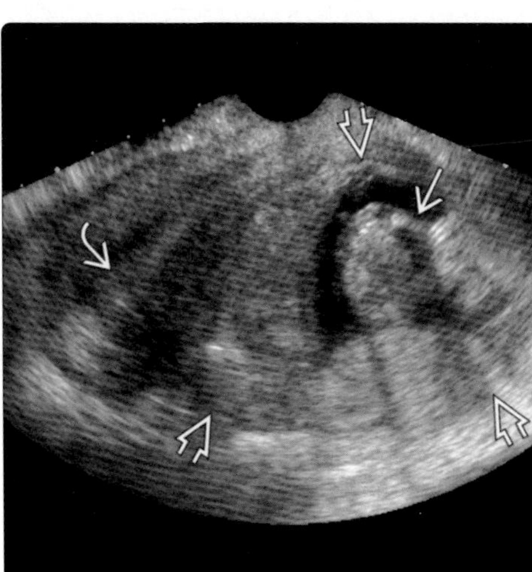

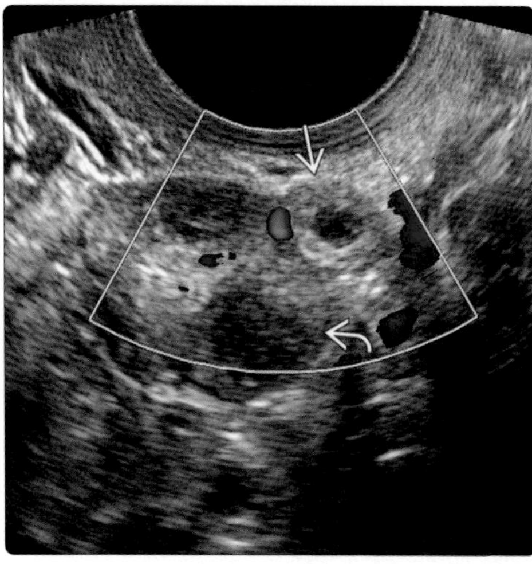

(Left) *Sagittal transvaginal US shows an abdominal ectopic ➔, which has implanted in the posterior cul-de-sac. The membranes implant on surrounding peritoneal structures ➔. Note the empty endometrial cavity ➔.* **(Right)** *An exophytic echogenic gestational sac ➔ with peripheral flow is seen on the surface of the ovary. The uterus was empty, and the patient had severe adnexal pain. An ovarian ectopic is typically rounder and more echogenic than a corpus luteum cyst ➔.*

PART VI
SECTION 2
Brain and Spine

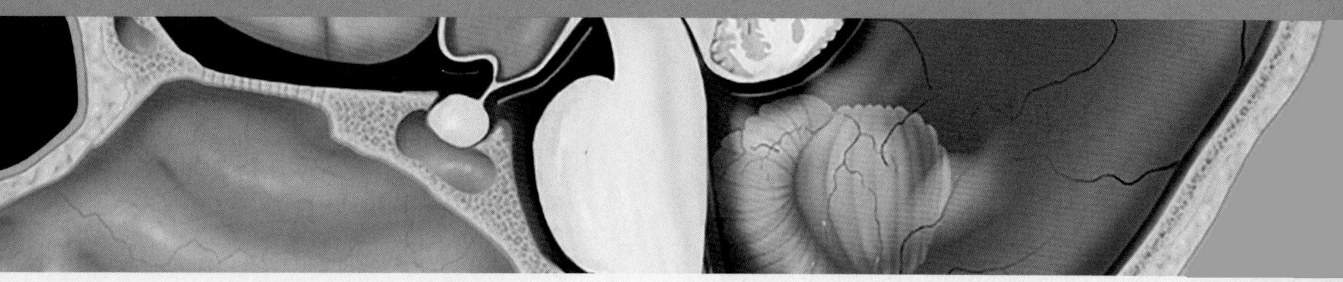

Anatomy and Approach

Brain

Spine

EMBRYOLOGY AND ANATOMY

Key Embryological Concepts

- Multiple processes occur during embryological development of brain and spine
- **Neurulation**: Ectodermal cells form midline neural plate in which folds develop then fuse to create a tube with openings at either end
  - Neurulation → neural tube + neural crest
    - **Neural tube** → brain, spinal cord
    - **Neural crest** → peripheral nerves, autonomic nervous system
- **Neuronal proliferation**: Neurons are "born" in ventricular zone; migrate peripherally to form white/gray matter
  - Glioblast cells provide metabolic/structural support to neurons; ependymal cells produce cerebrospinal fluid
- **Histogenesis**: Process of proliferation, migration, differentiation → development of mature cerebral cortex
  - Cerebral hemispheres formed by 11th week
  - Corpus callosum should be complete by 20 weeks
- **Neuronal migration**: Peak activity occurs from 11-15 weeks; majority of neurons in correct location by 24 weeks; continues up to 35 weeks
- **Myelination**: Occurs in orderly, predictable manner from caudal → cranial, deep → superficial, posterior → anterior
- **Operculization**: Development of insular cortex and infolding of sylvian fissures during weeks 11-28
- **Gyral and sulcal development**: Occurs in predictable fashion; continues through end of 35th week

Anatomy

- Standard scan planes
  - Transventricular: Axial image superior to thalami
    - Size, shape, and orientation of lateral ventricles, choroid plexus, falx
  - Transthalamic: Axial image at level of thalami, includes cavum septi pellucidi (CSP)
    - 3rd ventricle, CSP, cerebellar hemispheres
  - Transcerebellar: Oblique axial image at level of CSP, tipped to include posterior fossa structures
    - Cerebellar hemispheres, vermis, cisterna magna

SCANNING APPROACH AND IMAGING ISSUES

Protocol Advice

- Use highest resolution transducer possible
  - If fetus in cephalic presentation, use vaginal transducer for brain evaluation
  - If fetus in breech presentation, use vaginal ultrasound (US) for distal spine evaluation, particularly in late gestation, obese maternal habitus, or low fluid
  - 9-MHz linear transducer provides exquisite detail of accessible structures
- Image brain in more than axial planes; coronal and sagittal images can be obtained with transducer manipulation
  - 3D volume acquisition allows reconstruction of dataset to "create" true orthogonal image planes
- Use color Doppler to evaluate course of marker vessels
  - Normal anterior cerebral artery branches (callosomarginal and pericallosal) run along corpus callosum
- Fetal MR is a problem-solving tool that can be used to clarify abnormal US findings
- If distal spine looks abnormal, double check bladder, external genitalia, anal dimple
  - Common embryological precursor from caudal cell mass

Scanning Approach to Brain

- Head shape and size
  - Familial head size variants are common
  - Microcephaly usually associated with severe brain abnormalities
  - Macrocephaly may relate to hydrocephalus, megalencephaly, intracranial tumors
  - Head shape may be a key to a diagnosis
    - Cloverleaf: Thanatophoric dysplasia, lemon: Chiari malformation, strawberry: Trisomy 18
  - Cephaloceles are most commonly occipital but may be at other locations
- Midline
  - Falx cerebri creates midline linear echo bisecting cranium, separating cerebral hemispheres
    - Present in severe hydrocephalus, hydranencephaly
    - Absent in alobar holoprosencephaly
      - ▫ Variable posterior component in other forms of holoprosencephaly
    - On coronal images, midline echo continues from falx, lines up with CSP, 3rd ventricle
      - ▫ Subtle abnormality described as distortion of the interhemispheric fissure seen when anterior falx-deficient, medial surface gyri interdigitate across midline
  - CSP should be visible from 18-37 weeks
    - Box-like structure with bright linear echogenic walls surrounding an anechoic space, between frontal horns of lateral ventricles
    - Marker of normal midline development
    - By term, septi often fuse → septum pellucidum with obliteration of the cavum
  - Pitfall: Fornices, just caudal to CSP, create series of parallel black and white lines; do not form a box shape
- Ventricles
  - Lateral ventricles should be symmetric in size with butterfly wing configuration; parallel orientation is abnormal
    - Frontal horns are narrow, almost slit-like at term
    - Widest portion is ventricular atrium; confluence of body with occipital, temporal horns
    - Ventricular diameter measured at atrium, perpendicular to long axis of ventricle, inner edge to inner edge
      - ▫ Should always be ≤ 10 mm
- Cerebral hemispheres
  - Fissures and sulci develop as cortical mantle grows
    - Fissures are deeper infoldings than sulci with fixed position on cerebral surface
      - ▫ Sulci are shallower, more subject to individual variation
    - Interhemispheric fissure seats falx cerebri, traverses brain from anterior to posterior
    - Sylvian fissure initially appears as shallow indentation on lateral surface of brain (~ 18 weeks)

      - ▫ Indentation deepens, becomes "squared off," shaped like an open box (~ 24 weeks)
      - ▫ Eventually becomes covered by process of opercularization, which is not complete until term
  - Gestational age when sulcus/fissure should be seen
    - Sylvian: US at 18 weeks, MR at 24 weeks
    - Parietooccipital: US at 18 weeks, MR at 22-23 weeks
    - Calcarine: US 18 weeks, MR at 22-23 weeks
- Posterior fossa
  - Visually inspect occipital bone contour; cephaloceles may be quite small and subtle
  - Cisterna magna depth is measured in the midline, from posterior surface of vermis to inner table of calvarium
    - Should be < 10 mm throughout gestation
    - Linear echoes in the cisterna magna are thought to be vestigial remnants of the walls of the Blake pouch
  - Normal falx cerebelli bisects posterior fossa
    - If asymmetric position, look for space-occupying lesions (e.g., arachnoid cyst) or asymmetry of hemispheres (e.g., cerebellar hemihypoplasia)
  - Torcular Herophili marks confluence of transverse sinus with straight/superior sagittal sinuses
    - Enlargement of the cisterna magna (e.g., in Dandy-Walker malformation) causes torcular elevation
  - Normal cerebellum is composed of 2 rounded lobes joined in midline by vermis
  - Cerebellar vermis is more echogenic than hemispheres
    - On transcerebellar plane, transverse diameter of echogenic vermis is measured at level of 4th ventricle
    - On sagittal view, craniocaudal diameter can be measured at limits of a line drawn perpendicular to fastigial declive line
    - Tegmentovermian angle is angle between a line along dorsal brainstem surface parallel to tegmentum and a line along ventral surface of vermis
      - ▫ Normal angle is close to zero
      - ▫ Angle < 30 are likely due to Blake pouch cyst
      - ▫ Angle > 45° strongly associated with Dandy-Walker malformation
  - 4th ventricle (V4) assessment is an integral part of vermian evaluation
    - On axial views, V4 is quadrangular with anteroposterior diameter < transverse diameter
    - Fastigial point is the posterior, superior recess of V4
      - ▫ Forms an acute angle at apex of triangular-shaped V4 on sagittal view
    - Declive is cerebellar lobule just inferior to primary fissure
    - Fastigial declive line used as landmark for vermian measurement
  - Brainstem and pons
    - Normal pons creates a prominent bulge anterior to 4th ventricle on sagittal view
    - Biometric data available

Scanning Approach to Spine

- Check alignment in coronal and sagittal planes if possible
  - Coronal plane is best for scoliosis, sagittal plane best for kyphosis
  - If abnormal alignment look for hemivertebrae, block or butterfly vertebrae, spinal dysraphism
- Count segments particularly in lumbar region
  - Mild caudal regression syndrome can be missed as spine may taper where it ends
  - Check that all lumbar and sacral segments are present
- Assess relative size and ossification of vertebral bodies
  - Abnormal ossification and platyspondyly associated with skeletal dysplasia
- Check skin line; should see amniotic fluid between spine and uterine wall to ensure intact skin
  - Myeloschisis has no sac (unlike myelomeningocele), look for defect in skin echo
  - Closed neural tube defects not associated with Chiari malformation; need to look for subcutaneous mass
- Check position of conus
  - By 18 weeks, should be superior to L3/4, above L2/3 by term

Approach to Abnormal Findings

- Characterize abnormalities
  - Is an intracranial finding within the substance of the brain (intraaxial) or not (extraaxial)?
    - Differential diagnosis is different for intraaxial vs. extraaxial lesions
  - Is a mass cystic or solid?
    - If cystic, is it vascular? Use color Doppler!
    - If cystic, is it a developmental abnormality or a destructive process?
      - ▫ A porencephalic cyst **replaces** a focal area of brain destruction, arachnoid cyst is a space-occupying lesion **displacing** adjacent brain
      - ▫ A schizencephalic cleft is due to abnormal neuronal migration → local abnormality of brain architecture
  - Is a spine alignment fixed or variable? More likely to be structural if fixed
- Is the finding isolated?
  - Aneuploidy or syndrome more likely with multiple abnormalities

Imaging Pitfalls

- Normal structures mistaken for pathology
  - Yolk sac confused with cephalocele in 1st trimester
  - Rhombencephalon confused with posterior fossa cyst in 1st trimester
  - Fluid in ventricular atrium mistaken for choroid plexus cyst
  - Fornices mistaken for CSP
  - Rotation of vermis may be mistaken for vermian dysgenesis
- Unossified coccyx confused with dermal sinus
- Failure to recognize interrupted skin line in myeloschisis
- Failure to recognize vascular lesions; misdiagnosed as cystic mass unless color Doppler used

1ST-TRIMESTER EMBRYO

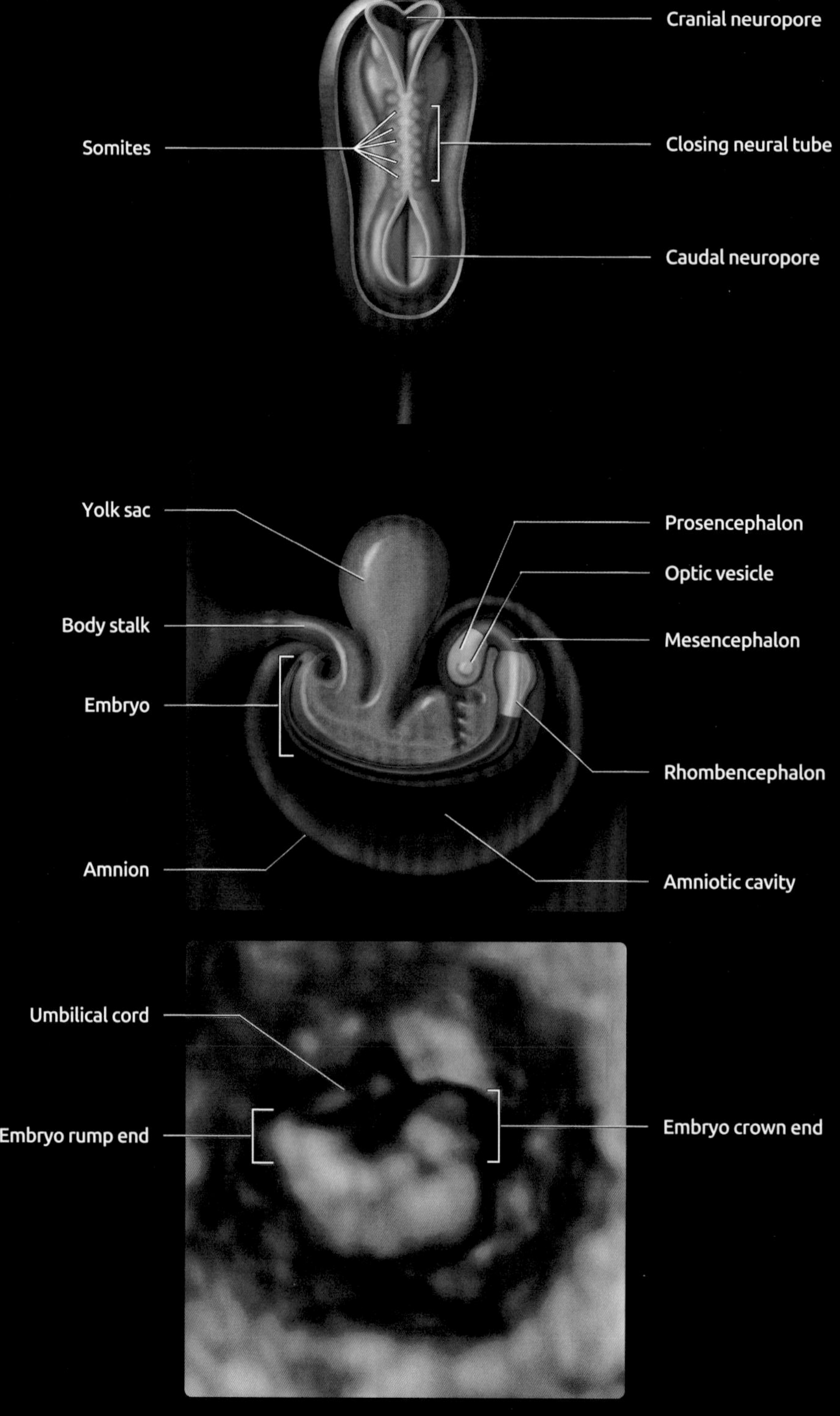

(Top) *The neural tube forms when the folds of the neural plate fuse to form a cylinder. It closes in a bidirectional manner. The cranial neuropore closes at day 24, while the caudal neuropore closes at day 25.* **(Middle)** *A series of vesicles develop at the same time the head end of the embryo enlarges and the flat embryonic disc becomes curved in profile and tubular in cross section. These are the precursors to the adult brain. The prosencephalon (green) gives rise to the forebrain, the mesencephalon (purple) to the midbrain, and the rhombencephalon (light blue) to the hindbrain.* **(Bottom)** *Surface-rendered 3D US of a 7-week embryo shows the external contour with a recognizable head end. The abdominal wall has closed, the yolk sac has detached, and the umbilical cord has formed. The torso is relatively small, and the limb buds have not yet developed, but as shown in the middle graphic, the neural tube within the embryo has already developed the precursors to the forebrain, midbrain, and hindbrain.*

1ST-TRIMESTER EMBRYO

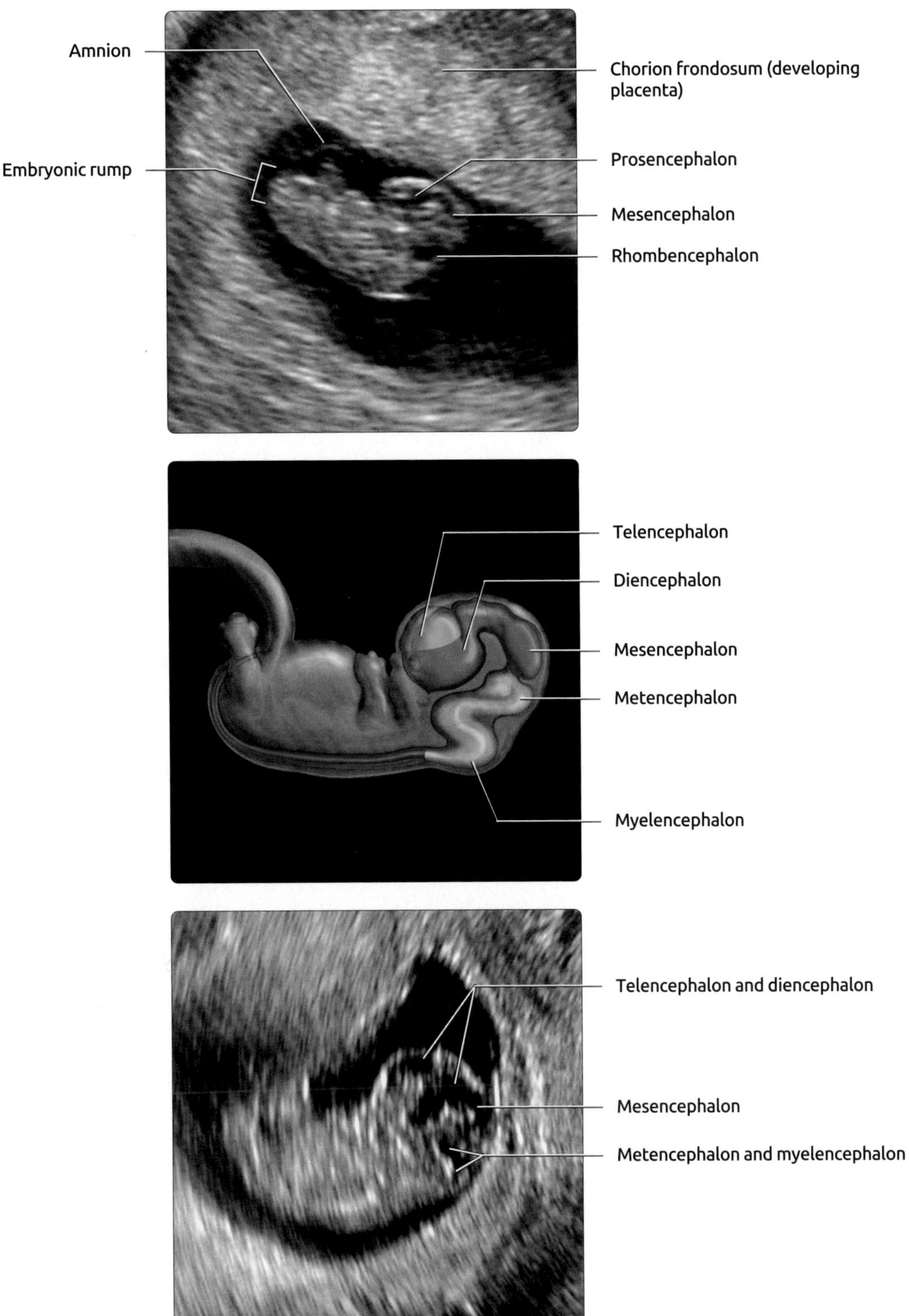

(Top) *This is a vaginal US of an 8-week, 2-day embryo in which the primitive brain vesicles are visible. This is a normal finding with high-resolution modern equipment and should not be mistaken for holoprosencephaly or other brain malformation.* **(Middle)** *With further embryonic growth, the prosencephalon gives rise to secondary vesicles, the telencephalon and diencephalon from which the cerebral hemispheres and thalamus develop. The mesencephalon elongates, while the rhombencephalon gives rise to the secondary vesicles, metencephalon, and myelencephalon. At this point, several flexures develop in the neural tube so that it adapts to the contour of the developing cranium.* **(Bottom)** *Another midline sagittal scan of a slightly older embryo, this time 9 weeks, 6 days, shows further neural tube growth with development of secondary vesicles and multiple flexures in the lengthening tube. Again, it is important to recognize that this is normal for gestational age.*

AXIAL IMAGES: 1ST-3RD TRIMESTER

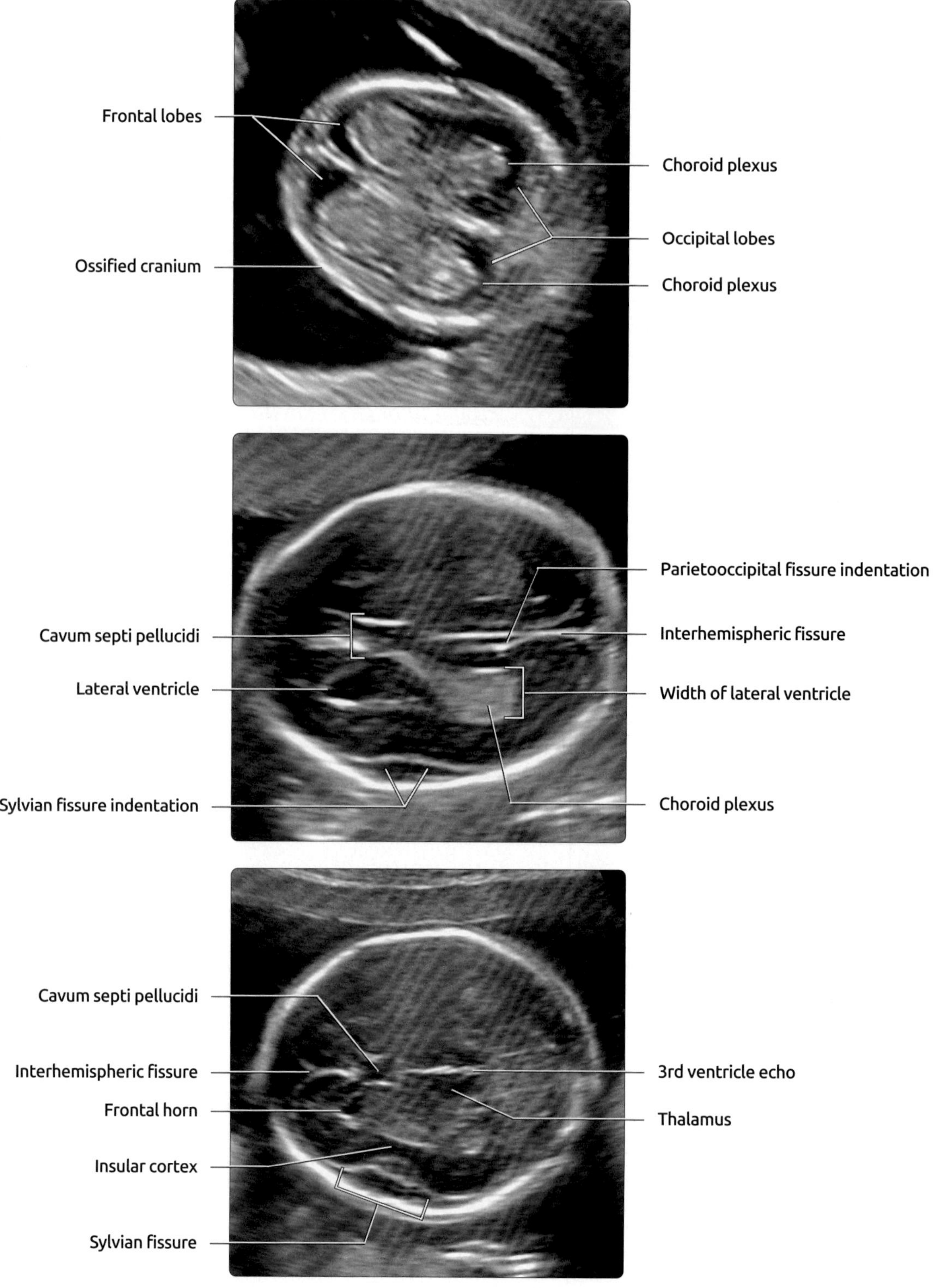

(Top) *At 12 weeks, the choroid plexus fills most of the ventricular cavity and the brain parenchyma is thin and smooth. The choroid plexus echogenicity and shape on an axial image gives rise to the butterfly sign in which the choroid forms the butterfly wings. This confirms 2 cerebral hemispheres. This is very reassuring to a patient who previously had a fetus with alobar holoprosencephaly.* **(Middle)** *At 18 weeks, the cerebral mantle is quite smooth with just the earliest "thumb print" indentation for the sylvian fissure and a tiny indentation at the site of the developing parietooccipital fissure. The latter marks the anatomic location at which the width of the lateral ventricle should be measured.* **(Bottom)** *The sylvian fissure is one of the easiest cortical indentations to see in the fetus. In this 20-week fetus, the sylvian fissure is seen as a groove on the surface of the brain; the walls create obtuse angles with the insular cortex. As the brain grows, the sylvian fissure deepens to a square shape that is then covered by the process of opercularization.*

AXIAL IMAGES: 1ST-3RD TRIMESTER

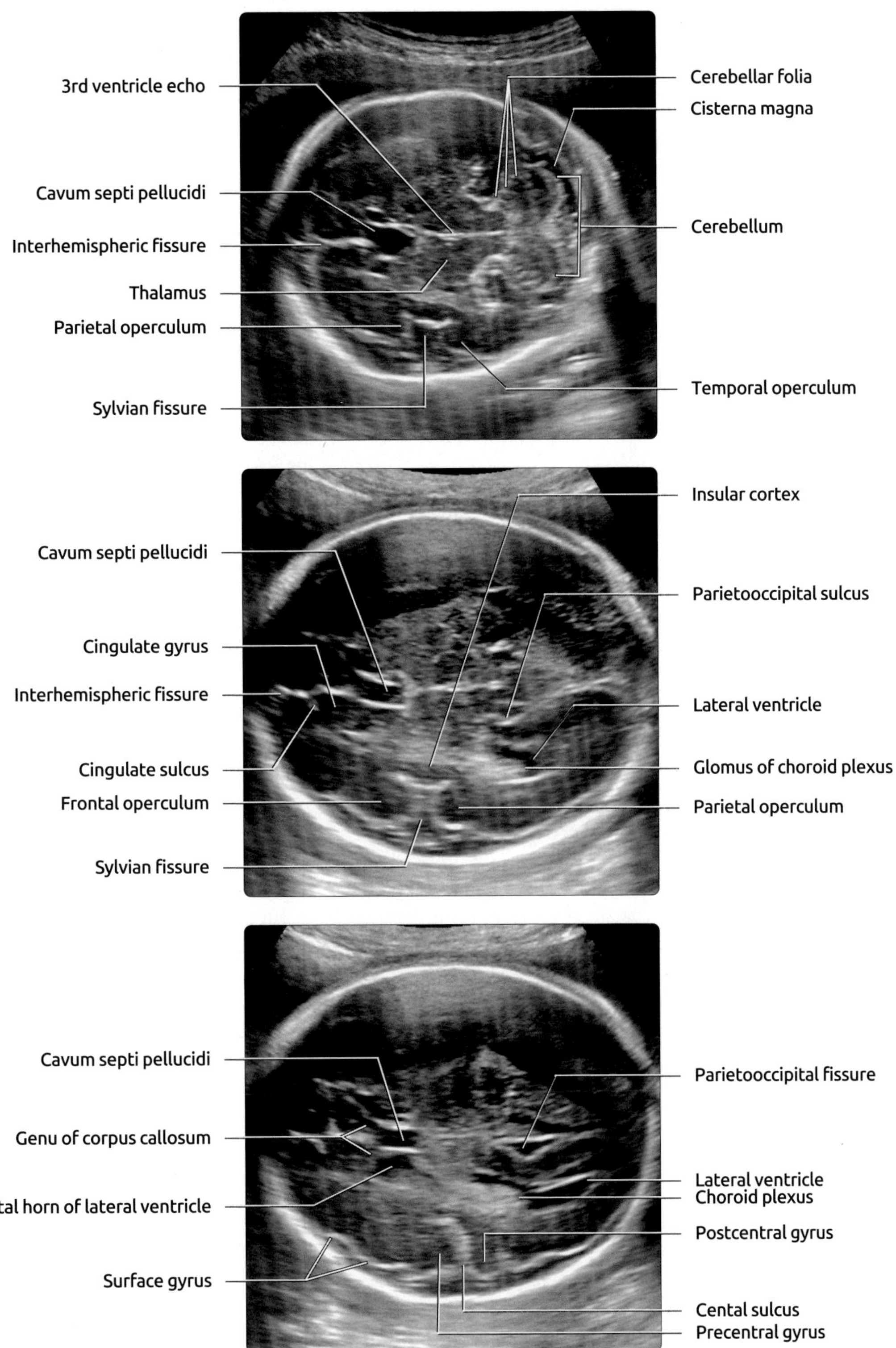

(Top) *As the brain grows and the surface becomes more convoluted, the sylvian fissure deepens and becomes square in profile, like an open box. This is well seen in this 25-week fetus. The temporal and parietal opercula are also now visible.* **(Middle)** *In this 28-week fetus, the opercula have enlarged and "closed the box" of the sylvian fissure. The floor of the box is the insular cortex and the lid of the box is composed of the frontal and parietal opercula. The sylvian fissure separates the parietal lobe superiorly from the temporal lobe inferiorly. The surface of the brain is becoming more convoluted with visible parietooccipital sulcus, cingulate sulcus, and shallow surface gyri.* **(Bottom)** *Even though the corpus callosum is best seen on direct sagittal view, the genu can be identified on the standard axial image obtained at the level of the cavum septi pellucidi (CSP). The genu of the corpus callosum forms the curved part of the so-called anchor complex in the normal anterior brain (the stem of the anchor is created by the interhemispheric fissure). This fetus is at 28 weeks of gestation. Note the increasing number of surface gyri that are now visible.*

PROBLEM SOLVING: CORONAL VIEW

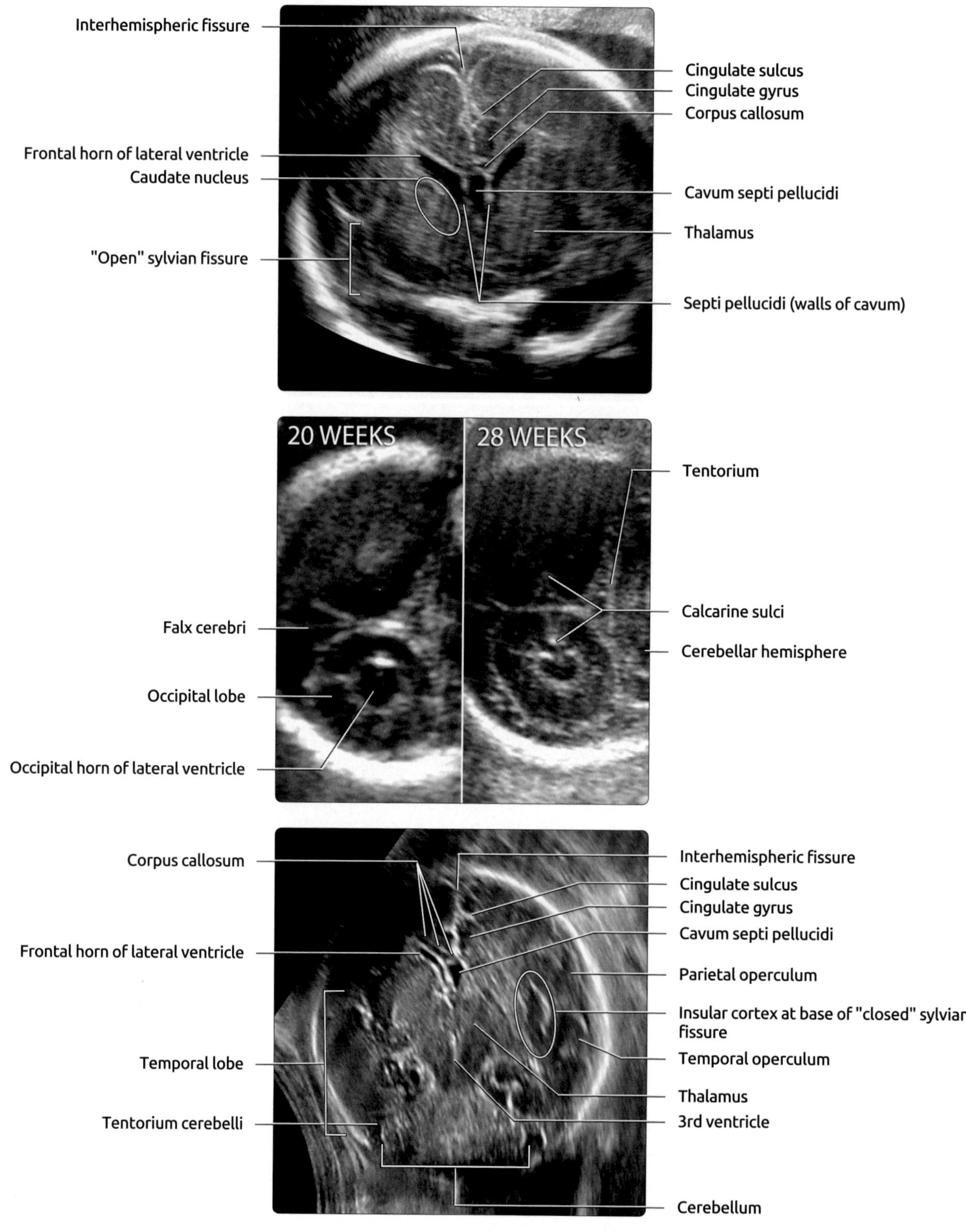

(Top) *A complete neuroanatomic survey requires multiplanar imaging. In this coronal image at 24-weeks gestation, the brain surface is still relatively smooth, but the corpus callosum and cingulate gyrus are well seen.* **(Middle)** *The calcarine sulcus develops on the medial surface of the occipital lobe branching from the parietooccipital sulcus. It is best seen on the coronal plane, since the US beam is then perpendicular to the plane of the sulcus. In this composite image, note how smooth the medial occipital cortex is at 20 weeks. By 28 weeks, the calcarine sulcus is easily visible in the same fetus.* **(Bottom)** *Later in the 3rd trimester (this is a 31-week fetus), the ventricles appear relatively small compared to scans at 20 and 24 weeks. The corpus callosum is thicker and easier to see. The cingulate gyrus and sulcus are well developed. Note that of the sylvian fissure is also complete at this gestational age.*

PROBLEM SOLVING: SAGITTAL VIEW

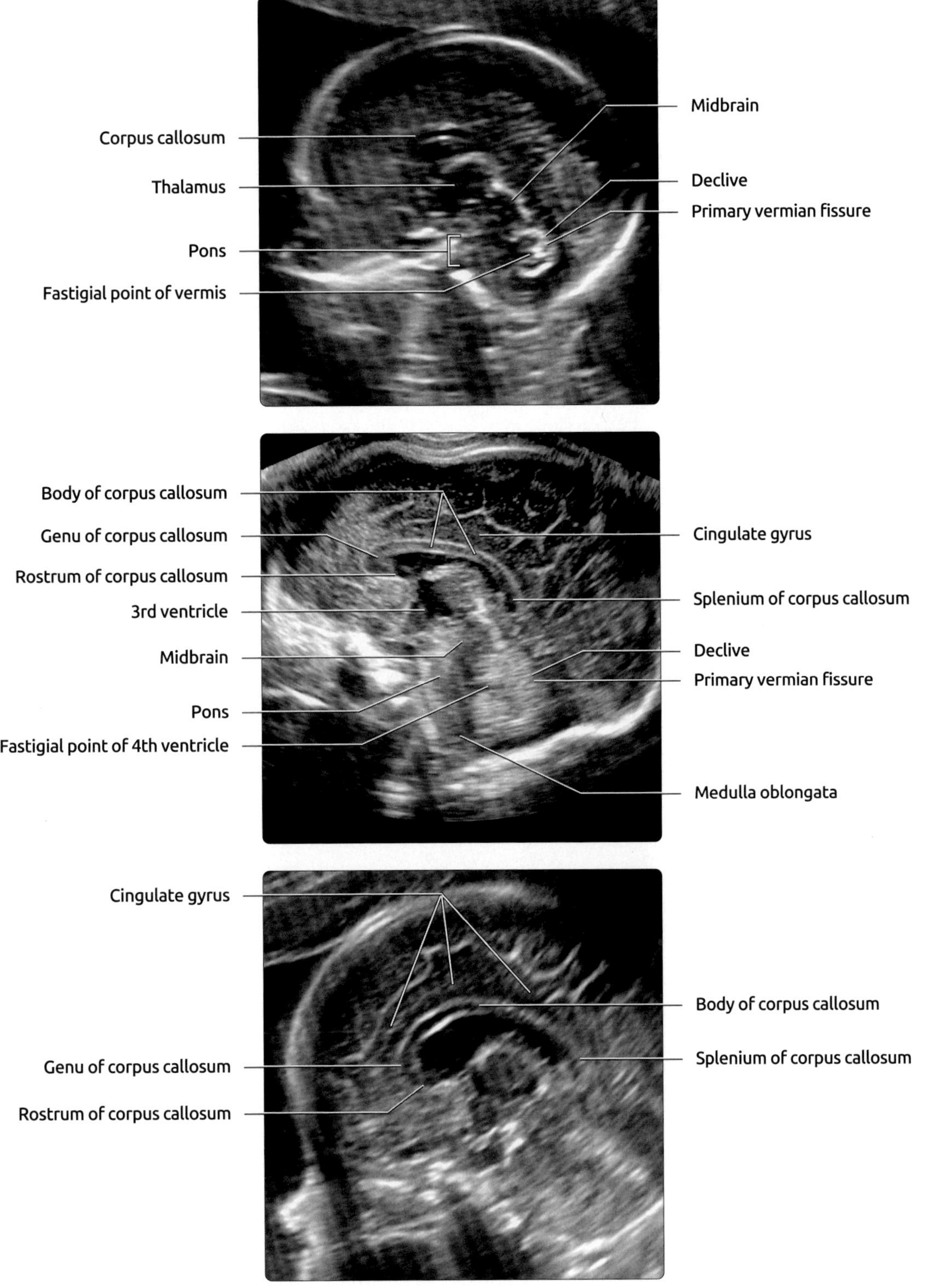

(Top) *A sagittal transabdominal US at 20 weeks shows normal midline structures very well. Although not a standard image in a 2nd-trimester scan, this is essentially the same plane as a profile view of the face. It can be used to verify presence of the corpus callosum if the CSP is difficult to see. It is also useful to assess the relationship of the vermis to the brainstem if there is concern for a posterior fossa cyst.* **(Middle)** *If the fetus is in cephalic presentation, transvaginal US in the 3rd trimester produces exquisite images of normal brain anatomy. In this image, the cingulate gyrus is seen running parallel to the body of the corpus callosum, which is seen in its entirety.* **(Bottom)** *A transabdominal, midline sagittal image at 31 weeks shows the entire corpus callosum as well as the cingulate gyrus, which is on the medial surface of the cerebral hemisphere and runs parallel to the curve of the corpus callosum. This gyrus is absent in agenesis of the corpus callosum, and the medial surface gyri are abnormally oriented creating a sunburst pattern radiating from the 3rd ventricle.*

PITFALLS

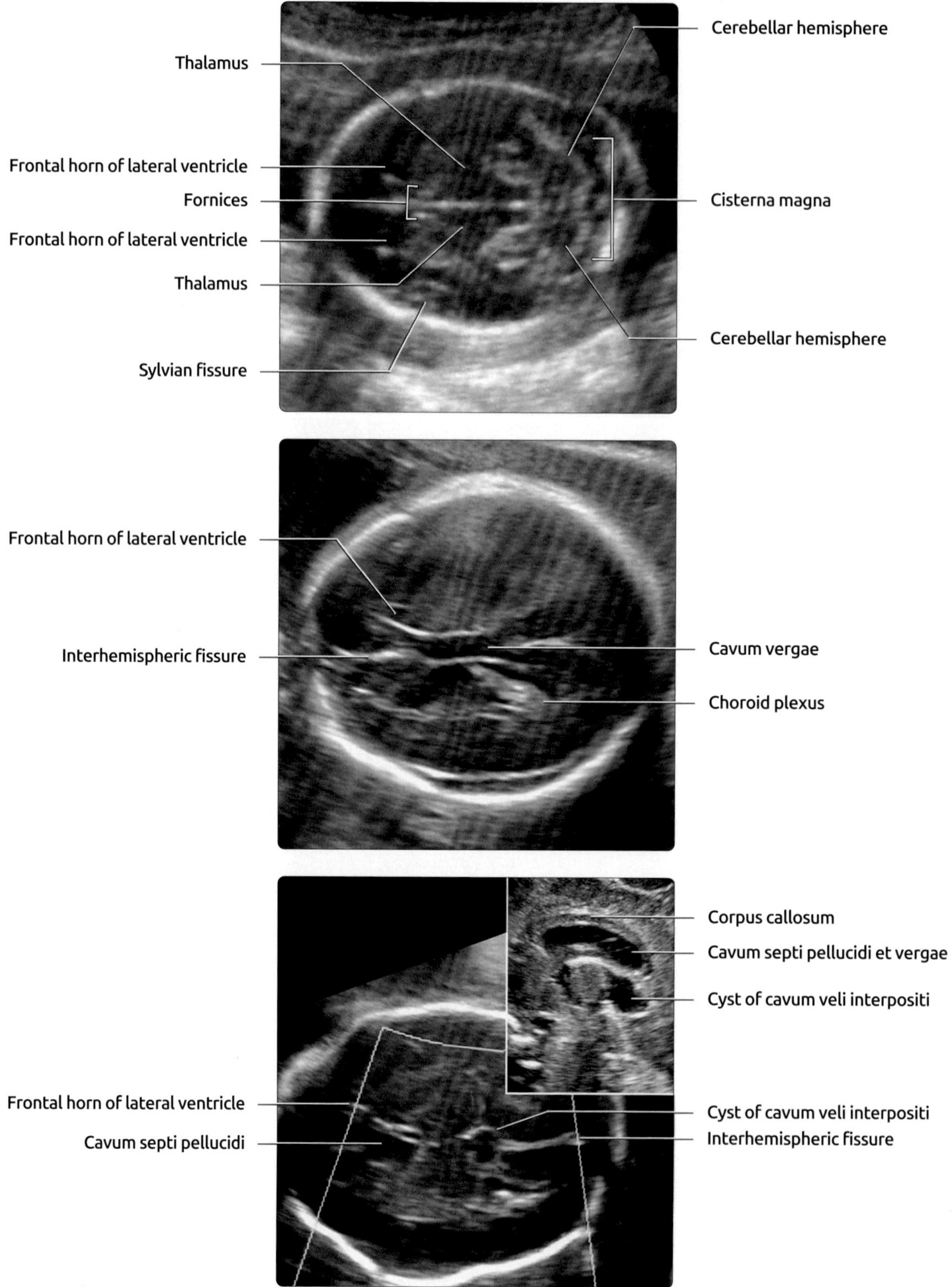

(Top) *This is an example of the fornices in an 18-week fetus. Unlike the CSP, which is a black box outlined by white lines, situated between the frontal homes of the lateral ventricles, the fornices create a series of parallel black and white lines. The fornices may be normal even when the cavum is absent. In some midline brain malformations, the fornices are fused, creating a single black structure that runs anterior to posterior in or above the 3rd ventricle.* **(Middle)** *The cavum vergae is a posterior extension of the CSP, posterior to the anterior columns of the fornix, anterior to the splenium of the corpus callosum. It is a benign anatomic variant and should not be confused with an interhemispheric cyst.* **(Bottom)** *The cavum veli interpositi extends below the splenium of the corpus callosum and the columns of the fornix and reaches as far forward as the foramen of Monro. Within it, a fluid-filled structure > 1 cm in axial measurement with outwardly bowed margins is described as a cavum veli interpositi cyst. The sagittal inset is a postnatal scan in the same case.*

CEREBELLUM

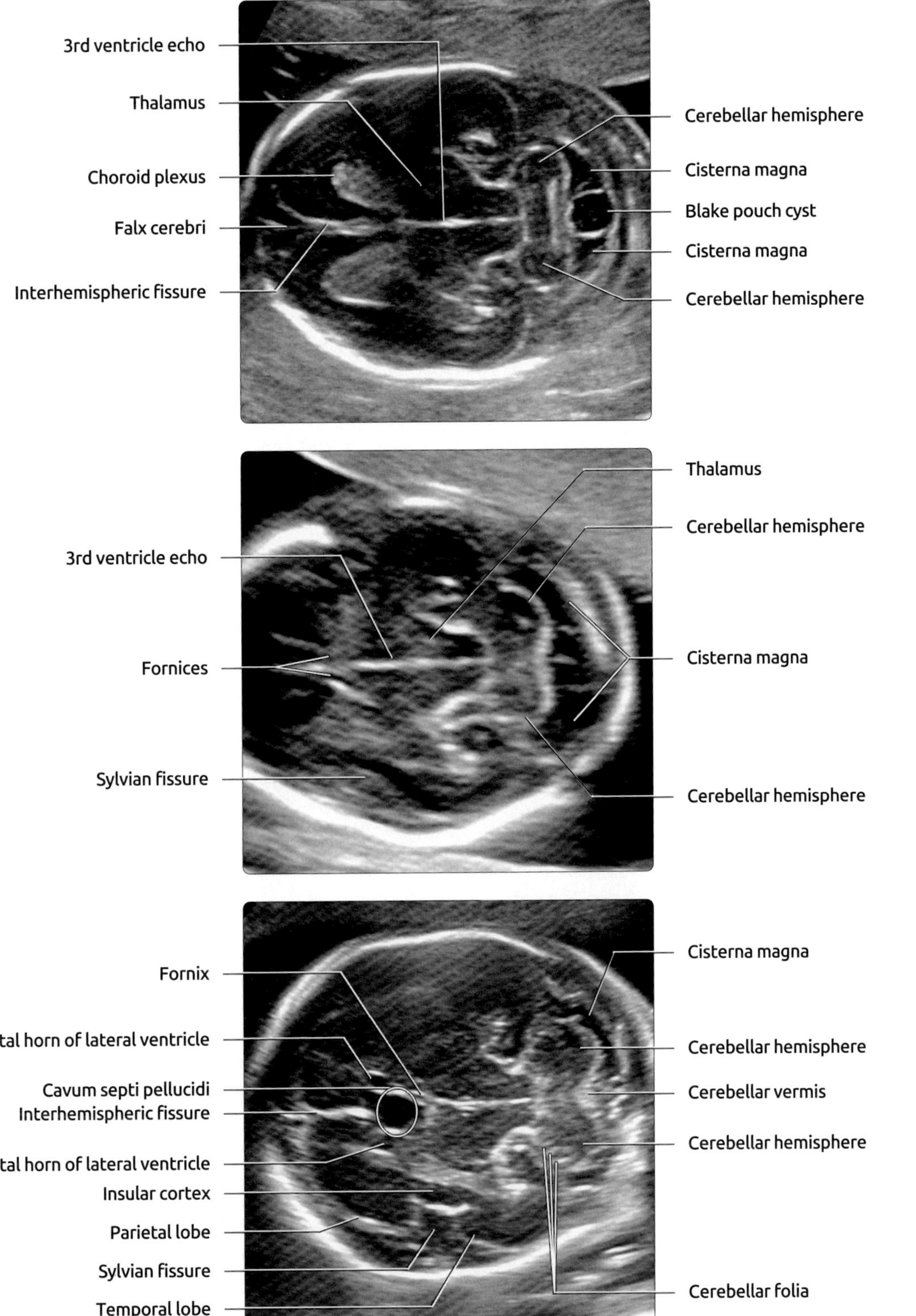

(Top) *This image of an 18-week fetus was obtained using a 9-MHz linear transducer. It shows a persistent Blake pouch in the posterior fossa. Note the biconvex walls and the anechoic contents of the cyst compared to the echogenicity of the fluid in the cisterna magna. Delayed fenestration of the foramina of Luschka and Magendie lead to the persistence of the Blake pouch. It is not the same as a Dandy-Walker malformation and carries an excellent prognosis. In this case, the finding resolved on follow-up, and the infant was normal at birth.* **(Middle)** *The posterior fossa structures are evaluated on the transcerebellar plane. For measurement of the nuchal fold and cisterna magna depth, the CSP is used as a landmark to confirm appropriate obliquity. This image includes the fornices, so it is slightly off axis. At 18 weeks, the hemispheres are round with relatively simple architecture.* **(Bottom)** *In this coronal view of a 25-week fetus, the brain surface is more convoluted. The sylvian fissure is deeper and square in profile, like an open box. The cerebellum is well seen in this projection, which may be used for posterior fossa evaluation when fetal head position precludes the axial oblique view. Note development of more cerebellar folia with increasing gestational age.*

SPINE

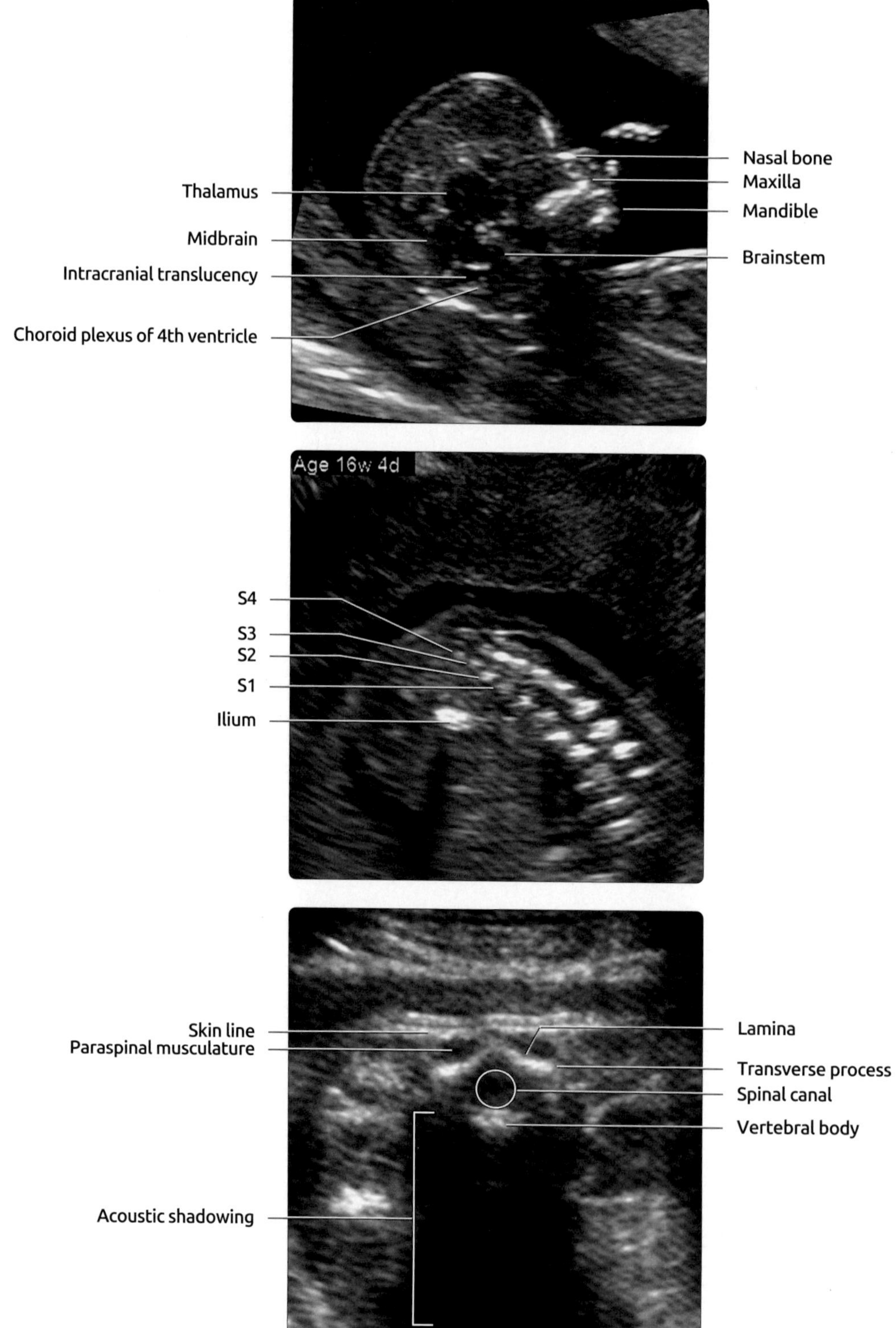

(Top) *Sagittal abdominal US at 13 weeks shows a normal thalamus, midbrain, and brainstem. The intracranial translucency (the future 4th ventricle) is seen between the brainstem and the choroid plexus of the 4th ventricle. Intracranial translucency assessment may play a role in early detection of open neural tube defects.* **(Middle)** *Vaginal transducers are higher MHz than abdominal transducers. Thus, although penetration is decreased, image quality is better. This diabetic patient had a child with severe caudal regression syndrome in her 1st pregnancy, which was complicated by poor diabetic control and no prenatal care. TVUS was used to confirm normal sacral development in this pregnancy.* **(Bottom)** *Ossification of the vertebrae increases with advancing gestational age. There is dense distal acoustic shadowing from the vertebral body in the 3rd-trimester fetus. The lamina are well seen coming together toward the spinous process and creating a teepee appearance. Axial sweeps through the entire spine are necessary to confirm normal laminae and to check the skin line.*

SPINE

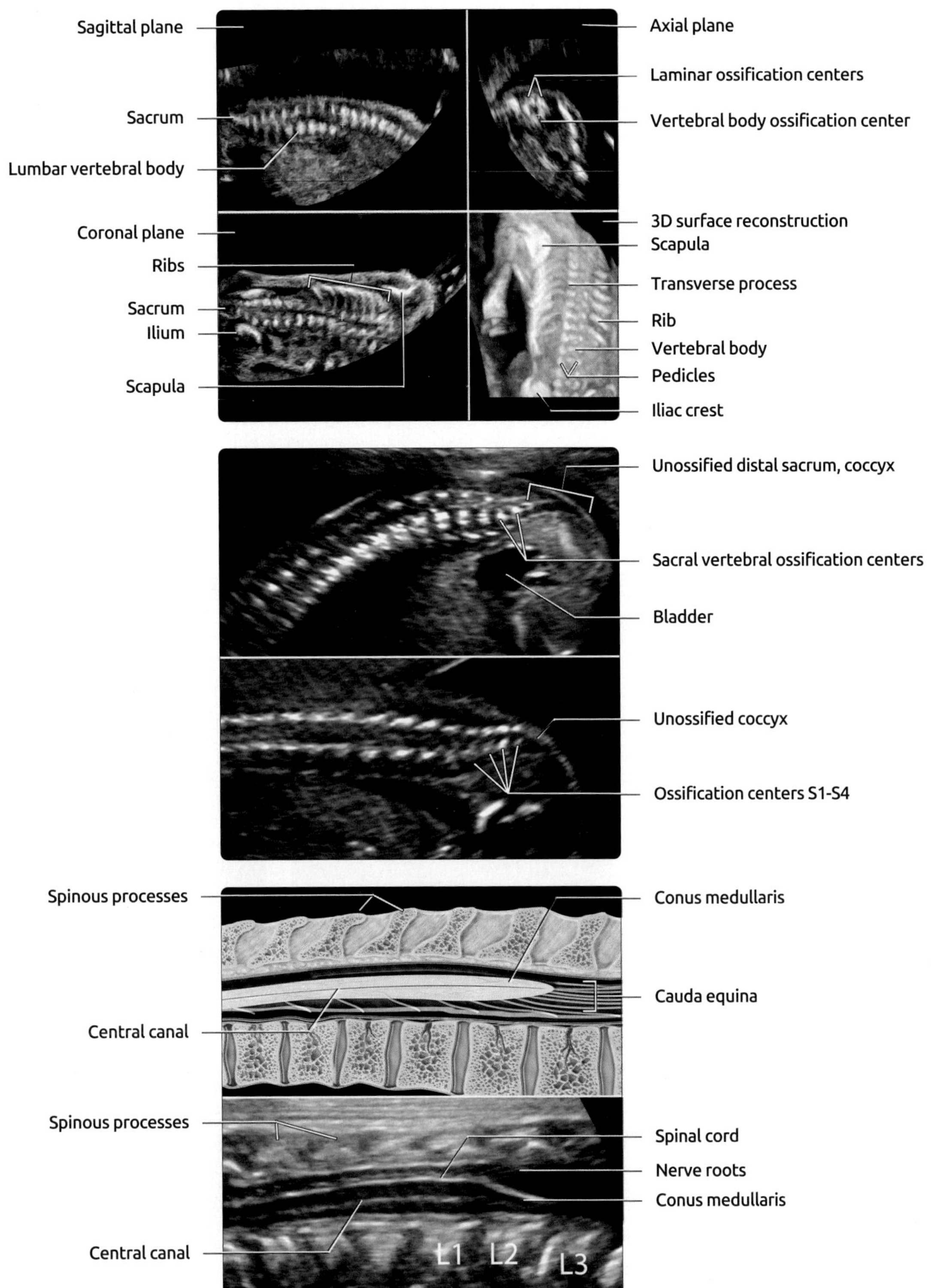

(Top) *3D US is ideal for assessment of the spine, as all 3 planes can be evaluated with a single-volume acquisition. 3D reconstruction using a bone algorithm renders a skeletal view.* **(Middle)** *Sagittal transabdominal US at 18 weeks (top) shows normal ossification and alignment of the lumbar spine. The coccyx and part of the sacrum are unossified, which is an expected finding. At 22 weeks (bottom), there has been more complete ossification. Ossification should be complete by 25 weeks.* **(Bottom)** *Sagittal graphic shows the normal appearance of the lumbar spinal column, conus medullaris, cauda equina, and central spinal canal. A correlative sagittal US of a fetal spine shows the normal hypoechoic appearance of the cord with a hyperechoic central canal. The lumbar portion of the spinal cord widens slightly compared to the thoracic portion. The normal cord ascends during gestation and should be at or above L3-L4 after 18 weeks and L1-L2 by 2 months of age.*

KEY FACTS

TERMINOLOGY

- Exencephaly is early manifestation of anencephaly before neural tissue has worn away

IMAGING

- No calvarium with absence of neural tissue above orbits
  - Neural tissue wears away during gestation until no organized neural tissue remains
  - Cranial defect covered by angiomatous stroma, which gives "lumpy" configuration in 2nd trimester
  - Often contiguous with cervical spine defect
- **Should be able to diagnose routinely at 10-14 weeks**
  - Neural tissue often still present (exencephaly)
  - Head has irregular, flattened, splayed appearance
- Proptotic eyes (described as frog-like appearance)
- Amniotic fluid often echogenic secondary to dissolved neural tissue
  - Polyhydramnios common later in pregnancy

TOP DIFFERENTIAL DIAGNOSES

- Amniotic band syndrome
  - Calvarium may be absent, but large amount of intact brain often remains
  - Look for other defects and presence of fine linear bands
  - Important distinction for counseling, as bands are sporadic and have no increased recurrence risk
    - Exencephaly, anencephaly has 2-5% recurrence risk, and preconceptual folic acid treatment needed for next pregnancy

SCANNING TIPS

- CRL < expected is not always due to incorrect dates
- Endovaginal scanning in 1st trimester for earlier diagnosis
  - May still be difficult diagnosis to make before 10 weeks
  - Visible tissue of exencephaly may be mistaken for normal brain, so examine cranial contour carefully
- Short-term follow-up for any case when head looks asymmetric or irregular

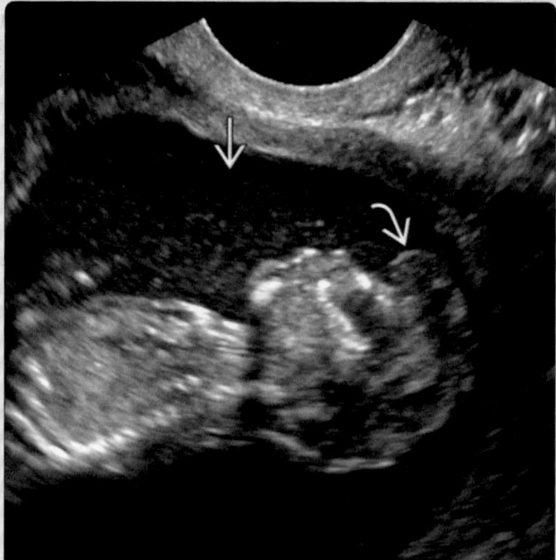

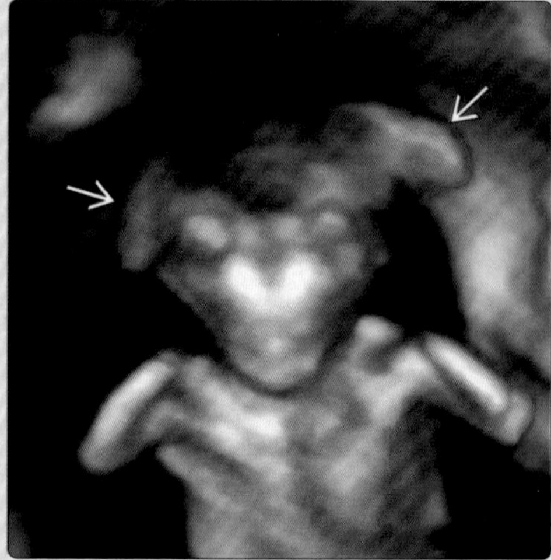

(Left) *Sagittal ultrasound of a 13-week fetus with exencephaly shows no normal cranium and a lobular, exposed brain ➡. As brain tissue erodes, the appearance changes from exencephaly to anencephaly. Note the increased echogenicity of the amniotic fluid ➡ from dissolving neural tissue.* **(Right)** *3D surface reconstruction in the same case confirms no cranium and splaying of remaining brain tissue ➡. This is a lethal malformation, which should be recognized in the 1st trimester.*

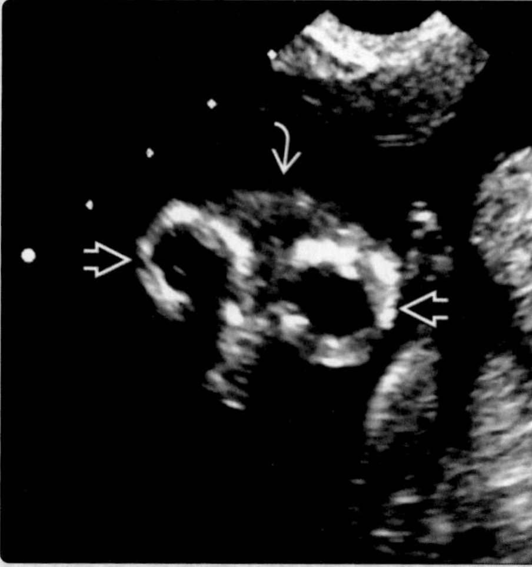

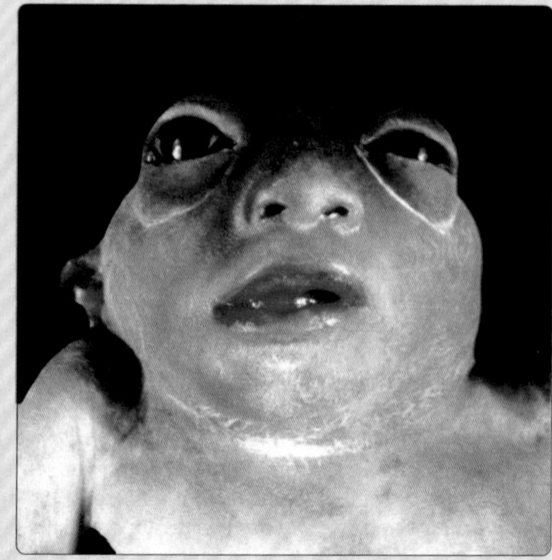

(Left) *By the 2nd trimester, the neural tissue has worn away, and there is now anencephaly. There is marked proptosis of the eyes (frog-like) ➡, and there is near-complete absence of neural tissue ➡ above the orbits.* **(Right)** *Autopsy photograph of an anencephalic fetus illustrates the classic proptotic, frog-like appearance of the eyes. This is secondary to shallow orbits and an abnormally formed skull base. The eyes themselves are normal in size.*

Cephalocele

KEY FACTS

TERMINOLOGY

- Defect in skull with protrusion of intracranial structures
  - Encephalocele: Cerebrospinal fluid (CSF), brain tissue, and meninges
  - Meningocele: Meninges and CSF

IMAGING

- Bony defect should be demonstrated
  - Occipital defect most common and is posterior midline
  - Parietal defect usually midline and higher
- Other CNS anomalies common, including ventriculomegaly (70-80%) and microcephaly (25%)

TOP DIFFERENTIAL DIAGNOSES

- Amniotic band syndrome
  - May cause cranial defect and cephalocele
  - Other body parts often affected, especially extremities
- Cystic hygroma: Cranium intact
  - Septated cystic neck mass; hydrops common
  - In early pregnancy, cystic hygroma often misdiagnosed as cephalocele and vice versa

PATHOLOGY

- Associated with multiple syndromes
- Meckel-Gruber most common genetic disorder
  - Encephalocele, polydactyly, polycystic kidneys

SCANNING TIPS

- Always image from several directions to exclude edge artifact, which may mimic calvarial defect
- Use endovaginal sonography in 1st trimester if any suggestion of irregular head contour transabdominally
- Look carefully for bands as possible cause
  - Roll patient to side to see if fetus remains in fixed position
- Look carefully for other anomalies, which may identify specific syndrome

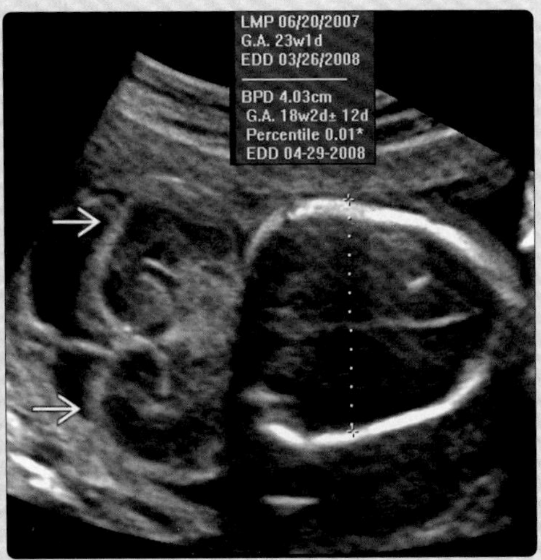

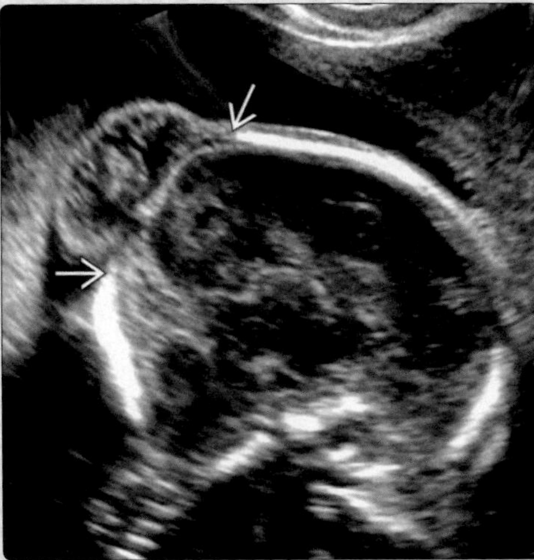

(Left) *Axial US through the fetal brain shows large amounts of cerebrum ➔ in the cephalocele with marked reduction in BPD measurement indicating microcephaly. When a large amount of cerebral tissue is herniated, as in this case, the prognosis is poor.* **(Right)** *Sagittal view of a calvarial defect ➔ is shown. The transvaginal technique provides high-resolution images; 3D volume acquisition is also helpful, as orthogonal planes can be reconstructed from the volume data set.*

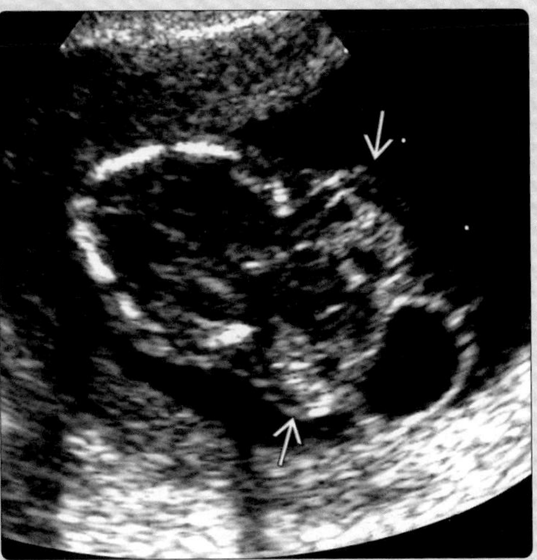

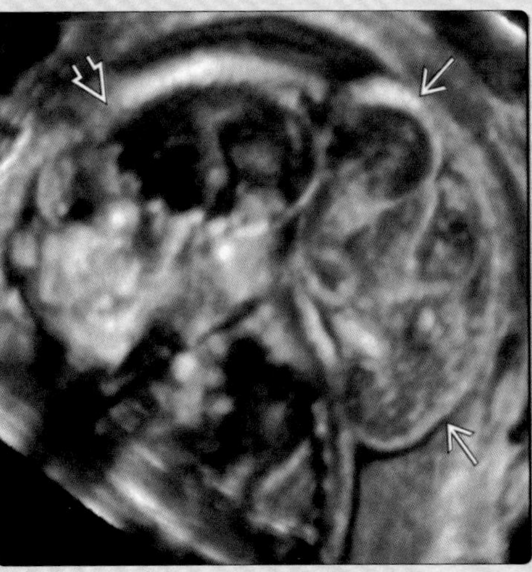

(Left) *Axial transvaginal US shows a large encephalocele ➔. Cephaloceles may be identified in the 1st trimester, and any head irregularity on a transabdominal scan should be further investigated with endovaginal sonography. Genetic counseling should be offered, as cephaloceles may be seen with multiple genetic syndromes, most commonly Meckel-Gruber syndrome.* **(Right)** *3D reconstruction shows dramatic sloping of the forehead ➔, indicating microcephaly with most of the brain contained within the cephalocele ➔.*

Holoprosencephaly

KEY FACTS

TERMINOLOGY

- Alobar holoprosencephaly (HPE) implies complete or nearly complete lack of cerebral hemisphere separation

IMAGING

- 1st trimester: Absent butterfly sign
  - Both choroids normally seen as "butterfly wings"
- 2nd/3rd trimester
  - Absent midline structures, fused thalami
  - Monoventricle: Crescent-shaped, centered on midline
  - Dorsal cyst: Distended 3rd ventricle as fused thalami prevent normal CSF flow

TOP DIFFERENTIAL DIAGNOSES

- Hydranencephaly (falx is present)
- Aqueductal stenosis (falx is present)

PATHOLOGY

- Chromosomal abnormalities in 25-50%, mostly trisomy 13
- Infants of diabetic mothers have 1% risk

SCANNING TIPS

- Be vigilant at time of nuchal translucency screening as can make diagnosis of alobar HPE
- Use vaginal ultrasound if limited brain visibility on abdominal imaging
- Use 3D US to characterize facial anomalies
  - Facial malformations of any kind should trigger very careful evaluation of brain
  - Cyclopia, hypotelorism, absent nose, proboscis, midline cleft all associated with HPE, trisomy 13
- Look at head shape; normal head is oval in cross section
  - If head is round in all scan planes, look for brain malformation
- Look for additional findings of trisomy 13
  - Echogenic kidneys, polydactyly, cardiac anomalies, omphalocele
  - Growth restriction, which is often early onset

(Left) *Axial ultrasound at 20 weeks shows absent midline structures, a monoventricle ➡, and a continuous anterior rind of cerebral tissue ⇒. These are characteristic findings of alobar holoprosencephaly (HPE). Absence of the falx differentiates alobar HPE from other causes of a fluid-filled cranium.* **(Right)** *Axial transabdominal ultrasound in a different case at 17 weeks shows the characteristic monoventricle ➡, continuous mantle of brain ➡, and fused thalami ➡.*

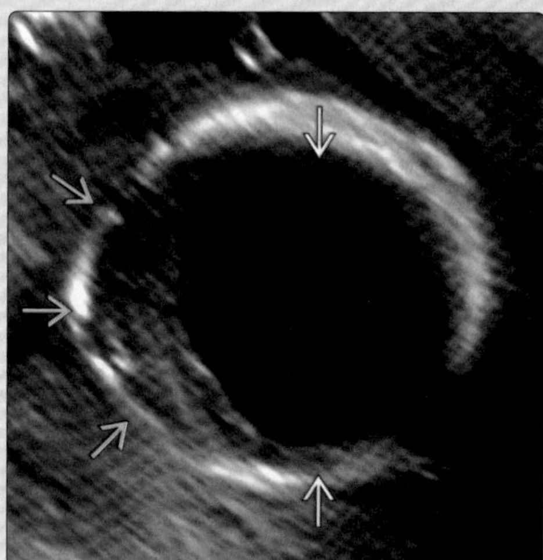

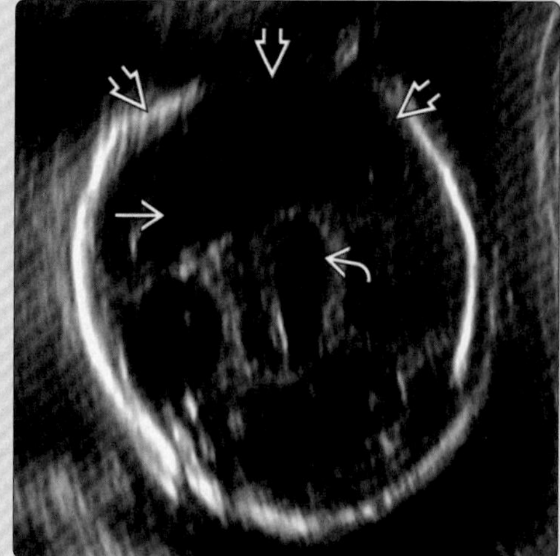

(Left) *Coronal transvaginal ultrasound in the 3rd trimester shows a continuous mantle of noncleaved cerebral cortex ➡ above the fused thalami ➡. These are characteristic findings in alobar HPE.* **(Right)** *Coronal section through the brain of similar case of alobar HPE demonstrates no evidence of an interhemispheric fissure with fusion of the rudimentary hemispheres ➡ across the midline. The central monoventricle ⇒ is horseshoe-shaped. (From Osborn's Brain.)*

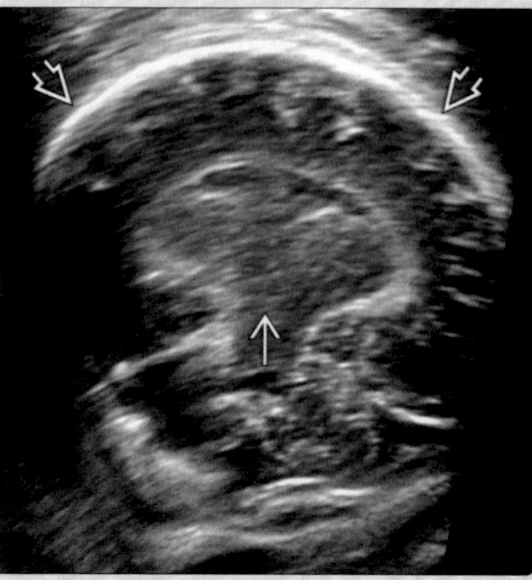

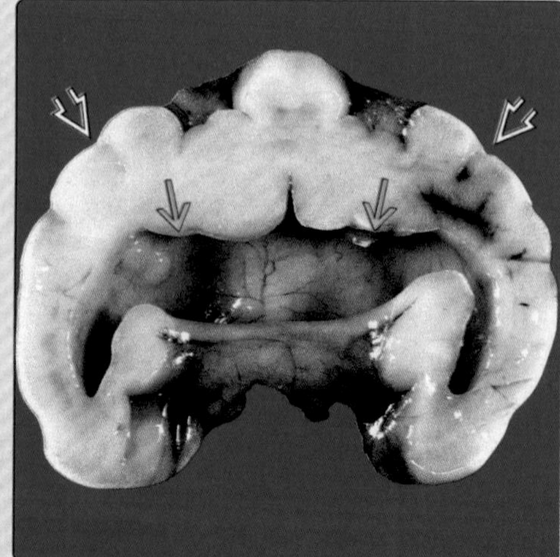

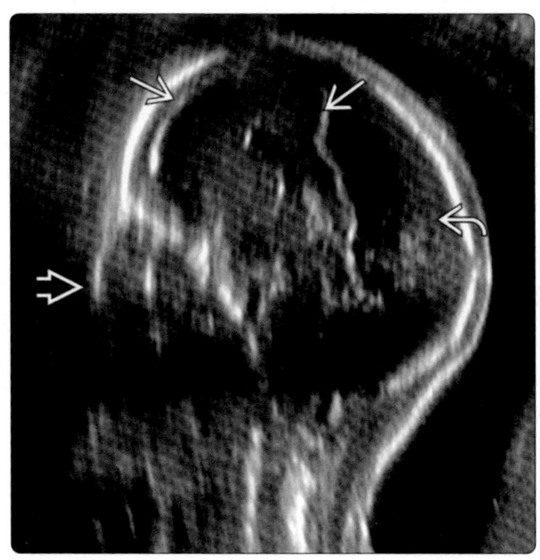

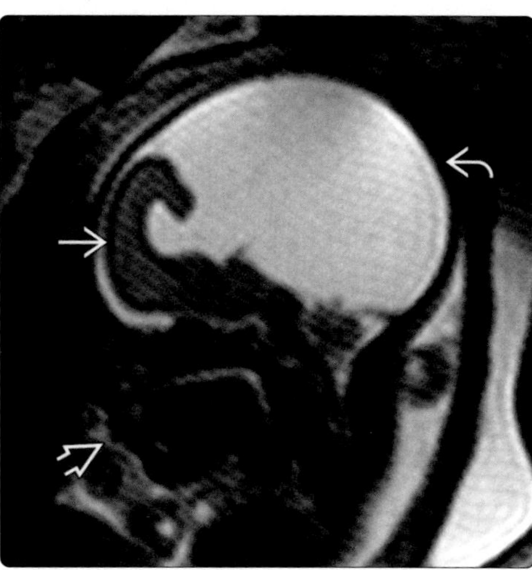

(Left) *Sagittal ultrasound of a 2nd-trimester fetus shows the abnormal brain tissue ➡ in alobar HPE "cupping" a dorsal cyst ↩. The dorsal cyst is thought to be an expansion of the posterior and dorsal portions of the 3rd ventricle because the fused thalami block normal egress of cerebrospinal fluid. Note the abnormal, flat profile ⇨.* **(Right)** *Sagittal T2WI MR scan shows similar "cup" brain morphology ➡ with abnormal brain surrounding a large dorsal cyst ↩. The profile ⇨ is normal in this case.*

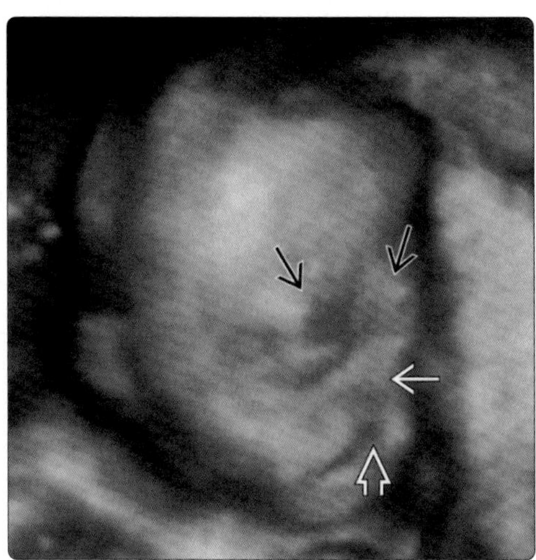

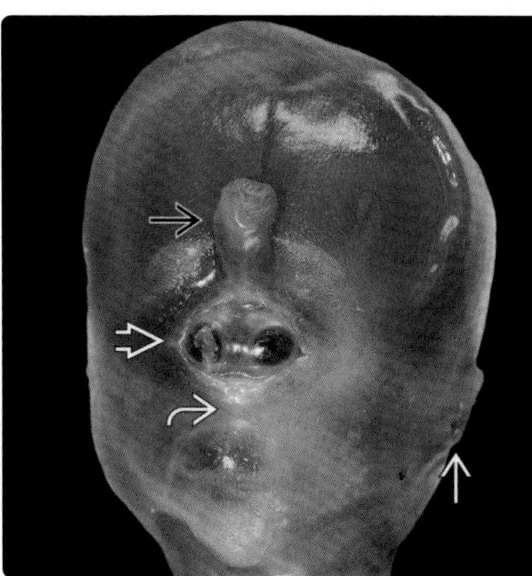

(Left) *3D ultrasound of the face shows midline cleft lip ⇨, severe hypotelorism ➡, and an abnormal, flattened nose ➡ in a fetus with premaxillary agenesis associated with ALHPE. Remember "the face predicts the brain" and any facial abnormality should trigger a careful evaluation of the brain.* **(Right)** *Autopsy image following termination of pregnancy for trisomy 13 shows a proboscis ➡, cyclopia with a single orbit ⇨, absent philtrum ↩, and low-set ears ➡.*

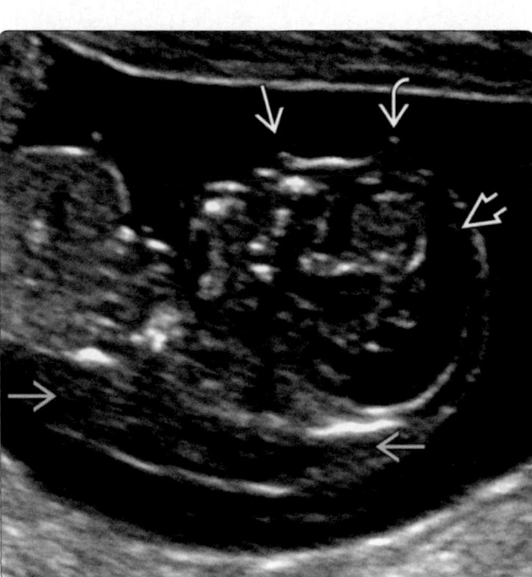

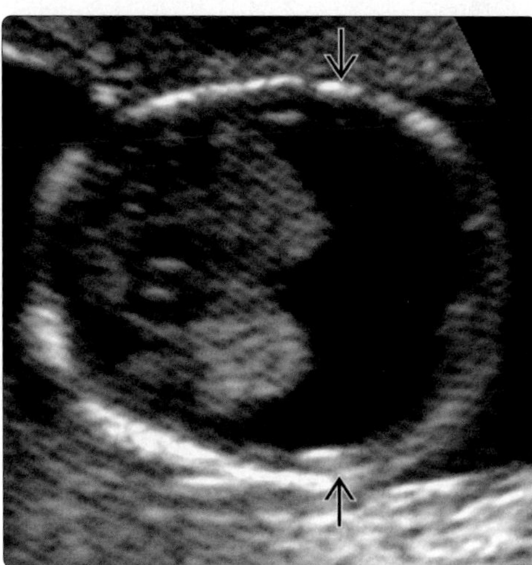

(Left) *Parasagittal ultrasound obtained at the time of 1st-trimester screening shows an abnormal profile ➡, a small proboscis ⇨, monoventricle ➡, and thick nuchal translucency ↩.* **(Right)** *Axial TVUS at 12 weeks shows a monoventricle ➡ and lack of expected midline structures. TVUS was performed as the brain looked odd at the time of NT screening. Chorionic villus sampling in this case revealed triploidy. Attention to detail allows early diagnosis of this severe brain malformation; alobar HPE is considered lethal.*

KEY FACTS

TERMINOLOGY

- Complete absence of corpus callosum (CC)
- May be partially present but abnormal (dysgenesis)

IMAGING

- Mild ventriculomegaly often 1st clue
- **Absent cavum septi pellucidi (CSP)**
  - CSP: Anechoic, box-shaped midline structure between frontal horns of lateral ventricles
  - Do not mistake paired fornices for CSP
- Axial plane
  - Absent CSP, **teardrop-shaped ventricles (colpocephaly)**, parallel lateral ventricles
  - May see associated interhemispheric cyst or lipoma
- Coronal plane
  - Absent CSP, Texas longhorn morphology to anterior horns of lateral ventricles, nonvisualization of CC
- Midline sagittal plane
  - Absent or abnormal CC
  - Radial, spoke-wheel, sunray appearance of medial gyri radiating to 3rd ventricle
  - Abnormal vertical course and branching of anterior cerebral artery
    - Normally pericallosal branch parallel to CC, callosomarginal parallel to cingulate gyrus

TOP DIFFERENTIAL DIAGNOSES

- Mild ventriculomegaly: Ventricles have normal shape

SCANNING TIPS

- Scan in all 3 planes in any fetus with absent CSP
- Look at shape of ventricles: Colpocephaly strongly associated with callosal abnormalities
- Look for AVID complex
  - **A**symmetric **v**entriculomegaly, **i**nterhemispheric cyst, **d**ysgenesis of CC
- ACC seldom isolated; look for other anomalies in brain (50%) and body (60%)

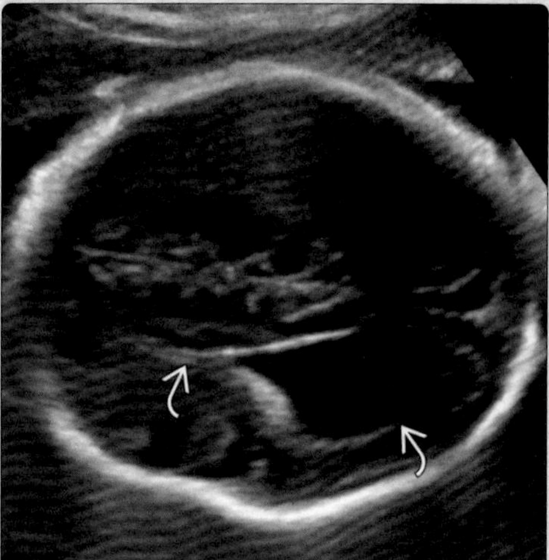

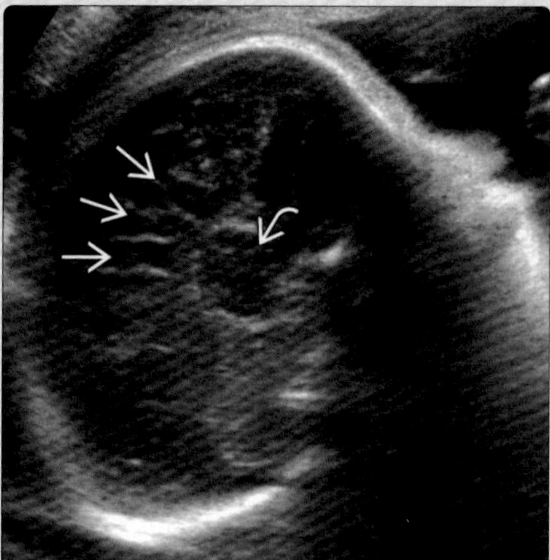

(Left) *Axial brain US shows teardrop-shaped lateral ventricles, pointed in the front and wide in the back. This is known as colpocephaly, which is strongly associated with agenesis of the corpus callosum and helps to distinguish it from hydrocephalus of another etiology.* **(Right)** *Sagittal US shows radially oriented gyri converging on the 3rd ventricle. Use color Doppler in this plane to look for abnormal course/branching of anterior cerebral artery into pericallosal and callosomarginal branches.*

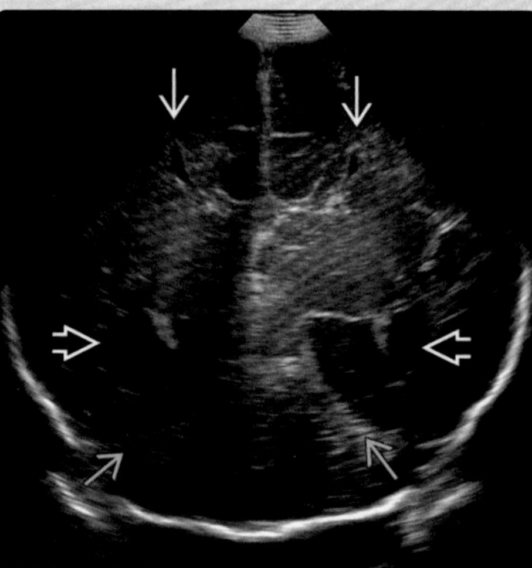

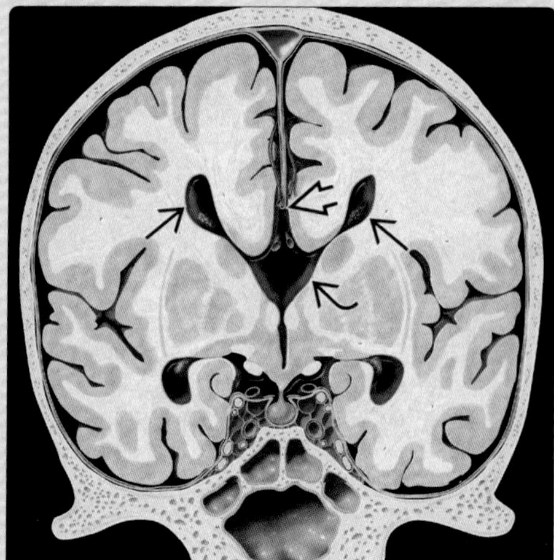

(Left) *Coronal oblique neonatal head US shows the typical Texas longhorn appearance of the anterior horns and the dilated occipital horns of colpocephaly. Tentorium is noted. Coronal views in the fetus appear the same. If presentation is cephalic, TVUS provides excellent detail.* **(Right)** *Coronal graphic shows callosal agenesis with widely spaced lateral ventricles. The 3rd ventricle is elevated and is contiguous superiorly with the interhemispheric fissure.*

KEY FACTS

TERMINOLOGY

- Choroid plexus cysts (CPC) are unilocular cysts usually located in the posterior thick portion of choroid plexus

IMAGING

- CPC are most often incidental isolated findings
  - Almost all resolve by 32 weeks
  - Might be large, multiple, or bilateral
  - Not associated with aneuploidy in low-risk patients
- CPC may be seen in trisomy 18 (T18)
  - Anomalies and growth restriction almost always present
    - Cardiac and extremity anomalies common
  - CPC > 10 mm associated with mild ↑ risk for T18
  - Multiple and bilateral CPC do not ↑ risk for T18

TOP DIFFERENTIAL DIAGNOSES

- Intraventricular hemorrhage
  - Blood clot adherent to choroid might mimic CPC
  - Echogenic ventricular wall, ventriculomegaly
- Choroid plexus papilloma (rare)
  - Vascular mass, ventriculomegaly

DIAGNOSTIC CHECKLIST

- Is patient low risk for aneuploidy? Has she had testing?
  - Cell-free DNA test results (best)
  - Maternal serum biochemistry results
  - Consider genetic counseling if patient has had no testing
- Follow-up to show CPC resolution is not necessary

SCANNING TIPS

- Do detailed scan of fetus when CPC is seen
  - Extra cardiac views
    - Outflow and inflow tract views
  - Extra extremity views
    - Open hands, normal feet
- Scan in multiple planes to show cyst located in choroid
  - Large cysts may be mistaken for ventriculomegaly
  - Normal fluid-filled atria may mimic CPC

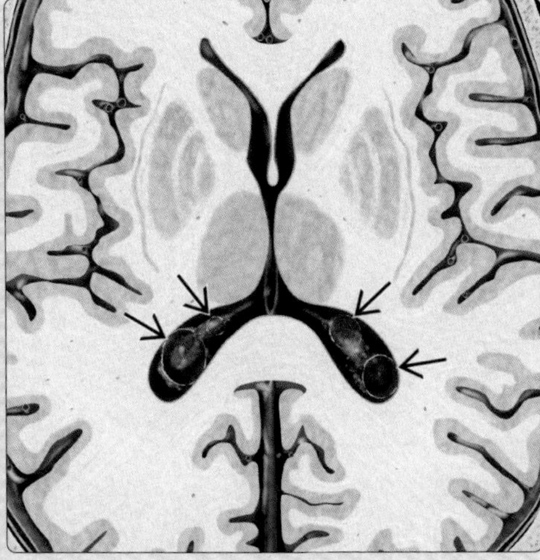

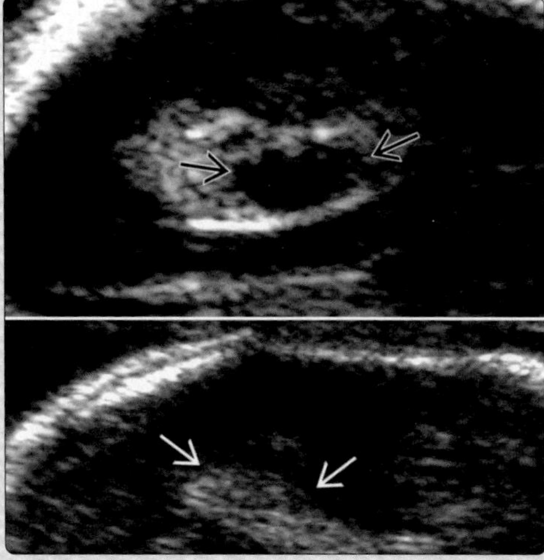

(Left) *Graphic representation of CPC ⇒ occurring in the posterior, thick portion of the choroid plexus (glomus of choroid) is shown. The choroid plexus produces cerebrospinal fluid, and CPCs are considered "entrapment cysts".* **(Right)** *Top image shows a small right CPC ⇒ at 20 weeks. The bottom image shows a normal CP ➡ at 28 weeks in the same fetus. Almost always, CPCs resolve by the 3rd trimester. An isolated CPC in a low-risk patient is not associated with aneuploidy and follow-up to show resolution is not necessary.*

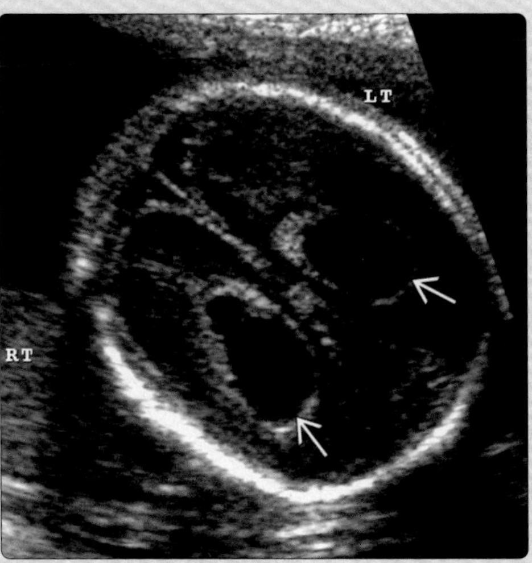

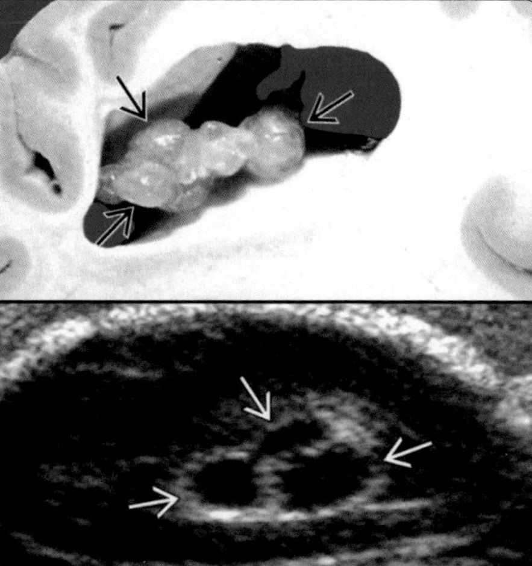

(Left) *Bilateral, symmetrical, large CPCs ➡ can mimic ventriculomegaly when imaged in the axial view. Large CPCs can fill the atria of the lateral ventricles, the same area measured for ventricular diameter.* **(Right)** *Gross pathology of clustered CPC ⇒, top image, matches the US finding of clustered CPCs ➡ from another case. Clustered cysts are common and resolve with advancing pregnancy. They do not increase the patient's risk for aneuploidy if she is a low-risk patient.*

Arachnoid Cyst

KEY FACTS

TERMINOLOGY

- Cerebrospinal fluid collection enclosed within layers of arachnoid membrane (i.e., extraaxial location inside skull but outside brain)

IMAGING

- Usually single, extraaxial, thin walled, smoothly marginated, avascular, anechoic
  - 2/3 supratentorial (i.e., adjacent to cerebral hemispheres)
  - 1/3 in posterior fossa (i.e., adjacent to cerebellum)
- Exerts mass effect displacing adjacent brain parenchyma or major cerebral vessels
- Underlying brain sonographically normal in majority of cases, but adjacent calvarium may be thinned, scalloped

TOP DIFFERENTIAL DIAGNOSES

- Porencephalic cyst: Replaces destroyed brain
- Schizencephaly
  - Cleft in brain substance, wedge-shaped rather than round, absent cavum
- Interhemispheric cyst/AVID
  - **A**symmetric **v**entriculomegaly with **i**nterhemispheric cyst and **d**ysgenesis of corpus callosum
- Dandy-Walker malformation
  - Posterior fossa cyst in continuity with 4th ventricle

SCANNING TIPS

- Always check Doppler in apparent cyst to rule out vascular malformation
  - Vascular lesions have worse prognosis
- Monitor for growth of cyst (occurs in ~ 20% of cases)
  - Rarely, may exhibit rapid growth and cause obstructive hydrocephalus
- Look for other abnormalities
  - Prognosis good if isolated abnormality
- > 90% discovered after 20-weeks gestation

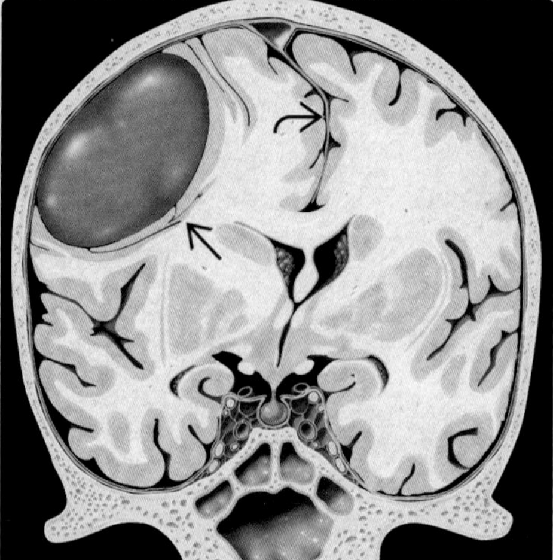

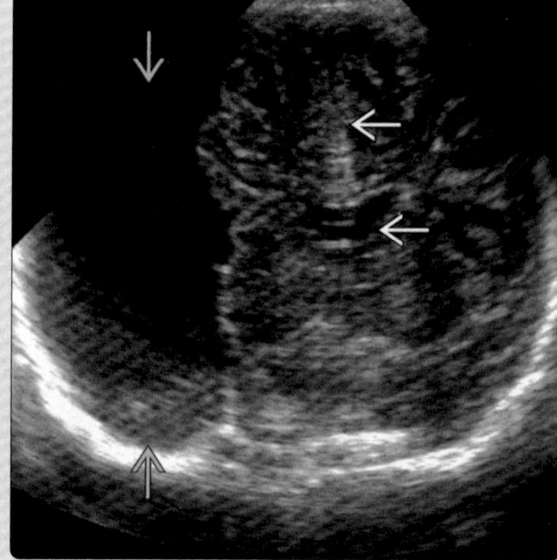

(Left) *Coronal graphic shows the effect of an extraaxial (i.e., outside the brain) arachnoid cyst. The cyst buckles the normal gray/white matter interface ➔ and displaces and compresses underlying normal brain. If large, the cyst may cause shift of vessels &/or the midline structures ➔.* **(Right)** *Neonatal head US shows a large arachnoid cyst ➔ in the sylvian fissure compressing the normal brain and causing mild shift of the midline ➔ (i.e., it is exerting mass effect).*

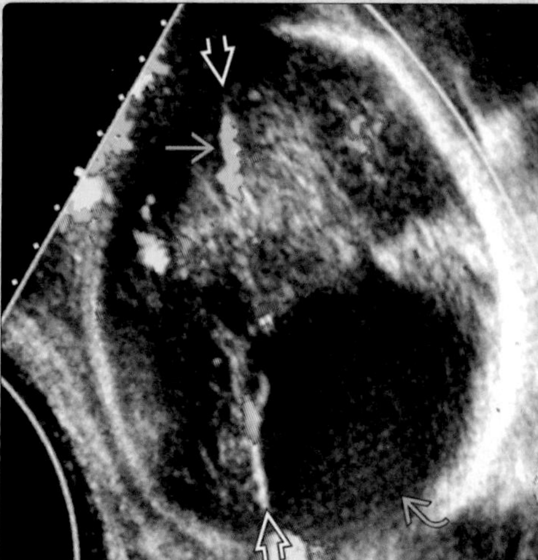

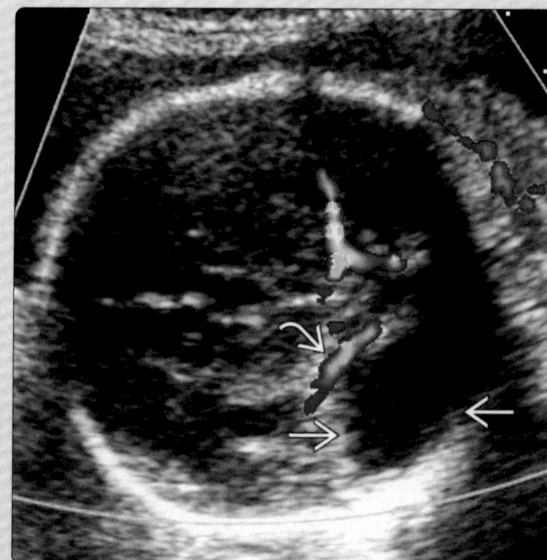

(Left) *Axial color Doppler US shows an avascular, simple cyst ➔ typical of an arachnoid cyst. The normal vessels are visible. Note the mass effect with midline shift ➔ and displacement of the anterior cerebral arteries ➔.* **(Right)** *Coronal color Doppler US shows an avascular cystic lesion ➔ at the skull base. Note mass effect with superior displacement of the ipsilateral middle cerebral artery ➔. This helps differential an arachnoid cyst from porencephaly, which replaces destroyed brain. Porencephaly does not have mass effect.*

KEY FACTS

TERMINOLOGY

- Narrowing/occlusion at aqueduct of Sylvius (between 3rd and 4th ventricles), causing obstructive hydrocephalus

IMAGING

- Moderate to severe ventricular dilatation (> 15 mm)
  - May be extreme with macrocephaly
- Dangling choroid: Choroid does not fill ventricle
  - When severe, upside choroid may fall through dilated foramen of Monroe into dependent ventricle
- Normally formed posterior fossa: Cerebellum may be compressed by supratentorial ventriculomegaly
- Male fetuses with X-linked form have adducted thumbs
  - Thumbs curled into palm of hand

TOP DIFFERENTIAL DIAGNOSES

- Holoprosencephaly: Single communicating ventricle, absent falx
- Hydranencephaly: Parenchyma destroyed, no cortical mantle

CLINICAL ISSUES

- Developmental delay in up to 90%, severe in X-linked form

SCANNING TIPS

- Posterior fossa images of critical importance to rule out other causes of ventriculomegaly
  - Normal in aqueductal stenosis, although can be compressed if hydrocephalus is severe
  - Often abnormal with other malformations
- Document gender and carefully image hands in males looking for adducted thumbs (X-linked hydrocephalus)
- Carefully assess for remaining cortical mantle
  - Differentiates aqueductal stenosis from destructive lesions or other congenital malformations
  - Use endovaginal probe if head is cephalic
  - Doppler to look for flow in compressed parenchyma

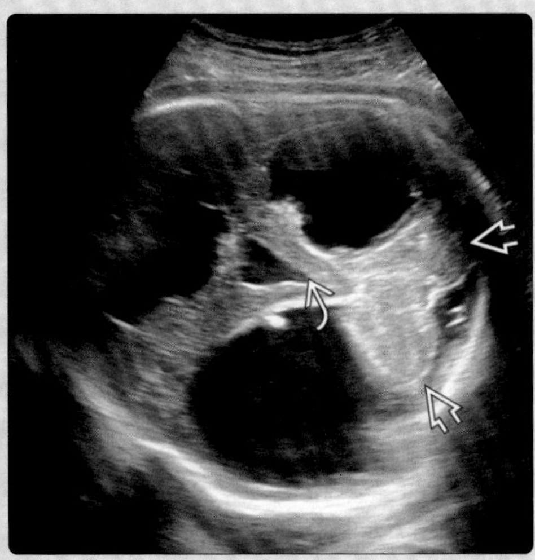

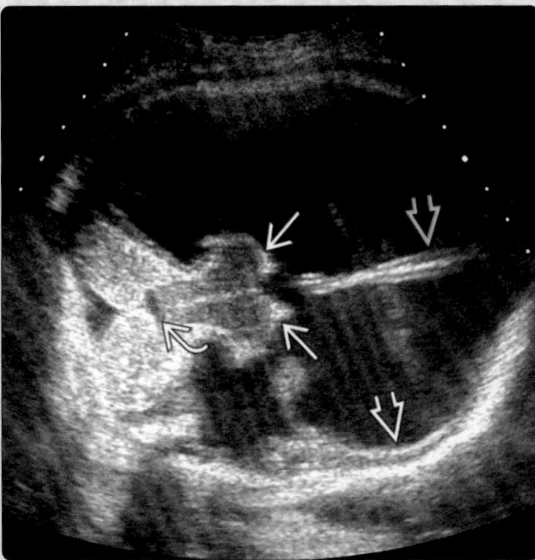

(Left) *Coronal oblique US of the brain at 29 weeks shows severe hydrocephalus with the enlarged 3rd ventricle "funneling" to a point ➡ at the aqueduct of Sylvius. The cerebellum ➡ is normal, an important feature of aqueductal stenosis (AS).* **(Right)** *Coronal oblique US in a more severe case shows an intact midline ➡, a thin rind of cerebral cortex ➡, & severe hydrocephalus. Thalami ➡, cerebellum, & 4th ventricle ➡ are normal. An intact cerebral cortex distinguishes AS from hydranencephaly.*

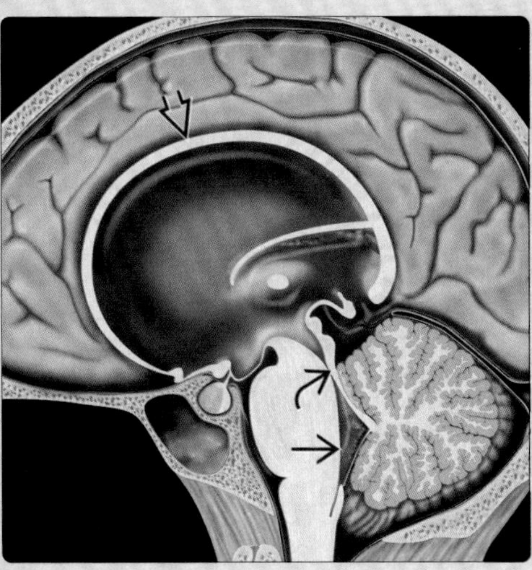

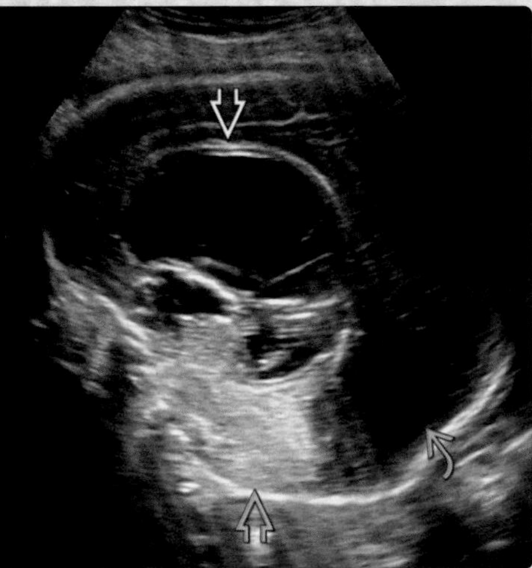

(Left) *Sagittal midline graphic of AS shows marked hydrocephalus, a stretched (thinned) corpus callosum ➡, and funnel-shaped, narrowed cerebral aqueduct of Sylvius ➡. Note the normal 4th ventricle ➡.* **(Right)** *Midline sagittal US of a fetal brain at 29 weeks shows a similar appearance with a stretched corpus callosum ➡. A portion of the dilated occipital horn is seen ➡. The mass effect of the supratentorial ventricular dilatation is compressing the cerebellum ➡.*

Chiari 2 Malformation

KEY FACTS

TERMINOLOGY

- Hindbrain compression with cerebellar herniation through foramen magnum
- Open spina bifida present in almost every case

IMAGING

- Posterior fossa compression is key finding
  - Small or obliterated cisterna magna (CM)
  - Cerebellum loses normal bilobed morphology
    - Only finding with mild compression
  - Banana sign when severe compression
    - Cerebellum wraps around midbrain
- Ventriculomegaly (often progressive)
  - 55% at diagnosis and > 90% at delivery
- Frontal bone concavity (lemon sign) is nonspecific finding that often resolves in 3rd trimester
- Loss of intracranial translucency can be finding at time of nuchal translucency screening

TOP DIFFERENTIAL DIAGNOSES

- Aqueductal stenosis
  - Progressive ventriculomegaly with macrocephaly
  - CM not obliterated
- Small cerebellum from other causes
  - Cerebellar hypoplasia: Small bilobed cerebellum
  - Rhombencephalosynapsis: Globular cerebellum

CLINICAL ISSUES

- Associated with aneuploidy
- ↑ maternal serum α-fetoprotein on quad screen results
- Newborn needs immediate postnatal ONTD surgery
- 80% need ventriculoperitoneal shunt

SCANNING TIPS

- Do not wait for banana sign to suspect Chiari 2
  - Obliteration of CM is best clue
- Look meticulously for spina bifida when Chiari 2 seen
  - Might be subtle and without sac

(Left) *Sagittal view of Chiari 2 malformation shows the hallmark findings of hindbrain herniation ➡ and a lumbar meningomyelocele ➡. Chiari 2 is almost always seen in conjunction with open neural tube defect.* **(Right)** *A detailed hindbrain view shows a small posterior fossa with herniated cerebellum ➡, compressed 4th ventricle ➡, and diminished cisterna magna ➡. These compressive forces lead to ventriculomegaly. Associated findings include agenesis or dysgenesis of the corpus callosum ➡ (dorsal portion missing here).*

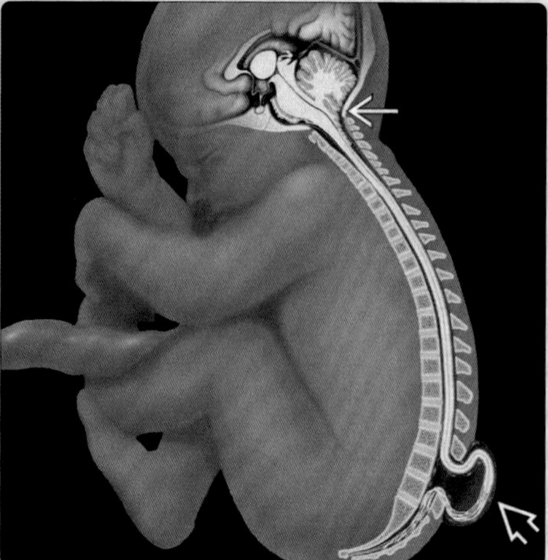

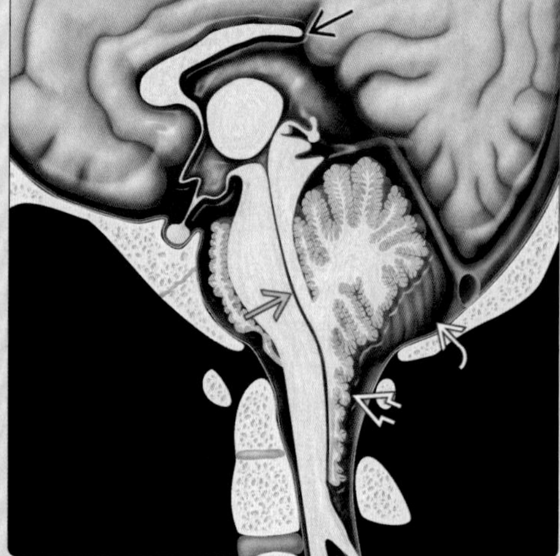

(Left) *Posterior fossa view in this 18-week fetus shows the banana sign. The cerebellum (calipers) has lost its normal bilobed morphology. The hemispheres ➡ are curved and "hug" the midbrain ➡, giving the cerebellum the shape of a banana.* **(Right)** *Ventriculomegaly is seen in the same fetus. The choroid is dangling ➡, and the lateral ventricle measures > 10 mm. Ventriculomegaly is often the 1st finding noticed with Chiari 2 malformation.*

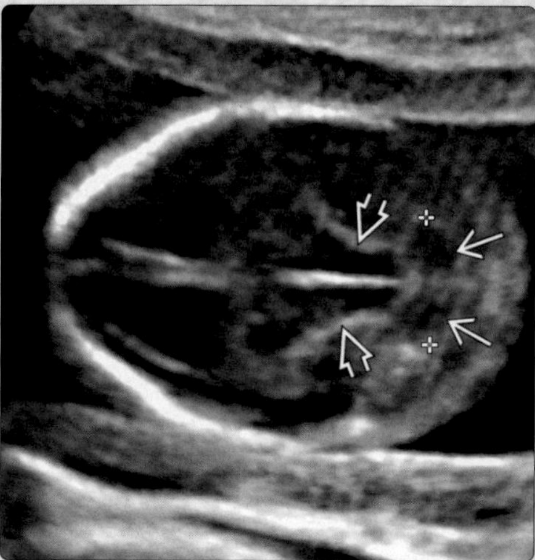

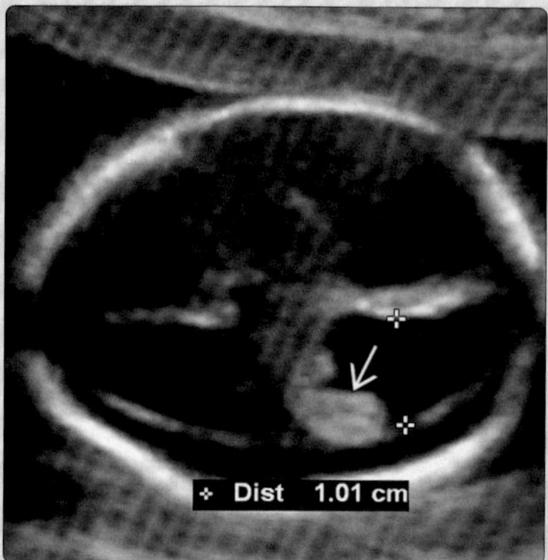

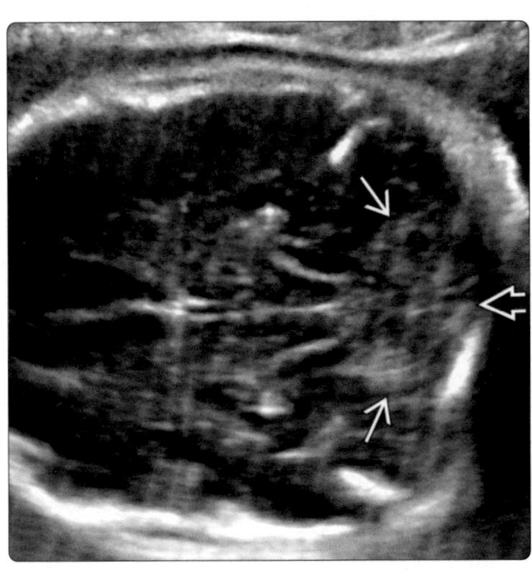

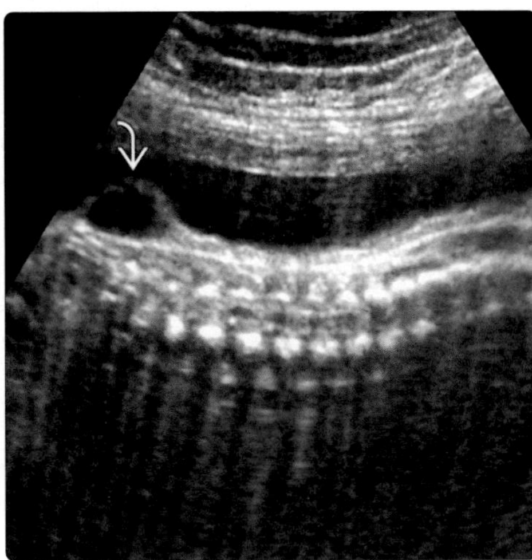

(Left) *In this fetus with Chiari 2, the normal fluid-filled cisternal magna is obliterated ➡. The cerebellum ➡ is mildly flattened by the occiput and has lost its bilobed shape. In addition, there was no ventriculomegaly. The findings in this case are subtle and exemplify that the loss of the cisterna magna is a significant finding.* **(Right)** *Sagittal US of the spine in the same fetus shows a small sacral meningocele sac ➡ from an open neural tube defect.*

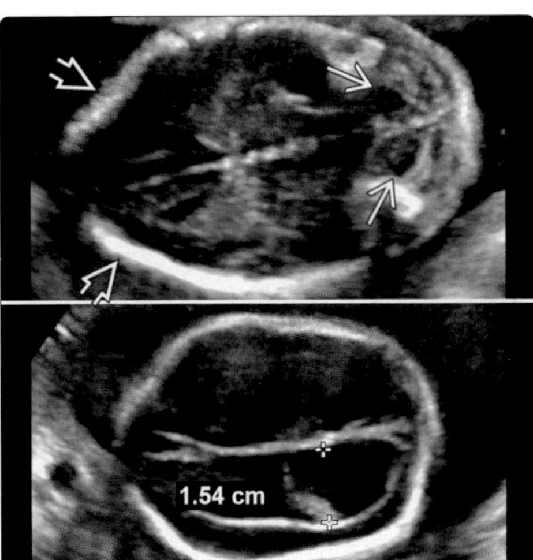

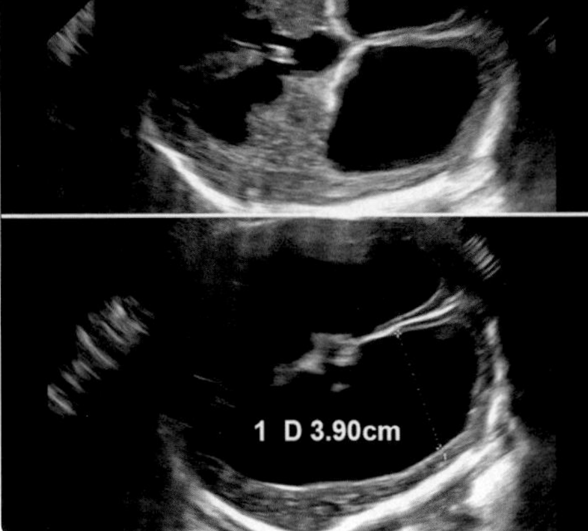

(Left) *Classic features of Chiari 2 on routine axial views of the midgestation fetal brain include cerebellar compression (banana sign when severe) ➡, frontal bone concavity (lemon sign) ➡, and ventriculomegaly (calipers).* **(Right)** *On follow-up in the 3rd trimester in the same patient, the frontal concavity has resolved, and the ventriculomegaly has worsened. Progressive ventriculomegaly is common with Chiari 2 due to progressive compressive pressure on the 4th ventricle.*

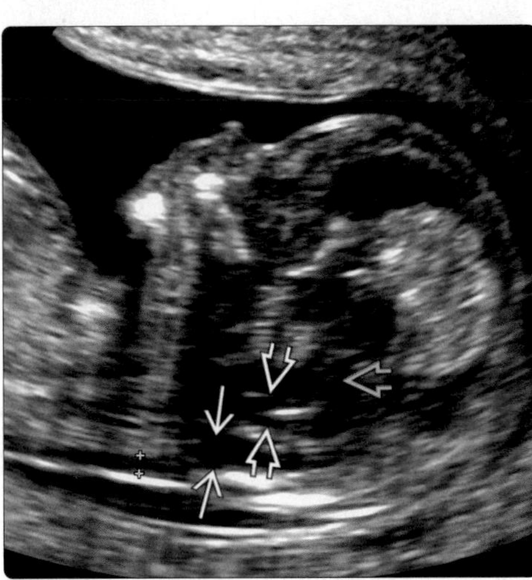

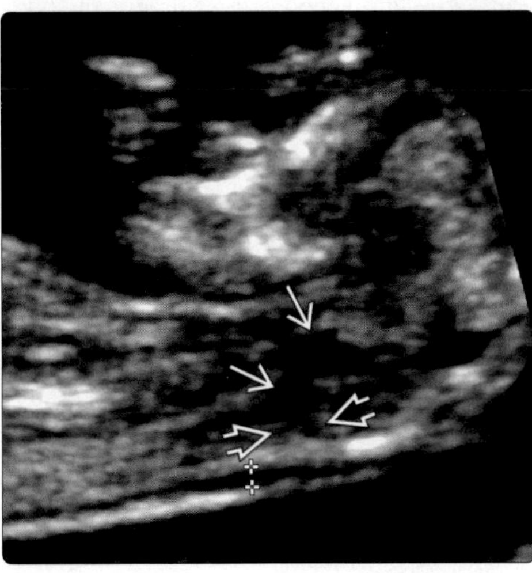

(Left) *In this normal 13-week fetus, the normal intracranial translucency (IT) ➡ is the 4th ventricle, located behind the hypoechoic brainstem ➡. The future cisterna magnum ➡ is a 2nd lucency dorsal to the IT. The nuchal translucency is the most superficial translucency (calipers) in the skin.* **(Right)** *In this 12-week fetus with spina bifida, the IT and cisterna magna are obliterated ➡. The brainstem ➡ is inferiorly and dorsally displaced ("kinked"). Follow-up US at 16 weeks confirmed Chiari 2 and spina bifida.*

Dandy-Walker Malformation

KEY FACTS

TERMINOLOGY

- Classic Dandy-Walker malformation
  - Cerebellar vermis is completely or partially absent
  - Cystic dilatation of 4th ventricle (4V)
  - Enlarged posterior fossa with elevated tentorium
    - Tentorium is roof of posterior fossa and separates cerebellum from occipital lobe

IMAGING

- 4V dilated and communicates directly with cisterna magna
- Posterior fossa cyst (often quite large)
  - Elevates tentorium (seen best on sagittal view)
- If partial vermis present, it is rotated and displaced superiorly
- Ventriculomegaly is common feature
- ~ 70-90% have additional anomalies
  - Other brain anomalies common (above tentorium)
- Fetal MR is additive (better sagittal view, other brain anomalies)

TOP DIFFERENTIAL DIAGNOSES

- Persistent Blake pouch cyst
  - Vermis is elevated but otherwise normal
- Mega cisterna magna
  - Cerebellum otherwise normal
- Arachnoid cyst
  - Mass effect on otherwise normal cerebellum

CLINICAL ISSUES

- Aneuploidy in ~ 50%
- Associated with syndromes

SCANNING TIPS

- Try 3D to obtain multiplanar sagittal view if not able to see this plane by 2D ultrasound
- Use transvaginal ultrasound if fetus is cephalic
- Measure vermis length on sagittal view
- Measure cerebellar diameter for any anomaly in posterior fossa

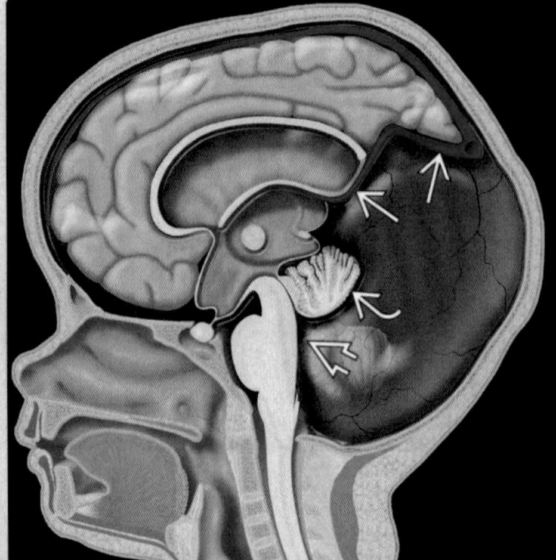

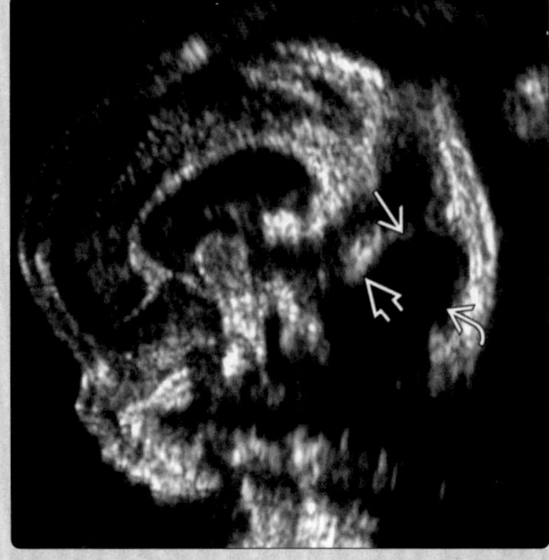

(Left) *Graphic shows a superiorly rotated vermian remnant ➡, an uncovered 4th ventricle ➡ communicating with a posterior fossa cyst, and elevation of the tentorium ➡. These are the requisite findings of a classic Dandy-Walker malformation (DMW).* **(Right)** *A sagittal brain view of this fetus shows a posterior fossa cyst ➡, a superiorly rotated vermian remnant ➡, and elevation of the tentorium ➡. Of note, however, the sagittal view of the posterior fossa is not always feasible with 2D ultrasound.*

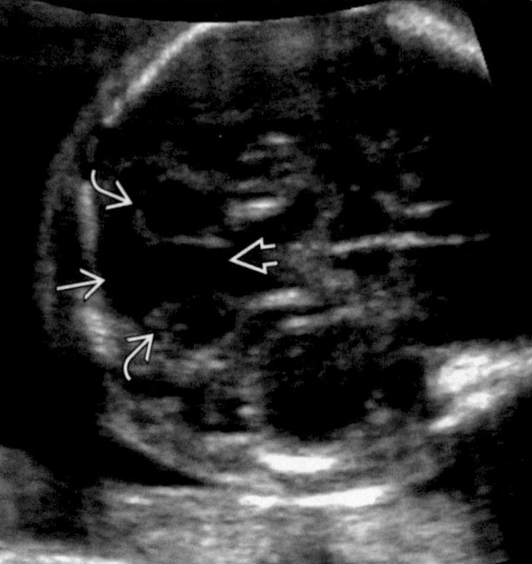

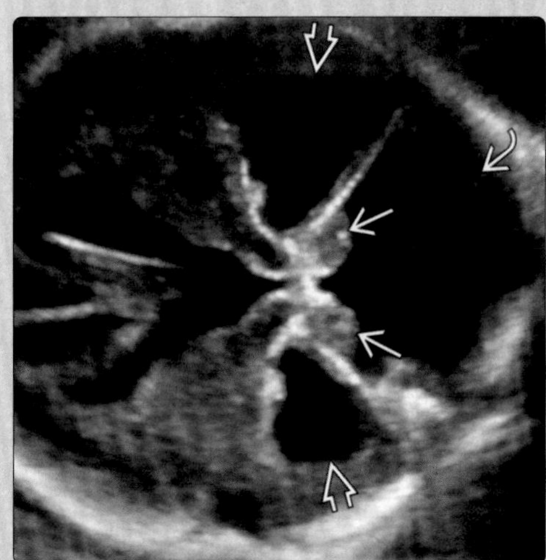

(Left) *Axial standard view of the posterior fossa in this fetus with DWM shows splaying of the cerebellar hemispheres ➡ and an absent vermis leading to communication between the cisterna magna ➡ and the 4th ventricle ➡.* **(Right)** *In a more severely affected fetus, the cerebellar hemispheres are small and splayed ➡. The dorsal cyst is large ➡ and there is ventriculomegaly ➡. These are the classic findings on the routine posterior fossa view.*

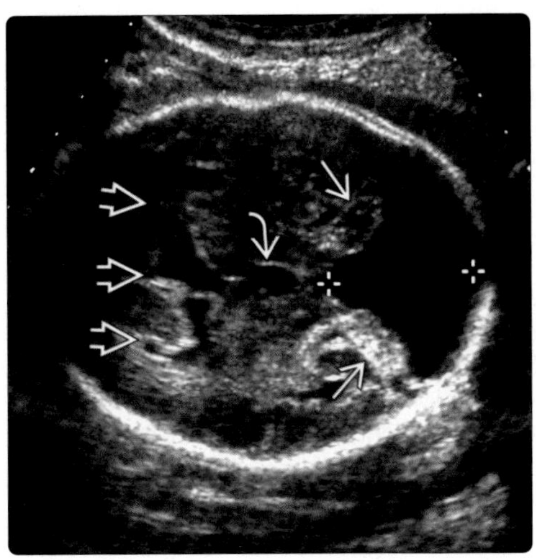

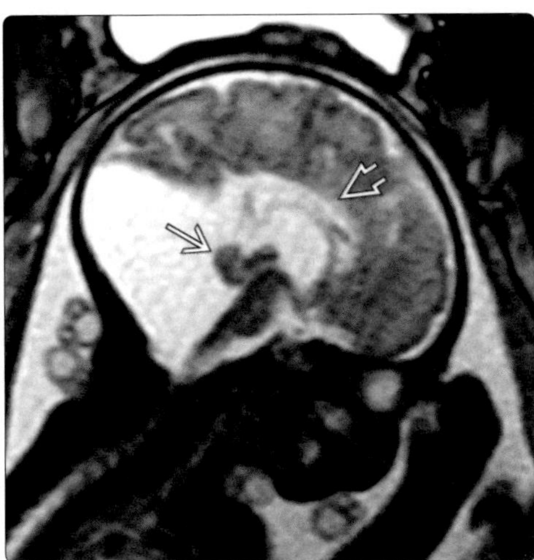

(Left) *Axial ultrasound of the posterior fossa shows splayed cerebellar hemispheres with absent vermis and large posterior fossa cyst (calipers), typical for DWM. However, also note a dilated 3rd ventricle and trident appearance of the frontal horns, ventricular shape findings typical for agenesis of the corpus callosum (CC).* **(Right)** *MR in a different case shows rotation of vermian remnant and dysgenesis of the CC. Many fetuses with DWM have additional anomalies, often involving other areas of the brain.*

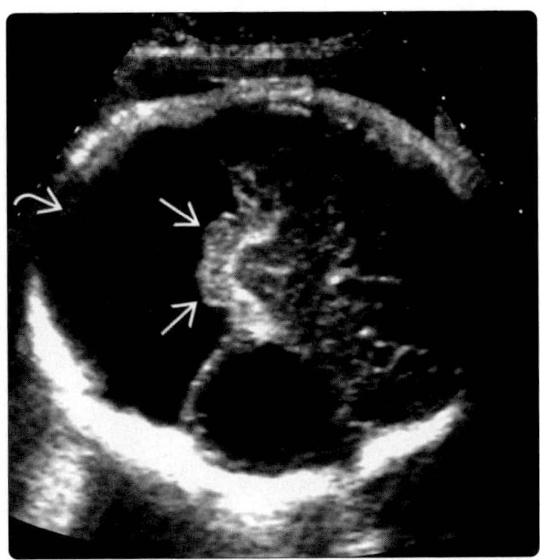

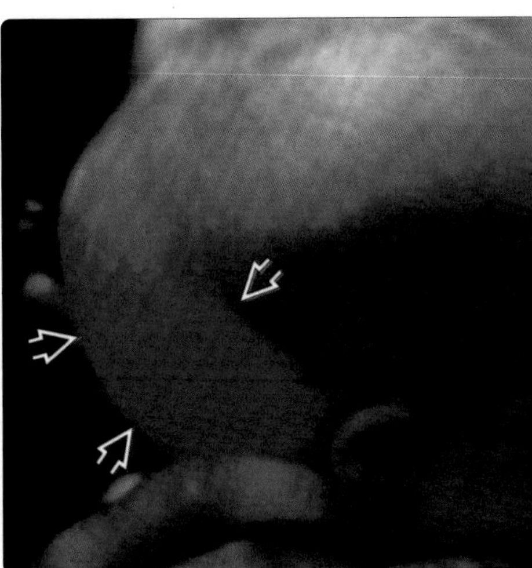

(Left) *Axial ultrasound shows 2 very small cerebellar hemispheres with lack of normal foliation and an enlarged posterior fossa from a large cyst.* **(Right)** *Transillumination of an infant's skull with a flashlight shows light traveling through a fluid-filled enlarged posterior fossa, unobstructed by normal cerebellum. These are examples of severe cerebellar hypoplasia associated with severe DWM.*

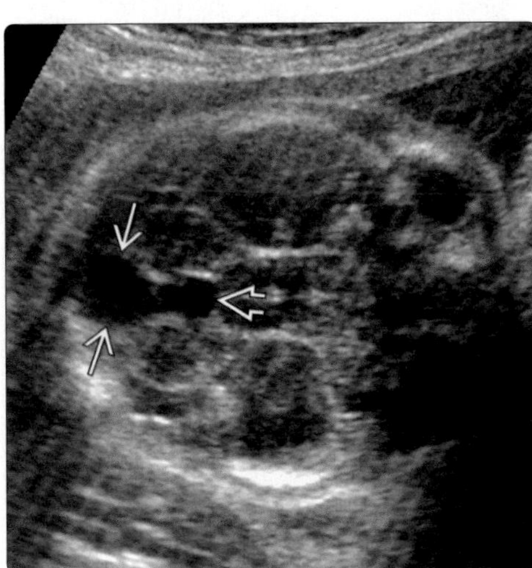

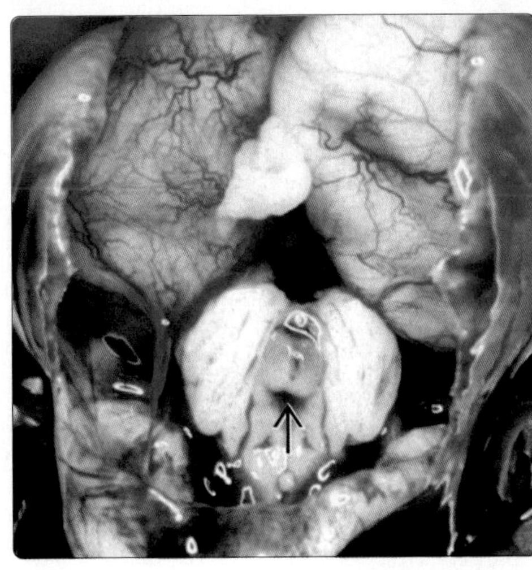

(Left) *The classic key hole appearance of partial or complete vermian absence on routine posterior fossa view is secondary to cystic dilation of the 4th ventricle and communication with the distended cisterna magna.* **(Right)** *Autopsy photograph of an early 2nd-trimester fetus shows cystic bulge of the 4th ventricle between the cerebellar hemispheres, confirming a prenatal diagnosis of DWM. The absence of the vermis allows for this "ballooning" cystic distention of the 4th ventricle.*

Mega Cisterna Magna

KEY FACTS

IMAGING

- Cisterna magna (CM) measures > 10 mm on routine posterior fossa view
- Cerebellar hemispheres and vermis otherwise normal
- Most often normal variant : < 20% with other findings

TOP DIFFERENTIAL DIAGNOSES

- Cerebellar hypoplasia: CM big because cerebellum is small
- Blake pouch cyst: Dilation of posterior medullary vellum
  - Cyst rotates vermis superiorly
  - Axial view mimics mega CM
- Anomaly of vermis
  - Dandy-Walker malformation
    - Absent vermis + ventriculomegaly
  - Partial vermian dysgenesis
    - Superior vermis present, inferior vermis missing
- Arachnoid cyst of posterior fossa
  - Look for mass effect on dural folds, vermis, cerebellum

CLINICAL ISSUES

- Usually isolated incidental finding: Excellent prognosis
- Can be part of multiple anomalies seen with trisomy 18

SCANNING TIPS

- Steep scanning angle may cause false enlarged CM
  - Posterior fossa view with 15° dorsal angulation, not more
- Pay careful attention to cerebellum and vermis anatomy
  - Look for normal bilobed cerebellar morphology
  - Measure bicerebellar diameter
  - Consider cine sweep to show vermis is completely intact
- Consider 3D multiplanar imaging to show vermis in axial, coronal, and sagittal views
  - Can measure vermis length on coronal and sagittal views
  - Can see if vermis is elevated off midbrain on sagittal view
- Turn on color Doppler to prove increased lucency behind cerebellum is not from vascular malformation

(Left) *Axial ultrasound shows the cisterna magna is enlarged ➡. Note the dural folds are in a normal central position ➡ without mass effect to suggest arachnoid cyst. Doppler ultrasound excludes a vascular anomaly, such as vein of Galen malformation.* **(Right)** *The cisterna magna is measured from the vermis to the inner table of the occipital bone (calipers). As seen in this case, a measurement > 1.0 cm is considered enlarged.*

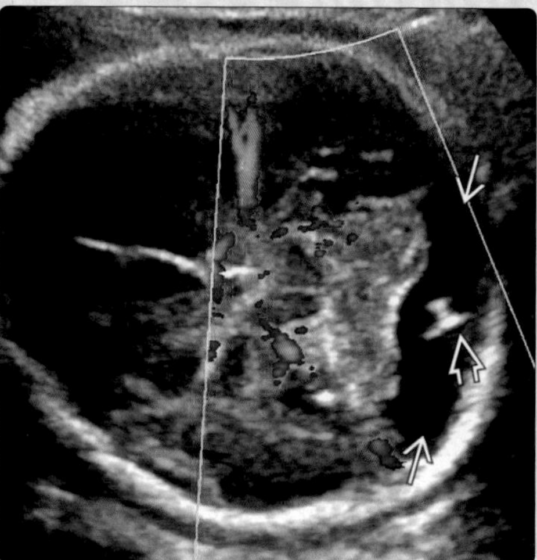

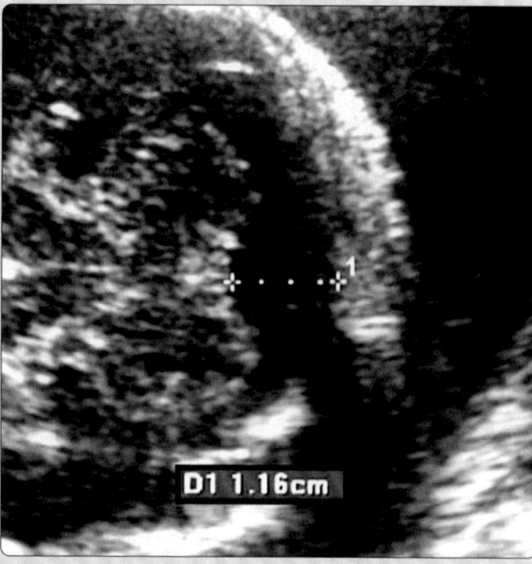

(Left) *Sagittal ultrasound of the posterior fossa in a fetus with enlarged cisterna magna ➡ shows a normal echogenic triangular cerebellar vermis ➡. The vermis length can be measured in this plane.* **(Right)** *Sagittal T2WI fetal MR shows the sagittal posterior fossa anatomy to better advantage and helps illustrate the anatomy of the sagittal view seen with ultrasound. The cisterna magna is enlarged ➡, but the vermis ➡ is normal, not elevated or deficient.*

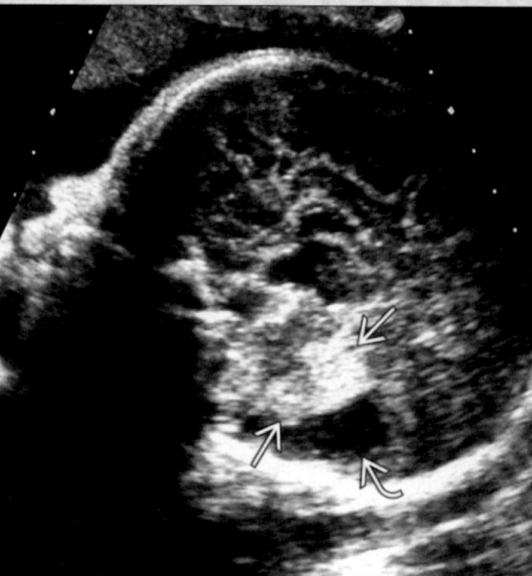

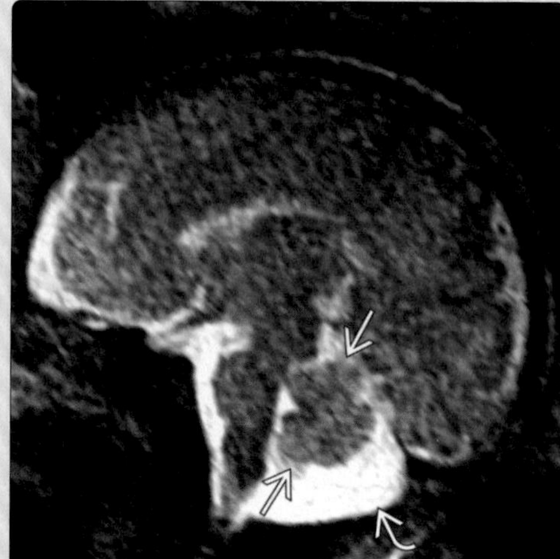

KEY FACTS

TERMINOLOGY

- Vein of Galen aneurysmal malformation (VGAM) is deep cerebral arteriovenous fistula

IMAGING

- Elongated midline cystic structure
  - Extends from area behind 3rd ventricle posteriorly toward occiput
  - Drains via straight sinus or superior sagittal sinus
- Flow on color Doppler with arterialized venous flow on pulsed wave tracing
- Other brain findings include both destructive (e.g., porencephaly) or developmental (e.g., migrational) lesions
- Serial US utilized to evaluate for developing hydrops or intracranial parenchymal damage

TOP DIFFERENTIAL DIAGNOSES

- Arachnoid cyst: May have similar grayscale appearance but no flow on color Doppler

CLINICAL ISSUES

- Up to 80% of fetal cardiac output may be diverted to cerebral circulation
- Presence of any associated finding confers poor outcome
  - High mortality; survivors with neurologic or cardiac impairment
  - Most common associated findings include cardiomegaly (66.7%) and ventriculomegaly (38.9%)
  - Even mild cardiomegaly correlated with poor outcome
- Better prognosis for isolated VGAM without other findings
- At birth, vascular shunt usually increases
  - Cessation of flow to low-resistance placenta

SCANNING TIPS

- **Always use color and pulsed Doppler for any cystic-appearing brain mass**
- Perform detailed views of brain parenchyma
  - High-flow state "steals" blood from surrounding developing brain, resulting in ischemic damage

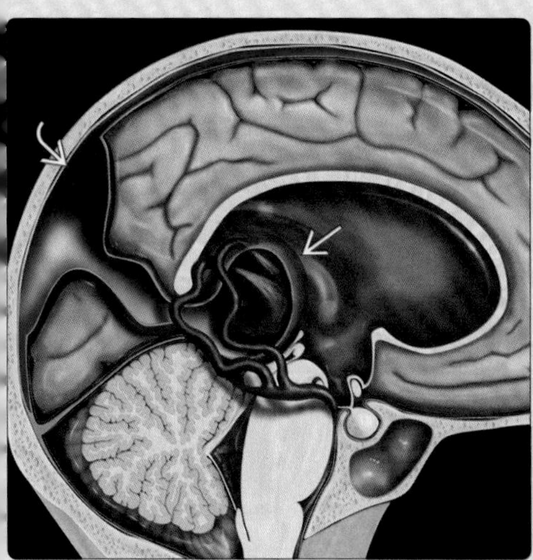

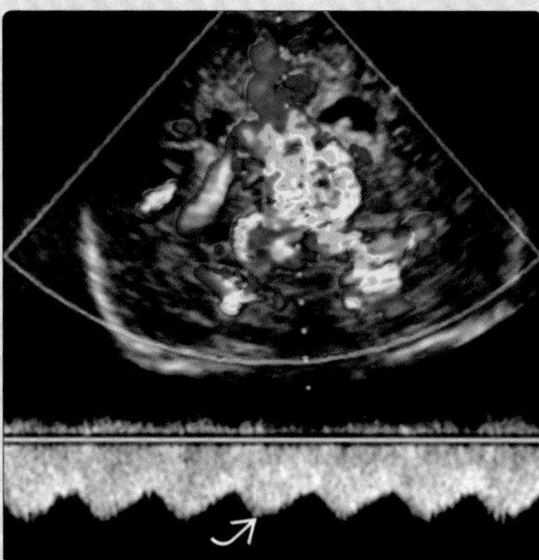

(Left) *Sagittal graphic depicts a large VGAM. There is an arteriovenous malformation with swirling blood within the aneurysm ➡. In this example, it drains into the superior sagittal sinus ➡.* **(Right)** *Postnatal color Doppler US shows turbulent flow within the venous drainage of the VGAM. There is arterialization of the venous waveform ➡ typical of high flow through a fistula. Up to 80% of fetal cardiac output may be diverted to the brain. This high-flow state eventually leads to cardiac decompensation.*

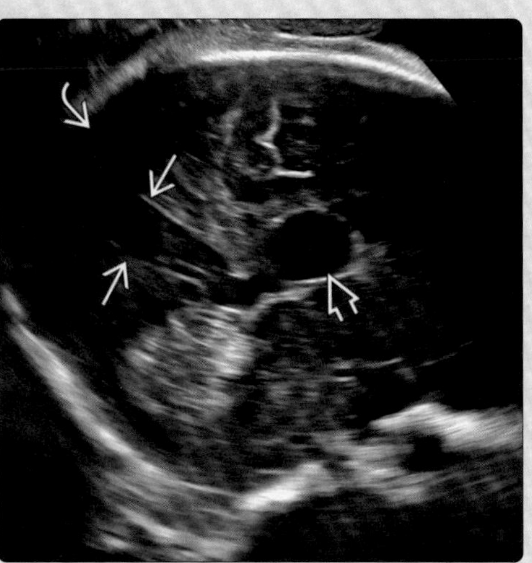

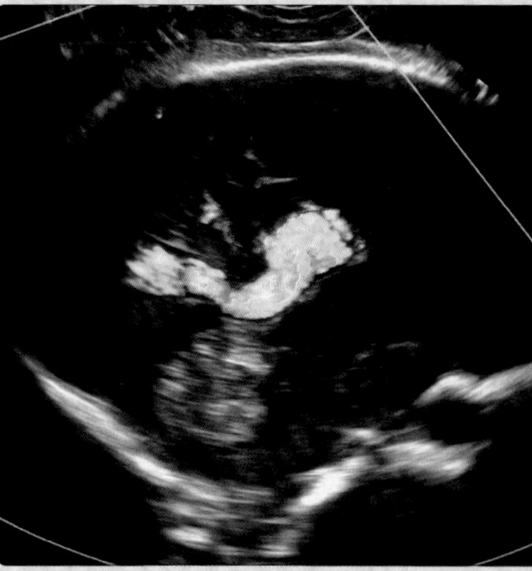

(Left) *Sagittal US (similar to the graphic) of an incidentally noted hypoechoic, midline mass ➡ in the 3rd trimester shows it elongates posteriorly ➡ toward the superior sagittal sinus ➡.* **(Right)** *Color Doppler US in the same plane confirms the VGAM, with turbulent flow, as typically seen within a fistula. VGAM is most commonly detected in the 3rd trimester. Subsequent evaluation for signs of high-output cardiac failure should be performed. A detailed evaluation of the brain should be done looking for any evidence of ischemic changes.*

KEY FACTS

TERMINOLOGY

- **Encephalomalacia**: Brain ischemia or inflammation
- **Porencephaly**: Focal destruction of brain tissue
- **Hydranencephaly**: Complete destruction of cerebral hemispheres

IMAGING

- Intracranial bleeding has variable appearance
  - Nonperfused intracranial mass of varying echogenicity
    - Initially echogenic, iso- to hypoechoic over time
  - Irregular, bulky choroid plexus due to adherent clot
  - Echogenic, irregular ependyma (ventricular lining)
  - Fluid-fluid level in ventricles
- Hydrocephalus from obstructed CSF flow due to ependymal thickening and layering clot
- Normal landmarks may be obscured by clot or tissue injury
- Porencephaly develops at site of parenchymal bleed
  - Resorption of clot/damaged tissue leaves anechoic parenchymal cyst connected to adjacent ventricle

TOP DIFFERENTIAL DIAGNOSES

- Intracranial tumor may be confused with clot but has internal blood flow and shows rapid growth
- Holoprosencephaly may be confused with hydranencephaly but falx is missing; face often abnormal

SCANNING TIPS

- Any echogenic material in frontal horns is suspicious for clot
  - Choroid plexus does not extend anterior to caudothalamic groove
- High-resolution transvaginal US if cephalic presentation
  - Features may be very subtle, especially if associated with acute hypotensive episode
    - Maternal trauma, abruption, post fetal intervention, after monochorionic twin demise
  - Assess at time of injury and again within 7-10 days
    - Signs of encephalomalacia take time to develop
- Use color Doppler to look for vascular malformation as potential cause

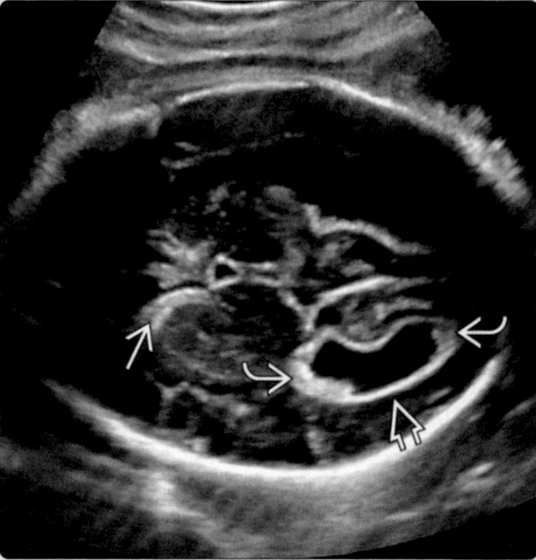

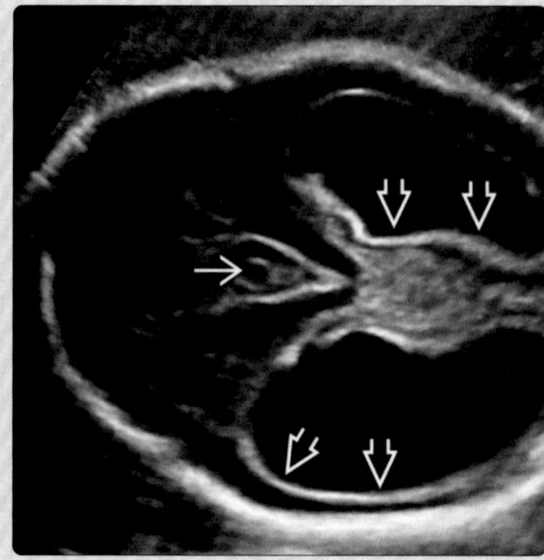

(Left) *Axial US in a subtle case of intracranial hemorrhage shows echogenic material in a nondilated frontal horn ➡, echogenic debris ➡ in the occipital horn, and thick, echogenic ependyma ➡ lining the ventricles.* **(Right)** *Axial US of the brain in a 3rd-trimester fetus shows obvious hydrocephalus with clot in the dilated 3rd ventricle ➡. Also note the thickened echogenic ependyma ➡, a common finding resulting from inflammation and irritation of the ependyma by blood breakdown products.*

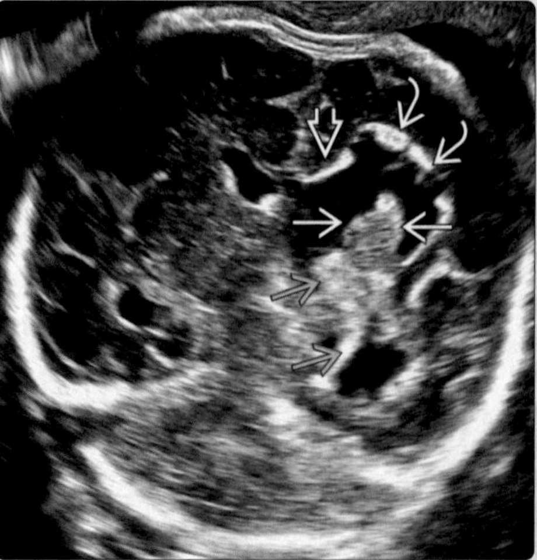

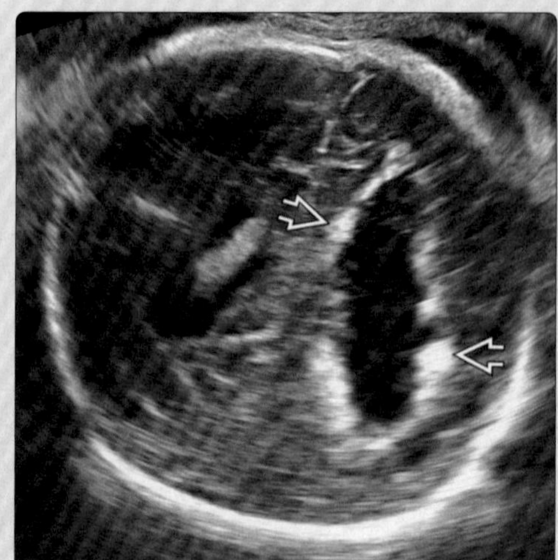

(Left) *Coronal TVUS in a 3rd-trimester fetus shows hypoechoic clot ➡ adherent to the more echogenic choroid plexus ➡. The lateral ventricle is dilated and irregular in shape with ependymal thickening ➡ and nodular debris at an area of developing porencephaly ➡.* **(Right)** *Coronal TVUS angled more posteriorly in the same fetus confirms nodular ependymal thickening ➡ and ventricular dilation. Postnatal MR confirmed parenchymal thinning from ischemia (encephalomalacia) and (focal destruction) porencephaly.*

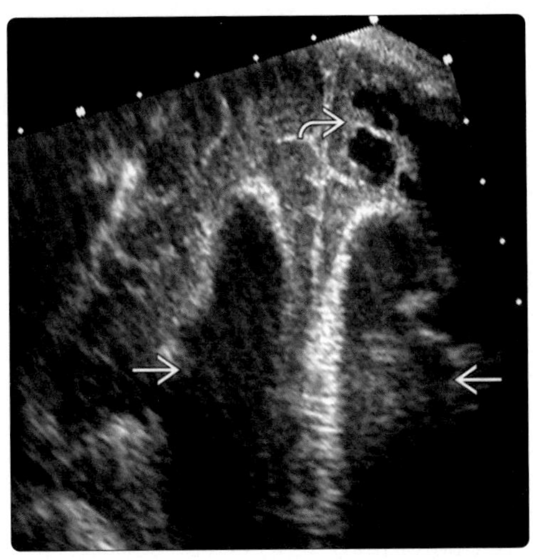

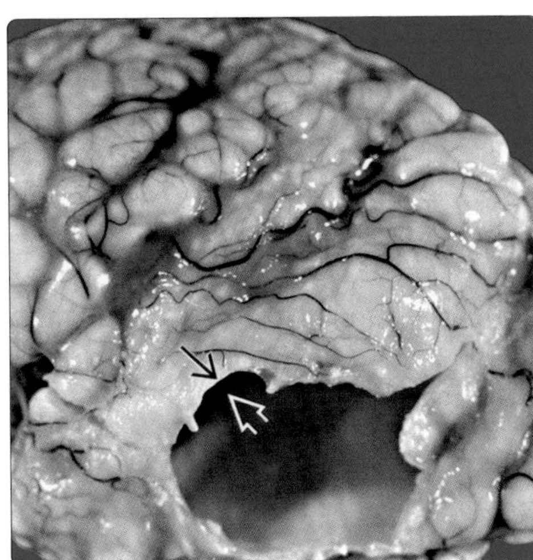

(Left) *Axial oblique US in this 3rd-trimester fetus shows ventriculomegaly ➡ and a porencephalic cyst ➡ formation in the left frontoparietal area. Fetal MR confirmed extensive intracranial hemorrhage and porencephaly in this case.* **(Right)** *Autopsy image shows a porencephalic cyst in the temporal lobe. It is a CSF-filled cavity that extends from the temporal horn to the brain surface ➡. The cyst is lined with gliotic white matter ➡, which is the equivalent to scar tissue in the brain. (Courtesy J. Townsend, MD.)*

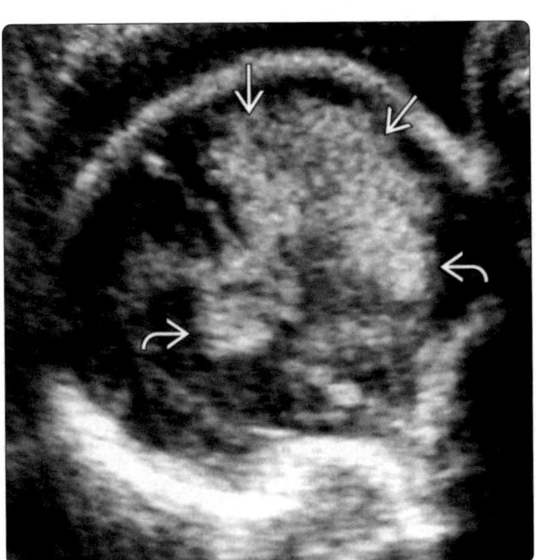

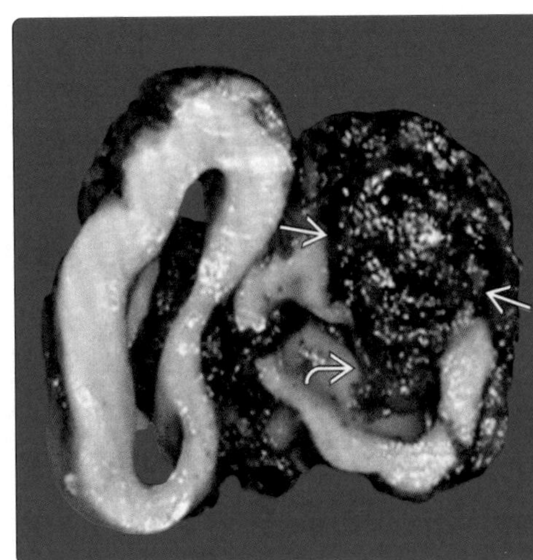

(Left) *Coronal US shows severe intracranial hemorrhage with echogenic clot filling the ventricles ➡ and extensive periventricular hemorrhagic infarction ➡ on the left. This is the equivalent of a grade 4 germinal matrix hemorrhage in a preterm infant. This fetus survived demise of a monochorionic twin but expired shortly after delivery.* **(Right)** *This is a coronal section from an autopsied brain showing both intraventricular clot ➡ and periventricular hemorrhagic infarction ➡. This case was associated with a vascular malformation.*

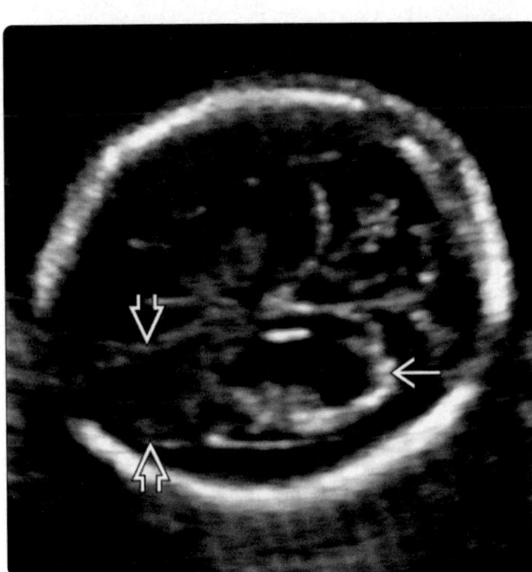

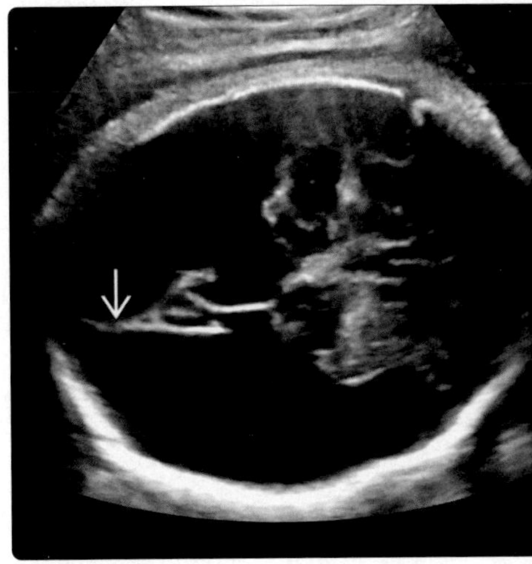

(Left) *Axial US in the survivor of a monochorionic twin pair with demise of one at 23 weeks shows clot is present in the anterior horn ➡, and there is ventriculomegaly with thickening of the ependymal lining ➡.* **(Right)** *Axial US at 37 weeks in the same case shows minimal residual brain tissue, consistent with evolution of intracranial hemorrhage and encephalomalacia to full-blown hydranencephaly (note the intact falx ➡). The head measurements were small, as is typically seen with a destructive process.*

Absent Cavum Septi Pellucidi

KEY FACTS

TOP DIFFERENTIAL DIAGNOSES

- **Agenesis of corpus callosum (ACC)**
  - Axial: Teardrop-shaped ventricles (colpocephaly)
  - Coronal: Texas Longhorn frontal horns
  - Sagittal: Loss of anterior cerebral artery branch pattern into pericallosal artery running along cingulate gyrus
- **Schizencephaly**
  - Grey matter-lined, wedge-shaped defect extending from ventricle to brain surface
  - Lateral ventricle tented toward side of defect
- **Septooptic Dysplasia (SOD)**
  - Frontal horns communicate: Flat top shape on coronal view
  - Attempt to use ocular globes as window to optic nerves in bony orbit
- **Holoprosencephaly spectrum**
  - Often small head with abnormal round shape
  - Incomplete falx (deficient anteriorly in semilobar)
  - Fused fornices described as sign of lobar HPE
  - Sylvian fissures anteriorly displaced, meet on brain surface in syntelencephaly (middle interhemispheric fissure variant of HPE)
  - **Isolated septal deficiency**
    - Diagnosis of exclusion, final diagnosis will be postnatal with normal ophthalmology exam and endocrinology work-up

SCANNING TIPS

- Cavum septi pellucidi (CSP) is marker of normal midline development
- Absent CSP should trigger complete neurosonogram with high-resolution transducers and multiplanar images
- **Incorrect scan plane is common**
  - CSP is box-shaped anechoic space with echogenic walls that interrupts midline echo between frontal horns
  - Differentiate from paired fornices: Parallel black and white lines without intervening fluid-filled space

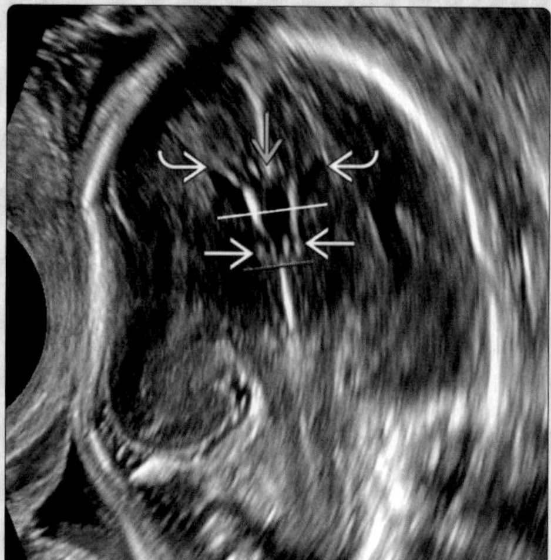

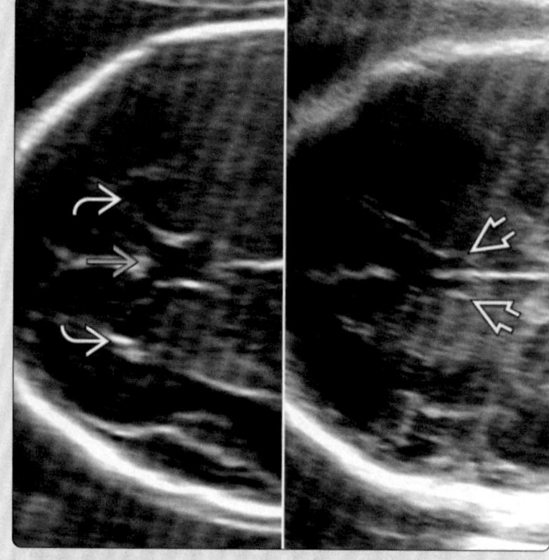

(Left) *Coronal TVUS shows the cavum septi pellucidi (CSP) ➡ between the frontal horns ➡. The roof of the CSP is formed by the corpus callosum (CC). The standard axial biparietal diameter image is obtained at the plane of the white line. The fornices ➡ are visible just inferior to the CSP.* **(Right)** *Axial US along the plane of the white line shows the CSP ➡ and frontal horns ➡. A similar image inferiorly, along the plane of the red line, shows the paired fornices ➡. These should not be mistaken for the CSP.*

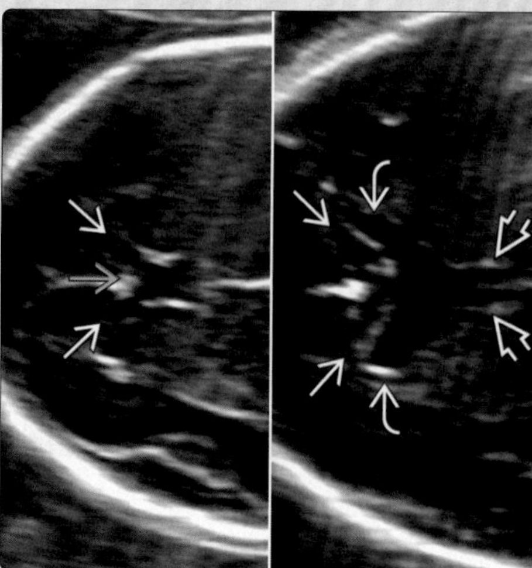

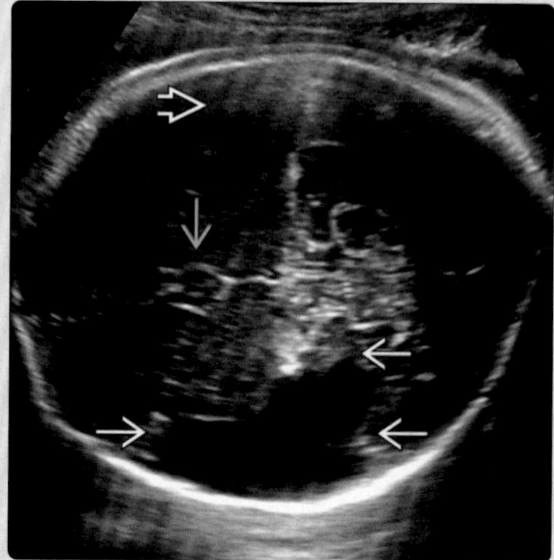

(Left) *Axial US (left) shows normal CSP ➡. On the right, the fornices ➡ are not fused, and the genu of the CC ➡ is normal, but the anterior horns ➡ communicate across the midline due to absent CSP. Final diagnosis was SOD.* **(Right)** *Axial 3rd-trimester US shows a wedge-shaped defect ➡ extending from the ventricles to skull. The fornices ➡ are visible, but there was no normal CSP. This is typical of open lip schizencephaly. Reverberation in the near field ➡ obscures detail; use multiple scan planes to look for bilateral defects.*

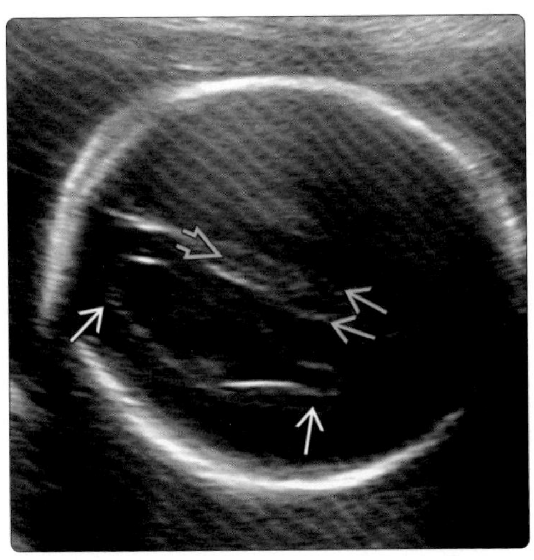

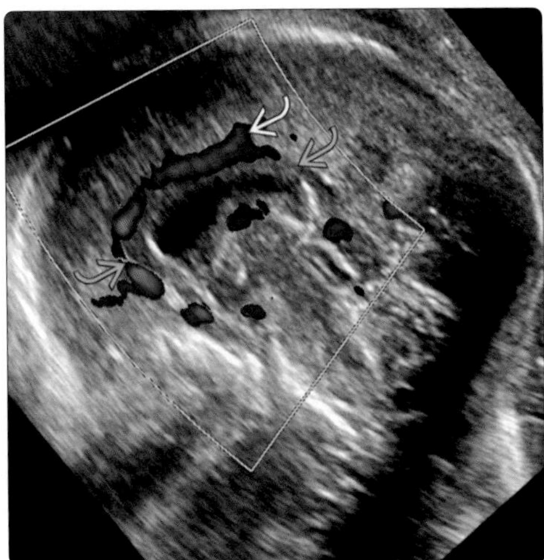

(Left) *Axial brain US in a fetus with absent cavum shows classic colpocephaly (i.e., teardrop shape of the ventricles) ➡ in ACC. Note the 3-line appearance as the medial hemispheric walls ➡ are visible mildly displaced from the falx ➡.* **(Right)** *Sagittal US with color Doppler shows the normal pericallosal artery ➡ running along the cingulate gyrus, which only forms if the CC ➡ is present. This fetus had absent CSP with normal CC and cerebral cortex. Prenatal diagnosis of SOD was confirmed at birth.*

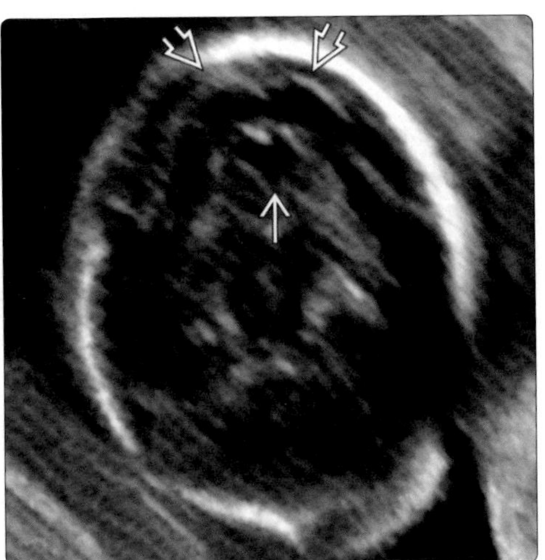

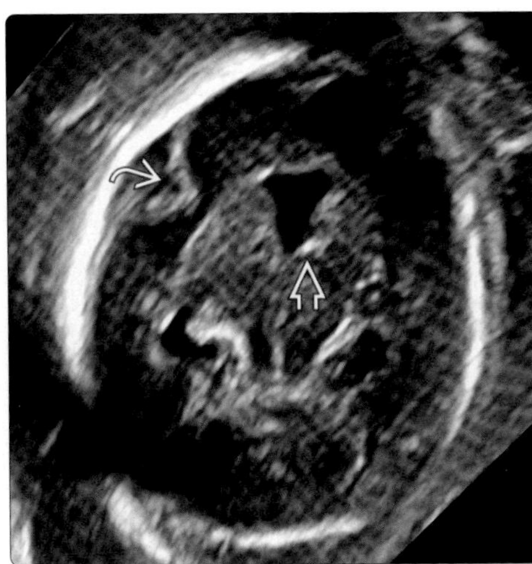

(Left) *Axial oblique US in an early 2nd-trimester fetus shows continuity of the cerebral cortex across the midline ➡. There is no anterior falx and the anterior "space" ➡ is not the cavum; it is fused, abnormal frontal horns in semilobar holoprosencephaly.* **(Right)** *Axial oblique US at 25 weeks shows anterior displacement of the sylvian fissure ➡ in association with absent cavum and fused frontal horns ➡ in a fetus with syntelencephaly.*

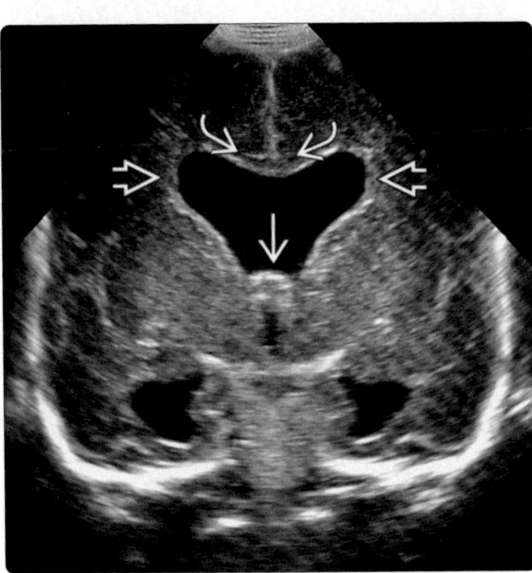

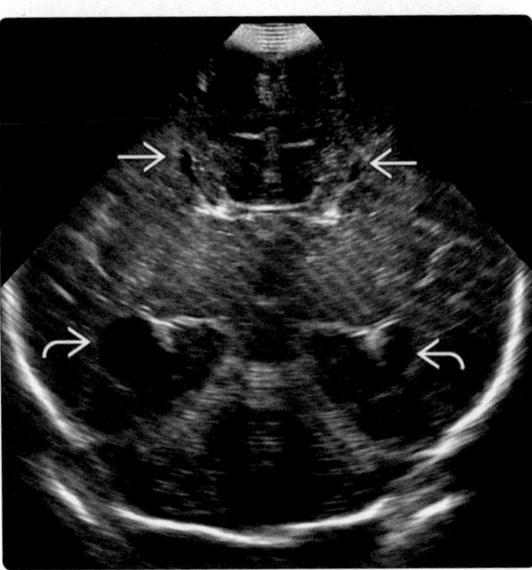

(Left) *Neonatal head US shows absent CSP and ventricular communication ➡ across the midline, thin CC ➡, and fused fornices ➡ (solid structure running anterior to posterior in roof of 3rd ventricle). MR confirmed the diagnosis of lobar holoprosencephaly by demonstrating a gyrus in continuity across the midline.* **(Right)** *Oblique coronal neonatal head US shows typical Texas Longhorn frontal horns ➡ and colpocephaly with dilated occipital horns ➡ in an infant with a fetal diagnosis of ACC.*

Spina Bifida

KEY FACTS

TERMINOLOGY

- Open spina bifida (bone and skin defect ± sac)
  - Meningomyelocele: Sac + neural elements
  - Meningocele: Sac with fluid only
  - Myeloschisis: No sac (cord directly exposed)
- Closed spina bifida: Skin-covered defect

IMAGING

- Level: Lumbosacral > thoracic > cervical
- Transverse view best for seeing dorsal element divergence
- Longitudinal views and 3D best for evaluating level
- Myelomeningocele: Complex cystic mass (most common)
- Meningocele: Anechoic cystic mass
- 20% are myeloschisis (subtle): No sac, cord is part of defect
- Chiari 2 brain findings with open spina bifida
- Tethered cord (cord seen at level of defect)
- Associated anomalies: Club feet, scoliosis
- Closed spina bifida: Chiari 2 absent or minimal

CLINICAL ISSUES

- ↑ maternal serum α-fetoprotein (msAFP)
- Associated maternal folate deficiency
  - From maternal metabolic gene defect
  - Preconception high-dose folic acid for next pregnancy
- 4% aneuploidy rate when isolated (14% if other anomalies)
- Prognosis depends on level and presence of hydrocephalus
  - 80% require ventricular shunting or bypass of hindbrain compressive obstructive hydrocephalus (from Chiari 2)
  - Only 17% with normal continence

SCANNING TIPS

- Look carefully at spine if cisterna magna is compressed (Chiari 2 is almost never isolated)
- Use last rib to determine T12 and count inferiorly to determine level of spina bifida
- If sac covering looks thick, follow it laterally to see if it is contiguous with skin (closed defect)

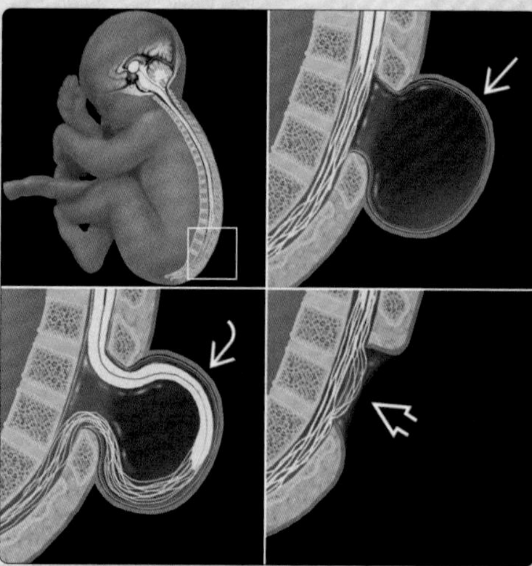

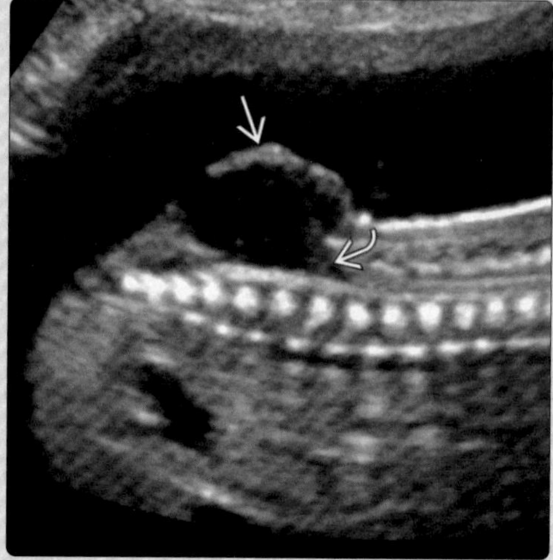

(Left) *Graphic shows open spina bifida classification. Meningoceles → contain only cerebrospinal fluid, while myelomeningoceles → also contain neural elements (most common). The neural tube defect is uncovered (no sac) in myeloschisis → and contains the spinal cord or nerve roots. Also, the cord is tethered to the defect.* **(Right)** *Sagittal view of the lumbosacral spine at 18 weeks shows a cystic mass →, which communicates with the spinal canal →. The finding is classic for open spina bifida with sac.*

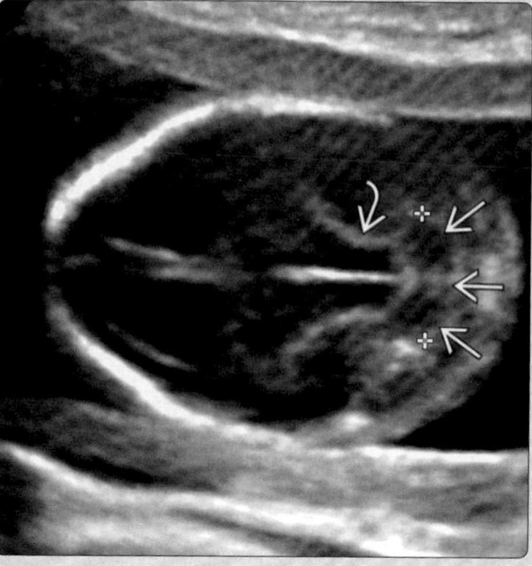

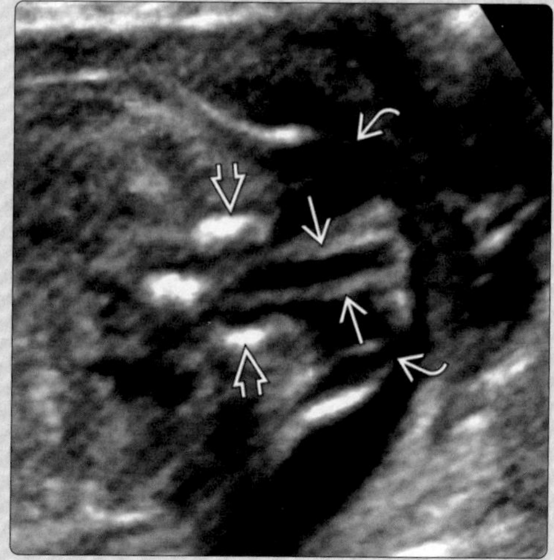

(Left) *In this 18-week fetus, an axial view through the posterior fossa shows hindbrain compression. The cerebellum (calipers →) wraps around the midbrain →, taking on the typical banana shape described with Chiari 2 malformation.* **(Right)** *Axial view of the lumbar spine in the same fetus shows neural elements → extending through splayed dorsal spine ossification centers (arches) → and into the myelomeningocele sac →. Chiari 2 is highly associated with open spina bifida.*

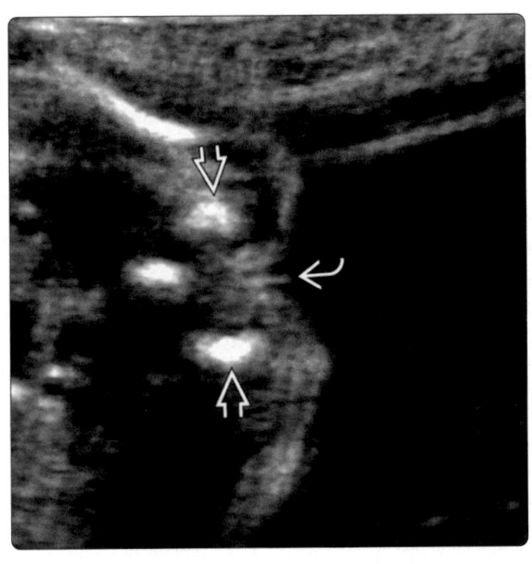

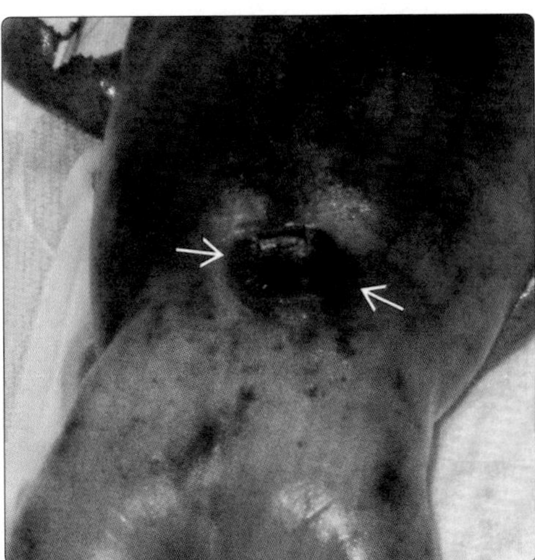

(Left) *Axial view through the spine of an 18-week fetus shows divergent dorsal spine ossification centers ➡ and a skin defect with linear echoes ➡ but no sac. The spinal cord itself is part of the neural elements in myeloschisis (open spina bifida without a sac).* **(Right)** *A clinical photograph of myeloschisis shows the skin defect ➡, exposure of neural elements, and no sac. Myeloschisis can be subtle on ultrasound, and it's the presence of Chiari 2 findings in the brain that alerts the sonographer to look carefully for an open spine defect.*

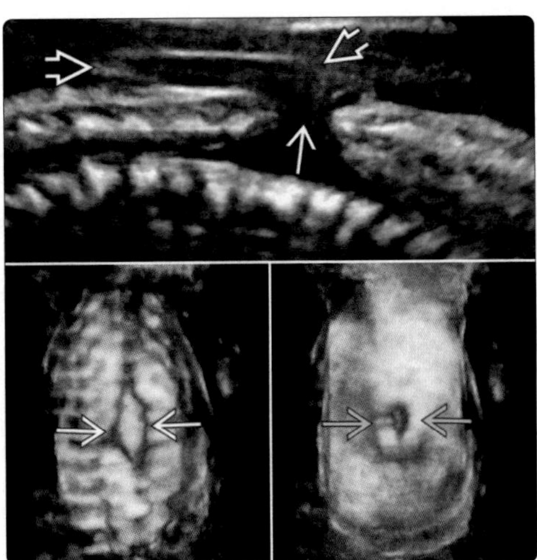

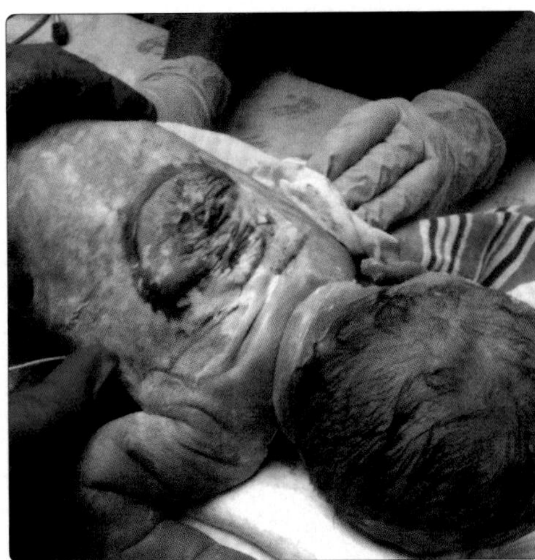

(Left) *3D multiplanar and bone-/soft tissue-rendered views show a midthoracic spinal defect ➡ with a sac ➡. The skin-rendered 3D view (bottom right) shows the skin defect ➡. The fetus had typical Chiari 2 findings in the brain.* **(Right)** *The postnatal clinical photograph after cesarean delivery shows the thoracic myelomeningocele sac. The most common location for spina bifida is lumbosacral. However, spina bifida can occur in the cervical and thoracic spine as well.*

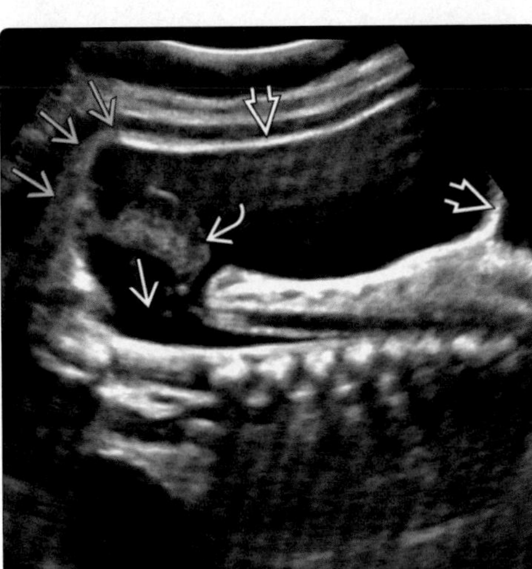

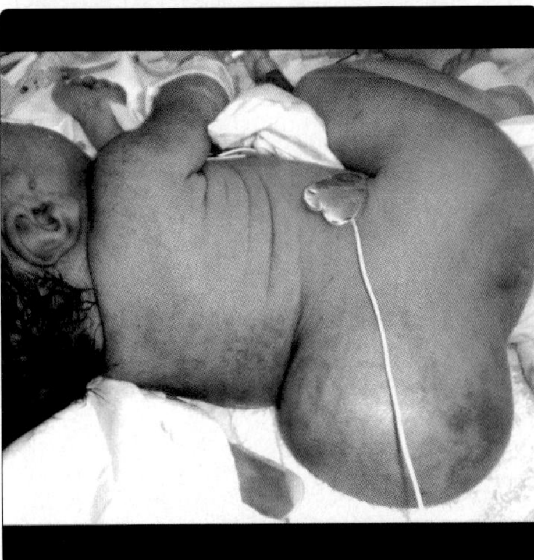

(Left) *In this case of a large lumbosacral meningomyelocele, there is a bone defect ➡ with neural tissue in the sac ➡. However, the covering "membrane" ➡ is thick, echogenic, and contiguous with the fetal skin ➡. This finding and the absence of Chiari 2 malformation led to the correct diagnosis of a skin-covered closed spina bifida.* **(Right)** *Clinical photograph after delivery shows the skin-covered myelomeningocele.*

KEY FACTS

TERMINOLOGY

- Malformation complex characterized by varying degrees of developmental failure involving sacral and lumbar vertebrae and corresponding segments of spinal cord
  - Abnormal innervation affects lower extremity development

IMAGING

- 1st-trimester US findings
  - Short crown-rump length
  - May have increased nuchal translucency
- 2nd- and 3rd-trimester US findings
  - Abrupt termination of spine on longitudinal views
    - Looks as if spine has been rubbed out
  - Because of absent sacrum, iliac wings are approximated or fused (shield appearance)
  - Lower extremity contractures and muscle wasting
    - Crossed-legged tailor or Buddha pose
- GI and GU anomalies common and often severe
- Open neural tube defect in up to 50%
- Congenital heart disease in 24%

CLINICAL ISSUES

- 1% of infants born to diabetic mothers have caudal regression sequence (CRS)
- 12-16% of infants with CRS have diabetic mothers
- Clinical outcome determined by level of defect
  - Neurogenic bladder, motor deficits common in survivors

SCANNING TIPS

- Always check for spine ossification centers in axial scan plane at level of iliac wings
  - Sacrum not well ossified until mid-2nd trimester
  - Mild cases easy to miss
- Can be seen at time of nuchal translucency exam
  - Should specifically target in any diabetic mother
  - Perform transvaginal exam looking for contour abnormalities of lower spine

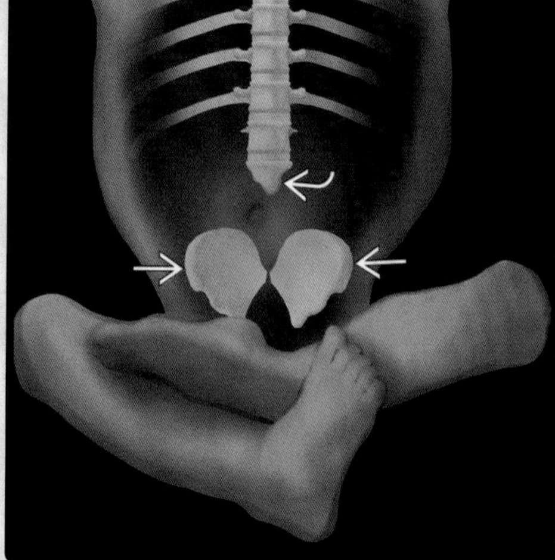

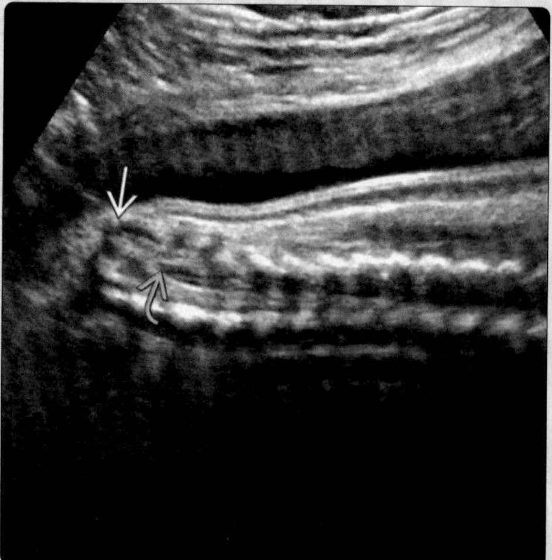

(Left) *Graphic illustrates several features of caudal regression sequence (CRS), including abrupt termination of the spine, absence of the sacrum, and medial positioning of the iliac wings. The pelvis is foreshortened, and there is abnormal lower extremity positioning (crossed-legged tailor or Buddha pose) with muscle wasting.* **(Right)** *Coronal view of the spine at 32 weeks shows abrupt termination at L2. The conus of the spinal cord is seen ending above that point.*

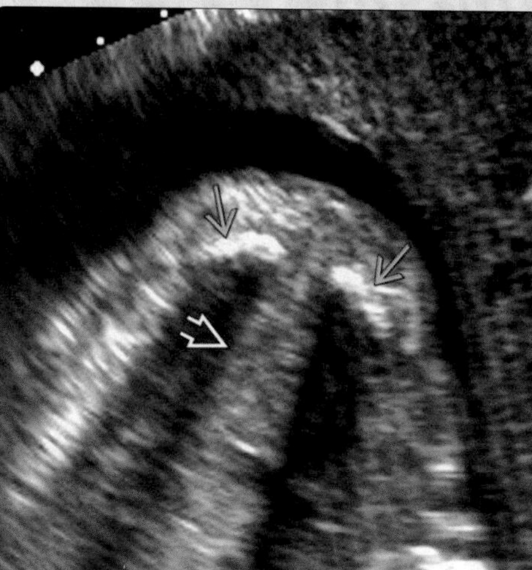

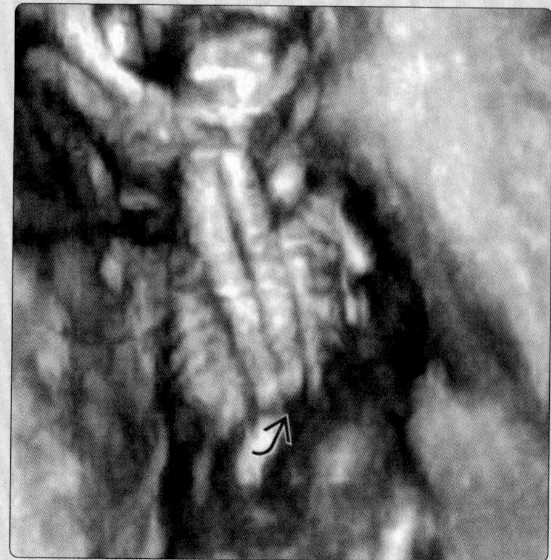

(Left) *Axial transvaginal ultrasound of the fetal pelvis shows absence of the sacrum; note the lack of shadowing as there is no bone to reflect the ultrasound beam. This creates a shield appearance of the iliac wings as they are brought closer together.* **(Right)** *3D ultrasound of the fetal spine at 20 weeks shows abrupt termination at the 12th thoracic vertebra in a severe case of CRS. Other abnormalities are common, including GI, GU, open neural tube defects, and cardiac anomalies.*

KEY FACTS

IMAGING

- Exophytic mixed cystic/solid mass extending from sacrum
  - Variable size but often large, with potential for extremely rapid growth
  - Commonly extends into pelvis and abdomen
- Solid tumors may have significant arteriovenous shunting
  - Color Doppler essential to evaluate vascularity
  - Scan every 1-3 weeks depending on size, vascularity, impending hydrops, and complications
- Calculate tumor volume:fetal weight ratio (TFR)
  - Tumor volume: Tumor length x width x depth x 0.523
  - Divide by estimated fetal weight
  - TFR > 0.12 prior to 24 weeks has poor prognosis

TOP DIFFERENTIAL DIAGNOSES

- Myelomeningocele in differential for cystic SCGT
  - Sac contains meninges + neural elements
  - Splayed posterior spinal ossification centers
  - Chiari 2 malformation of brain

CLINICAL ISSUES

- Large, solid, vascular tumors have high mortality and morbidity; better outcome for cystic tumors
- Prognosis significantly worse for fetus than neonate
  - Fetal diagnosis 30-50% mortality

SCANNING TIPS

- Carefully assess for intrapelvic extension as it is part of surgical classification
- Try to measure tumor in same plane each time
- Evaluate for signs of impending cardiovascular compromise
  - Tumor growth, amniotic fluid index, placental thickness
  - Any signs of developing hydrops (skin edema, pleural or pericardial effusion, ascites)
- Early vascular signs of high cardiac output state
  - Increased cardiothoracic ratio (> 50%)
  - Inferior cava diameter > 1 cm
  - Increase descending aortic velocity (> 120 cm/s)
- Look for complications: Tumor rupture/hemorrhage

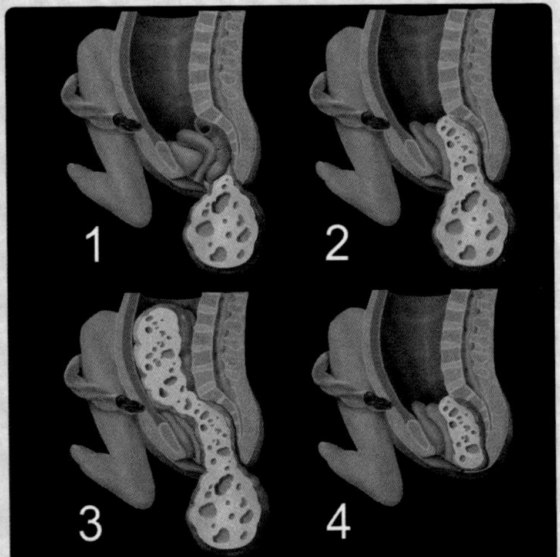

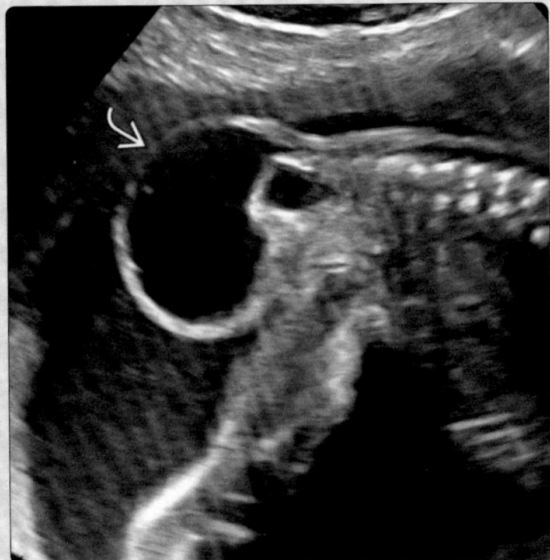

(Left) *Graphic shows the surgical classification of sacrococcygeal teratoma (SCGT). Type 1 is predominately external with minimal presacral component; type 2 extends into the presacral space; type 3 extends up into the abdomen; and type 4 is completely internal.* **(Right)** *This sagittal US of the distal spine at 18 weeks shows a predominately cystic SCGT ➔. This remained stable throughout gestation, and the prenatal course was uncomplicated. A cystic SCGT generally has a good prognosis.*

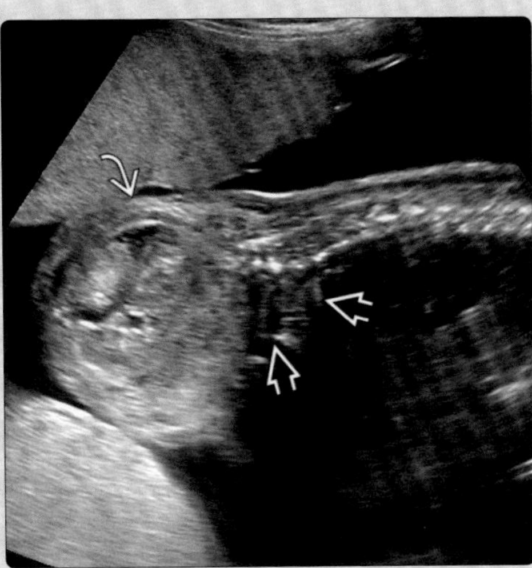

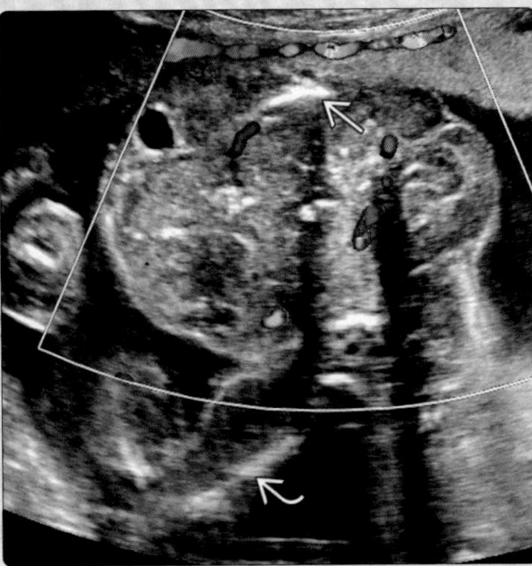

(Left) *As a comparison, here is an example of a solid SCGT ➔ of similar size in a 19.5-week fetus. Note the extension into the presacral space ➔.* **(Right)** *In 4 weeks time, there was dramatic growth (note the size of the leg for comparison ➔). This mass shows several classic features of a teratoma, including internal vascularity and calcifications ➔. Solid tumors may show very rapid growth and have a much more guarded prognosis. This fetus developed hydrops with intrauterine fetal death at 26 weeks.*

PART VI
SECTION 3
Face and Neck

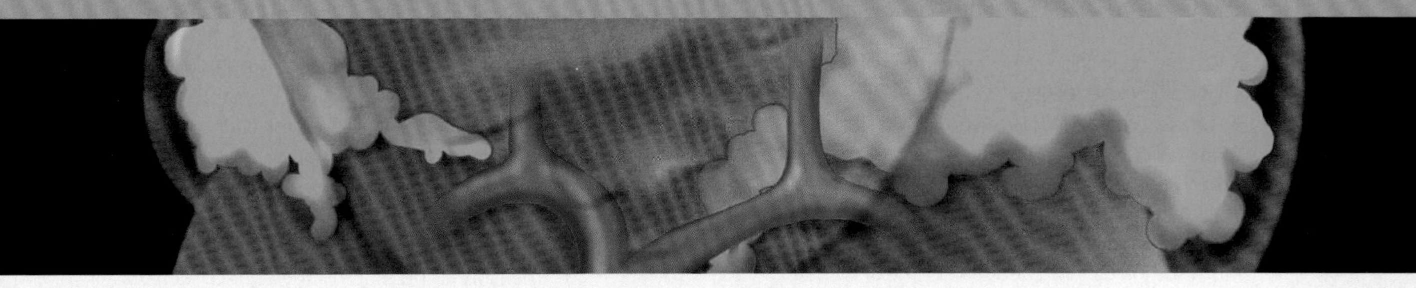

Anatomy and Approach

Face and Neck Lesions

EMBRYOLOGY AND ANATOMY

Overview

- For patient, her family, and her support system, imaging of fetal face is one of most anticipated parts of ultrasound exam
  - Studies have shown that seeing fetal face improves bonding experiences
- 3D ultrasound is additive to show both normal and abnormal anatomy
  - With single 3D view, like photograph, everyone can immediately recognize face
- Much of face and neck anatomy routinely seen in midgestation can also be seen at time of nuchal translucency screening

Key Embryology Concepts

- Right and left upper lip, maxilla, and nostrils start as separated plates of tissue (placodes)
  - Placodes migrate medially and fuse
  - Failure to fuse leads to cleft lip, cleft palate, nose deformities, and midface hypoplasia
- Bony palate has separate front portion (primary palate) and paired side and back portions (secondary palate) that also have to migrate together and fuse
  - Failure to fuse leads to bony and soft tissue cleft palate
- Jaw growth, ear development, and posterior soft tissue palate development occur together and are linked
  - If mandible is small, ears are often low set
  - Extremely small mandible is almost always associated with soft tissue palate defect
    - Very hard to see with ultrasound
    - Soft tissue palate is more easily seen with fetal MR

SCANNING APPROACH AND IMAGING ISSUES

Standard Views of Fetal Face

- **Nose and lips view**
  - Technique: Angle transducer to obtain coronal view of nose and mouth (snout view)
  - Structures seen
    - Intact upper lip
    - Normal rounded nares and nostrils
  - **Pitfalls**
    - If including bony maxilla, then too far back
- **Profile view**
  - Technique: Angle transducer exactly midline and sagittal
  - Structures seen
    - Full nasal bone, forehead, maxilla, mandible
  - **Pitfalls**
    - Erroneous short or absent nasal bone because angle of beam is "shooting" down length of nose
      - Take image when fetal neck position is neutral (not looking straight up)
      - Ultrasound beam should be near 90° to nasal bone
    - Short nasal bone because not true sagittal
    - Fetal head is tucked down so chin looks small
- **Orbits (eyes)**
  - Technique: Axial view through orbits
  - Structures seen: Orbits, lens of eyes
  - **Pitfalls**
    - Central hyaloid canal/artery (thin line extending from lens to dorsal orbit) not to be confused with anomaly
    - Off-axis view may make one orbit look small
- **Nuchal fold** (measure 16-20 weeks)
  - Technique: Standard angulated (< 15°) view through posterior fossa includes neck skin
    - Measure from outer skull to skin/fluid interface
  - Structures seen
    - Nuchal skin (should be < 6 mm)
    - Additional posterior fossa structures include cerebellum, vermis, cisterna magna
  - **Pitfalls**
    - Overangulation causes false thickened nuchal fold (measuring too much of lower neck skin)
    - Including skull in measurement

Additional Views (Detailed Exam)

- **Maxilla**
  - Sagittal view: Box-like and without disruption
    - Any disruption > 2 mm suggests cleft palate
    - Appearance of flattened midface is abnormal
      - Measure maxilla-nasion-mandible angle (MNM)
  - Axial view: Show curved intact anterior maxilla
- **Mandible**
  - Sagittal view: Frontal margin only slightly behind maxilla front margin
    - Measure MNM angle if profile is abnormal
  - Axial view: Measure jaw index if mandible is small
- **Ears**
  - Coronal, sagittal, 3D views best to show ear position
    - Top of ear at medial eye level
  - Normal ear length is ~ 1/3 biparietal diameter
- **Thyroid**
  - Axial view: At level of maximum diameter of gland
    - Fluid-filled central airway and peripheral neck vessels flank thyroid gland
  - Measure thyroid circumference: Compare to published normative data

Role of 3D Ultrasound

- Multiplanar capacity allows for evaluation of normal anatomy in challenging fetal position cases
  - Example: Coronal view of face is obtainable but profile is not because of fetal position
    - Obtain 3D volume in coronal plane and manipulate images in orthogonal planes to get good profile view
- Better evaluation of facial anomalies
  - Cleft lip/palate
    - Soft tissue views show extent of defect to family and maxillofacial team
    - Palate defects seen best with multiplanar views and bone rendered views
  - Ear anomalies seen best with 3D
    - Helix anomalies, deficient ear
    - Ear position on face
  - Complex face anomalies and facial characteristics associated with syndromes
    - More easily identified with photograph-like 3D images than with multiple 2D views in different planes

ANATOMY OF FACE AND NECK

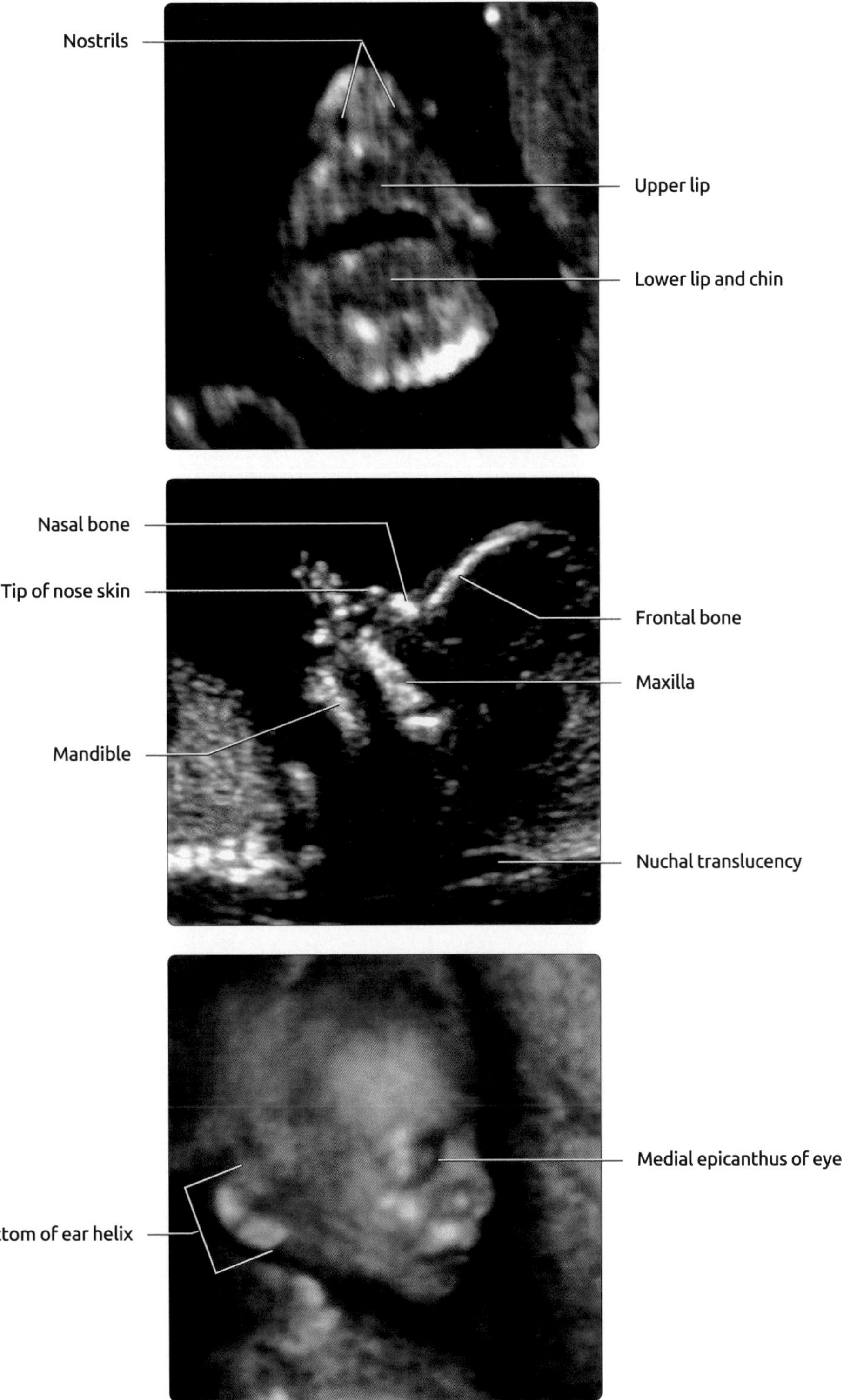

(Top) *Frontal ultrasound through the soft tissue of the fetal nose and lips shows the nares, nostrils, intact upper lip, and part of the lower lip and chin. Documentation of the nose and lips with this view is considered part of the routine anatomy scan at midgestation.* **(Middle)** *High-resolution, midsagittal face and neck view of a 12-week fetus presenting for nuchal translucency (NT) assessment shows important anatomy in addition to the normal NT. The normal nasal bone is as bright as the frontal bone and is seen separately from the nasal skin. In addition, the normal profile view seen here includes a normally shaped frontal bone, a box-like maxilla, and a normal-sized mandible. Cleft palate, abnormal calvarium, flat midface, and small chin can be diagnosed at the time of NT scan.* **(Bottom)** *3D ultrasound profile view in this fetus includes the nose, eye, and ear and shows a normal face. The top of the ear helix should be at the same height as the medial epicanthus of the eye. 3D ultrasound is the best modality to look at ear shape. In addition, most patients enjoy seeing the soft tissue rendered normal fetus images in which they can easily identify "the baby."*

FETAL FACE MEASUREMENTS

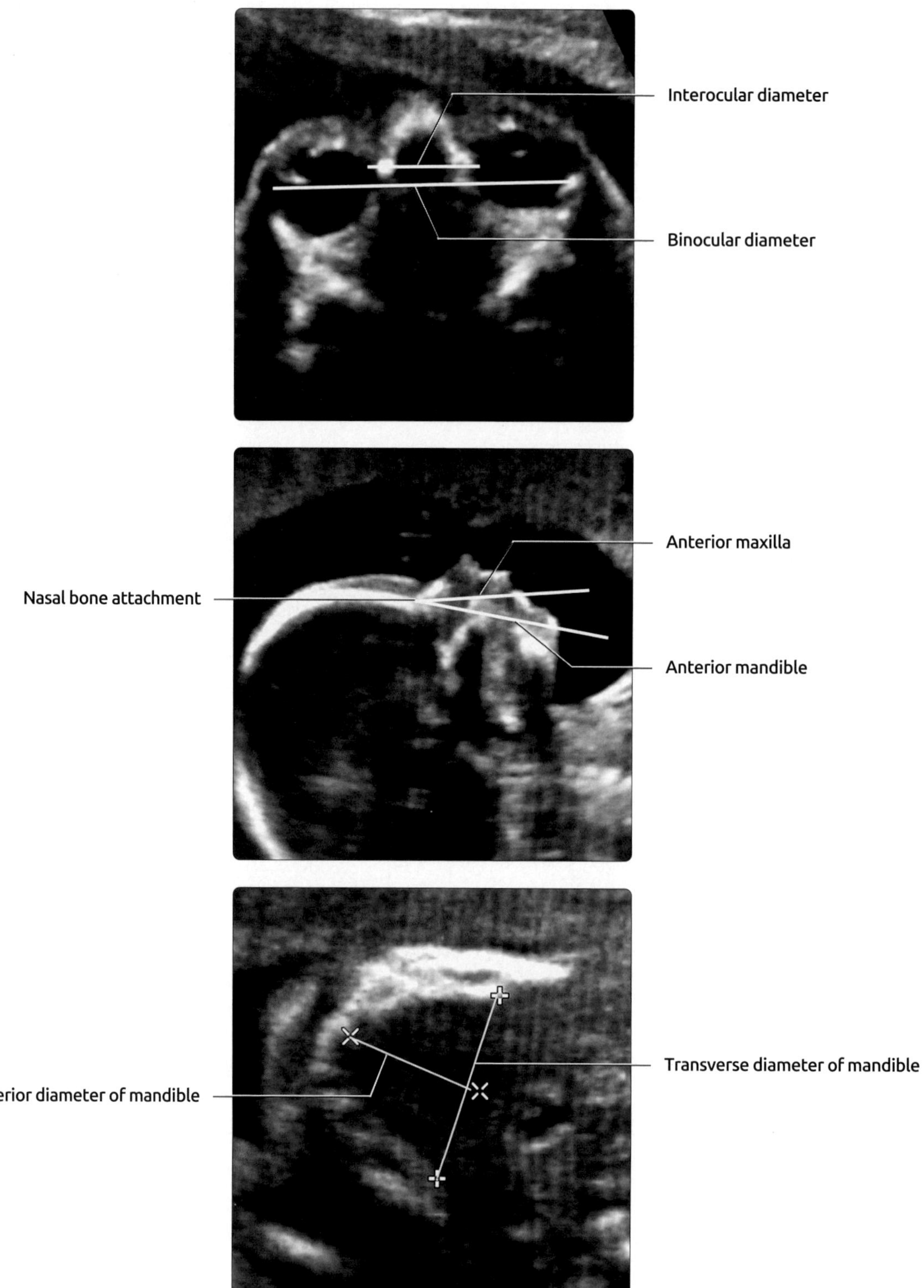

(Top) *If the eyes appear to be too close or too far apart, orbit measurements can be obtained and compared with published tables. The binocular diameter and the interocular diameter can be measured easily. By "eyeballing" it, a 3rd eye should fit between the 2 normal eyes.* **(Middle)** *The maxilla-nasion-mandible (MNM) angle is the angle formed between a line from the nasal bone attachment at the skull to the front of the maxilla and a line from the same nasal point attachment to the front of the mandible. Normal MNM angle is consistently near 13.5° (5th percentile to 95th percentile range: 10.4°-16.9°). MNM > 95th percentile suggests a small chin (micrognathia). MNM < 5th percentile suggests a flat midface. These measurements are not routinely obtained but recommended if midface or mandible anomalies are suspected.* **(Bottom)** *If a small chin (hypognathia or micrognathia) is suspected on the profile view, an axial view through the body of the mandible can be used to measure the transverse and anterior-posterior diameter of the mandible. The jaw index can be calculated (AP diameter/BPD x 100) and compared with published gestational age normative data.*

EMBRYOLOGY OF LYMPHATIC DISORDERS

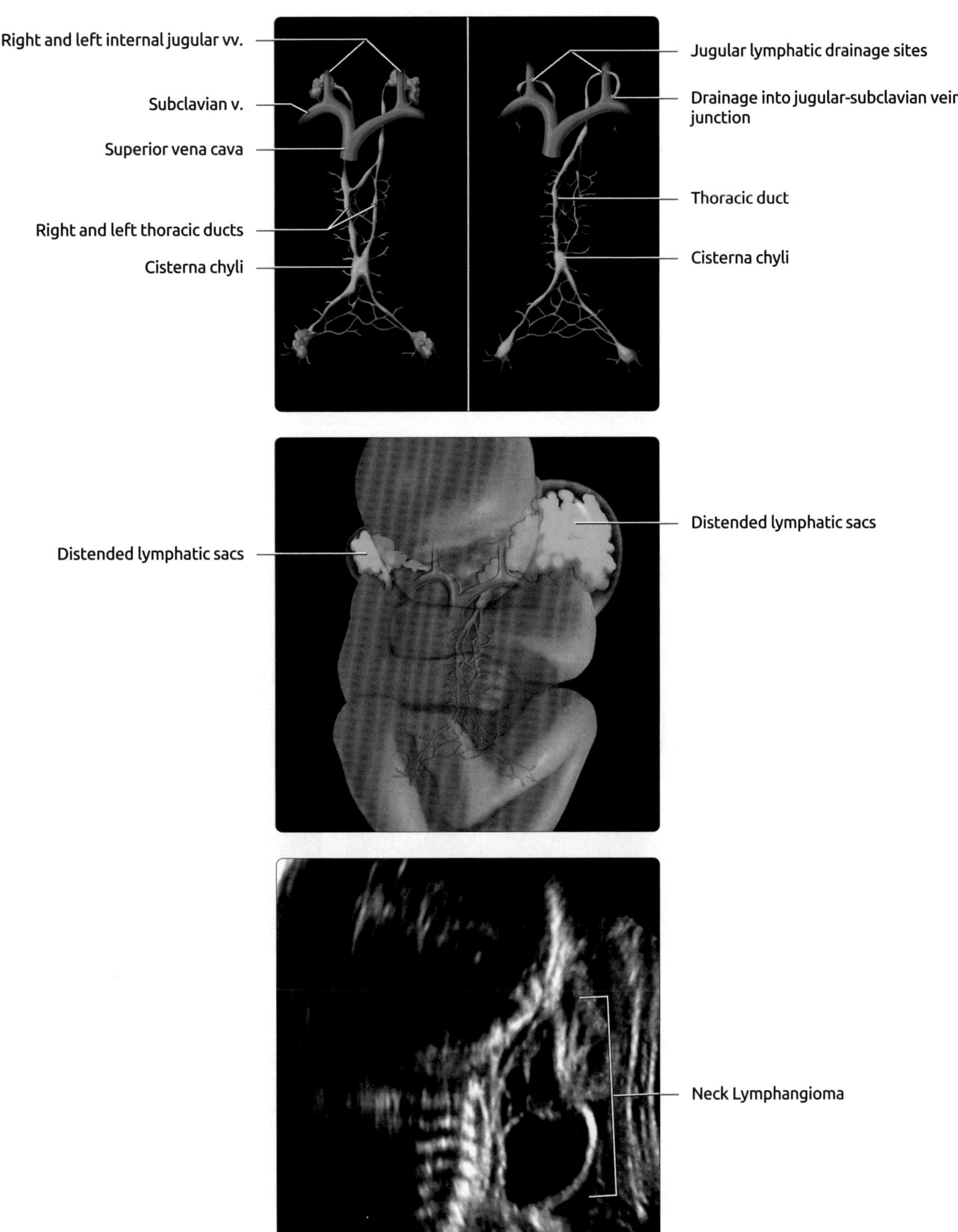

(Top) *Graphic of the lymphatic system at 7 weeks (left) and 17 weeks (right) shows that, originally, there are paired thoracic ducts. Portions involute, resulting in a thoracic duct in the chest that crosses the midline. Upper body lymphatic drainage occurs mostly at the venous connection near the jugular-subclavian vein junction.* **(Middle)** *Graphic of lymphatic obstruction shows massively distended jugular lymph sacs because the connection of jugular drainage sites to the venous system failed. When this happens symmetrically in the neck, the fetus will develop cystic hygroma. Focal or asymmetric drainage blockages will lead to focally dilated lymphatic channels and lymphangioma. These "masses" are usually large and are most often in the neck, axilla, and chest, although they can also involve the trunk and lower extremities.* **(Bottom)** *In this fetus with a left anterolateral neck lymphangioma, the lymphatic/venous connection anomaly was localized to the left jugular/lymphatic drainage site. The rest of the fetus was normal. Unlike cystic hygroma, this anomaly is not associated with chromosome defects and has less chance of developing additional fluid drainage problems leading to hydrops.*

Cleft Lip, Palate

KEY FACTS

TERMINOLOGY

- Cleft lip (CL) occurs ± cleft palate (CP)
  - > 80% of fetuses with CL also have CP
- Variable classifications, best to be descriptive about defects
  - Unilateral (right or left), bilateral, midline
  - Complete CL: Defect extends to nose (nares)
  - Incomplete CL: Cleft does not extend to nares
- Primary palate: Front of palate (alveolar ridge)
- Secondary palate: Back of palate (soft + hard palate)

IMAGING

- Unilateral CL + CP is most common type
  - CL extends to nose and flattens nares
  - Seen best on standard coronal nose-lip view
- Bilateral CL/CP
  - Alveolar ridge becomes mass-like and bulges forward
  - Profile view best to see premaxillary protrusion
- Midline CL/CP: Central lip and palate defect
  - Flat midface and nose
- Isolated CP without CL is highly associated with small chin
  - Palate defect is deep (posterior to alveolar ridge)
- 3D ultrasound helpful for making specific diagnosis
  - Helps family and maxillofacial team prepare
- Associations: Aneuploidy, brain, and cardiac anomalies
  - Trisomy 13, trisomy 18, > 200 syndromes
  - More likely with midline and bilateral CL/CP

SCANNING TIPS

- Best to obtain 3D volume from profile view
  - Use soft tissue post processing to determine if CL extends to nares and their appearance (often flattened)
  - Use axial plane and bone postprocessing coronal images to best evaluate palate defect
- When chin is small, look for fluid extending from mouth to nasal cavity posteriorly (soft tissue palate defect)
- Scan carefully for other anomalies, especially brain and heart

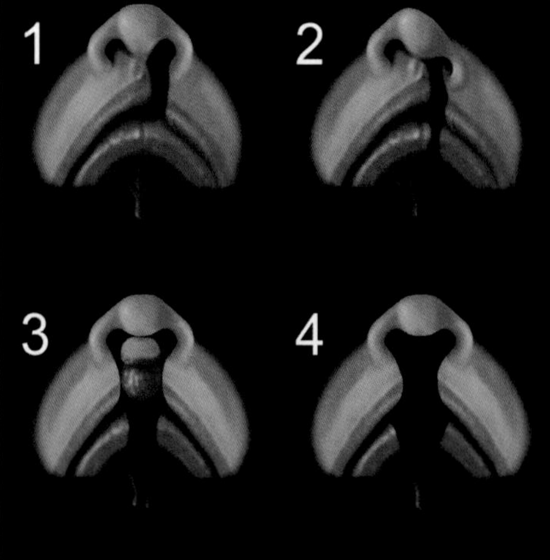

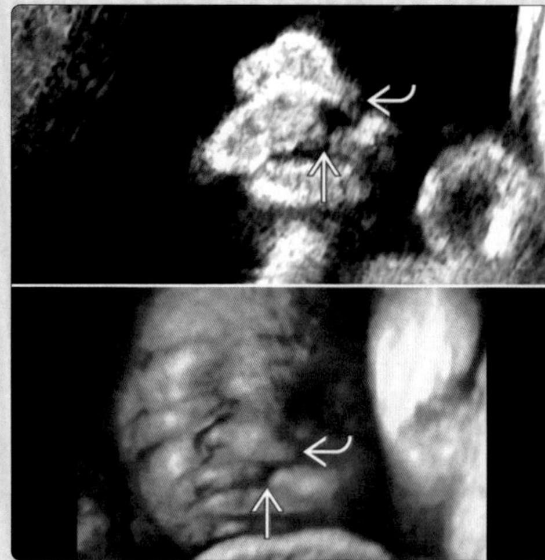

(Left) *Graphic shows the different types of cleft lip (CL) and cleft palate (CP) defect. 1 is CL without CP (most subtle type and not frequently seen in utero), 2 is unilateral CL with CP (most common type seen in utero), 3 is bilateral CL and CP, and 4 is midline CL/CP.* **(Right)** *Angled coronal nose/mouth view (top) and 3D surface-rendered view (bottom) show a unilateral CL ➡. The flattened naris ➡ is seen best with 3D. This fetus also had CP. Treatment includes multiple surgeries and presurgical nasal alveolar molding.*

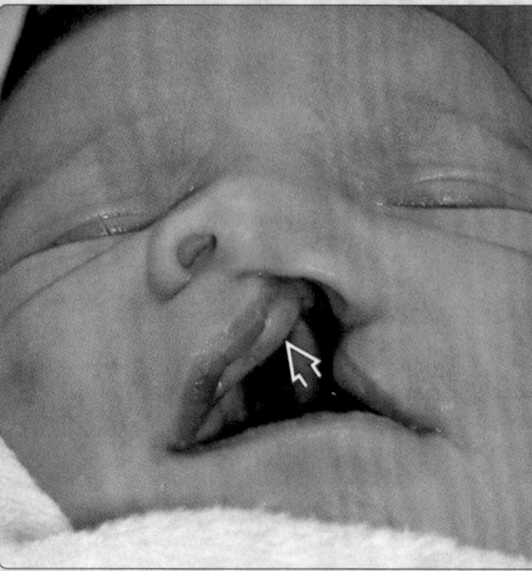

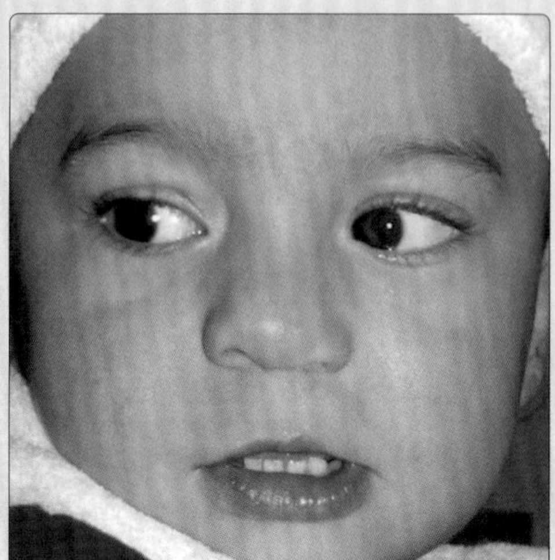

(Left) *Clinical photograph of a child with unilateral complete CL and CP demonstrates the defect extending to the nose, flat naris, and the palate defect involving the anterior alveolar ridge ➡ (and beyond).* **(Right)** *Clinical photograph of the same child after lip and palate repair demonstrates minimal deformity. Further lip or nasal revisions in adolescence may be performed. Modern surgical techniques yield excellent results. Most children need at least 2 operations and many need speech therapy.*

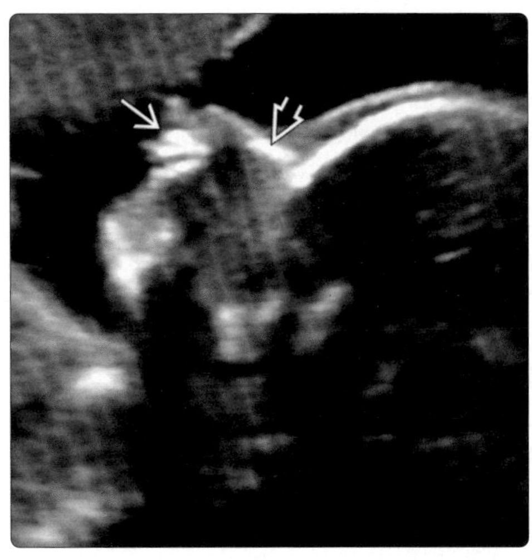

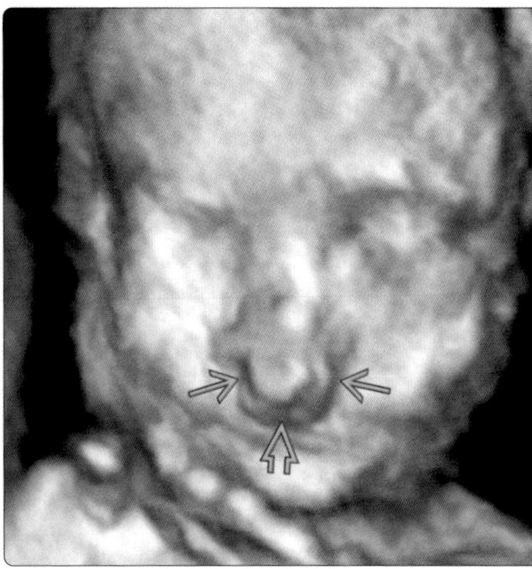

(Left) *Profile view of a 2nd-trimester fetus with bilateral CL/CP shows the classic premaxillary protuberance ➡ beneath the nose (nasal bone ➡). Premaxillary "mass" is a hallmark finding of bilateral CL with CP and should not be confused with a true mass. Protrusion of the alveolar ridge, flanked by bilateral clefts, causes this appearance.* **(Right)** *3D surface-rendered image in the same fetus at 20 weeks, confirms bilateral CL ➡ and mass-like premaxillary protrusion ➡. The karyotype results were normal.*

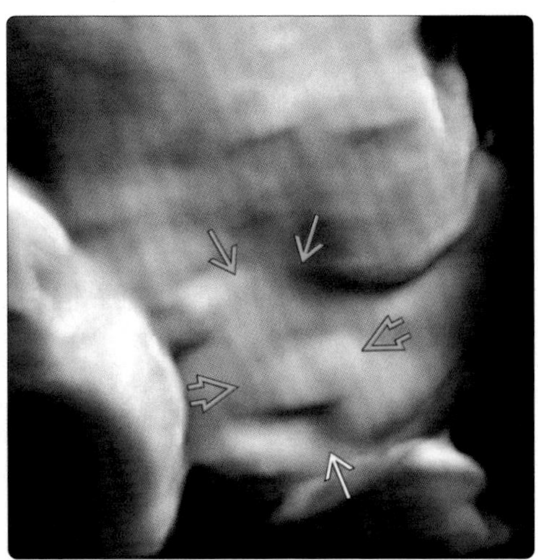

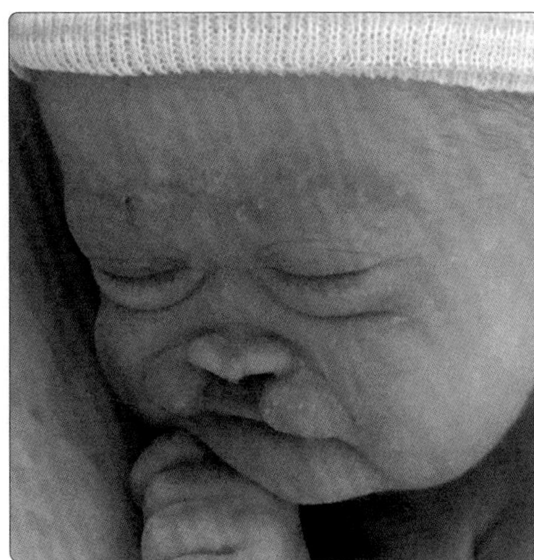

(Left) *3D surface-rendered image of the face shows a midline CL ➡, flat nose ➡ with fused nares, and close-set eyes ➡. The fetus also had a severe brain anomaly (alobar holoprosencephaly).* **(Right)** *Photograph of the child after delivery confirms the prenatal diagnosis. Midline CL/CP is highly associated with midline brain anomalies, usually on the holoprosencephaly spectrum. Both defects are associated with trisomy 13. This child's karyotype results were normal.*

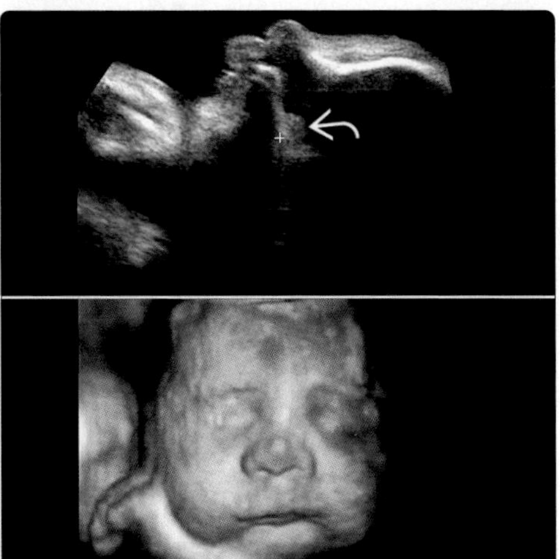

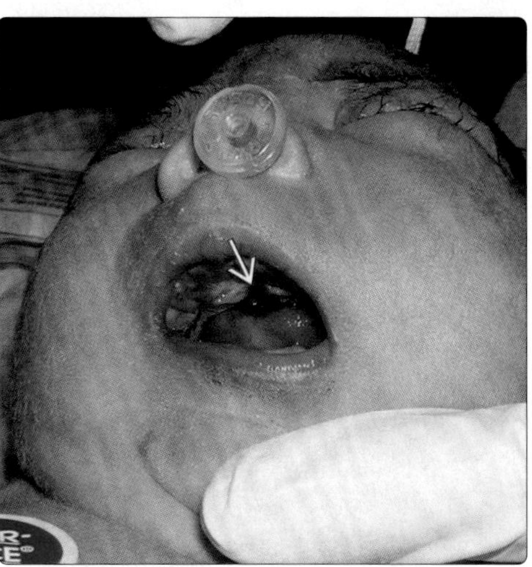

(Left) *3D face and multiplanar profile views of a fetus with small chin shows CP. The surface-rendered view (bottom) shows a small chin and an intact upper lip; however, the tongue ➡ and a sliver of amniotic fluid extends into the nasal cavity through a posterior palate defect.* **(Right)** *Postnatal photograph from the same case shows the posterior palate defect ➡. A nasal airway is placed because of the resultant airway obstruction. Hypognathia is strongly associated with dorsal palate defect (often difficult to see in utero).*

Cystic Hygroma

KEY FACTS

TERMINOLOGY

- Cystic lymphatic disorder involving **back and side of neck** causing multiseptated fluid-filled mass

IMAGING

- Cystic hygroma (CH) is typically large
  - **Multiple internal septations** is key to diagnosis
  - Different than isolated ↑ nuchal translucency because of size and septations
- Associated with hydrops
  - Hydrops defined as fluid in 2 anatomic areas
  - CH counts as 1 area: Additional findings include pleural effusion, ascites, skin edema beyond neck
  - CH and hydrops can be diagnosed in 1st trimester
- Highly associated with aneuploidy and syndromes (2/3)
  - Turner syndrome (monosomy X): Most common
  - Trisomy 21: 2nd most common
  - Others: Trisomy 18, trisomy 13, Noonan syndrome, other syndromes

TOP DIFFERENTIAL DIAGNOSES

- Body/trunk lymphangioma
  - Less likely to cause hydrops, not associated with aneuploidy
- Occipital encephalocele: Calvarial defect + brain anomaly
- Cervical teratoma: Solid and cystic mass

CLINICAL ISSUES

- CH + hydrops is grim finding, high mortality rates
- Small isolated CH may resolve
- Genetic counseling recommended for all cases

SCANNING TIPS

- Use high-resolution probe to look for septations
- Large CH may mimic pocket of amniotic fluid
  - Move patient to move fetus away from uterine wall
- CH may be only "tapable" pocket of fluid for amniocentesis, karyotype is possible with this technique

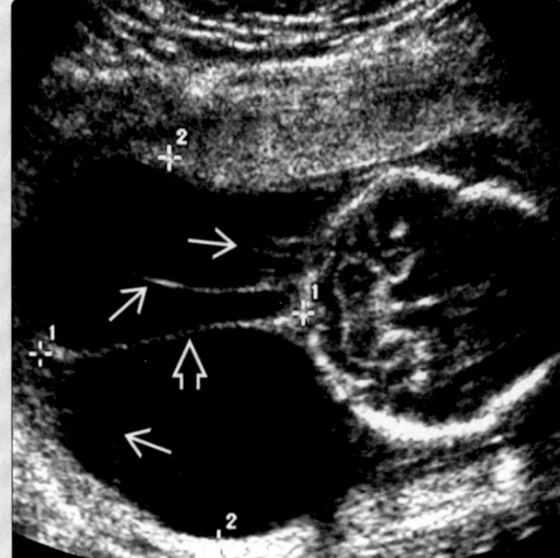

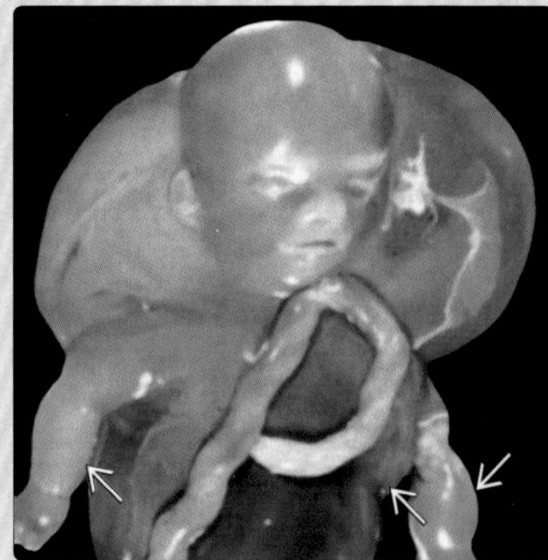

(Left) *The cystic hygroma (CH) (calipers) in this fetus is larger than the fetal head. It contains multiple thin septations ➡. The midline septation ➡ is the nuchal ligament. Oligohydramnios was also present. If fluid for genetic testing is desired, and there are no other accessible fluid pockets, the CH can be sampled for testing.* **(Right)** *Postmortem photograph of a fetus with Turner syndrome shows a large CH as well as body wall and extremity edema ➡. CH, hydrops, and Turner syndrome are common associations.*

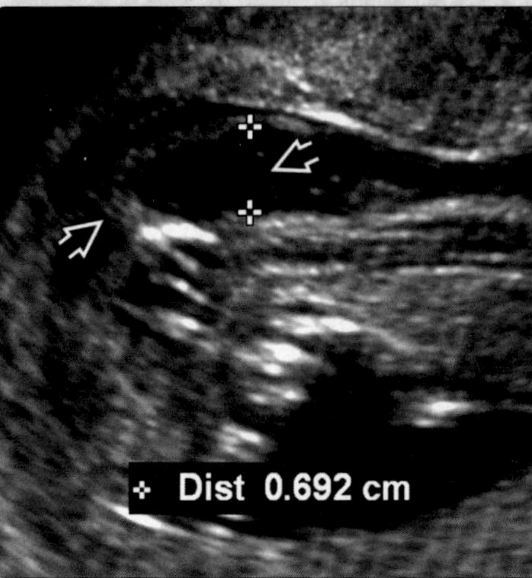

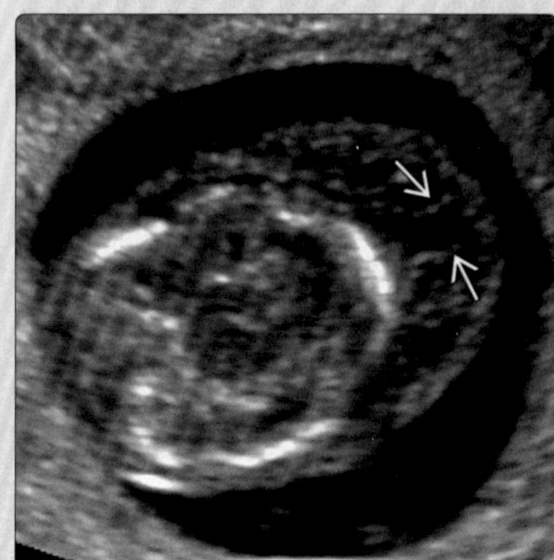

(Left) *A large nuchal translucency (NT) of 6.9 mm is seen in this 12-week fetus. Note the presence of thick and thin septations ➡, allowing for a more accurate diagnosis of CH, rather than simply increased NT.* **(Right)** *High-resolution axial view through the posterior neck in the same fetus shows more thin septations ➡. The patient chose to have CVS instead of maternal serum screening. The results were positive for an unbalanced translocation.*

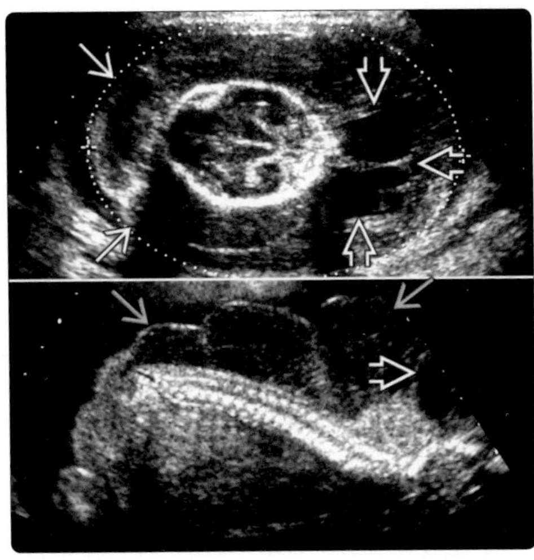

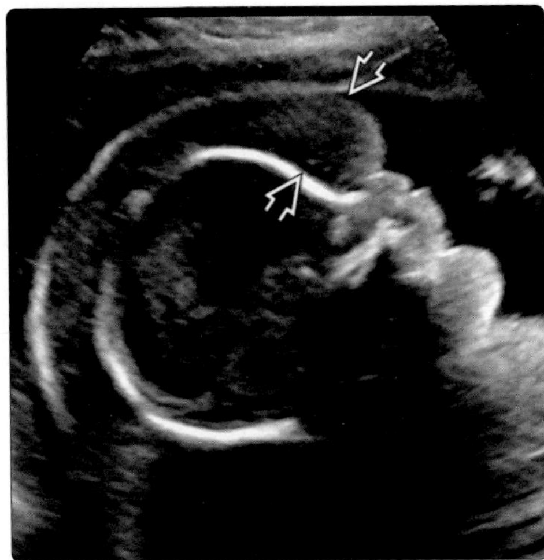

(Left) *Axial (top) and sagittal (bottom) images of the fetal head (top) and back (bottom) show marked skin thickening extending to the front of the calvarium* ➡ *and down the back* ➡*, as well as a nuchal CH* ➡ *in a fetus with trisomy 21. The extent of lymphedema in this case is unusually severe.* **(Right)** *A profile view in another fetus with a CH shows marked scalp and facial edema/anasarca* ➡*. The fetus developed worsening hydrops at 30 weeks, and the newborn died shortly after delivery.*

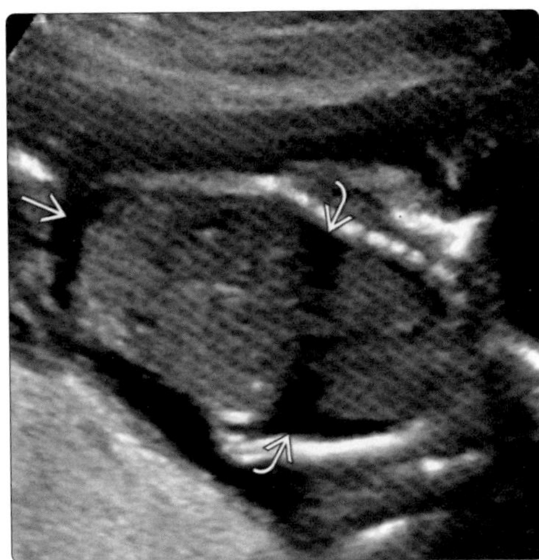

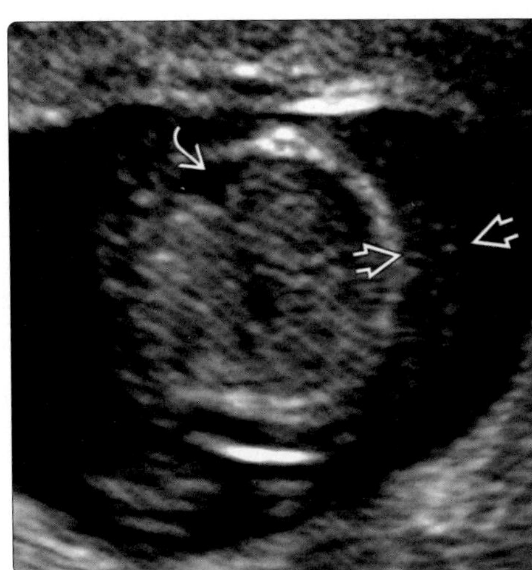

(Left) *Coronal view of the chest and abdomen in a fetus with CH detected at the time of NT screening, shows ascites* ➡ *and pleural effusions* ➡*. These findings may be subtle in the 1st trimester.* **(Right)** *Axial image through the body, in another 1st-trimester case, shows anasarca* ➡ *and ascites* ➡*. Development of hydrops is a very bad prognostic sign with a high rate of in utero demise.*

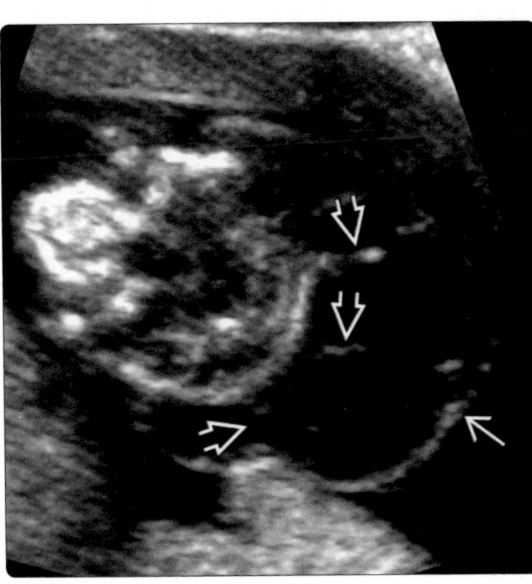

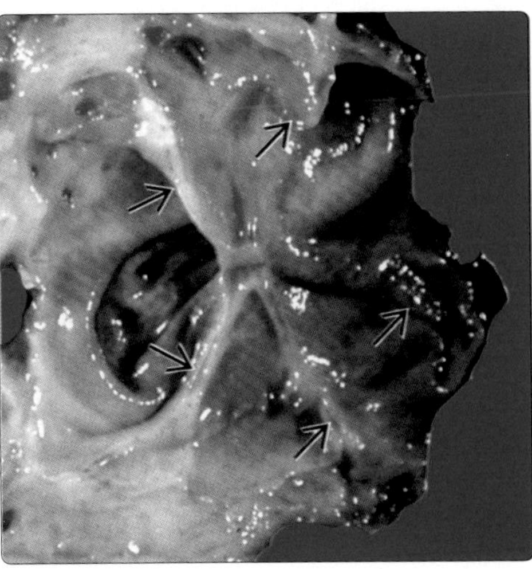

(Left) *Ultrasound shows an early 2nd-trimester CH. Axial view through the posterior neck shows a cystic mass* ➡ *with septations* ➡*.* **(Right)** *Gross pathology of a CH shows multiple internal septations* ➡*. CHs are smooth cystic masses of dilated lymphatic sacs lined by a single layer of flattened endothelium.*

PART VI
SECTION 4
Chest

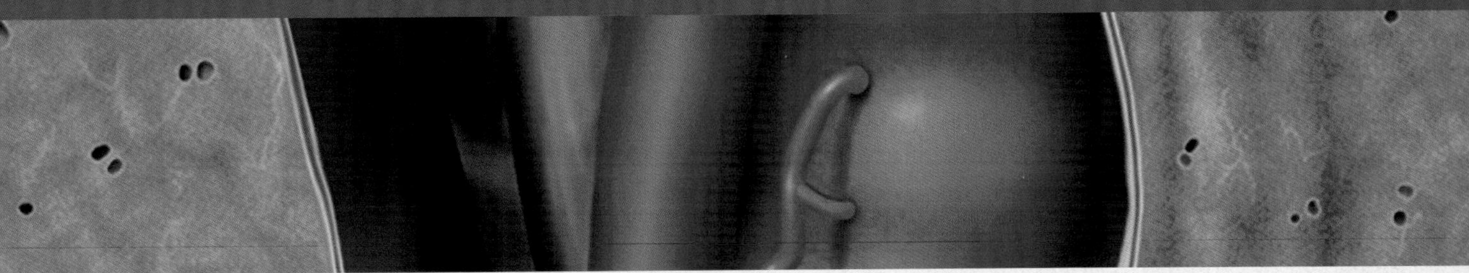

Anatomy and Approach

Chest Lesions

EMBRYOLOGY AND ANATOMY

Overview

- **Trachea** separates from foregut and developing esophagus
  - Failure to separate results in tracheoesophageal fistula
- **Lungs** go through several stages of development from primitive bronchi to alveoli capable of respiration
  - Until alveoli develop (~ 25 weeks gestational age) fetus would not be able to breath if delivered
  - Adequate intrathoracic volume required for normal pulmonary development
    - Intrathoracic masses (especially diaphragmatic hernia) and chest wall abnormalities (e.g., skeletal dysplasias) restrict space for lung growth
  - Amniotic fluid and fetal breathing also required for normal lung development; oligohydramnios has severe adverse effect on lung development
- **Diaphragm** development is complex with 4 embryologic structures which must fuse; failure of fusion results in a congenital diaphragmatic hernia (CDH)

SCANNING APPROACH AND IMAGING ISSUES

Techniques and Sonographic Appearance

- Required chest views include: 4-chamber heart, outflow tracts, and diaphragm
  - Evaluation of lungs is not specified but are generally well seen when obtaining required views
- **Heart** occupies ~ 1/3 of intrathoracic area
  - **Cardiothoracic ratio** is calculated by dividing cardiac circumference by thoracic circumference (TC); normal being ~ 50%
  - Increased ratio usually indicates cardiomegaly but may also occur when chest is small
- **Lungs** are initially similar to liver in echogenicity but become more echogenic with advancing gestation
  - Any aberration in this homogeneous echotexture raises suspicion for mass
- **Diaphragm** appears as a thin, arched, hypoechoic band
  - Best imaged in sagittal plane; need to assess both sides completely moving from chest wall to chest wall during real-time scanning
    - Most CDHs occur posteriorly; if only viewed in anterior coronal plane, a CDH may be missed
- **Thymus** may be prominent in 3rd trimester
  - Above the heart and is hypoechoic compared to lungs with a slightly reticular appearance
  - Look for **thy-box** to confirm it is not a chest mass
    - Color Doppler of superior mediastinum, at level of 3-vessel view, shows thymus between internal mammary arteries creating box appearance
- Fetal breathing is essential for normal lung development and is one component of biophysical profile

Approach to Fetal Chest Mass

- The following questions form a framework for evaluation of the fetal chest; specific diagnoses will be discussed in other chapters
- **Is the chest normal in size?**
  - A TC is not generally performed unless there is concern that the chest is small (e.g., skeletal dysplasia)
    - Performed at level of 4-chamber view with soft tissues excluded
  - Can compare to expected value for gestational age or as a ratio with the abdominal circumference (AC)
    - TC:AC ratio is stable throughout gestation with normal being > 0.8
    - Enlarged chest size is unusual but is a prominent feature of congenital high airway obstruction sequence (CHAOS)
- **Is the axis of the heart deviated?**
  - Any shift in cardiac axis is highly suspicious for a thoracic mass or, alternatively, a cardiac defect
  - While a normal axis rules out most significant chest masses, small masses may not deviate axis
- **Where is the stomach?**
  - Absence of the normal abdominal stomach bubble is a cardinal sign of a left-sided CDH (stomach in chest)
  - Important to note, however, that a left-sided hernia may contain only bowel &/or liver, with stomach remaining below diaphragm
  - With a right-sided CDH, stomach remains in the abdomen but is often more midline than normal
- **Is the mass cystic or solid?**
  - Although there is overlap in the 2 differentials [congenital pulmonary airway malformation (CPAM) and CDH may look either cystic or solid], this is the starting point for forming a differential diagnosis
- **If cystic, is it a simple cyst or a complex cystic mass?**
  - Simple cyst is more likely to be a foregut duplication cyst, while a complex cystic mass is more likely to be a CDH, macrocystic CPAM, or lymphangioma
  - Do not confuse an effusion with a cystic mass; lung will float within an effusion and have a wing-like appearance, while a cystic mass will displace and compress lung
- **If solid, what does the Doppler show?**
  - CPAM: Vascular supply from pulmonary circulation
  - Sequestration: Prominent feeding vessel from aorta
  - CDH containing liver will show hepatic and portal veins
- **Where is the mass?**
  - Sequestrations are almost always at left lung base (or below the diaphragm), while CPAMs are more variable in location, occurring equally on both sides
  - Bilateral chest masses are less common but include bilateral CPAMs, bilateral CDHs, or CHAOS
- **Does the mass extend beyond the chest wall?**
  - Lymphangiomas are primarily in subcutaneous tissues, with secondary intrathoracic involvement
  - Teratomas can be locally aggressive and erode through chest wall
- **Is there hydrops?**
  - Development of hydrops is a poor prognostic sign and may warrant clinical intervention (e.g., cyst drainage, in utero resection, early delivery); all chest masses should be monitored carefully for developing hydrops
- **Are there other anomalies?**
  - CDH has a high association with chromosomal anomalies, other structural anomalies, and syndromes
  - Especially important to carefully evaluate the heart
  - Because the cardiac axis is often distorted, it may be more difficult to adequately evaluate, and a dedicated fetal echo may be warranted

LUNGS, DIAPHRAGM, & THYMUS

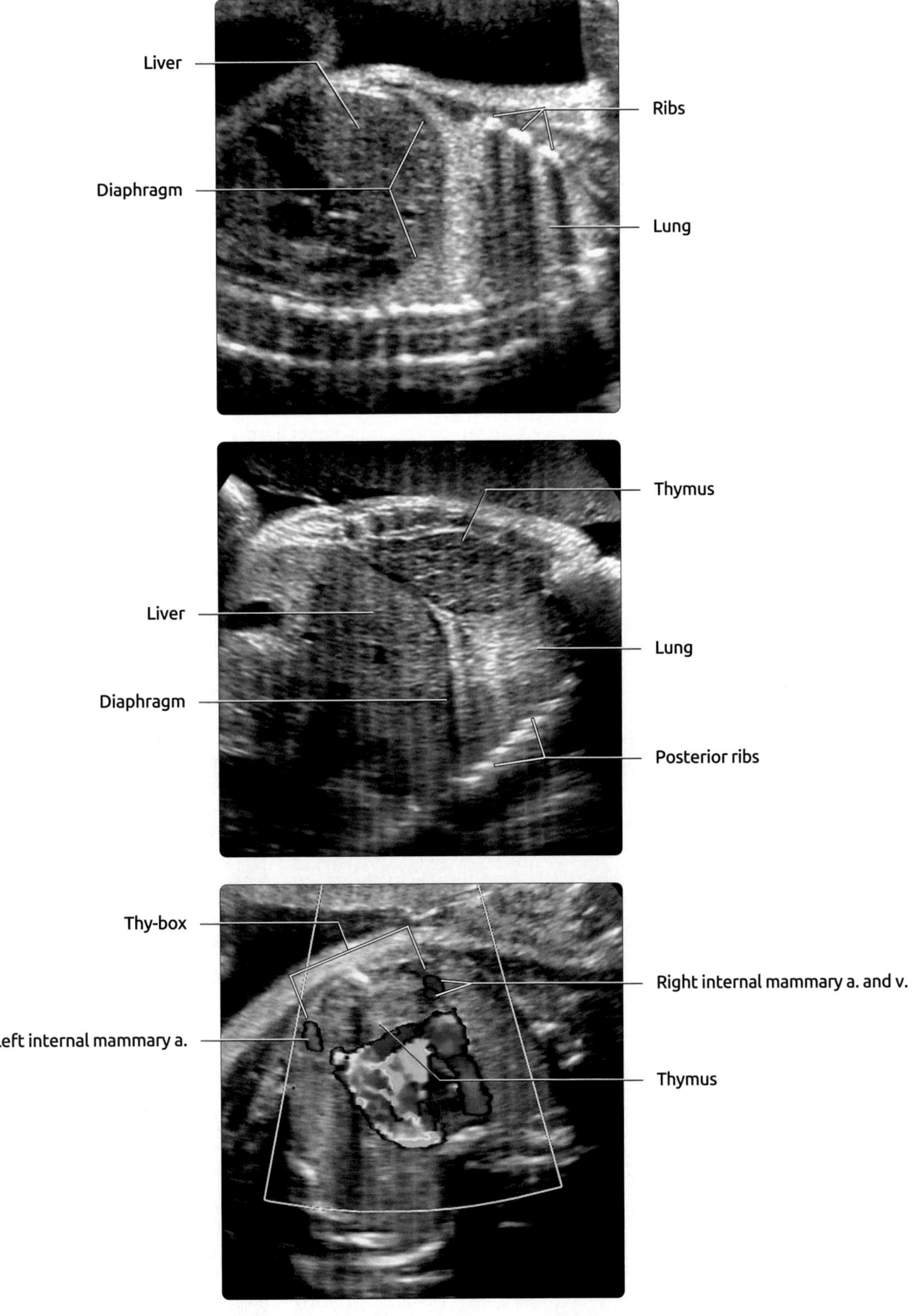

(Top) *Sagittal ultrasound of the fetal chest shows the diaphragm, which is a thin, hypoechoic, muscular band. The diaphragm is best evaluated in this projection to ensure it has been seen in its entirety.* **(Middle)** *Sagittal ultrasound of the fetal chest in the 3rd trimester shows the fetal thymus. It is hypoechoic when compared to the lungs and has a slightly reticular appearance. The thymus is often quite prominent in a fetus and should not be confused with a lung or mediastinal mass.* **(Bottom)** *Axial color Doppler ultrasound of the superior mediastinum at the top of the outflow tracts shows the thy-box. The internal mammary arteries, branches of the subclavian arteries, flank the thymus and create a box appearance. Thymic measurements can be taken if there is a suspicion for hypoplasia, as in 22q11 deletion (DiGeorge) syndrome.*

Congenital Diaphragmatic Hernia

KEY FACTS

IMAGING

- Congenital diaphragmatic hernias (CDH) are most commonly left sided (80-90% of cases) through posterior foramen of Bochdalek
  - Stomach usually in chest
  - Deviation of heart toward right chest wall
  - 80-85% contain herniated liver (liver up)
    - Liver up confers poorer prognosis
- Right-sided hernias all contain liver ± gallbladder ± bowel
- Be suspicious of bilateral hernias when stomach is in chest but little mediastinal shift
- **Calculate lung:head ratio (LHR)**
  - Area of lung contralateral to CDH divided by head circumference (all measurements done in mm)
    - Trace periphery of visible lung to calculate area
    - < 1.0 high mortality; significant morbidity in survivors
    - 1.0-1.4 extracorporeal membrane oxygenation usually required
    - > 1.4 better outcomes
- Associated abnormalities in up to 50% of cases
  - Structural anomalies (especially cardiac), aneuploidy, and many syndromes all reported

SCANNING TIPS

- Confirm CDH findings are real
  - Oblique axial image may simulate CDH
  - Check ribs; if multiple ribs seen, axis is incorrect
- Imperative to view entire diaphragm in sagittal plane
  - Coronal view of anterior diaphragm may be normal
- Higher frequency transducers helpful for differentiating herniated bowel vs. liver
  - Use color looking for hepatic and portal veins
- Document stomach position
  - More posterior position suggests liver also herniated
  - From least to most aberrant: Anterior left chest (likely no liver herniation), midposterior left chest, retrocardiac right chest

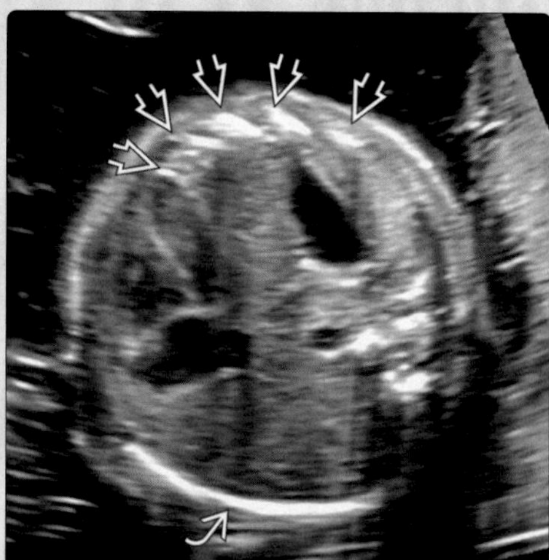

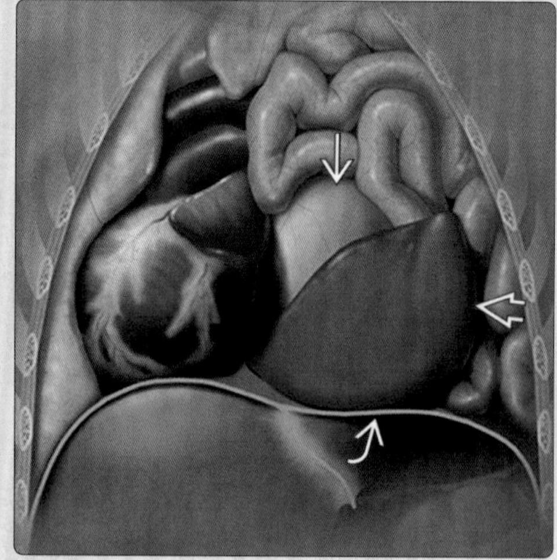

(Left) *This incorrect scan plane creates the erroneous appearance of a CDH. Note there is a single rib on the downside ➡ and multiple ribs ➡ on the upside, indicating this image is severely obliqued.* **(Right)** *Graphic of a liver-up, left-sided CDH shows the left lobe of the liver ➡ pushing the stomach posteriorly ➡. Note that the anterior diaphragm ➡ remains intact, stressing the importance of the sagittal plane when evaluating the diaphragm. If viewed only in the anterior coronal plane, a CDH could be missed.*

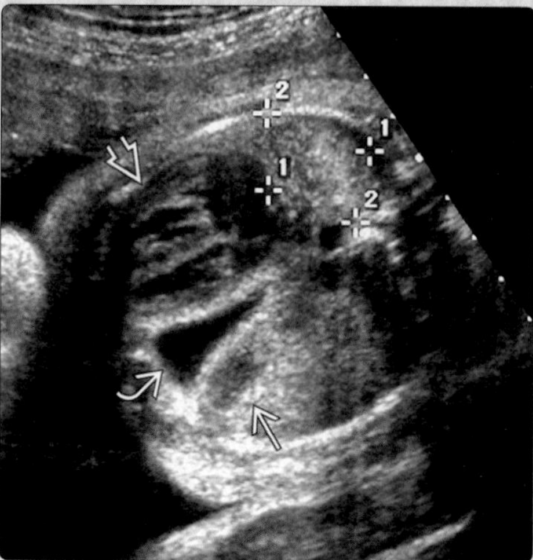

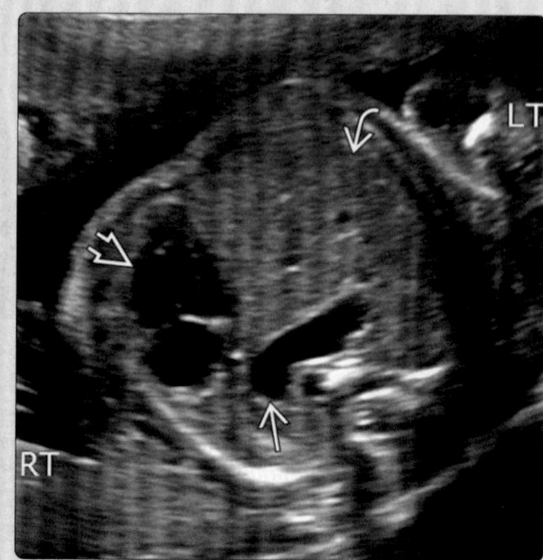

(Left) *Axial ultrasound at the level of the heart ➡ shows both the stomach ➡ and bowel ➡ are herniated into the chest cavity. The anterior position of the stomach suggests the liver is not herniated (liver down). Always evaluate the contralateral lung (calipers).* **(Right)** *Axial ultrasound through the chest shows the heart ➡ abutting the right chest wall. The stomach is posterior, crosses the midline, and has a retrocardiac portion ➡. The posterior location indicates significant liver herniation ➡.*

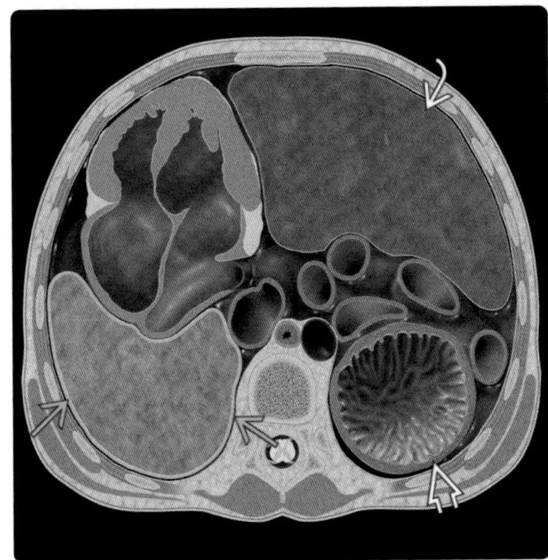

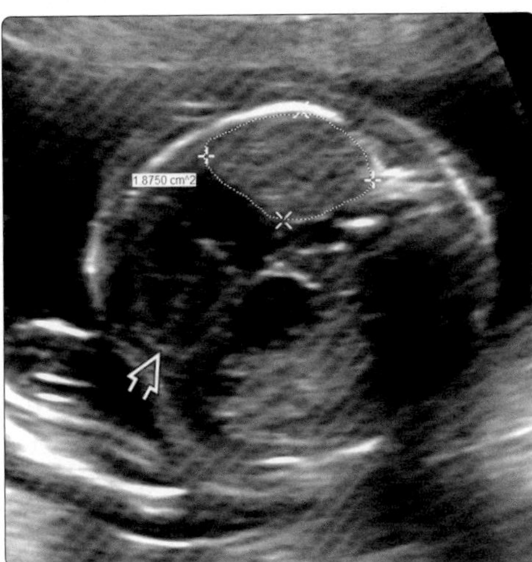

(Left) *This graphic shows a left-sided CDH with the liver up ➡ and the stomach pushed posteriorly ➡. The area of the contralateral lung should be traced ➡ to calculate the LHR.* **(Right)** *The lung area should be taken at the level of the 4-chamber view ➡. It can be calculated by either tracing the area or multiplying the longest diameters (calipers). The tracing method is preferred, as the area can be overestimated by as much as 45% using the longest diameters. This would erroneously make the LHR better than it truly is.*

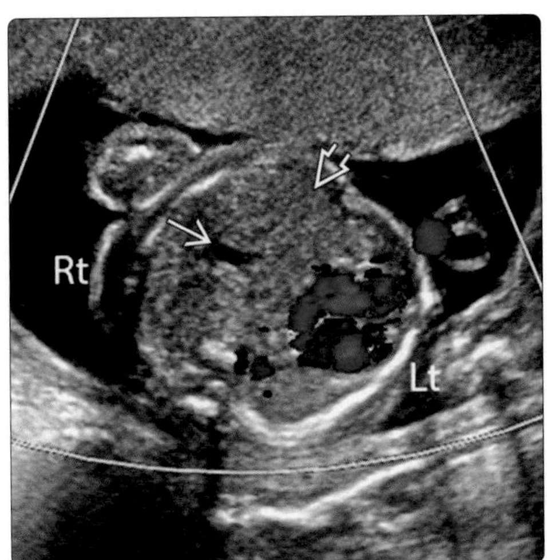

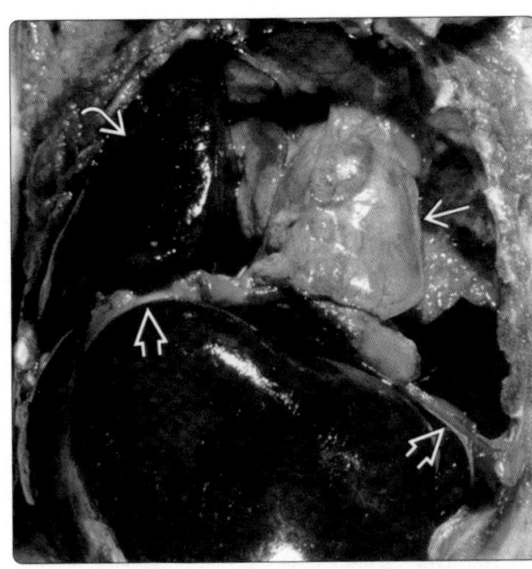

(Left) *Right-sided hernias are less common, occurring in 10-15% of cases. The liver ➡ is always herniated ± bowel ± gallbladder. Color Doppler allows differentiation of the gallbladder ➡ from hepatic vessels. The stomach will be located below the diaphragm but may be more centrally located as it is pulled toward the midline by the hernia.* **(Right)** *Autopsy photograph of a right-sided CDH shows liver ➡ within the right hemithorax (heart ➡). Note the anterior diaphragm ➡ is intact.*

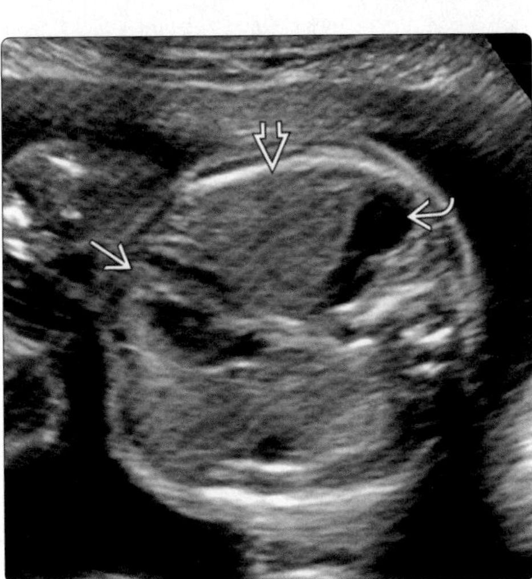

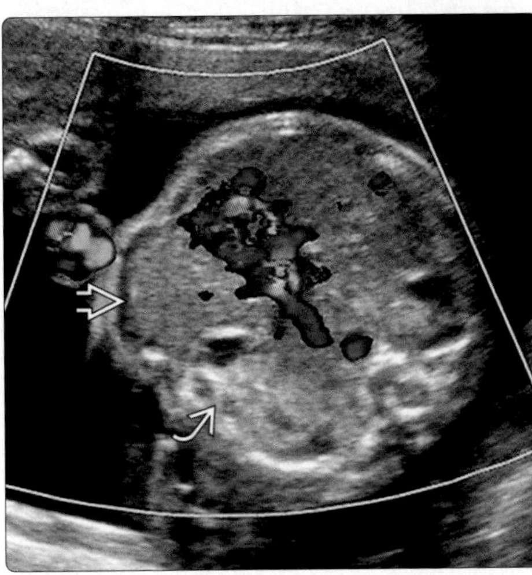

(Left) *Axial ultrasound through the chest shows what was initially thought to be a left-sided hernia with the stomach ➡ and liver ➡ in the chest, but it is very important to note the cardiac position ➡, which is midline and not pushed to the right.* **(Right)** *A color Doppler ultrasound slightly higher shows there is a liver ➡ and bowel ➡ on the right side as well. A midline location of the heart is an important clue that the CDH is bilateral, an almost uniformly lethal diagnosis.*

Congenital Pulmonary Airway Malformation (CPAM)

KEY FACTS

IMAGING

- Variable appearance from solid-appearing (microcystic) to complex cystic mass (macrocystic)
  - **Macrocystic**: 1 or more cysts ≥ 5 mm
    - May have single large cyst
  - **Microcystic**: Cysts < 5 mm (appears homogeneously echogenic)
- No side predilection, more common at lung bases
- Vascular supply from pulmonary artery
- Monitor frequently for hydrops
  - Ascites, from mediastinal compression, may be 1st sign
  - Follow closely until growth stabilizes

TOP DIFFERENTIAL DIAGNOSES

- Bronchopulmonary sequestration
  - Should see obvious feeding vessel from aorta
- Congenital diaphragmatic hernia
  - Dilated bowel loops can appear like macrocystic CPAM

CLINICAL ISSUES

- Stable lesions may be watched without intervention
  - Often decrease in size or completely regress ("disappearing" CPAM)
- Microcystic CPAMs often stabilize and begin regressing at 26-28 weeks but are more prone to cause hydrops
- Macrocystic CPAM may grow throughout pregnancy
- Hydrops significantly impacts prognosis
  - Near 100% mortality with hydrops if untreated
  - Mortality has declined significantly with steroid administration

SCANNING TIPS

- Ensure diaphragm intact, ruling out diaphragmatic hernia
- Color Doppler evaluation essential for any chest mass to look for source of feeding vessel
- Look carefully for signs of developing hydrops

(Left) *Axial US of the fetal chest at the level of the right ventricular outflow tract ➡ shows a large, uniformly echogenic lung mass ➡ having mass effect with shift of the heart ➡ to the right. The primary differential is a microcystic CPAM vs. a sequestration, so the next step is evaluation of the blood supply.* **(Right)** *Color Doppler US just below the prior image in the same patient shows a feeding vessel ➡ from the pulmonary artery, not the aorta ➡, confirming that this is a CPAM.*

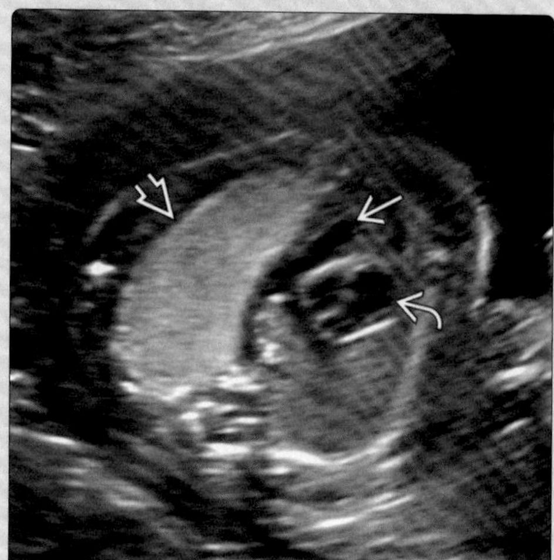

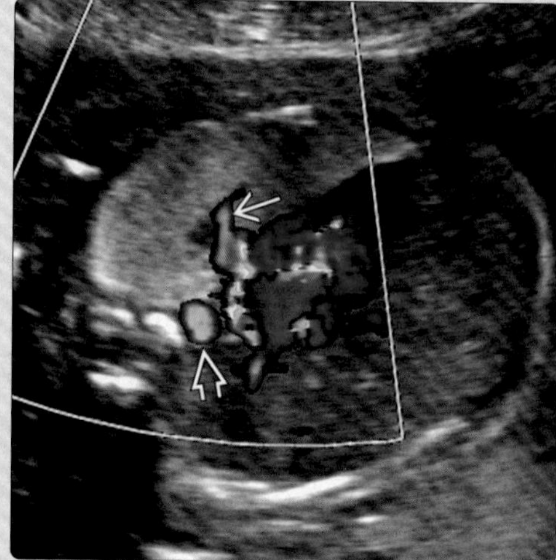

(Left) *Sagittal US of a macrocystic CPAM at 20 weeks shows a mixed cystic and solid mass filling the right hemithorax. The diaphragm is flattened and partially everted ➡. More importantly, there is ascites ➡. Developing hydrops portends a very poor prognosis, so the patient was treated with steroids.* **(Right)** *The same fetus 4 weeks later shows improvement with resolution of the ascites and a normal domed contour of the diaphragm ➡. Note the cysts of varying sizes ➡ scattered throughout the mass.*

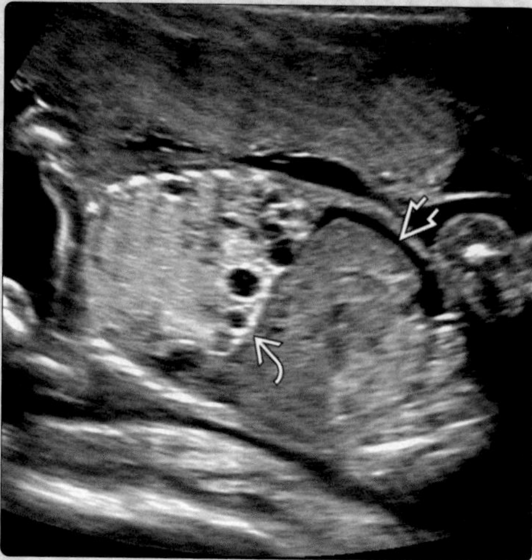

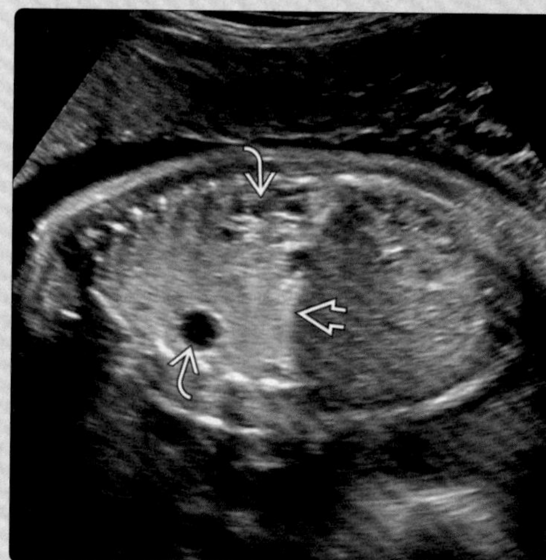

KEY FACTS

TERMINOLOGY

- Bronchopulmonary tissue that does not connect to tracheobronchial tree or pulmonary arteries

IMAGING

- Homogeneously echogenic lesion adjacent to diaphragm
  - Typically triangular and well defined but can fill hemithorax and be difficult to differentiate from compressed lung
- Color Doppler key: Prominent feeding vessel from aorta
- 85-90% in chest; 90% left sided
- 10-15% subdiaphragmatic
  - Stomach is displaced anteriorly by echogenic mass
  - Separate from adrenal gland
  - Has prominent feeding vessel from aorta just like those in chest
- Unilateral pleural effusion (same side as BPS) in 6-10%
  - May cause tension hydrothorax shifting heart and compressing mediastinal structures

TOP DIFFERENTIAL DIAGNOSES

- Congenital pulmonary airway malformation (CPAM)
  - Microcystic (echogenic) CPAM has similar appearance
  - Vascular supply from pulmonary arteries, not aorta
- Neuroblastoma: Most common differential consideration for subdiaphragmatic sequestration
  - More often on right
  - Often cystic with no feeding vessel

CLINICAL ISSUES

- 10-20% of fetal lung masses
- Associated anomalies reported in up to 50%
  - Most commonly associated with congenital diaphragmatic hernia but is often missed
- Excellent prognosis when isolated finding

SCANNING TIPS

- Use color Doppler on every chest mass looking for blood supply

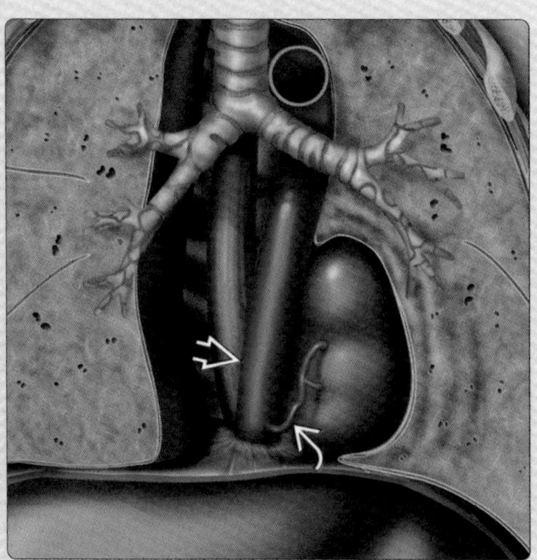

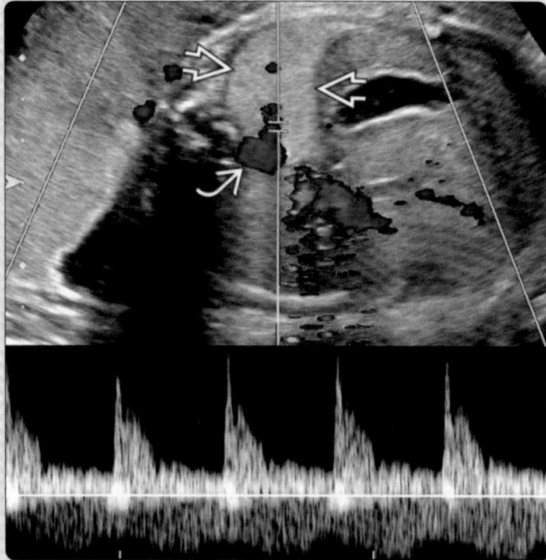

(Left) *Graphic shows a BPS at the left lung base. The vascular supply ➡ is from the aorta ➡. It is sequestered from the surrounding lung, and there is no communication with the tracheobronchial tree.* **(Right)** *Oblique axial image through the left lung base shows a uniformly echogenic lung mass ➡. A large feeding vessel is seen coming from the aorta ➡. A tracing from this vessel (below) shows the classic aortic waveform with a sharp, rapid upstroke.*

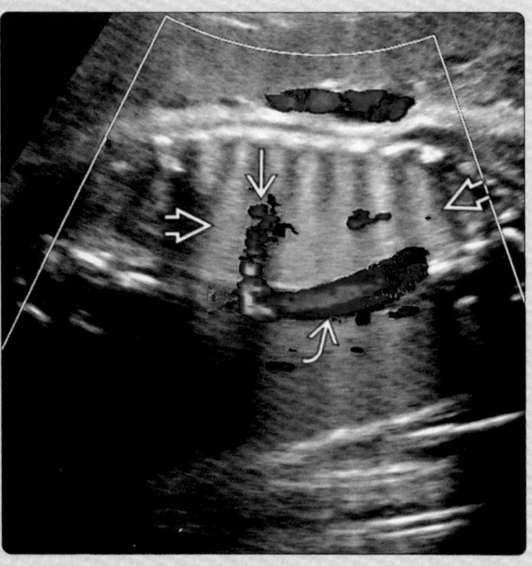

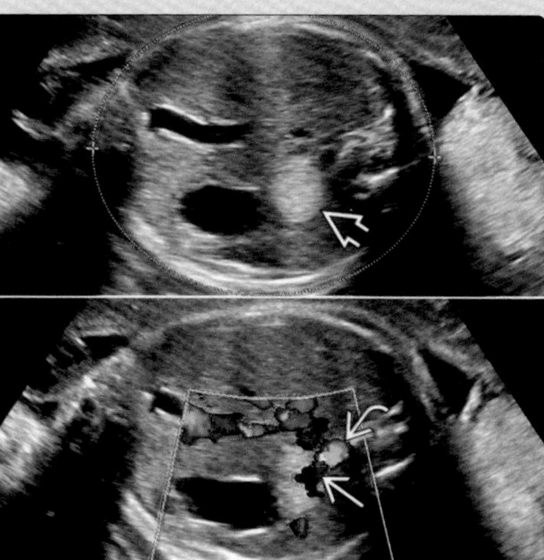

(Left) *A coronal US of the chest shows a large, left-sided mass ➡ that was only slightly more echogenic than the lung. Color Doppler is extremely helpful in situations like this as the feeding vessel ➡ is usually easy to find. Note the aorta ➡ is being bowed to the right by the mass.* **(Right)** *Axial abdominal images show an echogenic mass ➡ posterior to the stomach with a large feeding vessel ➡ off the aorta ➡. Also try to document a separate adrenal gland. Both features help differentiate a subdiaphragmatic BPS from a neuroblastoma.*

PART VI
SECTION 5
Heart

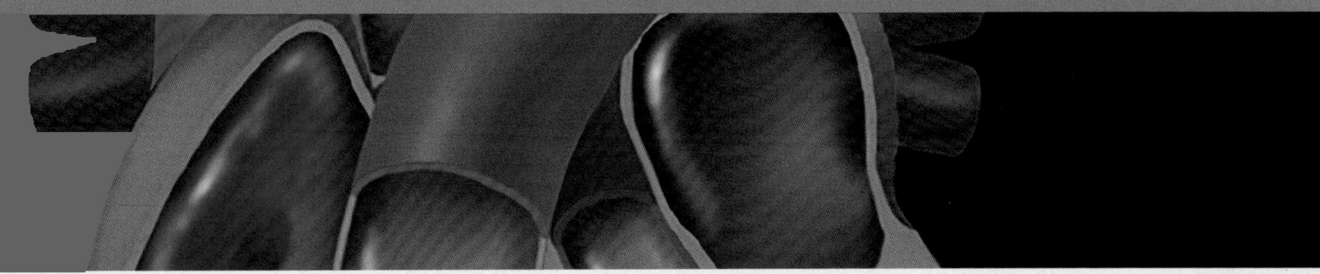

Anatomy and Approach

Heart Defects

EMBRYOLOGY AND ANATOMY

Embryology

- Primitive heart tube begins **contracting** around 4th embryonic week
- Primitive heart tube from caudal to cranial ends of embryo
  - Sinus venosus, primitive atria, primitive ventricles, bulbus cordis, truncus arteriosis
- Primitive heart tube grows, loops, and undergoes septation in complex series of events that result in
  - 4 chambers: Right and left atria, right and left ventricles (RV, LV)
  - 2 arterial outflows: Aorta (Ao) to body, pulmonary artery (PA) to lungs
  - Venous inflow from pulmonary circulation to left atrium (LA) via pulmonary veins, from systemic circulations to right atrium (RA) via superior and inferior vena cava (IVC)

Normal Anatomy

- Cardiac apex is directed left, axis of 45° (± 15°)
- 2 atria and 2 ventricles ~ equal in cavity size, wall thickness
  - RA identified by confluence with superior and IVC
  - LA identified by confluence with pulmonary veins
  - RV identified by moderator band, septal attachments of tricuspid valve
    - RV should be anterior ventricle
  - LV is smooth walled; mitral valve has attachments to free wall only
    - LV should be posterior ventricle
  - Both ventricles reach apex and contract equally
- 2 atrioventricular (AV) valves
  - Tricuspid valve belongs to RV, should separate it from RA
  - Mitral valve belongs to LV, should separate it from LA
  - Tricuspid valve is apically displaced on interventricular septum compared to mitral valve
- Together with AV valves, atrial and ventricular septa form "crux" of heart
- Atrial septum ~ 1/2 length of ventricular septum
  - Atrial septum has defect [foramen ovale (FO)] allowing oxygenated blood from placenta to enter LA
- Ventricular septum thins from muscular to membranous at level of crux
- 2 **great arteries**; Ao, main PA
  - Ao gives rise to head and neck vessels some distance from valve at apex of arch
    - Aortic arch has a tight curve candy cane shape, lies superior to ductal arch
  - PA branches into right, left PAs, ductus arteriosus shortly after valve
    - Ductal arch has broad and flat hockey stick shape, no branches, inferior to aortic arch
- Arteries cross each other as exit heart, PA anterior to Ao
- Both arches should have antegrade flow (same direction on color Doppler images)

Fetal Circulation

- Arteries move blood **away** from heart
  - Ao takes blood to brain and body
  - **Umbilical arteries** carry blood away from heart to placenta
  - Main PA takes blood from RV to body via ductus arteriosus, only small volume to lungs as gas exchange in fetal life occurs in placenta
- Veins take blood **toward** heart
  - **Umbilical vein** brings oxygenated blood back to heart, from placenta
  - Superior vena cava (SVC) and IVC bring deoxygenated blood from head/body to RA
- Oxygenated blood preferentially tunneled by ductus venosus to IVC then through FO → LA → LV → Ao → brain
- Distribution of cardiac output is very different in fetus compared to adult
  - **Ductus arteriosus** connects PA to descending Ao, bypassing lungs
  - Oxygenated RV blood directed to body
  - Fetal combined cardiac output is 55% RV, 45% LV

Neonatal Circulation

- Onset of breathing increases oxygen in lungs → PAs dilate → decreased pulmonary arterial resistance
- Cutting umbilical cord closes low-resistance arterial connection to placenta → increased systemic arterial resistance
- End result is increased flow in PA with decreased flow across ductus arteriosus, which closes
- Pulmonary veins bring oxygenated blood from lungs to LA
- ↑ venous return to LA → ↑ pressure → FO closes
- End result is complete separation of pulmonary and systemic circulations
  - Retrograde filling of obstructed/atretic outflow tract is possible in fetus as ductus connects Ao and PA
  - Duct closure at birth → complete circulatory collapse in "duct dependent" congenital heart disease
  - Infants need prostaglandin infusion to keep ductus open until definitive treatment

SCANNING APPROACH AND IMAGING ISSUES

Standard Views

- 4-chamber: Axial image through fetal chest with single C-shaped ribs on either side
- Left ventricular outflow tract (LVOT)
  - Transducer rotated toward fetal right shoulder to elongate ascending Ao
- Right ventricular outflow tract
  - Angled image at 90° to LVOT, so Ao is seen in circular cross section, with PA long axis branching to ductus running toward spine and right PA branch running toward right lung

Additional Views (Detailed Exam)

- 3 vessel view (3VV)
  - Oblique axial image directly cranial from 4-chamber view to show SVC, Ao, PA
  - Vessels in straight line, increasing in size from SVC to PA
- 3 vessel trachea view (3VT)
  - Slight tilt of transducer to left from 3VV to show confluence of aortic and ductal arches as V shape with apex to left of spine and trachea
- Aortic arch view
  - Sagittal oblique image to show candy cane shape of Ao with head and neck vessels coming off apex

- Bicaval view
  - Parasagittal image to right of midline to show confluence of IVC, SVC with RA

Approach to the Fetal Heart

- Check situs
  - Fetus in cephalic presentation with spine to maternal right has its left side closest to maternal abdominal wall
    - Stomach and cardiac apex should be on fetal left; this is normal or situs solitus
    - If stomach and cardiac apex are on fetal right, it is situs inversus; good prognosis
    - If heart and stomach are located on opposite sides, heterotaxy or situs ambiguous is present with very high likelihood of complex congenital heart disease
- Check cardiac axis
  - Angle between a line from spine to sternum and line along axis of interventricular septum
    - Normal axis is ~ 45°; range is 30-60°
    - Line from spine to sternum should pass through LA and RV
  - Abnormal axis/position
    - Associated with conotruncal heart disease, heterotaxy syndromes
    - Chest masses push heart away from abnormal side
    - Lung or lobar hypoplasia pulls lung toward abnormal side
- Check heart size
  - Normal heart circumference ~ 1/2 of chest circumference
  - Normal heart area ~ 1/3 of chest area
  - Increased ratio occurs with cardiomegaly or when chest is small (e.g., skeletal dysplasia, pulmonary hypoplasia)
  - **Cardiac causes of cardiomegaly**
    - Cardiomyopathy, arrhythmia
    - Ebstein anomaly → RA markedly enlarged → increased heart circumference
  - **Noncardiac causes of cardiomegaly**
    - Volume overload due to shunting from tumors, vascular malformation, or in recipient twin in twin-twin transfusion syndrome
    - High output in anemia or in pump twin in twin reverse arterial perfusion
- Look for pericardial effusion
  - Trace fluid along 1 ventricular wall is normal
    - Significant effusion measures > 2 mm, surrounds atria and ventricles
- Check for chamber symmetry
  - If asymmetric, which chamber is abnormal?
    - RV enlargement is seen with aortic coarctation, premature ductal constriction
    - RV may be very thick walled in fetus with pulmonary atresia/intact ventricular septum
    - LV enlargement can be seen with critical aortic stenosis
- Look for cardiac "mass"
  - Most common is isolated echogenic focus in LV; soft marker for trisomy 21; of no consequence if cell-free DNA screening is low risk
  - Rhabdomyoma: Homogenous hyperechoic, variable size and number
    - If multiple, almost 100% association with tuberous sclerosis
- Check FO flap
  - Should open into LA as oxygenated blood from placental return streams from RA to LA
  - Atrial septal aneurysm describes redundant flap
    - Extends at least halfway across LA, moves during cardiac cycle
    - May be associated with premature atrial contractions
- Check area behind LA
  - Increased distance between Ao and LA → increased suspicion for anomalous pulmonary venous return
    - Esophagus may be seen in 3rd trimester; varies in size with fetal swallowing
    - Normal azygos vein may be seen in 3rd trimester (venous flow, vertical orientation, smaller than Ao)
  - "Twig" sign describes stick-like appearance caused by confluence of anomalous veins posterior to LA, anterior to Ao on 4-chamber view
- Check great vessels
  - Abnormal 3VV
    - Only 1 artery suggests **truncus arteriosus** or **pulmonary or aortic atresia**
    - If only 2 vessels seen, is arterial vessel large?
      - Large artery with SVC suggests **truncus**
      - Normal artery with SVC suggest **transposition** (both arteries present but abnormally located so not both visible on 3VV plane)
    - 4 vessels suggest persistent left SVC
  - Small ascending Ao suggests **coarctation** or **interrupted aortic arch**
  - Parallel great vessels most commonly due to **transposition of great arteries**
- Check rate and rhythm
  - Normal rate is 120-160 beats per minute
  - Normal rhythm is 1:1 transmission of atrial contraction to ventricular contraction
  - Obtain M-mode with beam directed through 1 atrium and 1 ventricle
  - If arrhythmia, obtain separate atrial/ventricular rates
  - For pulse wave evaluation of rhythm, place sample volume at junction of aortic and mitral valves
    - Inflow to ventricle across mitral valve → atrial rate on one side of baseline
    - Outflow from ventricle across aortic valve → ventricular rate on other side of baseline
  - Color M-mode superimposes directional information on M-mode tracing
    - Easier to separate atrial from ventricular rate

Key Points

- Normal 4-chamber view only detects 50-55% of congenital diaphragmatic hernias
  - Detection improves to 80-84% with addition of outflow tract views
- Limbs of V on 3VT view should both show antegrade flow on color Doppler

FETAL CIRCULATION

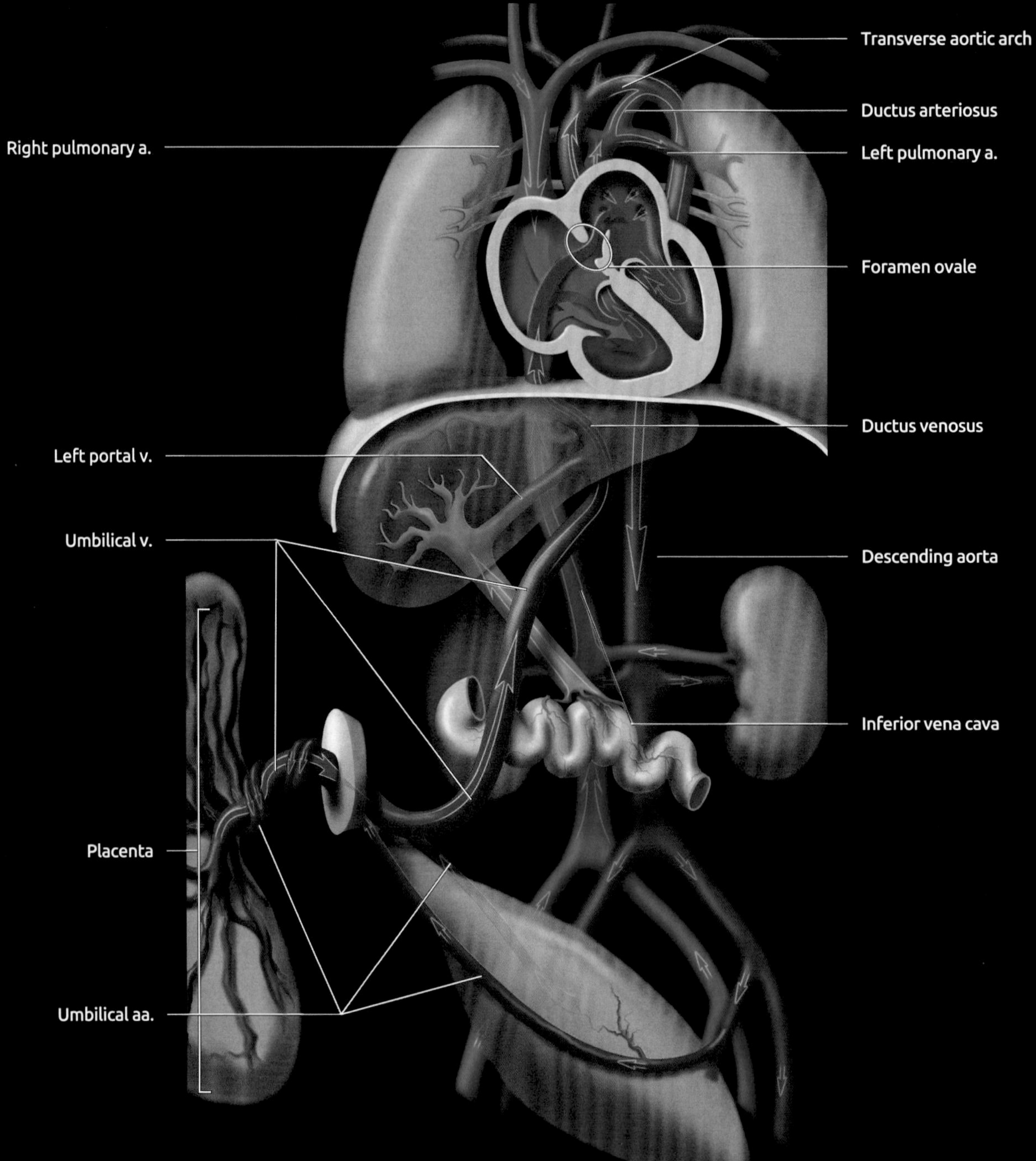

In the fetus, blood is oxygenated by the placenta and returns to the heart via the umbilical vein. This highly oxygenated blood (red) shunts through the ductus venosus and streams across the foramen ovale to the left side of the heart. This shunting allows the most oxygenated blood to perfuse the coronary arteries and the brain. Deoxygenated blood (blue) returns to the (RA) right atrium via the superior vena cava (SVC) and inferior vena cava (IVC. This blood preferentially flows to the right ventricle, which pumps a small amount to the pulmonary arteries, but the majority is shunted across the ductus arteriosus to the descending aorta. Reversed flow across the ductus is associated with duct dependent congenital heart disease.

FETAL CIRCULATION

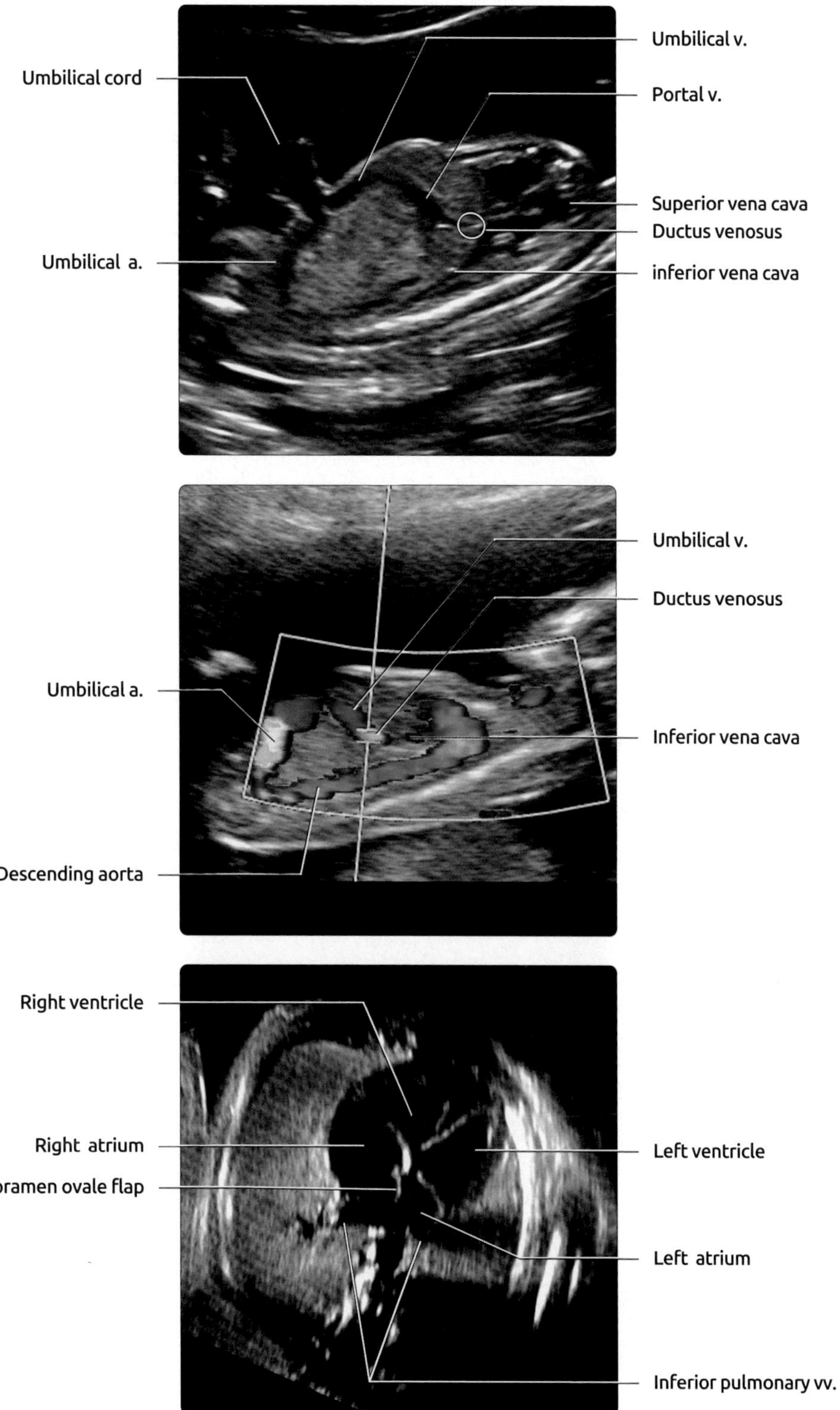

(Top) *Sagittal view shows the sonographic correlate of the vessels of fetal circulation illustrated in the graphic. The umbilical arteries run to the placenta via the cord insertion site. Oxygenated blood returns from the placenta via the umbilical vein, which runs along the free edge of the falciform ligament to reach the liver, ductus venosus, and the heart.* **(Middle)** *Color Doppler at 14-weeks shows the umbilical vein anastomosing with the left portal vein after it enters the liver. The oxygenated blood it carries is preferentially shunted through the ductus venosus to reach the IVC and then the RA. The umbilical arteries carry blood toward the umbilicus, the vein carries blood away, hence the different flow directions seen with color Doppler.* **(Bottom)** *Oxygenated blood from the placenta is funneled into a jet as it traverses the ductus venosus. This jet preferentially flows across the foramen ovale to the left atrium, pushing the foramen ovale flap into the left atrium.*

STANDARD VIEWS

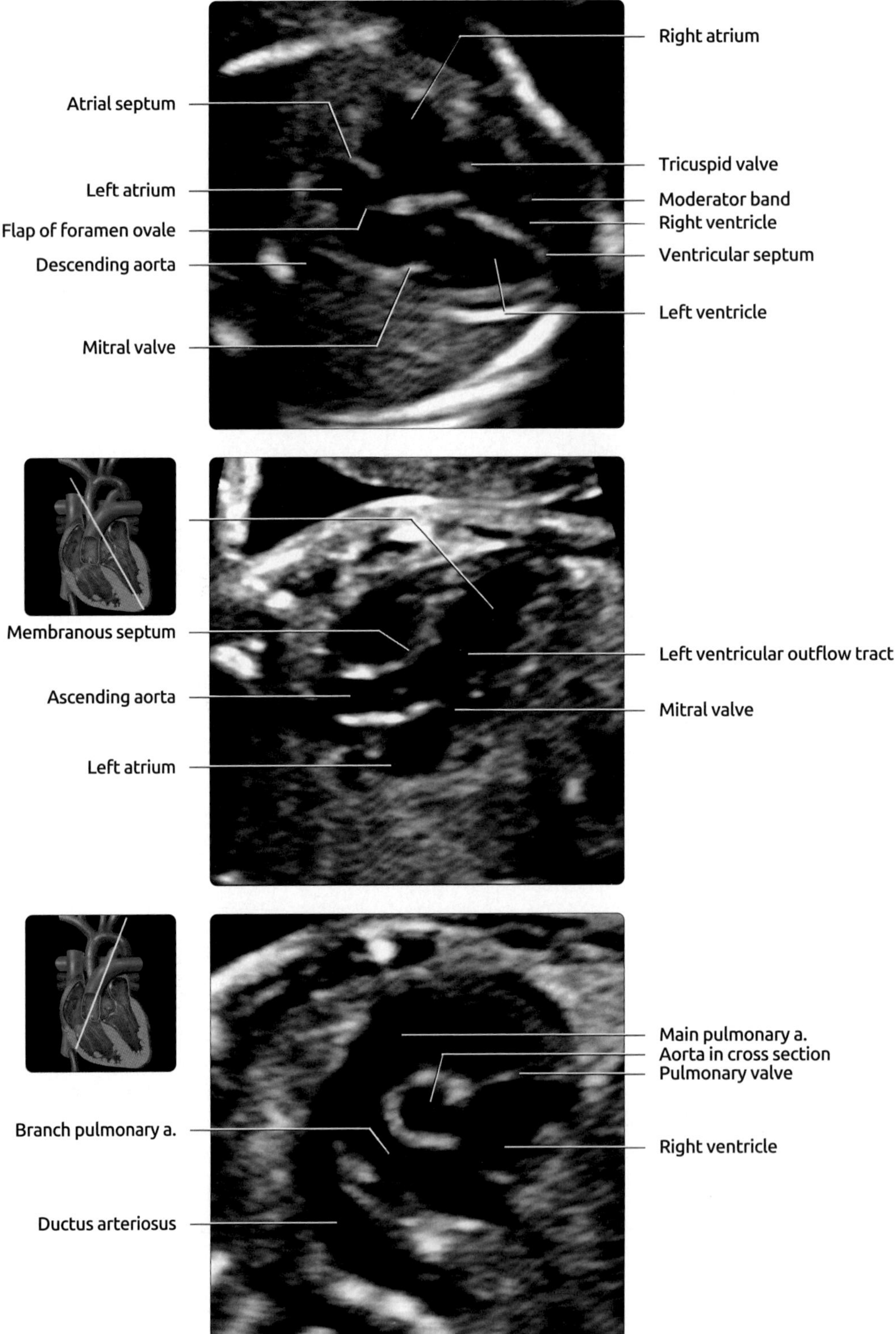

(Top) *This is a zoomed-in 4-chamber view using the machine cardiac setting, which creates more contrast to bring out the fine details of the cardiac structures. The ventricles are symmetric and apex forming. The mitral and tricuspid valve leaflets are visible as is the foramen ovale flap. The atria are symmetric in size, and the descending aorta is the only structure visible behind the left atrium.* **(Middle)** *The left ventricular outflow tract view is the best view to evaluate the membranous ventricular septum. A defect in this area may simply be an isolated perimembranous ventricular septal defect but may also be found in association with right ventricular outflow tract or conotruncal lesions, such as tetralogy of Fallot or double outlet right ventricle.* **(Bottom)** *This is the standard right ventricular outflow tract view, which is a short-axis view at the level of the aortic valve. It allows one to lay out the main pulmonary artery and the ductus arteriosus as it runs posteriorly, toward the spine, to join the descending aorta.*

OUTFLOW TRACTS, ADDITIONAL VIEWS

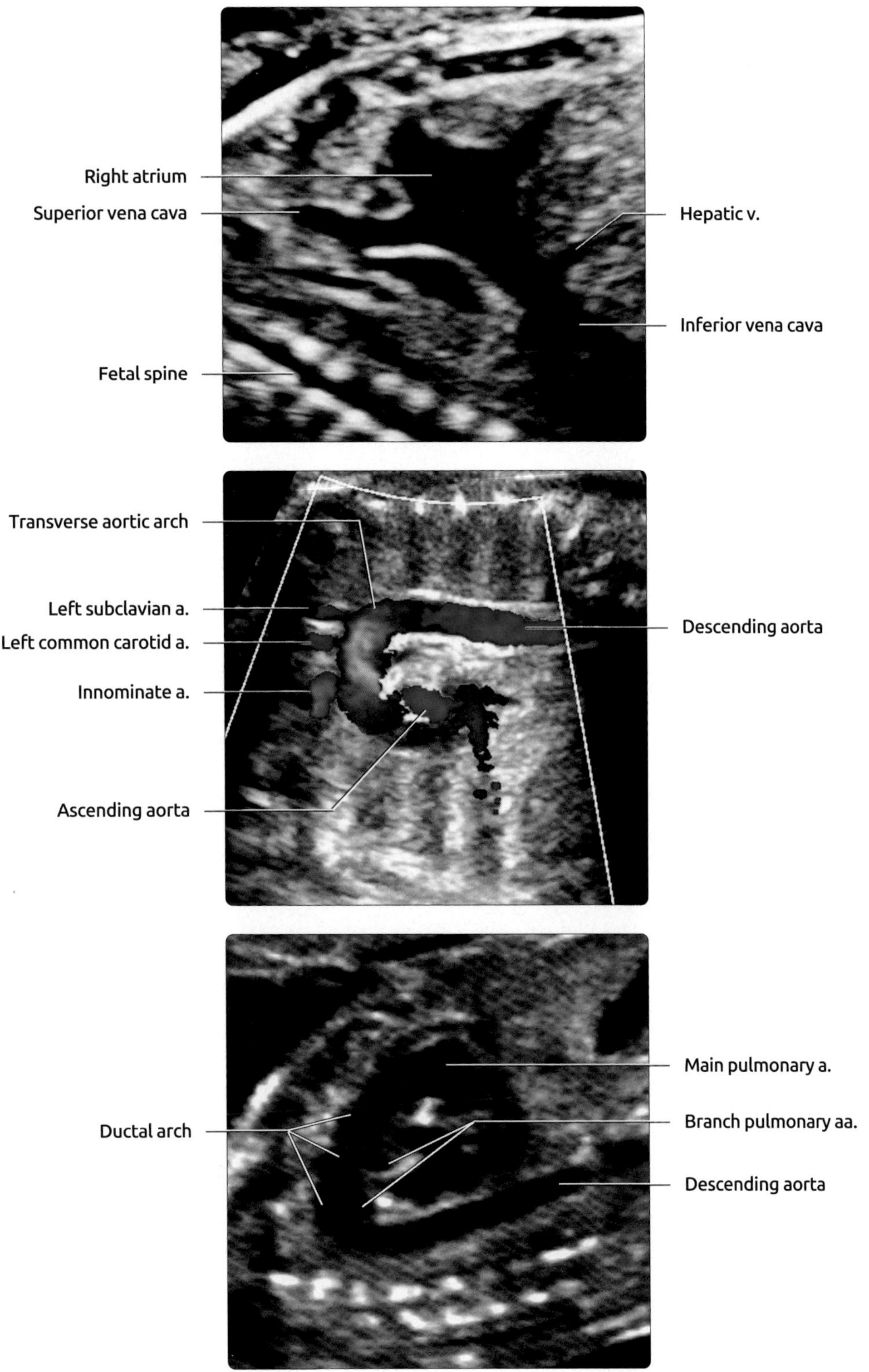

(Top) *The bicaval view demonstrates systemic venous return to the RA. Note the hepatic vein (HV) confluence with the IVC. In azygous continuation of the IVC, the HVs may drain directly to the RA but are small and should not be mistaken for the IVC. In azygous continuation of the IVC, a large azygous vein is seen posterior to the heart on the 4-chamber view.* **(Middle)** *Color Doppler of the aortic arch shows the entire thoracic aorta. Flow superiorly, toward the head, is visible in the head and neck vessels arising from the apex of the arch. Also note the color change as flow wraps around the transverse arch.* **(Bottom)** *Unlike the aortic arch view, the ductal arch view is not required for the detailed anatomy scan. The ductal arch is flatter and broader than the aortic arch, and no vessels arise from its apex. The ductus arteriosus diverts a substantial portion of right ventricular output to the torso, bypassing the lungs. Gas exchange in the fetal circulation takes place in the placenta.*

THREE VESSEL, THREE VESSEL TRACHEA VIEWS

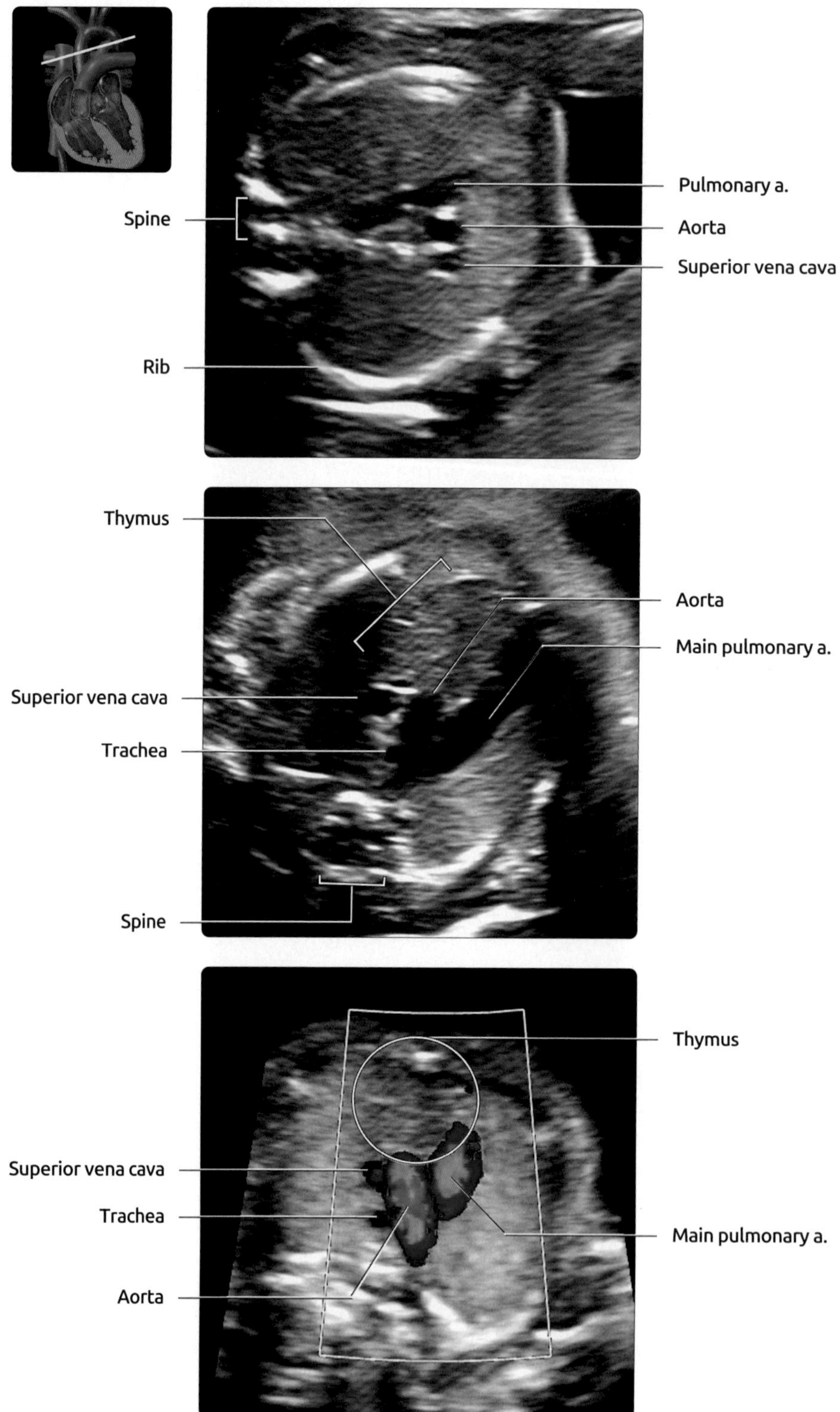

(Top) *The 3-vessel view shows the main pulmonary artery continuing as the ductus arteriosus, which is directed straight posteriorly toward the spine. The pulmonary artery is larger than the aorta, which is, in turn, larger than the SVC. Note that the vessels all line up anteriorly. Abnormal findings include a change in this alignment, a change in the size gradient, or a change in the number of vessels.* **(Middle)** *This is the 3-vessel trachea view in which the ductal and aortic arches are visualized as they join to form the descending aorta. The confluence creates a V shape with the apex of the V posterior and to the left of the trachea and the spine.* **(Bottom)** *In this 3-vessel trachea view with color, the trachea remains black as it is fluid filled but not a vascular structure. The limbs of the V are the same color, indicating normal flow direction. In duct-dependent congenital heart disease, there may be retrograde filling of one of the great vessels, so the limbs of the V will be different in color.*

CARDIAC RATE AND RHYTHM

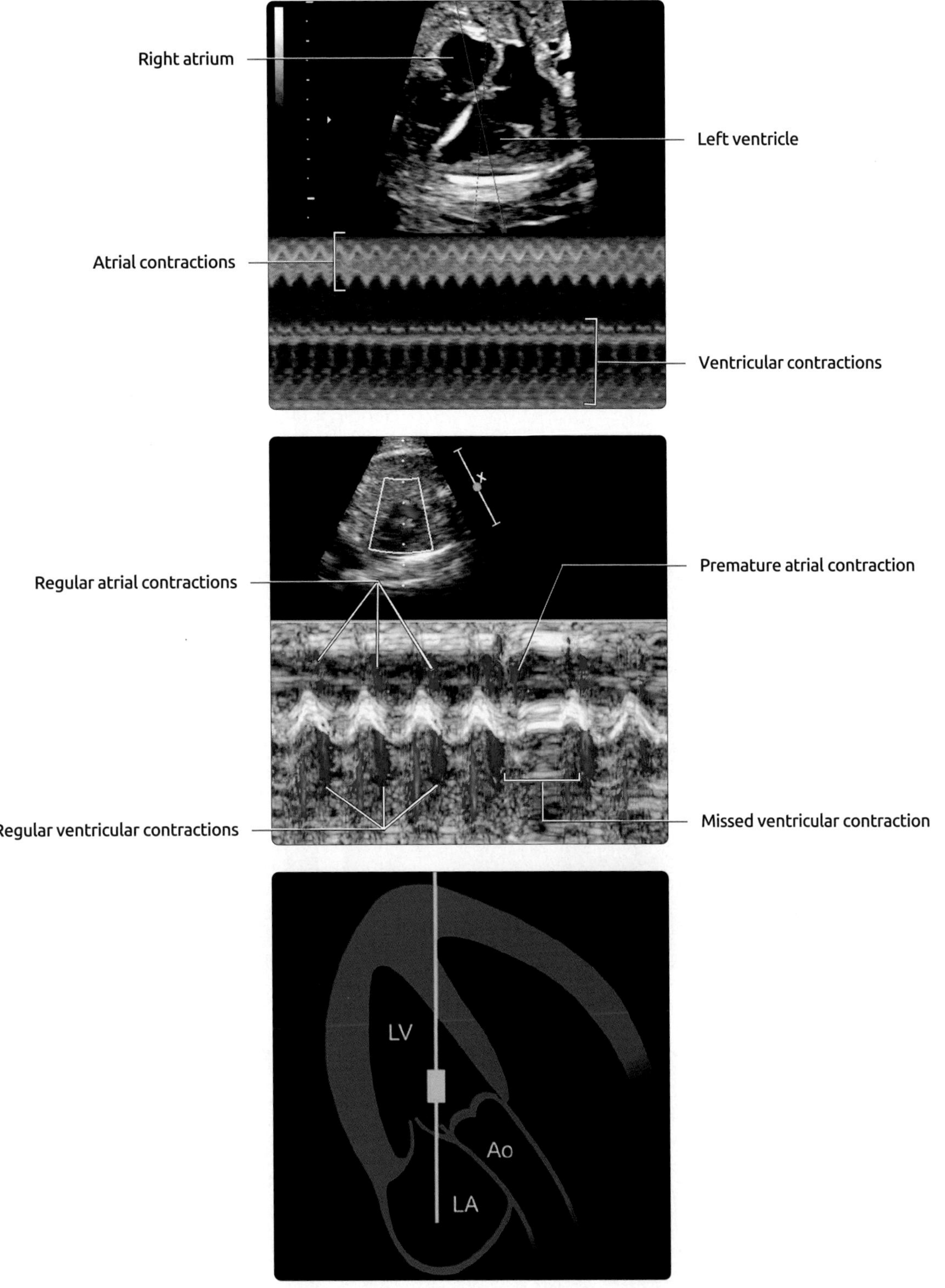

(Top) *Image shows the static line through the RA and the left ventricle with the atrial contractions on top and the ventricular contractions on the bottom and 1:1 conduction in a patient with supraventricular tachycardia.* **(Middle)** *This is a color M-mode in which directional information is superimposed on the M-mode tracing. After a series of regular atrial beats, there is a premature atrial contraction; this is blocked and therefore not transmitted to the ventricle where there is a gap or a missed beat. This most commonly presents as an irregular heart rate on auscultation.* **(Bottom)** *The graphic demonstrates cursor placement for Doppler assessment of cardiac rate and rhythm. The sample volume is placed at the junction of the aortic and mitral valves. Inflow to the ventricle across the mitral valve is toward the transducer (above baseline) and represents the atrial rate. Outflow from the ventricle across the aortic valve is away from the transducer (below baseline); it represents the ventricular rate.*

Atrioventricular Septal Defect

KEY FACTS

TERMINOLOGY

- Central cardiac defect involving atrial (ASD) and ventricular (VSD) septal defects, atrioventricular (AV) valves, and conducting system
  - **Balanced**: Right and left ventricles are equal in size
  - **Unbalanced**: Majority of flow to 1 ventricle so unequal size

IMAGING

- Missing crux (central portion) of heart on 4-chamber view
  - Normally atrial and ventricular septa meet at crux of heart and AV valves are separate and distinct
  - Tricuspid insertion normally 1-2 mm offset (toward apex) from mitral insertion
  - In atrioventricular septal defect (AVSD), usual offset of AV valves is absent
- Single AV valve makes straight line across heart in systole
- Appears as large central defect in diastole

SCANNING TIPS

- Use cine/video clips and color Doppler in all fetal heart evaluation
  - Look for flow through VSD, AV valve regurgitation
- Check ventricular size: Asymmetry suggests unbalanced defect
- Slow heart rate suggests heart block, so check situs, look for additional features of heterotaxy syndromes
  - Look at vessels behind heart on 4-chamber view
    - Azygos continuation of inferior vena cava (2 vessels present; aorta and dilated azygos vein)
    - Anomalous pulmonary venous return (tubular vascular confluence posterior to atria, anterior to descending aorta)
- **Look for features of trisomy 21**
  - ~ 50% of fetal AVSD cases have trisomy 21
  - Thick nuchal fold, rhizomelic limb shortening, duodenal atresia, echogenic bowel, pelviectasis, clinodactyly

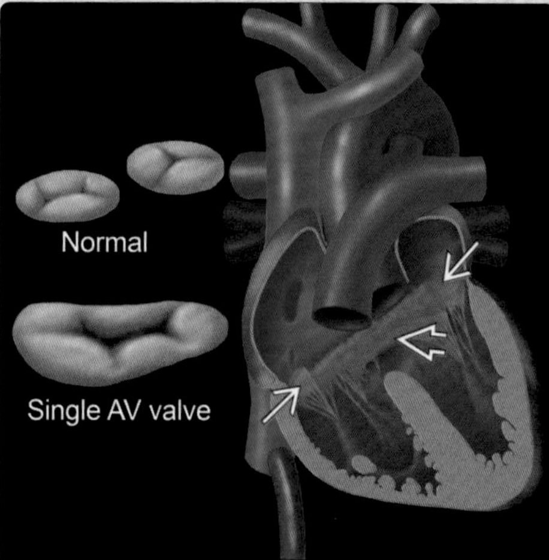

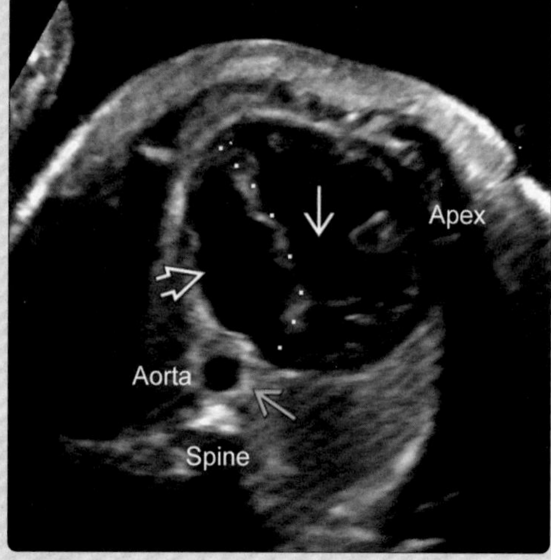

(Left) *AVSD graphic shows both ASD & VSD creating a defect in the crux of the heart ➡. Instead of the normally separate tricuspid & mitral valves, a single AV valve ➡ straddles the central defect.* **(Right)** *Four-chamber view shows a large VSD ➡, no atrial septum ➡, & a single AV valve (dots) spanning both ventricles that are similar in size, indicating a balanced AVSD. The aorta should be the only structure behind the heart on this view. Look for azygos continuation of the IVC ➡ or anomalous pulmonary veins in heterotaxy.*

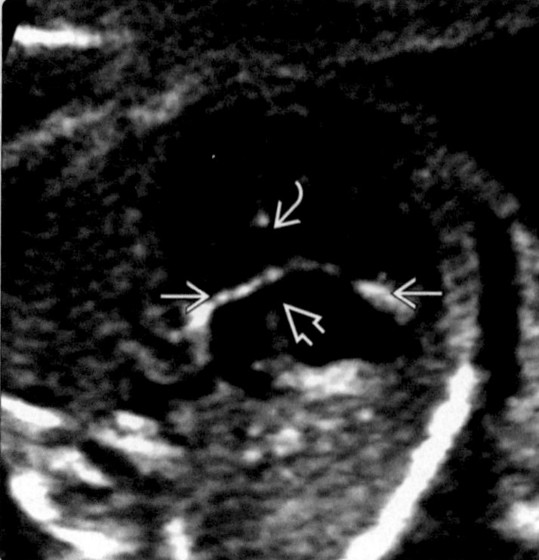

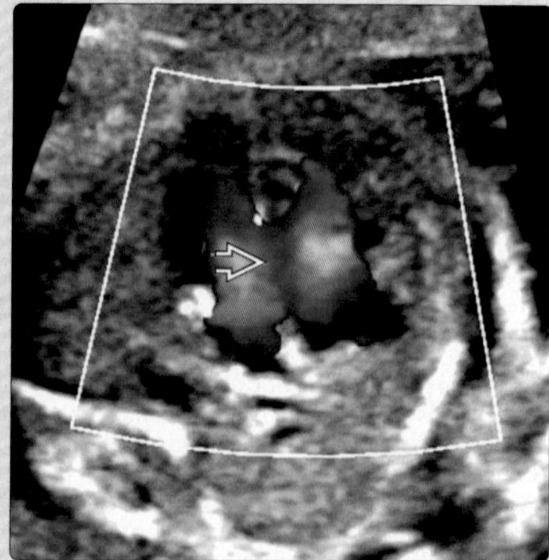

(Left) *Four-chamber view shows a balanced AVSD with a single common AV valve ➡ in the systole and contiguous atrial ➡ & ventricular ➡ septal defects. The usual offset of the valves on the ventricular septum is absent.* **(Right)** *Color Doppler US in diastole shows blood filling the entire AVSD ➡. The crux of the heart is missing, & there is complete mixing of oxygenated and deoxygenated blood. Approximately 50% of AVSD cases have trisomy 21, so carefully look for other associated findings.*

Ventricular Septal Defect

KEY FACTS

TERMINOLOGY

- Ventricular septal defects (VSD) classified according to location
  - Membranous: Defect in outflow tract of left ventricle, immediately below aortic valve
  - Muscular: Defect in muscular portion of septum, anywhere from cardiac apex to base
  - Outlet: Defect in outflow tract of right ventricle, below pulmonary valve
  - Inlet: Located posterior and inferior to membranous septum, beneath septal leaflet of tricuspid valve

IMAGING

- Small muscular ventricular septal defects may not be visible on grayscale or color Doppler

TOP DIFFERENTIAL DIAGNOSES

- Atrioventricular septal defect
  - Large VASD as well as VSD
  - Missing crux (middle) of heart
  - Single atrioventricular valve

SCANNING TIPS

- **Signal dropout at membranous-muscular junction of septum potential pitfall**
  - Try to image perpendicular to ventricular septum
- Look for echogenic dot at edge of defect
  - Normally no echo at site of transition from muscular to membranous septum
- Confirm on long-axis view if seen on apical 4-chamber view and vice versa
- Look for septal continuity with aortic annulus in left ventricular outflow tract view to exclude membranous VSD
- Use color Doppler to confirm blood flow across defect
- Obtain dedicated fetal echo
  - Associated cardiac abnormalities present in 50%

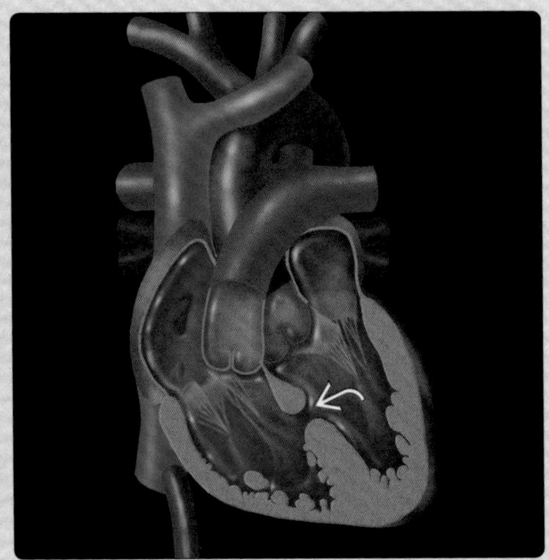

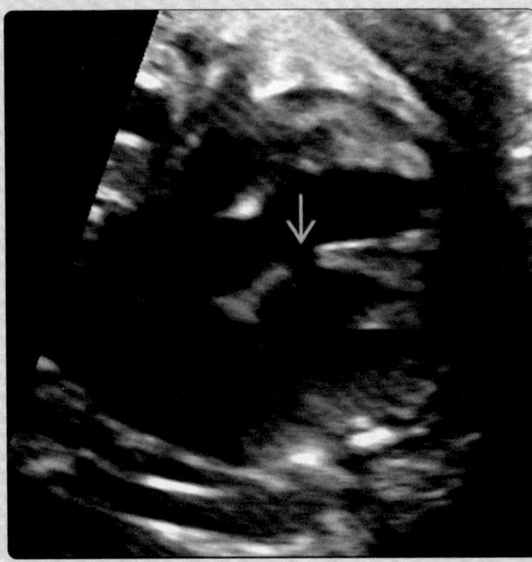

(Left) *Graphic shows a midmuscular ventricular septal defect (VSD)* ➡. **(Right)** *A large muscular VSD* ➡ *is noted in the midventricular septum. Always try to scan perpendicular to the septum. There is often signal dropout if scanning parallel to the septum, and a VSD can be erroneously diagnosed. Also use color Doppler to look for flow across the defect. Even with good technique a small VSD may be missed.*

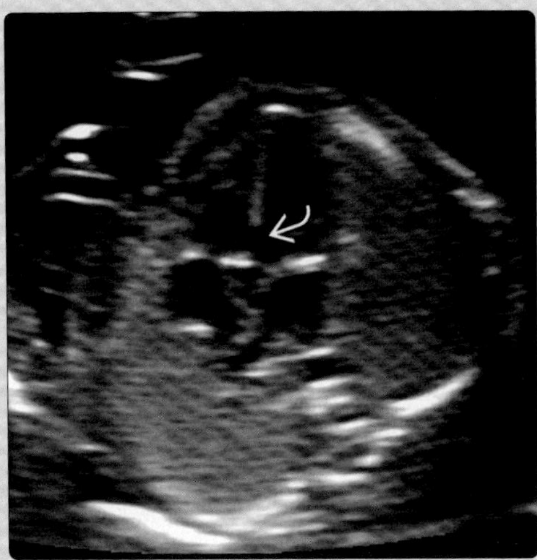

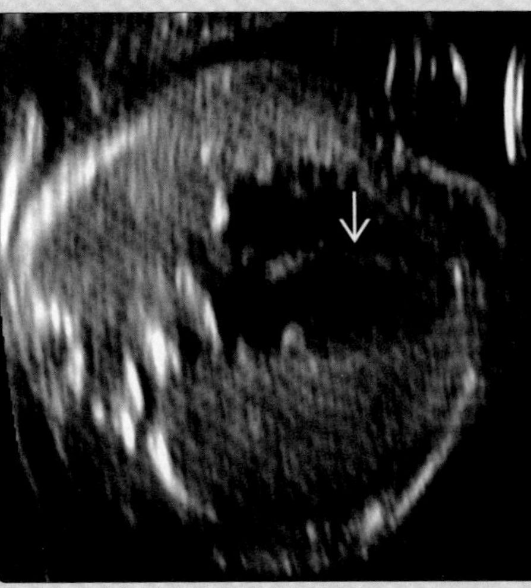

(Left) *Apical 4-chamber view in an 18-week fetus shows an area of signal dropout* ➡ *at the junction of the ventricular and membranous septa simulating a VSD.* **(Right)** *In the same case a few minutes later, moving the transducer so that the ultrasound beam is perpendicular to the septum* ➡*, it is clear that the septum is intact. Color Doppler can be used to confirm that there is no flow across the septum.*

KEY FACTS

TERMINOLOGY

- Apical displacement of septal and posterior tricuspid valve leaflets
- Coaptation point of tricuspid valve (i.e., where valve leaflets fit together) is lowered into right ventricle (RV)
  - Low valve coaptation point causes "atrialization" of RV
  - Right atrium (RA) is large; functional RV is small

IMAGING

- Tricuspid valve dysplasia + leaflet malposition → tricuspid regurgitation
- Tricuspid regurgitation → right atrial enlargement
  - Right atrial enlargement can be severe by 3rd trimester
  - Creates wall-to-wall heart appearance
- Atrialization of ventricle → small functional RV
  - Pulmonary artery often small or atretic

CLINICAL ISSUES

- In utero mortality rate is 45%

SCANNING TIPS

- Check for offset of valves on 4-chamber view of every fetal heart scan
  - Tricuspid leaflet should be more apically inserted than mitral
  - Mean mitral valve-tricuspid valve distance in 2nd trimester is 2.8 ± 0.9 mm
  - Mean mitral valve-tricuspid valve distance in 3rd trimester is 4.6 ± 1.1 mm
- Abnormal offset of tricuspid valve is key to making diagnosis of Ebstein anomaly
- At 18-20 weeks, RA enlargement may not be dramatic
  - If abnormal offset, bring patient back for follow-up
- Use Doppler (color ± pulsed wave) to look or tricuspid regurgitation
- Use 3-vessel view to assess size of outflow tracts, as pulmonary artery is often small
- Look for other abnormalities
  - Ebstein anomaly has been described in trisomy 21, 18

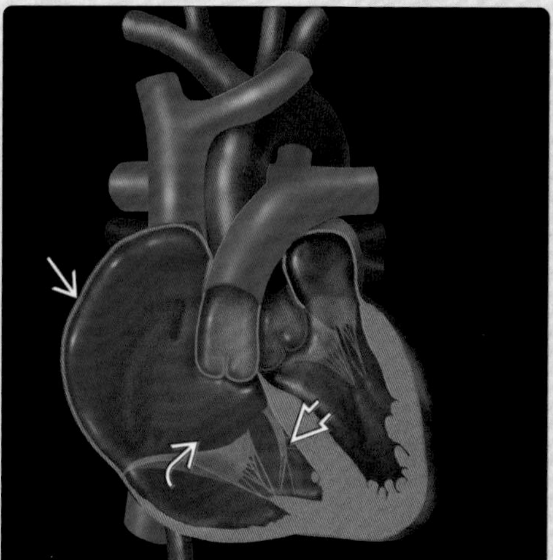

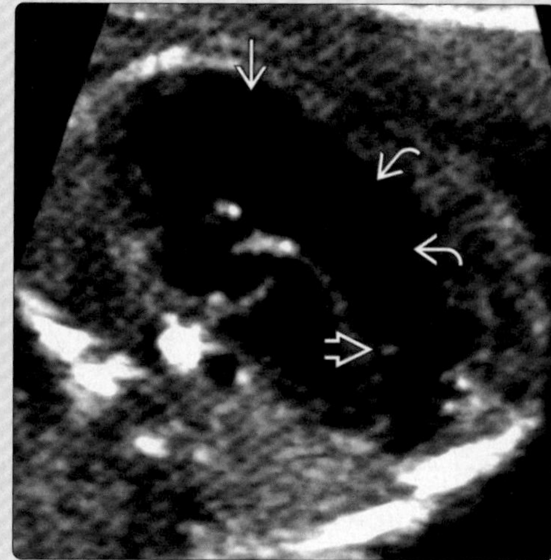

(Left) *Graphic of Ebstein anomaly shows a large right atrium ➡, which includes the "atrialized" inlet portion of the right ventricle ➡. Note the downwardly displaced and attached septal leaflet of the tricuspid valve ➡.* **(Right)** *Four-chamber (4C) view shows a massively dilated heart filling thorax, the "wall to wall" heart. The axis is abnormal at almost 90°. Septal leaflet ➡ of the tricuspid valve is downwardly displaced almost to apex of the heart resulting in a large atrialized portion of the RV ➡ in continuity with the RA ➡.*

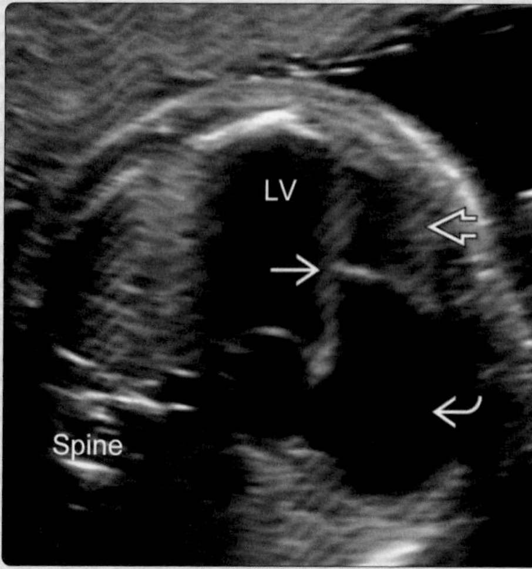

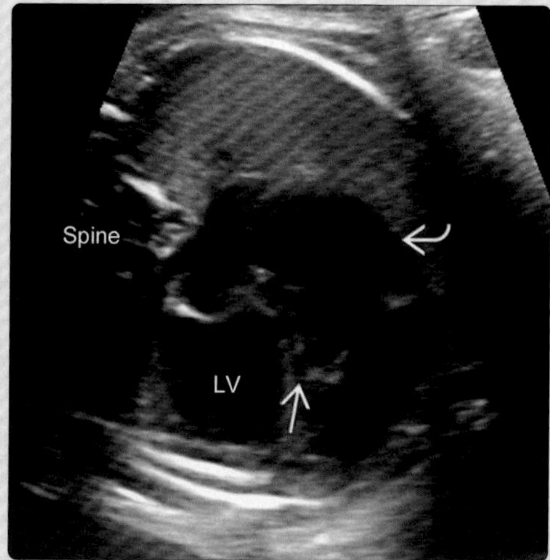

(Left) *4C view shows apically displaced septal tricuspid valve leaflet ➡, a key finding in Ebstein anomaly. The right atrium ➡ is large, and the functional RV ➡ is small. The heart is large, filling more than 1/2 the area of the chest (LV = left ventricle).* **(Right)** *4C view shows mild right atrial ➡ enlargement without distortion of the cardiac contour. On a still image, it might be read as normal but the septal tricuspid valve leaflet ➡ is apically displaced, indicating Ebstein anomaly. Always watch valve movement in real time.*

Hypoplastic Left Heart

KEY FACTS

TERMINOLOGY

- Hypoplasia of left heart syndrome (HLHS) associated with
  - Mitral stenosis/atresia
  - Aortic stenosis/atresia
  - Hypoplastic ascending aorta and coarctation

IMAGING

- Left ventricle (LV) small or nonexistent, not apex forming
  - Spherical, not bullet-shaped, decreased contraction
  - May be brightly echogenic indicating endocardial fibroelastosis
- Right ventricle (RV) is dilated with good function
  - Enlarged from extra blood flow, may wrap around LV
- Interatrial septum bowed from left atrium (LA) toward right atrium (RA) signifying direction of blood flow
  - Normal fetal circulation is flow of oxygenated blood across foramen ovale from RA → LA
- Ascending aorta and transverse arch are very small
  - Arch does not fill by forward flow from LV, fills retrograde from ductus arteriosus and RV
  - Retrograde filling of aortic arch = ductal dependence after delivery
    - Infant will need intensive care with prostaglandin infusion at delivery, which keeps ductus arteriosus open
    - These cases need to deliver in tertiary-level hospital

SCANNING TIPS

- Check every 4-chamber view for ventricular symmetry
  - Both ventricles should be apex forming
- Look at foramen ovale flap on 4-chamber view
  - Flap should open into RA
- Use 3-vessel view to compare size of outflow tracts
  - In HLHS, aorta (Ao) is small, pulmonary artery (PA) is large
- Use 3-vessel trachea view with color Doppler
  - If Ao, PA are different colors, there must be retrograde filling of 1 great vessel (i.e., duct dependence)

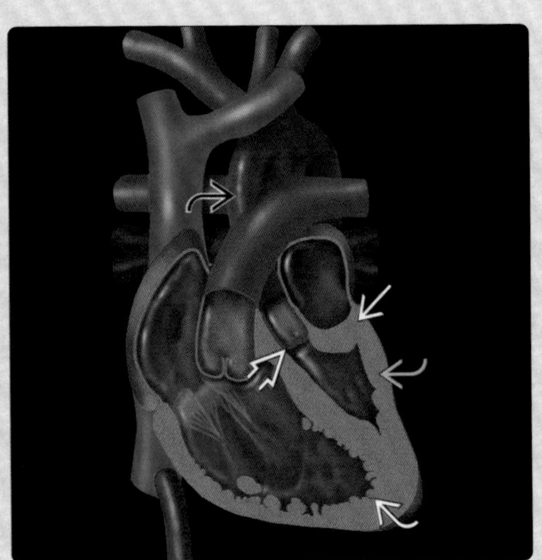

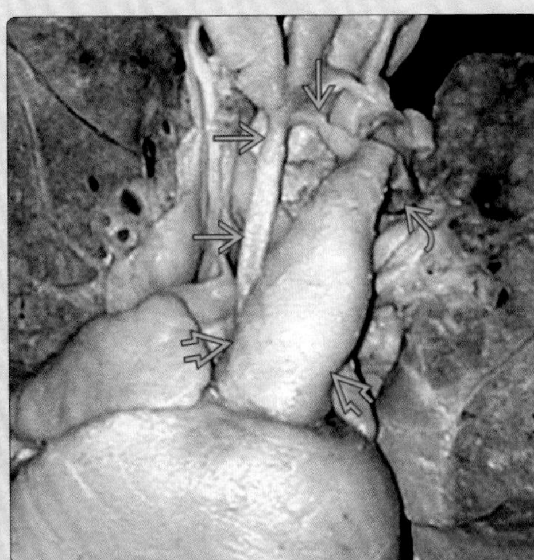

(Left) *Graphic shows hypoplasia of left heart syndrome. There is mitral ➡ and aortic ➡ valve atresia as well as asymmetry of ventricular sizes. The larger right ventricle (RV) is apex forming ➡ and wraps around the smaller left ventricle (LV) ➡. The ascending aorta ➡ is hypoplastic.* **(Right)** *Gross pathology shows a hypoplastic ascending aorta and transverse arch ➡, and a very large main pulmonary artery ➡ with continuation to the descending aorta via the ductus arteriosus ➡.*

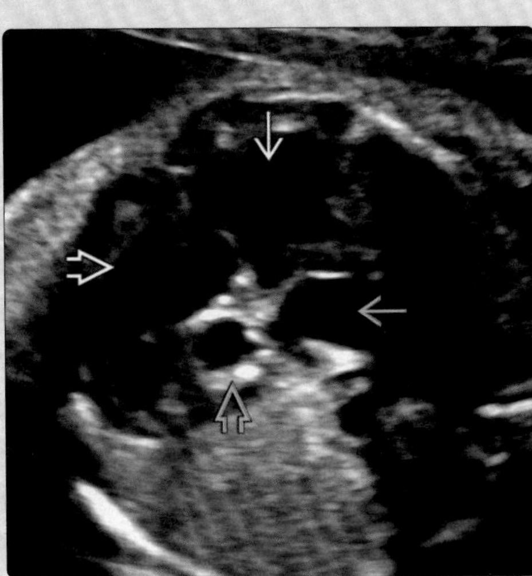

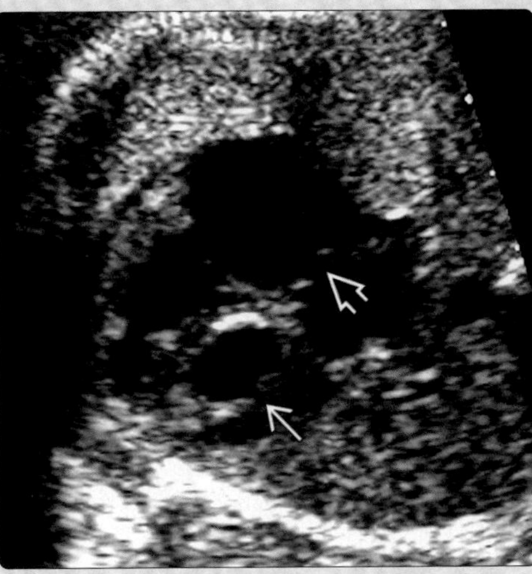

(Left) *Four-chamber view shows a classic picture of hypoplastic left heart. The right atrium ➡ and RV ➡ are large. The left atrium ➡ and LV are small ➡. The LV myocardium is much brighter than the rest of the myocardium, consistent with endocardial fibroelastosis.* **(Right)** *4-chamber view shows a thick-walled, small LV ➡, which does not reach the apex. The foramen ovale flap ➡ opens into the right atrium, indicating left to right shunting at the atrial level.*

Tetralogy of Fallot

KEY FACTS

TERMINOLOGY

- Congenital heart disease with 4 components
  - Right ventricular outflow tract (RVOT) obstruction
  - Right ventricular hypertrophy
  - Ventricular septal defect (VSD)
  - Aorta overrides or straddles VSD

IMAGING

- **95% of affected fetuses have normal 4-chamber view**
- **Outflow tract assessment is key to making diagnosis**
- Normal cardiac axis is 35-45°
  - Abnormal axis may be only sign of conotruncal heart disease on 4-chamber view
- RVOT obstruction
  - Anterior deviation of infundibulum (part of interventricular septum) at level of outflow tracts
  - Pulmonary valve (PV) usually abnormal
  - Pulmonary artery (PA) small with stenotic PV
  - PA and branches markedly enlarged if absent pulmonary valve (APV)
    - Back and forth flow across PV seen with color Doppler
- Aorta overrides large VSD

SCANNING TIPS

- Careful evaluation of outflows in any fetus with abnormal cardiac axis
- Use 3-vessel view to compare sizes of aorta and PA
  - Aorta is large in tetralogy of Fallot (ToF)
  - PA is huge in ToF with APV
- Look for other abnormalities
  - ToF associated with trisomies 21,18,13
  - Look for fetal thymus (absence suggests 22q11 deletion syndrome)
  - ToF may be component of syndromes such as VACTERL
    - Vertebral, anorectal, cardiac, tracheoesophageal, renal, limb anomalies

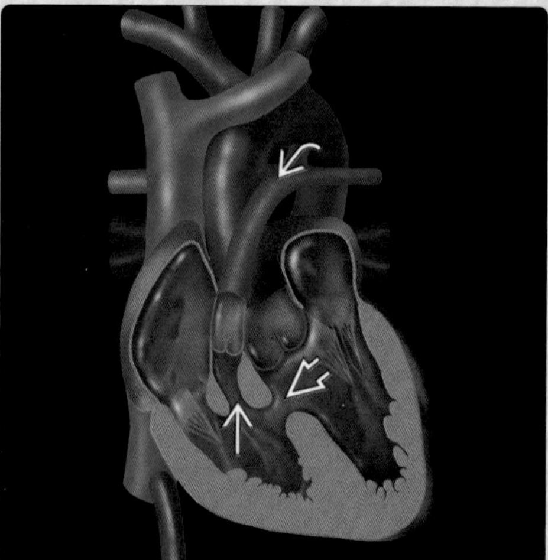

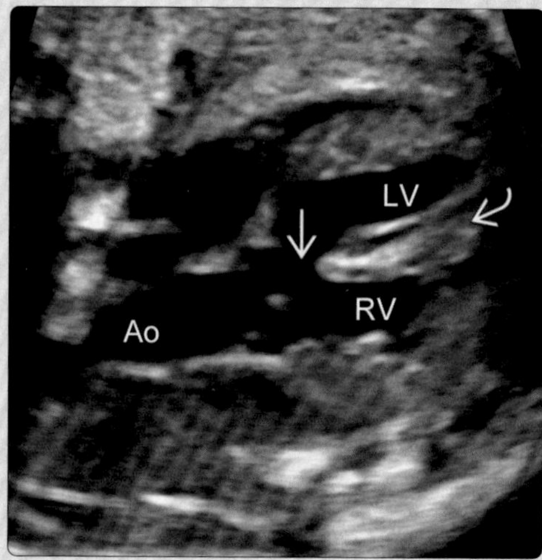

(Left) *Graphic shows pulmonary artery (PA) hypoplasia ➡ as the pulmonary outflow tract ➡ is narrowed by the anterior deviation of the infundibulum (i.e., interventricular septum inferior to the outflow tracts). The VSD ➡ allows for mixing of blood between right and left sides of the heart.* **(Right)** *Outflow view shows a VSD ➡ with the aorta (Ao) overriding the ventricular septum ➡. This is a classic finding in tetralogy of Fallot but is not diagnostic as a truncus also overrides a VSD. (RV: Right ventricle; LV: Left ventricle.)*

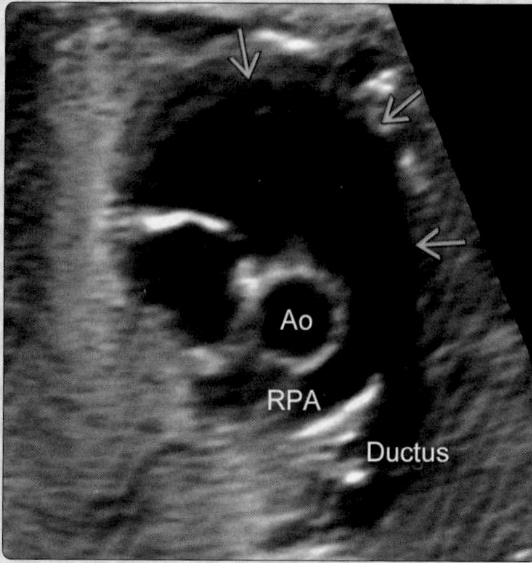

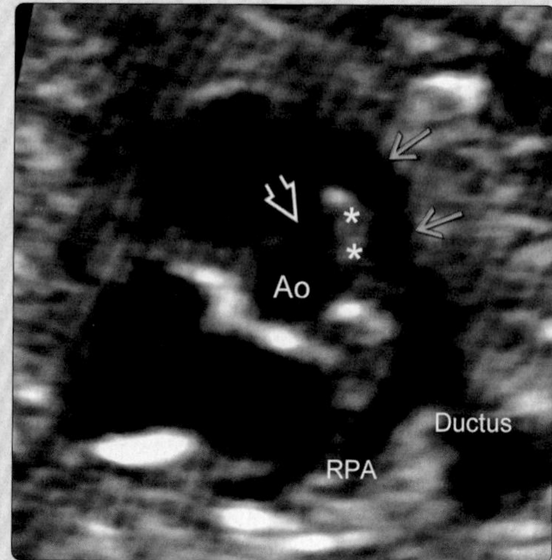

(Left) *Normal RVOT view shows the PA ➡ in long axis as it encircles the aortic root (Ao), which is seen as a circle in cross section. The ductus and right PA branch (RPA) are seen in this view.* **(Right)** *RVOT view in tetralogy of Fallet (ToF) shows a large VSD ➡ making the circle of the Ao incomplete. Anterior/superior deviation of the infundibulum (asterisks) decreases the size of the RVOT ➡. This is the picture you want to get to confirm ToF in the setting of a VSD with an overriding aorta. (RPA = right pulmonary artery.)*

KEY FACTS

TERMINOLOGY

- Ventriculoarterial discordance (arteries are switched)
  - Aorta arises from right ventricle (RV), pulmonary artery (PA) arises from left ventricle (LV)

IMAGING

- **4-chamber view is normal in TGA: Outflow tract assessment is key to making diagnosis**
  - Outflow tracts parallel as they exit heart
  - PA arises from LV, bifurcates early
    - Left ventricular outflow tract obstruction in 25%
  - Aorta arises from RV, gives rise to arch/head and neck vessels
    - Coarctation of aorta in 5%
- Ventricular septal defect (VSD) in 40-45%

TOP DIFFERENTIAL DIAGNOSES

- Double-outlet RV
  - Only other diagnosis with parallel outflow tracts

CLINICAL ISSUES

- **Postnatally TGA is lethal without treatment**
  - Must detect on prenatal scan for appropriate planning

SCANNING TIPS

- Never assume vessel from LV is aorta: Verify by showing head and neck branches
- Never assume vessel from RV is PA: Verify by showing early division into branch PAs
- If parallel outflow tracts are seen
  - Identify LV, RV, look for VSD
  - Differentiate aorta from PA
  - Look for outflow tract obstruction
- If only 2 vessels visible on 3-vessel view
  - Superior vena cava (SVC) + normal-sized vessel → transposition of great arteries
    - Both great arteries are present but aligned abnormally so not visible on same axial plane
  - SVC + large vessel → truncus

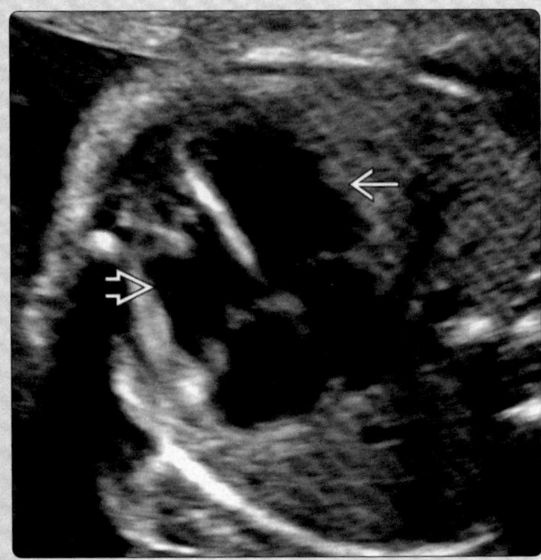

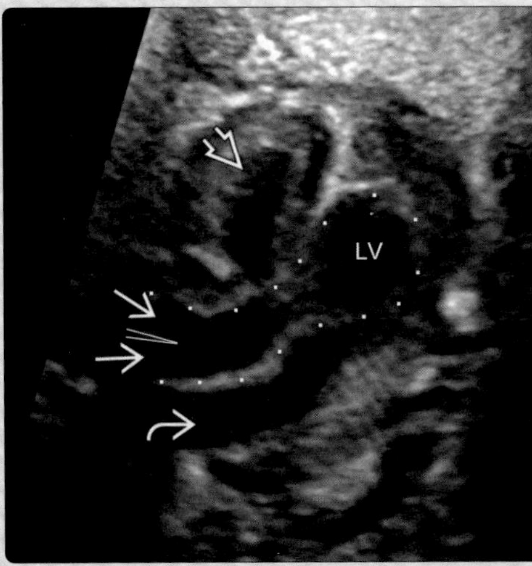

(Left) *Four-chamber view in a fetus with TGA looks normal. The RV is anterior ➡, the LV posterior ➡, and the ventricular septal defect (VSD) is not visible. Without real-time video clips and outflow tract assessment, significant congenital heart disease will be missed.* **(Right)** *The outlet view shows parallel outflow tracts with the branching pulmonary artery ➡ coming off the posterior, smooth-walled LV. The aorta ➡ came off the anterior, trabeculated RV, which is identified by the presence of the moderator band ➡.*

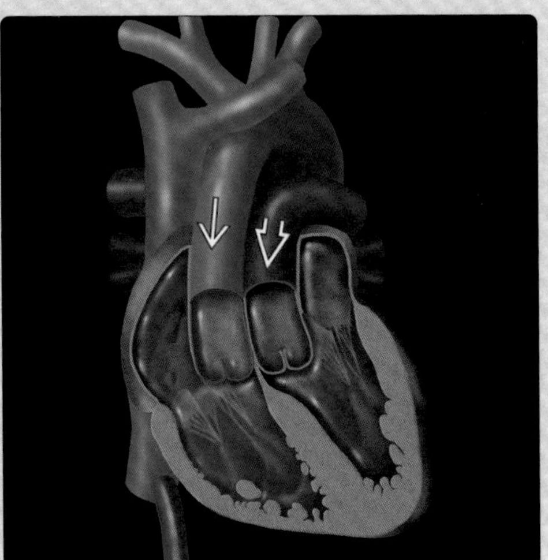

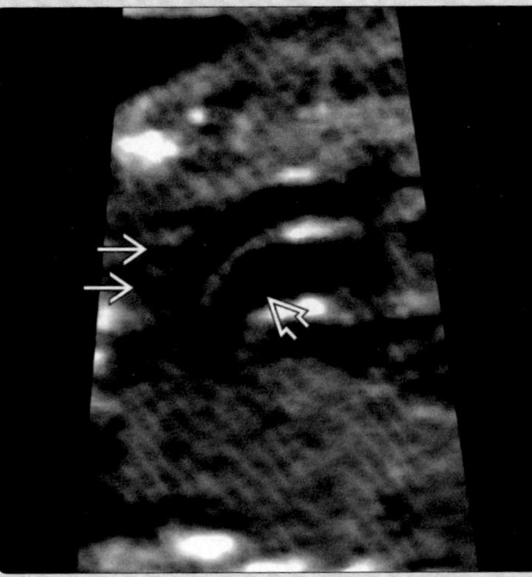

(Left) *Graphic shows the aorta ➡ arising from the RV and the pulmonary artery ➡ arising from the LV in simple transposition without a VSD. The great arteries are parallel as they exit the heart rather than crossing as they normally do.* **(Right)** *Outflow view shows parallel great vessels exiting the heart. The aorta is identified by the head and neck branches ➡ and arose from the anterior RV. The pulmonary artery ➡ arose from the LV.*

Truncus Arteriosus

KEY FACTS

TERMINOLOGY

- Single vessel (truncus) exits from heart giving rise to both aorta and pulmonary artery

TOP DIFFERENTIAL DIAGNOSES

- Other malformations with large vessel overriding VSD
  - Tetralogy of Fallot (will have 2 outflow tracts, aorta overrides)
  - Double-outlet right ventricle (will have 2 outflow tracts, parallel as exit heart)

SCANNING TIPS

- **4-chamber view can look normal: Outflow tract assessment is key to making diagnosis**
  - Look for single great vessel arising from heart
  - Pulmonary artery (PA) coming from proximal branch of single vessel is diagnostic
- If great vessel is noted overriding VSD, look at branch pattern
  - **Truncal vessel gives rise to both head and neck vessels and PAs**
- If great vessel is noted overriding VSD, look at valve leaflets
  - > 3 leaflets = truncal valve
  - Look for associated stenosis, regurgitation
- If only 2 vessels visible on 3 vessel view
  - Superior vena cava (SVC) + large vessel → truncus
  - SVC + normal-sized vessel → transposition
- Evaluate for other anomalies; if present, they impact prognosis
  - Right-sided aortic arch in 21-36%; interrupted aortic arch in 10-19%
  - Extracardiac anomalies in 21-30%
  - Look for features associated with 22q11 deletion (DiGeorge syndrome)
    - Absent thymus, bulbous nasal tip, broad nasal bridge, micrognathia
    - Long slender fingers, toes

(Left) *Graphic shows a single vessel ➡ arising over a ventricular septal defect (VSD) ➡. The pulmonary artery ➡ branches shortly after it exits the heart, and the head and neck vessels arise from the apex of the same vessel. This is characteristic of truncus arteriosus.* **(Right)** *Gross pathology shows a ventriculoseptal defect ➡ with a single common trunk ➡ leaving the heart. A left-sided branch ➡ gives rise to a pulmonary artery.*

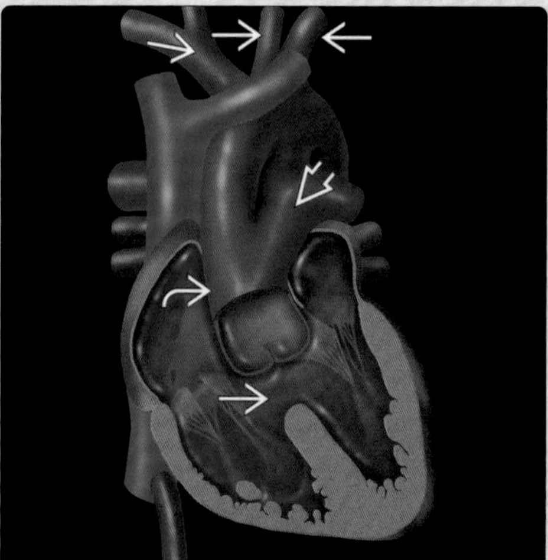

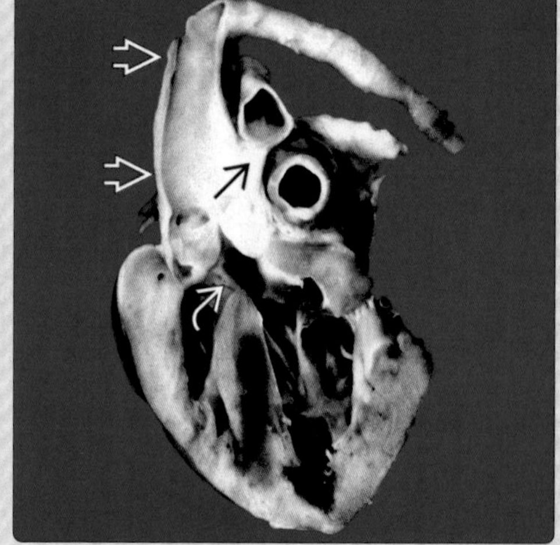

(Left) *Echocardiogram shows a large VSD ➡ with the truncus straddling both ventricles. The main pulmonary artery ➡ is an early branch of the truncus (RV: Right ventricle; LV: Left ventricle).* **(Right)** *Outlet view shows a single great vessel, the truncus (T), exiting the heart. It gives rise to the pulmonary artery (PA) and the aorta (Ao), which is identified by the presence of a head and neck vessel ➡. Note the thick, dysplastic truncal valve ➡.*

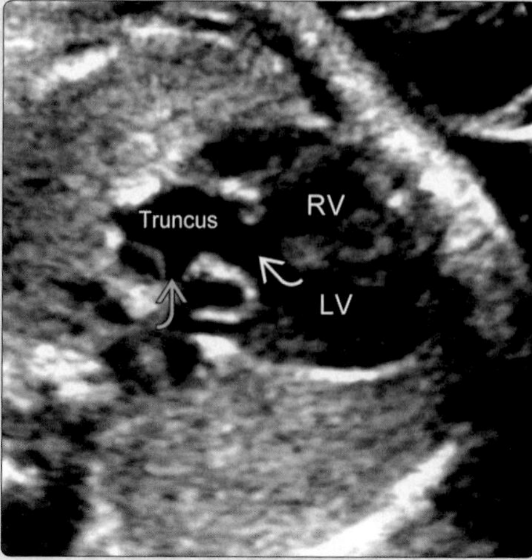

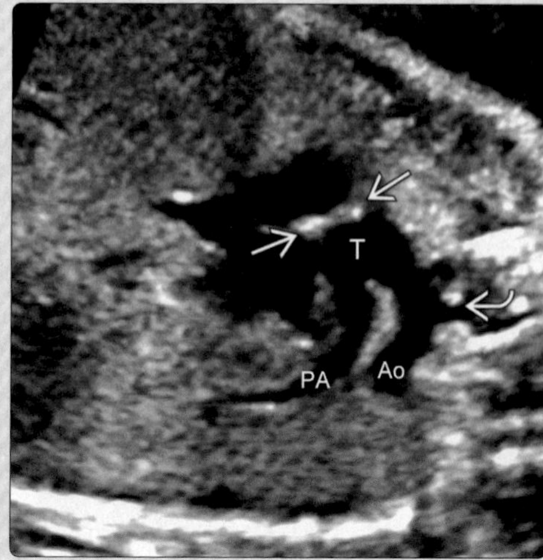

Rhabdomyoma

KEY FACTS

TERMINOLOGY

- Congenital, benign cardiac tumor composed of abnormal muscle cells

IMAGING

- Well-defined, homogeneous, hyperechoic, intracardiac mass
  - May be solitary but more typically multiple
  - Most common in ventricles but can be anywhere
- Rhabdomyomas less likely to cause pericardial effusions than other cardiac tumors

TOP DIFFERENTIAL DIAGNOSES

- Echogenic cardiac focus
  - Majority in left ventricle, associated with papillary muscle
  - Small, very echogenic (similar to bone)
- Pericardial teratoma
  - Pericardial, not myocardial
  - Heterogeneous, mixed cystic/solid mas, calcifications

CLINICAL ISSUES

- 75-80% of infants with cardiac rhabdomyomas have tuberous sclerosis (TS)
  - Almost 100% with multiple cardiac masses

SCANNING TIPS

- When cardiac mass is identified
  - Assess location
  - Look for additional masses
  - Check for rhythm abnormalities
  - Look for signs of hydrops
- Obtain formal fetal echocardiogram
  - Monitor cardiac function
  - Watch for development of valve obstruction or regurgitation
- Look carefully for brain findings seen in TS
  - Subependymal nodules cause subtle irregularity along lateral ventricular walls

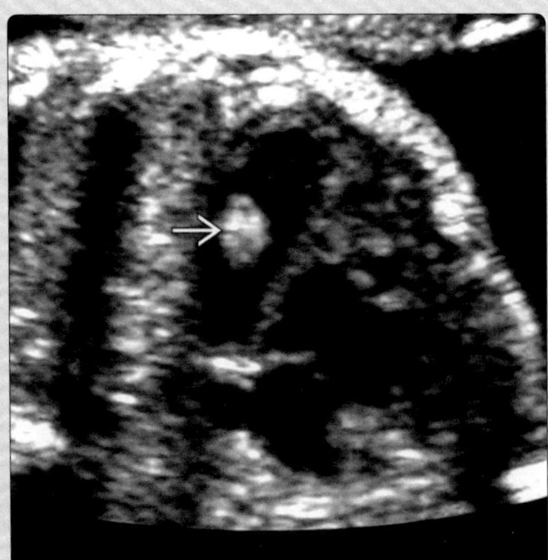

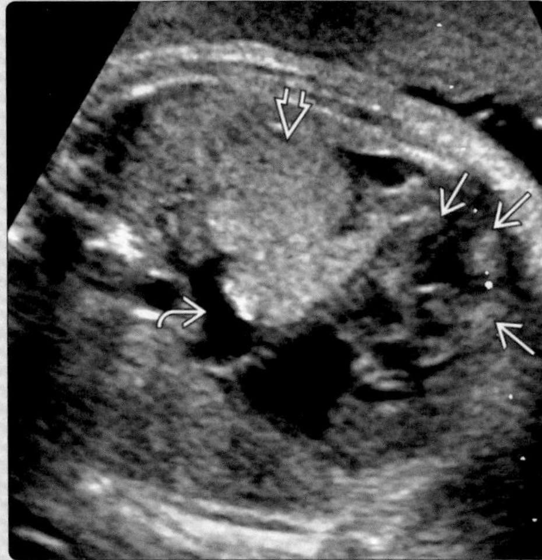

(Left) *Fetal echocardiogram shows a small, hyperechoic, well-defined mass ➡ involving the papillary muscle of the left ventricle. This was a solitary lesion, and the fetus was otherwise normal.* **(Right)** *A very large, echogenic mass ➡ fills the left ventricular cavity and appears to protrude into the left atrium ➡, raising concern for obstruction to flow across the mitral valve. Multiple small masses are also seen in the right ventricle ➡ in this patient with tuberous sclerosis.*

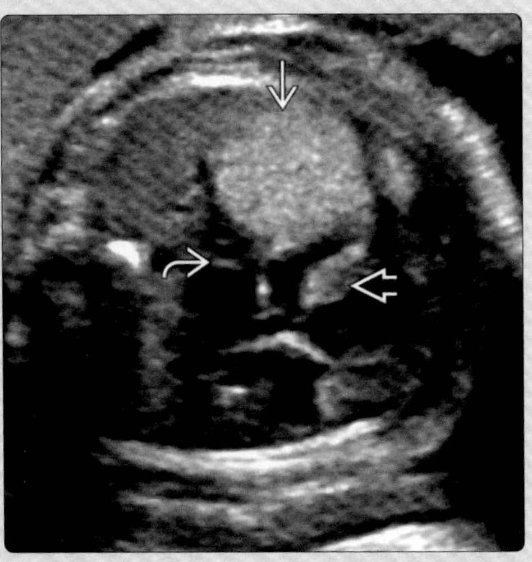

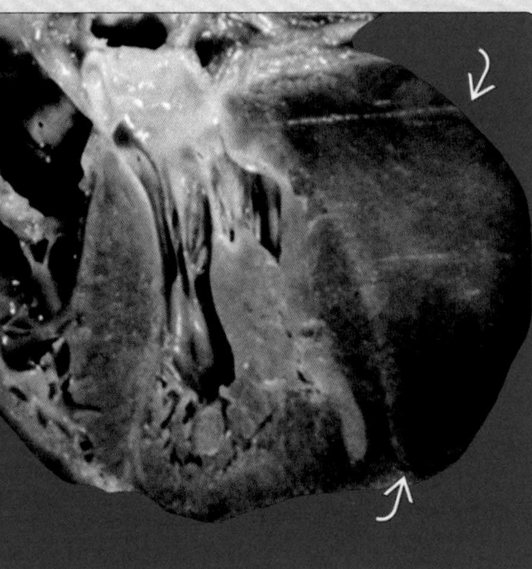

(Left) *Four-chamber view of the fetal heart shows a very large mass ➡ at the apex of the left ventricle, which almost completely obliterates the cavity. The mitral valve ➡ almost seems to be attached to it. There is an additional mass in the septum ➡. These are consistent with rhabdomyomas.* **(Right)** *Gross pathology from a different, but similar, case shows a rhabdomyoma ➡ causing dramatic left ventricle wall thickening.*

PART VI
SECTION 6

Abdominal Wall and Gastrointestinal Tract

Anatomy and Approach

Abdominal Wall Defects

Bowel Abnormalities

Hepatobiliary Abnormalities

EMBRYOLOGY

Bowel Development

- Gastrointestinal (GI) tract forms from 1 straight tube
  - **Foregut**: Forms esophagus, stomach, and duodenum
  - **Midgut**: Small intestine and colon up to splenic flexure
    - Connected to yolk sac
    - Portion that lengthens and loops around superior mesenteric artery (SMA)
  - **Hindgut**: Descending colon, sigmoid, rectum, and upper anal canal
    - Caudal end of hindgut terminates in **cloaca**
      - Cloaca (Latin for sewer) is common chamber with early communication between the urinary, GI, and reproductive tracts
- **Physiologic herniation**
  - Length of midgut increases rapidly and is greater than body can accommodate so it herniates into base of umbilical cord
  - It rotates 90°counterclockwise around axis of SMA and returns to the abdomen after total rotation of 270°
  - Abdominal wall closes around base of cord (umbilical ring)
  - Physiologic hernia is commonly seen on early 1st trimester scans but the **bowel should be back within the abdomen by 12 weeks gestational age**
  - An **omphalocele** results from failure to complete physiologic herniation or close umbilical ring
- **Rectum** forms when urorectal septum divides cloaca into rectum posteriorly and urogenital sinus anteriorly
  - Cloacal membrane ruptures by beginning of 8th week, creating anal opening
  - Urogenital sinus will divide to form bladder and in females, the vagina

SCANNING APPROACH AND IMAGING ISSUES

Techniques and Sonographic Appearance

- American Institute of Ultrasound in Medicine (AIUM) scan of the abdomen requires documentation of stomach, kidneys, bladder, umbilical cord insertion site, and umbilical cord vessel number
  - Diaphragm, esophagus, small intestine, colon, gallbladder, and liver should also be examined but is not required as part of the standard midtrimester scan
- **Stomach** is seen as a fluid-filled structure in the left upper quadrant and is one of the 1st organs identified
  - Document heart and stomach are on same side, and it is anatomic left of fetus (normal situs)
    - Opposite sides are seen in **heterotaxy syndromes**
  - Changes in size and shape during exam
  - Fluid may intermittently be seen to enter the duodenal bulb but should never persist
    - A persistently dilated duodenum is never normal and suspicious for **duodenal atresia**
- Fluid must be visualized on **both sides of the umbilical cord insertion** in a transverse section of the fetal abdomen
  - Stimulation of fetal movement may be necessary to create a more favorable acoustic window, especially in 3rd trimester when the fetal knees are often tucked up against abdominal wall
- **Normal cord contains 2 arteries and 1 vein**
  - May be visible at cord insertion site, but easiest way to confirm is color Doppler showing umbilical arteries on either side of bladder
- **Diaphragm** appears as a thin, arched, hypoechoic band
  - It is imperative that it be completely imaged from front to back, which is best done in the sagittal plane
  - If viewed only in the anterior coronal plane, a congenital diaphragmatic hernia (CDH) may be missed
- **Esophagus** is not normally seen on fetal imaging, but a blind-ending, fluid-filled pouch may be seen in the fetal neck in esophageal atresia
  - Use color Doppler to ensure that the fluid-filled structure is between the neck vessels
- **Bowel**
  - In early 2nd trimester, often appears as intermediate echogenicity "filler" between the solid organs, bladder, and stomach; higher frequency transducers may show distinct bowel loops
  - Normal **meconium-filled colon** often prominent near term
  - **Anal dimple** best seen on an axial view of perineum
    - Anal mucosa is echogenic and surrounded by hypoechoic muscles of the anal sphincter, creating a target or doughnut appearance
- Fetal **liver** is relatively large and extends across the upper abdomen with the left lobe anterior to stomach
  - Major contributor to the abdominal circumference (AC)
  - Both portal and hepatic veins seen on color Doppler
  - **Gallbladder** may be seen, especially in the 3rd trimester, and should not be confused with an abdominal cyst

Approach to the Abdominal Wall

- **Is the abdominal wall intact?**
  - **Gastroschisis** (most common abdominal wall defect) is generally located to the right of the umbilical cord insertion and is not covered by a membrane
    - Small bowel is the most commonly extruded organ, although stomach, large bowel, and other structures may also be involved
  - **Omphalocele** involves extrusion of bowel into the base of the umbilical cord
    - Covered by a membrane; umbilical cord inserts on this membrane
    - May rarely rupture; in these cases, it may be difficult to distinguish from gastroschisis
  - Defects may also occur in more unusual locations
    - Low, suprapubic mass may be associated with **bladder or cloacal exstrophy**
      - Both will have absent bladder, but cloacal exstrophy will also have extruded bowel described as appearing like an elephant trunk
    - Supraumbilical defect associated with diaphragmatic and cardiac abnormality is seen in **pentalogy of Cantrell**
    - Other unusual or bizarre abdominal wall defects may be seen in cases of **amniotic bands or body stalk anomaly**
- **Is the fetus freely mobile?**
  - In **body stalk anomaly**, the fetus is "stuck" to the placenta, and the umbilical cord is absent or very short

- A fetus entrapped within **amniotic bands** may also be tethered in one position
  - Look for strands of membrane or other defects, such as unusual facial or cranial clefts

Approach to the Gastrointestinal Tract

- **Is the abdomen normal in size?**
  - Per AIUM guidelines, the **AC** is measured at the skin line on a true transverse view at the level of the junction of the umbilical vein, portal sinus, and fetal stomach
  - AC is utilized with other biometric parameters to calculate the fetal weight/average gestational age
  - **AC below the normal range**
    - Generally, the most affected parameter in growth restriction
    - May also measure small when normal abdominal contents are outside the abdomen (e.g., gastroschisis, omphalocele) or up in the chest (i.e., CDH)
  - **AC above the normal range**
    - Macrosomic fetus of a diabetic mother
    - Overgrowth syndromes, such as Beckwith-Wiedemann, may also exhibit increased AC size, primarily due to enlarged kidneys and liver
    - AC often increased in fetuses with large abdominal masses, dilated bowel, or distended bladder
- **Is the stomach normal?**
  - A fluid-filled stomach should reliably be identified after 14 weeks
    - If not seen, short-term follow-up required to confirm its presence or absence
    - Ensure that it is not in an abnormal location, such as within the chest in a CDH
  - **Small/absent stomach**
    - Esophageal atresia ± tracheoesophageal fistula
      - Look for blind-ending pouch in neck
      - Will have significant polyhydramnios by 3rd trimester
    - May be seen in cases of decreased swallowing (e.g., neurologic disorder)
  - **Large stomach**
    - Often a transient finding or may be seen in evolving, distal GI obstructions
    - **Double bubble** sign (dilated stomach and duodenum) is seen in **duodenal atresia**
- **Is there an abdominal mass?**
  - Masses should be characterized as to their location and appearance (cystic, solid, or complex; vascular or nonvascular) to narrow the differential diagnosis
  - **Cystic masses** in the abdomen are relatively common
    - Many of these are related to the urinary tract and include cystic kidneys, lower urinary tract obstruction, and ovarian cysts
    - GI causes include
      - **Bowel atresia**: Look for peristalsis
      - **Meconium pseudocyst**: Irregular cystic mass, which forms after bowel perforation; look for other sequelae, including peritoneal calcifications
      - **Enteric duplication cyst**: Look for gut signature
      - **Mesenteric cysts/lymphangioma**
      - Persistent **cloaca** occurs when genitourinary tract and colon never separate
  - **Solid masses** are less common; the differential diagnosis starts with the organ of origin
    - The most common liver mass is a **congenital hemangioma**, which usually has prominent vascularity
    - Bulk of a **sacrococcygeal teratoma** is exophytic but may extend into pelvis/abdomen
      - Rarely may be only intrapelvic with no external component
    - **Fetus-in-fetu** is a mixed solid/cystic mass and is often quite large
      - Calcifications common; bones and vertebrae may be seen
- **Are there calcifications in the abdomen?**
  - Calcifications **on the surface of the liver** are actually in the peritoneum
    - These correlate strongly with intrauterine bowel perforation
    - Look for associated echogenic or dilated bowel loops, small amounts of ascites, &/or meconium pseudocysts to add weight to this diagnosis
  - Calcification **in the liver parenchyma** concerning for infection, most commonly **cytomegalovirus**
  - Calcifications **in the bowel lumen** indicate admixture of meconium and urine in the setting of abnormal distal bowel and bladder development
    - These "meconium marbles" roll within the bowel lumen with peristalsis
    - Look carefully for the anal dimple to detect associated anal atresia
- **Does the bowel appear echogenic?**
  - A high-frequency transducer may give the false impression of echogenic bowel
    - Confirm the finding is persistent with a lower frequency transducer (< 5 MHz)
  - Bowel is not abnormal unless it is **as bright as bone**
  - Fetal **ingestion of blood** from a recent bleed is a common benign cause and resolves spontaneously
  - Evaluate for pathologic causes, including **aneuploidy, infection, cystic fibrosis**, and early bowel abnormalities, such as **atresia**, before the bowel becomes dilated
  - May be seen in **bowel ischemia** in association with severe growth and hemodynamic stress as in twin-twin transfusion
- **Is there ascites?**
  - Care should be taken to differentiate true ascites from **pseudoascites**, a potential pitfall created by the hypoechoic abdominal wall musculature
  - Ascites may be 1st sign of **impending hydrops**
    - Look for other evidence of hydrops (pleural and pericardial effusions and skin edema)
  - Chest masses may compromise venous and lymphatic return and cause isolated ascites without generalized hydrops
  - May also result from **perforation of an abdominal viscus**, either bowel or bladder

PHYSIOLOGIC HERNIATION

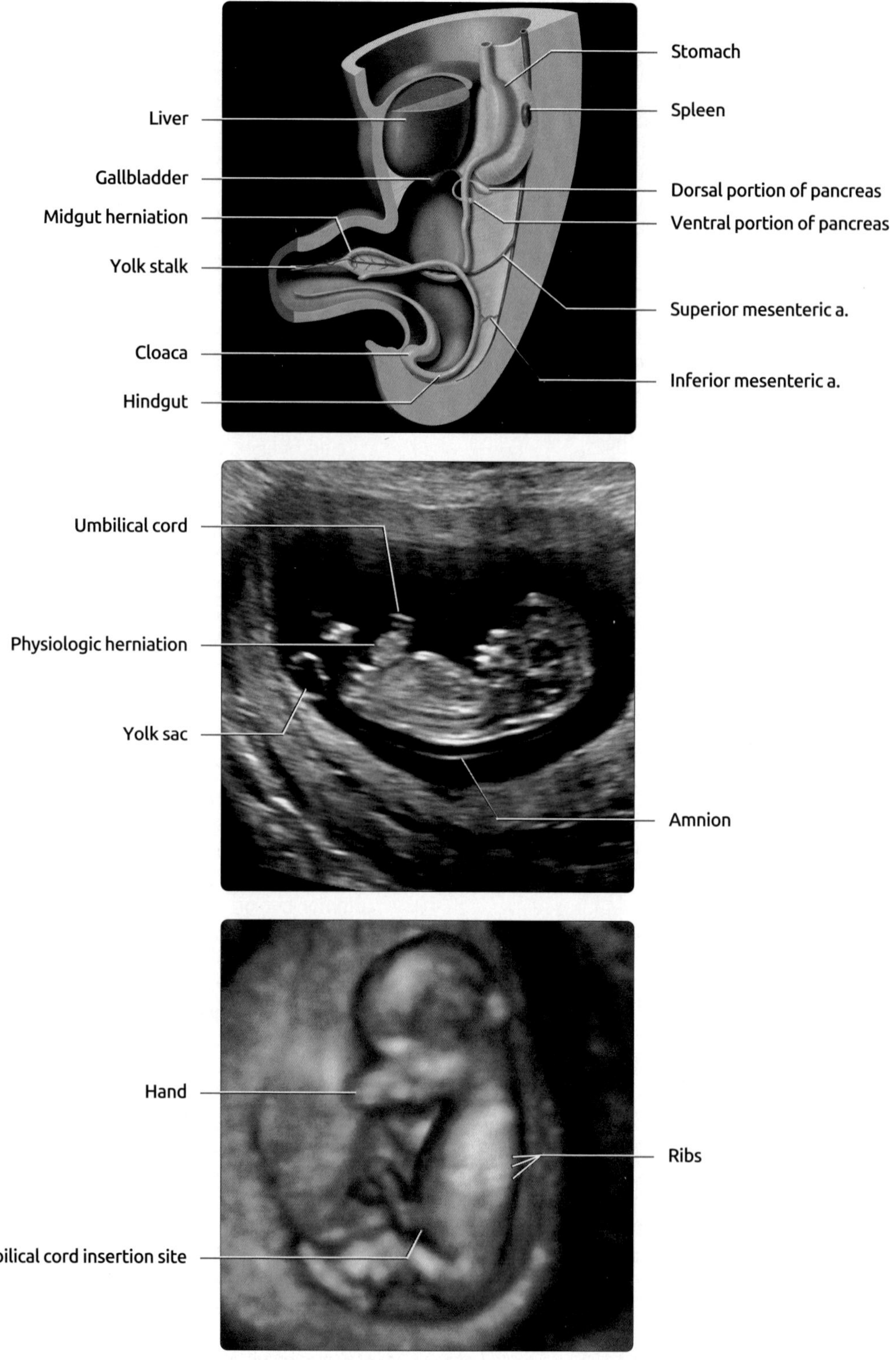

(Top) *Sagittal graphic at ~ 5 weeks gestational age shows the developing gastrointestinal tract. The length of midgut increases rapidly and is greater than the body can accommodate, so it herniates into the base of the umbilical cord. It rotates 90° counterclockwise around the axis of the superior mesenteric artery and returns to the abdomen after a total rotation of 270°. The abdominal wall then closes around the base of the cord (umbilical ring). Failure of the bowel to return or incomplete closure of the abdominal wall results in an omphalocele.* **(Middle)** *Sagittal US of a 10-week fetus shows normal physiologic herniation of bowel. Do not mistake this normal appearance for an omphalocele.* **(Bottom)** *3D US at 12 weeks shows a normal cord insertion site with bowel having completely returned to the abdomen. Persistence of herniation after 12 weeks is abnormal.*

ABDOMINAL ANATOMY

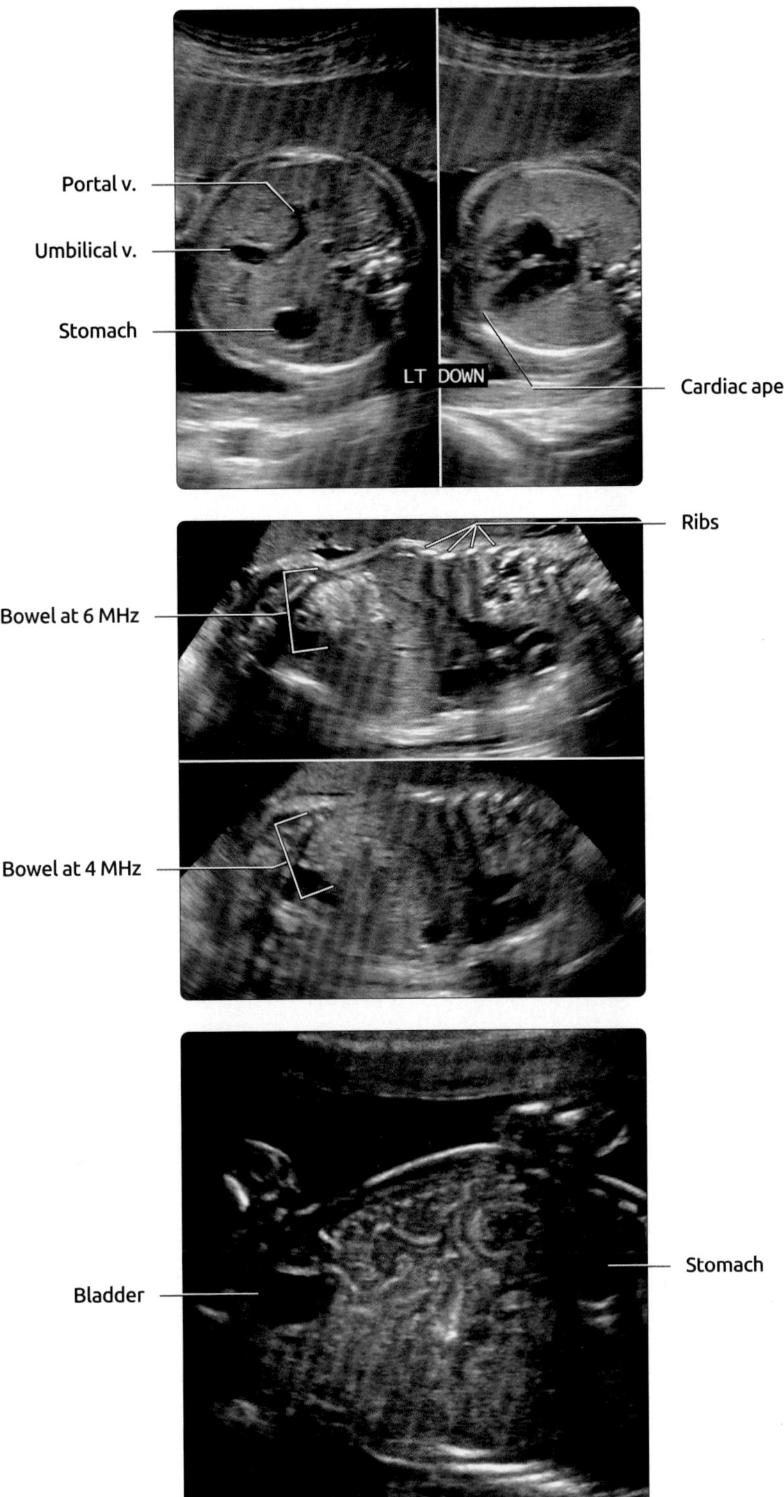

(Top) *The 1st step in fetal evaluation should be to determine which is the anatomic left and right of the fetus. This fetus is in cephalic presentation with the spine to the maternal left; therefore, the left side is down, and both the cardiac apex and stomach are on the same side (situs solitus). This is also the correct level for the abdominal circumference (AC) measurement with the umbilical vein and portal vein forming a C shape.* **(Middle)** *Composite shows the importance of transducer frequency. The bowel at 6 MHz (top) looks echogenic, but at 4 MHz (bottom), it does not. High frequencies provide much more detail (note you can see individual bowel loops) but be aware that the bowel may appear hyperechoic. To be considered abnormal, bowel should be bright as bone. Note that it is much less echogenic than the nearby ribs.* **(Bottom)** *High-resolution US of the bowel at 19 weeks shows the tubular morphology with the gut signature of hypoechoic muscular walls and hyperechoic mucosa.*

ABDOMINAL ANATOMY

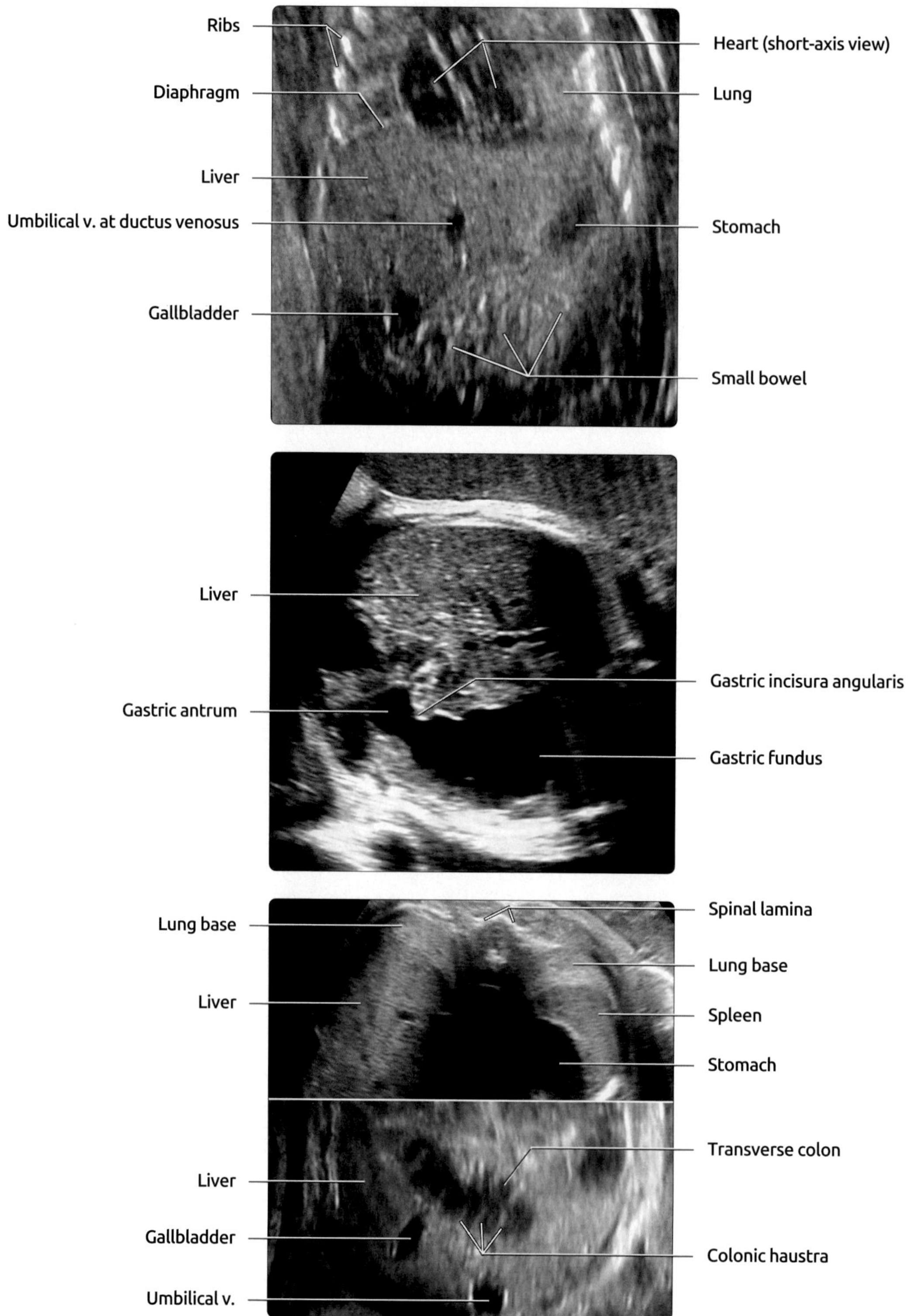

(Top) *Coronal US in a 20-week fetus shows the anatomy of the upper abdomen.* **(Middle)** *Oblique axial US shows the incisura angularis, a muscular indentation along the lesser curve of the stomach near the pylorus. This needs to be recognized as normal and not confused with the duodenum leading to the erroneous diagnosis of duodenal atresia. With real-time observation, the stomach is seen to contract and change shape during fetal swallowing.* **(Bottom)** *Subtle differences in echogenicity allow the identification of the various organs, as shown in this composite image of a 3rd-trimester fetus. The upper oblique axial image shows the lungs are mildly hyperechoic compared to the liver and spleen. Changes in echotexture often provide clues regarding a pathologic process in a given organ. The lower image is an oblique coronal US of the transverse colon. US can show detailed anatomy, such as the colonic haustra.*

ABDOMINAL ANATOMY

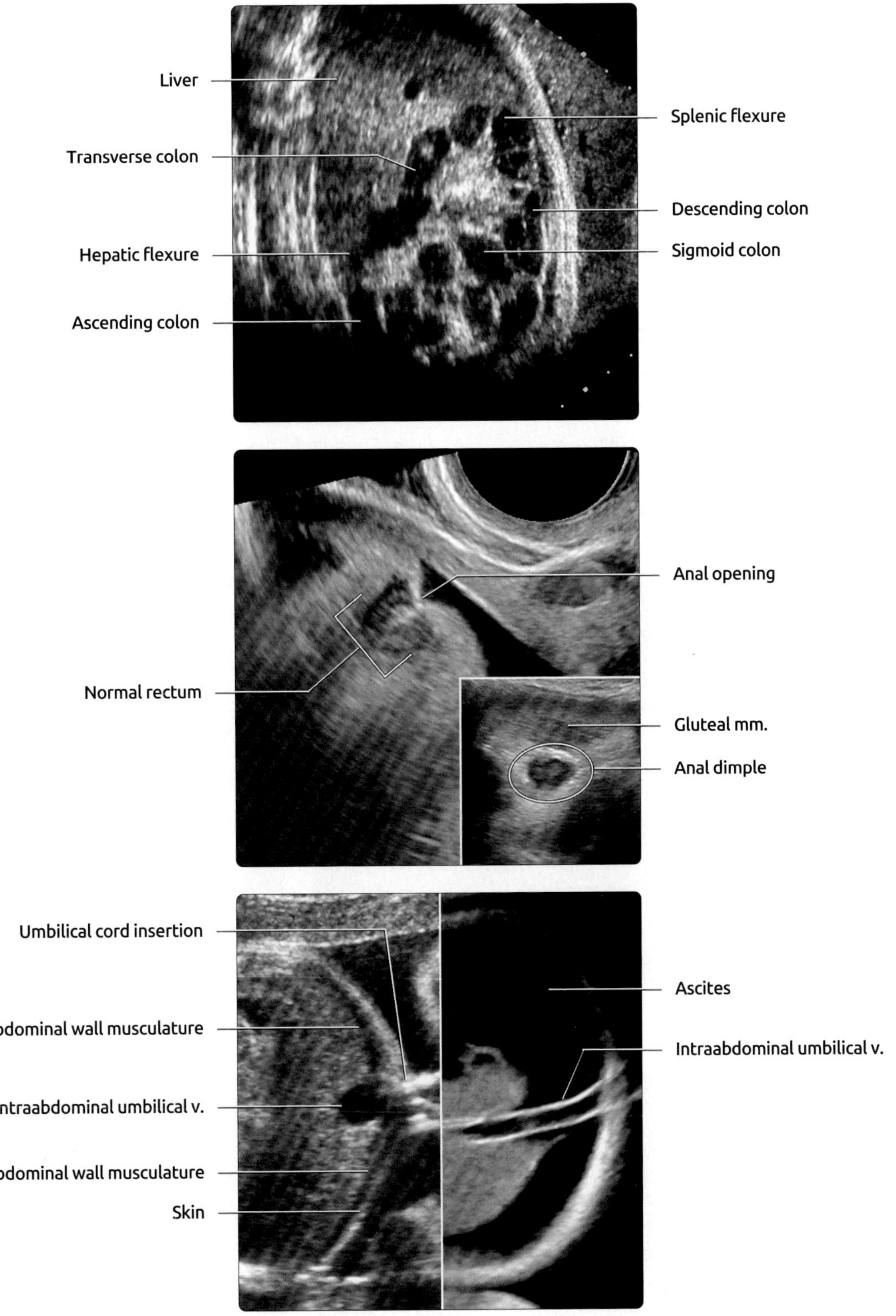

(Top) *Coronal US of a late 3rd-trimester fetus shows meconium within the colon. The colon can appear quite prominent in the late 3rd trimester and should not be confused with a pathologic process.* **(Middle)** *Transvaginal US in a breech presentation fetus shows a coronal view of the anorectal complex in detail. There is a normal external indentation at the anal sphincter with the muscular layered appearance of the rectal wall and hyperechoic mucosa. Axial US of the perineum (insert) shows the anal dimple having a doughnut or target appearance created by the hypoechoic wall surrounding the hyperechoic mucosa.* **(Bottom)** *Axial US shows an example of pseudoascites (left) created by the hypoechoic abdominal wall musculature. Note that the hypoechoic line stops abruptly at the cord insertion site and does not surround the intraabdominal portion of the umbilical vein. Compare to the case of true ascites (right) from a bladder rupture, where fluid clearly outlines both sides of the umbilical vein.*

Omphalocele

KEY FACTS

TERMINOLOGY

- Membrane-covered midline abdominal wall defect with herniation of abdominal contents into base of cord

IMAGING

- Liver + small bowel is most common type (large defects)
- Bowel-only type is smaller and more likely missed
- Omphalocele membrane is peritoneum + amnion
  - Mostly thin membrane but can also be cystic
- Umbilical cord inserts onto membrane (not always central)
  - Color Doppler best to show cord insertion site
- Ascites is common
- Membrane rupture is complication

TOP DIFFERENTIAL DIAGNOSES

- Normal physiologic bowel herniation
  - Bowel returns by 12 weeks
- Gastroschisis
  - Defect to right of normal cord insertion

CLINICAL ISSUES

- 25-30% with associated anomalies
  - Cardiac defects common
- Chromosomal abnormalities in 30-40%
  - Bowel-only omphalocele with highest risk
- Syndromes associated with omphalocele
  - Beckwith-Wiedemann syndrome: Big tongue, macrosomia, large &/or horseshoe kidneys
  - Pentalogy of Cantrell: Part of heart in omphalocele sac
  - OEIS complex: **O**mphalocele, bladder **e**xtrophy, **i**mperforate anus, **s**pine anomaly
- Survival as high as 80-90% if normal chromosomes, no syndromes, and no other significant anomalies

SCANNING TIPS

- Evaluate abdominal wall cord insertion site at time of nuchal translucency screening
- Consider sac rupture if ascites suddenly resolves
- Consider formal echocardiogram in all cases

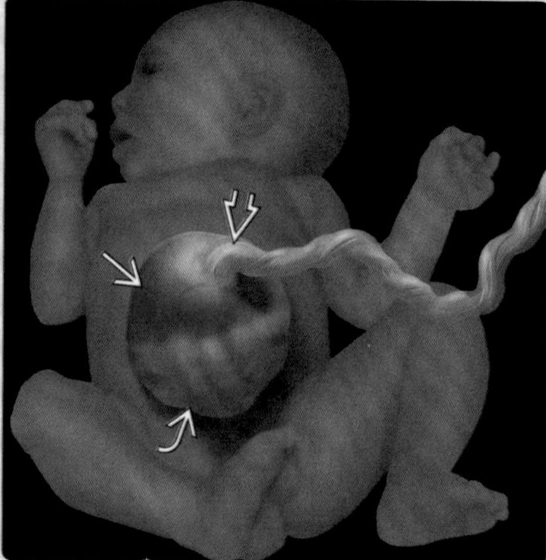

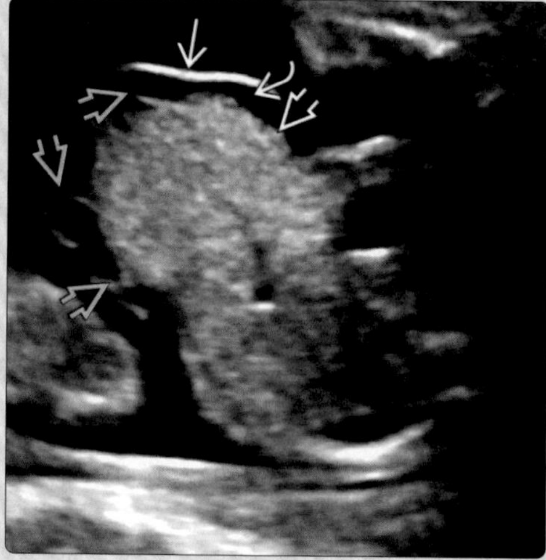

(Left) *Graphic shows the most common type of omphalocele. A midline abdominal wall defect with herniated small bowel ➡ and liver ➡ is covered by a membrane. The umbilical cord inserts directly onto the sac ➡.* **(Right)** *In this fetus with liver-containing omphalocele, the membrane ➡ and liver ➡ are seen well because of the presence of ascites ➡. Also, there are some septations/cysts associated with the membrane ➡, not uncommon since the membrane is peritoneum and amnion and can be thickened or cystic.*

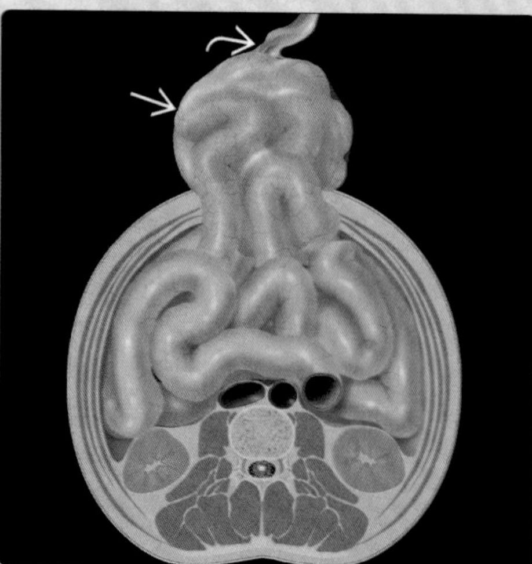

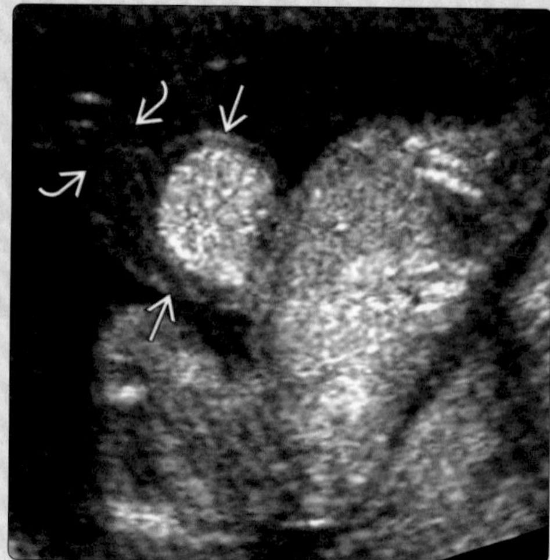

(Left) *The less common type of omphalocele contains only small bowel. This graphic shows the membrane-covered defect, eviscerated small bowel ➡, and umbilical cord insertion upon the membrane ➡.* **(Right)** *Sagittal view of a 15-week fetus shows the umbilical cord ➡ inserting upon a bowel-only omphalocele ➡. The bowel is not free floating (as would be expected in gastroschisis) since it is confined by a membrane. Also, physiologic bowel herniation can only look like this in fetuses < 12 weeks.*

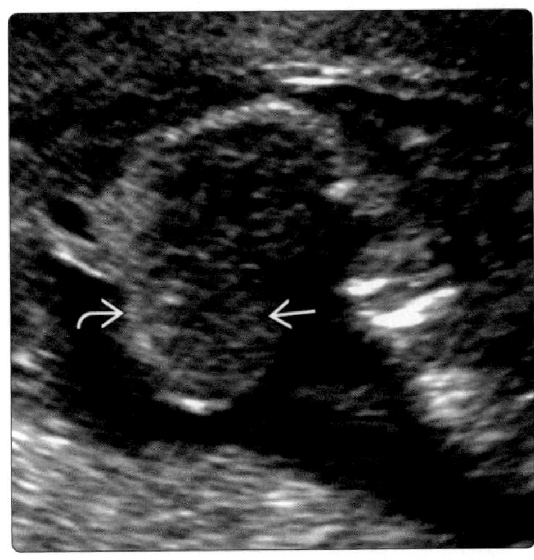

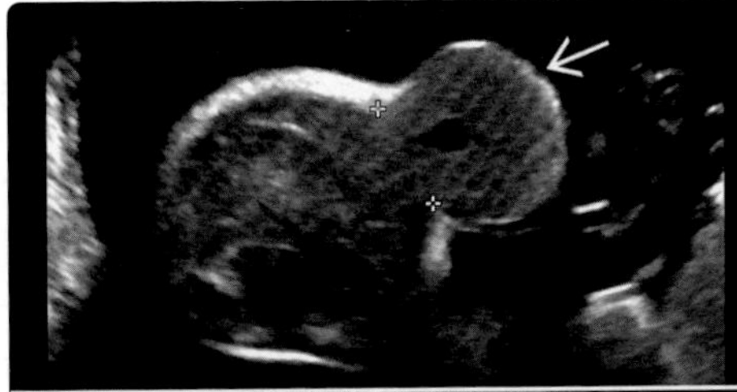

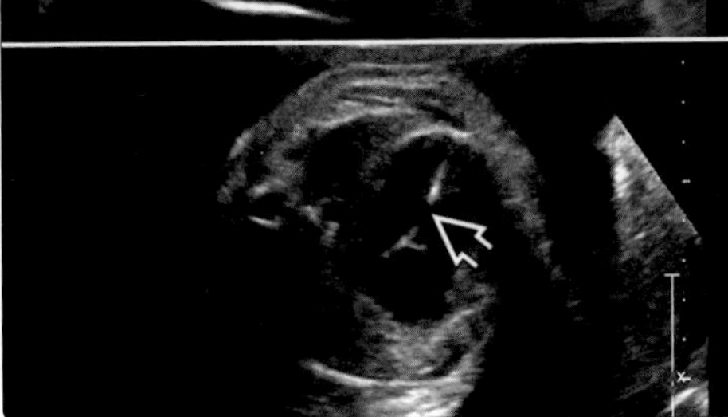

(Left) *An omphalocele was diagnosed in this fetus presenting for nuchal translucency assessment. Note that the herniated liver ➡ is more hypoechoic than the bowel ↪. The liver should never be outside of the abdominal cavity, regardless of gestational age.* **(Right)** *This fetus with an abdominal wall defect (calipers) and eviscerated liver ➡ also had a cardiac defect (note the large ventricular septal defect ⇨). Omphalocele is associated with aneuploidy and cardiac defects.*

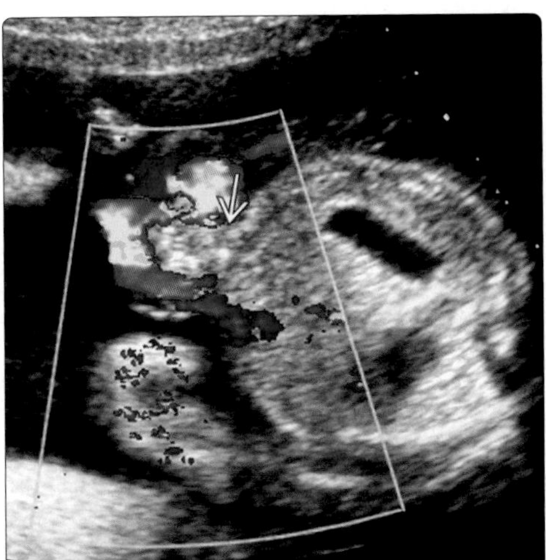

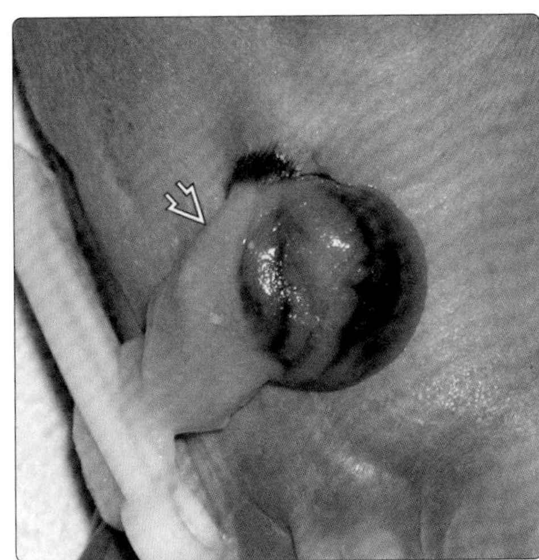

(Left) *Axial US shows a small omphalocele ➡ containing only bowel in a fetus with multiple anomalies, including a heart defect. Suspicion for aneuploidy is highest with bowel-only omphalocele. Also, these are the cases most likely to be missed because of their smaller size.* **(Right)** *Clinical photograph shows a small omphalocele containing only bowel (no liver) in a stillborn with trisomy 13. The umbilical cord inserts at the apex of the small defect ⇨.*

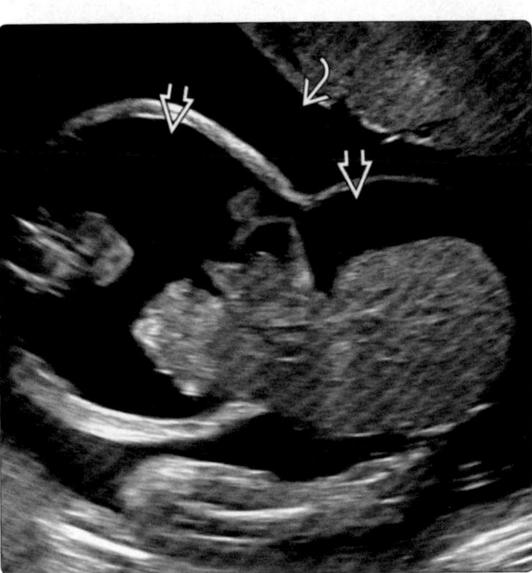

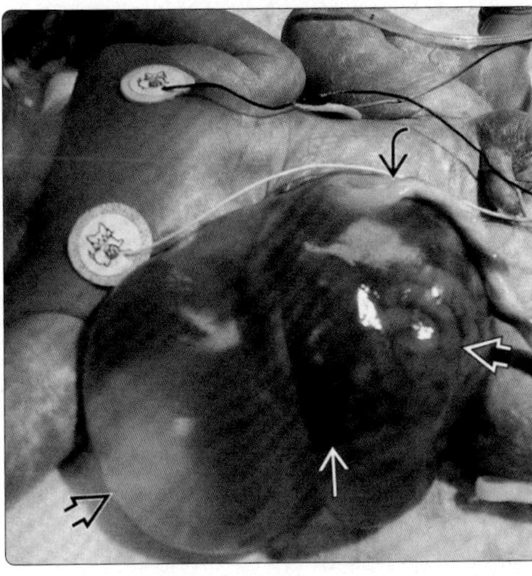

(Left) *This fetus with a large omphalocele also has a large amount of ascites ⇨ and polyhydramnios ↪, features typical for "giant" omphalocele (defect > 5-6 cm, containing most of the liver).* **(Right)** *This newborn with a giant omphalocele has a small bowel ↪, liver ➡, and a large amount of ascites ⇨ in the sac. The cord inserts on the sac ⇨ but is to the side. These omphaloceles are also at risk for rupture, either in utero or during delivery (most often performed by C-section).*

Gastroschisis

KEY FACTS

TERMINOLOGY

- Bowel herniates through right-sided abdominal wall defect next to normal umbilical cord insertion site
- Newborn classification of gastroschisis
  - Simple: Isolated, no other bowel anomalies
  - Complex: Bowel atresia, necrosis, perforation, volvulus
- Difficult to predict complex gastroschisis in fetus

IMAGING

- Free-floating bowel, no covering membrane
- Bowel dilatation (> 7-10 mm)
  - Bowel outside of fetus is often dilated and not predictive of bowel pathology
  - Dilated bowel inside fetus more concerning
  - > 14-mm bowel diameter most concerning for atresia
- Associations: Growth restriction, oligohydramnios
- Can make diagnosis in 1st trimester
  - Fetal bowel should be back in abdomen by 12 weeks

TOP DIFFERENTIAL DIAGNOSES

- Bowel-only omphalocele
  - Bowel not free-floating, covered by membrane
  - Cord insertion is not normal: Inserts on omphalocele sac
- Amniotic band syndrome and body stalk anomaly
  - Multiple fetal defects

CLINICAL ISSUES

- Associated with young maternal age
  - Not associated with aneuploidy
- Survival for simple gastroschisis approaches 100%
- Complex gastroschisis mortality rates 28-50%

SCANNING TIPS

- Color Doppler shows cord insertion site best
- Note appearance of bowel wall
  - Thick, echogenic, matted bowel wall is more concerning
- Biophysical profile surveillance later in gestation
  - 5% risk of intrauterine fetal demise

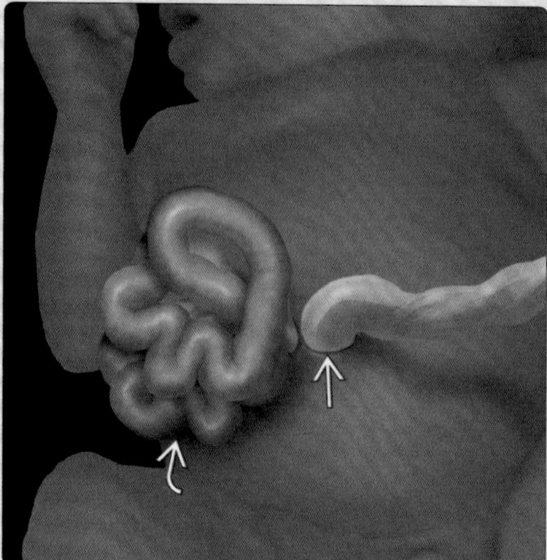

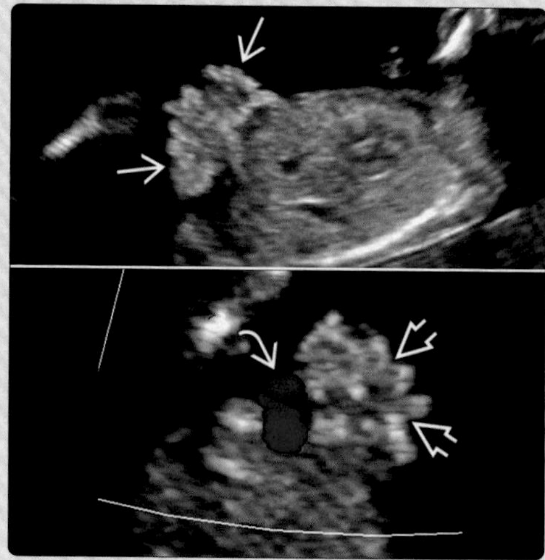

(Left) *Graphic of gastroschisis shows an abdominal wall defect with bowel herniation ➡. The defect is to the right of the umbilical cord insertion site ➡.* **(Right)** *Normal early bowel herniation returns to the abdomen by 12 weeks, and gastroschisis can be diagnosed early. In this 13-week fetus, there is bowel outside of the abdomen ➡. Amniotic fluid separates several loops of bowel ➡, proving "free-floating" bowel not covered by a membrane. The cord insertion site on the abdominal wall ➡ is seen well with color Doppler.*

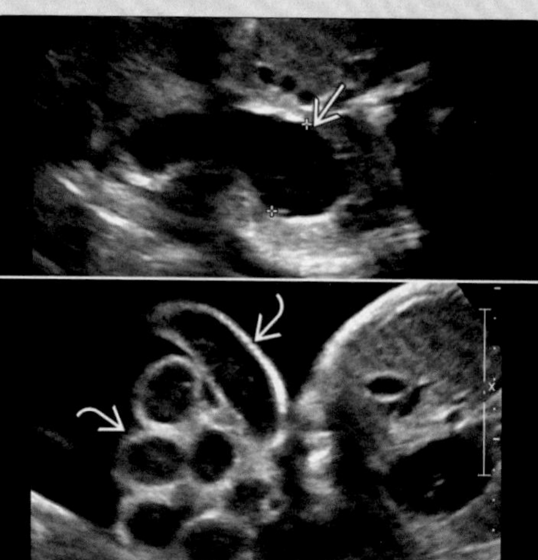

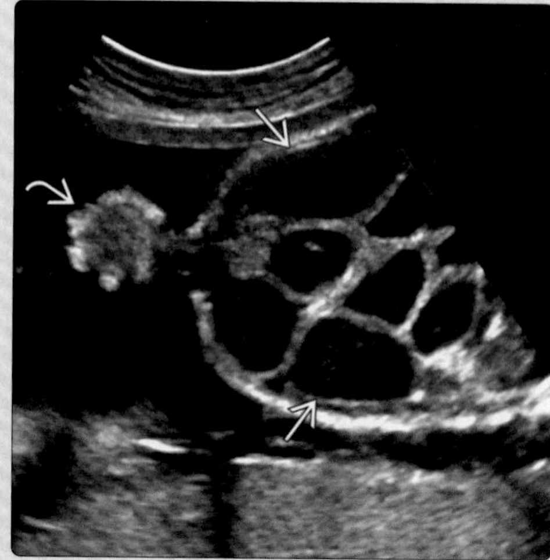

(Left) *The fetal stomach ➡ is partially outside of the body in this fetus with gastroschisis and dilated bowel ➡. The intraabdominal bowel was otherwise normal. Extraabdominal bowel dilatation is often seen and does not predict outcomes.* **(Right)** *In this fetus with gastroschisis, the bowel inside the abdomen is markedly dilated ➡, and the bowel outside is decompressed ➡. Intraabdominal bowel distention is more concerning for bowel pathology, such as bowel atresia and ischemia.*

KEY FACTS

TERMINOLOGY

- Lethal malformation characterized by attachment of viscera to placenta with short or absent umbilical cord

IMAGING

- Gross distortion with complete loss of anatomic landmarks
- Abnormal fetus inseparable from placenta
- Large thoracoabdominal wall defect without covering membrane; often complete evisceration
- Absent/very short umbilical cord
  - Vessels seen running from placental surface to fetal torso
- Scoliosis, often severe
- Limb defects may be present but not major feature as is often seen with amniotic bands
- Head usually unaffected
- Body stalk anomaly is most likely diagnosis with severe abdominal wall defect (AWD), scoliosis, and "stuck" fetus

TOP DIFFERENTIAL DIAGNOSES

- In other severe defects, AWD fetus will not be attached to placenta (amniotic bands, pentalogy of Cantrell)

SCANNING TIPS

- Be vigilant at time of nuchal translucency screening
  - Early diagnosis allows earlier/safer termination of pregnancy
- Use 3D US to help define anatomic relationships
- Color Doppler often useful to clarify confusing anatomy and look for umbilical cord
  - Identify fetal vascular landmarks (e.g., iliac bifurcation, renal arteries)
- In fetus with large AWD, look for free-floating loops of cord
  - Absent or short cord = body stalk anomaly
  - Normal cord makes amniotic bands more likely
    - Roll patient, look for delicate bands as fetus "floats" away from placenta

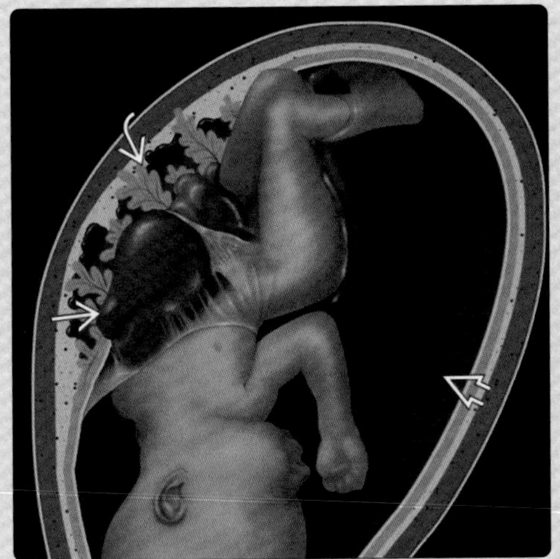

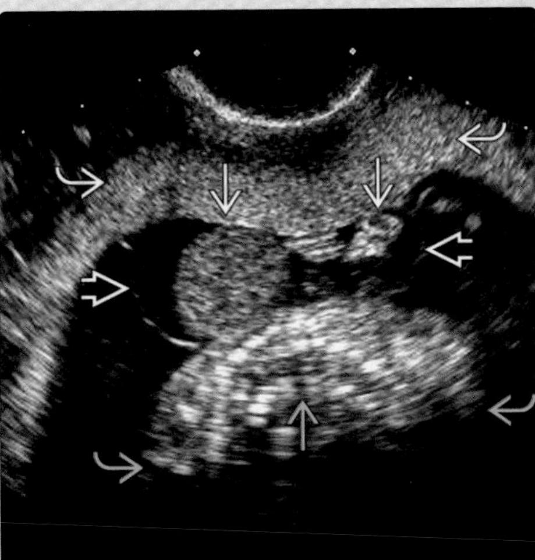

(Left) *Graphic shows a large abdominal wall defect (AWD) with viscera ➡ attached to placenta ➡. Scoliosis results from fetal tethering. The upper part of the fetus is inside the amniotic cavity ➡ while lower parts are in the extraembryonic coelomic cavity. There is no normal umbilical cord.* **(Right)** *On TVUS most of the torso ➡ is in amniotic cavity. Viscera ➡ are in extraembryonic coelomic space anchoring fetus to the placenta ➡, causing scoliosis ➡. The amnion ➡ (not a band) is visible at the edges of the AWD.*

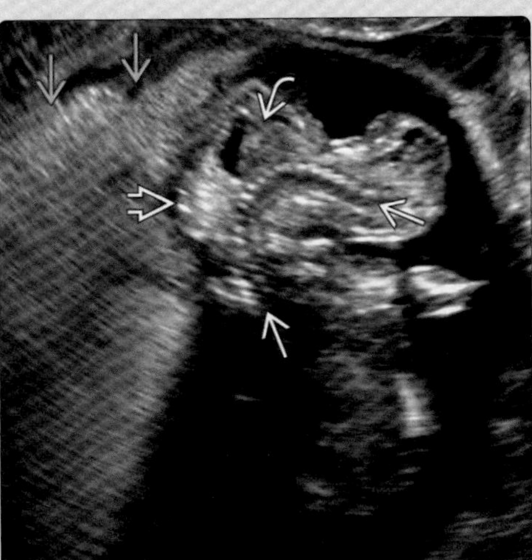

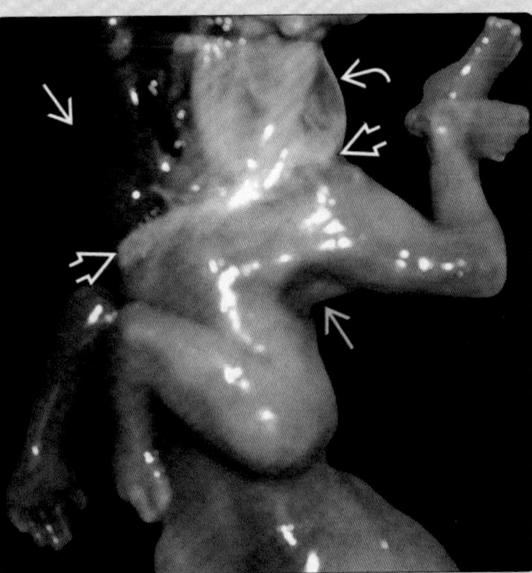

(Left) *TVUS at 13 weeks shows severe scoliosis ➡ with the spine bent into a U shape and evisceration of the liver ➡ and bowel ➡, which are adherent to the placenta ➡.* **(Right)** *Autopsy image presented in a similar orientation shows severe scoliosis ➡ and evisceration of liver ➡ and bowel. The amnion ➡ reflects off the edges of the large AWD ➡ so that the peritoneal cavity is open and adherent to the placental surface.*

Bladder Exstrophy

KEY FACTS

TERMINOLOGY

- Failure of closure of lower abdominal wall resulting in exposed bladder

IMAGING

- Inability to demonstrate fluid-filled bladder
- Soft tissue mass/nodular contour of lower anterior abdominal wall due to exposed posterior bladder wall
- Normal fluid

TOP DIFFERENTIAL DIAGNOSES

- Absent bladder
  - Renal anomalies or other conditions with low/absent urine production are associated with oligo/anhydramnios
  - If associated with oligohydramnios in monochorionic twin, may indicate twin-twin transfusion syndrome
- Cloacal exstrophy
  - Absent fluid-filled bladder, imperforate anus
  - Bowel herniation through abdominal wall defect → elephant trunk sign

SCANNING TIPS

- Red flag for this diagnosis is normal amniotic fluid without visible bladder
  - Obtain midline sagittal image through torso for abdominal wall contour
  - Check cord insertion site; inferiorly displaced in bladder exstrophy
  - Evaluate for genital anomalies, which are common in both males and females
  - Look for anal dimple on axial image of perineum
- Do not confuse cystic pelvic structures with bladder
  - Normal bladder fills and empties repeatedly during scan
  - Umbilical arteries encompass bladder as they course from internal iliac arteries to umbilicus
- Use 3D surface-rendered ultrasound images to clarify anatomy

(Left) *Axial oblique US shows the umbilical arteries ➡. The bladder, normally seen as a fluid-filled structure between them, was never visible in this case, even though the kidneys and amniotic fluid volume were normal. The spine ➡ is shown for orientation.* **(Right)** *Sagittal US shows an irregular contour to the lower anterior abdominal wall ➡ inferior to the cord insertion site ➡ (which is inferiorly displaced). The bladder is not seen as a fluid-filled structure in the expected location ➡. Bladder exstrophy was confirmed at delivery.*

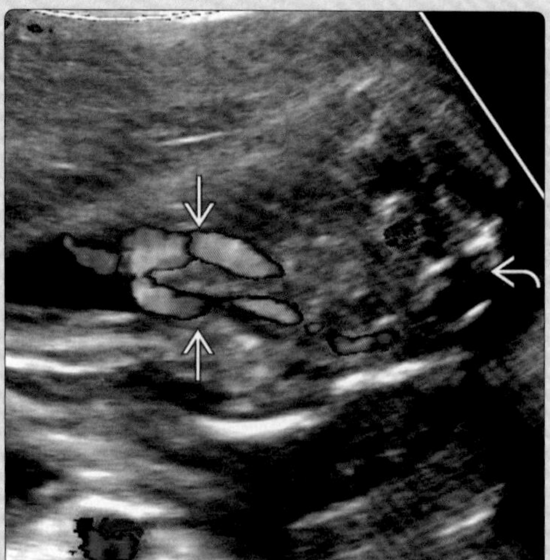

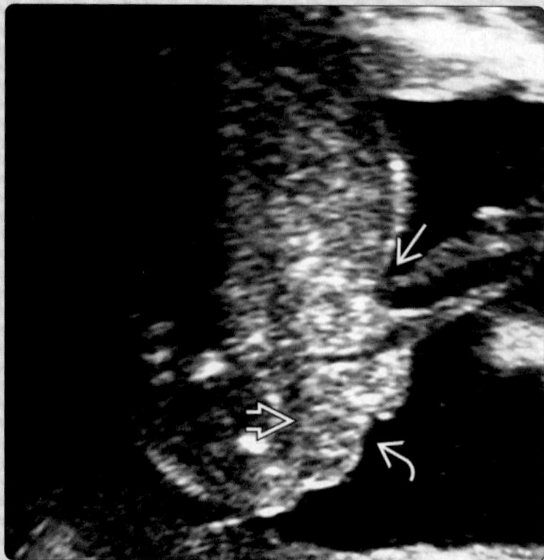

(Left) *3D US shows a normal scrotum ➡ and anus ➡. The everted bladder mucosa ➡ creates a lower abdominal wall mass, and there is an associated bifid penis ➡. The cord inserts low ➡ at the apex of the defect.* **(Right)** *Clinical image shows low cord insertion ➡, everted bladder ➡, and abnormal penis ➡ inferior to the prostate gland ➡. The abnormal genitalia and everted bladder create the "lumpy bumpy" abdominal wall on US. The scrotum ➡ is normal; passage of meconium ➡ indicates patent anus.*

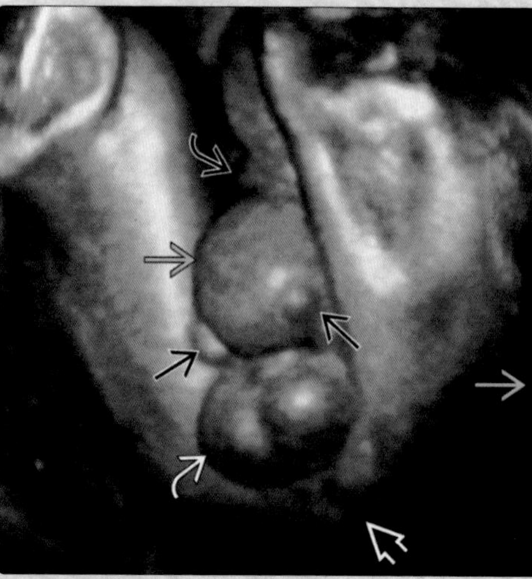

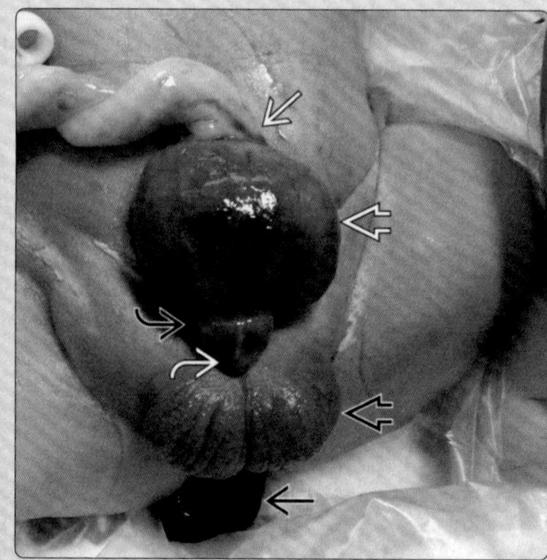

Esophageal Atresia

KEY FACTS

TERMINOLOGY

- Esophagus atresia (EA) often associated with tracheoesophageal fistula (TEF)

IMAGING

- **Small or absent stomach bubble**
  - Often difficult to define when stomach is "small"
  - Stomach size varies in same fetus over several hours
  - Because fetuses breathe amniotic fluid, small amount of fluid may get into stomach if there is TEF
    - Complete absence suggests no TEF
- **Pouch sign**
  - Transient filling of proximal esophagus with swallowing
- Fetal growth restriction seen in up to 40%
- Polyhydramnios rarely develops before 20 weeks
  - Fetal swallowing not important part of amniotic fluid dynamics until that time
- Risk for aneuploidy (trisomy 13 and 21)
- > 50% have other anomalies
- VACTERL (vertebral anomalies, anal atresia, cardiac malformation, TEF/EA, renal anomalies, limb malformations) association in 30%

SCANNING TIPS

- US is poor in detecting EA before onset of polyhydramnios
  - Must have high degree of suspicion and perform follow-up scans in setting of small stomach
- Perform focused exam looking specifically at neck and upper chest for esophageal pouch when stomach is small
  - Pouch will expand with fetal swallowing
  - Distinguish from normal hypopharynx anatomy
    - Trachea should be easily identified as separate nondistensible structure, relatively thicker wall, and connected to epiglottis
    - Esophagus located more posterior than trachea
  - Determine location of distal end of pouch
    - Termination in neck worse prognosis than termination in mediastinum

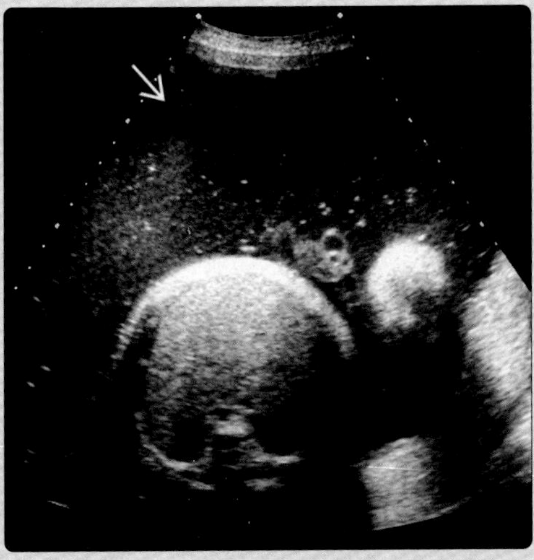

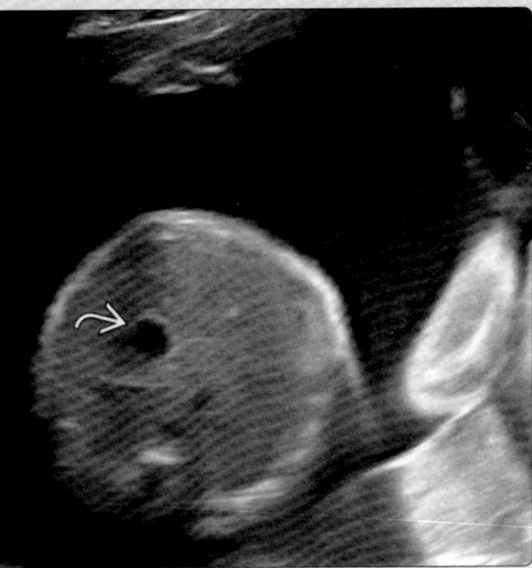

(Left) *Axial US through the upper abdomen in a 3rd-trimester fetus shows no stomach bubble. There is also marked polyhydramnios ➡. No fluid was identified in the stomach throughout gestation, which is suspicious for EA without TEF.* **(Right)** *At 24 weeks, the stomach of this fetus appears small ➡ and was persistently small over multiple scans. The additional finding of polyhydramnios led to a suspicion for EA. A small amount of fluid may get into the stomach if a TEF is present.*

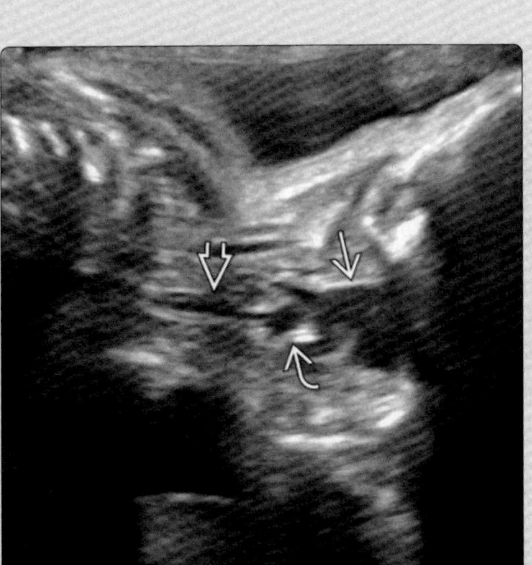

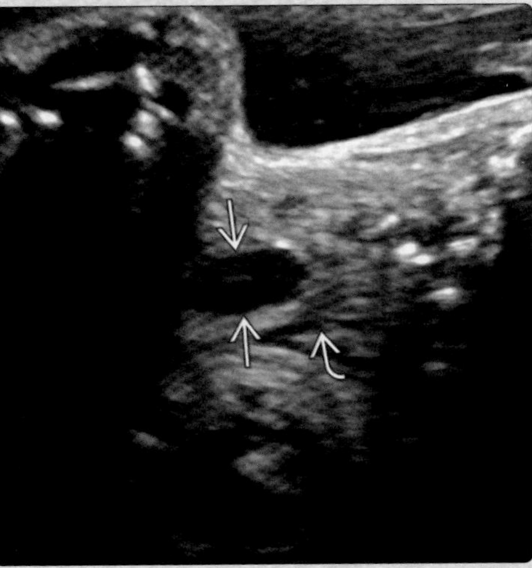

(Left) *Focused imaging of the neck at 32 weeks in the same case shows the normal fluid-filled hypopharynx ➡, epiglottis ➡, and proximal trachea ➡. The esophagus will be just posterior to these structures.* **(Right)** *A plane just posterior to the prior image shows an anechoic pouch at the point of esophageal atresia ➡. Real-time imaging showed this blind-ending pouch expanded and contracted with fetal swallowing. Note the adjacent carotid artery ➡ provides an anatomic landmark.*

Duodenal Atresia

KEY FACTS

IMAGING

- **Double bubble**: Fluid-filled stomach and duodenum
- Persistent fluid in duodenum is always abnormal
- Hyperperistalsis of stomach on real-time imaging
- Fetal regurgitation may intermittently decompress stomach
- Polyhydramnios; may be severe in 3rd trimester

TOP DIFFERENTIAL DIAGNOSES

- Distal atresias (jejunal, ileal, colonic, anal) will all have multiple dilated loops of bowel
- Abdominal cysts
  - None will communicate with stomach
  - Polyhydramnios not feature

CLINICAL ISSUES

- Duodenum most common site of intestinal obstruction
- 30% of duodenal atresia (DA) cases have trisomy 21
- 5-15% of trisomy 21 cases have DA
- Overall mortality is 15-40%
  - Dependent on associated abnormalities
- Isolated defect in liveborn; 95% survival with prompt surgical treatment
- 50-70% of DA cases have other anomalies
  - Cardiac and other GI malformations are most common

SCANNING TIPS

- Continuity with stomach confirms diagnosis
  - May be better demonstrated in coronal plane if stomach is severely distended
  - Peristalsis with thick gastric folds easily identified on real-time scanning
- Look for other findings of T21
  - Cardiac malformations: Atrioventricular septal defect, ventricular septal defect, tetralogy of Fallot
  - Markers: Nuchal thickening, short femur/humerus, absent/hypoplastic nasal bone, mild ventriculomegaly, echogenic bowel, echogenic cardiac focus, pelviectasis

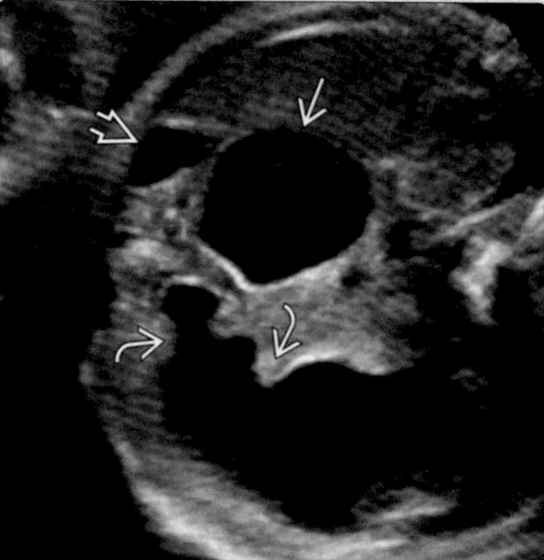
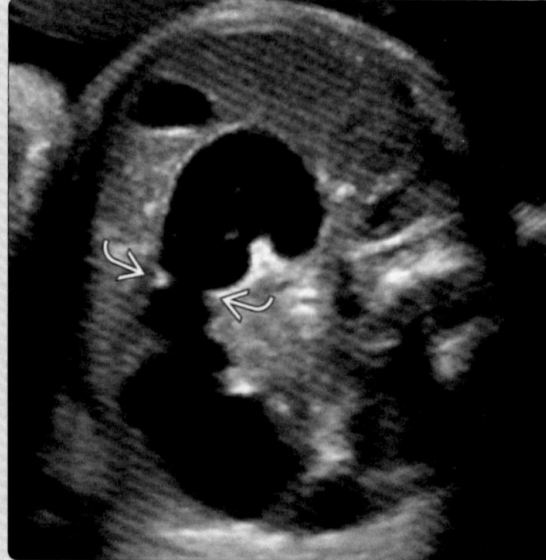

(Left) *Third-trimester ultrasound shows a dilated stomach with prominent gastric folds ➡. The duodenal bulb is markedly enlarged ➡, and polyhydramnios was present. The gallbladder ➡ is displaced by the duodenal bulb. Noninvasive prenatal testing showed trisomy 21.* **(Right)** *Use real-time imaging to connect the stomach with the dilated duodenum via an open pylorus ➡, excluding an abdominal cystic mass. Hyperperistalsis and fluid motion through the pylorus can also be seen on real-time imaging.*

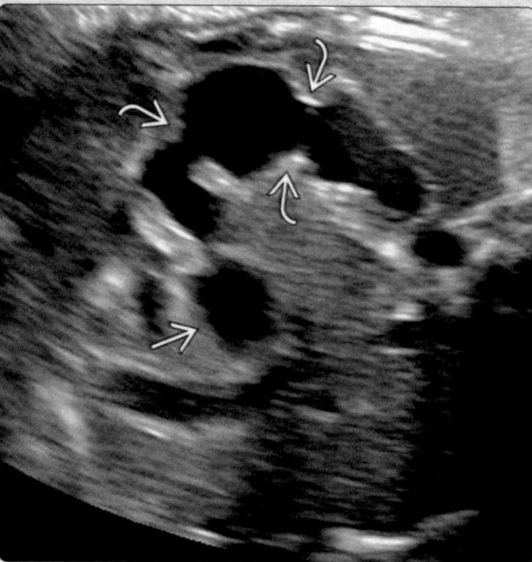
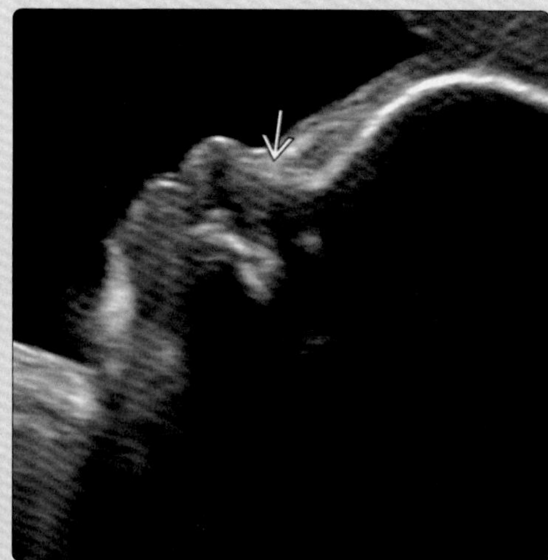

(Left) *In this case of duodenal atresia, multiple focal gastric contractions ➡ reflecting hyperperistalsis are demonstrated. The dilated duodenal bulb ➡ is also shown. Real-time scanning showing fluid moving across the pylorus is key to confirming the diagnosis. Severe associated polyhydramnios was present.* **(Right)** *Profile view of the same fetus at 34 weeks was easily obtained due to the polyhydramnios and shows an absent nasal bone ➡. Postnatal exam confirmed trisomy 21.*

KEY FACTS

IMAGING

- Dilated, fluid-filled loops of bowel progressively enlarge
  - Triple bubble for proximal jejunal atresia
  - Sausage-shaped bowel loops
- Normal small bowel < 7-mm diameter
- Echogenic bowel in 2nd trimester may be 1st sign of atresia
- Hyperperistalsis of obstructed segments in real time
- Polyhydramnios more likely with proximal atresia
  - Usually develops after 26 weeks
- At risk for perforation and meconium peritonitis
  - More common with ileal obstruction

TOP DIFFERENTIAL DIAGNOSES

- Meconium ileus: Meconium impaction in distal ileum
  - Often indistinguishable from atresia
  - High association with cystic fibrosis
    - Testing for cystic fibrosis is recommended in all cases of distal obstruction
- Anal atresia: Very difficult to distinguish large from small bowel in fetus
  - Absent anal dimple (target sign) is key
- Ureterectasis: Tubular appearance may be mistaken for bowel; often has dilated bladder

SCANNING TIPS

- Determining point of obstruction is difficult, especially when multiple loops are dilated, but look for clues
  - Must rule out anal atresia as repair is more complicated
    - Obtain sonographic views of perineum looking for normal rectum and anal dimple (target sign)
  - Jejunal atresia: Greater bowel dilatation, more likely to have enlarged stomach and polyhydramnios
  - Ileal atresia: Less distensible with earlier perforation, usually not associated with polyhydramnios
- Follow for complications: Polyhydramnios, increasing bowel dilatation, perforation (meconium peritonitis)

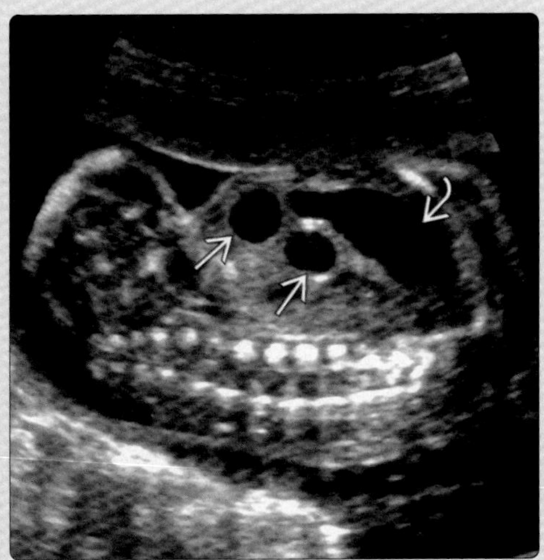

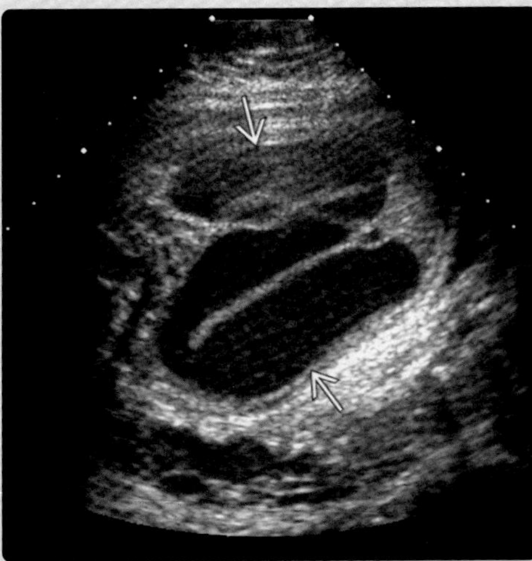

(Left) *Sagittal ultrasound through the fetal abdomen shows a triple bubble in this case of proximal jejunal atresia. Two dilated loops of small bowel ➡ as well as the stomach ⮫ are seen. Stomach distention and polyhydramnios are more common with proximal obstructions.* **(Right)** *Axial oblique ultrasound shows echogenic, fluid-filled loops of bowel creating a tubular sausage-like appearance ➡. Active peristalsis was noted during the exam.*

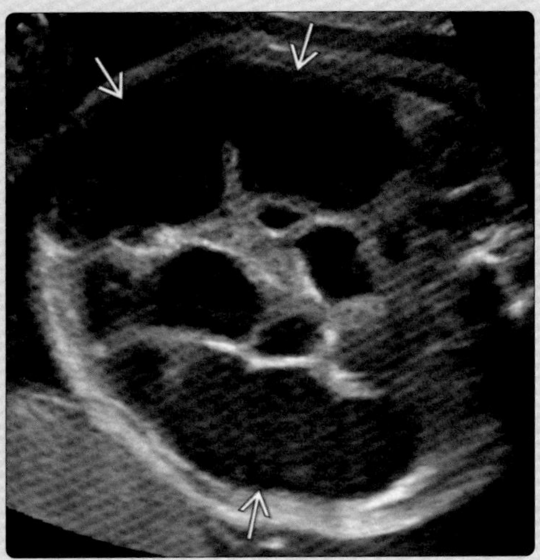

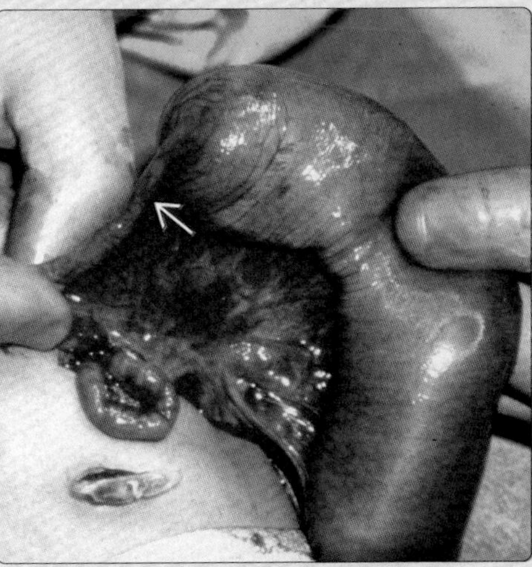

(Left) *Axial abdominal ultrasound of a fetus at 33 weeks shows marked bowel distention. There was marked continual bowel peristalsis on real-time imaging with distention up to 2.8 cm ➡. Hypoechoic debris (succus entericus) fills the bowel lumen. Given the marked distention without perforation, jejunal atresia was correctly diagnosed.* **(Right)** *Intraoperative photograph shows the very dilated jejunum terminating at a fibrous cord ➡.*

Meconium Peritonitis, Pseudocyst

KEY FACTS

TERMINOLOGY

- Chemical peritonitis due to intrauterine bowel perforation

IMAGING

- Intraperitoneal calcifications in 85%
  - May be only finding if early perforation has healed
- Implants on peritoneal surfaces
  - Best seen along liver capsule
  - May also be in scrotum (meconium periorchitis)
- Ascites secondary to both spilled contents and inflammatory response
- Meconium pseudocyst results from walled-off perforation
  - Irregular, often angular, thick walls
- Dilated bowel seen when meconium peritonitis is secondary to obstruction
- Bowel anomalies at risk for perforation: Atresias (distal at greater risk than proximal), meconium ileus, volvulus
- Bowel may not be dilated when perforation is secondary to ischemia

CLINICAL ISSUES

- Genetic counseling for cystic fibrosis
- Spontaneous in utero closure of perforation may occur with no long-term sequelae

SCANNING TIPS

- Examine liver carefully
  - Calcifications are on capsular surface with meconium peritonitis, while infection causes intraparenchymal calcifications
- Try to determine cause of perforation
  - Dilated bowel makes primary intestinal abnormality most likely; look for bowel peristalsis
  - Nonperistalsing, dilated loops concerning for volvulus with ischemia; ischemic bowel then perforates
- Frequent follow-up scans after initial diagnosis
  - May worsen with increasing bowel dilation and abdominal distention
  - May resolve completely with no sequelae

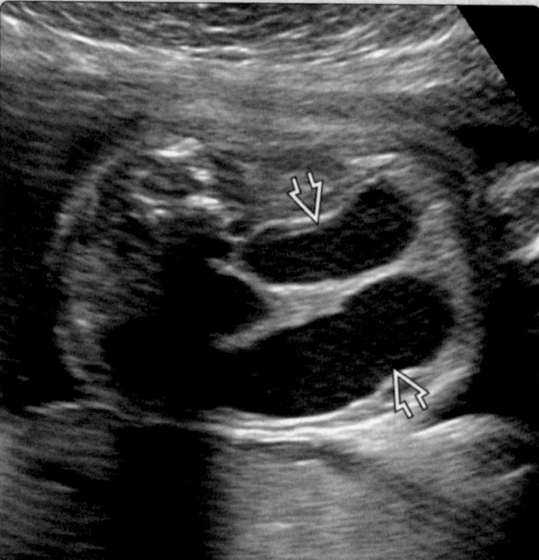

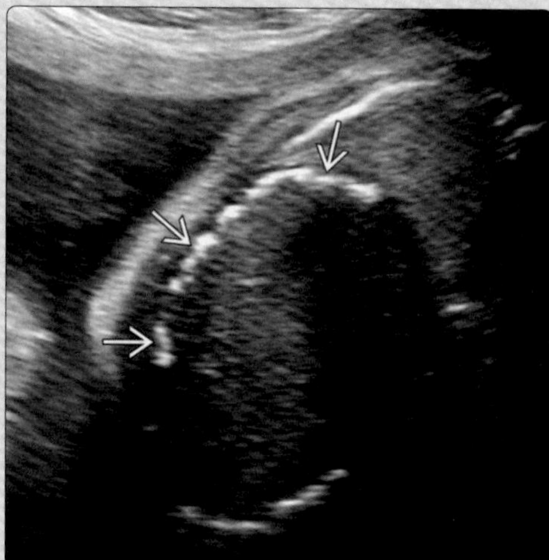

(Left) *This 29-week fetus with ileal atresia shows multiple dilated loops of small bowel ➾.* **(Right)** *There was no ascites, but a sagittal image through the liver in the same case shows calcifications along the capsule ➡, indicating prior perforation with meconium peritonitis. Bowel atresia is a significant risk factor for perforation. It is very important to ensure that the calcifications are on the liver capsule and not in the parenchyma, as would be seen with infection.*

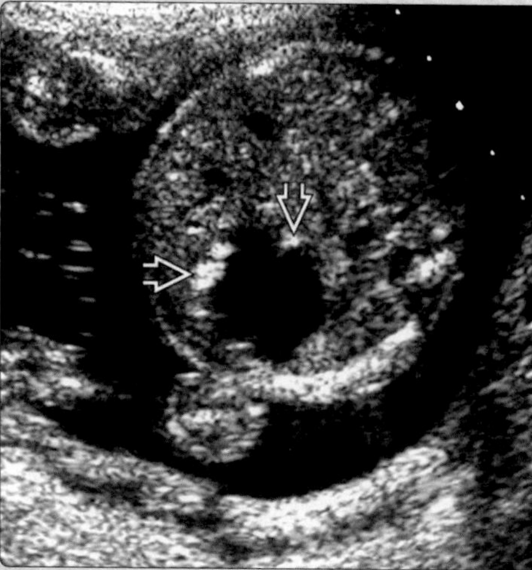

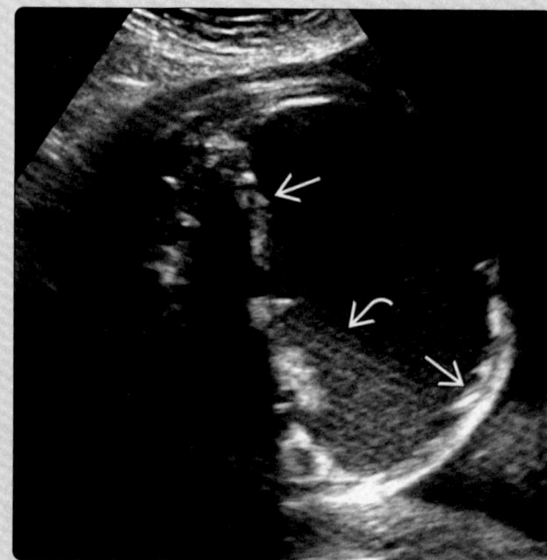

(Left) *Axial ultrasound of an 18-week fetus shows an irregular abdominal cyst with bright calcifications along the periphery ➾. This resolved on follow-up scans. A postnatal radiograph showed right upper quadrant calcifications but was otherwise normal, as was the physical exam. This is typical of an early perforation, which has healed.* **(Right)** *In contrast, this is a very large pseudocyst in a 22-week fetus. Note the hyperechoic irregular walls ➡ and a layering debris level ↶. Surgery showed a midjejunal perforation from an internal hernia with volvulus.*

KEY FACTS

IMAGING

- **Inability to demonstrate normal anal dimple or target sign**
- Normal appearance
  - Axial: Hyperechoic mucosa within hypoechoic muscular ring
  - Coronal: Hyperechoic mucosal stripe between hypoechoic walls, extending to perineum
  - No other appearance is proof of normal anorectal development; should be demonstrable from 20 weeks
- Dilated, fluid-filled distal bowel is late manifestation; not seen at time of 2nd-trimester survey
  - U- or V-shaped bowel in presacral space without extension to perineum
- Polyhydramnios unusual
  - Unlike proximal small bowel atresias

SCANNING TIPS

- Remember that colon is often prominent in 3rd trimester
  - Normal caliber ≤ 18 mm
- 3D data sets can be obtained to demonstrate rectum in sagittal and coronal planes
- Look for calcified meconium enteroliths
  - Results from mixture of meconium and fetal urine within bowel lumen if fistula between colon and bladder
  - Look for echogenic "marbles" moving within bowel
- Look for other abnormalities as anal atresia is seldom isolated
  - VACTERL association (**v**ertebral, **a**nal atresia, cardiac, **t**racheo-**es**ophageal, **r**enal and **l**imb anomalies)
  - Cloacal exstrophy
    - Abdominal wall defect, absent bladder, often spine abnormalities
  - Cloacal malformation
    - Female fetus, distended vagina, small bladder
- Take dedicated views of rectum/anus when any bowel, spine, or genital abnormality is present

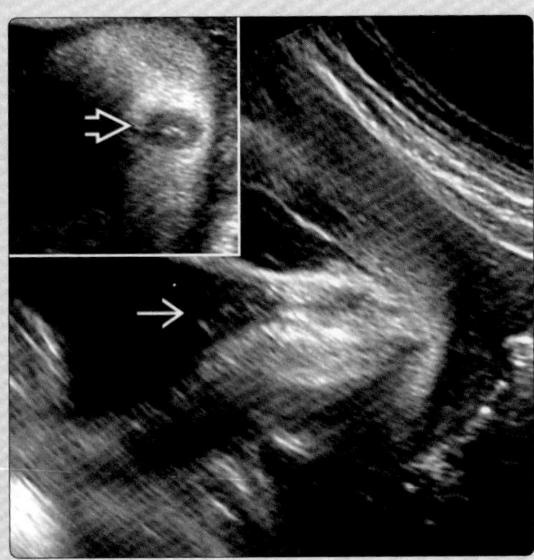

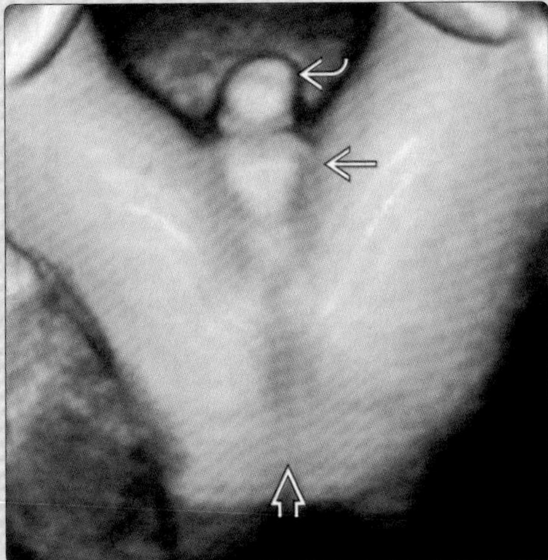

(Left) *Axial view of the perineum of a fetus with multiple anomalies shows the labia majora ➡ but no evidence of an anal dimple in the expected location. A normal anal dimple (target sign) ➡ is shown in the inset.* **(Right)** *3D US surface reconstruction shows undescended testes ➡ (empty scrotum); short, curved penis ➡; and absence of an anal opening in the natal cleft ➡. Anal atresia is often associated with genital and distal spine abnormalities. Look for the anal dimple when evaluating fetal sex.*

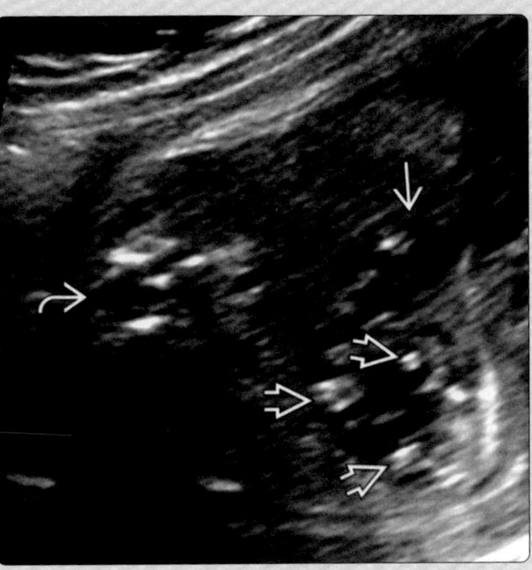

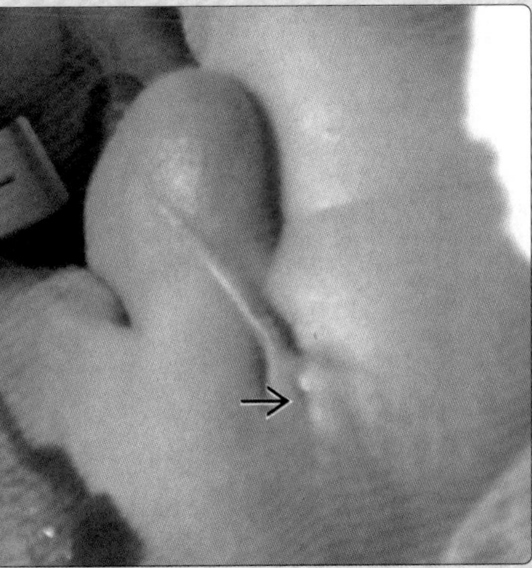

(Left) *Axial abdominal US in the 3rd trimester shows "marbles" ➡ of calcified meconium in the dilated transverse colon ➡. They were freely mobile during real-time scanning. This only occurs when meconium mixes with urine (e.g., vesicocolic fistula in addition to anal atresia). Note the lumbar spine ➡.* **(Right)** *Clinical photograph in an infant with multiple anomalies detected on prenatal US confirms anal atresia ➡. In this case, the final diagnosis was VACTERL association.*

Cloacal Malformation/Urogenital Sinus

KEY FACTS

TERMINOLOGY

- Cloaca is single cavity present in early embryonic development when bladder, genital tract, and bowel are all connected
- Spectrum of abnormal anatomy is related to timing of developmental arrest
  - Range from **urogenital sinus** (2 perineal openings) to cloacal dysgenesis (no perineal opening)
  - **Classic cloaca** defined as coalescence of urethra, vagina, and hindgut into common channel draining through single perineal orifice (exclusively in females)

IMAGING

- Most common presentation is cystic pelvic mass in female fetus; "cyst" is grossly dilated vagina (hydrocolpos)
- Uterine and vaginal duplication is observed in ~ 80% of cases in which hydrocolpos is present
  - Vaginal duplication creates linear septation within conical fluid collection
- Abnormal perineum; absent anal dimple
- High percentage have additional abnormalities, most commonly genitourinary, bowel, and lumbosacral

SCANNING TIPS

- Vagina is most distended structure and appears as cystic pelvic mass
  - Scan in coronal plane looking for vertical septum
  - Even if no septum is present, may still see fluid-debris level (vaginal secretions ± meconium mixing with urine)
- **Do not confuse with bladder**
  - Bladder may be compressed by distended vagina
  - Be very suspicious if female fetus is sent for "urethral atresia"; far more likely to be cloacal malformation
- When any lower GI or GU abnormality is suspected, perform high-resolution images of perineum looking for abnormal genitalia and absent anal dimple
  - If abnormal, highly suspicious for cloacal malformation even if no cystic mass is present

(Left) *Sagittal graphic shows a common channel (cloaca) ➡ with hydrocolpos ➡ compressing the rectum and bladder. The distended vagina is the most obvious finding on US and may be confused with the bladder.* **(Right)** *Coronal US through the pelvis of a female fetus shows fluid-fluid levels ➡ representing layering debris in obstructed, duplicated vaginas (note the linear septum ➡). Debris results from the mixing of urine with vaginal secretions ± meconium. This is the most specific finding for a cloacal malformation.*

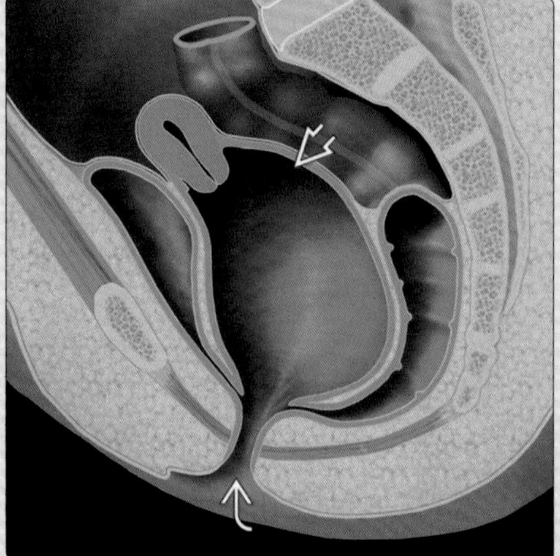

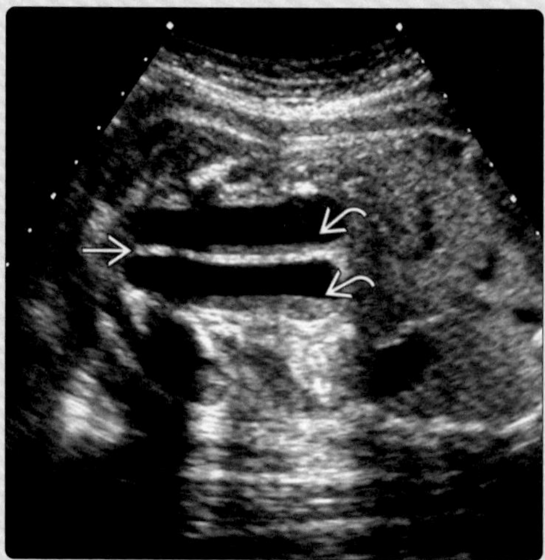

(Left) *Transabdominal US of the fetal perineum shows no evidence of an anal dimple in the expected location ➡. The labia are seen anteriorly ➡, which did not appear normal during real-time scanning.* **(Right)** *The inset shows the abnormal labia. There was no anal opening. With the labia spread, a single orifice is identified ➡, which is diagnostic of a cloaca. This opening represents the common channel draining the bladder, vagina, and rectum.*

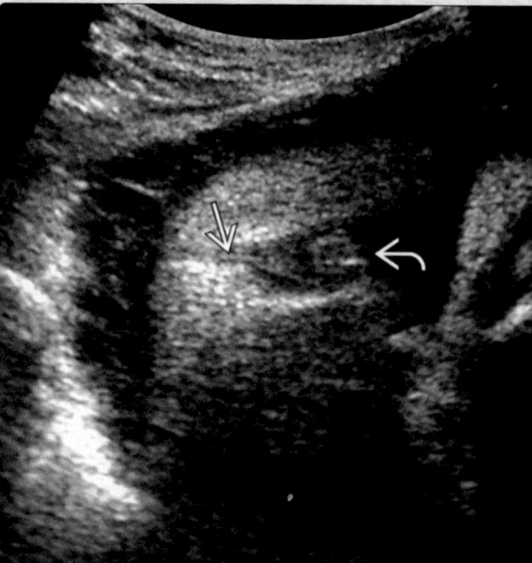

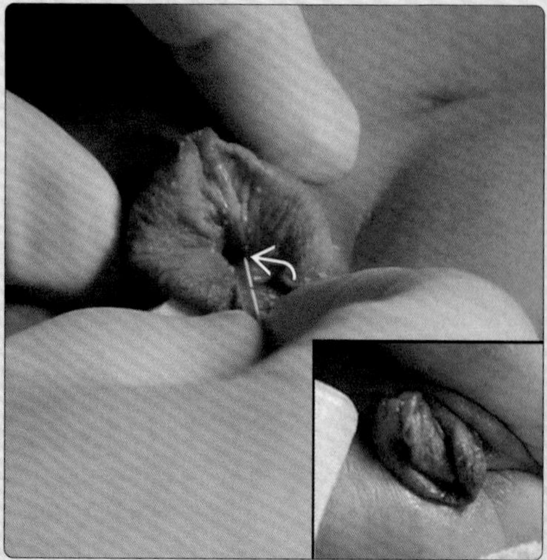

Choledochal Cyst

KEY FACTS

TERMINOLOGY

- 5 types, but cystic dilation of common bile duct (CBD) is most common type seen in utero

IMAGING

- Upper abdominal cyst associated with liver
  - Represents markedly dilated CBD
- Adjacent to but separate from gallbladder
- Color Doppler shows relationship to porta hepatis
  - Helps rule out vascular mass or vascular malformation
- Look for connections to hepatic ducts
  - Coronal view is best
- Cyst grows with advancing pregnancy

TOP DIFFERENTIAL DIAGNOSES

- Umbilical vein varix: Color Doppler shows flow
- Gallbladder duplication: Sac-like, less tubular
- Liver cyst: Can occur anywhere in liver
- Liver tumors: Often solid or mixed cystic/solid

CLINICAL ISSUES

- Most often incidental finding at time of anatomy scan
- 1/3 of all cases are from Japan
  - 1:1,000 incidence in Asia
  - 1:100,000 incidence outside Asia
- Treatment and prognosis
  - Better outcome with early diagnosis and treatment
    - Untreated leads to cholestasis, biliary cirrhosis, and liver failure
  - Surgical resection with biliary-bowel anastomosis

SCANNING TIPS

- Look for gallbladder in every case with liver anomaly
  - Can be routinely seen in 2nd trimester
  - Do not confuse choledochal cyst with gallbladder
- 3D ultrasound may be helpful
  - Multiplanar images to look at all margins of cyst for biliary connections

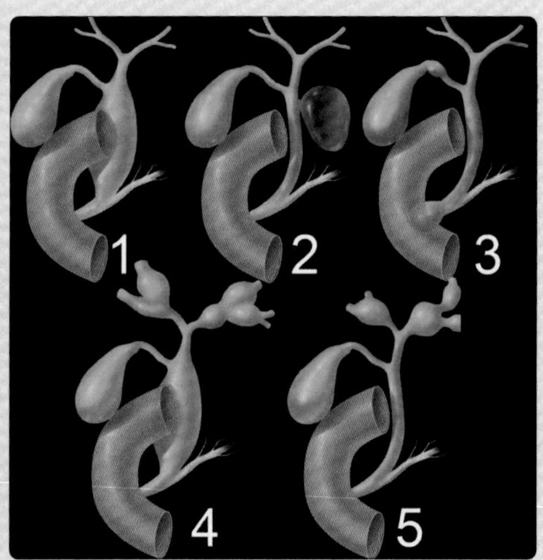

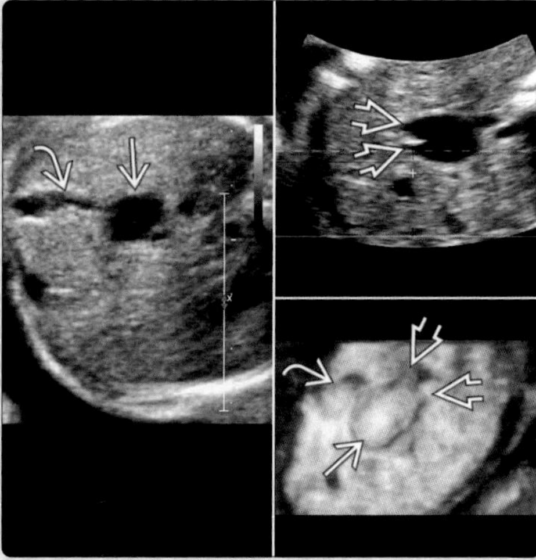

(Left) *There are 5 different types of congenital choledochal cyst (Todani classification). However, cystic dilatation of the common bile duct (CBD), type 1, is the type seen in utero 80-90% of the time.* **(Right)** *Multiplanar and 3D images in a 25-week fetus with a choledochal cyst show a cyst ➡ next to the gallbladder ➡ on the axial view. The cyst communicates with dilated right and left hepatic ducts ➡, seen best on coronal views. These are key findings for the diagnosis.*

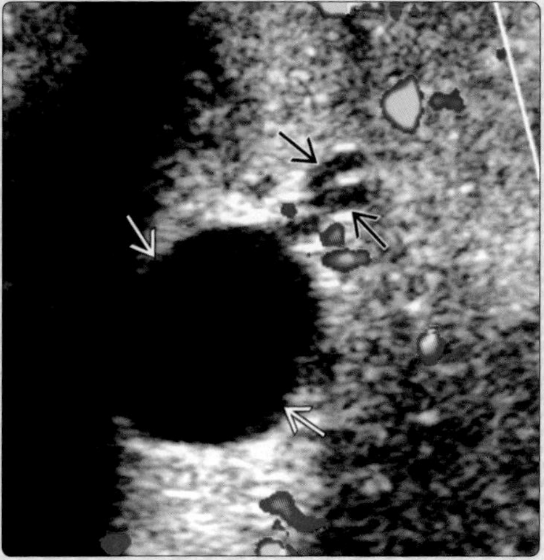

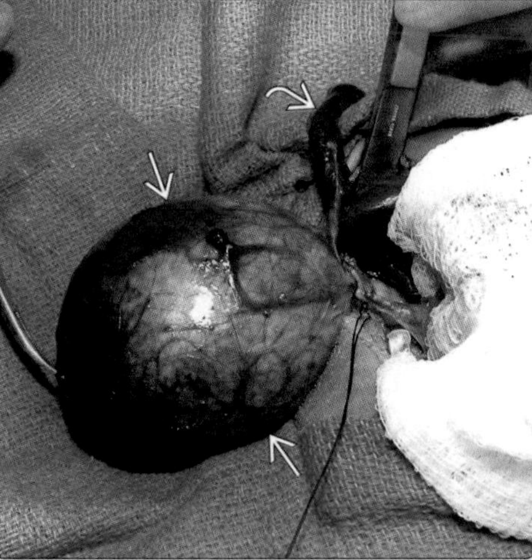

(Left) *Coronal oblique color Doppler US in a fetus with a choledochal cyst shows the cyst (dilated CBD) ➡ communicating with dilated bile ducts ➡. That is the most specific finding for making the diagnosis. This cyst grew throughout the pregnancy, which is typical.* **(Right)** *Intraoperative photograph of a child shows a large choledochal cyst ➡ next to the gallbladder ➡. Definitive treatment for choledochal cyst is cyst resection and biliary diversion.*

PART VI
SECTION 7

Genitourinary Tract

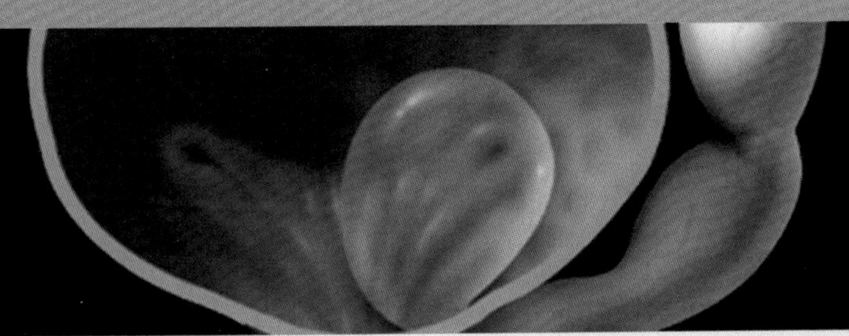

Anatomy and Approach

Kidneys and Bladder

Adrenal

Genitalia

EMBRYOLOGY AND ANATOMY

Kidney Formation

- Kidney development undergoes a complicated series of formation and regression of primitive renal structures
- Final kidney is formed from interaction of the ureteric bud and specialized mesoderm, the metanephric blastema
  - **Ureteric bud** induces **metanephric blastema** to form nephrons
  - In turn, metanephric blastema induces ureteric bud to bifurcate into developing calyces
- Anomalies resulting in failure of ureteric bud to interact appropriately with metanephric blastema
  - **Renal agenesis**
    - Failure of ureteric bud to come into contact with metanephric blastema; no kidney is formed
  - **Multicystic dysplastic kidney**
    - Ureteric bud does not signal appropriate development so there is disorganized stromal expansion and cyst formation

Renal Ascent

- Early in development, the kidneys lie close together low in pelvis with renal hila facing anteriorly
- Mechanism for "ascent" to final retroperitoneal flank position is not completely understood, but caudal embryonic growth is likely major contributing factor
- Blood supply changes as kidneys "recruit" arterial blood supply from iliac arteries and aorta
  - New, more superior arterial branches form as inferior branches involute
- With ascent, renal pelves rotate medially ~ 90°
- Ascent complete by 9 weeks when kidneys come into contact with adrenal glands
- **Anomalies related to abnormal ascent**
  - **Renal ectopia** (e.g., pelvic kidney)
    - Kidney usually low in position with abnormal rotation
  - **Crossed-fused ectopia and other fusion abnormalities**
    - Embryonic fusion prior to ascent leads to various appearances
  - **Horseshoe kidney**
    - Inferior poles fuse
    - Become "stuck" under inferior mesenteric artery
  - **Accessory renal arteries**
    - Persistence of normally transient renal arteries during ascent

Bladder

- The bladder forms from the **cloaca** (Latin for sewer), which is common chamber with early communication between urinary, gastrointestinal, and reproductive tracts
  - It is divided by the urorectal septum into **urogenital sinus** anteriorly and **rectum** posteriorly
  - Urogenital sinus divides into bladder and in females, the vagina
  - Failure to divide results in a **cloacal malformation**, 1 common communicating chamber between bladder, vagina, and rectum
    - The vagina is often septated, which may be an important clue to the diagnosis

SCANNING APPROACH AND IMAGING ISSUES

Techniques and Sonographic Appearance

- American Institute of Ultrasound in Medicine requires documentation of the kidneys, bladder, and amniotic fluid volume (a reflexion of fetal urine output) in all 2nd- and 3rd-trimester fetuses
  - Evaluation of fetal sex is only required when medically indicated
  - These are considered the minimum requirements; if any anomaly is suspected, a detailed examination should ensue
- Components of the genitourinary tract include the **kidneys, ureters, bladder, urethra, adrenal glands, internal and external genitalia**
  - Knowledge of the normal developmental appearance of each of these structures is needed in order to recognize pathologic processes
- **Kidneys** can be identified by 12- to 14-weeks gestation using endovaginal sonography; internal architecture can be resolved as early as 16-18 weeks
  - External renal contour is lobular (fetal lobulation), a finding that may persist into adulthood
  - Cortex around the periphery is intermediate in echogenicity with hypoechoic medullary pyramids arranged symmetrically around the renal pelvis
    - **Do not confuse normal hypoechoic pyramids with dilated calyces**
  - Normative data is available for all renal dimensions, but a rule of thumb is the length in mm approximates the fetal gestational age in weeks
  - The renal circumference:abdominal circumference ratio is stable throughout pregnancy with values from 0.27-0.30
    - When you look at the abdomen in axial plane, kidneys should never take up more than 1/3 of the area
- To obtain an accurate measurement of the **anterior-posterior renal pelvis diameter (APRPD)**, it must be measured perpendicular to the pelvis at the 12 o'clock or 6 o'clock position
  - Normal measurements are < 4 mm from 16-27 weeks and < 7 mm from 28 weeks to term
  - If the APRPD measures larger than normal, or there is calyceal dilation or parenchymal changes, then follow-up is required
- **Color Doppler**
  - Used to identify the bladder between umbilical arteries and **document 2 umbilical arteries**
    - Many renal anomalies are associated with a single umbilical artery
  - Crucial when questioning **renal agenesis**
    - Potential pitfall is lumbar or adrenal arteries, which can appear quite prominent and be mistaken for renal arteries
- **Normal adrenal gland has a characteristic ice cream sandwich appearance** with hyperechoic medulla (the ice cream filling) surrounded by hypoechoic cortex
  - Triangular or Y-shaped and relatively large, when compared with the kidney
- **Fetal sex** is not required in low-risk pregnancies but is often the most pressing question for parents

- Preferred term is "sex" not "gender," which is self-identified
- At 12-14 weeks, the genital tubercle has a similar appearance in males and females
  - May look at "**the angle of the dangle**," which points caudally in females and cranially in males, but it is wise to avoid committing to sex unless clearly identified
- If sex identification remains indeterminate (i.e., possible disorder of sexual development), a careful search should begin for other anomalies, which would suggest a syndrome or aneuploidy

- **Amniotic fluid volume** is evaluated in every 2nd- and 3rd-trimester study and can be assessed subjectively (shown to be very accurate when performed by an experienced sonographer) or semiqualitatively by measuring fluid pockets
  - **Maximum (or deepest) vertical pocket (MVP)** measurement is anterior to posterior distance of the largest fluid pocket void of fetal parts and umbilical cord
    - "Vertical" implies the measurement is obtained with the transducer perpendicular to the maternal abdomen
    - Oblique measurements are not reproducible and may lead to errors in assessment of fluid volume
    - Normal is 2-8 cm with < 2 cm indicating oligohydramnios and > 8 cm polyhydramnios
  - **Amniotic fluid index (AFI)** measurement is the sum of the MVPs in 4 quadrants
    - Use color Doppler to exclude umbilical cord from measurement
    - AFI varies with gestational age, but values of 5-20 cm are the general normal range

Approach to the Abnormal Urinary Tract

- **Is it really the urinary tract?**
  - Peritoneal boundaries are not clear in the fetus, so care must taken in deciding what organ system is involved
    - A dilated tubular structure may be either ureterectasis or obstructed bowel
    - A **solid mass** may be coming from the kidney (e.g., mesoblastic nephroma), adrenal gland (e.g., neuroblastoma), or separate from both (e.g., extralobar sequestration)
- **Are there 2 kidneys? If so, where are they?**
  - If both kidneys are absent (**bilateral renal agenesis**), there will be anhydramnios by mid-2nd trimester
    - **Kidneys are not a major contributor to amniotic fluid until 16-weeks gestation**, so may see normal fluid before that time
    - Adrenal glands are very prominent early in gestation and may be confused with kidneys
      - Later in gestation, they have a lying-down appearance, lacking the normal triangular configuration
  - If there is normal fluid beyond 16 weeks, at least 1 kidney must be present
    - Evaluate renal fossa carefully, and if there is only 1 kidney, begin a careful search to see if the other is absent (i.e., unilateral renal agenesis) or in an aberrant location (e.g., pelvic kidney, crossed-fused ectopia)
- **Is the renal size and echogenicity normal?**
  - **Increased renal size and echogenicity** may be seen in autosomal recessive polycystic kidney disease, Meckel-Gruber syndrome, or in association with aneuploidy, typically trisomy 13
  - Differential diagnosis for **unilateral renal enlargement** includes: Unilateral renal agenesis with compensatory hypertrophy, cross-fused ectopia, duplicated renal collecting system, and renal vein thrombosis
- **Are anechoic structures renal cysts or hydronephrosis?**
  - Real-time evaluation is key
  - If they connect centrally with the renal pelvis, explore **causes of hydronephrosis** [e.g., ureteropelvic junction obstruction, ureterovesical obstruction, and lower urinary tract obstruction (LUTO)]
  - If they do not connect, the differential diagnosis is that for **multiple discrete cysts** (e.g., multicystic dysplastic kidney, cystic dysplasia from obstruction)
- **Is the bladder normal in size?**
  - Bladder should fill and empty during the course of a scan
    - Always check the bladder at the beginning and end of exam to make sure the observation of too big or too small bladder is persistent
  - An **absent bladder** is most commonly due to failure of urine production, in which case, look for bilateral renal anomalies
    - Can also occur with decreased renal perfusion (e.g., fetal growth restriction, donor twin in twin-twin transfusion)
    - If the bladder is never seen, but there is normal amniotic fluid, then consider **bladder exstrophy** (bladder is open on anterior abdominal wall with urine continuously leaking into amniotic fluid)
      - Scan the abdominal wall looking carefully for irregularity; cord insertion site is often lower than normal
  - If the bladder is distended and fails to empty (i.e., LUTO), **posterior urethral valves (PUV)** and **prune-belly syndrome** should be considered
    - Perform focused scan on bladder base looking for a dilated posterior urethra, which creates the classic keyhole appearance of PUV
    - In a female fetus, consider a **cloacal malformation** if there is a persistent fluid-filled structure in the pelvis
      - The distended structure is actually the vagina and not the bladder
      - Look for a fluid-debris level, which is mixing of urine, vaginal secretions, and meconium
      - Look for a vertical vaginal septum, which is present in many cases
- **Are the genitalia normal?**
  - Anomalous/ambiguous-appearing genitalia can be seen in disorders of sexual development
    - Disorders of sexual development in XY fetus
      - Hypospadias (most common), epispadias, cryptorchidism ± penile anomaly
    - Disorders of sexual development in XX fetus
      - Congenital adrenal hyperplasia is most common cause
  - Associated with aneuploidy (e.g., trisomy 13, trisomy 18, triploidy) and syndromes (e.g., Smith-Lemli-Opitz, Prader-Willi)
    - Always look for other anomalies

URINARY TRACT ANATOMY

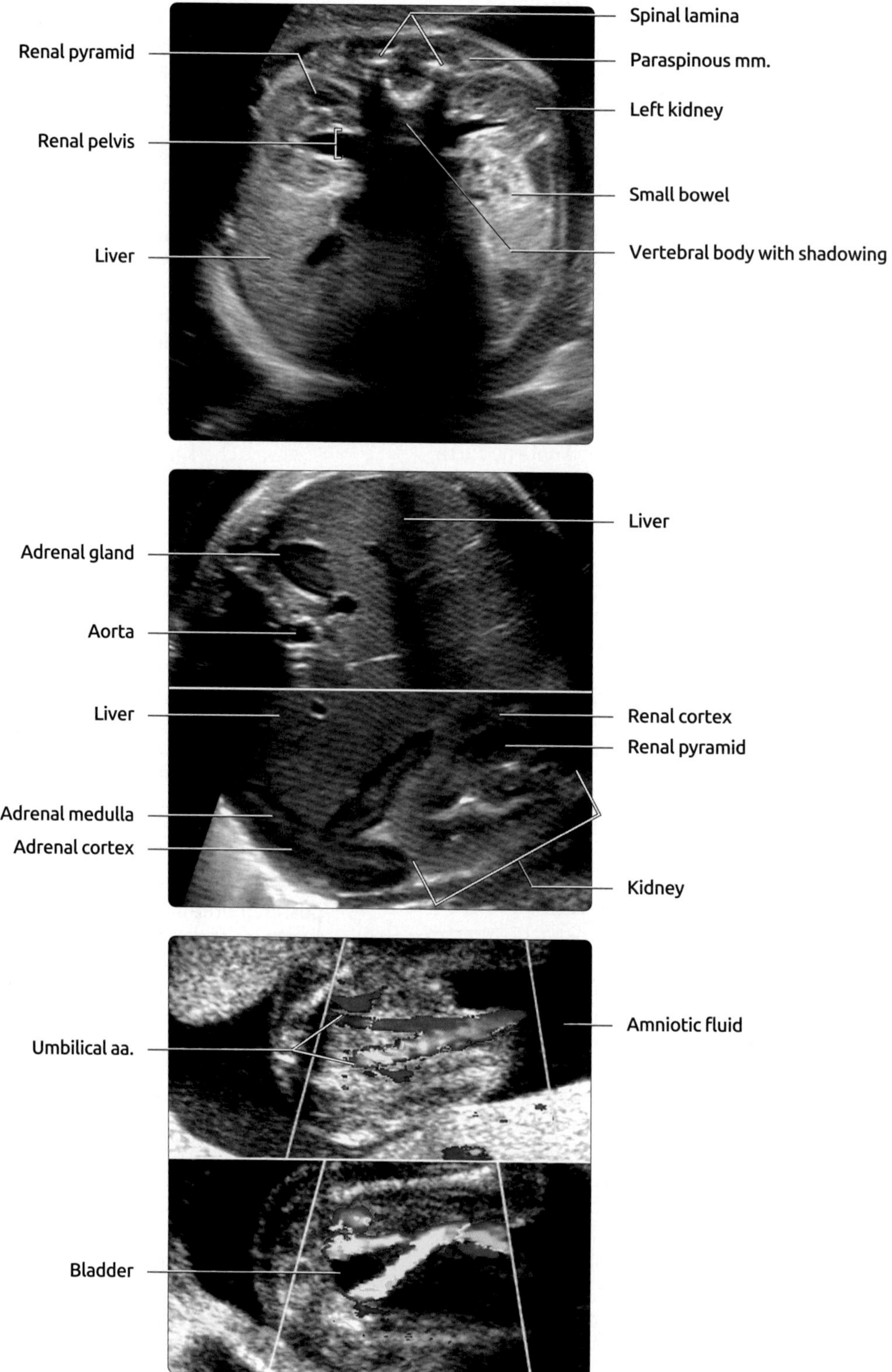

(Top) *This axial US is through the renal fossa with the spine at the 12 o'clock position. This is the best position to measure the anterior-posterior renal pelvis diameter. Do not confuse the normal hypoechoic renal pyramid for a dilated calyx.* **(Middle)** *This is a composite image of an axial fetal (top) and sagittal newborn (bottom) right adrenal gland. The fetal adrenal gland is 10-20x larger than the adult adrenal gland relative to body size. It is often quite prominent on fetal imaging and is recognized by its ice cream sandwich appearance with a hyperechoic medulla and hypoechoic cortex. It has an angular shape with a Y or tricorn hat configuration.* **(Bottom)** *Axial color Doppler US (top) shows 2 umbilical arteries. This is the anatomic landmark for the fetal bladder, but none was seen. Normal amniotic fluid and kidneys (not shown) make an anomaly unlikely. Another color Doppler US 7 minutes later (bottom) shows the bladder starting to fill, confirming that this fetus is indeed normal. The bladder should fill and empty during the course of a scan. Always check the bladder at the beginning and end of the exam to ensure the observation of "too big" or "too small" is persistent.*

URINARY TRACT ANATOMY

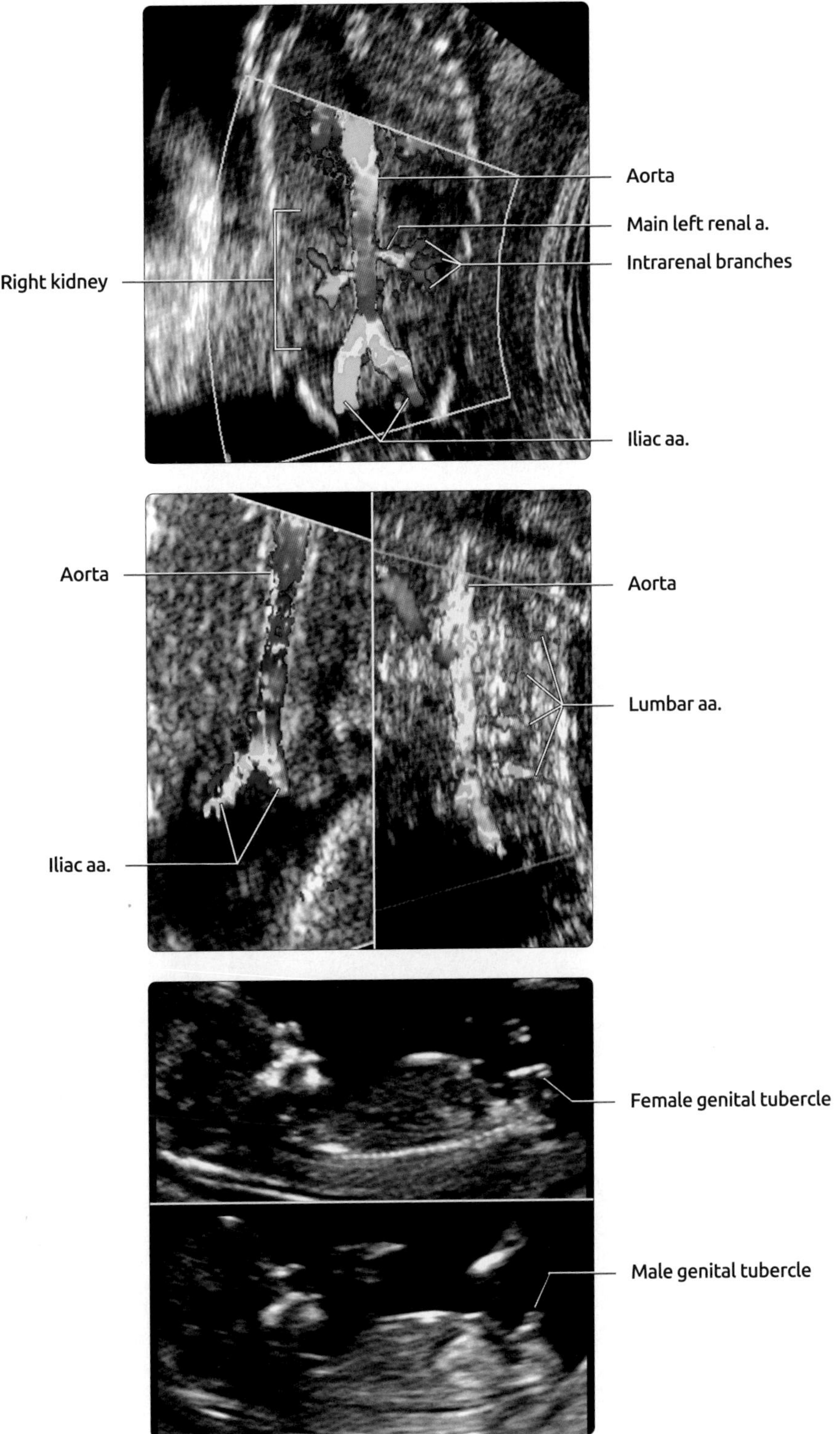

(Top) *Coronal color Doppler US of the fetal abdomen shows normal renal vasculature.* **(Middle)** *Color Doppler can be very helpful in evaluating urinary tract anomalies, especially to look for renal arteries in the setting of possible renal agenesis. In this coronal US of the aorta (left), no renal arteries are seen. It is important to be aware of potential pitfalls. When the transducer is angled posteriorly (right), multiple lumbar arteries are seen. One of these could be easily confused with a renal artery. Understanding normal anatomy and attention to detail is imperative in making the correct diagnosis.* **(Bottom)** *Sagittal views of the genital tubercle at 13 weeks in a female (top) and male (bottom) fetus show the difference in angle between the sexes. In the female fetus, the genital tubercle points caudally (down), while in the male fetus, it points cranially (up). This is the so-called "angle of the dangle" and has a reported accuracy of 90-95% at 12-14 weeks gestation; however, it is best not to commit unless findings are clear.*

Urinary Tract Dilation

KEY FACTS

TERMINOLOGY

- Urinary tract dilation (UTD) risk stratification system
  - A is for antenatal in UTD classification system
    - A1 = low risk for postnatal uropathy
    - A2-3 = increased risk for postnatal uropathy
  - P1, P2, and P3 for postnatal findings

IMAGING

- Measure anterior-posterior renal pelvis diameter (AP RPD)
  - Best technique is with spine at 12 or 6 o'clock
- Normal AP RPD
  - < 4 mm from 16-27 wk and < 7 mm when ≥ 28 wk
- **UTD A1 = isolated mild renal pelvis distention**
  - AP RPD 4-7 mm at 16-27 wk; 7-10 mm when ≥ 28 wk
  - Associations: Aneuploidy, early obstruction/reflux
  - Follow-up at 32 wk to look for resolution or progression
- **UTD A2-3 criteria (need only 1 to make diagnosis)**
  - AP RPD > 7 mm at 16-27 wk; >10 mm when ≥ 28 wk
  - Dilated calyces regardless of AP RPD
  - Dilated ureter or abnormal bladder
  - Echogenic kidney (> liver or spleen)
  - Thin renal parenchyma
  - Oligohydramnios from genitourinary cause
- UTD A2-3 cases are more likely to progress

SCANNING TIPS

- Look carefully at morphology of genitourinary tract distention to best determine level of obstruction
  - Most common cause of upper tract obstruction is ureteropelvic junction obstruction
  - Most common cause of lower tract obstruction is posterior urethral valves (in male fetuses)
- Obtain image with kidney + liver/spleen
  - Consider cystic dysplasia if renal echogenicity > liver/spleen echogenicity
    - From postobstructive or primary cystic dysplasia
  - Look for small cortical cysts in all UTD cases

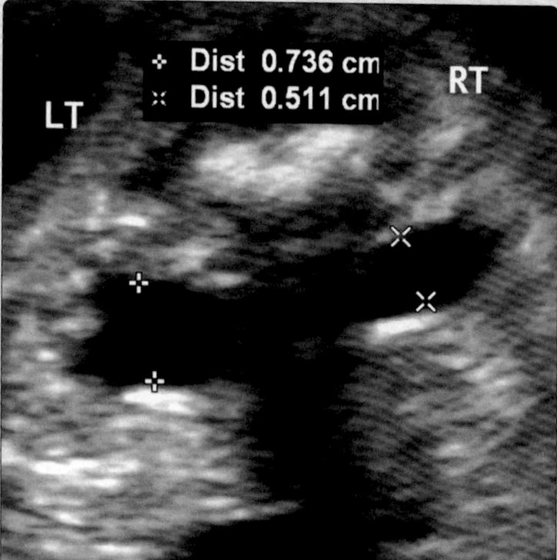

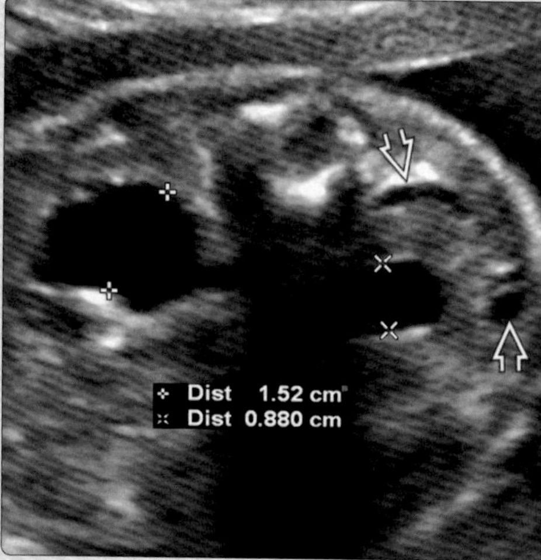

(Left) *In this 20-week fetus, AP RPD measures > 7 mm at < 28 weeks on the left, and therefore, the UTD classification is A2-3. The reason for this is 2-fold. The dilation is more severe and also, when the central pelvis is markedly "ballooned," the peripheral calyces may merge with the pelvis and not be seen separately.* **(Right)** *Bilateral ↑ AP RPD is seen in this 32-week fetus. The right renal pelvis is more dilated than the left; however, subtle cortical cysts ➡ are seen on the left, suggesting post-obstructive cystic dysplasia.*

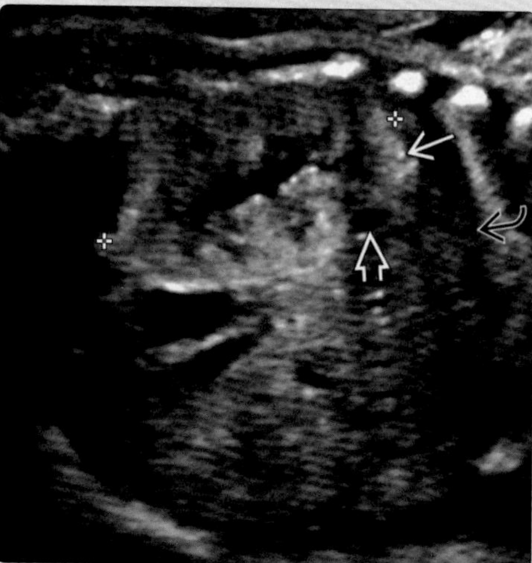

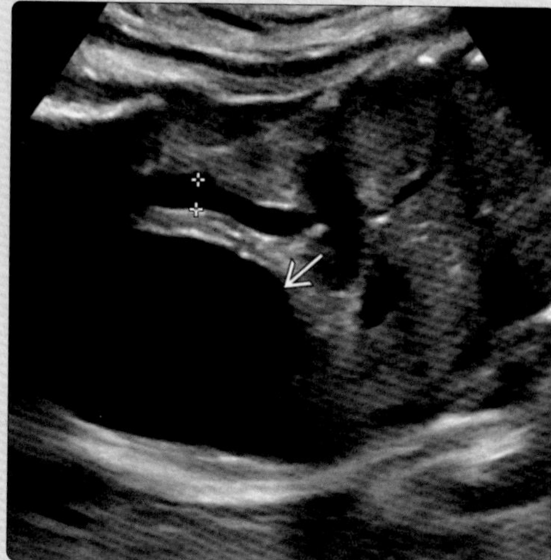

(Left) *Coronal ultrasound of the right kidney (calipers) shows that the renal echogenicity ➡ is greater than the liver echogenicity ➡ and there is a small cortical cyst ➡. Both kidneys had this appearance. The fetus was found to have a chromosome deletion associated with renal cystic dysplasia.* **(Right)** *A dilated ureter (calipers) is seen in this fetus with oligohydramnios and enlarged bladder ➡ from obstructing posterior urethral valves. Ureter dilation is always abnormal and can be serpiginous, mimicking bowel.*

KEY FACTS

TERMINOLOGY

- Duplicated kidney with separate upper and lower pole collecting systems
- Complete or partial duplication: Most in utero are complete

IMAGING

- 2 separate ureters drain upper and lower poles
- **Upper pole prone to obstruction**
  - Hydronephrosis and hydroureter
  - Ureter inserts into bladder lower and more medial than normal (ectopic insertion)
    - Creates ureterocele, which appears as cyst within bladder
- **Lower pole prone to reflux**
  - Variable and progressive hydronephrosis usually less than upper pole
- Bilateral duplication in 10-20%
- Severe obstruction may result in upper pole parenchymal cystic change, lower pole typically spared

TOP DIFFERENTIAL DIAGNOSES

- Ureteropelvic junction obstruction: Ureter not dilated, variable hydronephrosis

CLINICAL ISSUES

- Upper pole prone to infection and renal damage
- Most need early surgical repair

SCANNING TIPS

- Look carefully at all dilated renal calyx connections to renal pelvis when hydronephrosis present
- Look for 2 renal arteries when duplicationed
  - Coronal color Doppler view best
- If ureterocele in bladder, almost always duplicated kidney
  - Isolated simple ureterocele rare
- If renal duplication suspected but no ureterocele seen, wait and watch bladder fill and empty
  - Large ureterocele may mimic bladder and be missed

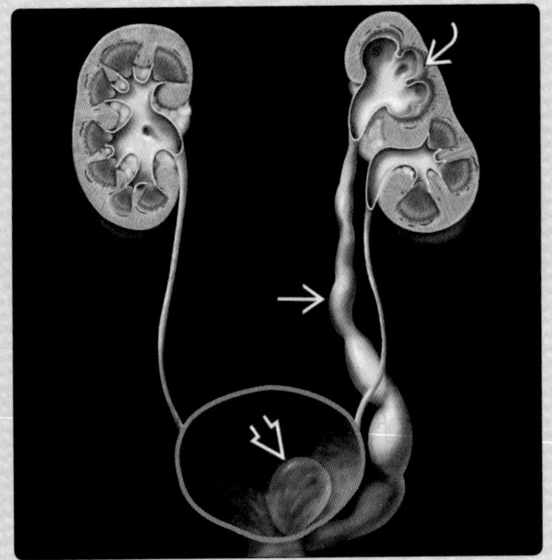

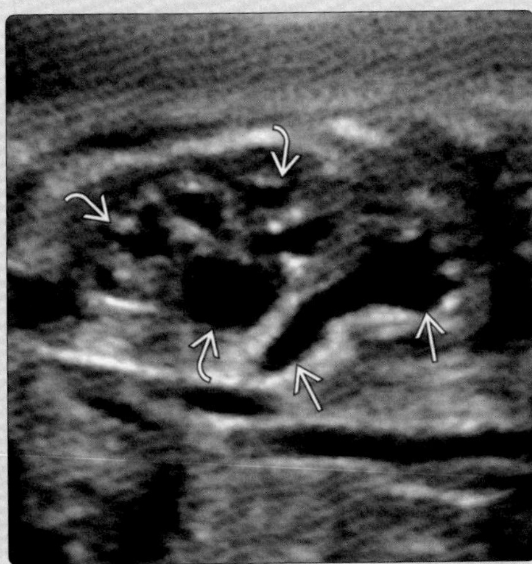

(Left) *Graphic of a duplicated left kidney shows upper pole collecting system ➔ and ureter ➔ dilatation because of ureterocele ➔ that herniates into the bladder lumen. That ureter inserts lower and more medial than normal. Reflux into the lower pole ureter also occurs, but the amount of distention is variable in utero.* **(Right)** *This 3rd-trimester fetus has a duplicated kidney. The upper pole collecting system and ureter ➔ are moderately distended. There is milder distention of the lower pole ➔ from reflux.*

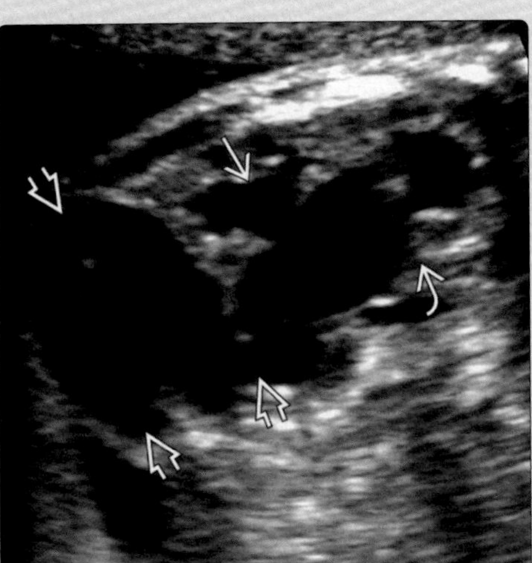

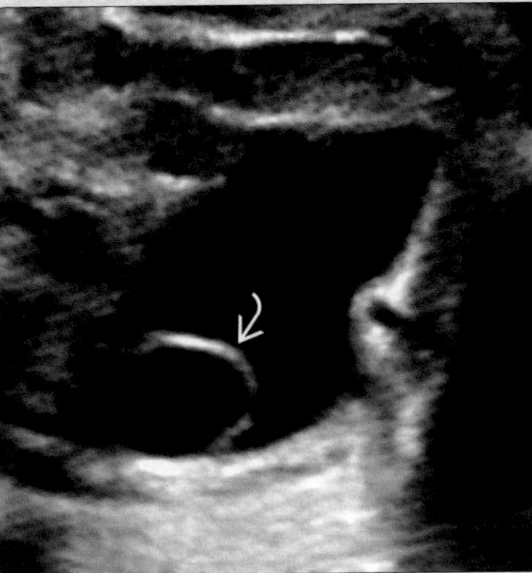

(Left) *Coronal oblique ultrasound of a duplicated kidney shows a markedly dilated upper pole collecting system ➔ compared to the lower pole collecting system ➔. The ureter associated with the upper pole is distended and serpiginous ➔, mimicking dilated bowel.* **(Right)** *In the fetal bladder, an ectopic ureterocele ➔ has a balloon-like appearance at the bladder base. Large ureteroceles can mimic the bladder if the bladder is empty and collapsed around the ureterocele.*

KEY FACTS

TERMINOLOGY

- Abnormality of renal fusion &/or ascent

IMAGING

- Horseshoe kidney (fused lower poles)
  - Isthmus = central bridging tissue
    - Isthmus is anterior to aorta
  - Often low lying: Isthmus "snags" on aortic vessels during ascent of fused kidneys from pelvis to flank
- Ectopic pelvic kidney
  - Failure of embryologic ascent from pelvis to flank
- Crossed-fused ectopia
  - Kidneys are fused and mostly in flank
  - Contralateral fused kidney often small, misshapen, and crosses midline (anterior to aorta)
- Associated kidney malrotation common with all renal developmental anomalies
  - Anterior renal pelvis, medial lower pole
- Associated obstruction and cystic dysplasia common
- Color Doppler shows highly variable blood supply
  - Low, multiple, anteriorly oriented renal arteries

TOP DIFFERENTIAL DIAGNOSES

- Renal tumor: Mimics cross-fused ectopia
- Pelvic mass: Mimics pelvic kidney

CLINICAL ISSUES

- More likely to have postnatal hydronephrosis, cystic dysplasia, urolithiasis
- Horseshoe kidney present in 1:400 (general population)
  - Associated with monosomy X (Turner syndrome)
  - VACTERL association

SCANNING TIPS

- Use color Doppler to find renal arteries
  - Ectopic renal arteries lead to ectopic kidneys
- Suspect renal development anomalies when renal pelvis is unusually rotated (anteriorly more often than posteriorly)
- Horseshoe kidney may be missed if isthmus is thin

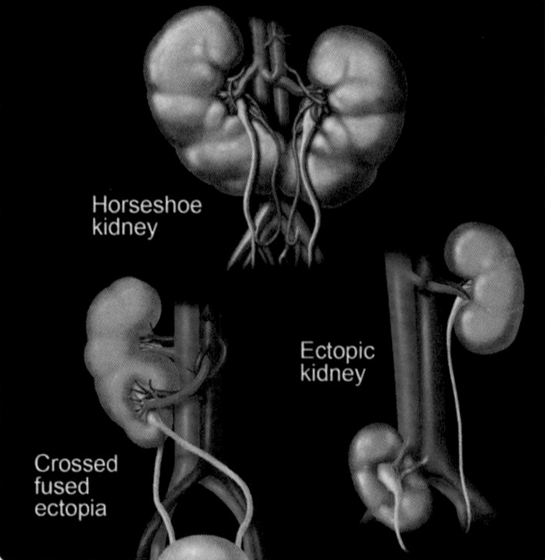

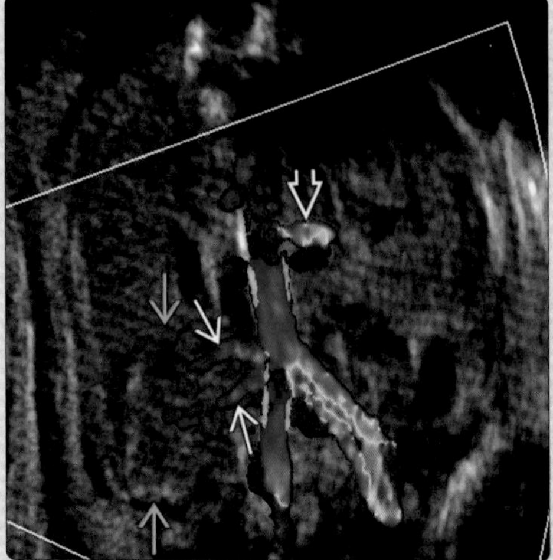

(Left) *Graphic drawings of renal development anomalies includes anomalies of renal tissue fusion (horseshoe and crossed-fused ectopia) and failure of normal renal ascent from the pelvis to the flank (ectopic pelvic kidney).* **(Right)** *Coronal color Doppler US of the aorta, iliac arteries, and renal arteries shows one renal artery ➡ in normal position, in the upper abdomen, and the other is bifid ➡ in the pelvis and associated with an ectopic pelvic kidney ⇨. The renal arteries can help find ectopic kidneys, often isoechoic with bowel.*

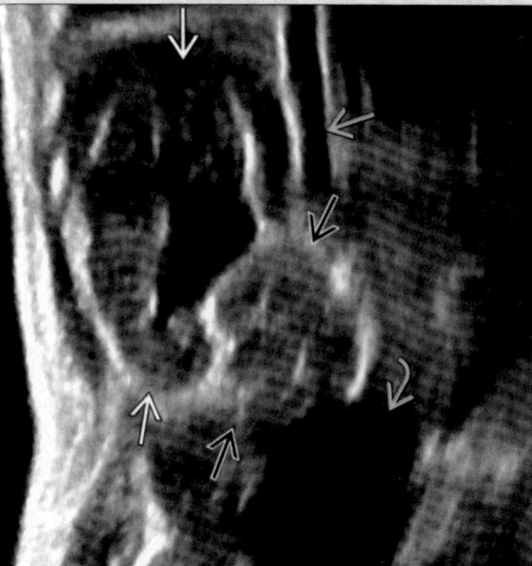

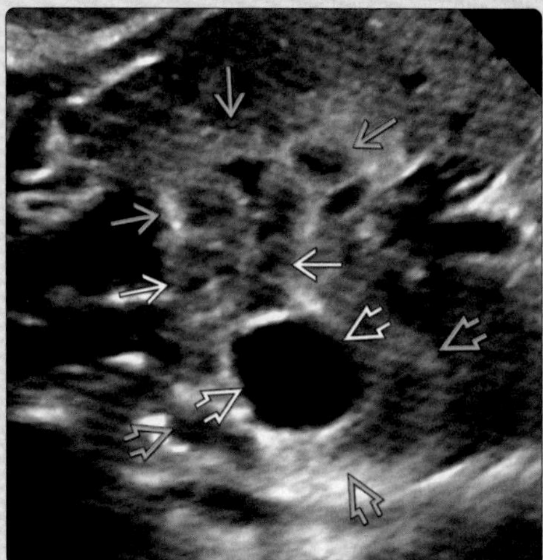

(Left) *Coronal US shows a right kidney ➡ in the normal position and an attached smaller left kidney ⇨ fused to the lower pole. Note how the cross fused ectopic kidney crosses the midline (note aorta ⇨) and touches the dome of the bladder ⇨.* **(Right)** *Coronal US shows a dilated left renal pelvis ➡ and a connecting isthmus of renal tissue ➡ between the lower poles of the right ⇨ and left ⇨ kidneys. Horseshoe kidneys are more prone to hydronephrosis.*

KEY FACTS

TERMINOLOGY

- Failure of kidneys to form

IMAGING

- No kidneys in renal fossa or anywhere else in fetus
- Adrenal glands are present and large, can mimic kidneys
    - Have ice cream sandwich appearance with hypoechoic cortex and hyperechoic medulla
    - Flattened, lying down appearance; lacks normal tricorn hat configuration
- Absent renal arteries
    - Best evaluated with coronal aorta color Doppler view
- No fluid-filled bladder
    - Best evaluated with axial pelvis color Doppler view showing no bladder between umbilical arteries
- No amniotic fluid in 2nd/3rd trimester (anhydramnios)
    - Normal or low-normal fluid might be seen before 16 wk
- Associated findings
    - Pulmonary hypoplasia from oligohydramnios
    - Limb deformities: Club feet, contractures
    - Facial anomalies: Micrognathia, low-set ears

TOP DIFFERENTIAL DIAGNOSES

- Other causes of severe oligohydramnios
    - Premature rupture of membranes
    - Severe growth restriction
    - Bilateral renal anomaly

CLINICAL ISSUES

- Bilateral agenesis is considered lethal anomaly
- Associated with aneuploidy and genetic syndromes

SCANNING TIPS

- Saline infusion may help with fetal anatomy evaluation
- Set color Doppler gain carefully so as not to "light up" lumbar arteries, which may mimic renal arteries
- Look for pelvic kidney when kidneys not seen in renal fossa
    - Renal artery may come off iliac artery

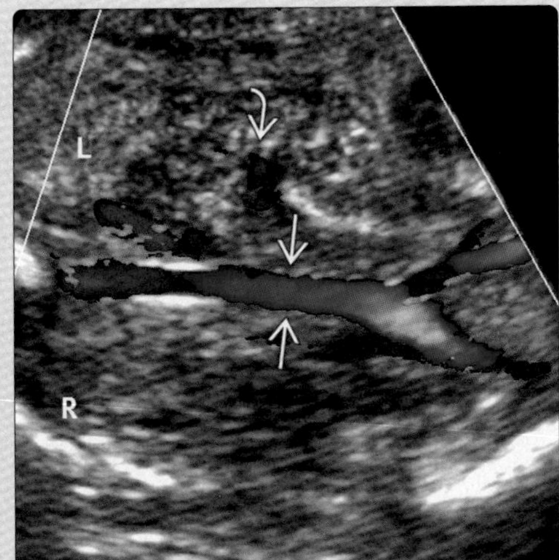

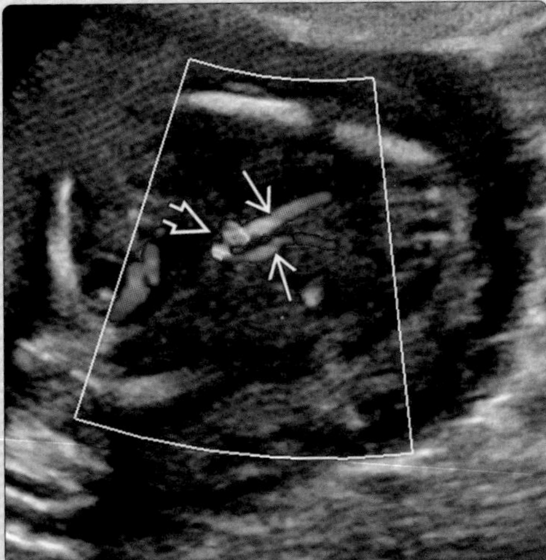

(Left) *No kidneys or measurable fluid was seen in this 18-week fetus with renal agenesis. Coronal color Doppler view of the aorta shows absent renal arteries. Part of the splenic artery is incidentally seen.* **(Right)** *Axial color Doppler view of the pelvis shows absence of a fluid-filled bladder. The umbilical arteries are seen as they travel from the cord insertion site to the iliac arteries (not shown). A fluid-filled bladder should be seen between the arteries.*

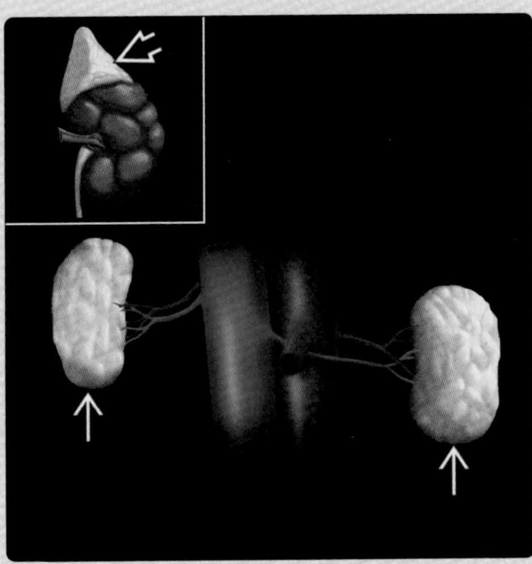

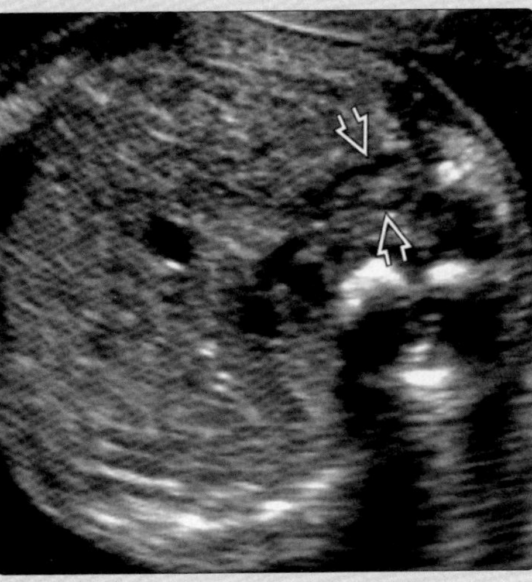

(Left) *The relatively large size of the normal fetal adrenal gland compared with the kidney (inset) is shown. With renal agenesis, adrenal glands lose their triangular shape and have a flattened appearance, filling the renal fossa, and potentially being mistaken for kidneys.* **(Right)** *Axial ultrasound after amnioinfusion shows no kidneys at the level of the renal fossa and a prominent adrenal gland. Note the ice cream sandwich appearance with a hypoechoic cortex and hyperechoic medulla.*

Echogenic Kidneys

KEY FACTS

IMAGING

- Multiple causes; can be isolated or syndromic
- **Autosomal recessive polycystic kidney disease** is single gene disorder
  - Large, diffusely hyperechoic kidneys most common
  - May see discrete cysts or areas of tubular ectasia
  - Sometimes just echogenic medullary pyramids
- **Obstructive cystic dysplasia**
  - Microscopic cysts develop due to chronic obstruction
  - Multiple interfaces → increased echogenicity
  - Macroscopic cortical cysts usually present
- **Trisomy 13**
  - Echogenic kidneys seen in 50%
  - Look for holoprosencephaly, cyclopia, proboscis, midline facial cleft, polydactyly, congenital heart disease
  - Early-onset fetal growth restriction
- **Meckel-Gruber syndrome**
  - Triad of findings: 2 needed to make diagnosis
    - Renal cystic dysplasia in > 90%
    - Encephalocele in 60-80%
    - Polydactyly in 55-75%

SCANNING TIPS

- Echogenic kidneys are brighter than liver
- Use high-resolution transducer to look for subtle cystic change/tubular ectasia
- Use vaginal transducer for better resolution in 1st trimester or with breech presentation
- If fluid is low, verify that membrane rupture has been ruled out: Relative contraindication to transvaginal ultrasound (TVUS) due to risk of introducing infection
- Look for other anomalies, more likely syndromal diagnosis
- Oligohydramnios may cause pulmonary hypoplasia
  - Measure chest:heart ratios to document small chest size
  - Normally, heart circumference is 1/2 of chest; heart area is 1/3 of chest

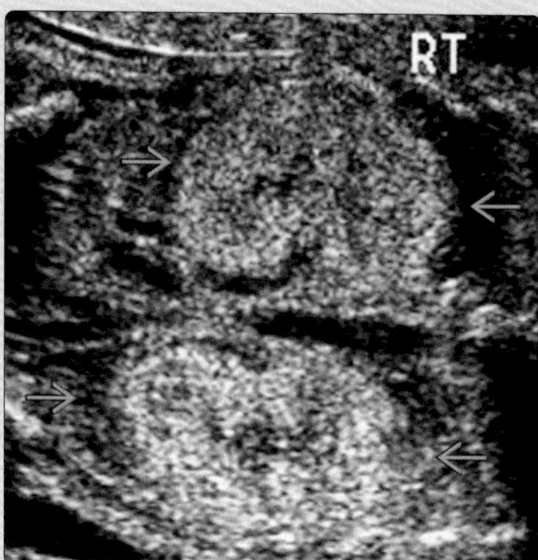

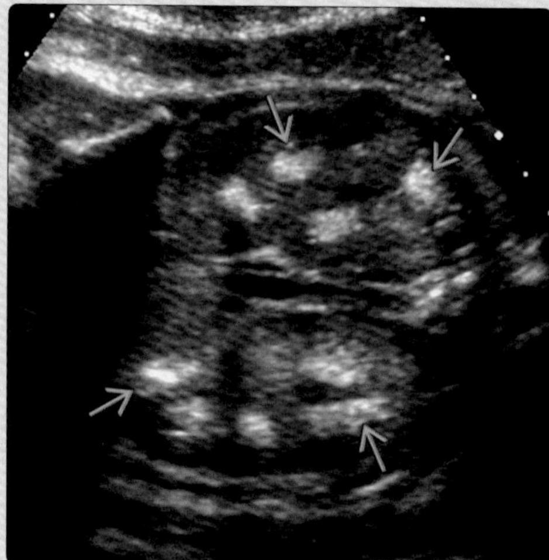

(Left) *Coronal US in the 2nd trimester shows large, echogenic kidneys ➡. The left measured 3.7 cm (> 90th percentile for gestational age). In this case, amniotic fluid volume was normal throughout pregnancy, and the diagnosis of autosomal recessive polycystic kidney disease (ARPKD) was established at birth.* **(Right)** *Coronal US in the 3rd trimester shows another appearance of ARPKD with echogenic pyramids ➡ in large kidneys. Oligohydramnios was present in this case as well.*

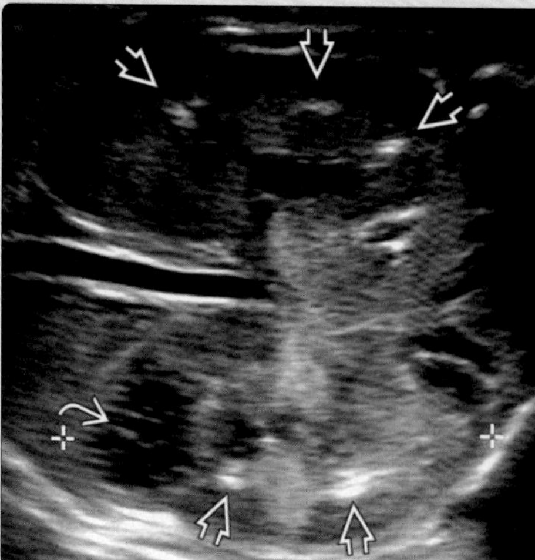

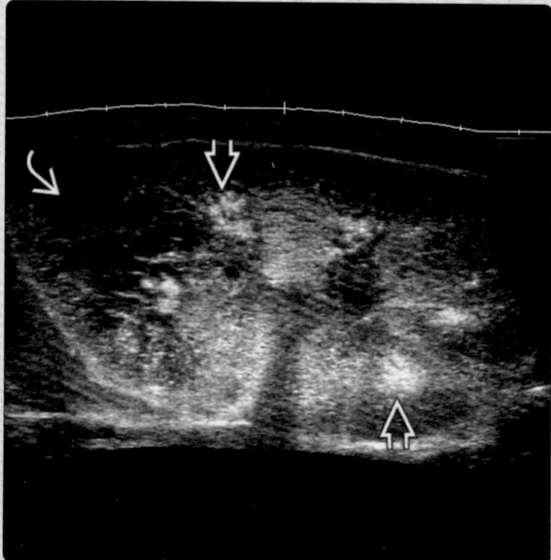

(Left) *Coronal US at 31 weeks shows another sonographic pattern of focal tubular ectasia ➡ in the left upper pole of a fetus with ARPKD. The kidneys are very large (calipers measure a 9-cm left kidney), and the medullary pyramids ➡ are echogenic.* **(Right)** *Extended field-of-view US of the left kidney after delivery confirms the fetal observations of echogenic pyramids ➡ and focal, upper pole tubular ectasia ➡.*

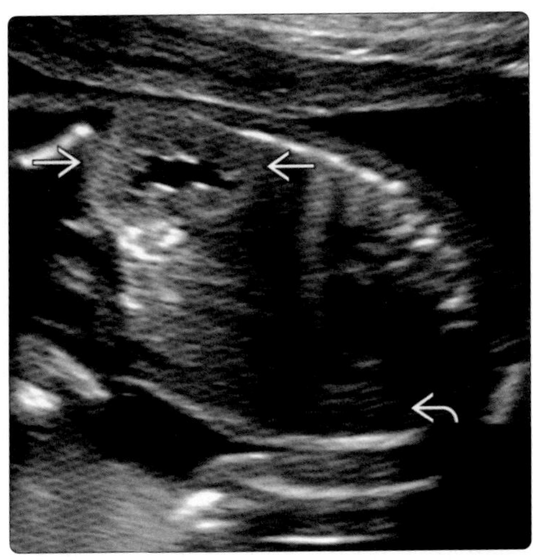

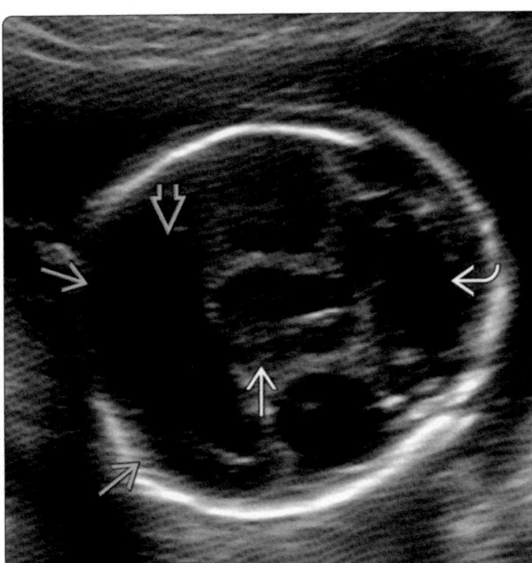

(Left) *Parasagittal US in a fetus with multiple anomalies shows a large, echogenic kidney* ➡ *and a left, liver-up diaphragmatic hernia* ➡. *Amniocentesis revealed trisomy 13.* **(Right)** *Axial oblique US through the fetal brain shows a monoventricle* ➡ *with a continuous rind of cerebral tissue* ➡ *anteriorly and partly fused thalami* ➡. *These are features of alobar holoprosencephaly, a hallmark anomaly in trisomy 13. The posterior fossa cyst* ➡ *was part of an associated Dandy-Walker malformation.*

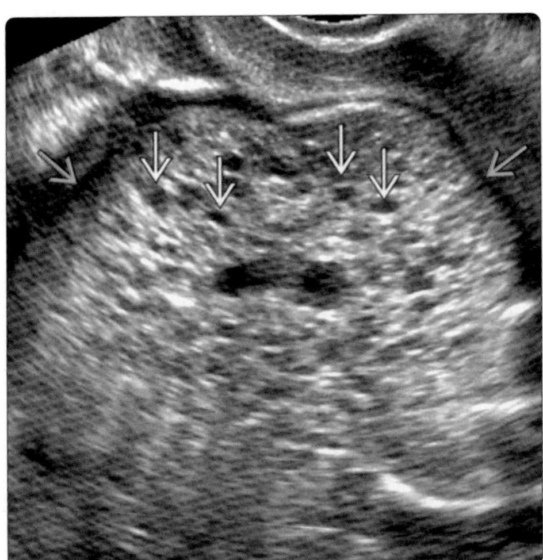

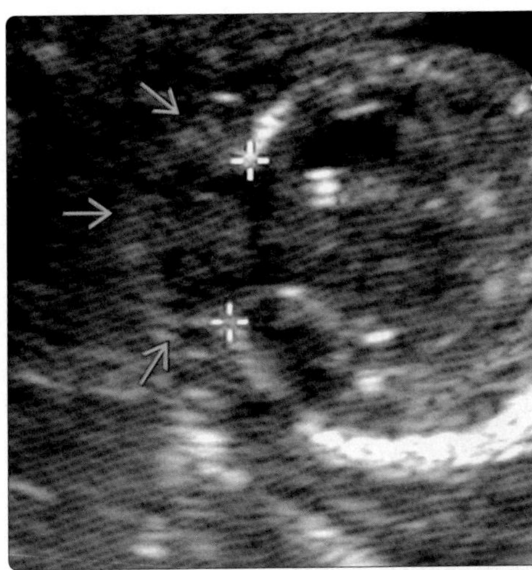

(Left) *TVUS performed for further assessment of severe oligohydramnios and large echogenic kidneys shows innumerable microcysts* ➡ *throughout the kidney* ➡. *Other abnormalities were present, and the final diagnosis was Meckel-Gruber syndrome.* **(Right)** *Meckel-Gruber syndrome may be recognized in the 1st trimester before oligohydramnios limits acoustic access. TVUS at the time of nuchal translucency screening shows an occipital calvarial defect (calipers) and a posterior cephalocele* ➡.

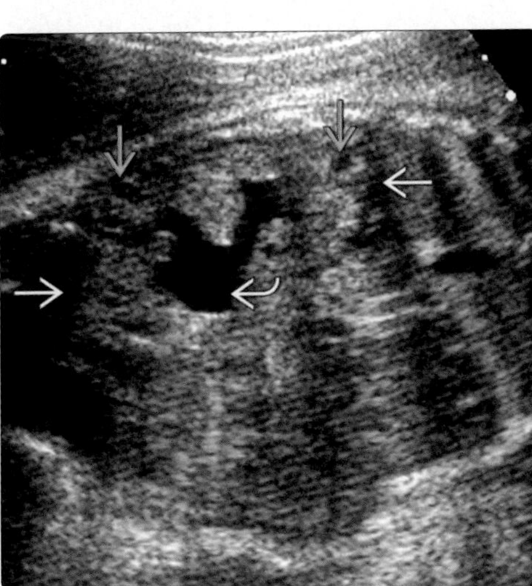

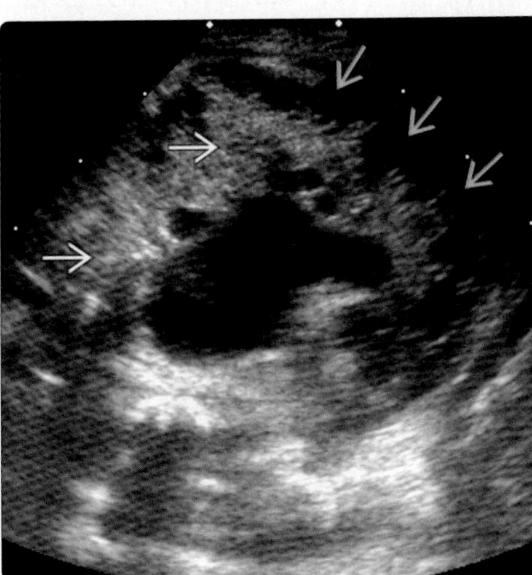

(Left) *Third-trimester US shows almost no amniotic fluid, an echogenic kidney* ➡ *with some visible cysts* ➡, *and a dilated collecting system* ➡. *The other kidney looked similar. This is the typical appearance of obstructive cystic dysplasia.* **(Right)** *Coronal US of the neonate's kidney on the 1st day of life shows more detail and confirms diffuse cystic dysplasia with macroscopic cortical cysts* ➡ *and echogenic parenchyma* ➡. *The infant had severe renal impairment secondary to bladder outlet obstruction.*

Ureteropelvic Junction Obstruction

KEY FACTS

IMAGING

- Obstruction at ureteropelvic junction (UPJ) leads to renal pelvis and calyceal distention
- Renal pelvis dilated, elongated, and bullet-shaped
  - Can extend into pelvis and touch bladder
    - Can mimic dilated ureter
  - Normal anterior-posterior (AP) renal pelvis diameter
    - 16 weeks to 27 weeks, 6 days: AP diameter < 4 mm
    - 28 weeks to term: AP diameter < 7 mm
- Dilated calyces can mimic parenchymal cysts
  - Look for connection to renal pelvis
- Postobstructive renal cystic dysplasia if severe
  - ↑ renal echogenicity ± renal cysts
- Bladder and amniotic fluid normal if unilateral process
- Associations often determine prognosis
  - Contralateral renal abnormality in 25%
  - Bilateral UPJ obstruction in 10%
  - Extrarenal anomalies in 10%
- UPJ may progress rapidly; even mild renal pelvis AP diameter distention (4-7 mm) needs follow up at 32 weeks

CLINICAL ISSUES

- Most common significant cause of hydronephrosis
- Variable outcomes
  - Many resolve spontaneously and need no treatment
  - May need surgery (pyeloplasty)
  - ↑ risk of renal impairment if prenatal AP diameter ≥ 10 mm
- Prognosis excellent if unilateral

SCANNING TIPS

- Use cine sweeps to show all calyces connect to renal pelvis
- Massively dilated renal pelvis may cross midline
- Beware that normal renal parenchymal pyramids can mimic dilated calyces
- Scan complete length of kidney, rule out duplicated kidney with only upper pole obstruction

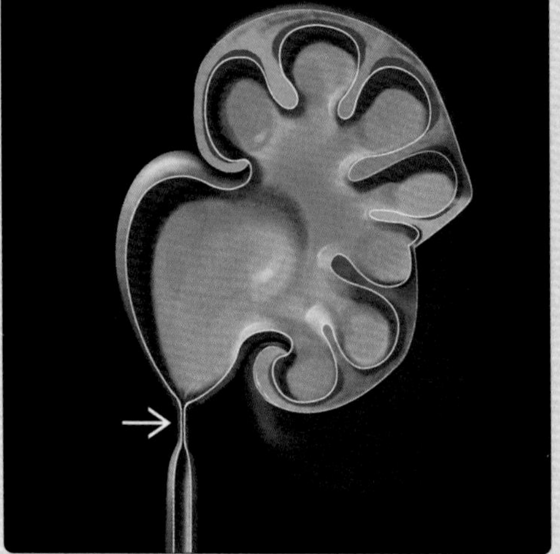

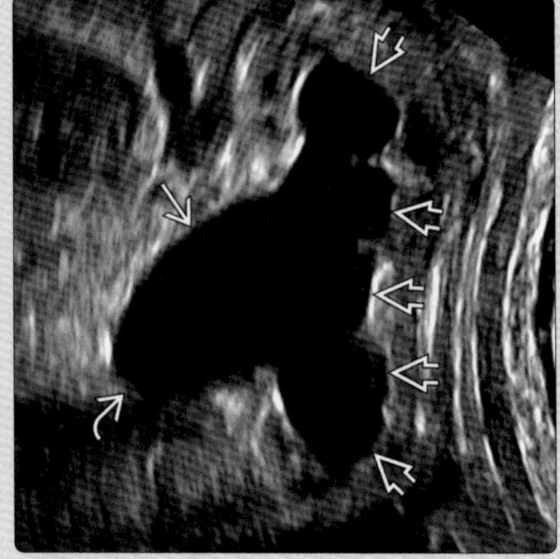

(Left) *Graphic shows focal narrowing at the ureteropelvic junction (UPJ) ➡ causing renal pelvis and calyceal dilation. Notice the abrupt transition between the distended renal pelvis and the ureter.* **(Right)** *Coronal ultrasound of a fetus with UPJ obstruction shows the classic bullet-shaped renal pelvis. The distended renal pelvis ➡ is elongated and ends abruptly at the UPJ ↗. The calyces are markedly dilated and blunted ➡. The renal pelvis may extend to the level of the bladder and should not be mistaken for a dilated ureter.*

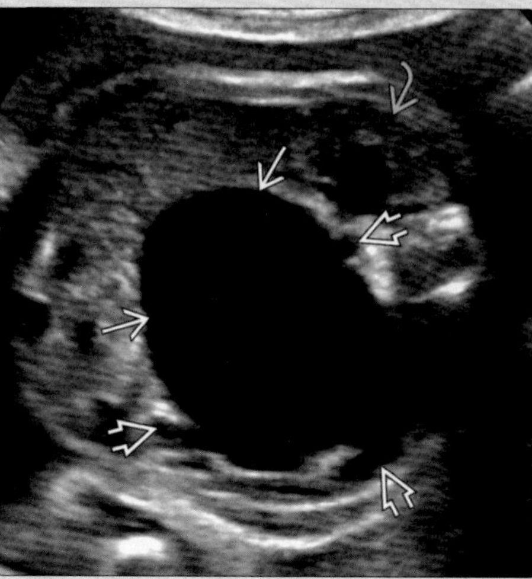

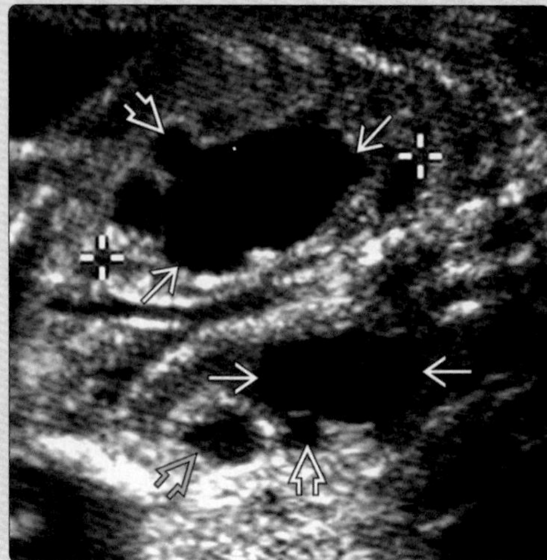

(Left) *In this 32-week fetus presenting for follow-up for mild bilateral pelviectasis at 20 weeks, the left renal pelvis is massively dilated ➡ and crosses the midline. Cystic out-pouchings peripherally are dilated calyces ➡. The left parenchyma is extremely thin as well. The right kidney ↗ is normal (AP diameter < 7 mm).* **(Right)** *Bilateral UPJ obstruction is seen in this case. The renal pelves ➡ communicate with the calyces ➡. Dilated calyces can mimic parenchymal cyst when this communication is not shown well ➡.*

Obstructive Renal Dysplasia

KEY FACTS

TERMINOLOGY

- Definition: Genitourinary tract obstruction (at any level) causing renal parenchymal destruction

IMAGING

- **Progression: Urinary tract dilation (UTD) → ↑ renal echogenicity → small peripheral cortical cysts → large cysts**
  - Findings are variable depending on stage of progression
- Compare kidney echogenicity with liver echogenicity
  - Normal kidney echogenicity ≤ liver echogenicity
  - Abnormal kidney echogenicity > liver echogenicity
  - Cortical cysts are always abnormal finding
- Variable appearance of UTD
  - Depends on level and age of obstruction
- Variable amniotic fluid volume (unilateral vs. bilateral)
- Most common causes of obstructive renal dysplasia (ORD)
  - Severe ureteropelvic junction obstruction
  - Posterior urethral valves in male fetus

TOP DIFFERENTIAL DIAGNOSES

- Multicystic dysplastic kidney
  - Can look exactly like late ORD
- Non-ORD
  - Echogenic kidneys without UTD
- Autosomal recessive polycystic kidney disease
  - Large echogenic kidneys is key finding
  - Without UTD and without visible cysts

SCANNING TIPS

- Look carefully for small cortical cysts in kidneys with significant hydronephrosis
- Look for unilateral loss of corticomedullary differentiation (CMD) as early finding
  - Note that CMD is not always seen in fetus
- Measure contralateral kidney to see evidence for compensatory hypertrophy
  - Contralateral kidney compensates for abnormal kidney and is considered "super kidney"

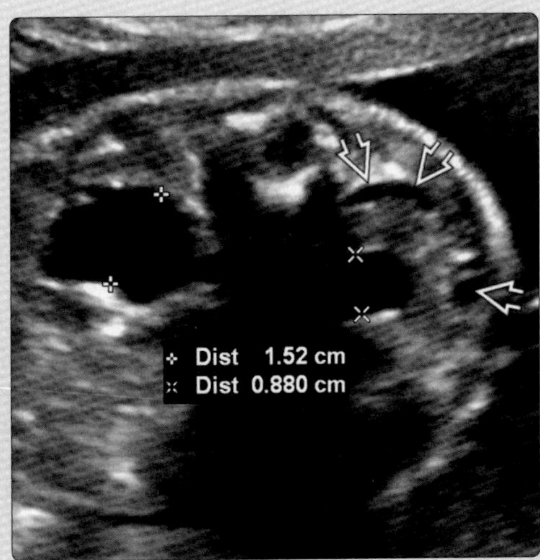

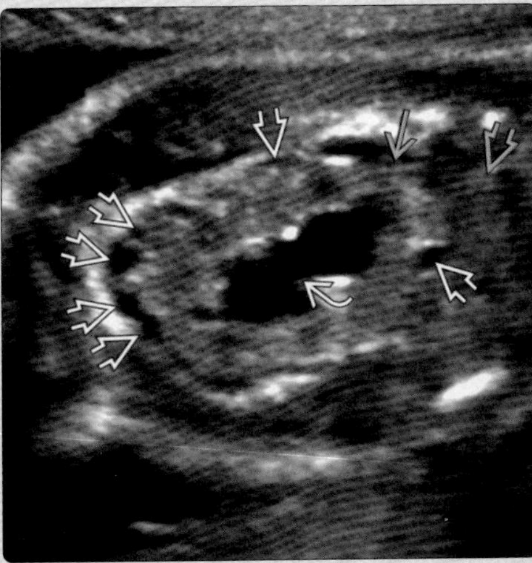

(Left) *In this fetus with bilateral renal pelvis dilation, the right renal pelvis dilation (x calipers) is less than the left (+ calipers). However, subtle subcortical cysts ➡ are seen, suggesting the obstruction has caused renal dysplasia on the right.* **(Right)** *Coronal view through the kidney shows hydronephrosis ➡, increased renal echogenicity ➡ (when compared with the liver ➡), and small cortical cysts ➡ (called rosary bead sign when lined up).*

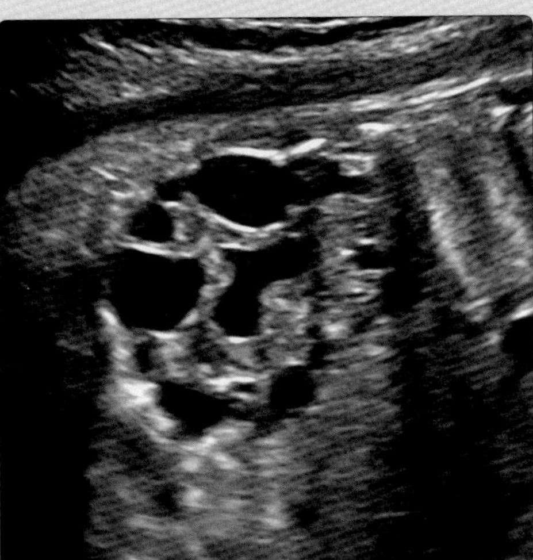

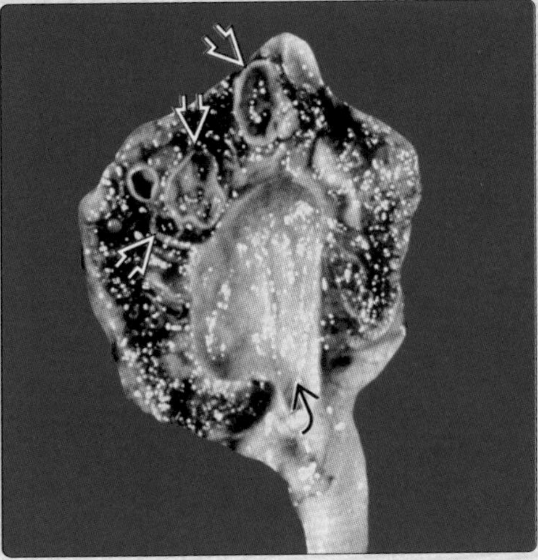

(Left) *In the 3rd trimester of the same fetus with bilateral ureteropelvic junction obstruction, the cortical cysts have increased in size and further parenchymal cysts have formed. This progression is typical for this diagnosis.* **(Right)** *Gross pathology of obstructive renal dysplasia shows renal pelvis distention ➡ and variable-sized cysts ➡ within the dysplastic renal parenchyma. The kidney is small and dysplastic from longstanding obstruction. Renal size is variable with obstructive renal dysplasia, especially during fetal life.*

Multicystic Dysplastic Kidney

KEY FACTS

TERMINOLOGY

- Multicystic dysplastic kidney (MCDK): Renal cystic dysplasia

IMAGING

- **Multiple noncommunicating cysts in kidney**
  - Intervening renal tissue is sparse and abnormal
  - Large kidney size in 90%
  - Often lose normal kidney reniform shape
- Bilateral MCDK in 20%
  - Severe oligohydramnios or anhydramnios
  - Grim prognosis from pulmonary hypoplasia
- Contralateral renal anomaly (non-MCDK) in 1/3
- MCDK pelvic kidney can mimic dilated bowel/pelvic mass
- MCDK can be partial (upper or lower pole only)
- Other nonrenal anomalies in 5%
- Role of surveillance
  - Evaluate contralateral kidney and amniotic fluid
  - MCDK can enlarge dramatically (↑ hydrops risk)

TOP DIFFERENTIAL DIAGNOSES

- Obstructive cystic dysplasia
  - Early hydronephrosis → late renal parenchymal cysts
  - Can look identical to MCDK in late phase
- Ureteropelvic junction obstruction
  - Dilated calyces mimic cysts

CLINICAL ISSUES

- MCDK most often does not function
- MCDK tends to grow in fetal life and then involute

SCANNING TIPS

- Contralateral renal evaluation is essential
  - Large contralateral kidney suggests compensatory hypertrophy and is good prognosticator
    - Measure renal length and look up in published tables
  - Look carefully for hydronephrosis, cysts, ↑ renal echogenicity
- Clue to pelvic MCDK is lack of normal kidney in flank

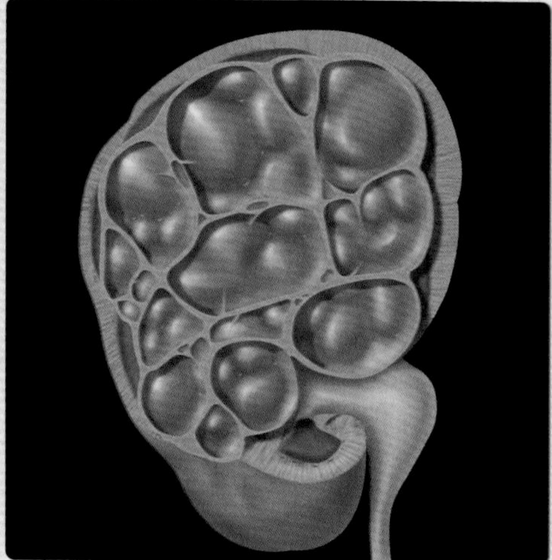

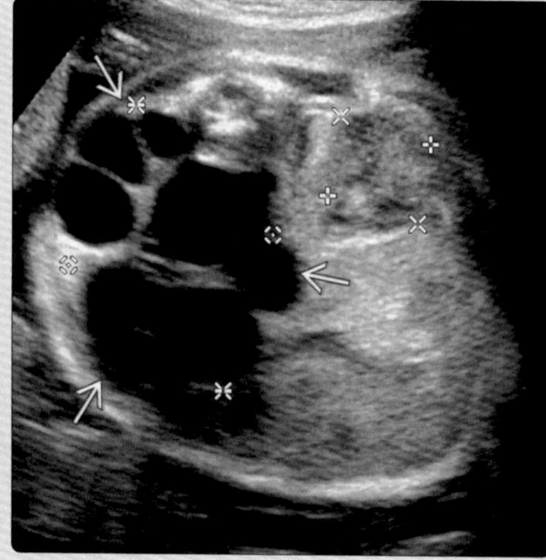

(Left) *Graphic of multicystic dysplastic kidney (MCDK) shows cysts of variable size have replaced the renal parenchyma. The cysts usually completely replace kidney, but MCDK can be segmental with some normal remaining parenchyma, as shown in the lower pole.* **(Right)** *Axial US shows a massively enlarged MCDK ➡, which crosses the midline, extends to anterior abdominal wall, and has lost its reniform shape. Compare size with normal contralateral kidney (calipers). MCDK kidneys often grow in fetal life but atrophy after birth.*

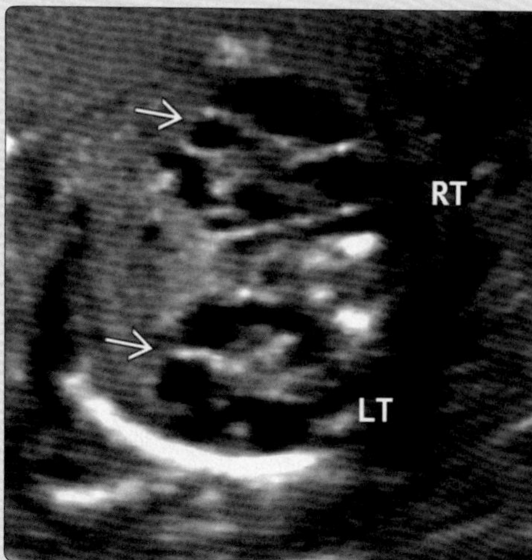

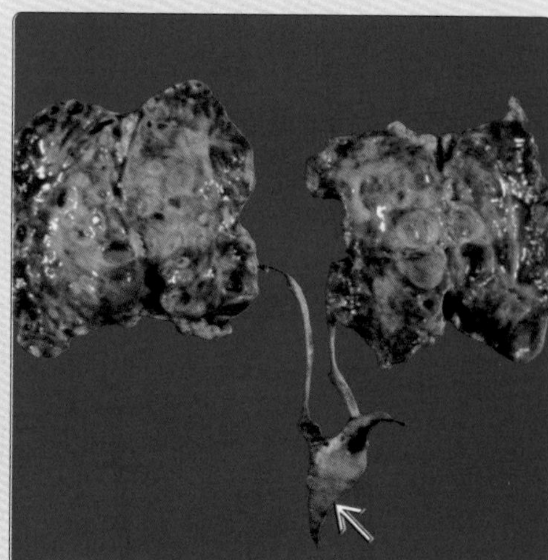

(Left) *Axial US through the kidneys at the time of anatomy scan at 20 weeks shows bilateral MCDK. The renal parenchyma is almost completely replaced by cysts ➡. Also, there is no measurable amniotic fluid. Prognosis is grim because of lack of fluid and secondary severe pulmonary hypoplasia.* **(Right)** *Gross pathology of bilateral MCDK (kidneys are bisected in the coronal plane) shows innumerable cysts. MCDKs do not function, and therefore, the bladder ➡ is atretic. Bilateral MCDK is almost always fatal.*

KEY FACTS

IMAGING

- Exclusively in male fetuses
- Bladder often grossly dilated, filling entire abdomen and increasing abdominal circumference
- Distended bladder "funnels" into urethra
  - **Keyhole sign** from dilated posterior urethra
- Small, bell-shaped chest
- Hydronephrosis/hydroureter
- Rupture → urinoma or urinary ascites
- Oligohydramnios or anhydramnios in severe cases
- Kidneys may show signs of obstructive renal dysplasia

TOP DIFFERENTIAL DIAGNOSES

- Cloacal malformation seen exclusively in females
  - Dilated, fluid-filled vagina can mimic bladder
- Prune-belly syndrome

CLINICAL ISSUES

- Most common cause of fetal lower urinary tract obstruction
- Variable degree of fetal renal damage, directly affects long-term outcomes and survival (overall mortality: 25-50%)
- May tap fetal bladder and assess urine electrolytes
  - Intervention (e.g., vesicoamniotic shunt) may be considered in cases with good prognostic markers

SCANNING TIPS

- If bladder appears large, check several times during exam to see if it decompresses
  - Likely normal if otherwise normal urinary tract and normal amniotic fluid
- Determine sex
  - May be difficult in setting of oligohydramnios
  - If female, what appears to be a dilated bladder may actually be vagina
- Obtain focused images of bladder base to evaluate for dilation of posterior urethra (keyhole)
- Evaluate kidneys for signs of renal parenchymal damage
  - Increased echogenicity, small cortical cysts, atrophy

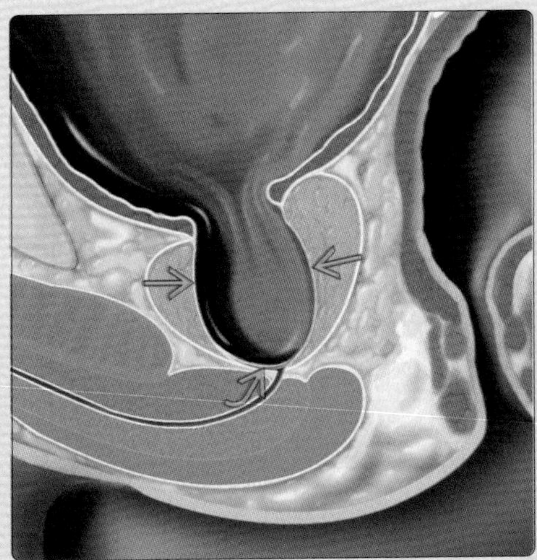

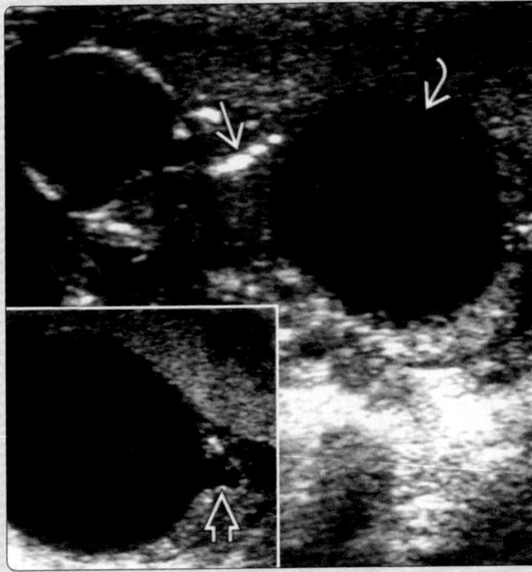

(Left) *Sagittal graphic shows the bladder funneling into a dilated posterior urethra* ➡*. The valve forms a thin membrane* ➡*, blocking antegrade flow of urine and creating a lower urinary tract obstruction (LUTO).* **(Right)** *US at 15 weeks shows gross distention of the bladder* ➡*, with severe oligohydramnios and a small, bell-shaped chest* ➡*. The inset shows dilatation of the posterior urethra* ➡*, the keyhole sign. This is the "key" to the diagnosis and differentiates posterior urethral valves from other causes of LUTO.*

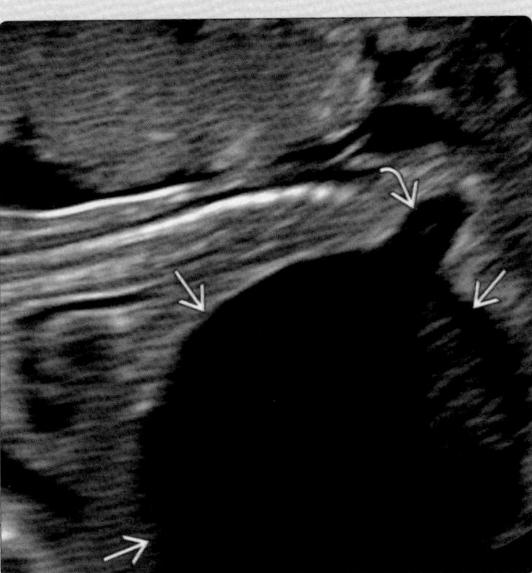

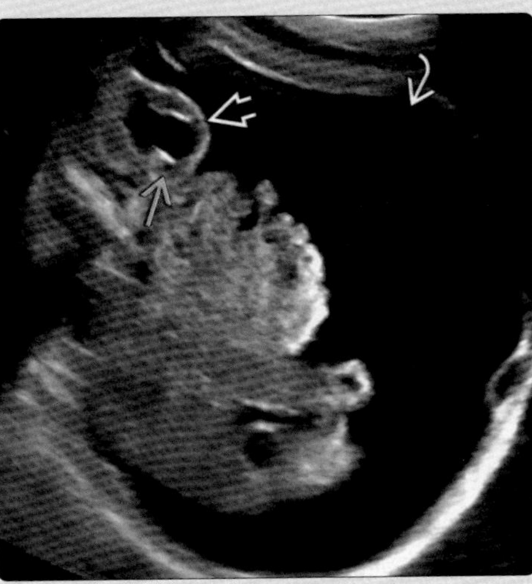

(Left) *The dilated posterior urethra* ➡ *at the base of the dilated bladder* ➡ *results in a keyhole sign. Always scan the bladder base carefully looking for this finding.* **(Right)** *When bladder distention is severe, rupture can occur, resulting in urinary ascites* ➡*, sometimes massive, as in this case. The visible kidney is abnormal with thinned parenchyma* ➡ *and small scattered cysts* ➡*. These findings are characteristic of obstructive renal dysplasia and are a poor prognostic sign.*

Prune-Belly Syndrome

KEY FACTS

TERMINOLOGY

- Disorder characterized by 3 principle components
  - Dramatic collecting system dilatation
  - Deficiency of abdominal musculature
  - Cryptorchidism (undescended testes)

IMAGING

- Gross dilatation of bladder, ureters, and renal pelves
- Urethral dilation without obvious point of obstruction
- Scan genitalia: Look for undescended testes
- Oligohydramnios often present

CLINICAL ISSUES

- Almost all cases are male fetuses
- Prognosis dependent on severity of oligohydramnios (results in pulmonary hypoplasia) and renal damage
- Postnatal flaccid, "doughy" abdomen from lack of musculature
- ~ 1/2 of patients surviving infancy will develop chronic renal disease

SCANNING TIPS

- Difficult to differentiate from posterior urethral valves (PUV); look for following differentiators
- Prune-belly syndrome (PBS) does not have dilated posterior urethra
  - **No keyhole sign** as seen with PUV
  - Entire urethra may be dilated
- Ureters and kidneys always dilated with PBS
  - May be normal with PUV
- Bladder wall is thin with PBS
  - Often thickened and trabeculated with PUV
  - May be difficult to see when bladder is dilated but pay particular attention if bladder is tapped
- Scan genitalia looking for undescended testes
  - Important feature of PBS

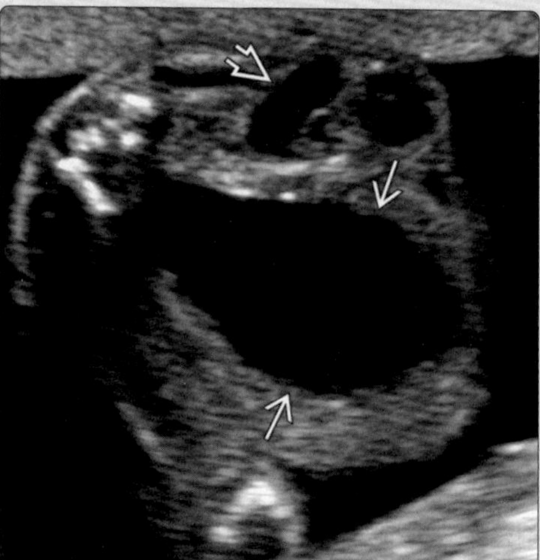

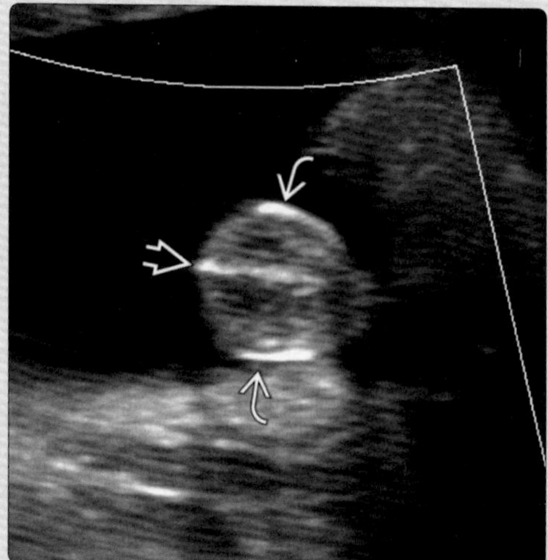

(Left) *At 21-weeks gestation, the bladder is already markedly enlarged ➡, extending well into the abdomen with adjacent hydroureter ➡. Note the absence of a keyhole sign, which is usually seen with posterior urethral valves.* **(Right)** *After 28-weeks gestation, the testes should be descended into the scrotal sac. When prune-belly syndrome is suspected, careful evaluation of the scrotum will show an empty sac ➡ with a lack of the typical echogenic oval testes. The median raphe of the scrotum ➡ is noted.*

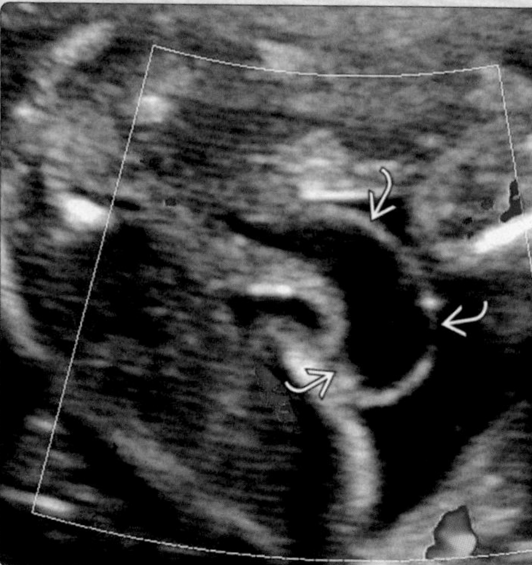

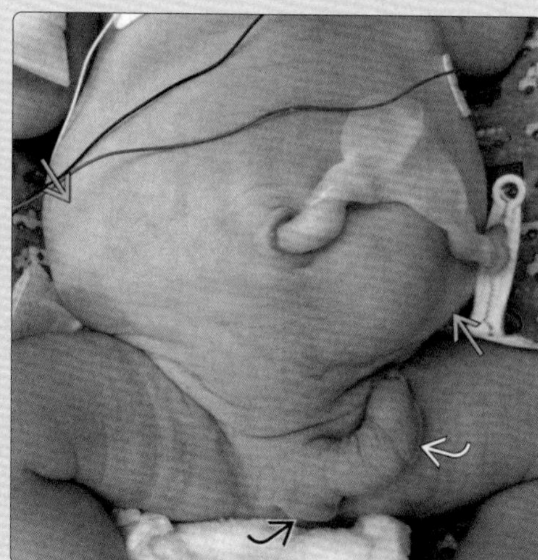

(Left) *One key finding that can help distinguish prune belly from posterior urethral valves is a dilated anterior urethra. In this fetus, an axial view through the perineum shows a massively distended penile urethra ➡.* **(Right)** *Postnatal clinical photo of the same fetus shows abdominal wall laxity ➡ due to deficiency of the abdominal wall musculature. This appearance gave rise to the name prune-belly syndrome. There is distended penis due to the dilated urethra ➡ and undescended testes (empty scrotal sac) ➡.*

KEY FACTS

IMAGING

- > 90% of fetal cases arise in adrenal gland
- May be solid, cystic, or mixed
  - Cystic appearance may represent involuting tumor and is excellent prognosis
- Calcification may be present but less common than in pediatric age group
- Liver most common location for metastases; may form discrete nodules or be diffusely infiltrating
- Look for placental metastases especially if maternal symptoms of preeclampsia

TOP DIFFERENTIAL DIAGNOSES

- Extralobar sequestration may present as suprarenal mass
  - Left-sided mass; separate normal adrenal gland
  - Dominant feeding vessel from aorta
- Adrenal hemorrhage much more common in pediatric population but has been reported in utero
  - No flow on Doppler; will involute over several weeks

CLINICAL ISSUES

- Variable fetal course
  - May resolve spontaneously, remain stable, or rarely progress to hydrops and even death
- Most fetal neuroblastomas have both favorable stage and biologic markers and have excellent prognosis

SCANNING TIPS

- Must perform careful, focused, high-frequency exam looking for normal adrenal gland
  - No normal adrenal gland supports neuroblastoma
  - If present, sequestration is more likely
- Assess vascularity with color Doppler
  - Some flow but no dominant feeding vessel
- Careful examination of liver for metastases
  - Diffusely infiltrating metastases are difficult to diagnose
  - Be suspicious when hepatomegaly or hydrops is present
- Close follow-up as may either grow or regress
- Monitor for hydrops

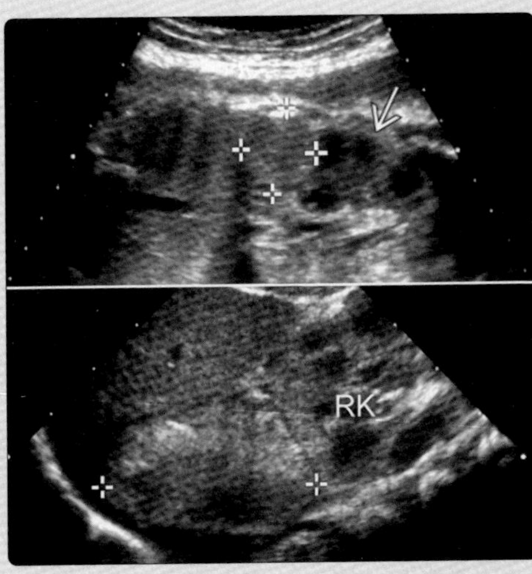

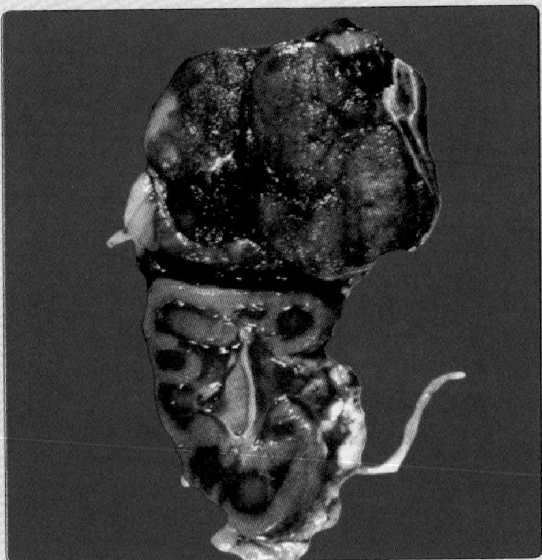

(Left) *Coronal ultrasound of the fetal abdomen (top) shows a solid, echogenic mass (calipers) above the right kidney ➡. Sagittal ultrasound after delivery (bottom) confirms a solid, suprarenal mass (calipers).* **(Right)** *Photograph of the surgical specimen shows the adrenal mass compressing the upper pole of the kidney. Most fetal neuroblastoma is low risk and has both a favorable stage and biologic markers. Current treatment recommendations are for a more conservative approach, with many being followed rather than resected.*

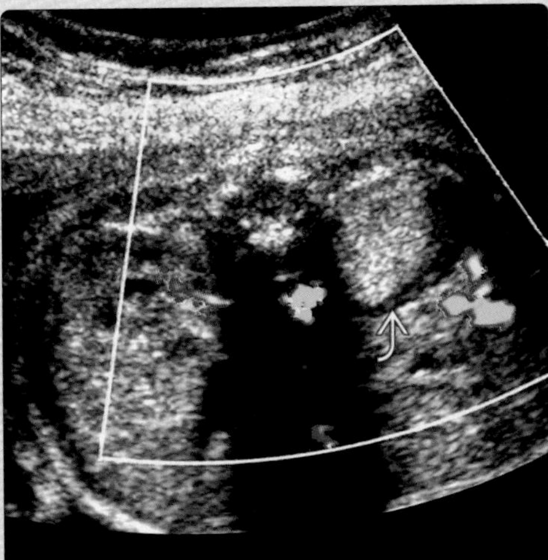

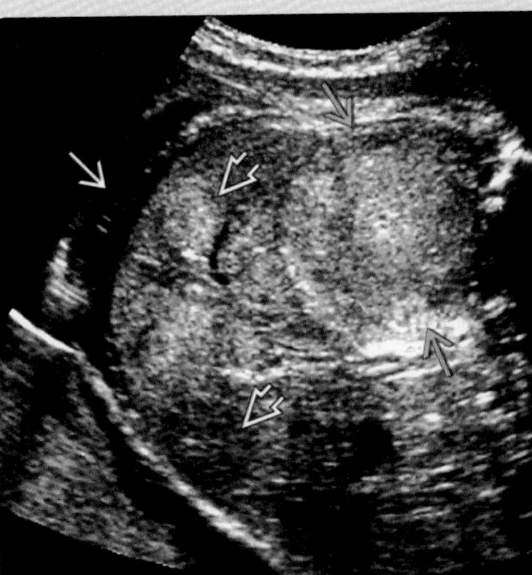

(Left) *Axial color Doppler US shows an echogenic mass in the left renal fossa (the left kidney was displaced inferiorly). A thin rim of normal adrenal cortex remains ➡. It is important to interrogate the mass with color Doppler to rule out a feeding vessel, as would be seen with a sequestration.* **(Right)** *Axial US shows an adrenal mass ➡. In addition, the liver is heterogeneous, with several discrete metastases ➡ and ascites ➡. Solid tumors are more likely to metastasize than cystic ones.*

KEY FACTS

TERMINOLOGY

- Disorders of sexual development (DSD)
- Most common DSD if karyotype is XY (male)
  - Hypospadias: Urethra opens on underside of penis
  - Epispadias (less common): Urethra opens on top of penis
  - Cryptorchidism: Empty, small scrotum
    - Often with small or abnormal penis
- Most common DSD if karyotype is XX (female)
  - Clitoromegaly ± congenital adrenal hyperplasia (CAH)
    - CAH causes virilization
  - Prominent or fused labia (less common)

IMAGING

- Hypospadias
  - Penis ends bluntly instead of normal taper
    - Lateral echogenic lines at tip = prepuce folds
  - Penis may be small and curved upward (chordee)
  - Tulip sign: Small, curved penis between scrotal folds
- Epispadias: Small, bifid penis
  - Associated with bladder extrophy
- Clitoromegaly (mimics small penis)
  - Associated prominent or fused labia mimic scrotum
  - CAD association: Adrenal glands may be large or normal

CLINICAL ISSUES

- Sex of fetus from genetic testing is key to diagnosis
- Some aspect of DSD seen in 1-2% of all live births
- Hypospadias in 1:200-250 males
- CAH is autosomal recessive (25% recurrence risk)
- Aneuploidy association: Trisomy 13, triploidy, trisomy 18
- Associated anomalies in 1/2 (most upper urinary tract)

SCANNING TIPS

- Do not assign sex at time of scan when DSD is suspected
- Pay attention to morphology of tip of phallus
- Look for testes in scrotum after 25 weeks
  - 97% descended by 32 weeks

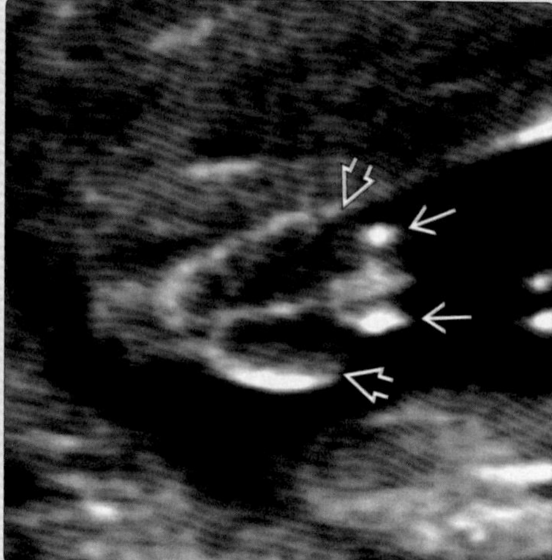

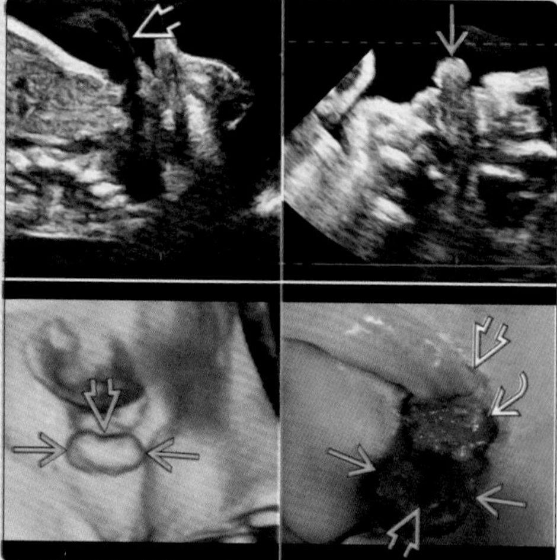

(Left) *Axial view of penis and scrotum of an XY fetus with tulip sign from hypospadias shows small penis with blunt tip and echogenic prepuce folds ➡ tucked between small scrotum ➡ without testes. The karyotype information is key to the diagnosis.* **(Right)** *Ultrasound with 3D reformatting and clinical picture of epispadias shows a small, broad, bifid penis ➡ with a cleft ➡. This fetus had bladder extrophy ➡ and low-lying cord insertion ➡ directly above the genitalia. These are hallmark findings for bladder extrophy.*

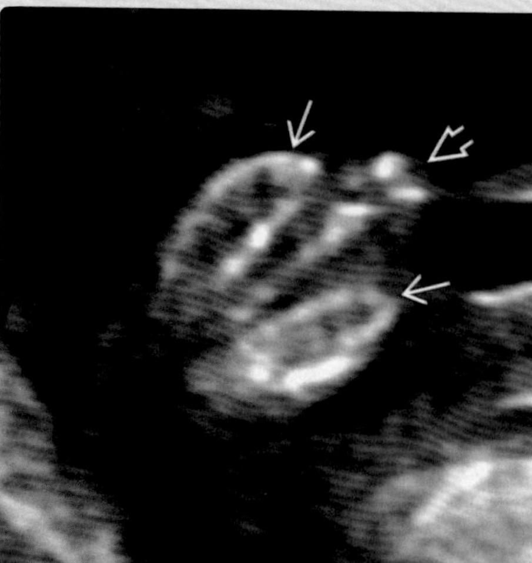

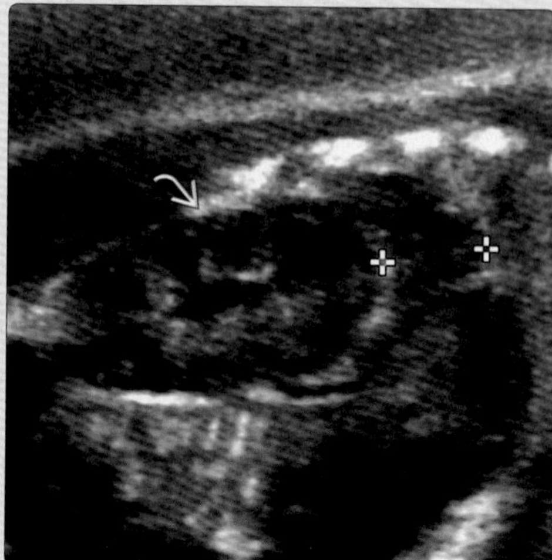

(Left) *Axial view through the perineum at the time of anatomy scan shows DSD. There are bilateral soft tissue mounds ➡ that may represent the labia or scrotum, and a central phallus ➡ that may be a clitoris or penis. Genetic testing showed XX, and therefore this represents clitoromegaly.* **(Right)** *Coronal view of the kidney ➡ and adrenal gland (calipers) in the same case shows an enlarged adrenal gland (normative data for adrenal size is available). This fetus has congenital adrenal hyperplasia, causing virilization.*

KEY FACTS

IMAGING

- Abdominal cyst in female fetus typically located in lower lateral abdomen or pelvis
  - Large cysts may extend into upper abdomen
- Well circumscribed, generally anechoic, unilocular, avascular with imperceptible walls
  - May have occasional septations
- Daughter cyst sign: Small follicle along wall of cystic mass
  - Highly specific for ovarian origin
  - 82% sensitive
- May be bilateral
- If cyst is seen before 3rd trimester, it is very unlikely that it is ovarian in origin
  - Fetal ovaries are too immature to respond to maternal/placental hormones before 3rd trimester

SCANNING TIPS

- Check fetal sex
  - **Ovarian cyst is most common cause of intraabdominal cyst in female fetus**
  - Male sex excludes diagnosis
- Confirm normal appearance of gastrointestinal and hepatobiliary systems
  - Use high-resolution transducer to characterize cyst wall
    - Layered gut signature in cyst wall is diagnostic of enteric duplication cyst
- Confirm normal urinary tract
  - High number of cystic abdominal masses are related to urinary tract
- Comment on size
  - Large cyst (> 6 cm) associated with increased risk of hemorrhage and torsion
- Consider torsion if
  - New fluid-fluid level
  - Previously anechoic or hypoechoic cyst becomes hyperechoic

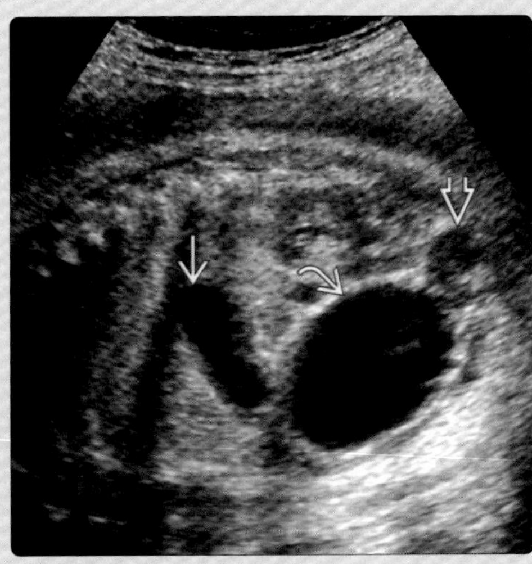

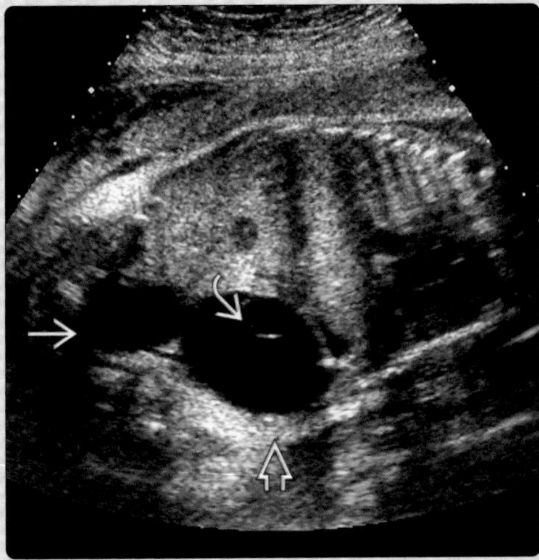

(Left) *Sagittal US shows a unilocular, simple cyst ➔ arising from the pelvis, anterior and superior to the bladder ➔ and inferior to the stomach ➔. The cyst was shown to be separate from the kidney and liver, and an ovarian cyst was suspected.* **(Right)** *Coronal US in a 3rd-trimester female fetus shows a large cyst ➔ above the bladder ➔. There is a smaller daughter cyst ➔ within the larger cyst. This is the most specific finding for an ovarian cyst.*

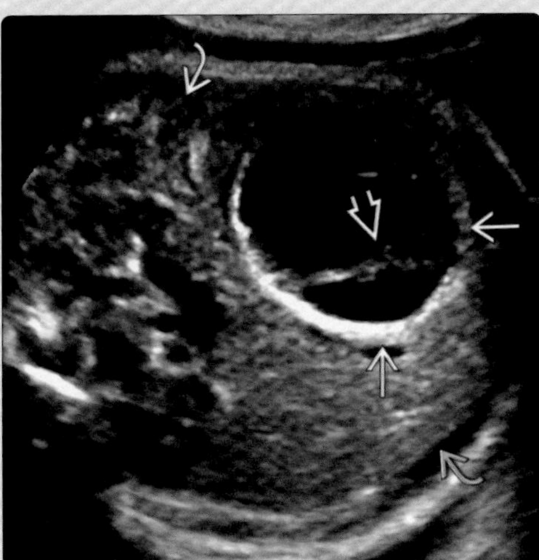

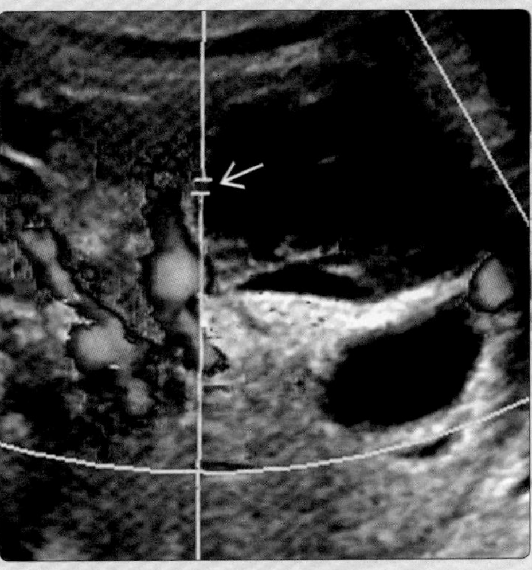

(Left) *Axial US in a 3rd-trimester female fetus shows a well-circumscribed, thick-walled cystic mass ➔ with internal amorphous echogenic material ➔. It is anterior to the kidney ➔ and well demarcated from the liver ➔.* **(Right)** *Power Doppler US shows flow in the wall of the mass ➔ (spectral Doppler not included). Despite this, at surgery, there was torsion and infarction of the ovary. Complex ovarian cysts are much more likely to have internal hemorrhage, which is strongly associated with torsion.*

PART VI
SECTION 8
Musculoskeletal

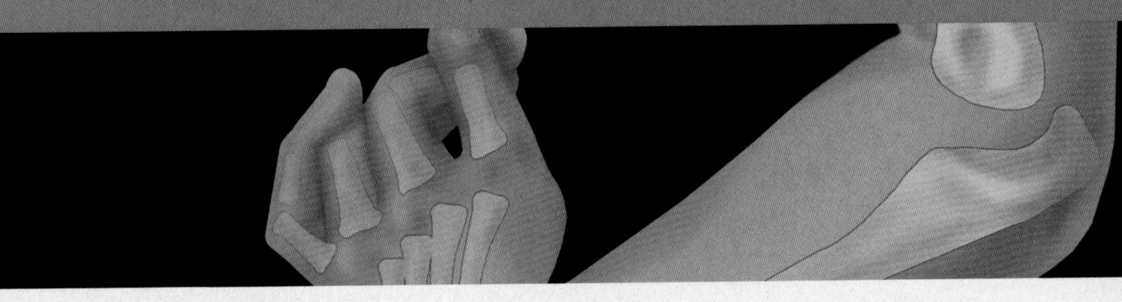

Dysplasias

Extremity Malformations

Achondrogenesis

KEY FACTS

TERMINOLOGY

- **Lethal skeletal dysplasia** with 3 clinical subtypes
  - Type IA (poorly ossified skull, unossified spine)
  - Type IB (poorly ossified skull, rib fractures)
  - Type II (normal skull ossification)

IMAGING

- Severe micromelia
  - All long bones are several standard deviations below mean for gestational age
- Disproportionately large head
  - Normal or deficient ossification depending on type
- Abnormal facies
  - Micrognathia, hypoplastic midface
- **Lack of vertebral ossification is hallmark finding**
- Short trunk with protuberant abdomen
- Short flared ribs, ± rib fractures depending upon type
- Polyhydramnios
- Hydrops in 1/3 of cases

SCANNING TIPS

- 1st-trimester endovaginal ultrasound in high-risk patient (autosomal recessive inheritance in some types)
  - Cystic hygroma; increased nuchal translucency common in 1st trimester
  - Can be diagnosed as early as 12-14 weeks based on limb appearances
- In any fetus with visually shortened long bones
  - Measure **femur:foot ratio**; if < 1, suggests skeletal dysplasia
  - Then, measure all long bones and compare to expected length for gestational age
- Other useful ratios in determination of lethal skeletal dysplasia
  - Femur length:abdominal circumference ratio < 0.16 suggests lethality
  - Chest circumference:abdominal circumference ratio < 0.8 suggests lethality

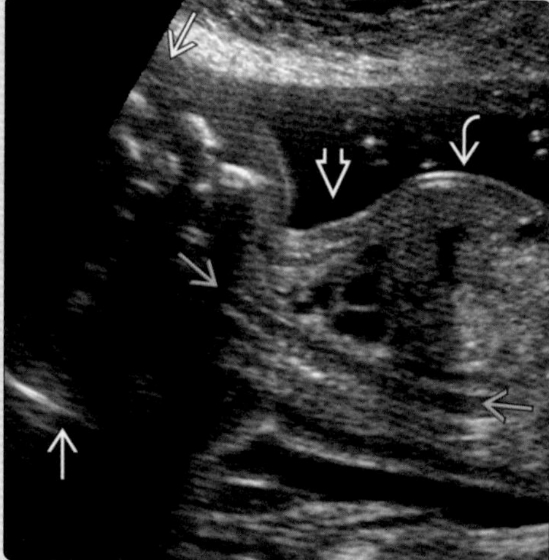

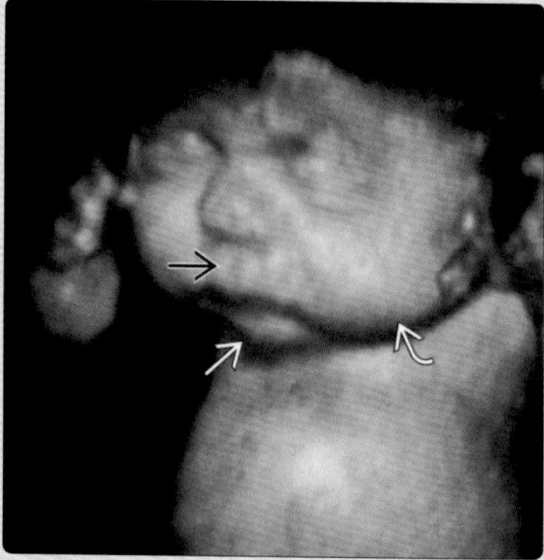

(Left) *Sagittal ultrasound of a 2nd-trimester fetus shows large head size ➡, very small chest size ➡, protuberant abdomen ➡, and complete lack of vertebral ossification ➡. These are typical findings of achondrogenesis with the lack of vetebral ossification being the most specific. Carefully evaluate the spine in all skeletal dysplasia cases.* **(Right)** *3D ultrasound shows the typical facial appearance late in the 2nd trimester. Micrognathia is striking ➡. Note the prominent cheeks ➡ and long philtrum ➡.*

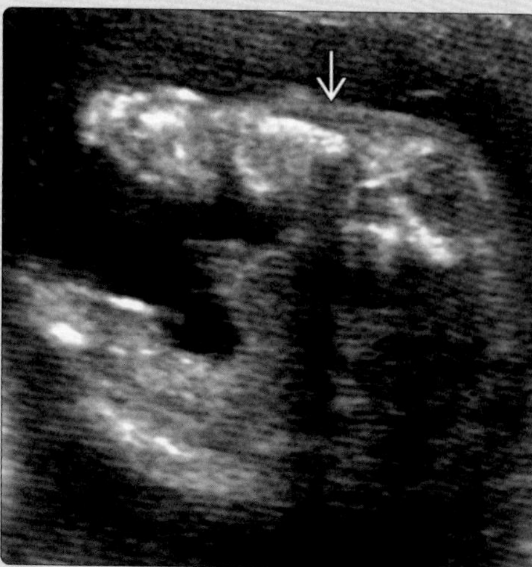

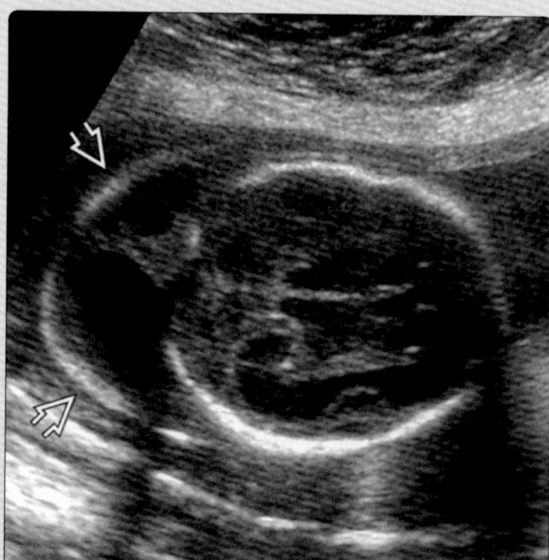

(Left) *Ultrasound of the legs shows severe micromelia ➡. Other images showed bilateral clubfeet. In any fetus with micromelia, the next steps include assessment of skull shape and ossification, long bone shape and ossification, and evaluation for fractures.* **(Right)** *Axial ultrasound shows normal shape and ossification of the calvarium. This is seen in type II achondrogenesis; the skull is underossified in type I. A cystic hygroma ➡ is a described association of several skeletal dysplasias.*

Achondroplasia

KEY FACTS

TERMINOLOGY

- Most common nonlethal skeletal dysplasia

IMAGING

- **Long bones**
  - Short limbs with normal ossification, no fractures
  - Rhizomelia: Proximal long bones (femur, humerus) more affected than distal long bones
  - Upper extremities more severely affected than lower
  - Femurs may show mild bowing but no angulation
  - Shortening often not present until late 2nd and 3rd trimester
- **Head and face**
  - Progressive macrocephaly with frontal bossing
  - Depressed nasal bridge with upturned nasal tip
- Chest normal to mildly bell-shaped
- Spine has prominent thoracolumbar kyphosis
- Trident-shaped hands with short fingers

CLINICAL ISSUES

- Autosomal dominant inheritance
  - If one parent has achondroplasia, fetus has 50% chance of being affected
- Over 80% of cases new mutations, so neither parent may be affected

SCANNING TIPS

- In any case of suspected skeletal dysplasia, pay particular attention to appearance and ossification of long bones
- Profile views and 3D images of face are very important to look for classic features
- Obtain sagittal views of spine to look for abnormal outward curvature (kyphosis)
- Need to follow-up at-risk fetuses (i.e., parent with achondroplasia)
  - Limb shortening and classic facial features may not be apparent at time of routine anatomy scan

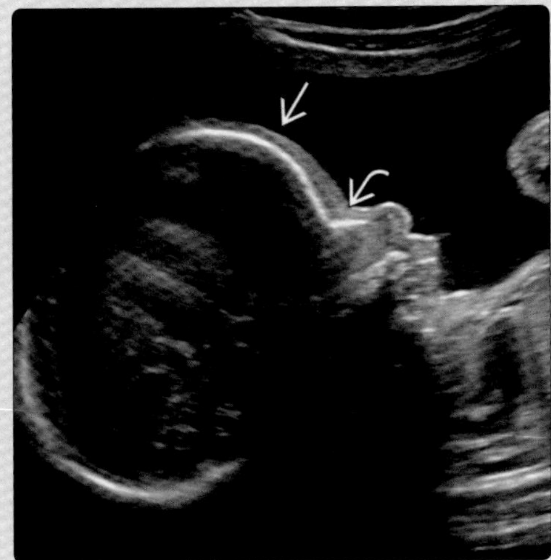

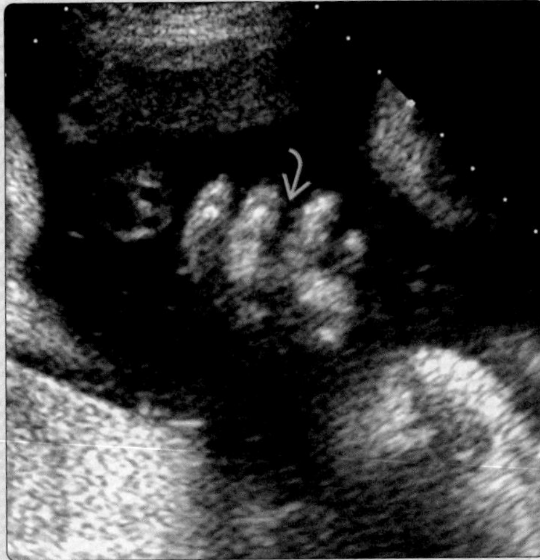

(Left) *Sagittal US shows the typical 3rd-trimester profile of a fetus with achondroplasia. Note the frontal bossing ➡ and the depressed nasal bridge ➡. The head circumference was > 95% for gestational age.* **(Right)** *Ultrasound shows the typical appearance of a trident hand of a fetus with achondroplasia. Note that all the fingers are of similar lengths and all the digits and are mildly splayed ➡.*

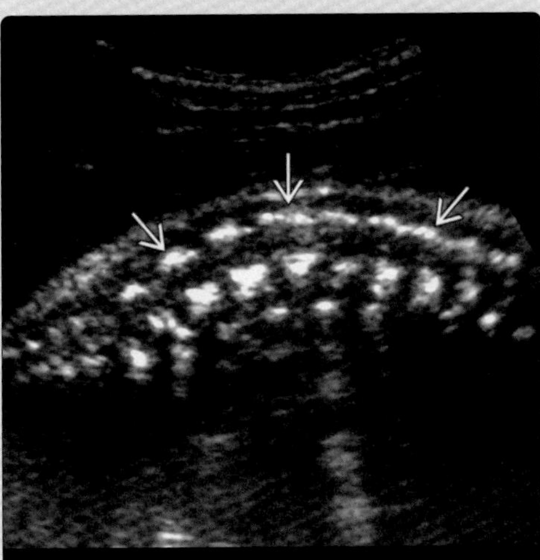

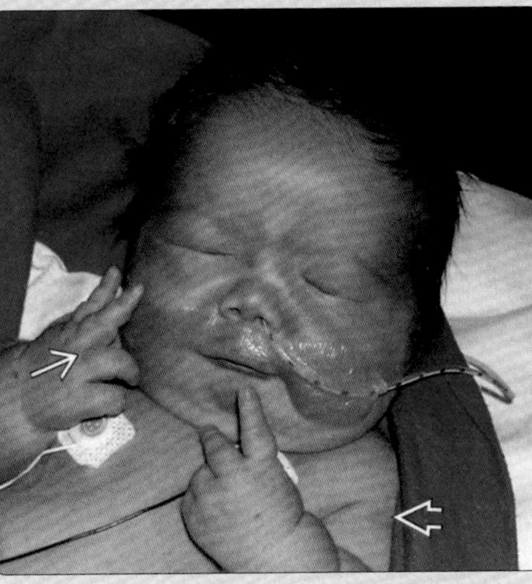

(Left) *Sagittal ultrasound shows the lower spine in a 3rd-trimester fetus with achondroplasia. There is a very prominent kyphosis of the lumbar spine ➡, a common finding in achondroplasia.* **(Right)** *Clinical photograph shows typical facial findings of achondroplasia with a flat midface, depressed nasal bridge, and upturned nasal tip. Note the trident hand ➡ and short humerus ➡. Long bone shortening was not significant until the 3rd trimester.*

Osteogenesis Imperfecta

KEY FACTS

TERMINOLOGY

- Genetically and clinically, heterogeneous group of connective tissue disorders presenting with osteoporosis and fractures
  - 90% of cases due to abnormalities in type I collagen
- Newer osteogenesis imperfecta (OI) nomenclature further subdivides 5 classic phenotypes
  - Type II (perinatal lethal OI) with most obvious in utero findings
- Presence of fractures distinguishes OI from most other skeletal dysplasias

IMAGING

- Long bone shortening/angulation secondary to fractures
- Callus formation gives bones crumpled appearance
- Poor mineralization especially noticeable in skull
  - Skull deformation from normal transducer pressure
  - Anatomy "seen too well" with no reverberation artifact
- Small chest with beaded (fractured) ribs

TOP DIFFERENTIAL DIAGNOSES

- Hypophosphatasia has generalized demineralization
  - Bones are thin and bowed but true fractures uncommon
- Achondrogenesis
  - Unossified spine is key finding, type 1A with rib fractures

SCANNING TIPS

- 1st-trimester endovaginal US in high-risk patients
  - Normal US does not exclude OI in high-risk patients
- Measure all long bones/assess for fractures
  - Severe shortening in perinatal lethal form
  - Pay special attention to femora
    - Less severe forms may present with apparently isolated bent femora
- Apply gentle pressure while scanning brain to look for flattening of calvarium
- Scan chest in coronal plane to look for beading of ribs
- Compare chest to abdominal circumference
  - Small chest → increased risk for pulmonary hypoplasia

(Left) *Longitudinal femoral US of a fetus with nonlethal osteogenesis imperfecta (OI) shows curvature of the femur ➡ and distal fracture with callus formation ➡. Autopsy photograph from a case of perinatal lethal OI shows severe crumpling of the femur. In general, fewer fractures are seen in the nonlethal forms of OI.* **(Right)** *Cranial US of a 3rd-trimester fetus with OI shows undermineralization with flattening of the skull ➡ with normal transducer pressure. Often, the brain is seen "too well" when the skull lacks normal ossification.*

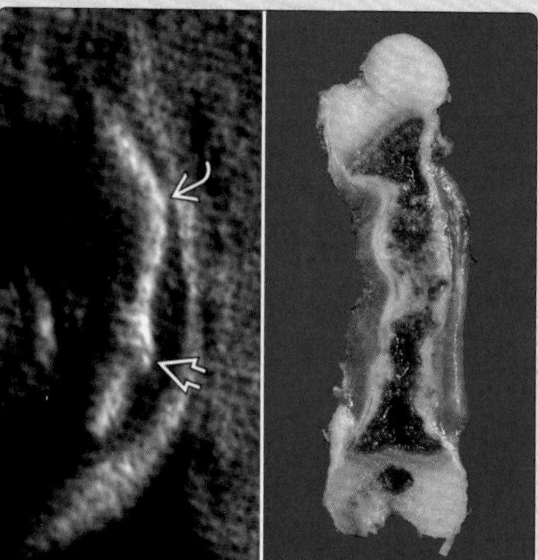

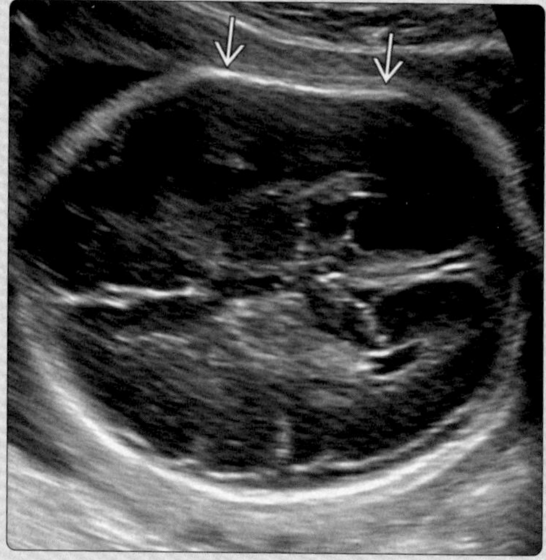

(Left) *Coronal US through the thorax and 1 upper extremity of a midtrimester fetus with OI shows a small chest ➡ and irregular, beaded ribs ➡ from multiple fractures. Note also the multiple fractures ➡ in the long bones of the arm.* **(Right)** *Frontal radiograph correlates with the findings seen on US. There are multiple rib fractures creating a beaded appearance. The arms and legs are short due to angulation and deformity resulting from the fractures ➡.*

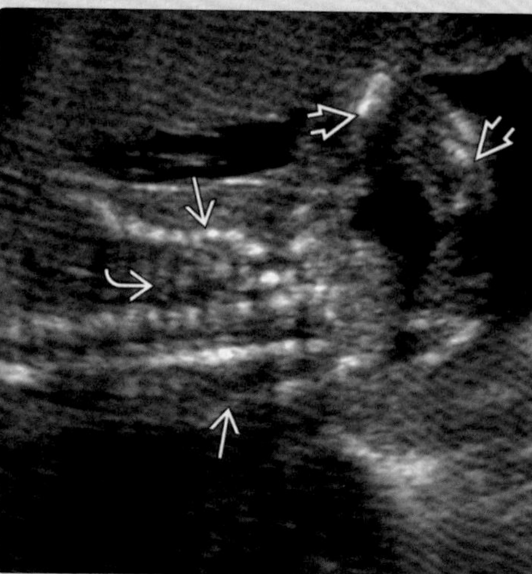

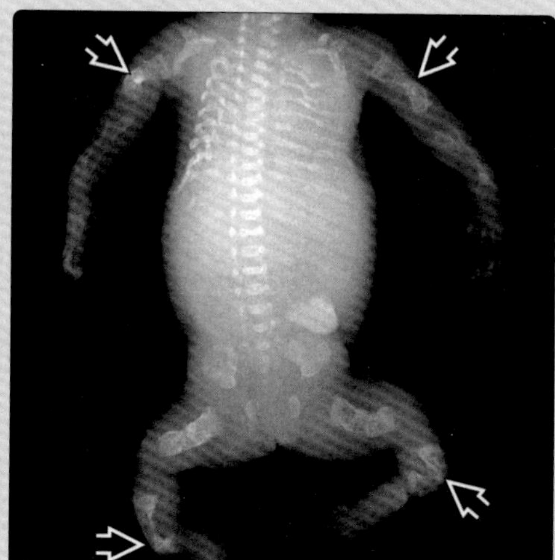

KEY FACTS

TERMINOLOGY

- **Lethal skeletal dysplasia**
  - Thanatophoric is Greek for death bearing
- Divided into 2 subtypes based on morphologic findings

IMAGING

- **Features seen in both TD1 and TD2**
  - **Micromelia**: All bones extremely short
    - Can be seen as early as 14 weeks
    - Becomes worse with advancing gestation
  - Bones normally ossified
  - Long bone bowing but no fractures
  - Chest small with short, straight ribs
  - Vertebral bodies flattened (platyspondyly) with exaggerated lumbar lordosis
  - Most have severe polyhydramnios by late 2nd trimester
- **TD type 1**
  - Femur more severely shortened and bowed
    - Telephone receiver appearance
  - Macrocephalic but relatively normal-shaped skull
- **TD type 2**
  - Distinctive cloverleaf-shaped skull (kleeblattschädel)

SCANNING TIPS

- Most important task in approaching skeletal dysplasia determining lethal vs. nonlethal
  - Lethal findings generally include micromelia and very small chest
- Obtain coronal and sagittal views of chest and abdomen
  - Abdomen will appear protuberant compared to chest
- Measure chest circumference and cardiothoracic ratio on 4-chamber view of heart
  - Heart may appear large but appearance actually because chest small
- Look carefully for more specific features
  - TD type 1: Very curved femur (telephone receiver)
  - TD type 2: Cloverleaf-shaped skull

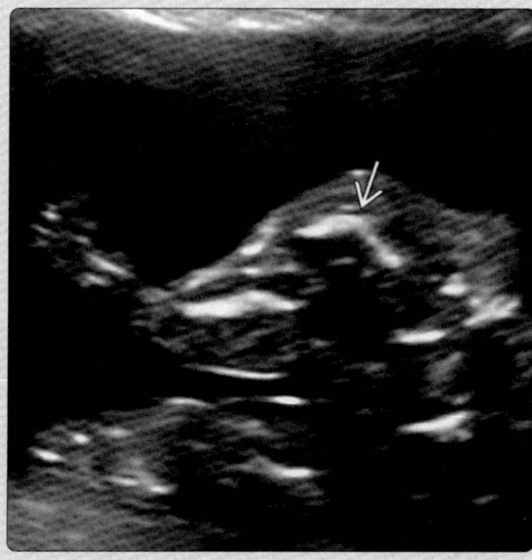

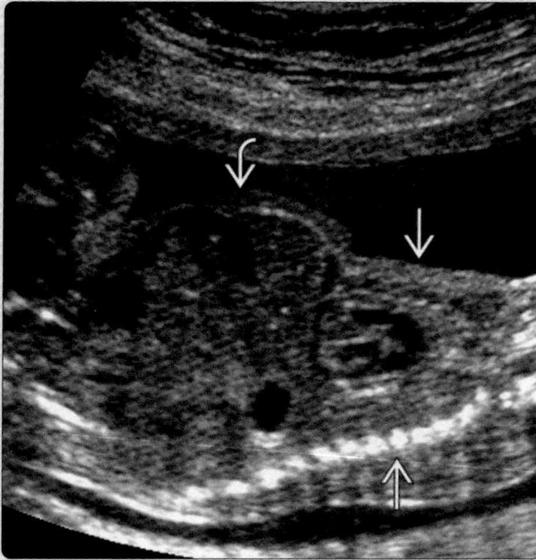

(Left) *Ultrasound shows the femur of a 2nd-trimester fetus with TD type 1. In addition to being very short, it is also bowed, which has been referred to as the telephone receiver appearance ➔.* **(Right)** *Sagittal ultrasound shows the small chest size ➔ when compared with the larger, more protuberant abdomen ➔ in a 3rd-trimester fetus with TD type 1. Chest findings are similar in both TD type 1 and 2, with pulmonary hypoplasia often being the cause of death.*

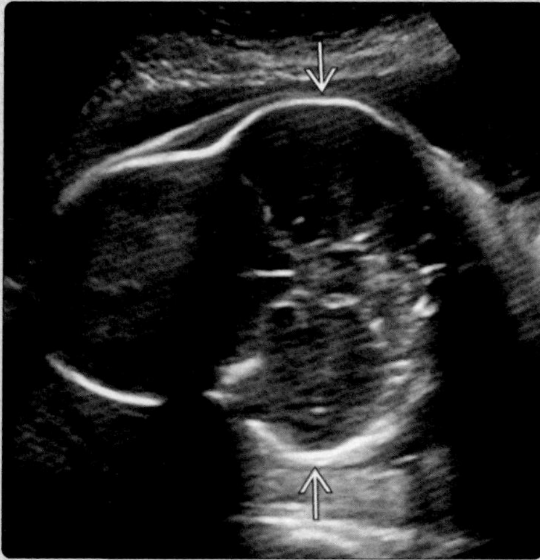

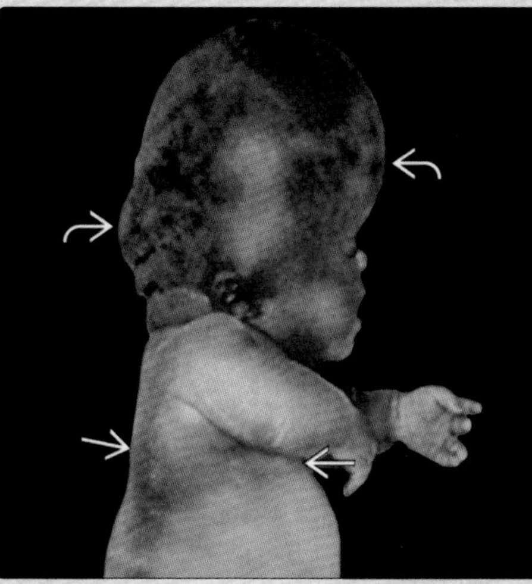

(Left) *Axial ultrasound in this 29-week fetus shows an abnormal skull configuration with bulging of the sides of the head at the skull base ➔. This is the cloverleaf skull (a.k.a. kleeblattschädel) typical of TD type 2.* **(Right)** *Clinical photograph of TD type 2 shows the cloverleaf skull shape ➔. The head is disproportionately large for the body. The chest is very small ➔. Note the short arms and fingers.*

KEY FACTS

TERMINOLOGY

- Clubfoot (talipes equinovarus)
  - Foot is turned in at ankle (varus)
  - Foot is pointed (equina)
- Rocker-bottom foot (congenital vertical talus)
  - Back of foot is convex (like bottom of rocking chair)
  - Toes are upturned

IMAGING

- Clubfoot: 2/3 bilateral
  - Frontal tibia/fibula view best to show turned-in foot
  - Plantar foot view shows short angulated foot
  - 2/3 are isolated: No other anomalies
  - Key associations: Spina bifida, arthrogryposis, aneuploidy, oligohydramnios
- Rocker-bottom foot: 2/3 bilateral
  - Sagittal view best to show morphology
  - Rarely isolated
  - Key associations: Aneuploidy (particularly trisomy 18), spine anomalies, arthrogryposis

CLINICAL ISSUES

- Clubfoot is most common musculoskeletal anomaly
  - 1-3:1,000 newborns
  - Prognosis depends on associated anomalies
  - Most do not need surgical correction
- Rocker-bottom foot requires more significant intervention

SCANNING TIPS

- 3D helps show severity
  - Bone-rendered views are additive
- Beware of transient foot position
  - Wait for feet to move away from uterus
  - Avoid 3rd-trimester diagnosis if possible
    - Higher false-positive rates
- Look carefully at spine, upper extremities, and fetal movement when lower extremity anomaly diagnosed

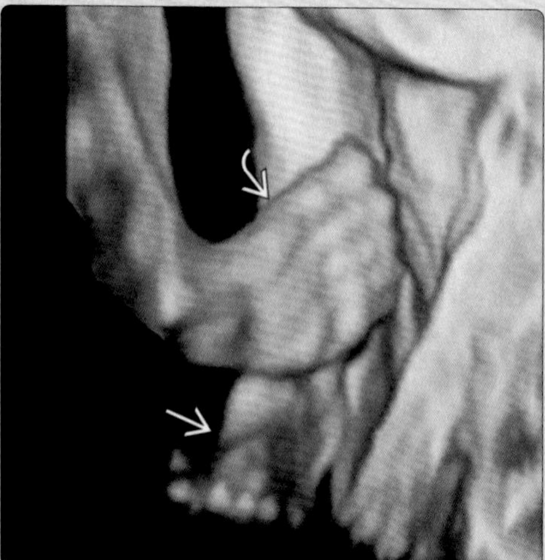

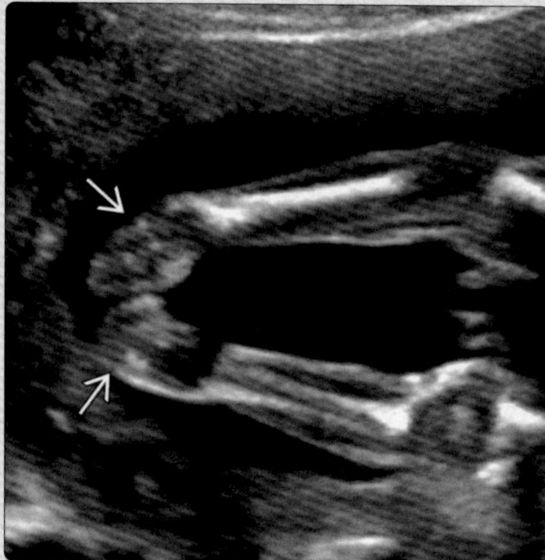

(Left) *In this case of isolated unilateral clubfoot at 24 weeks, 3D ultrasound shows a right inverted clubfoot ➢ and a normal left foot ➢. 3D images allow for better appreciation of the severity of the clubfoot and allows the patient and orthopedic team to truly see the anomaly.* **(Right)** *Frontal shin views in a 20-week fetus shows both feet turned inward ➢, classic varus deformity of clubfoot. The finding was isolated and genetic testing was not done. Bilateral isolated clubfoot does not increase risk of aneuploidy over unilateral.*

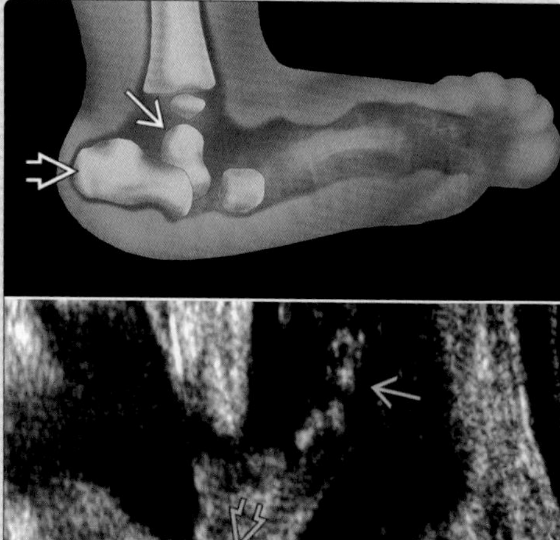

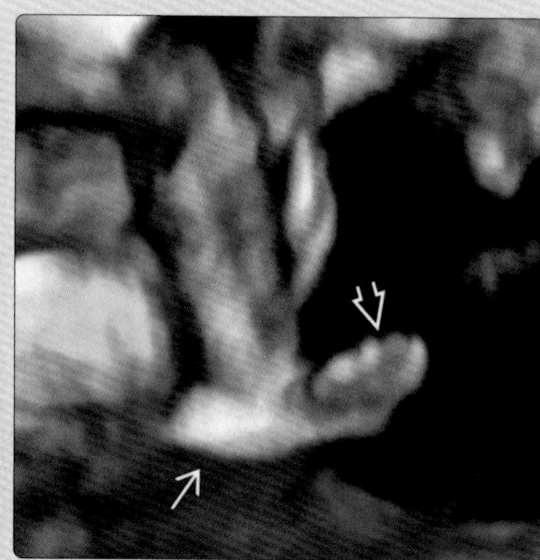

(Left) *Graphic shows a vertical talus ➢, which pushes the heel posteriorly ➢ and bows the sole, creating a rocker-bottom appearance. The correlative ultrasound shows the rocker-bottom heel ➢ and upturned toes ➢.* **(Right)** *3D ultrasound performed at the time of anatomy scan in a fetus with trisomy 18 shows classic morphology of rocker-bottom foot. The toes are upturned ➢ and the sole of the foot is convex ➢, giving the classic rocker-bottom heel. This fixed foot position is often easier to demonstrate with 3D than standard 2D ultrasound.*

KEY FACTS

TERMINOLOGY

- Spectrum of anomalies, including absence or hypoplasia of radius, radial carpal bones, &/or thumb

IMAGING

- Single forearm bone
- Radial deviation of hand
  - Fixed on prolonged scanning, not positional
- Abnormal thumbs: Use cine clips, 2D and 3D imaging
  - Absent or hypoplastic
  - Proximal implantation
  - Adducted (rolled onto palm)
  - Triphalangeal (normal thumb has only 2 phalanges)

SCANNING TIPS

- Distinguish from arthrogryposis, which also has abnormal hand position
  - Global lack of fetal movement
  - Abnormal positioning of hands and feet
  - All bones and digits present in arthrogryposis
- Look for other findings: 86% of patients with hypoplastic thumbs have other anomalies
  - Multiple anomalies increase likelihood of aneuploidy/syndrome
  - 44% have either Holt-Oram or VACTERL association
- Obtain formal fetal echocardiogram in all cases
  - Atrial septal defect is most common abnormality in Holt-Oram; very difficult fetal diagnosis
- Monitor for fetal growth restriction
  - Aneuploidy, especially trisomy 18
  - Cornelia de Lange syndrome (diaphragmatic hernia, abnormal facies)
  - Fanconi anemia (severe growth restriction, abnormal thumbs/eyes/kidneys)
- Use 3D US for facial detail/thumb morphology
  - May lead to specific syndromal diagnosis (e.g., Cornelia de Lange syndrome)

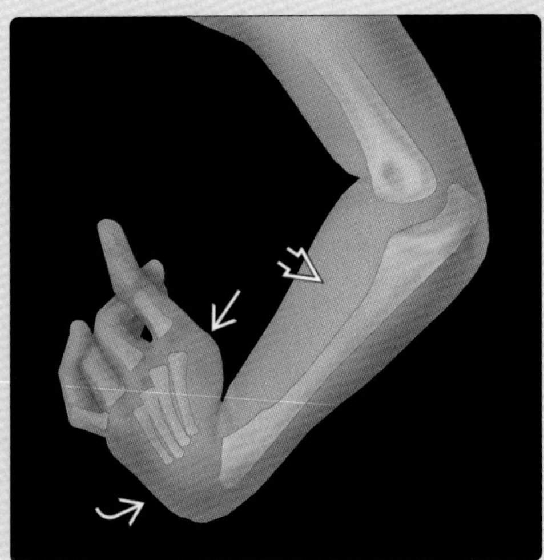

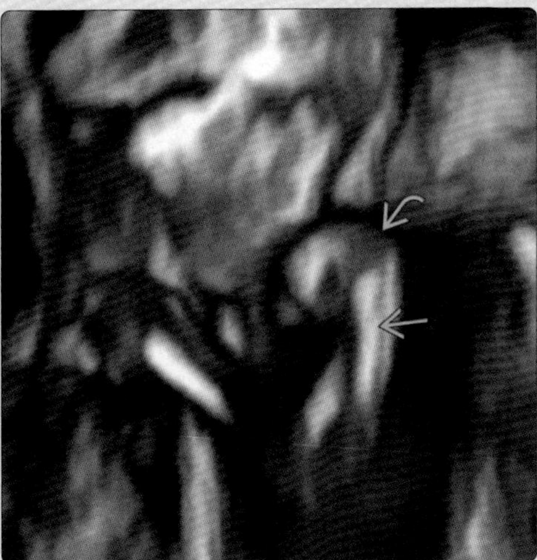

(Left) *Graphic illustrates the characteristic features of a radial ray malformation. The thumb may be absent ➡, malpositioned, hypoplastic, or triphalangeal. The hand position is often abnormal ➡. The hand is deviated toward the side of the radius, which is either absent ➡ or hypoplastic. The condition is also known as radial clubhand and radial dysplasia.* **(Right)** *3D ultrasound of a fetus with trisomy 18 and a radial ray malformation shows a single forearm bone (the ulna) ➡ with acute radial deviation of the hand at the wrist ➡.*

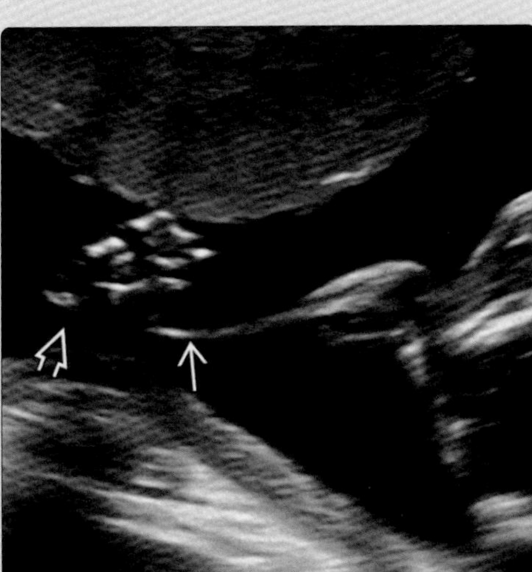

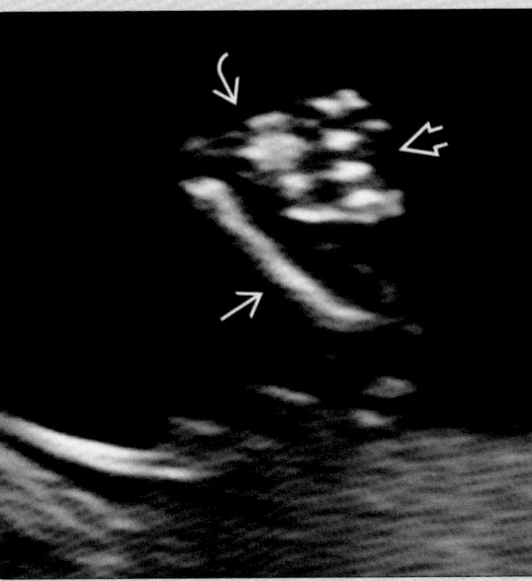

(Left) *Ultrasound of a fetus at 20 weeks with an isolated radial ray malformation is shown. The ulna is present ➡, but there is no radius. There is radial deviation at the wrist ➡ ("radial club hand"). There were 4 fingers but no thumb.* **(Right)** *Ultrasound at 14 weeks shows a single forearm bone ➡ and a sharply angled, radially deviated hand ➡ with 4 digits ➡ and absent thumb. Radial ray malformation can be detected in the 1st trimester. Cell-free DNA testing may be offered in this setting given the association with trisomy 18.*

Abnormal Hand

KEY FACTS

IMAGING

- **Polydactyly**
  - 1 or more extra digits or parts of digits
  - May be preaxial (thumb side) or postaxial (pinky side)
  - Nonsyndromal: May be isolated or familial
  - Syndromal: Common feature in multiple syndromes
  - Diabetes increases risk of preaxial polydactyly
  - Important feature of trisomy 13
- **Syndactyly**
  - Fusion of 1 or more digits; very easy to miss
  - Can be isolated but more often part of syndrome
  - Syndromic case may be extensive (mitten syndactyly)
  - Triploidy has characteristic fusion of 3rd and 4th digits
- **Clenched hand**
  - Trisomy 18; look for overriding 2nd finger
  - Feature of neuromuscular disorders (e.g., arthrogryposis)
- **Clinodactyly**
  - Radial deviation of distal 5th finger
  - 2-4% of normal fetuses have clinodactyly
  - Minor marker for trisomy 21
- **Split hand/foot malformation (ectrodactyly)**
  - Lobster claw deformity: Old term that should no longer be used
  - Deep median cleft with missing central phalanges and metacarpals/metatarsals with fusion of remaining digits
  - Creates deep cleft in midhand/foot
  - May involve only 1 or both hands/feet

SCANNING TIPS

- Easy to both under and over diagnose
- Use 3D ultrasound to aid in diagnosis
- Feet are also affected in many of these conditions but are harder to evaluate
  - Be suspicious of polydactyly when foot appears too wide
- Seldom isolated abnormality; carefully scan for other findings that would point to specific syndrome

(Left) *US of the hand of a fetus with trisomy 13 at 22-weeks gestation is shown. Postaxial polydactyly ➡ is noted with a small extra digit. An obvious bone is not seen. Postaxial polydactyly is one of the most common features in trisomy 13, in addition to severe brain, eye, cardiac, and genitourinary abnormalities.* **(Right)** *Clinical photograph of the hand shows a small extra digit ➡ attached to the 5th finger. This stillborn also had trisomy 13.*

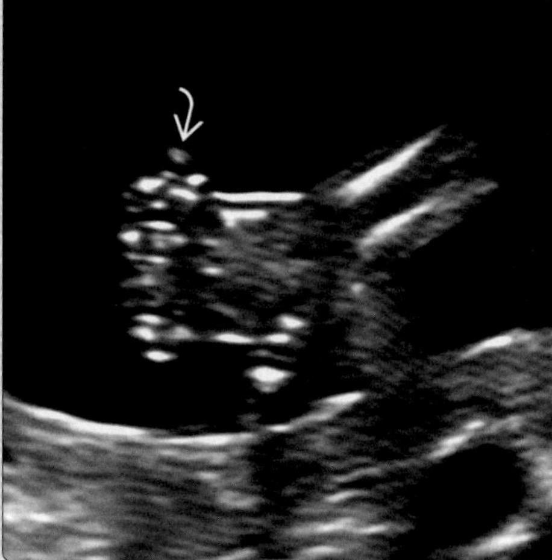

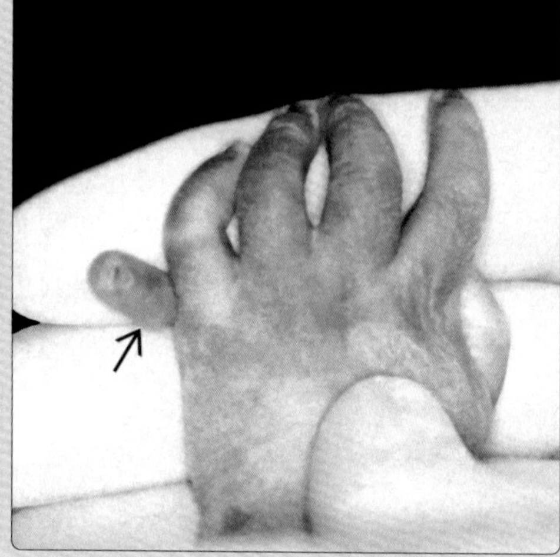

(Left) *3D US of the hand of a midtrimester fetus shows postaxial polydactyly ➡. Isolated polydactyly is usually autosomal dominant with variable penetrance. Family history is key to making the diagnosis.* **(Right)** *US and clinical photograph of a stillborn with triploidy shows the classic pattern of 3-4 syndactyly ➡. This is a typical feature of triploidy along with severe growth restriction and abnormal placenta. Isolated syndactyly is a difficult prenatal diagnosis to make and is frequently missed.*

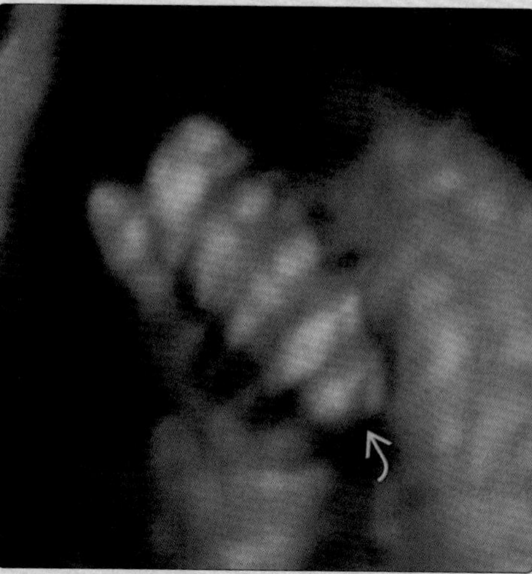

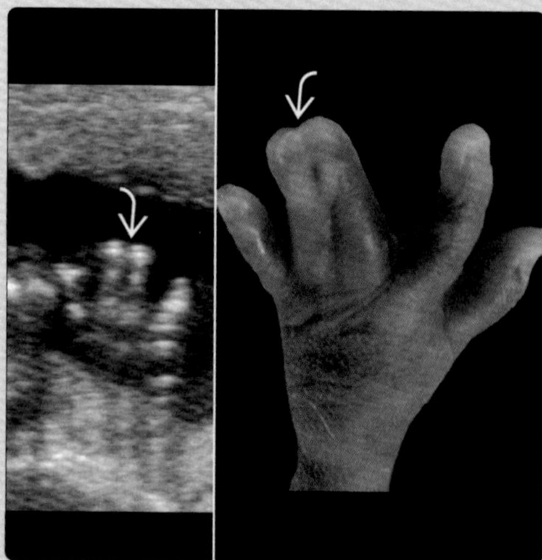

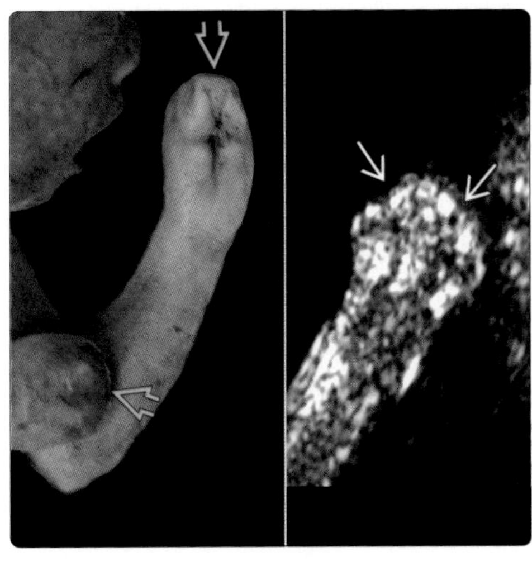

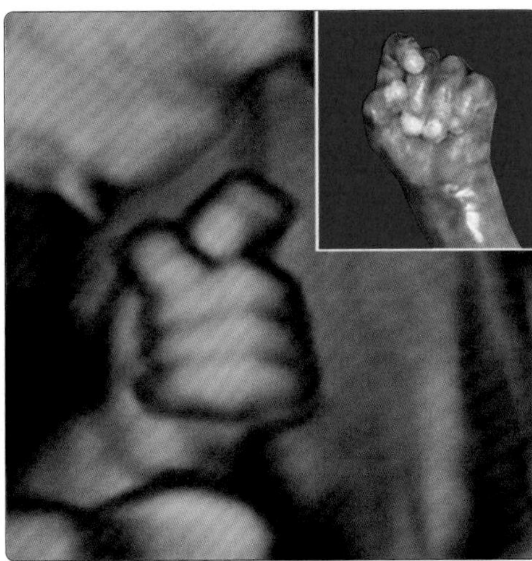

(Left) *Photograph and US of the hand in a case of Apert syndrome is shown. The US shows apparent absence of digits ➡. In fact, the digits are shortened and fused ➡ (mitten syndactyly) as shown in the gross photograph. When syndactyly is this severe, it is usually part of a syndrome, so look carefully for other findings.* **(Right)** *3D US and clinical photograph (inset) shows a clenched hand with overriding 2nd finger, typical of trisomy 18.*

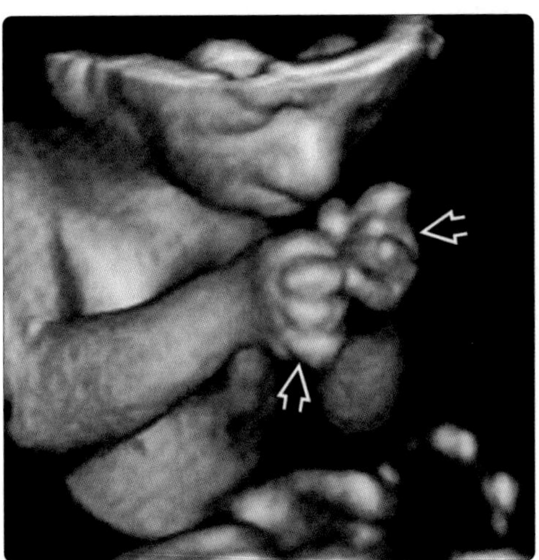

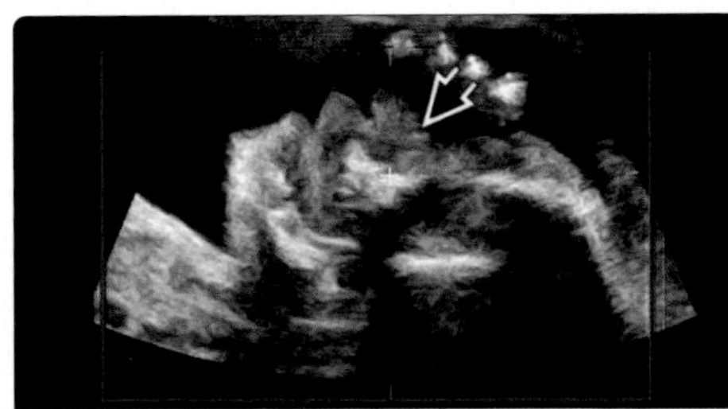

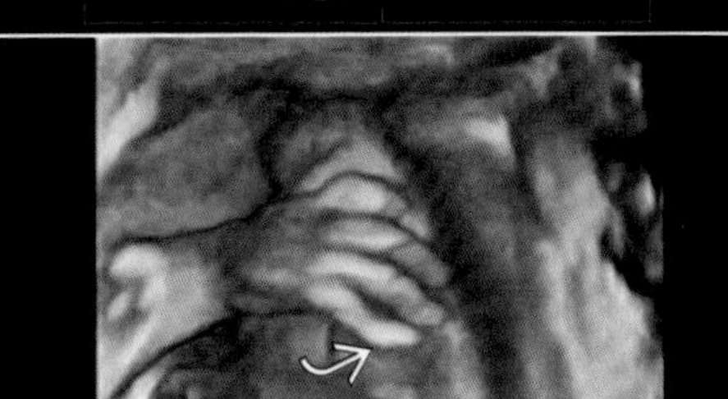

(Left) *3D US shows a fetus with arthrogryposis who had multiple findings, including overlapping clenched fingers ➡, polyhydramnios, clubbed feet, and micrognathia. These findings are common in fetuses with neuromuscular disorders.* **(Right)** *This fetus with trisomy 21 has an absent nasal bone ➡ and clinodactyly ➡. This case demonstrates the utility of 3D US. If you are not technically limited by position or fluid, always try to obtain 3D images to better evaluate the hands and feet whenever an abnormality is suspected.*

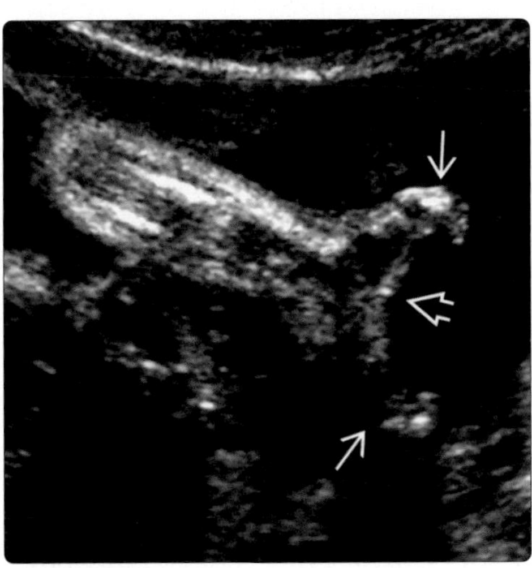

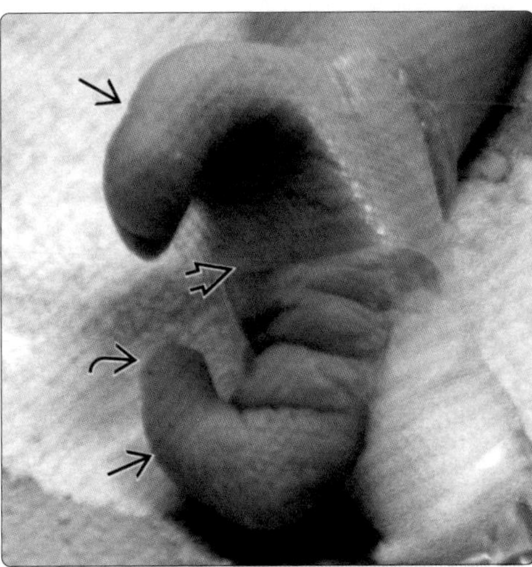

(Left) *US of a 3rd-trimester fetus shows the classic appearance of the split hand malformation. Note the wide cleft ➡ with 2 remaining digits ➡.* **(Right)** *Clinical photograph of the same infant at birth shows the striking appearance of the hand with 2 opposable digits ➡ and a large median cleft ➡ with central ray deficiency. In addition, the nails are quite hypoplastic ➡. 40% of individuals with split hand/foot have an associated syndrome, so further evaluation is required.*

PART VI
SECTION 9

Placenta, Membranes, and Umbilical Cord

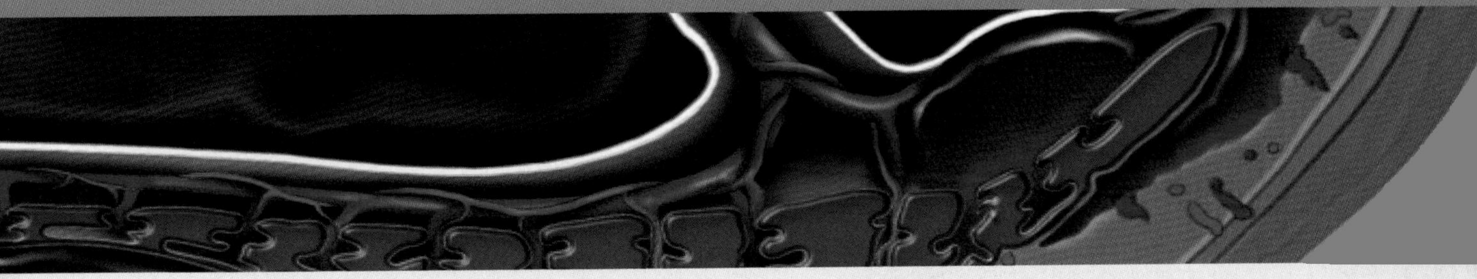

Placenta and Membrane Abnormalities

Umbilical Cord Abnormalities

Placental Abruption

KEY FACTS

TERMINOLOGY

- Placenta detachment
  - Most often partial and can see hematoma
- Categorized by location of abruption

IMAGING

- Marginal abruption (most common)
  - Hemorrhage from edge of placenta
- Retroplacental abruption (2nd most common)
  - Hematoma between placenta and uterus
  - May be confused for placentomegaly when acute
- Preplacental abruption (rare)
  - Hematoma on fetal surface of placenta
- Hematoma **appearance depends on age of blood**
  - Acute hematoma: Often isoechoic to placenta
  - Subacute hematoma: Hypoechoic to placenta
  - Resolving/chronic hematoma: Sonolucent

TOP DIFFERENTIAL DIAGNOSES

- Leiomyoma: Will see flow on color Doppler
- Focal myometrial contraction: Changes during scan

CLINICAL ISSUES

- Abruption is clinical diagnosis: Only 1/3 will have findings
- Risk factors: Trauma (particularly MVA), gestational hypertension, smoking, placenta previa, prior abruption

SCANNING TIPS

- Use color Doppler to differentiate isoechoic clot (no flow) from placenta
- Scan entire uterus
  - Hematoma may be distant from placenta edge
- Look for abruption and previa in all 2nd- and 3rd-trimester cases with vaginal bleeding or tender uterus
- Evaluate fetal heart rate early if new diagnosis of abruption
  - Stop scanning and call for help if bradycardia
  - Emergency cesarean warranted if viable fetus

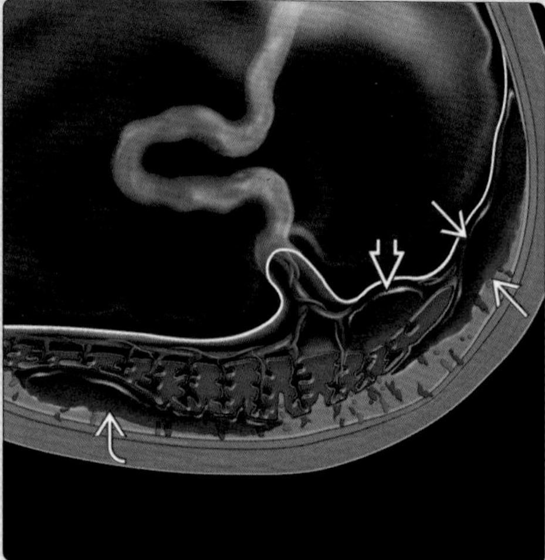

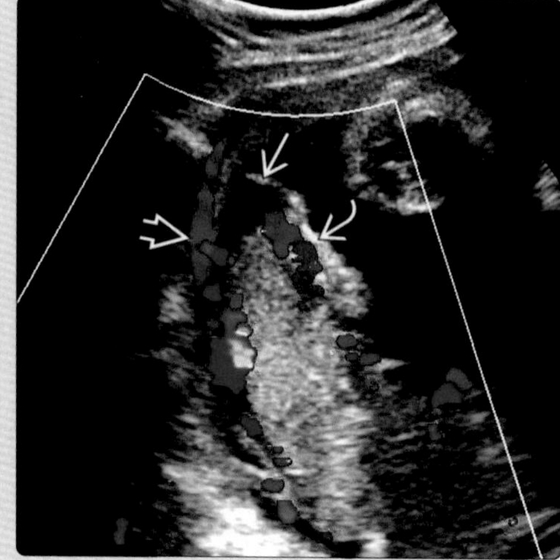

(Left) *Graphic shows placental abruption (PA) sites. Marginal PA ➡ occurs at the placental edge. Retro-PA ➡ occurs between the placenta and uterine wall, and pre-PA ➡ occurs in front of the placenta, between the placenta and membranes.* **(Right)** *In this example of a small marginal abruption, the edge of the placenta ➡ has been lifted off the uterine wall ➡. A small sonolucent hematoma is seen ➡, suggesting the abruption is old. Color Doppler shows flow in the placenta and uterus but not in the clot.*

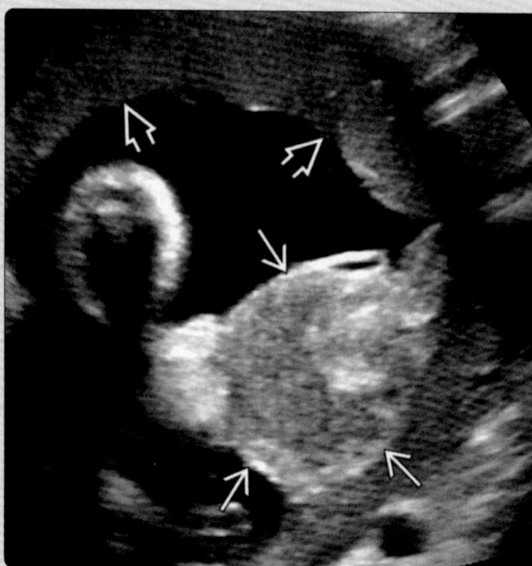

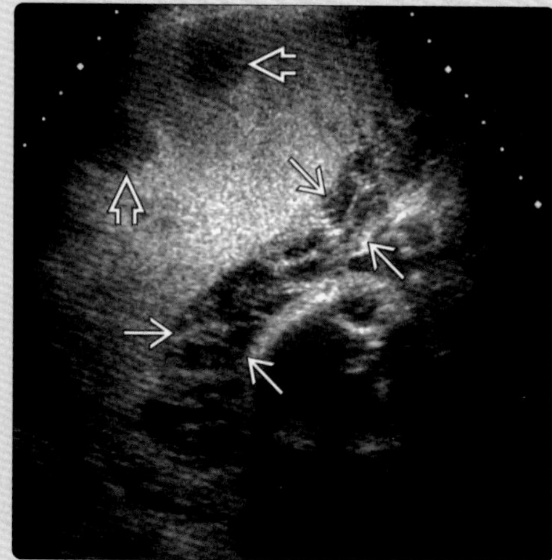

(Left) *A hematoma ➡ adjacent to an otherwise well-attached anterior placenta ➡ is from a marginal abruption. The clot is isoechoic to the placenta, implying a recent bleed. A lifted placental edge is not always seen, and the hematoma may be at a distance from the placental edge.* **(Right)** *Hematoma on the placental surface ➡ as well as focal retroplacental hematomas ➡ are seen in this case of extensive abruption. Pre-PA is rare and often presents in conjunction with marginal and retro-PA.*

Low-Lying Placenta and Previa

KEY FACTS

TERMINOLOGY

- **Placenta previa (PP)**: Placenta covers cervix internal os (IO)
- **Low-lying placenta (LLP)**: Placenta edge < 2 cm from IO
- Normal: Placenta edge 2 cm or more from IO
- Avoid "marginal" or "partial" PP (deemed confusing)

IMAGING

- Placental tissue near cervix is hallmark finding
  - Sagittal view is best
- Transvaginal US (TVUS) is essential for diagnosis
  - Best way to evaluate lower uterine segment (LUS)
  - Measure distance between placental edge and IO
  - Marginal placental vessels count as placenta
- Important associations
  - Morbidly adherent placenta (placenta accreta spectrum)
    - ↑ risk if prior cesarean section (C-section)
    - Greater risk if multiple prior C-sections
  - Vasa previa: Fetal vessels cross IO

TOP DIFFERENTIAL DIAGNOSES

- Overdistended maternal bladder: Pushes front and back of uterus together; mimics long cervix and low placenta
- Focal myometrial contraction: Shortens uterus, "pulls" placenta low
- Placental abruption: Isoechoic blood clot mimics placenta

CLINICAL ISSUES

- LLP or PP is seen in 2% of all midgestation studies
- > 90% will resolve: Follow-up at 32 and maybe 36 weeks
- C-section for PP, LLPs might deliver vaginally

SCANNING TIPS

- Scan whole uterus before determining placenta location
- TVUS if any placenta seen in LUS
- Use color Doppler: Find cord insertion, rule out vasa previa
- Move baby head out of pelvis
  - Put bed in Trendelenburg (head lower than feet)
  - 2nd person in room to push baby head up

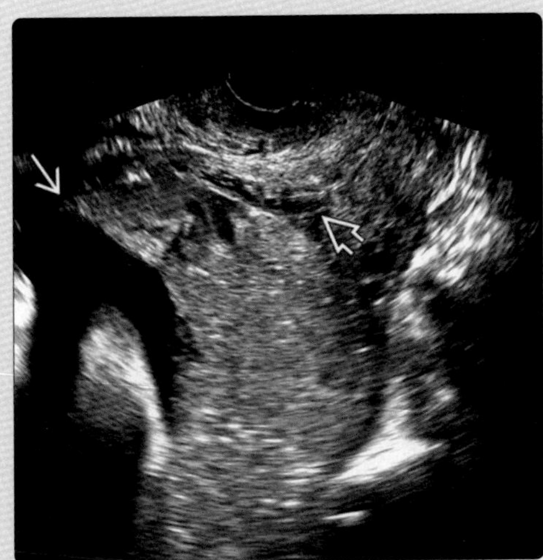

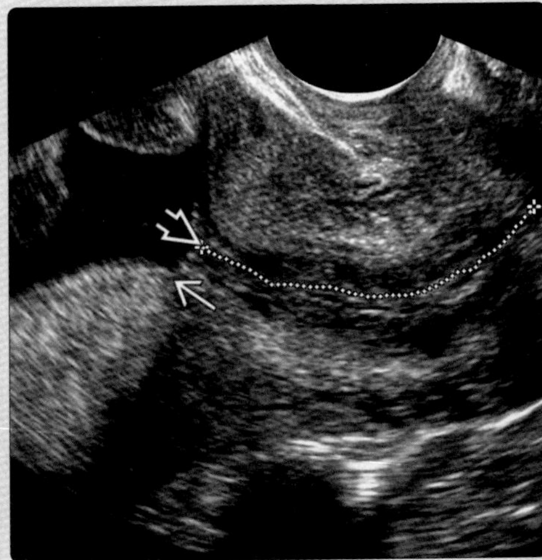

(Left) *Carefully performed transvaginal US shows the lower uterine segment best. Anterior edge of the placenta ➡ is several centimeters over the internal cervical os ➡. It is not surprising that this case of asymptomatic placenta previa (PP) did not resolve with advancing pregnancy.* **(Right)** *Transvaginal US of low-lying placenta (LLP) shows the placental edge ➡ close to, but not covering, the cervical os ➡. There is a 90% chance this will resolve with advancing pregnancy. Follow-up at 32 weeks was recommended.*

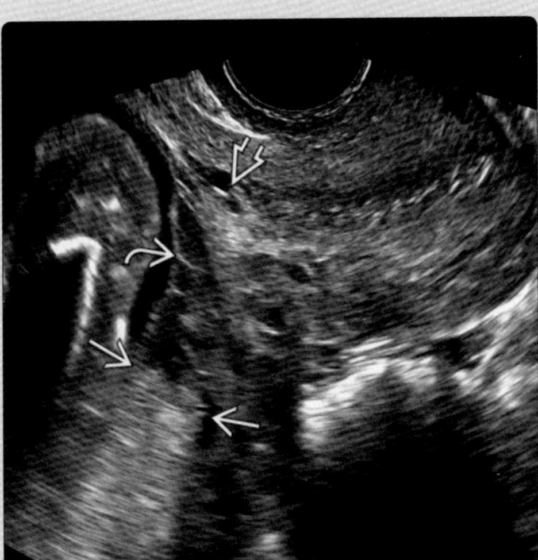

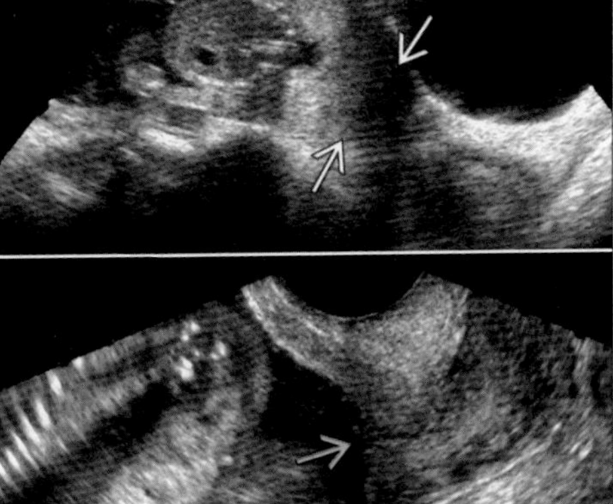

(Left) *In this patient with bleeding, the placenta parenchyma ➡ is > 2 cm from the internal os ➡; however, marginal sinus placental veins ➡ are located adjacent to the internal os. These vessels should be considered part of the placenta.* **(Right)** *(Top) A full bladder ➡ and myometrial contractions push the anterior and posterior uterine segment together ➡, mimicking previa. (Bottom) Transvaginal US in the same patient shows the internal os ➡ is clear of placental tissue. The placenta is not near the cervix at all.*

KEY FACTS

TERMINOLOGY

- Vasa previa (VP): Umbilical (fetal) vessels under membranes < 2 cm from internal os

IMAGING

- 90% associated with low-lying placenta
- Can occur in 2 different scenarios
  - Velamentous cord insertion
  - Vessels traveling over/near cervix between main placenta and accessory (succenturiate) lobes
- Transvaginal US + color Doppler are best tools
  - Pulse Doppler necessary to prove visualized vessels are fetal and not maternal in origin

TOP DIFFERENTIAL DIAGNOSES

- Low-lying placenta or placenta previa without VP
  - Maternal vessels near or cover os (not fetal)
  - Marginal sinus vessels of placenta often confused for fetal vessels

CLINICAL ISSUES

- Up to 50% mortality if VP is not diagnosed prenatally
  - Fetal hemorrhage because unprotected umbilical vessels prone to compression and tear
- Alternatively, 97-100% survival if VP is diagnosed prenatally

SCANNING TIPS

- Look for VP with color and pulse Doppler if low-lying placenta diagnosed
- Look for low succenturiate lobes
- Identify placental cord insertion in all cases
- Obtain pulsed Doppler when suspecting VP to prove it is same as fetal heart rate
- Beware of mimickers
  - Placental marginal vessels (along edge of placenta, not submembranous)
  - Uterine arterial or venous flow (deeper than VP vessels)
    - Arterial flow matches maternal heart rate; venous flow changes with maternal Valsalva

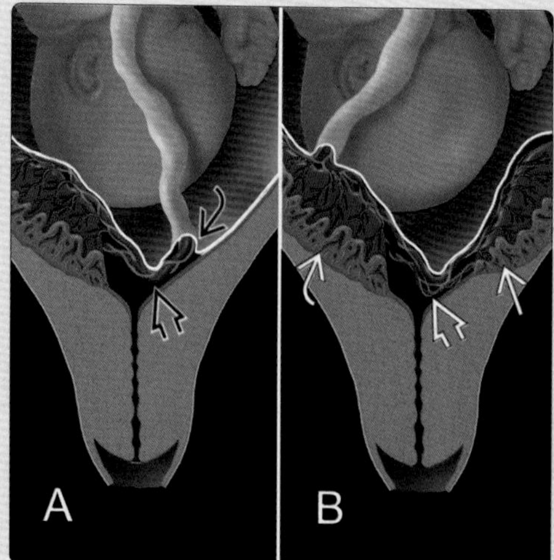

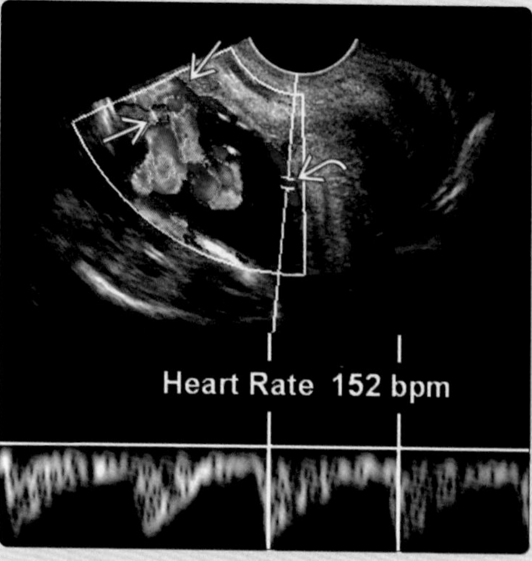

(Left) *Vasa previa (VP) can occur in 2 different ways. (A) A low-lying placenta with a velamentous cord insertion ➔ and fetal vessels ➔ crossing the cervical os is shown. (B) Fetal vessels ➔ traveling between the main placenta ➔ and an accessory (succenturiate) lobe ➔ are shown.* **(Right)** *Transvaginal US in this pregnancy with VP shows a lower uterine segment velamentous cord insertion ➔ and a subvelamentous fetal artery ➔ crossing the cervical internal os. Pulse Doppler US proves this is a fetal vessel.*

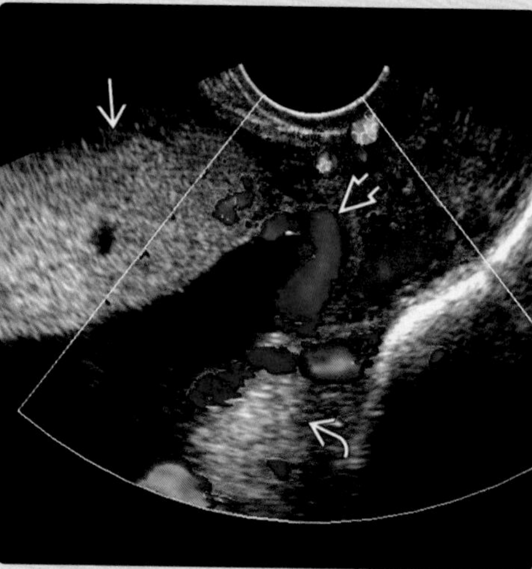

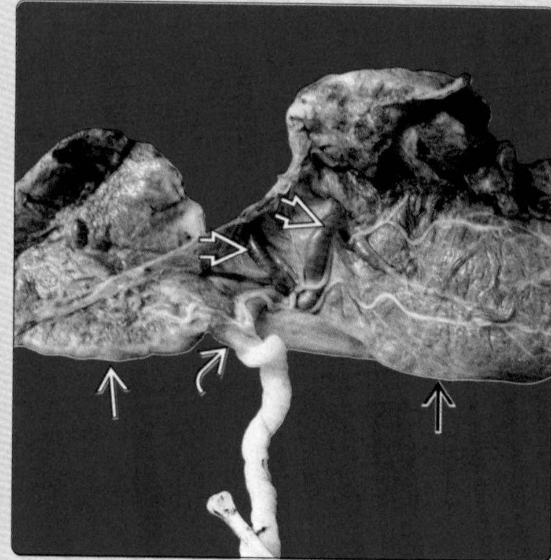

(Left) *In this case, transvaginal color Doppler US shows a low-lying anterior placenta lobe ➔ and a posterior accessory (succenturiate) lobe ➔ with communicating vessels ➔ crossing the internal cervical os. Failure to recognize this can cause catastrophic bleeding and fetal death at the time of delivery.* **(Right)** *The delivered placenta, in the same case, shows submembranous vessels ➔ and a cord insertion ➔, which is also velamentous and closer to the accessory lobe ➔ than the main lobe ➔.*

Succenturiate Lobe

KEY FACTS

TERMINOLOGY

- Succenturiate lobe (SL): 1 or more accessory placental lobes connected by submembranous fetal vessels

IMAGING

- 2 or more separate placentas
  - Color Doppler shows connecting vessels
- Find placental cord insertion
  - Might be on small placenta
  - Might be velamentous or marginal
- Risk for vasa previa if placental tissue in lower uterus
  - Crossing fetal vessels within 2 cm of internal cervical os

TOP DIFFERENTIAL DIAGNOSES

- Acute placental abruption
  - Isoechoic blood mimics smaller placenta
- Focal myometrial contraction
  - Contracted focus of muscle is echogenic

CLINICAL ISSUES

- Seen in 5-6% of all pregnancies
  - More common with twins and with in vitro fertilization
- ↑ risk for retained placenta after delivery
- SL with velamentous cord insertion has more complications
  - ↑ risk of growth restriction, ↑ risk for cord trauma

SCANNING TIPS

- Scan entire uterus before assigning placental location
  - Look for additional placental lobes
  - If 1 additional lobe seen, look for more
  - Look for vascular connections between lobes
    - Color Doppler to show connections
- Perform TVUS for any case in which any placental tissue or connecting vessels are suspected in lower uterus
  - Rule out vasa previa, low-lying placenta, and placenta previa of SL
  - Move fetal head to see internal os well

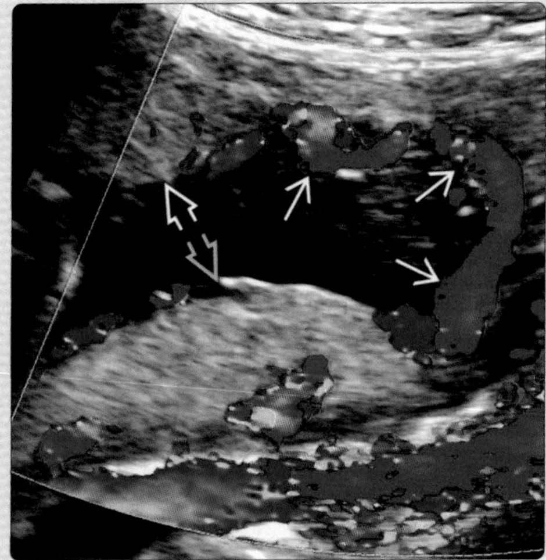

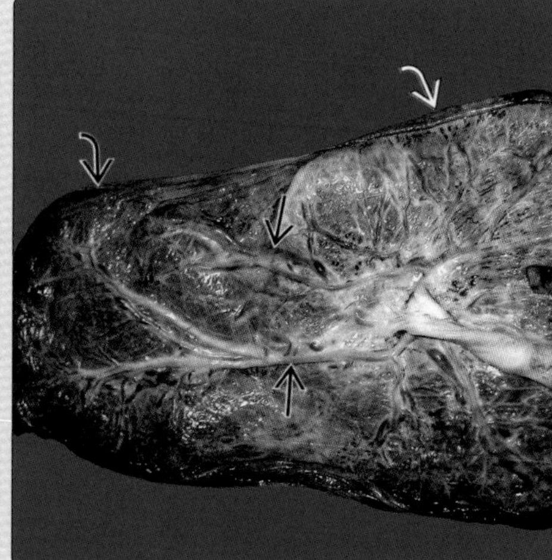

(Left) *Anterior ➔ and posterior ⇨ placentas are connected by submembranous communicating vessels ➔ carrying fetal blood. The main placental lobe in this case is posterior, and the anterior lobe is considered accessory (succenturiate).* **(Right)** *Gross pathology specimen of a main placental lobe ➔ and a succenturiate lobe ⇨ shows large connecting submembranous vessels ⇨. These vessels are prone to tear and injure if near the cervical os.*

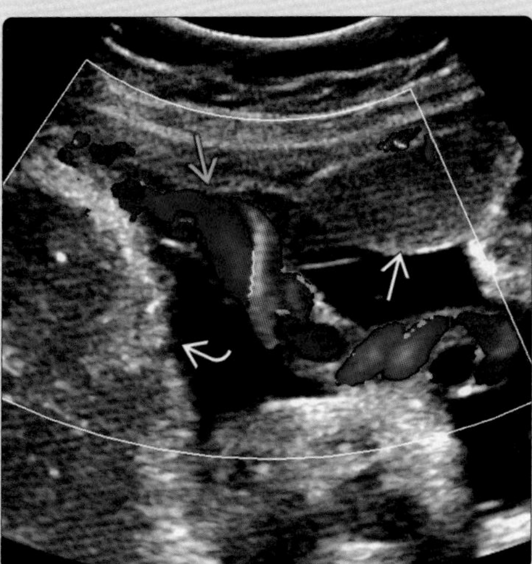

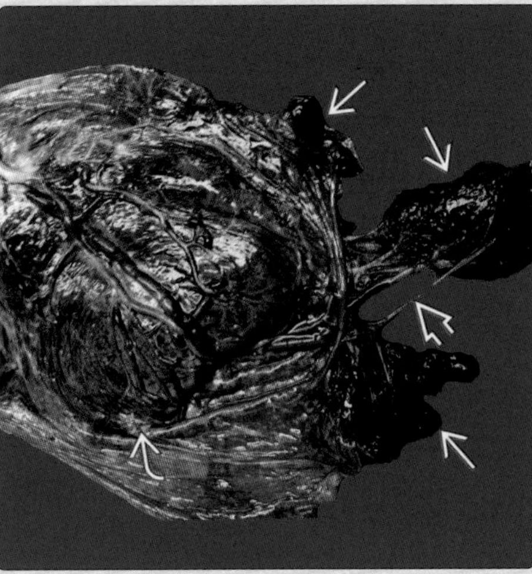

(Left) *Axial image shows a primary placenta ➔, a small adjacent succenturiate lobe ➔, and the umbilical cord inserting between the 2 ⇨. Velamentous cord insertion between placental lobes is not uncommon.* **(Right)** *Gross pathology of a placenta with several accessory lobes shows the main placental lobe ➔ connected by vessels to 3 small accessory lobes ➔. A vessel is even seen connecting 2 of the accessory lobes ➔. If any of these lobes are left behind, the patient will have symptoms from retained products of conception.*

Morbidly Adherent Placenta

KEY FACTS

TERMINOLOGY

- Extension of placental tissue beyond endometrial lining
- Described as morbidly adherent placenta (MAP), placental adhesive disorder, and abnormally invasive placenta
- Pathology subtypes of placenta accreta, increta, and percreta based on depth of myometrial invasion

SCANNING TIPS

- **Be familiar with normal appearance of placenta and placental/myometrial interface on US**
  - Normal pregnant uterus has inverted pear shape with smooth contour, no focal bulging
  - Normal placenta has uniform texture, intermediate echogenicity
  - Retroplacental hypoechoic zone or "clear zone" should be present over entire placental surface
  - Beware of excess transducer pressure and reverberation in near field mimicking loss of clear zone
- **Large, irregular, tornado-shaped placental vessels with turbulent flow are most sensitive US indicator of MAP**
- Multiple findings increase specificity
  - Look for loss of retroplacental "clear zone"
  - Look for uterine "bulge" (i.e., disruption of smoothly contoured, inverted pear shape)
  - Look for interruption of bladder wall/uterine interface
  - Look for "bridging vessels" extending beyond myometrium
  - Beware bladder varices as pitfall: Vessels in bladder mucosa **not** coming from placenta
- Have high index of suspicion for MAP in setting of placenta previa with prior cesarean section
- **Use highest resolution transducer to "walk the scar" and assess uterine wall**
  - Use high-MHz curved/linear transducer abdominally; use vaginal ultrasound for anterior placenta/previa
  - **Keep bladder partly full** during evaluation of uterine interface

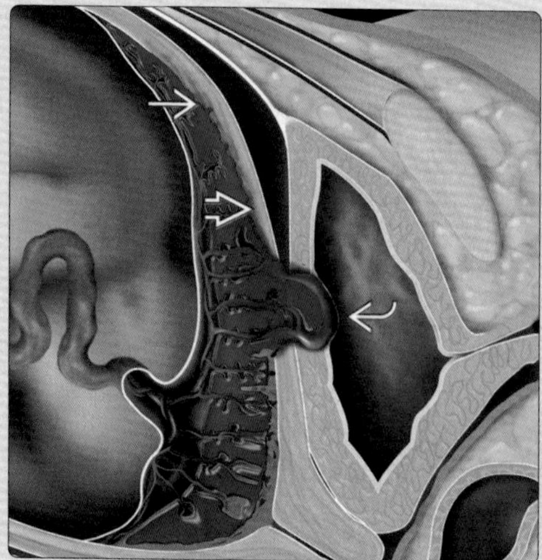

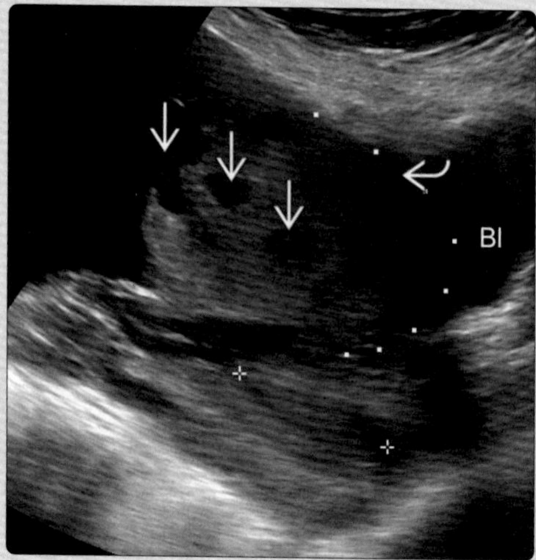

(Left) *Graphic illustrates progressively more abnormal placentation from accreta ➔ with chorionic villi attaching to the myometrium via defective decidua basalis, to increta ➔ with myometrial invasion, to percreta ➔ with myometrial breach and bladder invasion.* **(Right)** *Sagittal US in a patient with placenta previa and 7 prior sections shows a prominent myometrial bulge (dots), thick, inhomogeneous placenta with tornado vessels ➔, and loss of the subplacental hypoechoic zone ➔. Bl stands for bladder. Calipers measure the cervix.*

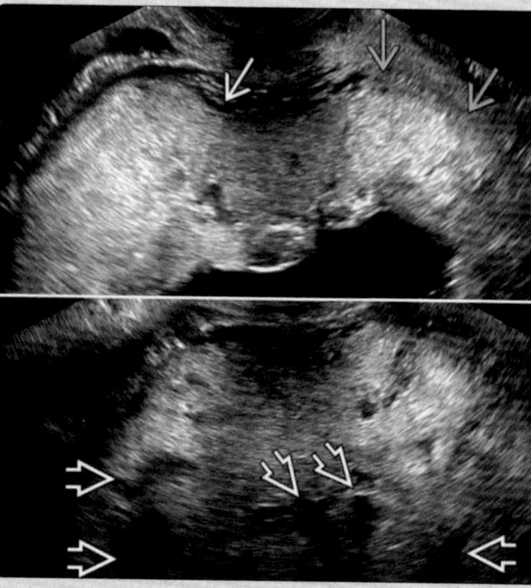

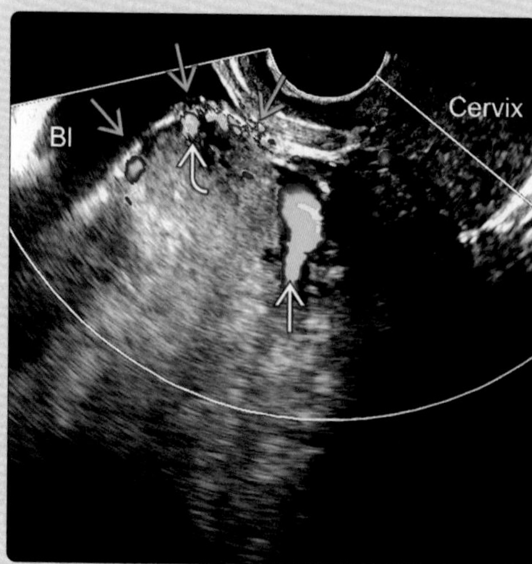

(Left) *TVUS is excellent for suspected MAP associated with placenta previa and prior cesarean section. The upper image shows a placental "bulge" ➔ and loss of the subplacental hypoechoic zone ⇨. The lower image shows a thick placenta with inhomogeneous echotexture and multiple lacunae ➔.* **(Right)** *Sagittal TVUS with color Doppler shows the placenta ⇨ bulging against the posterior bladder (Bl) wall with bridging vessels ➔ extending into the Bl. Note the tornado vessel ➔ within the placenta.*

KEY FACTS

TERMINOLOGY

- Membranes insert on fetal surface of placenta instead of along edge
  - Edges not "tacked down" & curl away from uterine wall

IMAGING

- Edge of placenta is rolled toward center
  - Amniotic fluid gets between rolled-up edge & placenta
- Turning longitudinally creates band or shelf appearance
  - **Edges of shelf attach to placenta**
- Cord insertion may be normal or marginal (vessels on edge)

TOP DIFFERENTIAL DIAGNOSES

- Many things create intrauterine linear echogenicities (ILE)
  - Key is to look where they attach
- Synechiae (amniotic sheets)
  - From uterine scar (covered by membranes)
  - Thick membrane attaches to uterine wall
  - Placenta may implant on synechiae
- Amniotic bands
  - From rupture of amnion
  - Thin membrane entangles fetus &/or umbilical cord
- Septate uterus (uterine duplication anomaly)
  - Septum is always at fundus
- Marginal placental abruption
  - Placental edge is lifted because of associated hematoma
  - No placental shelf

CLINICAL ISSUES

- Excellent prognosis if partial & isolated
- ↑ incidence of preterm delivery, abruption, growth restriction (if most or all of placental margin is involved)

SCANNING TIPS

- Look for sites of attachment whenever ILEs are seen
- Make sure fetus & cord are not involved with ILE, which would indicate amniotic bands
- Look for placental shelf when edge looks free floating

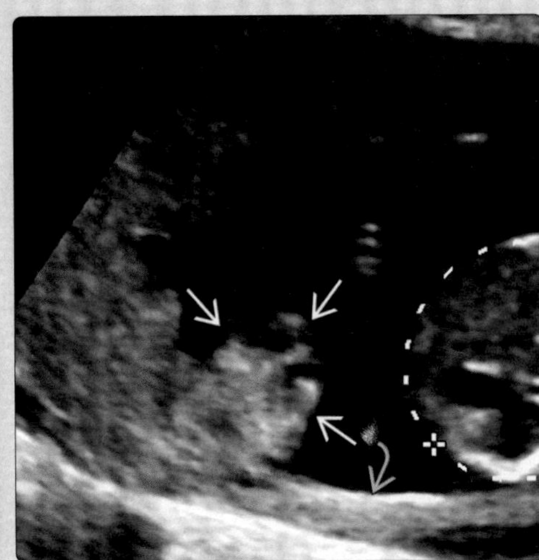

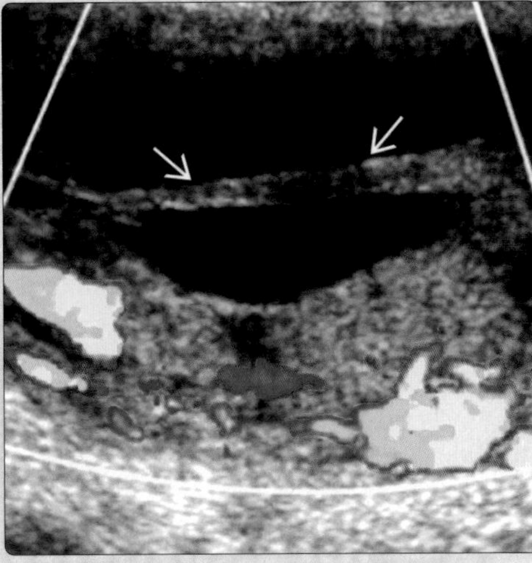

(Left) *In this 2nd-trimester case with circumvallate placenta, the placental edge ➡ is lifted off the uterine wall ➡ and curled inward.* **(Right)** *Longitudinal color Doppler US along the placental edge shows a placental shelf ➡. Amniotic fluid is between this curled edge and placenta. The thick band attaches on the placenta, not the uterus, and therefore can be differentiated from synechia. The key to differentiating intrauterine linear echogenicities is where the edges attach.*

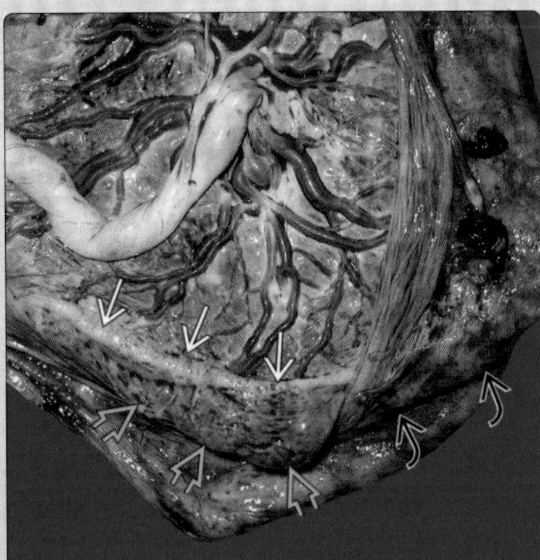

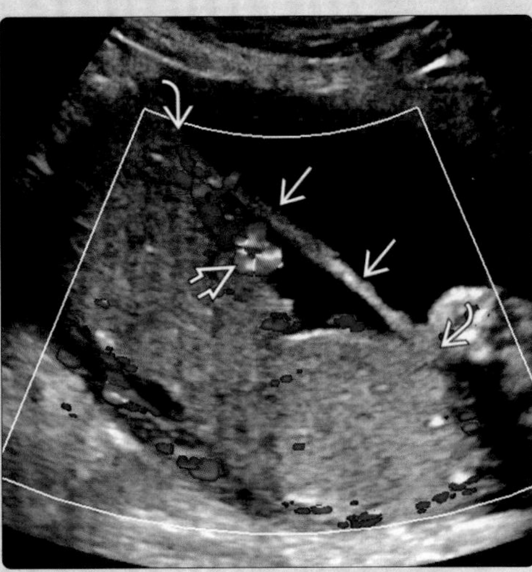

(Left) *Gross pathology shows membranes attached to the fetal surface ➡ of the placenta, several centimeters from the true edge ➡. Importantly, placental tissue growing along the membranes ➡ is lifted up, giving the rolled-placenta appearance on ultrasound.* **(Right)** *Axial color Doppler US shows a thick membrane ➡ (placental shelf) extending from placenta margin to placenta margin ➡. The cord insertion ➡ is also seen. The band is on the margin of the placenta and does not compress the cord.*

Marginal and Velamentous Cord Insertion

KEY FACTS

TERMINOLOGY

- **Marginal cord insertion (MCI)**
  - Umbilical cord inserts within 2 cm of placenta edge
- **Velamentous cord insertion (VCI)**
  - Umbilical cord inserts on membranes

IMAGING

- MCI: All branching vessels are on surface of placenta
- VCI: Cord inserts on membranes and at variable distance from placental margin
  - VCI vessels often diverge and travel separately beneath membranes toward placenta
    - This has been called "mangrove tree" sign
- VCI in lower uterine segment may cause vasa previa
- MCI can progress to VCI if placental margin absorbs
  - Reasons for peripheral atrophy include abruption and poor vascularity of placental margin

TOP DIFFERENTIAL DIAGNOSES

- Submembranous vessels from succenturiate lobe

CLINICAL ISSUES

- VCI incidence: 1-2% singleton, 7% dichorionic twins, up to 40% monochorionic twins
- VCI associated with ↑ risk for adverse perinatal outcome
  - Submembranous vessels not protected by Wharton jelly and are susceptible to injury
- MCI and VCI are associated with fetal growth restriction
  - 3rd trimester follow-up growth scan indicated

SCANNING TIPS

- Document placental cord insertion site in all cases
  - Especially multiple gestations (can see at time of nuchal translucency)
- Rule out vasa previa if VCI is in lower uterus
- Do not confuse surface fetal vessels for cord insertion
  - See convergence of vessels into true cord insertion

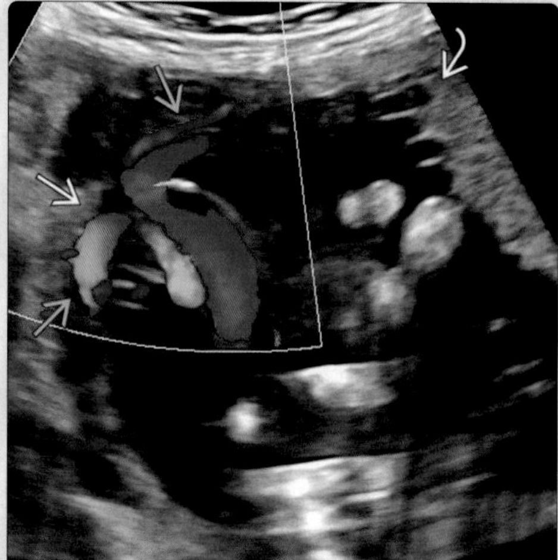

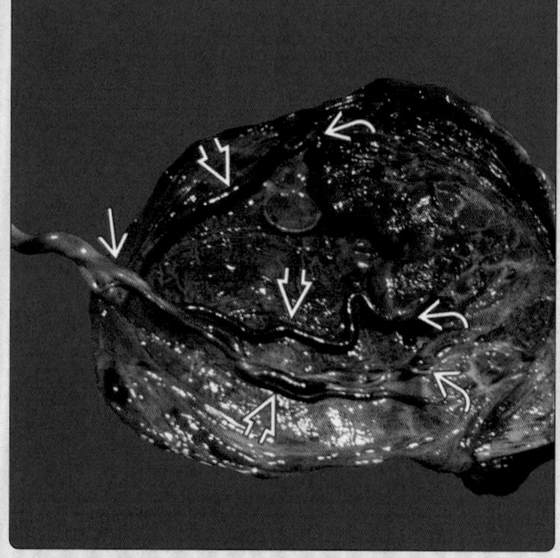

(Left) *In this case of velamentous cord insertion (VCI), the cord inserts directly on the uterine wall ➡ ~ 5 cm from the closest placental edge ➡, and the vessels splay upon insertion ➡.* **(Right)** *Gross pathology of VCI shows the cord inserts ➡ ~ 10 cm from the placental edge ➡. The cord divides on the membrane, and the splayed submembranous vessels ➡ are not protected by Wharton jelly as they travel to the placenta. Note the associated small placenta. VCI is associated with fetal growth restriction.*

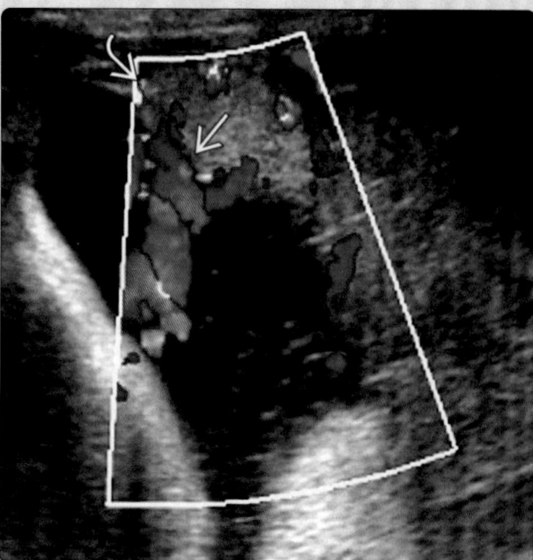

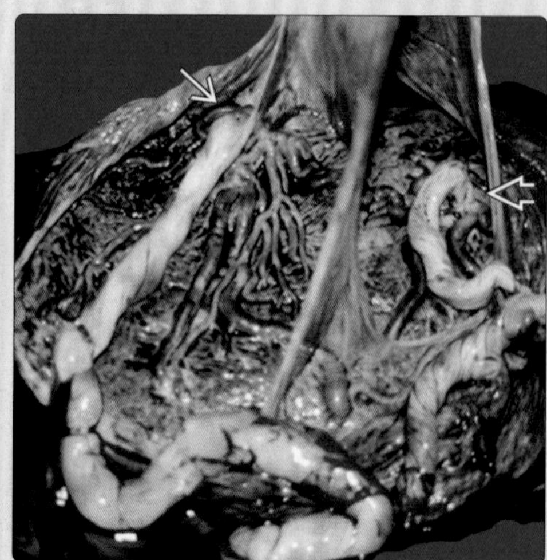

(Left) *In this case of marginal cord insertion (MCI), the umbilical cord ➡ inserts within 2 cm of the placental edge ➡. No submembranous fetal vessels were seen.* **(Right)** *Photograph of a monochorionic twin placenta complicated by discordant twin growth shows an MCI at the placental edge ➡ and a normal, more centrally located cord insertion ➡. MCI and VCI are often seen in twins and can be a cause of unequal placental sharing and discordant twin growth.*

KEY FACTS

TERMINOLOGY

- Reactive proliferation of placental tissue, not true neoplasm

IMAGING

- Most common on fetal side of placenta, near cord insertion
- Well-defined, hypoechoic mass
- Flow on color Doppler essential for making diagnosis
- Amount of flow in mass is quite variable
  - Flow through mass is from fetal circulation
  - Greater arterial flow increases risk of developing high-output cardiac failure and hydrops
  - Vascularity may be more important than size for predicting outcome
  - Vascularity may either increase or decrease as gestation progresses
- Masses ≥ 5 cm are considered large and are more likely to have complications
- Chorioangiomatosis may present as multiple small masses or diffusely heterogeneous placenta
  - More likely to cause complications
- Monitor for complications
  - Polyhydramnios common with large or multiple masses
  - Hydrops or fetal anemia from arteriovenous shunting
  - Fetal growth restriction

TOP DIFFERENTIAL DIAGNOSES

- Venous lakes and intervillous thrombi
  - No flow or swirling slow flow usually not visible on color Doppler

CLINICAL ISSUES

- Excellent prognosis if small and single
- Amnioreduction for polyhydramnios

SCANNING TIPS

- Evaluate all placental masses with color Doppler

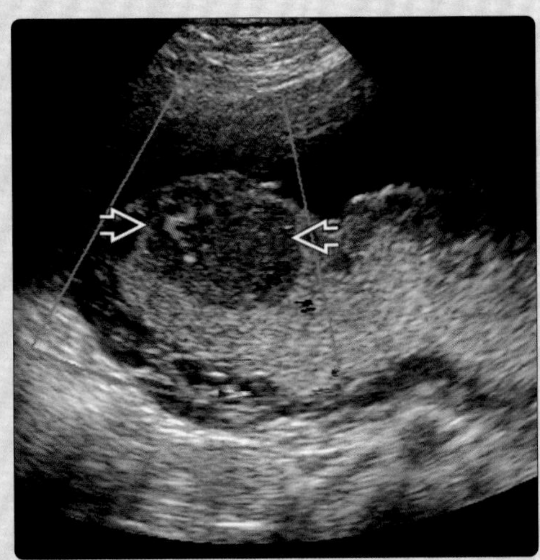

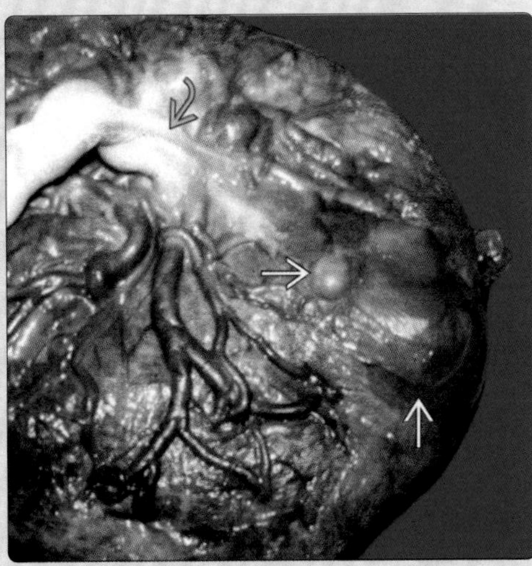

(Left) *Color Doppler ultrasound shows a well-defined, vascular, solid, hypoechoic mass ➡ on the fetal surface of the placenta. This is the typical appearance of a chorioangioma. Vascularity and size are the most important risk factors for complications. Most small masses remain asymptomatic, as was the case in this pregnancy.* **(Right)** *Gross pathology from a different case shows small chorioangiomas ➡ on the placental surface near the cord insertion ➡.*

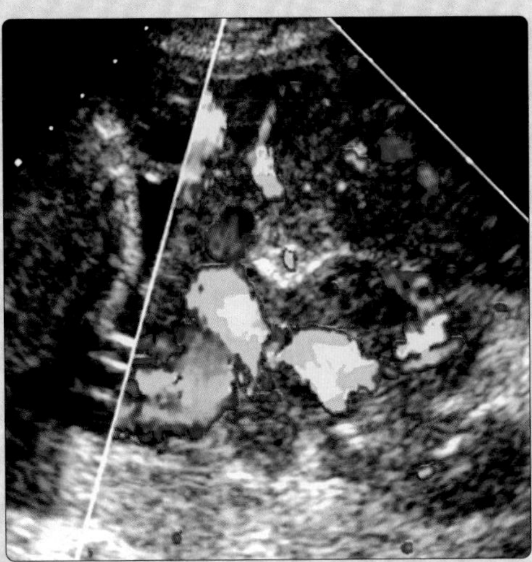

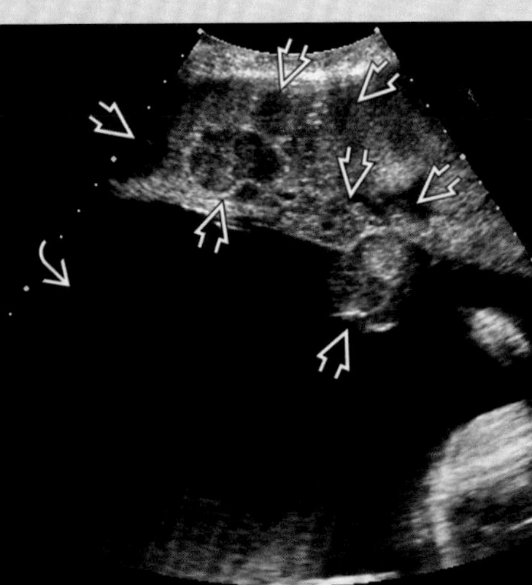

(Left) *Color Doppler ultrasound shows marked vascular flow in a large placental chorioangioma. The pregnancy was complicated by fetal hydrops and polyhydramnios.* **(Right)** *Grayscale ultrasound of the placenta shows multiple solid hypoechoic masses ➡ (chorioangiomatosis), which increase the likelihood of complications. There was severe polyhydramnios ➡, which required multiple amnioreductions.*

Single Umbilical Artery

KEY FACTS

TERMINOLOGY

- Umbilical cord with single umbilical artery (SUA) and 1 umbilical vein (UV) instead of 2 UAs and 1 UV
- Also referred to as 2-vessel cord

IMAGING

- Free loop of cord with 2 vessels instead of 3 vessels
- Color Doppler shows 1 UA adjacent to bladder
- SUA is most often isolated finding; however, it is associated with placental insufficiency (2x increased risk)
  - Fetal growth restriction, maternal hypertension
  - Placental anomaly association: Succenturiate lobe, velamentous cord insertion
- 1/3 with fetal anomalies: Renal and cardiac most common
- Aneuploid in 10% (trisomy 18 and 13, not trisomy 21)

CLINICAL ISSUES

- Common finding: 0.5-5.0% of all pregnancies
- Follow-up for fetal growth in 3rd trimester recommended when isolated SUA diagnosed in 2nd trimester
- Genetic counseling offered if not isolated or if SUA is diagnosed in patient at increased risk for fetus with aneuploidy or genetic syndrome

SCANNING TIPS

- Look for number of vessels in free loop **and** on color Doppler bladder view
  - Sometimes, 3 vessels present in free cord, but UAs fuse before entering fetus
- Look for SUA in 1st trimester if ↑ nuchal translucency
  - Increases risk of aneuploidy
- Consider diagnosis if 1 UA is smaller than the other
  - Hypoplastic UA is variant of SUA
  - Carries same risks and associations
- SUA is often larger than UA in a 3-vessel cord
  - Carries all fetal blood to placenta

(Left) *Axial US through a free loop of cord shows only 2 vessels. The umbilical artery (UA) ➔ has a thicker wall than the umbilical vein (UV) ➔.* **(Right)** *Long-axis color Doppler US of a free loop of cord shows a single UA (SUA) ➔. No other anomalies were seen, and fetal growth was normal. Isolated SUA is a common finding. Note that the SUA is almost the same diameter as the UV. This is not surprising, since the SUA is carrying all the fetal blood to the placenta.*

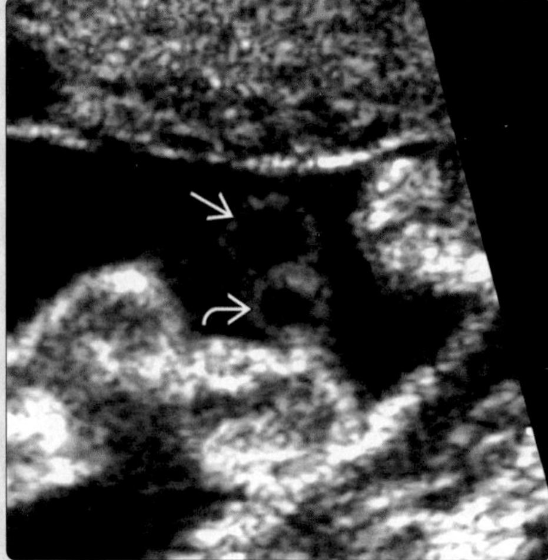

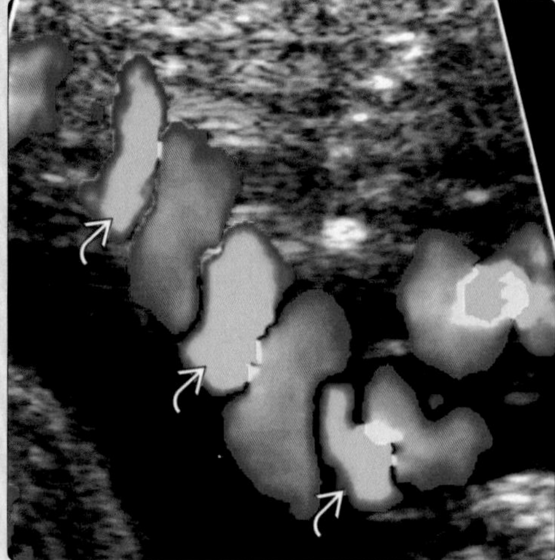

(Left) *SUA ➔ is seen adjacent to fetal bladder ➔ at the time of nuchal translucency (NT) screening in a 13-week fetus. In addition, NT was increased, and other anomalies were seen. Anatomy assessment at the time of NT screening is additive.* **(Right)** *Axial US of the fetal cord insertion site shows a small omphalocele containing small bowel ➔ and a 2-vessel cord ➔. Other anomalies were also seen, and amniocentesis results revealed trisomy 18. SUA is associated with aneuploidy but rarely is SUA the only finding in these cases.*

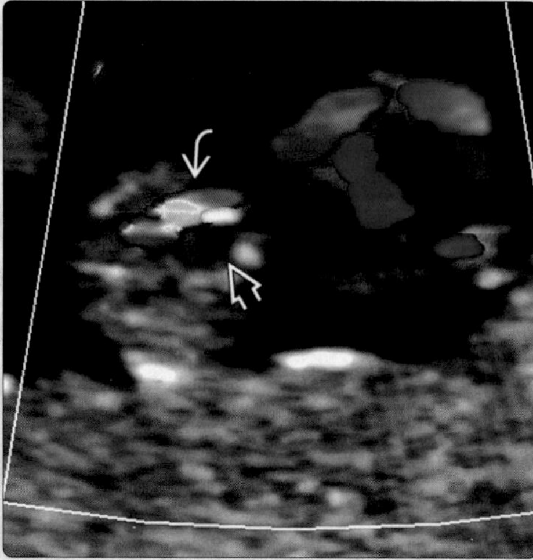

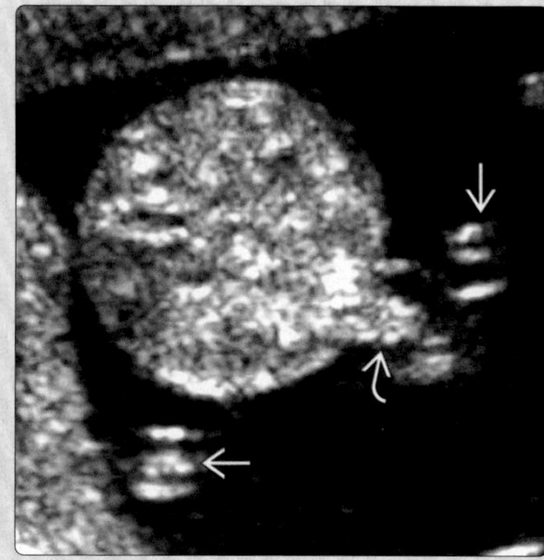

KEY FACTS

TERMINOLOGY

- Several definitions in use
  - Focal dilatation of umbilical vein (UV) > 9-mm diameter
  - Varix diameter 50% > intrahepatic portion of UV
  - UV diameter > 2 standard deviations above mean for gestational age

IMAGING

- Cyst-like space in upper abdomen with venous flow on Doppler
- Usually intraabdominal, extrahepatic
  - May be intrahepatic or even in free loops of cord
- Cord umbilical vein varix (UVV) is diagnosis of chance, as hard to systematically run length of cord in mobile fetus
  - Rupture of UVV in free loops may → fetal exsanguination

TOP DIFFERENTIAL DIAGNOSES

- Abdominal cysts (none show internal blood flow)
  - Choledochal cyst
  - Meconium pseudocyst
  - Ovarian cyst
  - Enteric duplication cyst
  - Urachal cyst
- Umbilical cord cysts (flow in surrounding umbilical vessels, not in cyst)

SCANNING TIPS

- If UVV seen, perform detailed anatomic survey
  - ~ 35% have other anomalies
  - Cardiovascular, renal most common
- Formal fetal echocardiogram as UVV may be 1st manifestation of elevated venous pressures
- Monitor for signs of impending hydrops
- Monitor varix size, presence of thrombus
- Monitor fetal growth
  - Increase surveillance if fetal growth restriction develops

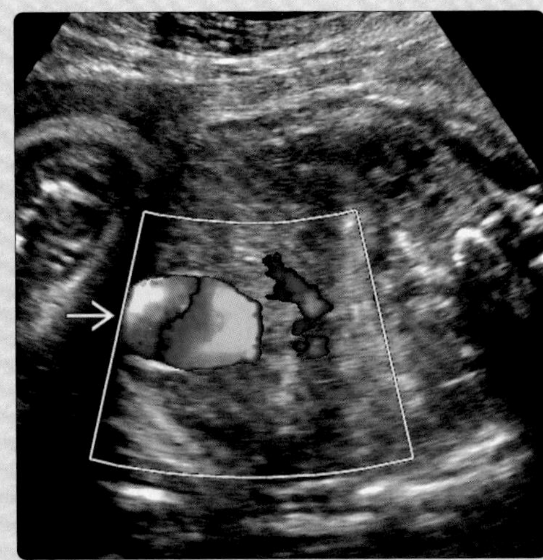

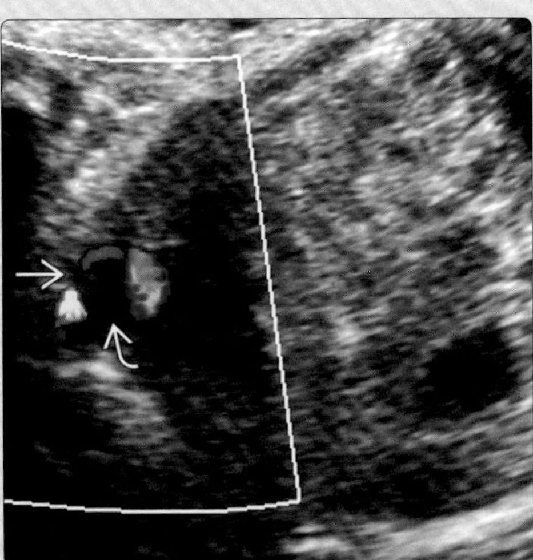

(Left) *Axial color Doppler US shows complete filling of a 13-mm umbilical vein varix (UVV) ➡. The swirling color is a manifestation of eddying flow as the blood from the normal-caliber umbilical vein enters the varix. Whether or not the degree of turbulence in the varix can be characterized by color Doppler is debatable.* **(Right)** *This case shows incomplete filling of a UVV ➡ due to partial thrombosis with clot ➡ filling ~ 1/2 of the varix. This occurred at 37 weeks and 1 day. The infant was delivered by cesarean section and did well.*

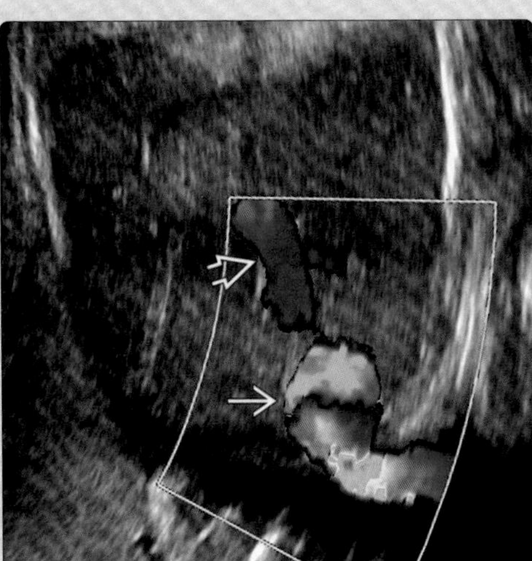

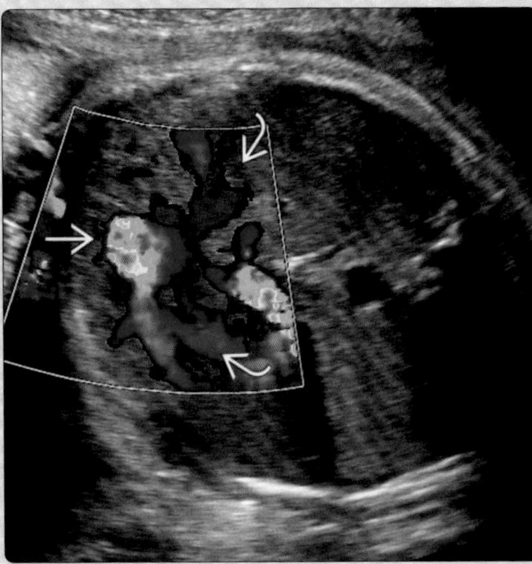

(Left) *Coronal color Doppler US nicely demonstrates the size of the varix ➡ in comparison to the size of the intrahepatic umbilical vein ➡.* **(Right)** *Axial color Doppler US shows enlargement of the portal veins ➡ in association with a UVV ➡. This suggests impaired venous circulation. There is a case report in which this finding was associated with progressive liver enlargement and resulted in intrauterine fetal demise. All testing was negative for liver disease, infection, and aneuploidy.*

PART VI
SECTION 10
Multiple Gestations

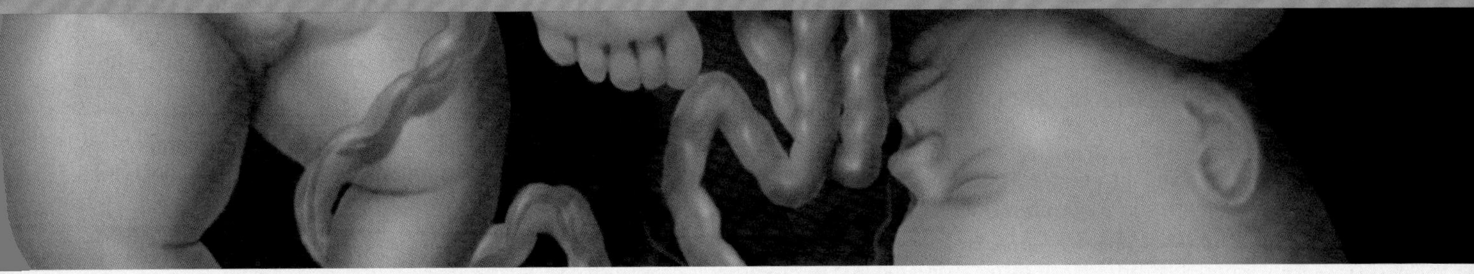

Chorionicity and Amnionicity in Twins

KEY FACTS

TERMINOLOGY

- **70% dizygotic**: 2 ova fertilized by different sperm; therefore, all are dichorionic
- **30% monozygotic**: Single ovum fertilized by single sperm, which then divides to produce twins
  - 30% dichorionic, 60-65% monochorionic diamniotic
  - 5-10% monoamniotic, < 1% conjoined

IMAGING

- Dichorionic 1st trimester: Thick echogenic chorion completely surrounds each embryo
  - 2 amniotic sacs, 2 yolk sacs (YS)
- Dichorionic 2nd/3rd trimester: Twin peak sign with wedge of chorionic tissue extending from placenta into base of intertwin membrane
  - Thick intertwin membrane, 2 separate placentas
- Monochorionic 1st trimester: Single thick chorion surrounds both embryos
  - Diamniotic: 2 YS, 2 amnions, 1 around each embryo
  - Monoamniotic: 1 YS, 1 amnion surrounds both embryos
- Monochorionic 2nd/3rd trimester must be same sex with single placental mass
  - Diamniotic: Thin membrane, T sign of membrane perpendicular to placenta
  - Monoamniotic: No membrane, cord entanglement

SCANNING TIPS

- **Use transvaginal US in 1st trimester to document chorionicity and amnionicity as chorionicity determines prognosis**
- Look for placenta/vasa previa, marginal/velamentous cord
- Monitor growth at least monthly
- Check fluid volume every 2 weeks in monochorionic twins to monitor for twin-twin transfusion
  - If diamniotic: Maximum vertical pockets on either side of membrane
  - Must rely on bladders/Doppler in monoamniotic
- Careful search for anomalies; increased risk in all twins

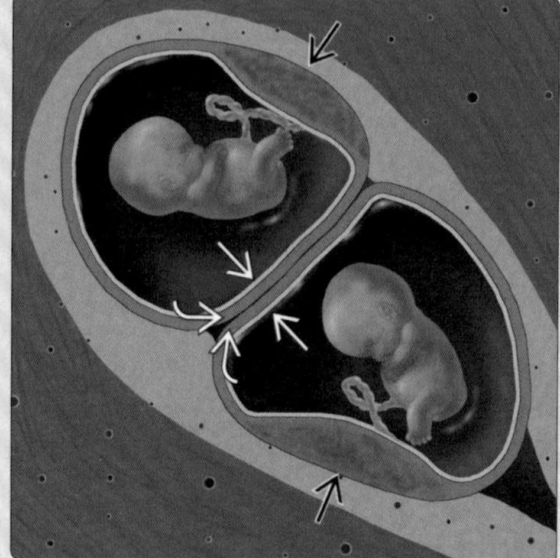

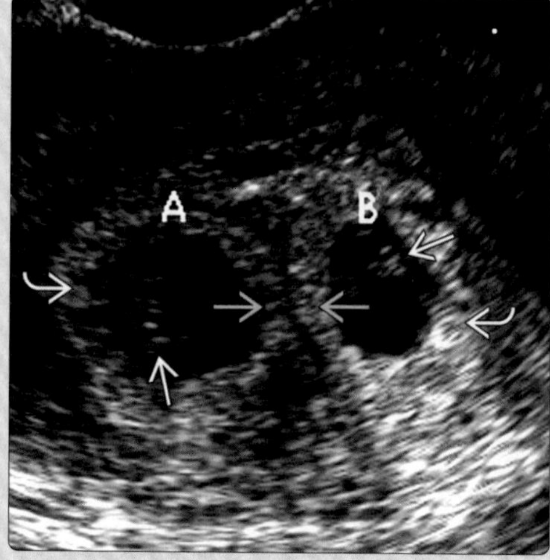

(Left) *Graphic of dichorionic twins shows a thick intertwin membrane composed of 2 thin layers of amnion ➡ and 2 thick layers of chorion ➡. The placentas ➡ are separate.* **(Right)** *Transvaginal ultrasound in the 1st trimester shows 2 thick, echogenic, chorionic sacs ➡, each surrounding an embryo ➡. The twin peak sign and thick membrane will develop as a result of apposition of the adjacent chorions ➡. This case illustrates the ease of determining chorionicity with vaginal sonography.*

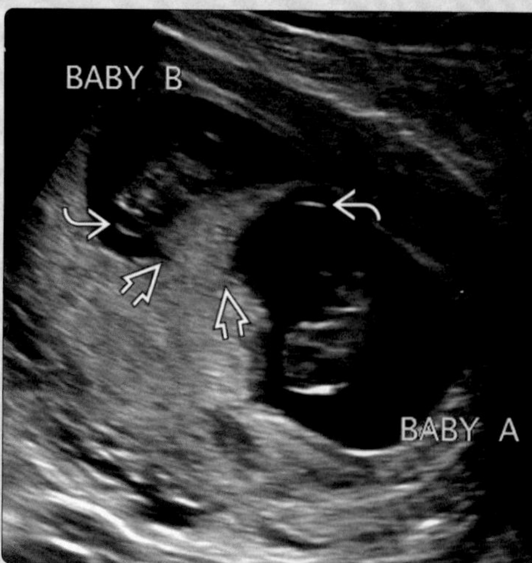

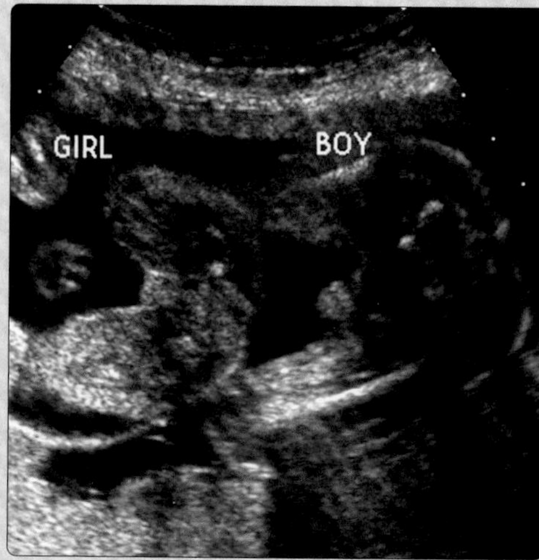

(Left) *Transabdominal ultrasound at a later gestational age shows 2 embryos with the delicate amniotic membranes ➡ barely visible inside the echogenic chorionic sacs. The twin peak sign is now visible ➡ where the broad-based triangle of chorion extends into the thick membrane. This is also sometimes called the lambda sign.* **(Right)** *Transabdominal ultrasound shows different fetal sex. These twins are therefore dizygotic and, by definition, must be dichorionic.*

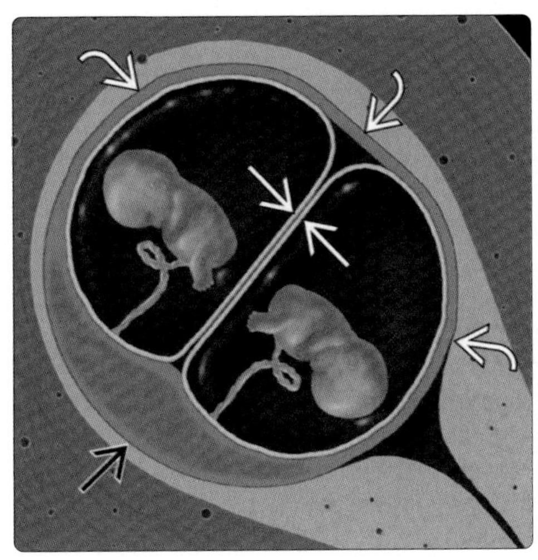

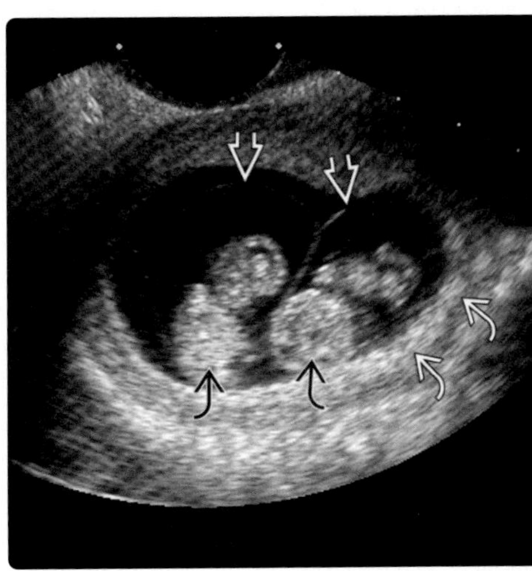

(Left) *Graphic of monochorionic diamniotic twins shows a thin membrane formed by the apposition of the 2 thin layers of amnion ➡. There is a single placenta ➡ and a single chorionic sac ➡.* **(Right)** *Transvaginal scan in the 1st trimester shows single chorion ➡ surrounding 2 embryos ➡, each of which is within its own thin amniotic sac ➡. Thus, this is a monochorionic diamniotic twin pregnancy. Monochorionic twins can be diamniotic or monoamniotic.*

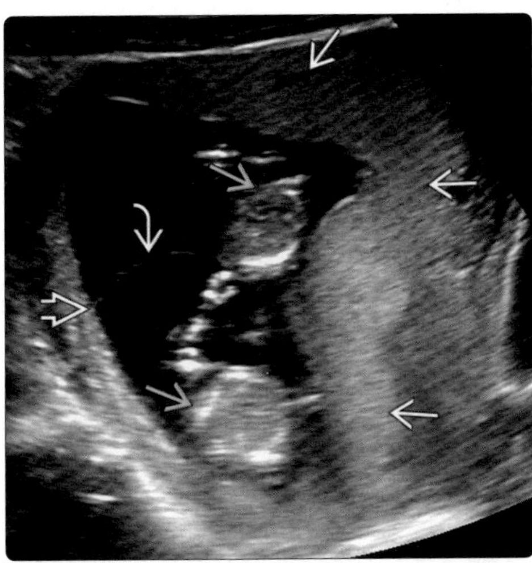

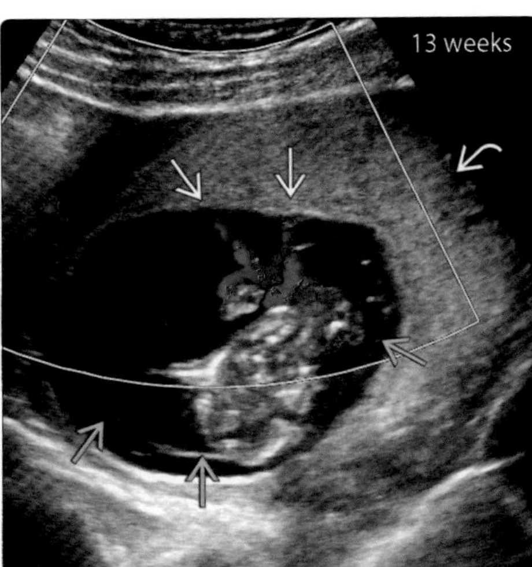

(Left) *TAUS at 13 weeks shows monochorionic diamniotic twins with a single placenta ➡ and 2 fetuses ➡ separated by a thin membrane ➡, which meets the uterine wall in a T-shaped configuration ➡ (as opposed to the lambda or twin peak configuration seen in dichorionic twins).* **(Right)** *In these monoamniotic twins, the umbilical cords ➡ are close to each other on the surface of a single placenta ➡. The cords are knotted together, and only a single amnion ➡ is visible. The other fetus was out of the scan plane.*

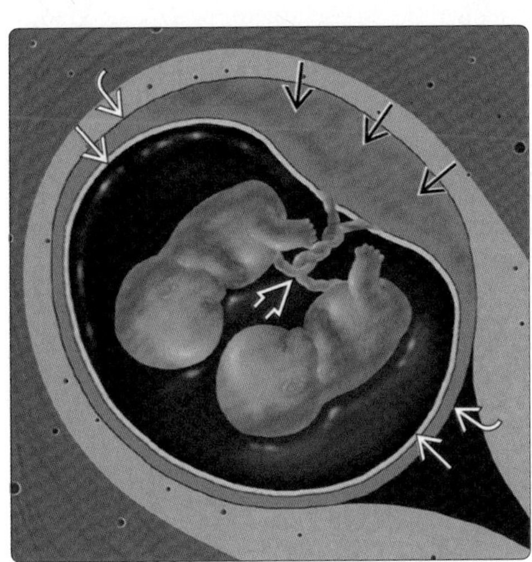

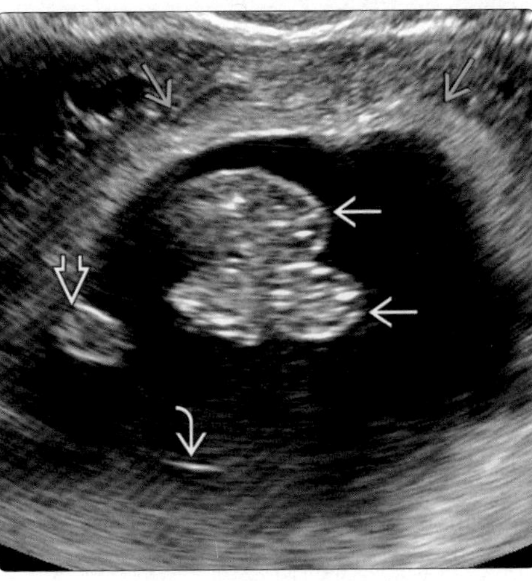

(Left) *Graphic illustrates monoamniotic twins with 2 embryos inside a single amniotic sac ➡, which is surrounded by a single chorion ➡. There is a single placenta ➡ and the umbilical cords are tangled ➡.* **(Right)** *TVUS in monochorionic monoamniotic twins shows 2 embryos ➡ surrounded by a single amnion ➡ and single chorion ➡. Note the single yolk sac ➡. Be sure to confirm that the embryos are separable (this may not be possible until late 1st trimester) to exclude conjoined twins.*

Twin-Twin Transfusion Syndrome

KEY FACTS

TERMINOLOGY

- **Monochorionic (MC) twin complication** caused by intrauterine transfusion of blood from donor twin to recipient twin via arteriovenous placental anastomoses

IMAGING

- Hallmark finding is oligohydramnios in 1 sac + polyhydramnios in other of diamniotic pair (difficult diagnosis in monoamniotic twins)
- **Donor** has oligohydramnios defined as maximum vertical pocket (MVP) ≤ 2 cm
  - **"Stuck twin"** describes severe oligohydramnios with donor twin "shrink-wrapped" to uterine wall
  - **Cocooning** describes severe oligohydramnios where donor twin, in tight cocoon of membranes, is suspended within pool of fluid from recipient twin
- **Recipient** has polyhydramnios defined as MVP ≥ 8 cm at < 20 weeks, > 10 cm at > 20 weeks
- Discordant twin growth not mandatory feature

SCANNING TIPS

- **Establish chorionicity and amnionicity in all multiple gestations in 1st trimester**
- All MC twins need growth monthly with fluid/bladder check every 2 weeks from 16 weeks gestation
- Check movement of any twin near uterine wall
  - "Stuck" or cocooned twin cannot extend extremities or change position
  - Change maternal position
  - Use high-resolution transducer to identify thin membrane reflected off head or between extremities
- Stage twin-twin transfusion syndrome (TTTS) when seen
  - Stage 1: Oligohydramnios/polyhydramnios
  - Stage 2: + absent bladder in donor
  - Stage 3: + abnormal umbilical artery Doppler with either absent (AEDF) or reversed end diastolic flow (REDF)
  - Stage 4: + hydrops
  - Stage 5: + demise of 1 twin

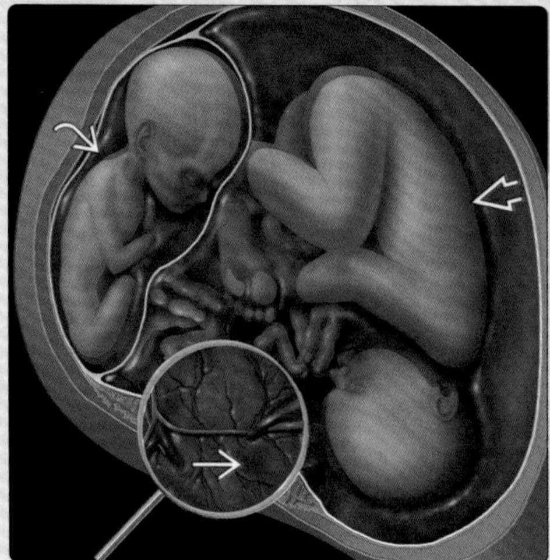

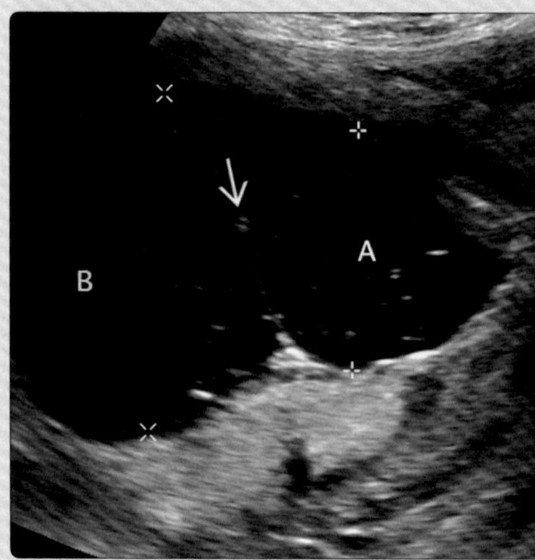

(Left) *Graphic shows discordant MC twins with a unidirectional AV shunt ➡ of deoxygenated blood from the oligemic, poorly grown donor ➡ with oligohydramnios to the hypervolemic recipient ➡ with polyhydramnios.* **(Right)** *At 17 weeks 5 days, there is asymmetric distribution of fluid around the thin intertwin membrane ➡. A difference of > 4 cm between maximum vertical pockets is concerning for developing TTTS. The combination of oligohydramnios (< 2 cm) and polyhydramnios (> 8 cm) is diagnostic.*

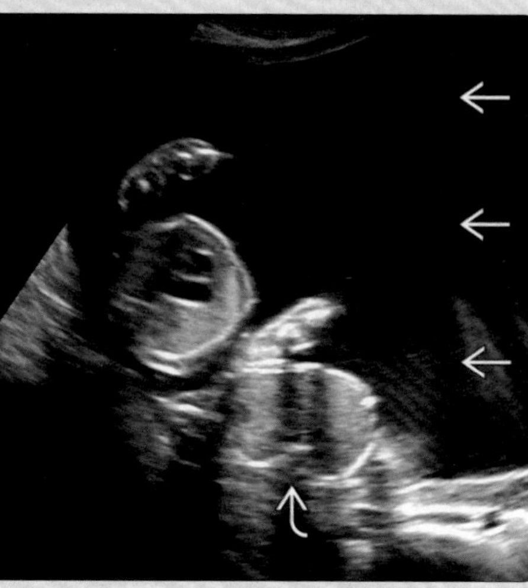

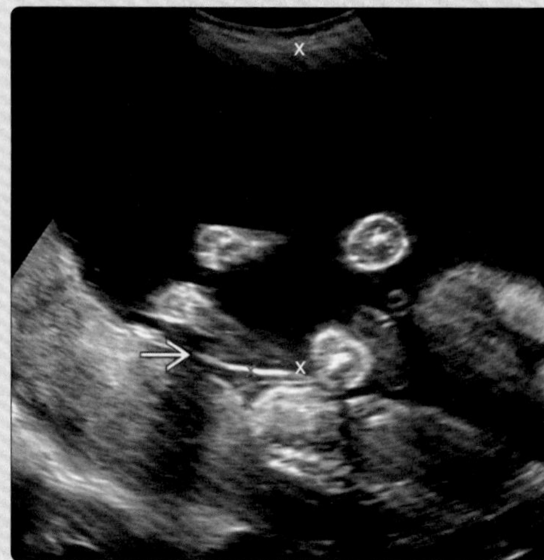

(Left) *Follow-up scan in the same case shows dramatic polyhydramnios ➡. The membrane is no longer visible because it is "shrink-wrapped" around the donor twin ➡, which was unable to move at all while the recipient twin was very active.* **(Right)** *Careful search showed the membrane ➡ and confirmed development of oligohydramnios (red x) and polyhydramnios (white x). The patient was referred for laser therapy. Unfortunately, her membranes ruptured a week after treatment.*

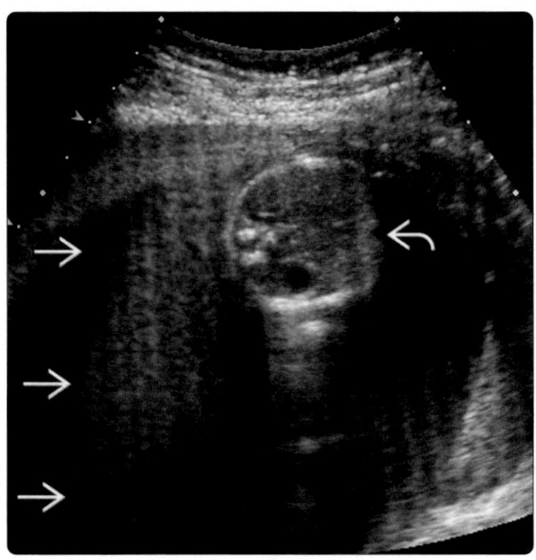

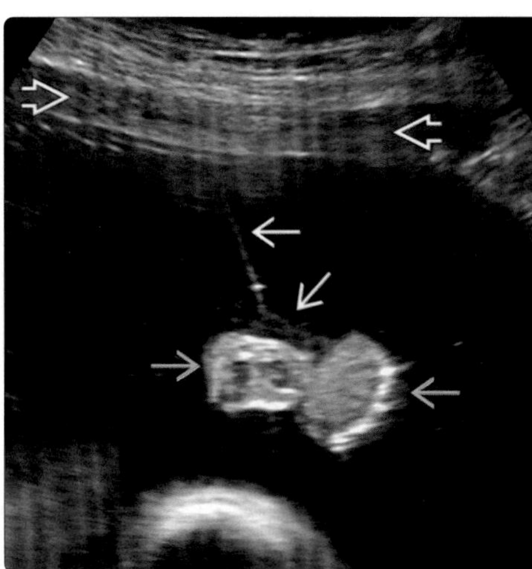

(Left) *Ultrasound shows polyhydramnios ➡ (recipient twin not included in image) and the "antigravity" appearance of the donor twin ➡ stuck to the anterior uterus. Use a high-resolution linear transducer to look for the membrane in this situation.* **(Right)** *Ultrasound shows a cocooned donor fetus. The feet ➡ are visible wrapped in a membrane sling ➡ that reflects back to the uterine wall ➡. The donor, suspended by and cocooned in the sling, floats in the large pool of the recipient's fluid.*

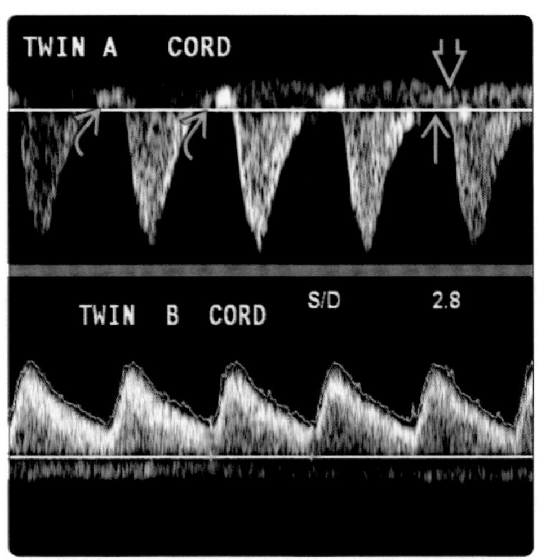

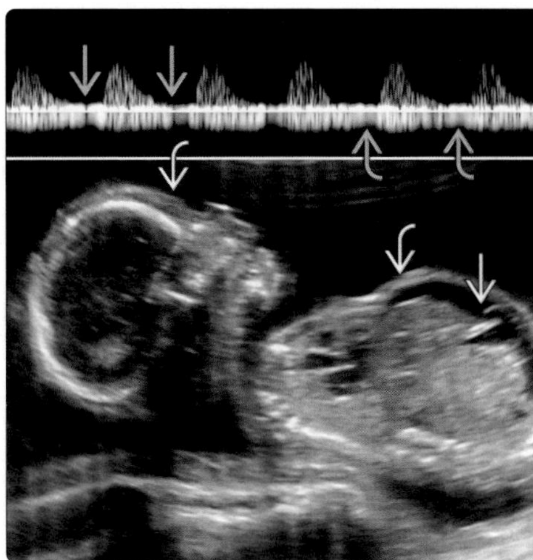

(Left) *Abnormal Doppler findings are used to stage TTTS. In this case, the donor (A) shows either absent ➡ or reversed ➡ end diastolic flow and pulsatile umbilical vein flow ➡. The recipient (B) has normal cord flow. This is stage 3 TTTS.* **(Right)** *Stage 4 TTTS implies hydrops. Continued shunting from donor to recipient causes volume overload, which eventually results in hydrops. Note the skin thickening ➡ and ascites ➡. Cord Doppler is abnormal with absent end diastolic flow ➡ and pulsatile umbilical vein flow ➡.*

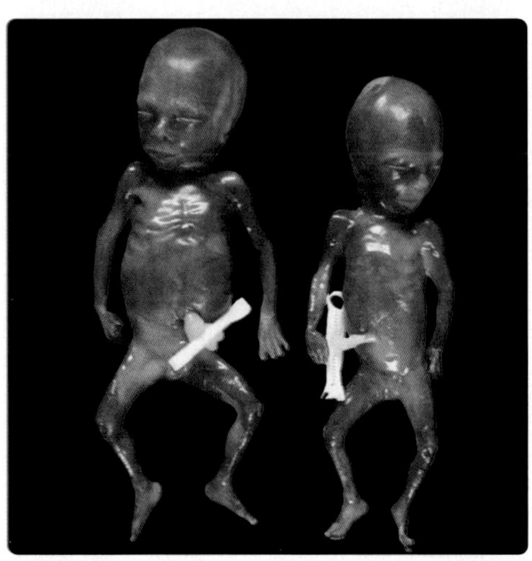

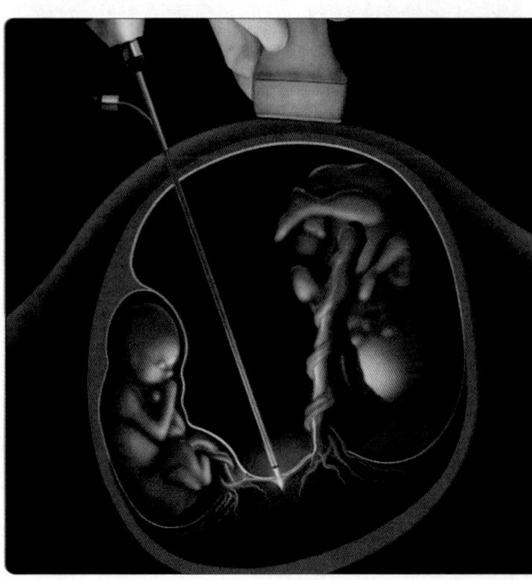

(Left) *If untreated, TTTS is often lethal, as in these 20-week twins; the recipient is on the left and the smaller donor twin is on the right. (From DP: Placenta.)* **(Right)** *Graphic illustrates endoscopic laser coagulation of the chorionic anastomoses that cause TTTS. It is important to recognize the condition as effective treatment is now available. Fluid checks at least every 2 weeks are essential for prompt diagnosis The placenta is accessed via the recipient's large sac. The "stuck" donor twin is seen on the left. (From DP: Placenta.)*

Discordant Twin Growth

KEY FACTS

TERMINOLOGY

- Discordant twin growth most commonly defined as 20% difference in estimated fetal weight (EFW) between fetuses
  - Percentage difference in EFW = EFW larger - EFW smaller/EFW larger x 100
- Abdominal circumference (AC) difference > 20 mm in 2nd/3rd trimester
- Ratio of large AC:small AC > 1.3 predicts severe birth weight discordance better than EFW

SCANNING TIPS

- Dizygotic twins are genetically different: 2 sperm + 2 ova = 2 unique zygotes; benign growth rate deviations may occur
- Monozygotic twins are genetically identical: 1 sperm + 1 ovum = 1 zygote that divides to create twins
  - Should have same growth potential: Discordant growth abnormal even in absence of growth restriction
- **Determine chorionicity and amnionicity in all multiples**
- Careful search for anomalies/signs of aneuploidy if crown rump length discrepancy
- Document placental cord insertion sites
  - **Velamentous cord insertion is marker for unequal placental sharing** in monochorionic (MC) twins
    - Associated with 13x increase in discordant birth weight
- Check placental implantation sites: ↑ risk growth restriction with implantation on septum/fibroids
- Use cord Doppler as part of fetal well-being assessment
  - Vascular connections occur in all MC placentas
  - Track flow in growth-restricted twin: **Reversed end-diastolic flow indicates high risk for demise**
  - Demise of 1 twin results in acute hypotensive event in surviving twin with ischemic injury to brain/myocardium
- **Check for twin-twin transfusion in MC twins with discordant growth**

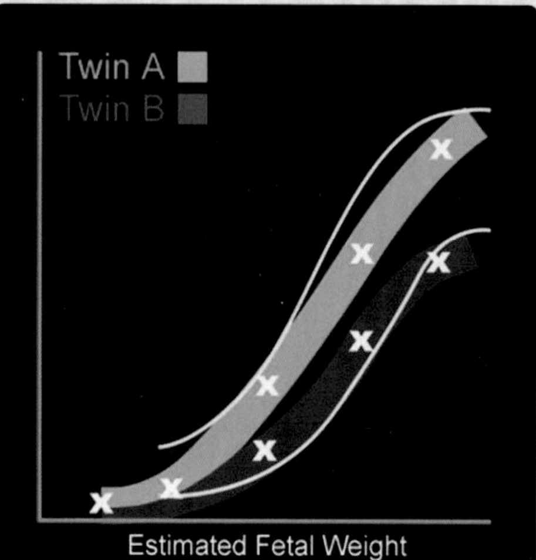

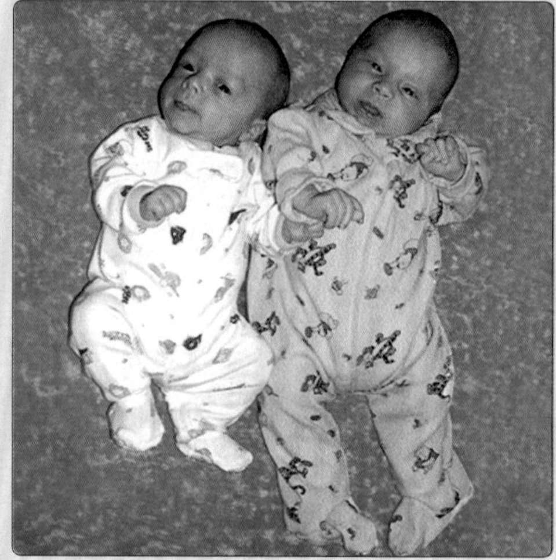

(Left) *Graphic demonstrates 3rd-trimester growth lag for twin B with the estimated fetal weight dropping below the 10th percentile, while twin A is normally grown. Yellow lines represent 10th and 90th percentiles of EFW vs. gestational age.* **(Right)** *Despite being delivered by emergency C-section at 36 weeks for growth restriction, low fluid, & abnormal Doppler, these monochorionic twins had no adverse consequences. At 11 months, there was a 5-lb weight difference, but both were healthy & developmentally normal.*

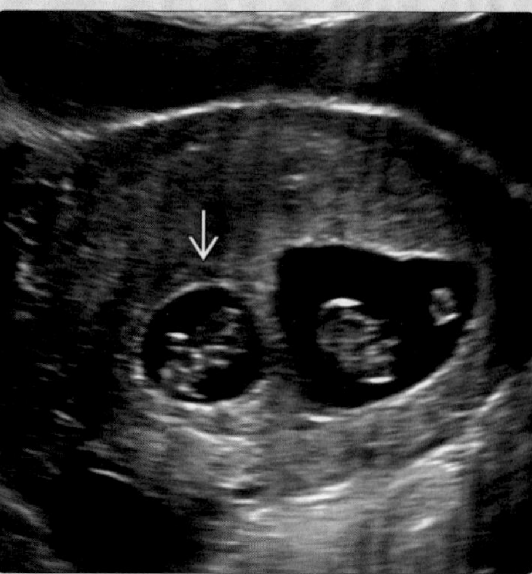

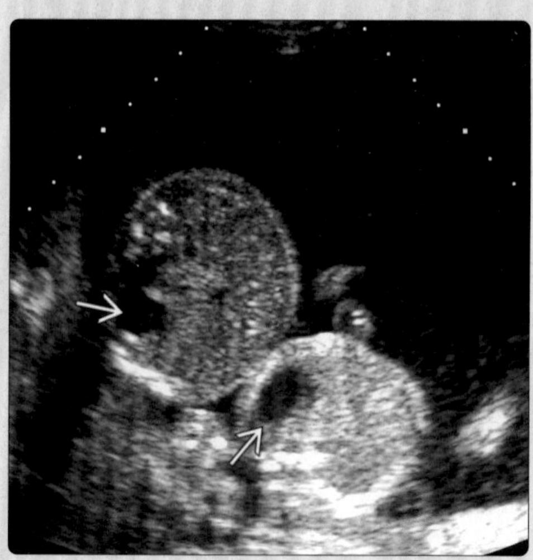

(Left) *1st-trimester US shows an obvious discrepancy in sac size in this dichorionic twin pair. The smaller twin ➡ looks "crowded." Neither aneuploidy nor anomalies were detected. Both infants were liveborn; this is an example of different growth potential in dizygotic twins.* **(Right)** *US shows monochorionic monoamniotic twins side by side (stomach bubbles ➡). Abdominal circumference of the superior twin is visibly larger than that of the inferior twin. Discordant growth is always abnormal in monochorionic twins.*

Twin Reversed Arterial Perfusion

KEY FACTS

TERMINOLOGY

- Anomalous twin [twin reversed arterial perfusion (TRAP) twin] perfused by deoxygenated blood from pump twin
- Blood enters fetus via umbilical artery (UA)
  - Reversed perfusion → selective development of torso/lower extremities
  - Lack of umbilical vein flow into heart → impaired/absent cardiac development

IMAGING

- **Must be monochorionic gestation**
- **Flow in UA of anomalous twin is toward fetus**
- TRAP twin anomalies are lethal
  - Dysmorphic fetus with edema and cyst formation in soft tissues
  - Usually recognizable torso and lower extremities
  - Rudimentary heart may exist
  - Often no identifiable cranial structures
  - Presence of upper extremities variable

SCANNING TIPS

- **You will never miss this diagnosis if you check direction of UA flow in anomalous twins**
- Careful search for anomalies of pump twin as intervention only indicated to salvage healthy pump twin
- Compare abdominal circumferences: Prognosis worse if ≥ 50% difference
- Monitor size of abnormal twin
  - Prolate ellipsoid formula (width x height x length x 0.523) most accurate
  - TRAP twin > 70% of pump twin → increased risk of pump twin compromise
- Monitor fluid volume: Polyhydramnios is poor prognostic indicator
- Look for signs of impending hydrops in pump twin
  - Tricuspid regurgitation
  - Abnormal flow in ductus venosus

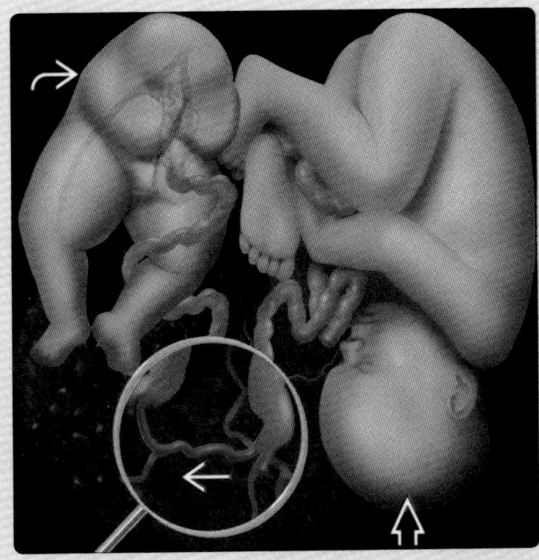

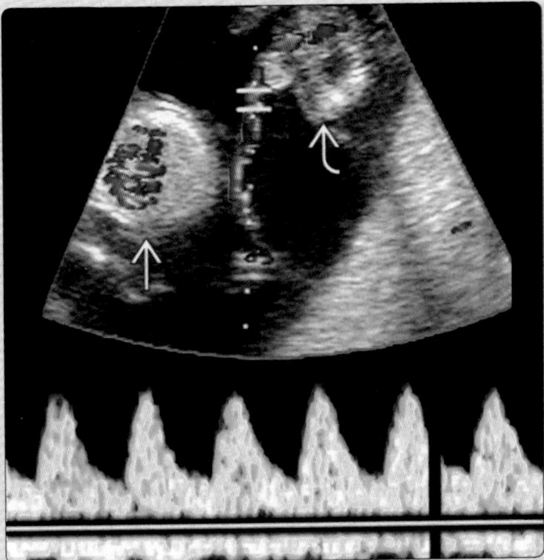

(Left) *Graphic depicts a normal twin ➡ perfusing an abnormal co-twin ➡ via an artery (deoxygenated blood) to artery placental anastomosis ➡. Abnormal circulation with selective perfusion of the lower extremities impairs development of the heart, torso, and head.* **(Right)** *Color Doppler ultrasound at 14-weeks gestation shows umbilical arterial flow toward the abnormal, edematous twin ➡. Reverse flow in the umbilical artery is diagnostic of TRAP. The normal pump twin ➡ is also visible.*

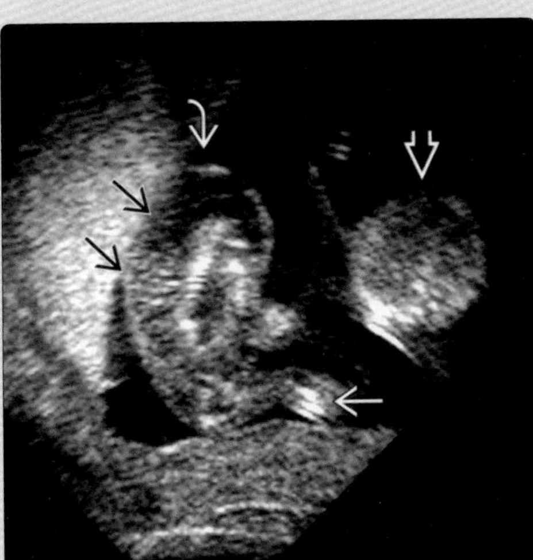

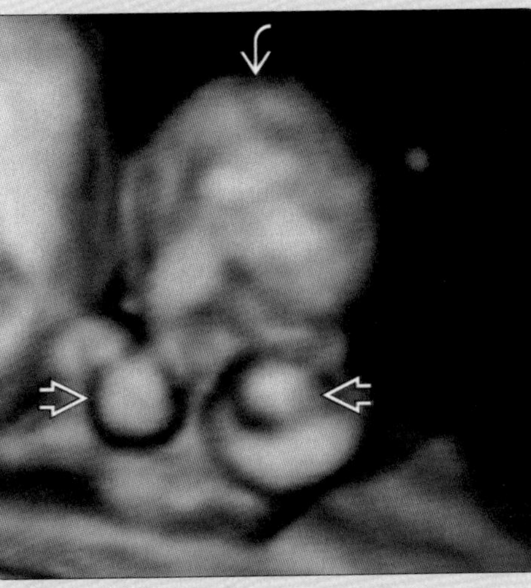

(Left) *Ultrasound shows a relatively well-developed TRAP twin with lower extremities ➡ but no cranial structures ➡. Note edema of torso ➡. The pump twin ➡ was structurally normal.* **(Right)** *3D ultrasound shows the abnormal morphology of the anomalous twin in TRAP. Abnormal lower extremities ➡ protrude from the amorphous soft tissue mass ➡ that represents the torso. No cranial structures or upper extremities are seen.*

Conjoined Twins

KEY FACTS

TERMINOLOGY

- Fetal fusion of variable degree
- Nomenclature
  - **Site of fusion + suffix "pagus"**
    - **Omphalopagus**: Abdomen fused from xiphoid to umbilicus, heart not involved
  - **Prefix "di" denotes separate parts associated with conglomerate structure**
    - **Dicephalus**: Conglomerate mass with 2 identifiable heads

IMAGING

- **Only occurs with monochorionic twinning**
  - Single placental mass
  - No intertwin membrane
  - **Fetuses inseparable, but relative position is not always constant**
  - Often hyperextension of cervical spines, unusual limb positioning
- Fused umbilical cords common
- Polyhydramnios in 50%

SCANNING TIPS

- Look for contiguous skin covering between fetuses for diagnosis of conjoined twins
  - Variable presentation does not exclude diagnosis
  - Connection may be extensive (e.g., thoracoomphalopagus) or quite small (e.g., ischiopagus)
- Use 3D US surface-rendered images to help parents understand anatomy
- Perform dedicated fetal echocardiography
  - High incidence of congenital heart disease
  - Acoustic access is better in utero than post delivery; fetuses stable on placental support
- Use color Doppler to assess shared organ blood supply
  - Omphalopagus twins: 80% share liver
  - Thoracopagus twins: 90% share pericardium, 75% share heart

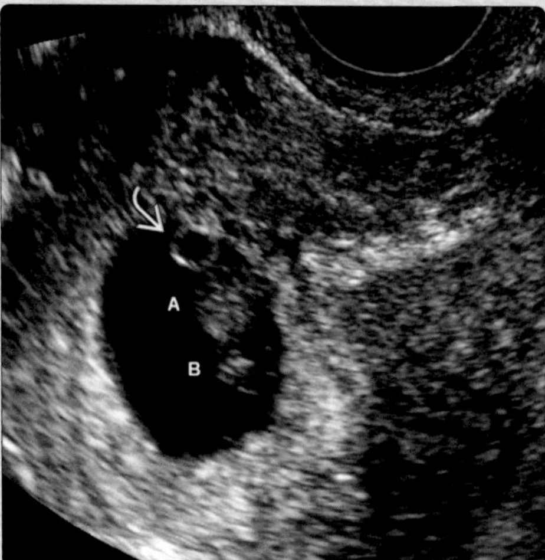

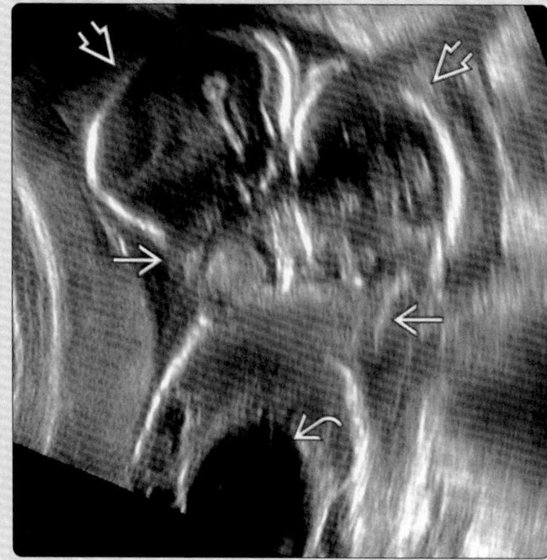

(Left) *Transvaginal US shows 2 embryos (A, B) and a single yolk sac ➙. The embryos were inseparable on prolonged inspection. Cardiac pulsations were visible in 2 separate areas. This pregnancy ended in spontaneous abortion before the type of conjoined twinning could be determined.* **(Right)** *Coronal oblique US shows 2 heads ➪ and necks ➡ on a single torso (i.e., dicephalus twins). As is so often the case, there are multiple anomalies, in this instance, bladder outlet obstruction ➙. This patient chose to terminate the pregnancy.*

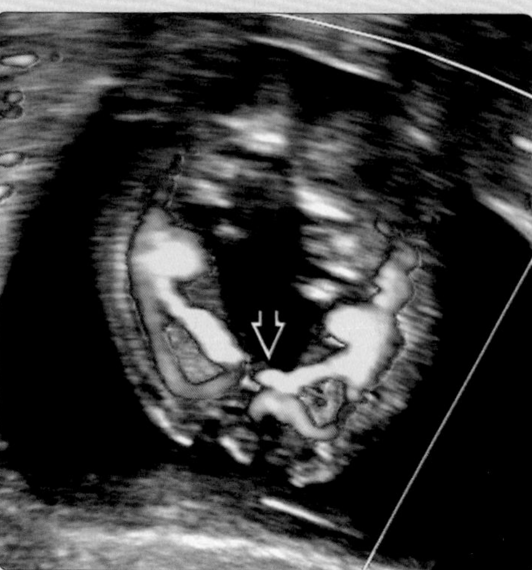

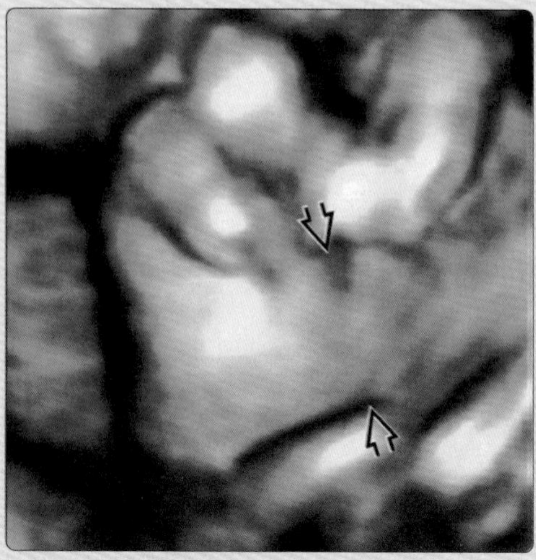

(Left) *Sagittal power Doppler US shows conjoined twins with a very narrow connecting bridge of tissue at the umbilical cord insertion site ➪. These twins would have been excellent candidates for separation, but intrauterine demise occurred within weeks of this scan.* **(Right)** *3D surface-rendered US demonstrates skin continuity ➪ across the abdomens of these omphalopagus twins. Monoamniotic twins may be very close to each other and appear to be hugging, but they will not have contiguous skin covering.*

KEY FACTS

TERMINOLOGY

- 3 or more embryos/fetuses with any combination of
  - Separate or shared chorionic sacs
  - Separate or shared amniotic sacs

IMAGING

- **Establishment of chorionicity is critical as it determines pregnancy management**

SCANNING TIPS

- Determine chorionicity and amnionicity in every multiple pregnancy
  - 1st trimester is best time; use transvaginal ultrasound (TVUS) for highest resolution
- Document fetal positions carefully
  - Vital for planned reduction of aneuploid fetuses
  - Essential to track individual fetal growth
- Measure nuchal translucency
  - Assumes greater importance in screening for aneuploidy
  - **Maternal serum screening and cell-free fetal DNA limited in multifetal gestations**
- Monthly scans for growth and fluid
  - More frequent follow-up with monochorionicity, anomalies, discordant growth or fluid
- Use maximum vertical pocket for each fetus to track fluid distribution
- Assess for complications of monochorionic placentation when present
  - Unequal placental sharing
  - Twin-twin transfusion syndrome
  - Twin reversed arterial perfusion
  - Conjoined fetuses
- **Check placental cord insertion for velamentous cord**
- Assess cervix with TVUS
  - Length: Definition and management of short cervix is controversial but best images obtained with TVUS
  - Placenta previa, low-lying placenta
  - **Always use color Doppler to look for vasa previa**

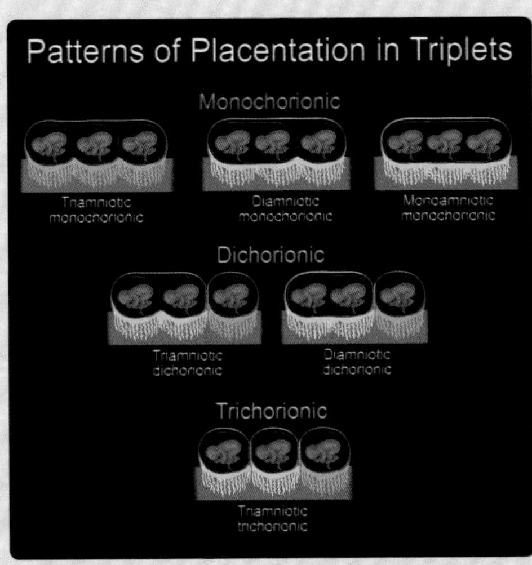

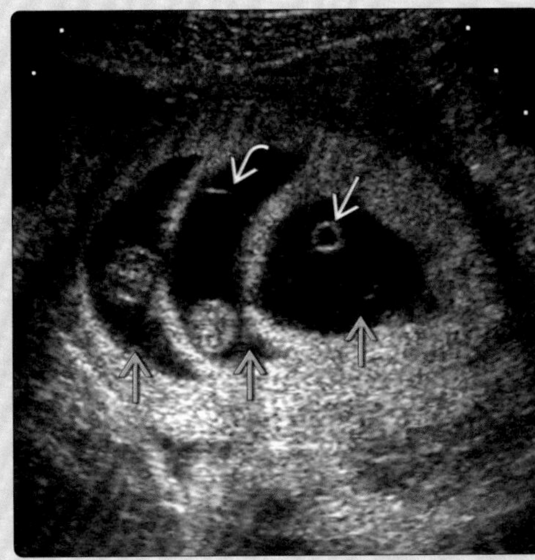

(Left) *Triplets may be monochorionic, dichorionic, or trichorionic with any combination of amniotic sacs. Monozygous triplets may be mono-, di-, or triamniotic. Dizygous triplets may be di- or trichorionic. Trizygous triplets must be trichorionic. Combinations of monozygous and polyzygous multiples are common. Multichorionic placentas may be separate or fused.* **(Right)** *TAUS shows 3 thick-walled sacs → in trichorionic triplets. All 3 embryos were visible in real time. Note the yolk sac → and amnion →.*

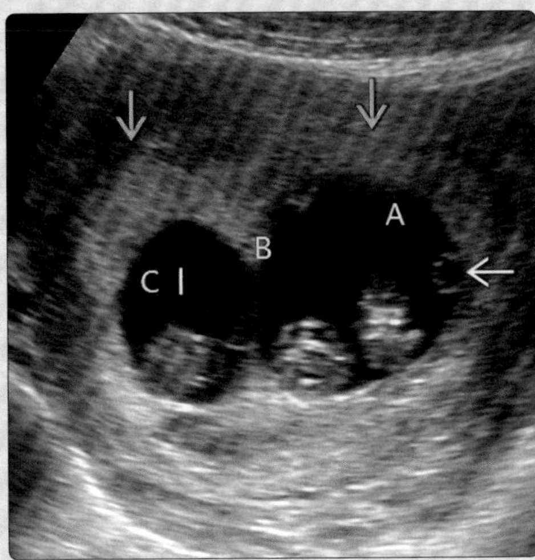

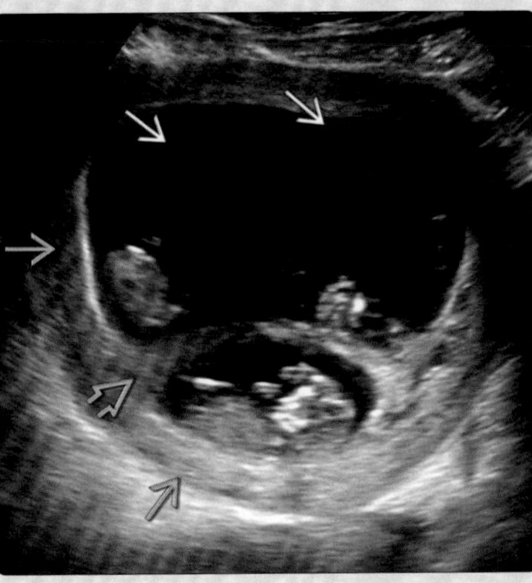

(Left) *TAUS shows 2 thick-walled sacs → indicating dichorionic triplets. With 1 yolk sac → and no membrane, there was concern that A and B were a monoamniotic pair. Vaginal US performed later in the study revealed a thin membrane proving diamnionicity. Final diagnosis was dichorionic, triamniotic triplets.* **(Right)** *TAUS shows 2 thick-walled sacs → with a twin peak sign → in dichorionic triplets. The fine, delicate amniotic membranes → are barely visible in the anterior sac. These are dichorionic triamniotic triplets.*

PART VI
SECTION 11
Aneuploidy

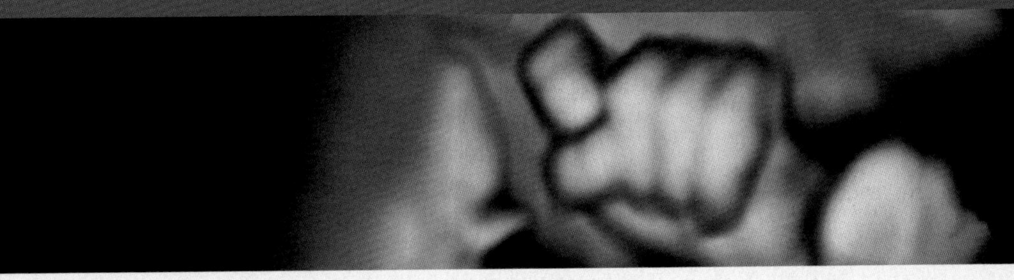

Trisomy 21

KEY FACTS

IMAGING

- **1st-trimester findings (11- to 14-week scan)**
  - ↑ nuchal translucency: ↑ fluid behind neck on midsagittal view
  - Absent nasal bone
  - Abnormal ductus venosus and tricuspid flow
- **2nd-trimester minor markers (15-22 weeks)**
  - ↑ nuchal fold thickness (≥ 6 mm)
  - Absent or small nasal bone
  - Short femur length/short humerus length
  - Echogenic bowel
  - Intracardiac echogenic focus
  - Renal pelvis dilatation
  - Mild lateral ventriculomegaly
- **Hallmark anomalies associated with trisomy 21**
  - Atrioventricular septal defect
  - Esophageal atresia (EA)
  - Duodenal atresia (DA)

TOP DIFFERENTIAL DIAGNOSES

- Turner syndrome: Cystic hygroma is hallmark anomaly
- Trisomy 18: Multiple anomalies
- Trisomy 13: Holoprosencephaly is hallmark anomaly

DIAGNOSTIC CHECKLIST

- Associated with advanced maternal age (≥ 35 years old)
- Cell-free fetal DNA (cfDNA) is best screening test
  - cfDNA detects 99.2% (0.1% false-positive rate)
- Maternal serum markers detect 95% (3-5% false + rate)
- Chorionic villus sampling and amniocentesis are true diagnostic tests

SCANNING TIPS

- Hepatomegaly/splenomegaly in 3rd trimester suggestive of fetal transient abnormal myelopoiesis or leukemia
- Polyhydramnios from EA or DA often in 3rd trimester
- Look at profile carefully (big tongue, flat midface)
- Ultrasound may be completely normal (40-50%)

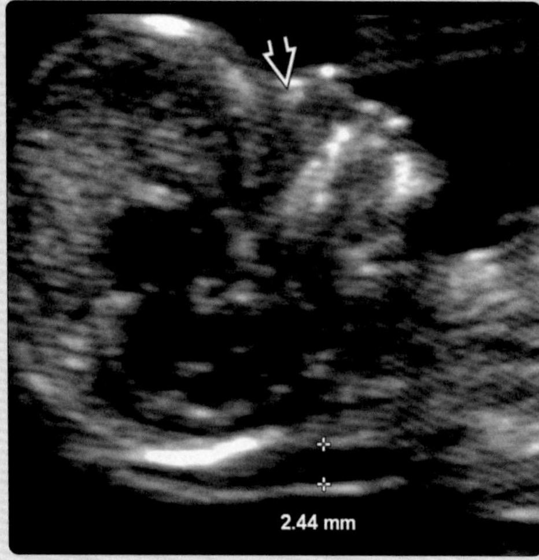

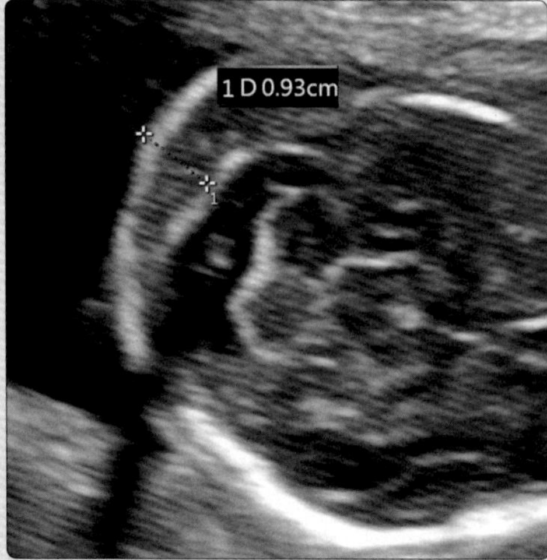

(Left) *In this 12-week fetus, the nuchal translucency (NT) (calipers) is greater than expected for the crown rump length. A faint nasal bone is present ➡. Maternal serum screen results were suspicious for trisomy 21 (T21) and amniocentesis in the 2nd trimester was performed, diagnostic for T21. The pregnancy was continued.* **(Right)** *Increased NT is fluid and may evolve into thickened nuchal fold (skin and subcutaneous tissue). Between 15-22 weeks, nuchal fold ≥ 6 mm is considered too thick as seen in this fetus with T21.*

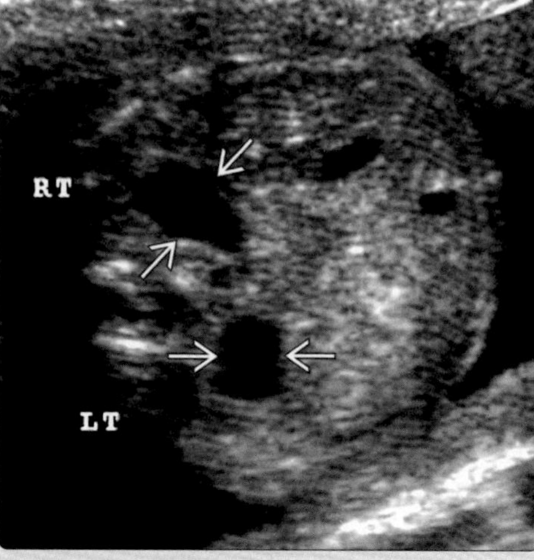

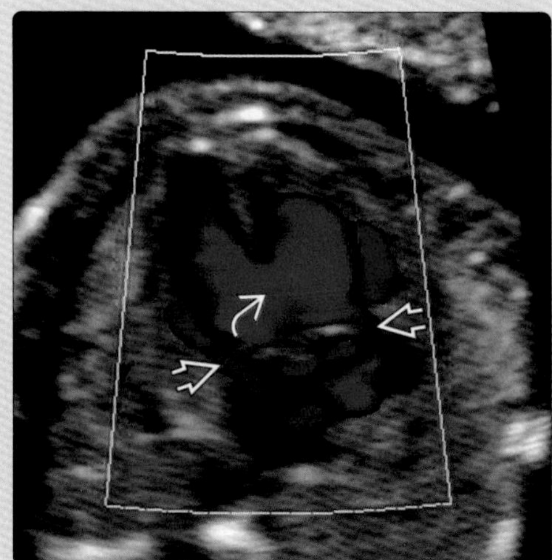

(Left) *Bilateral renal pelvis dilation ➡ (≥ 4 mm in midgestation) is seen in this 2nd-trimester fetus with T21. This finding is considered both a marker for aneuploidy and potential progressive hydronephrosis.* **(Right)** *In this fetus with T21, color Doppler 4-chamber view of the heart shows a large ventricular septal defect ➡ and mitral and tricuspid valves positioned at the same level ➡, typical findings of atrioventricular septal defect (AVSD). Up to 1/2 of the fetuses with AVSD have aneuploidy; most common diagnosis is T21.*

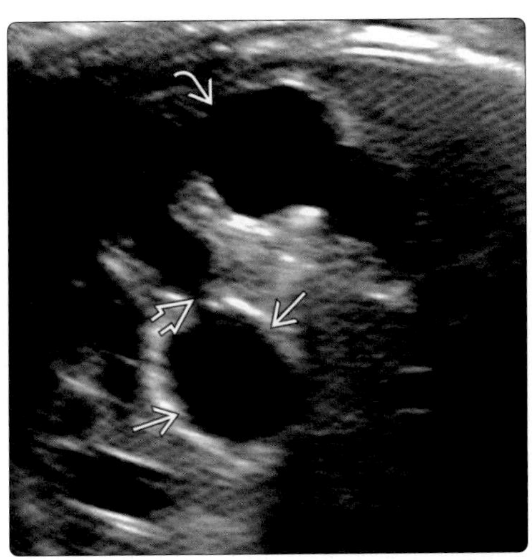

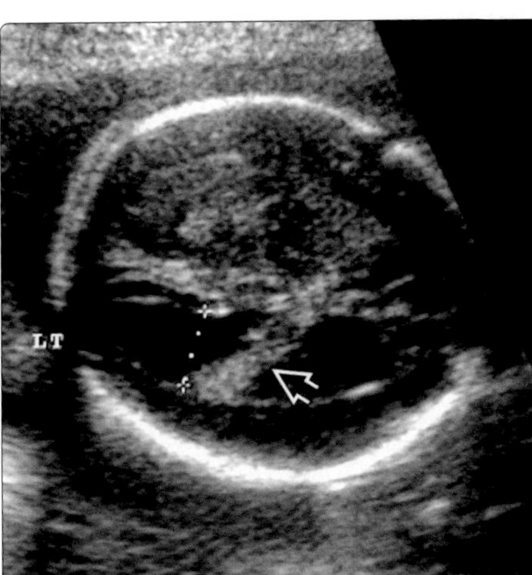

(Left) *The only finding in this fetus with T21 was duodenal atresia. The duodenum ➡ is dilated and ends abruptly. Seeing the pylorus ➡, connecting the dilated stomach ➡ to the duodenum, proves that the fluid-filled structure is the duodenum and not an abdominal cyst.* **(Right)** *Axial ultrasound shows mild lateral ventriculomegaly (10-12 mm dilation) in this fetus with T21. The choroid plexus ➡ dangles in the distended ventricle (calipers). Ventriculomegaly is a marker for aneuploidy as well as other brain anomalies.*

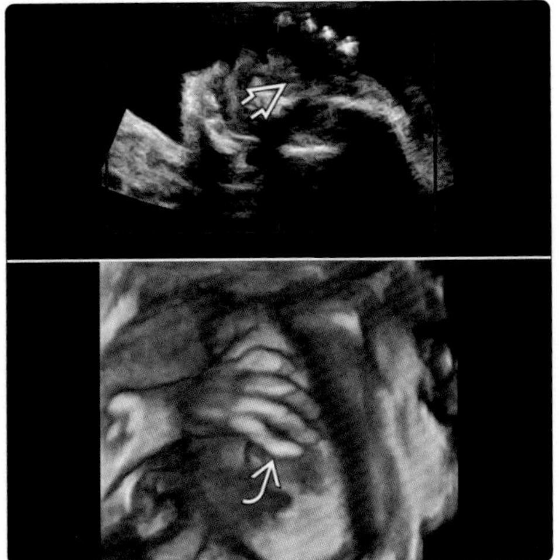

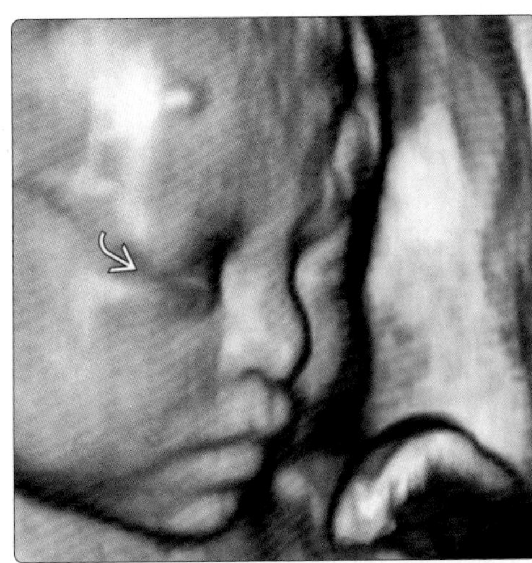

(Left) *This fetus with an absent nasal bone ➡ also has 5th finger clinodactyly (tip of finger turned inward because of short midfinger bone) seen best on the reconstructed 3D image ➡. Absent nasal bone is considered a strong marker and clinodactyly a soft marker for T21. Genetic testing should be offered when markers are seen.* **(Right)** *3D ultrasound of the face in a fetus with T21 shows classic features of flat midface and upslanted eyelids ➡. Macroglossia (large tongue) is another facial feature with T21.*

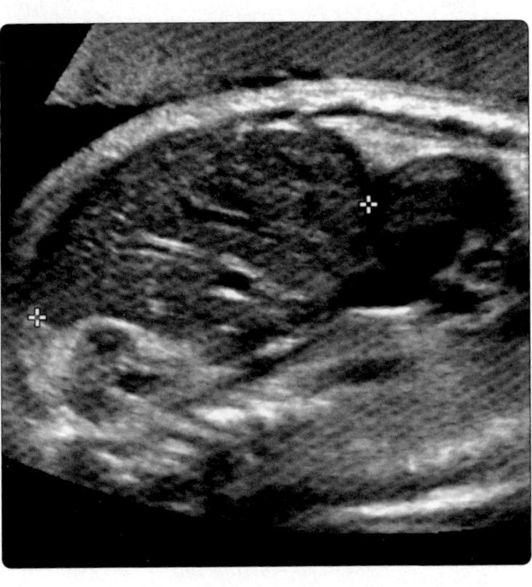

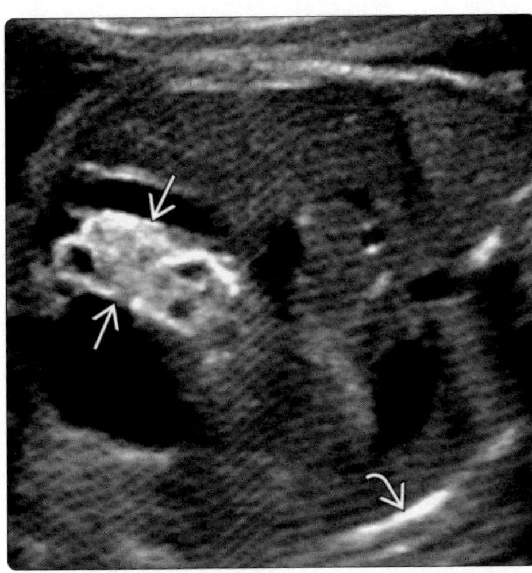

(Left) *In this 3rd-trimester fetus with T21, the liver is markedly enlarged (calipers measure liver length to look up in published tables). Fetuses with T21 are at risk for transient abnormal myelopoiesis (TAM) and leukemia, which present as hepatosplenomegaly. Increased monitoring is indicated when TAM is suspected.* **(Right)** *Echogenic bowel ➡ is another marker for T21. The bowel echogenicity is equal or greater than bone ➡. Other associations include fetal infection and cystic fibrosis.*

Trisomy 18

KEY FACTS

TERMINOLOGY

- Autosomal trisomy of chromosome 18 (T18)

IMAGING

- Hallmark finding: Multiple anomalies
  - No single anomaly is hallmark of T18
- Most cases with findings at time of nuchal translucency (NT)
  - ↑ NT, absent nasal bone, anomalies
- 2nd-trimester anomalies in almost all fetuses
  - Cardiac anomaly, omphalocele (often bowel only), diaphragmatic hernia, spina bifida, brain anomalies
  - Musculoskeletal anomalies
    - Radial ray, contractures (arthrogryposis), rocker-bottom feet (convex sole of foot)
    - Clenched hands + overlapping index finger
  - Markers are rarely isolated
    - Choroid plexus cysts (CPC), single umbilical artery, strawberry-shaped calvarium
- Fetal growth restriction: Early, progressive, and severe

TOP DIFFERENTIAL DIAGNOSES

- Trisomy 13: Holoprosencephaly is hallmark anomaly
- Triploidy: FGR and cystic placenta is hallmark
- Pena-Shokeir syndrome: Fetal akinesia/hypokinesia

CLINICAL ISSUES

- Associated with advanced maternal age
- Cell-free fetal DNA detection rate is 96%
- Maternal serum quadruple test with 80% detection
- 1/2 with intrauterine fetal demise (IUFD)
  - Ultrasound is poor predictor for IUFD
- 20% survive beyond 1 month, 5-10% beyond 1st year

SCANNING TIPS

- Obtain additional cardiac and extremity views if markers seen at time of anatomy scan
  - CPC will resolve regardless if fetus has T18 or not
- Structural anomalies at time of NT seen best with transvaginal ultrasound

(Left) *Multiple severe anomalies were seen at the time of anatomy scan in this 20-week fetus. On the sagittal view through the head, chest, and upper abdomen, an omphalocele ➡ and ventriculomegaly ➡ are seen.* **(Right)** *A ventricular septal defect ➡, abnormal heart axis ➡, and small left ventricle ➡ are also seen on the 4-chamber cardiac view. Not a single hallmark anomaly is associated with trisomy 18; however, the diagnosis should be suspected with multiple anomalies in different organ systems.*

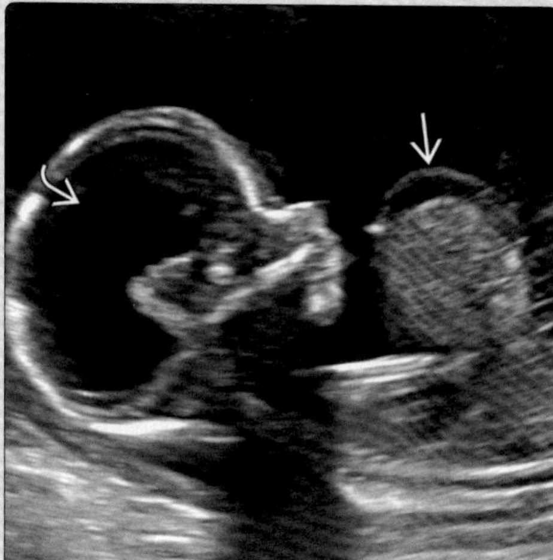

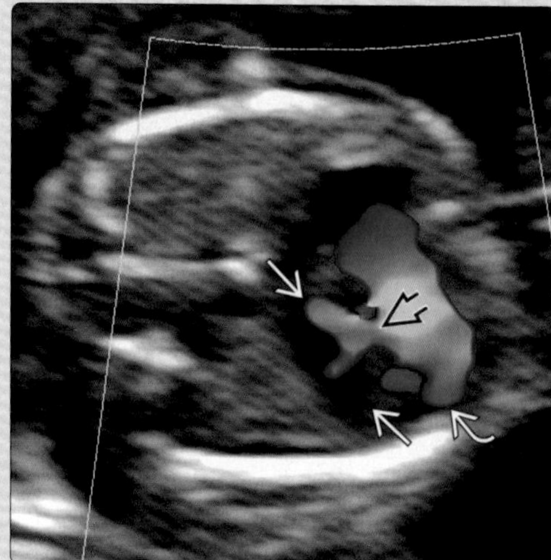

(Left) *3D ultrasound of a 3rd-trimester fetus with T18 shows a clenched hand with an overlapping index finger ➡. Multiple other anomalies were also present.* **(Right)** *Clinical photograph shows the typical hand position seen with T18. The hand is held clenched with overlapping fingers, and the index finger typically overlaps the other clenched fingers. Extremity contractures are a common feature of T18.*

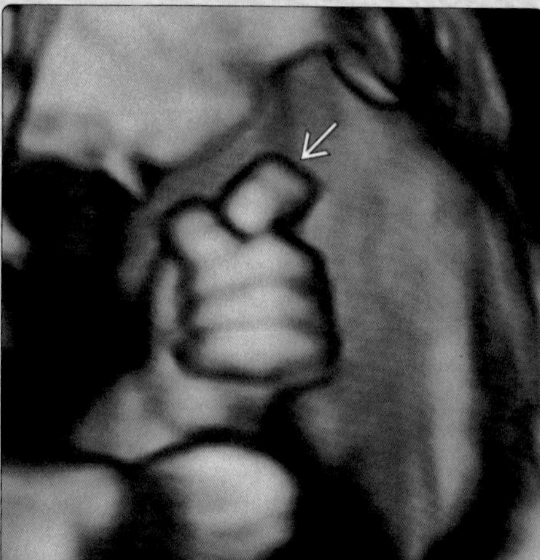

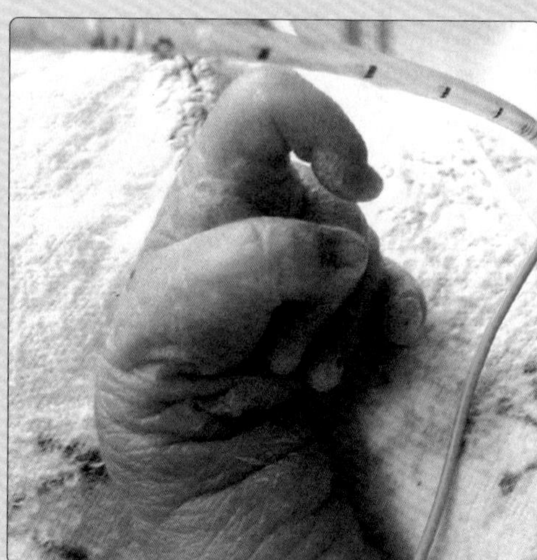

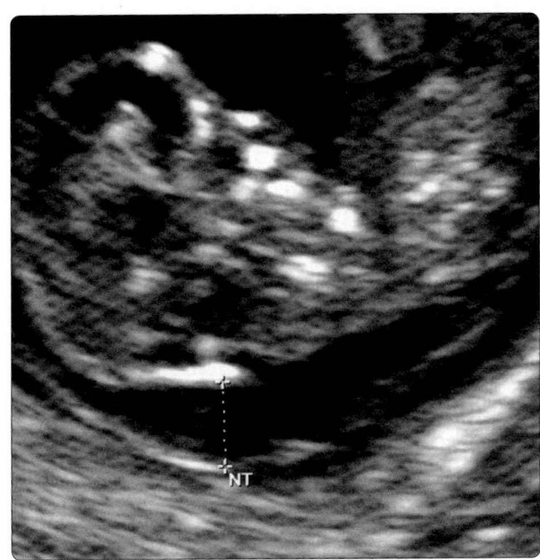

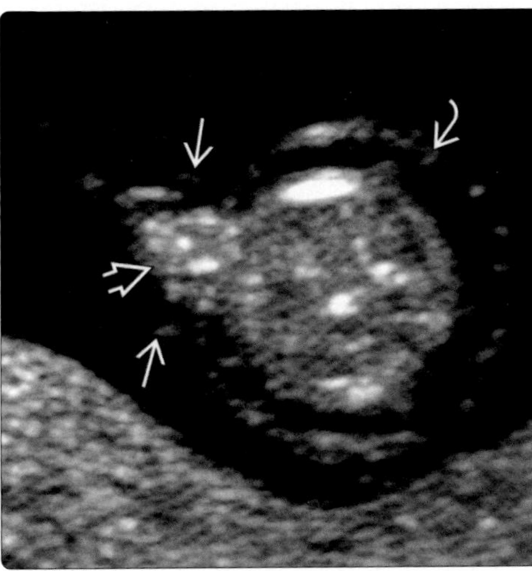

(Left) *Midline sagittal ultrasound shows a markedly increased nuchal translucency (calipers) in this 12-week fetus.* **(Right)** *Transverse view through the abdomen in the same case shows a bowel-containing omphalocele with a surrounding membrane and body wall edema. Anatomy scan at the time of nuchal translucency screening helps identify > 90% of fetuses with T18. Genetic testing via chorionic villus sampling is offered at this point (cell-free DNA testing is considered a screening test).*

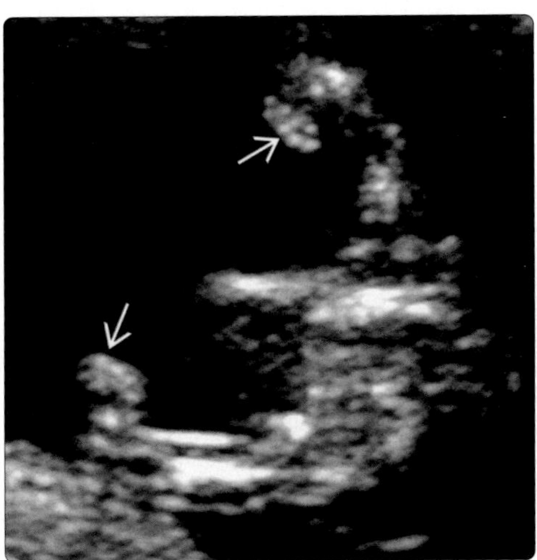

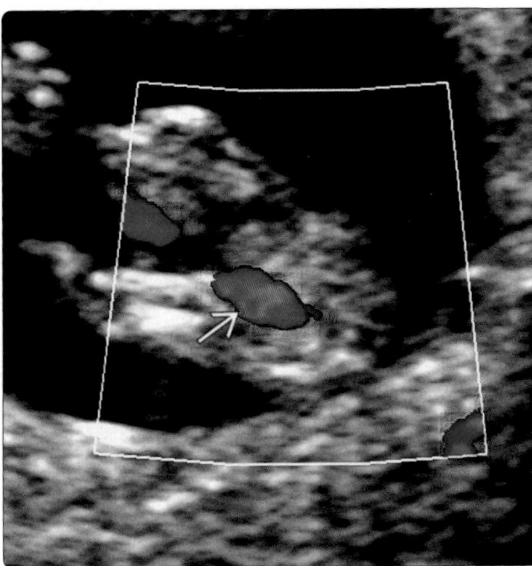

(Left) *Transverse ultrasound through the upper extremities at the time of nuchal translucency screening shows that the hands are both medially deviated, suggesting the diagnosis of bilateral radial ray malformation (radius short or absent and hand turned inward, often with missing thumbs).* **(Right)** *In addition, a single umbilical artery is seen in this fetus with T18. Chorionic villus sampling confirmed the diagnosis.*

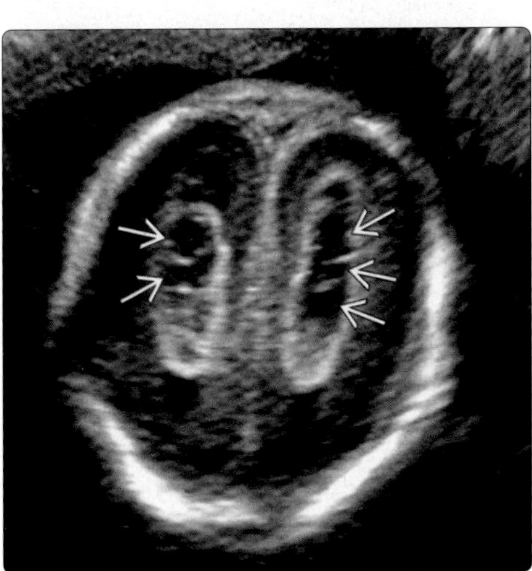

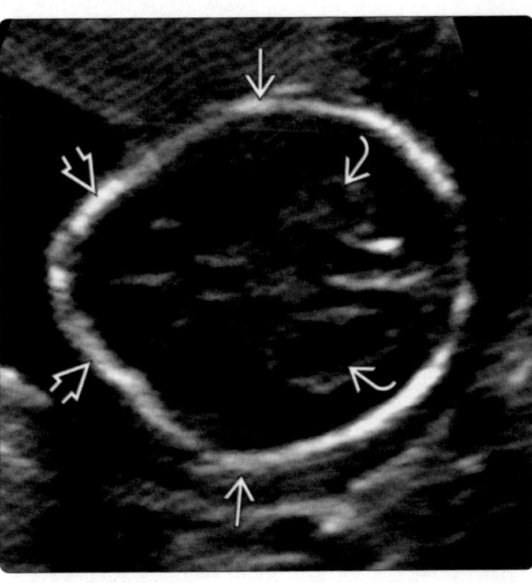

(Left) *The choroid plexus in this 2nd-trimester fetus shows multiple bilateral choroid plexus cysts (CPCs). CPCs are a marker for T18 but are most often incidental findings in normal fetuses, even when large and bilateral. This fetus had other anomalies.* **(Right)** *Strawberry-shaped calvarium is seen in this fetus with T18. The shape is because of frontal narrowing and midcalvarial widening (brachycephaly). The finding is often subtle. Bilateral CPCs were also present in this case.*

Trisomy 13

KEY FACTS

IMAGING

- Holoprosencephaly is hallmark anomaly
  - Spectrum of severity: Alobar, semilobar, lobar
  - Associated facial anomalies
    - Close-set orbits (hypotelorism), fused eyes (cyclopia)
    - Small nose, proboscis (tube-like and above orbits)
    - Cleft lip/palate: Midline or bilateral
- Cardiac defects in most cases
- Large echogenic kidneys
- Postaxial polydactyly: Extra finger or toe next to 5th digit
- Early fetal growth restriction commonly seen
- Detectable at time of nuchal translucency (NT) screening
  - ↑ NT, absent nasal bone, holoprosencephaly

TOP DIFFERENTIAL DIAGNOSES

- Holoprosencephaly without trisomy 13: Similar facial anomalies
- Trisomy 18: Also associated with holoprosencephaly
- Meckel-Gruber: Encephalocele, cystic kidneys, polydactyly

CLINICAL ISSUES

- Advanced maternal age at higher risk
- 3rd most common trisomy (after trisomy 21 and T18)
- Offer genetic testing when hallmark anomalies seen
  - Chorionic villus sampling, amniocentesis
    - Cell-free fetal DNA is for screening only
- Prognosis: 50% die in utero, 80% of live-born die 1st day of life, < 10% reach 1st birthday

SCANNING TIPS

- Look for falx at time of NT scan: Absent falx with fluid crossing midline suggests monoventricle of holoprosencephaly
- Profile view showing premaxillary protrusion at time of NT scan or midgestation is highly suggestive of bilateral cleft lip/palate
- If cavum septum pellucidum is absent, look for fused frontal horns (may be only finding of lobar holoprosencephaly)

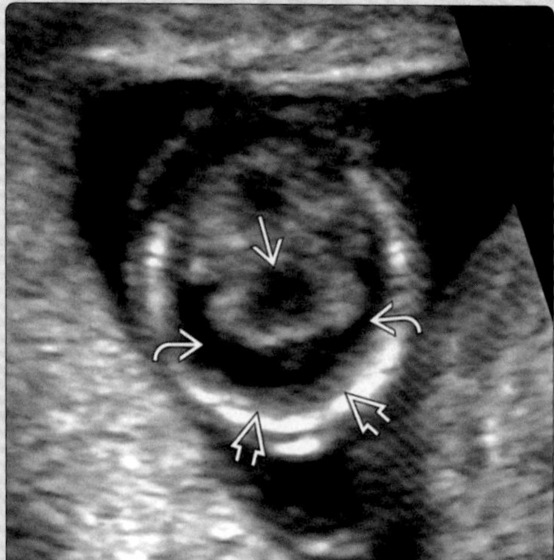

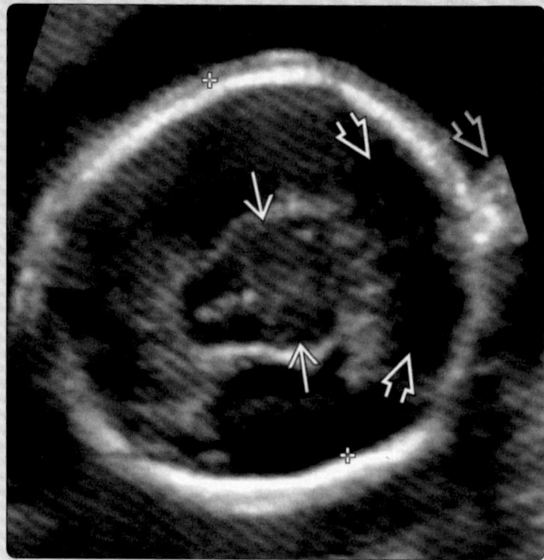

(Left) *Ultrasound of the brain at the time of nuchal translucency (NT) screening shows absent falx with monoventricle and thin anteriorly fused brain mantle across the midline. The thalamus is fused and "ball-like", classic findings of holoprosencephaly. The NT was also increased in this fetus.* **(Right)** *Similar features are seen in this 19-week fetus with holoprosencephaly. The thalamus is globular and fused. The falx is absent and the lateral ventricles are fused and cross the midline. Part of a proboscis is also seen.*

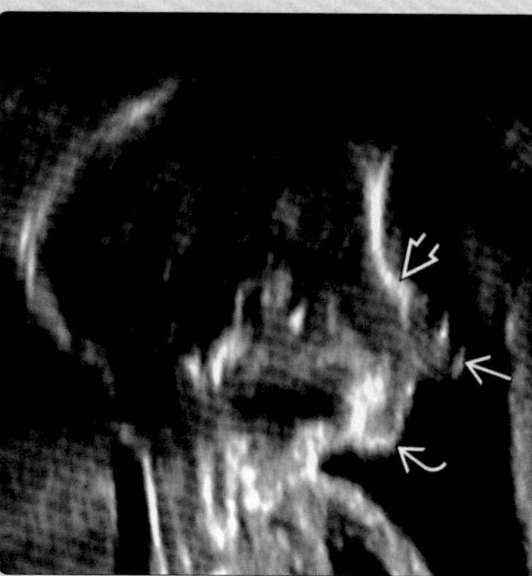

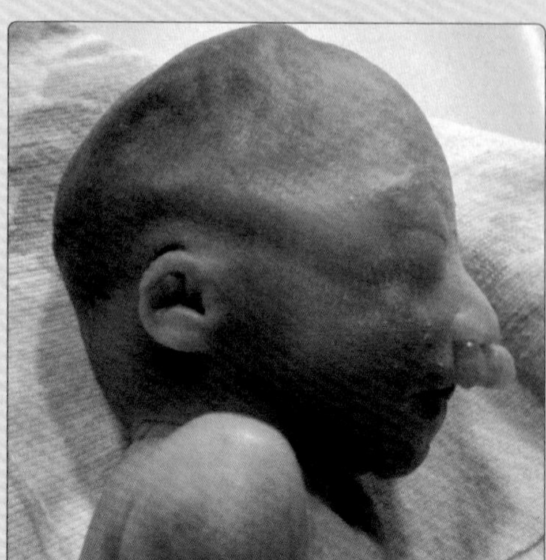

(Left) *Profile view of a 20-week fetus shows premaxillary protrusion of tissue caused by forward displacement of the anterior palate and soft tissue from bilateral cleft lip and palate. An otherwise normal nasal bone and chin are seen in this case.* **(Right)** *Clinical photograph of a fetus with trisomy 13 and premaxillary protrusion shows the excessive tissue beneath the nose, caused by bilateral cleft lip and palate. This tissue contains the anterior palate.*

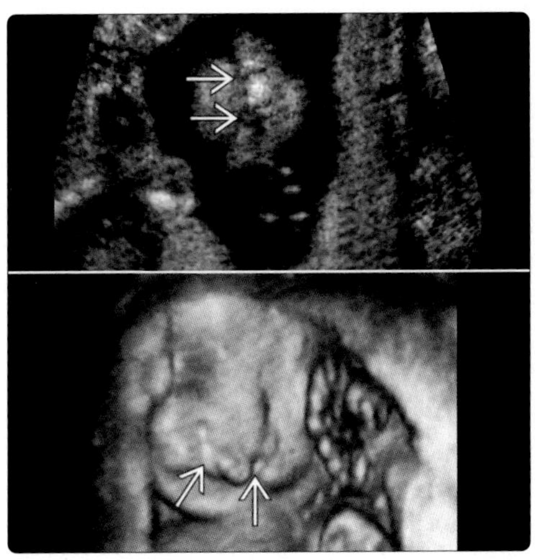

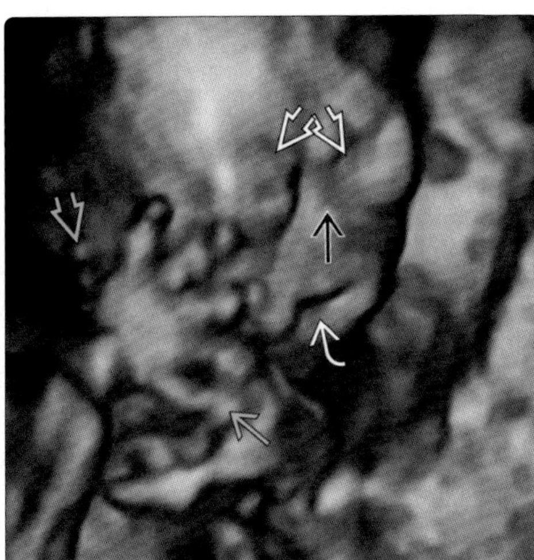

(Left) *Coronal multiplanar (top) and 3D surface-rendered (bottom) views of the fetal nose and lip show bilateral cleft lip ➡. The anterior palate plate, between the clefts, is dysplastic and prominent. On profile views, this part of the palate causes premaxillary protrusion.* **(Right)** *3D frontal face view in another case shows close-set eyes ➡, absent nose ➡, midline cleft lip ➡, and postaxial polydactyly ➡ (thumb ➡). Patients may better appreciate facial anomalies when 3D images are reviewed with them.*

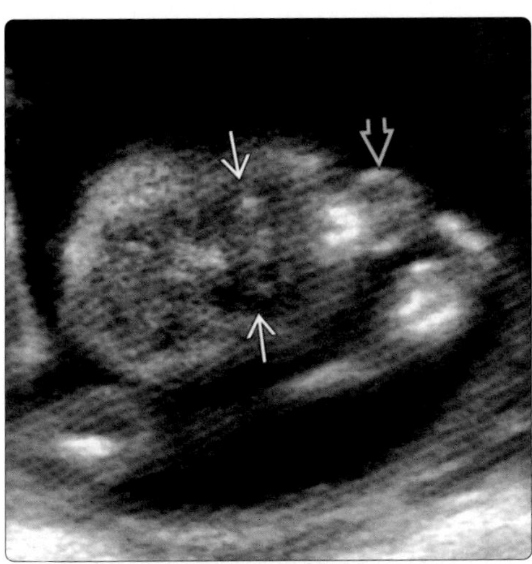

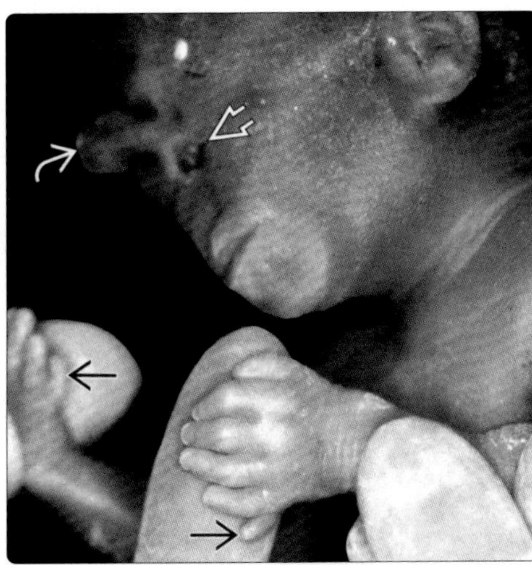

(Left) *Coronal ultrasound of the face shows small close-set eyes ➡ and a proboscis ➡, superior to the orbits. These facial features are never isolated findings.* **(Right)** *Clinical photograph of classic phenotypical features of trisomy 13 shows postaxial polydactyly ➡, proboscis ➡, and a single fused eye ➡ (i.e., cyclopia). The facial features are associated with holoprosencephaly, usually alobar.*

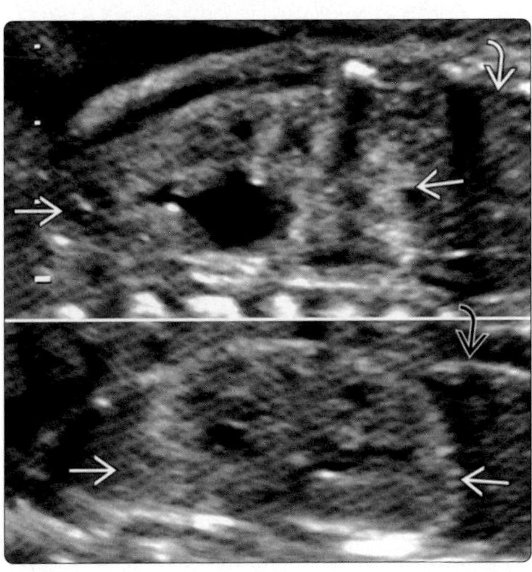

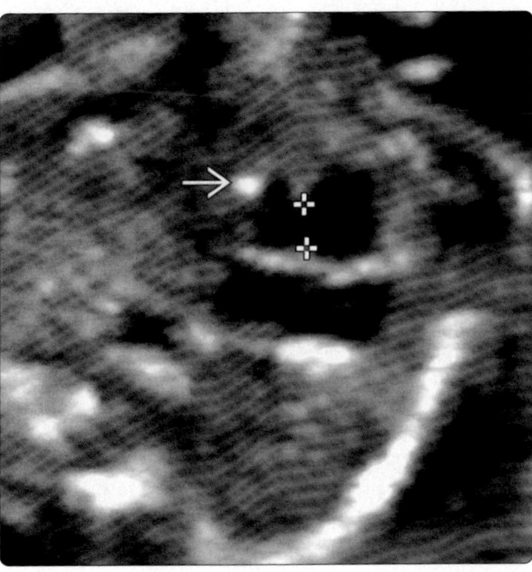

(Left) *Coronal ultrasound through the kidneys in a fetus with trisomy 13 shows bilateral enlarged echogenic kidneys ➡, a common finding with trisomy 13. Note the kidneys are more echogenic than liver ➡ and spleen ➡.* **(Right)** *Four-chamber heart view at 20 weeks shows an intracardiac echogenic focus (IEF) ➡ and a large ventricular septal defect (calipers). IEF is a common isolated finding in normal fetuses; however, IEF in conjunction with a cardiac defect is highly associated with trisomy 13.*

Turner Syndrome (45,X)

KEY FACTS

TERMINOLOGY

- Monosomy X is preferred term
- Definition: Complete or partial deficiency of X chromosome

IMAGING

- Cystic hygroma (CH) is hallmark finding
  - Large back of neck fluid collection with septations
    - CH is nuchal lymphangioma
    - Thin septations lateral + thick central nuchal ligament
  - 60% of fetuses with CH have monosomy X
- Associated nonimmune hydrops is common
  - Must see fluid in 2 cavities (CH counts as 1 area)
- Other associated anomalies
  - Hypoplastic left heart, coarctation of aorta
  - Horseshoe kidney
  - Short femur and humerus
- 1st-trimester findings in > 90% of cases
  - Typically very large nuchal translucency, CH, hydrops, normal nasal bone, reversed ductus venosus flow

TOP DIFFERENTIAL DIAGNOSES

- Noonan syndrome: Can look identical to Turner
- Trisomy 21: 2nd most likely diagnosis with CH
- Chest lymphangioma: Not associated with aneuploidy

CLINICAL ISSUES

- Very high in utero demise rates
- Cell-free fetal DNA: 89% detection rate
- Advanced maternal age not at higher risk
- Survivors variably affected
  - Webbed neck, broad chest, short limbs
  - Normal verbal IQ, delayed motor skills
  - Infertility, metabolic and autoimmune disorders

SCANNING TIPS

- Look for subtle left heart findings: Aorta smaller than pulmonary artery, mildly small left ventricle
- When massive, CH can mimic amniotic fluid (can tap CH for genetic testing)

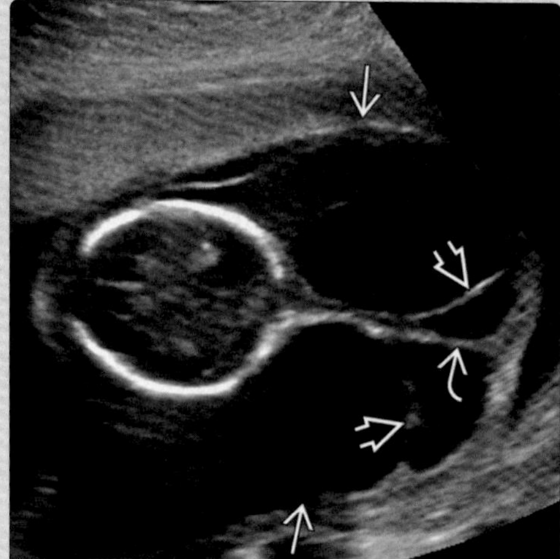

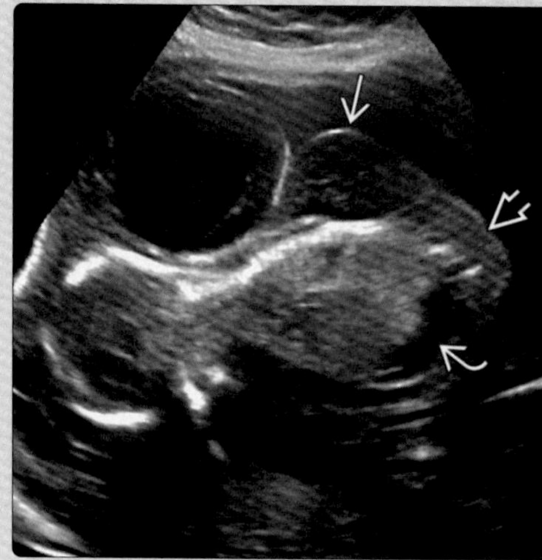

(Left) *This early 2nd-trimester fetus with monosomy X has a typical large cystic hygroma ➡. Multiple septations ➡ are seen in addition to the central nuchal ligament ➡.* **(Right)** *Sagittal view through the same fetus shows the extension of the cystic hygroma down the back ➡ as well as anasarca ➡ and ascites ➡. Hydrops is often associated with cystic hygroma and Turner syndrome. Prognosis is poor when these features are seen.*

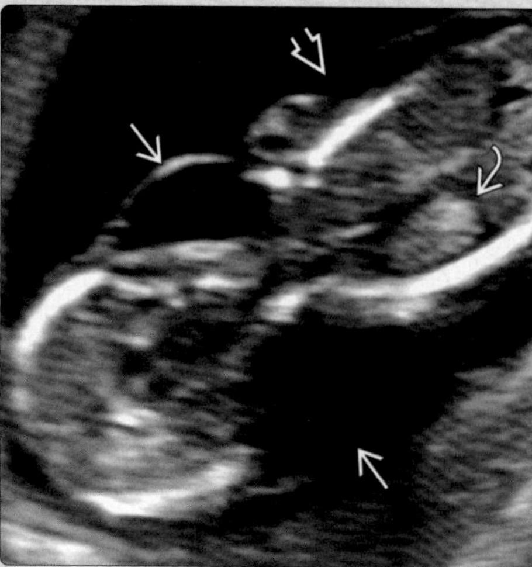

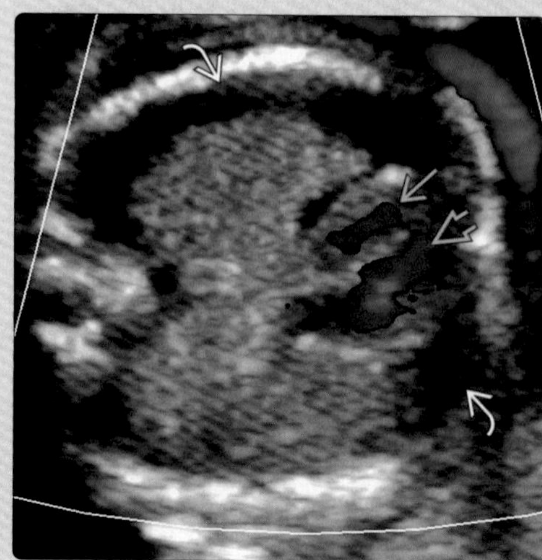

(Left) *Coronal view of a 12-week fetus at the time of nuchal translucency (NT) screening shows lateral neck fluid collections ➡, a trace amount of pleural fluid ➡, and skin edema ➡. Fetuses with monosomy X have the largest NT measurements.* **(Right)** *Axial view through the chest in a 2nd-trimester fetus shows pleural effusions ➡ and a small left ventricle ➡ compared to the right ➡. Aortic coarctation was diagnosed on a formal fetal echocardiography, commonly seen with monosomy X.*

KEY FACTS

TERMINOLOGY

- Synonym: Partial mole
- Definition: 69 chromosomes (instead of 46)
  - Most common is diandric triploidy (extra set is paternal)
  - Digynic triploidy if extra set is maternal

IMAGING

- 2 different appearances
  - Diandric triploidy
    - Large cystic placenta
    - Symmetric fetal growth restriction (FGR)
    - Ovaries enlarged with theca lutein cysts
  - Digynic triploidy
    - Normal or small placenta
    - Asymmetric FGR (large head, small body)
- Multiple other anomalies common
- Abnormal gestational sac in early 1st trimester
- Abnormal anatomy at nuchal translucency (NT) screening

TOP DIFFERENTIAL DIAGNOSES

- Twin molar pregnancy: Classic mole + normal fetus
- Placental hydropic/edema from failed pregnancy
- Placental mesenchymal dysplasia (can look identical)
  - Cystic placenta, associated with preeclampsia, FGR

CLINICAL ISSUES

- Definitive diagnosis with placental biopsy or amniocentesis
- Part of gestational trophoblastic disease spectrum
  - Variable hCG levels
    - High hCG associated with theca lutein ovarian cysts
  - Associated preeclampsia and placental abruption
- Triploidy considered lethal diagnosis
  - Most with intrauterine fetal demise
  - Lethal in neonatal period if live birth

SCANNING TIPS

- Look carefully for fetal anomalies when cysts seen in placenta, even at time of NT screening

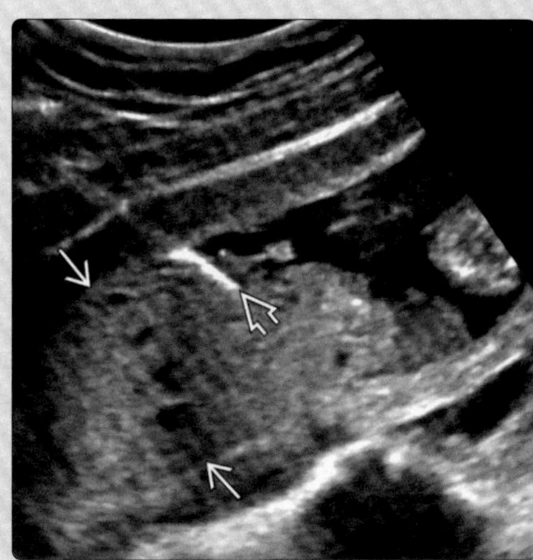

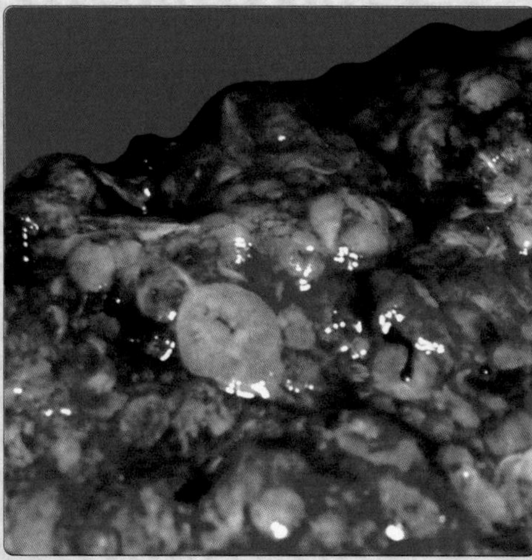

(Left) *Ultrasound-guided chorionic villus sampling is performed in this 13-week pregnancy with a thick cystic placenta ➔. The needle tip ➔ is seen within the placenta. Noninvasive testing cannot reliably detect triploidy, and placental biopsy is necessary for accurate diagnosis.* **(Right)** *Photograph of the placenta from a triploid pregnancy shows typical hydropic villi, which give the placental surface an irregular, cystic appearance. This placental phenotype is seen mostly with diandric triploidy (extra genetic material is paternal).*

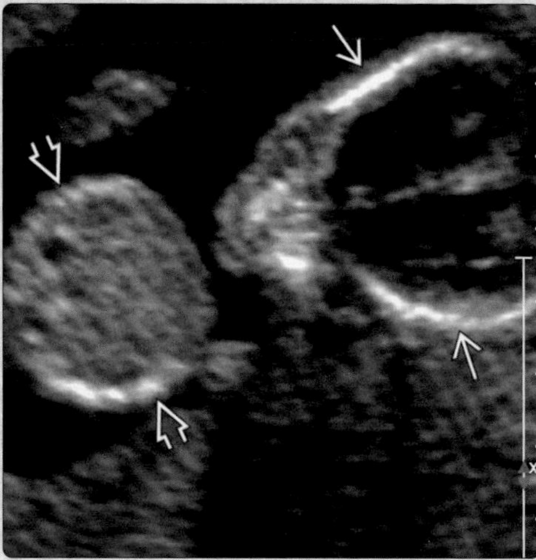

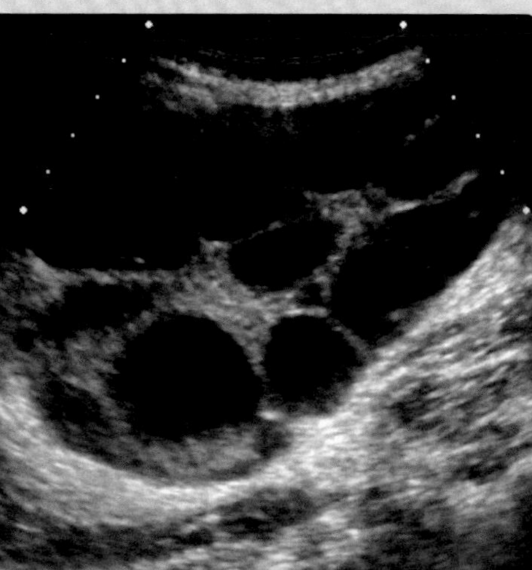

(Left) *Relative macrocephaly is seen in this early 2nd-trimester fetus with triploidy. The head ➔ is significantly larger than the abdomen ➔, although both were less than expected for gestational age.* **(Right)** *This ovary is enlarged and contains multiple enlarged follicles, typical for theca lutein cysts resulting from excessive levels of human chorionic gonadotropin hormone. The other ovary had a similar appearance.*

PART VI
SECTION 12
Syndromes and Multisystem Disorders

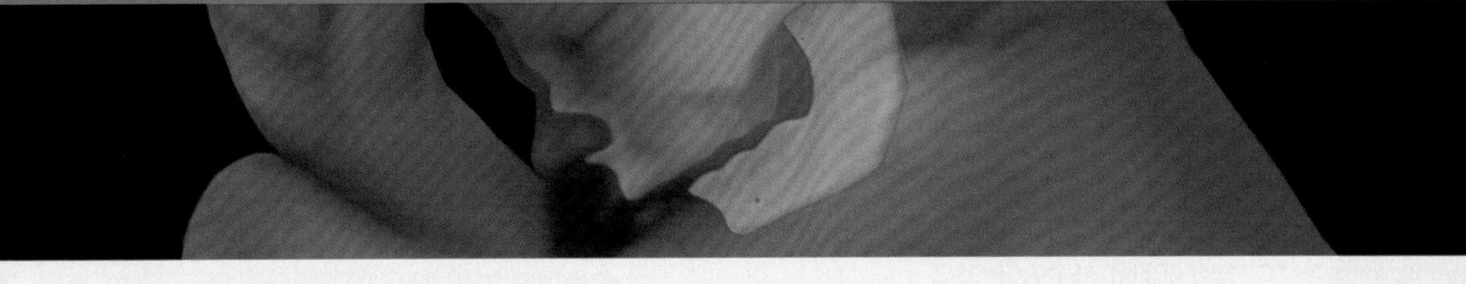

Amniotic Band Syndrome

KEY FACTS

TERMINOLOGY

- Controversial as to etiology, but simplest concept is entrapment of fetal parts by disrupted amnion

IMAGING

- Asymmetric distribution of bizarre "slash" defects is hallmark of syndrome
- Craniofacial deformities often severe; may look like anencephaly with singe orbit involvement
- Abdominal wall defects are large, complex, often with complete evisceration
- Extremities often involved

TOP DIFFERENTIAL DIAGNOSES

- Body stalk anomaly: Fetus stuck to placenta, short cord
- Developmental craniofacial and abdominal wall defects have defined anatomic distributions
  - Cephaloceles at suture lines (occipital most common)
  - Gastroschisis/omphalocele have characteristic appearance

CLINICAL ISSUES

- Defects range from minor to lethal

SCANNING TIPS

- Look for bands in any fetus with large abdominal wall or asymmetric craniofacial defect
- Amniotic band may be tightly adherent and difficult to see
  - Look for restricted movement of involved area
  - Changing maternal position may "float" fetus away from uterine wall, revealing short band
  - Use high-resolution transducer for detailed assessment in near field
- Edema of extremity distal to constricting band may progress to limb amputation
  - Use Doppler to check flow distal to constricting band
  - Abnormal, but present blood flow distal to band may identify cases suitable for fetal surgery

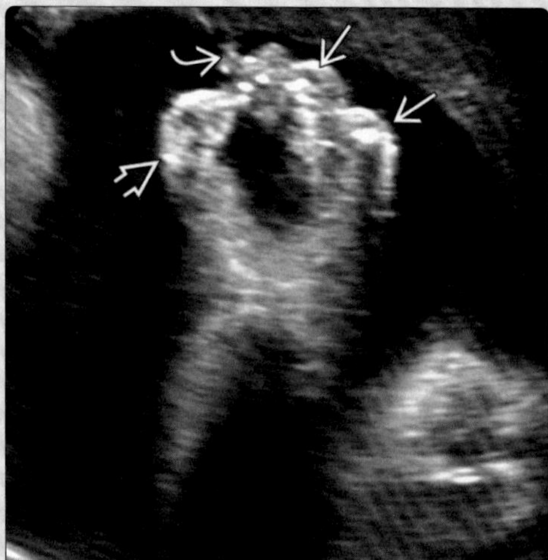

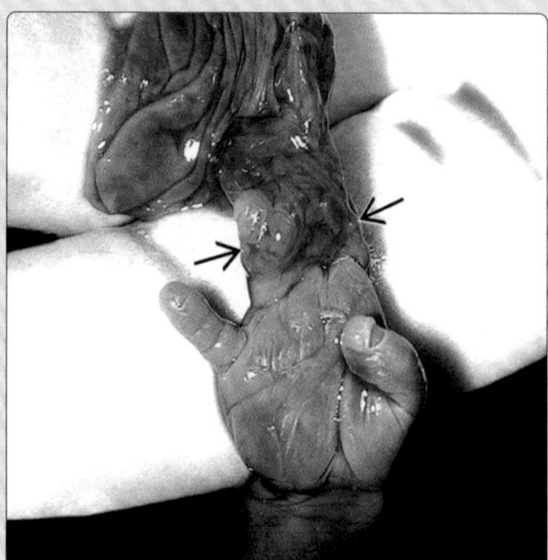

(Left) *US shows the fingertips ➡ tethered to each other (pseudosyndactyly) and to the thumb ➡ by a short band ➡, which was best seen on real-time evaluation. Remember to use cine clips and high-resolution transducers for focused assessment of bands.* **(Right)** *Gross pathology in a similar case shows the fingers trapped in a band ➡. As an isolated finding, this would be of little consequence, but, in this case, the only other area involved was the umbilical cord, which was occluded by a band, resulting in intrauterine fetal demise.*

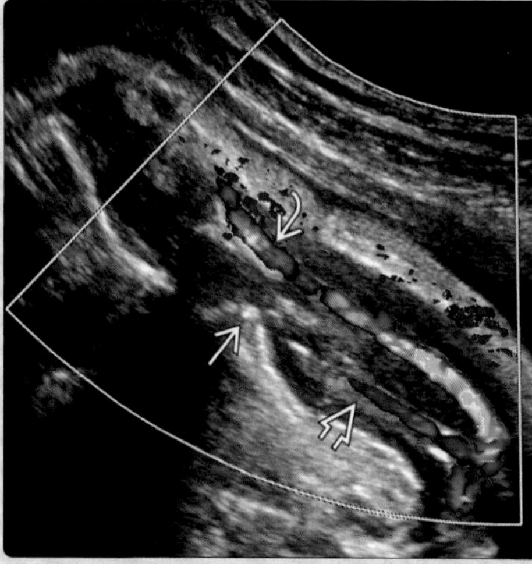

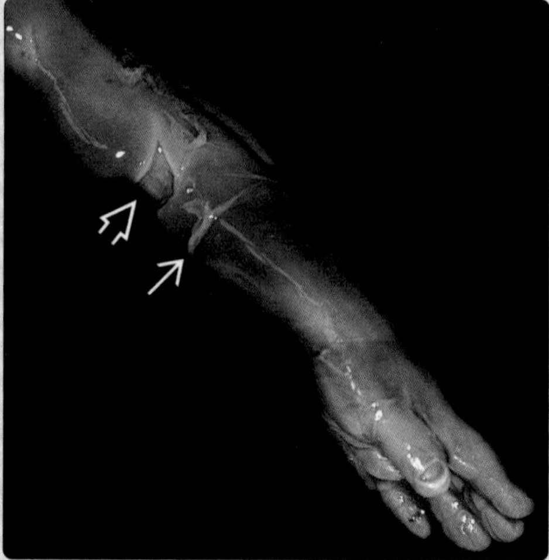

(Left) *Color Doppler US at 37 weeks shows a tight constriction band ➡ around the left calf with compromised flow in the posterior tibial artery ➡. The anterior tibial artery ➡ is unaffected with good flow distal to the constriction. The infant had only extremity involvement and has done well with plastic surgery.* **(Right)** *Gross pathology from a fatal case shows skin necrosis ➡ from a constriction band. Another band is seen encircling the forearm ➡.*

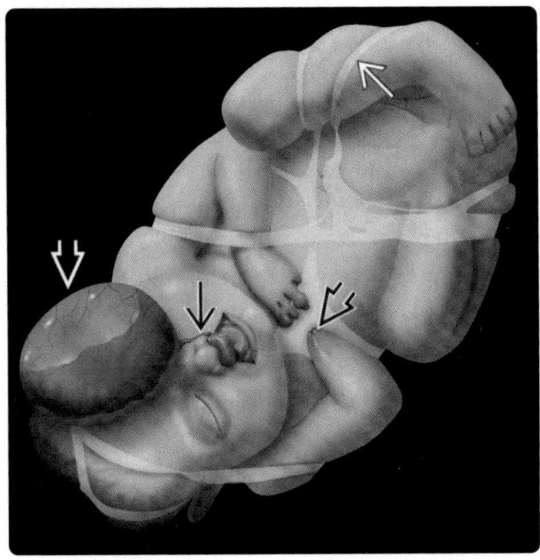

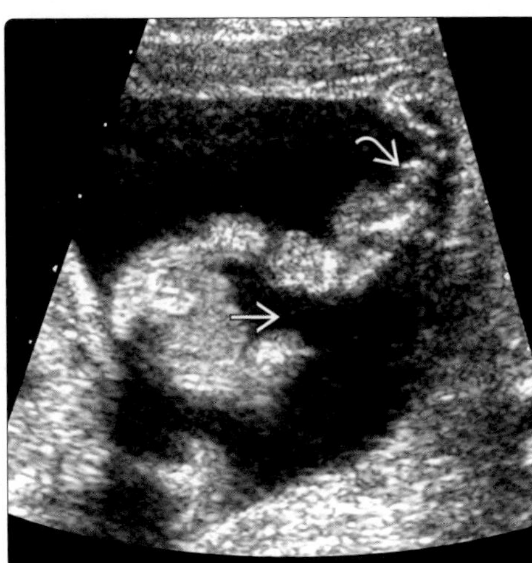

(Left) *Graphic shows various manifestations of amniotic band syndrome (ABS); these include deformations like extremity constriction ➡ or amputation ➡ and disruptions like facial cleft ➡ and cephalocele ➡. Cephaloceles and facial clefts are often asymmetric in ABS and do not follow expected embryological planes, like those of isolated cleft lip and palate .* **(Right)** *Coronal ultrasound shows a large, atypical facial cleft ➡ with a relatively thick band ➡ extending from the edge of the cleft to the uterine wall.*

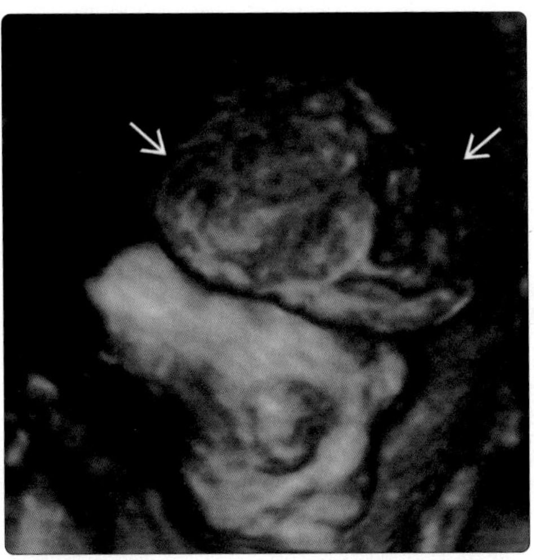

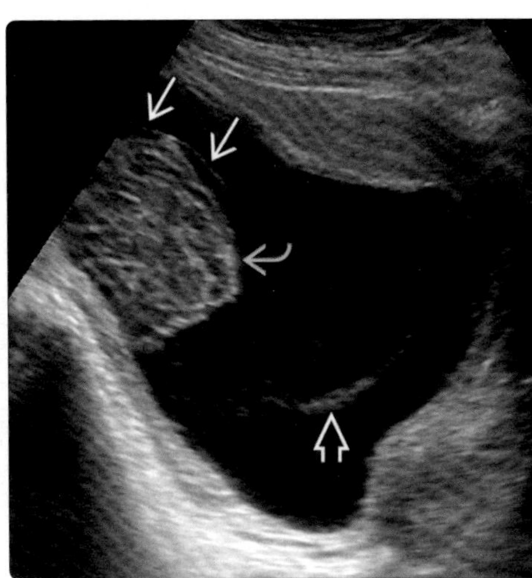

(Left) *3D ultrasound shows lack of a cranial vault, with exposed brain tissue ➡ above the face. Other images showed bands attached to the exposed brain. 3D images were very helpful in explaining this defect to the parents who did not appreciate the gravity of the findings on the 2D images. (Courtesy B. Oshiro, MD.)* **(Right)** *Oblique ultrasound in a similar case shows brain tissue ➡ that is not covered by skin or cranial bones but is attached to bands ➡, which are both draped over it and floating in the amniotic fluid ➡.*

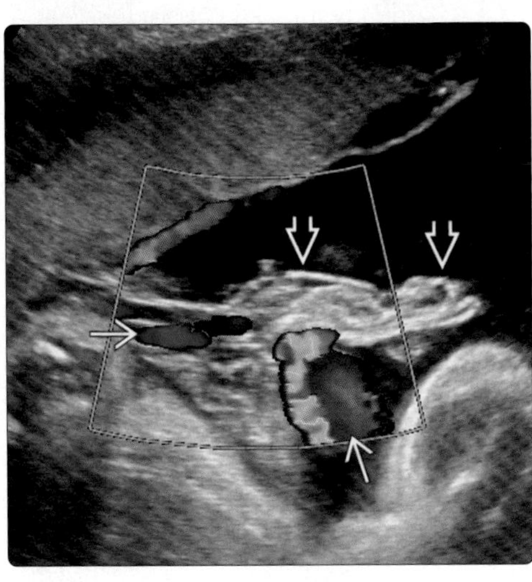

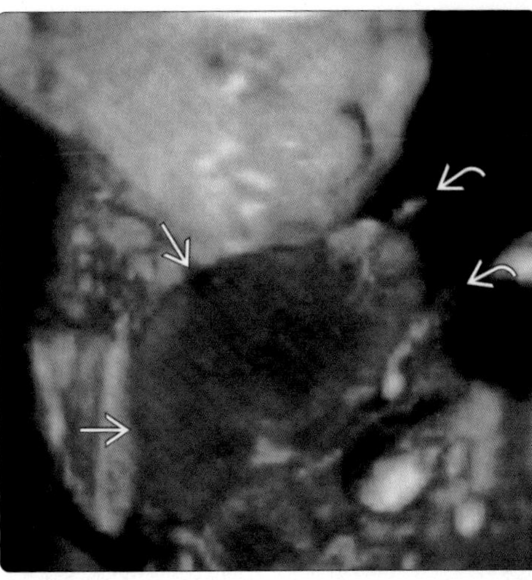

(Left) *Color Doppler shows a "clump" of umbilical cord loops ➡ near the placental cord insertion site with an adherent mass of bands ➡. The fetus was normal. Remember, not all bands cause destructive fetal defects. Due to the reported risk of cord avulsion in labor, the patient was delivered by cesarean section.* **(Right)** *3D reconstruction shows fetus with its chin resting on extruded liver ➡. Note the bands ➡ adhering to the edges of the abdominal wall defect and floating within the amniotic fluid.*

KEY FACTS

TERMINOLOGY

- Complex genetic disorder with principle features including **macrosomia, macroglossia, and omphalocele**

IMAGING

- Macroglossia most consistent finding
  - Persistent protruding tongue throughout exam with inability to close mouth
- Kidneys are large, but often normal echogenicity with hypoechoic pyramids preserved
- Hepatomegaly common
- Large abdominal circumference
  - Combination of nephromegaly and hepatomegaly
- Omphalocele, usually small
- Placental mesenchymal dysplasia, which appears as thickened, cystic placenta

TOP DIFFERENTIAL DIAGNOSES

- Macrosomia associated with maternal diabetes
  - Large size from increased subcutaneous fat, not organomegaly

CLINICAL ISSUES

- Increased risk in couples who have undergone various assisted reproductive technologies
- Increased frequency in monozygotic twins
- Airway difficulties; potentially life-threatening at delivery if macroglossia severe
- Increased risk of embryonal tumors in childhood, including Wilms tumor, hepatoblastoma, and neuroblastoma

SCANNING TIPS

- Ensure tongue is persistently protruded throughout exam
  - With macroglossia, fetus unable to retract tongue (tongue bigger than mouth)
- Be suspicious when omphalocele present and abdominal circumference large
- Measure kidneys and evaluate echogenicity
- Look at liver in coronal plane to get best impression of size

(Left) *Clinical photograph of a term infant with Beckwith-Wiedemann syndrome (BWS) shows several characteristic features of the disorder. Note the macrosomic appearance with protuberant abdomen ⇨ secondary to markedly enlarged liver and kidneys. There is macroglossia with the tongue protruding through the mouth ➔.* **(Right)** *3D US shows the face of a fetus with BWS at 32 weeks. Note the protruding tongue due to macroglossia ➔. It is important to confirm this is persistent throughout the exam.*

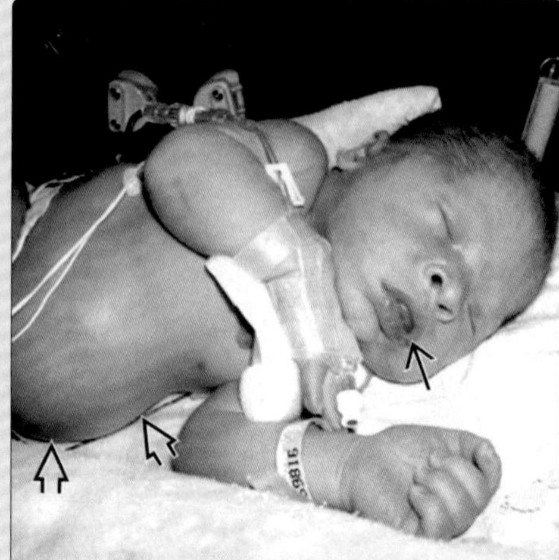

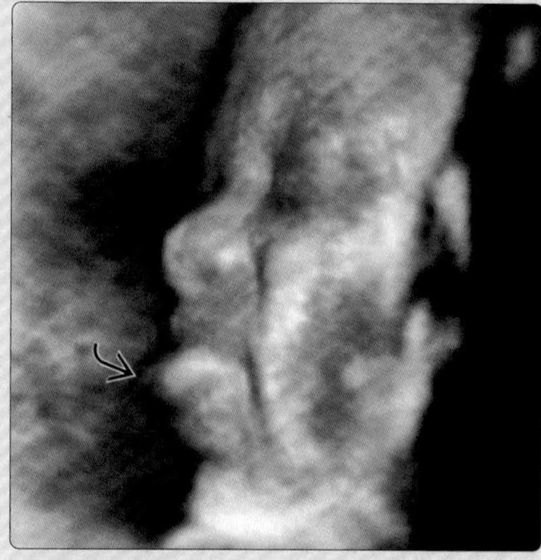

(Left) *Coronal US of a fetus with BWS at 32 weeks shows the characteristic finding of markedly enlarged kidneys (calipers). Although large, the overall appearance is relatively normal with hypoechoic pyramids ➔ seen in both kidneys.* **(Right)** *Axial US through the abdomen of a macrosomic fetus shows classic features of BWS, including an omphalocele ⇨, large kidneys ➔ (> 95th percentile for gestational age), and hepatomegaly ➔ with the liver extending into the pelvis on coronal views.*

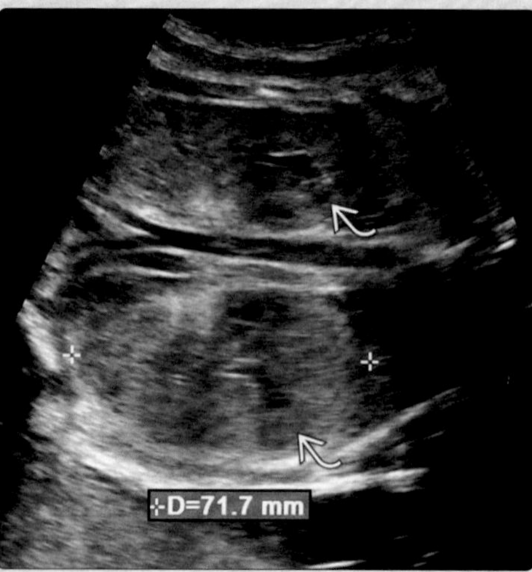

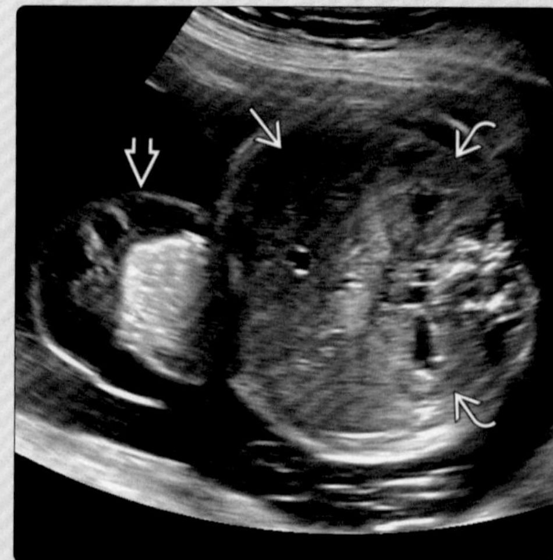

KEY FACTS

TERMINOLOGY

- Syndrome composed of **classic triad of findings**
  - **Renal cystic dysplasia** in 95-100%
  - **Encephalocele** or other central nervous system (CNS) abnormality in 90%
  - **Postaxial polydactyly** in 55-75%
- Should have at least 2 of 3 classic features

IMAGING

- Renal cystic dysplasia most consistent finding
  - Kidney appearance is variable
    - Most commonly grossly enlarged and echogenic but may be filled with macroscopic cysts
  - Renal size often massive, causing enlarged abdominal circumference
- Occipital encephalocele classic CNS finding (60-80%) but may have other malformations
  - Dandy-Walker malformation, microcephaly, holoprosencephaly, anencephaly
- Diagnosis can be made in 1st trimester
- Severe oligohydramnios or anhydramnios by 2nd trimester
  - Makes evaluation of polydactyly and other more subtle findings difficult

TOP DIFFERENTIAL DIAGNOSES

- Trisomy 13: Significant overlap in imaging features

CLINICAL ISSUES

- Oligohydramnios leads to pulmonary hypoplasia
  - Most stillborn or die within few hours
- Autosomal recessive with 25% recurrence risk for future pregnancies

SCANNING TIPS

- May first present with increased nuchal translucency
  - Use endovaginal US to search for anomalies if suspicious findings or positive family history
- When 1 finding seen (especially enlarged kidneys), carefully search for others

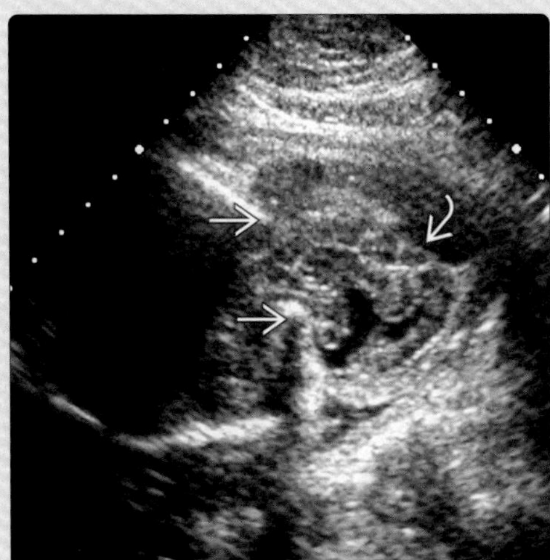

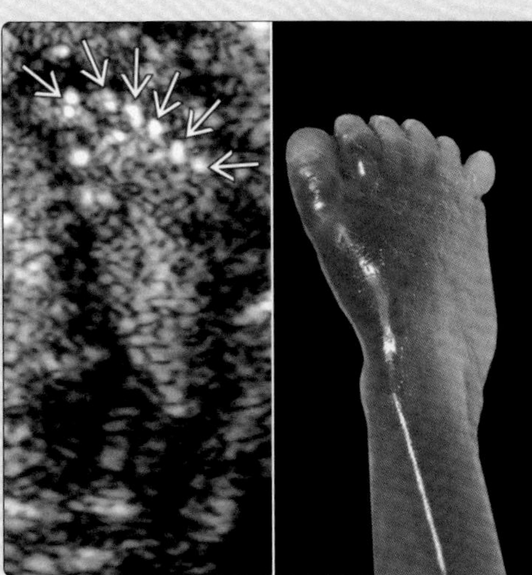

(Left) *Axial US of the fetal brain shows a posterior occipital calvarial defect ➡ with a large encephalocele ➡ in a fetus with Meckel-Gruber syndrome. There is also oligohydramnios secondary to renal dysplasia.* **(Right)** *Coronal US of the foot in the same case shows polydactyly ➡. Polydactyly is the least consistent finding in Meckel-Gruber syndrome and can be easily missed secondary to oligohydramnios. Postaxial polydactyly is confirmed on the autopsy picture.*

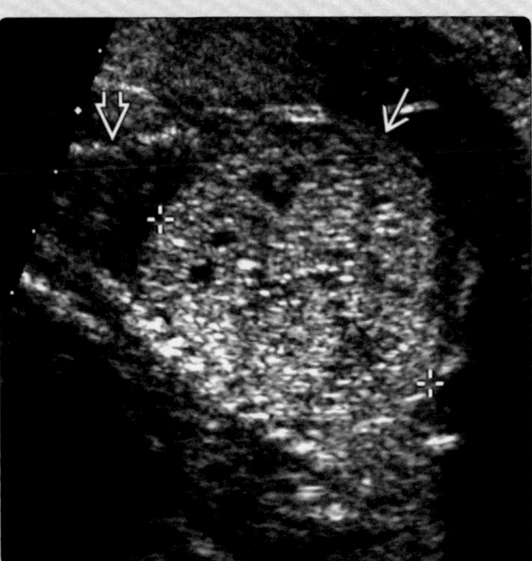

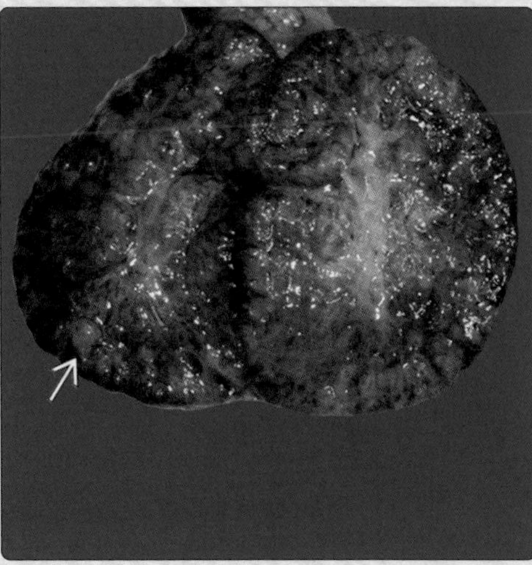

(Left) *Sagittal US shows a massively enlarged, echogenic kidney (calipers) with a few scattered macroscopic cysts. There are severe oligohydramnios, a small, bell-shaped chest ➡, and protuberant abdomen ➡.* **(Right)** *At autopsy the bisected kidney shows innumerable small cysts ➡ and complete lack of corticomedullary development. Cystic dysplasia is the most consistent finding in Meckel-Gruber syndrome with the kidneys often being massively enlarged, as in this case.*

Pierre Robin Sequence

KEY FACTS

TERMINOLOGY

- Mandibular hypoplasia with cleft palate and glossoptosis (backward and downward displacement of tongue)

IMAGING

- Severe micrognathia on midsagittal view in midtrimester
  - 1st-trimester diagnosis has been reported
- Specifically target palate to look for cleft when micrognathia is seen
  - Classic U shape seen on postnatal evaluation
- Polyhydramnios common in 3rd trimester

CLINICAL ISSUES

- ~ 65% of cases with other anomalies
  - Up to 30% mortality with severe defects
- Many syndromes have Pierre Robin sequence as component
- Airway obstruction due to glossoptosis may be life threatening
  - Airway protection critical in infants

SCANNING TIPS

- Usually micrognathia is obvious, but in questionable cases, measure maxilla-nasion-mandible (MNM) angle
  - MNM is angle formed between line from nasal bone attachment at skull to front of maxilla and line from same nasal point to front of mandible
  - MNM > 95th percentile is consistent with micrognathia
- Perform 3D ultrasound to enhance craniofacial evaluation
  - Palate defects seen best with multiplanar views and bone rendered views
- Specifically target palate during real-time evaluation
  - Try to obtain view in sagittal plane
  - Watch tongue and see if it thrusts upward through defect
- Careful evaluation of fetal anatomy given significant association with other anomalies and syndromes

(Left) *Graphic shows the typical U-shaped palatal defect seen in Pierre Robin ➔. Micrognathia ➔ is also a prominent feature of this condition. The position of the tongue within the small mandible prevents normal movement of the palatal shelves during embryogenesis, resulting in the cleft.* **(Right)** *3D ultrasound shows the face of a fetus with severe micrognathia ➔. Postnatally, the infant was found to have a U-shaped cleft palate typical of Pierre Robin sequence.*

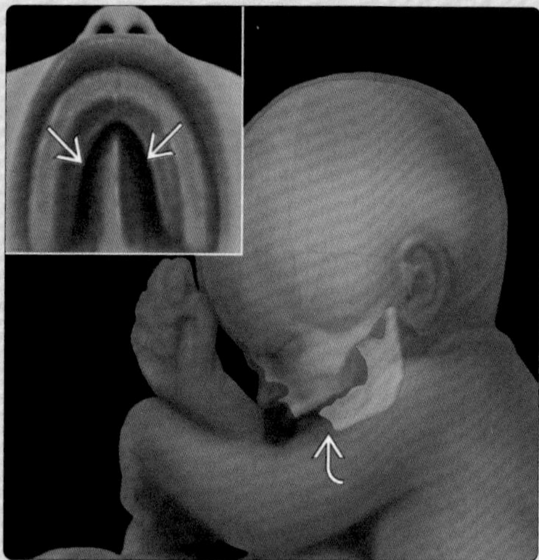

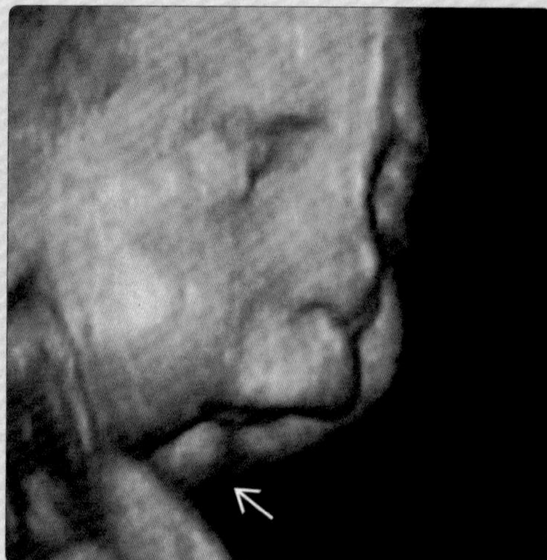

(Left) *Ultrasound of a 3rd-trimester fetus with significant micrognathia ➔ is shown. Although the palate is often difficult to image prenatally, preparation for possible airway compromise is important in this setting.* **(Right)** *Clinical photograph shows a newborn with severe micrognathia ➔ and a cleft palate typical of Pierre Robin. Note the foam pad ➔ under the neck for airway stabilization. Airway compromise due to an obstructing tongue is a concern in infants with this degree of micrognathia.*

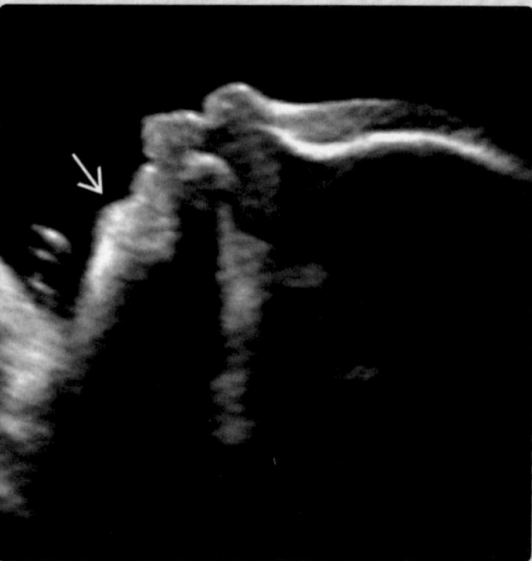

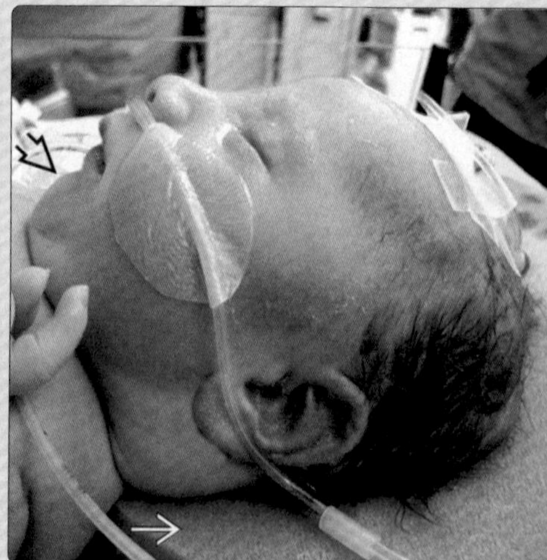

KEY FACTS

TERMINOLOGY

- Synonym: Mermaid syndrome
- Definition: Lower extremity fusion + other skeletal, gastrointestinal, and genitourinary abnormalities

IMAGING

- **Fused lower extremities** (variable amount of fusion)
  - Severe fusion may present as single lower extremity
- **Severe renal anomalies commonly seen**
  - Bilateral renal agenesis most common
  - Bilateral renal cystic dysplastic
  - Secondary anhydramnios is common
- Absence of normally tapered lumbosacral spine
- Single umbilical artery (SUA) goes directly to aorta
  - SUA is persistent vitelline artery → hypoperfusion of lower extremities, kidneys, abdominal organs
- Color Doppler findings in fetal abdomen
  - Absent renal arteries and aortic bifurcation (into iliacs)

TOP DIFFERENTIAL DIAGNOSES

- Caudal regression/dysgenesis syndrome
- VACTERL association
- Arthrogryposis with fixed lower limb posture

CLINICAL ISSUES

- Majority of cases lethal due to pulmonary hypoplasia
- ≥ 50% of diagnoses missed in utero because of poor visualization from anhydramnios
- Rare survivors with severe genitourinary and gastrointestinal anomalies

SCANNING TIPS

- Look for all expected bones of lower extremity in cases with no/low fluid
- Use color Doppler to show presence or absence of renal arteries when anhydramnios is present
- Follow SUA to its attachment in fetus
  - Normal umbilical artery attaches to iliac artery, not aorta

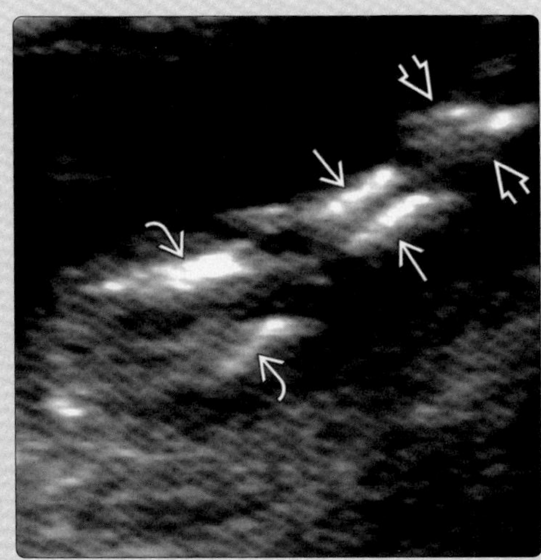

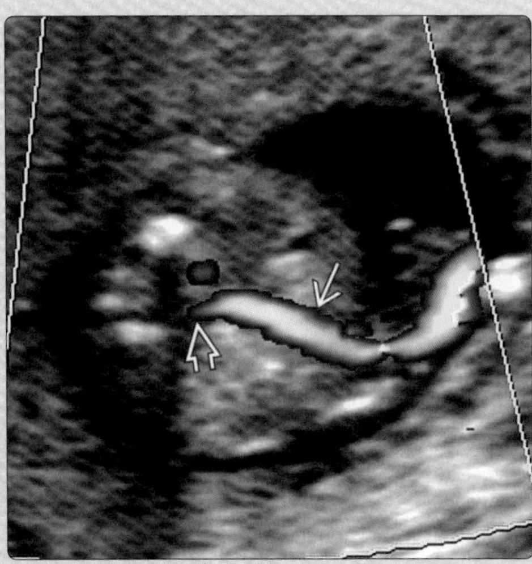

(Left) *Fused lower extremities are seen in a 13-week fetus with syrenomelia. There are 2 femurs ➡ and 2 midleg bones ➡ (should be 4). The feet are fused ➡ as well. Diagnosis of syrenomelia can be made at the time of the nuchal translucency scan. Later, there is usually no fluid, and anatomy may be more difficult to see.* **(Right)** *Color Doppler ultrasound in the same fetus shows a single umbilical artery ➡ that is midline and inserts directly into the aorta ➡. The umbilical artery is normally lateral to the bladder and inserts on the iliac artery.*

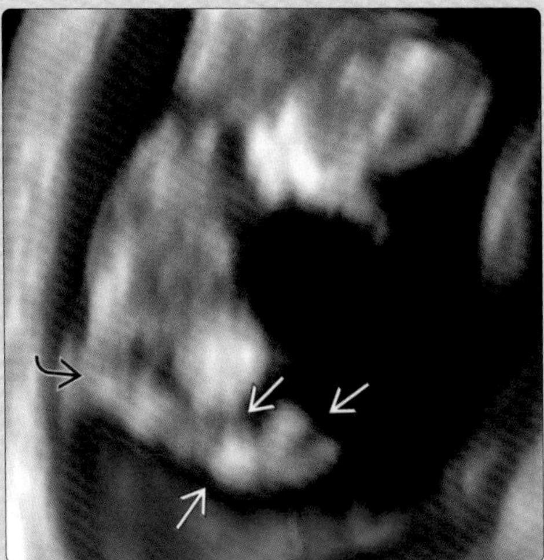

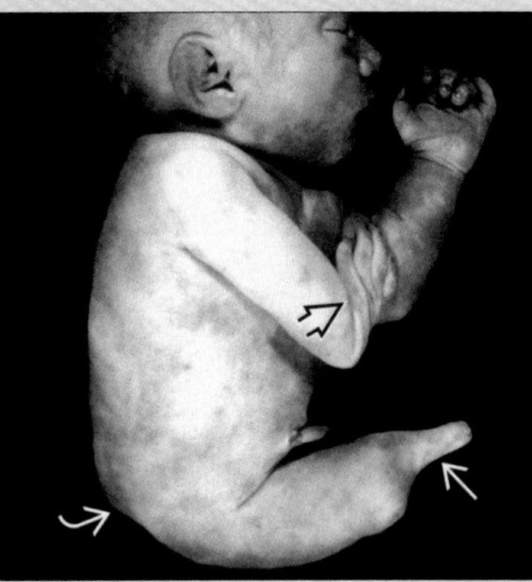

(Left) *3D ultrasound at 11 weeks shows short fused lower extremities ➡ and short torso from a truncated spine ➡.* **(Right)** *Clinical photograph of a newborn who died from pulmonary hypoplasia shows classic features of sirenomelia. The single fused lower extremity is evident ➡ as well as a unilateral radial ray defect ➡. The spine is truncated ➡. Spine and skeletal anomalies are associated with syrenomelia.*

KEY FACTS

IMAGING

- Nonrandom association of 6 core abnormalities
  - **V**ertebral defects
    - Hemivertebrae: Best demonstrated in coronal plane, scoliosis originates at hemivertebra(e)
    - Fusion of vertebral bodies or posterior elements (block vertebrae)
  - **A**nal atresia
    - Absent anal dimple
    - Dilated colon that does not reach perineum
  - **C**ardiac anomalies
    - Ventricular septal defect is most common defect in some studies
  - **T**racheoesophageal fistula with **e**sophageal atresia
    - Stomach absent or small, look for esophageal pouch in neck
    - Polyhydramnios usually late finding (3rd trimester)
  - **R**enal anomalies: Majority with structural renal defect also have anorectal malformation
    - Vesicoureteral reflux with additional structural defect (27%), unilateral renal agenesis (24%), multicystic dysplastic kidney (18%), duplicated collecting system (18%)
  - **L**imb defects: Usually bilateral upper limbs, may be asymmetric
    - Primarily radial ray malformation with hypoplasia/aplasia of radius with radial club hand or hypoplasia/aplasia of thumbs

SCANNING TIPS

- Perform systematic search for associated anomalies when 1 defect identified
  - Cardiac anomalies most common defect (~ 80%)
  - Esophageal atresia ± tracheoesophageal fistula in 50-60%

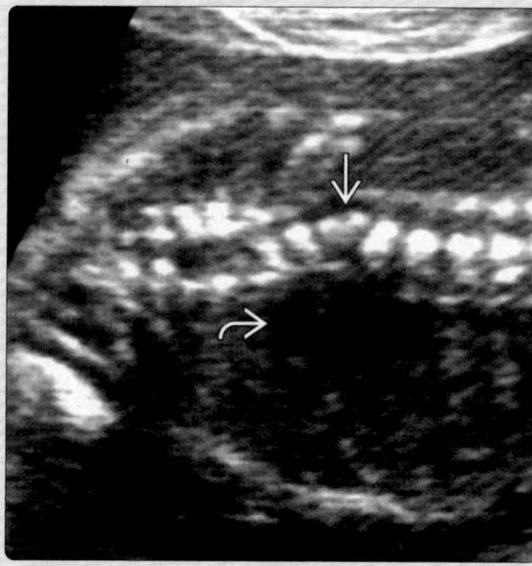

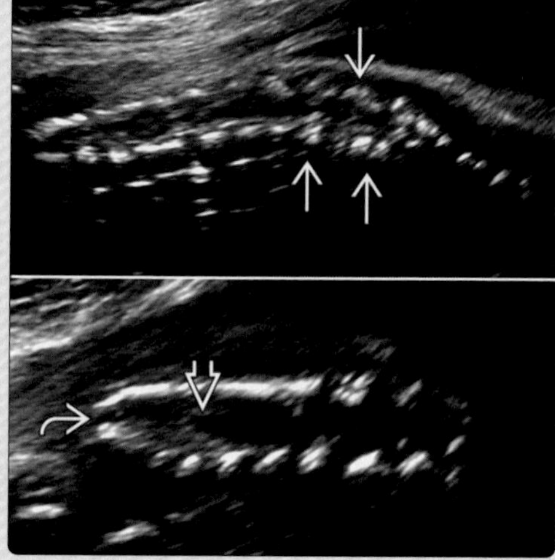

(Left) *Coronal US of the spine shows scoliosis secondary to fused vertebrae ➡. There is also a multicystic dysplastic kidney ➦. This finding was bilateral, resulting in severe oligohydramnios. Lack of amniotic fluid impairs anatomic visualization.* **(Right)** *Longitudinal images of the spine show "jumbled" vertebral bodies in the lower thoracic spine ➡, a short dysplastic sacrum ➦, and a tethered cord with the conus ➡ at the lumbosacral junction.*

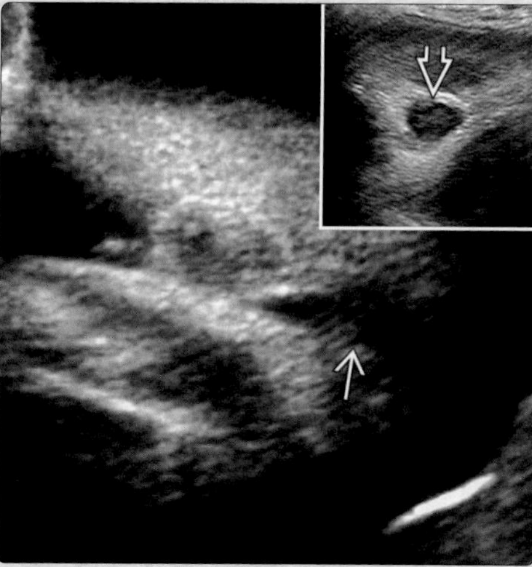

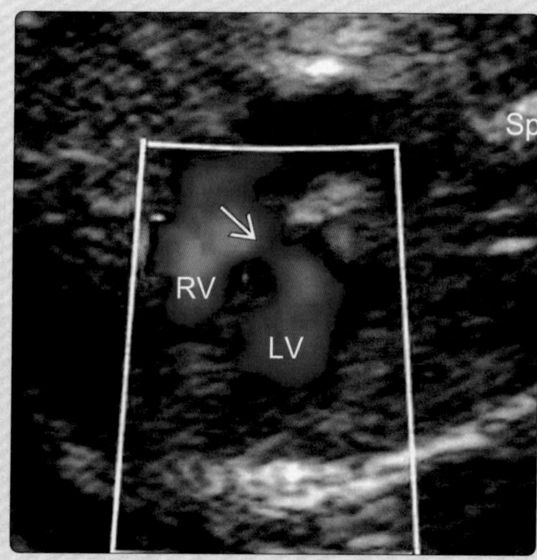

(Left) *The inset shows a normal anal dimple ➡ with a hypoechoic muscular wall surrounding the echogenic mucosa. Compare that to the appearance when the dimple is absent ➡ in this fetus with anal atresia.* **(Right)** *Color Doppler applied to the 4-chamber view of the heart confirms flow across a ventricular septal defect ➡. This fetus had many other findings culminating in a final diagnosis of VACTERL. Ventricular septal defect is the commonest cardiac defect [right ventricle (RV), left ventricle (LV), spine (Sp)].*

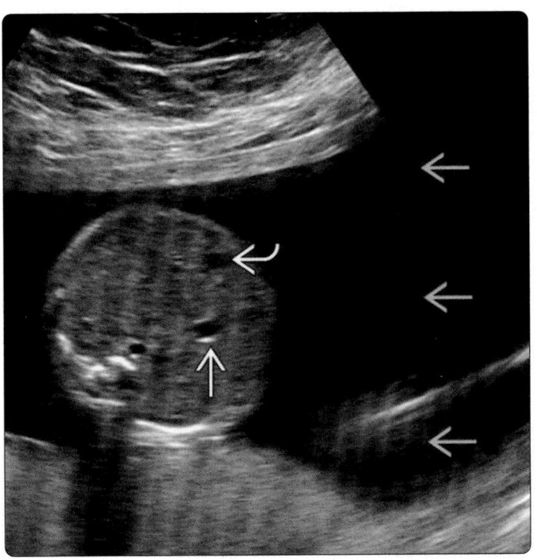

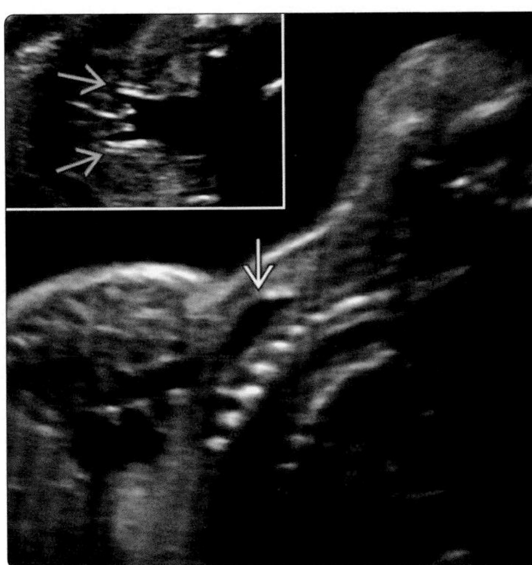

(Left) *Axial US through the fetal abdomen shows the gallbladder ➡ and umbilical vein ➡ but no fluid-filled stomach. This finding together with polyhydramnios is very concerning for esophageal atresia ➡.* **(Right)** *Sagittal US through the neck in the same fetus shows the dilated, fluid-filled esophageal pouch ➡ confirming the diagnosis. Color Doppler can be used to verify that this is not a vessel. The normal larynx is recognized by the piriform sinuses ➡ on a coronal view as shown in the inset.*

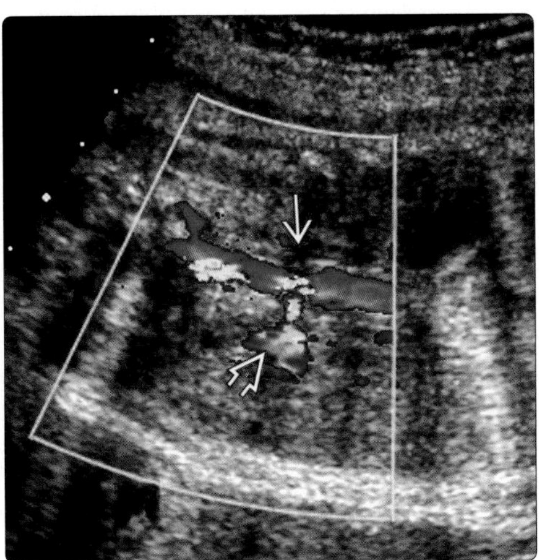

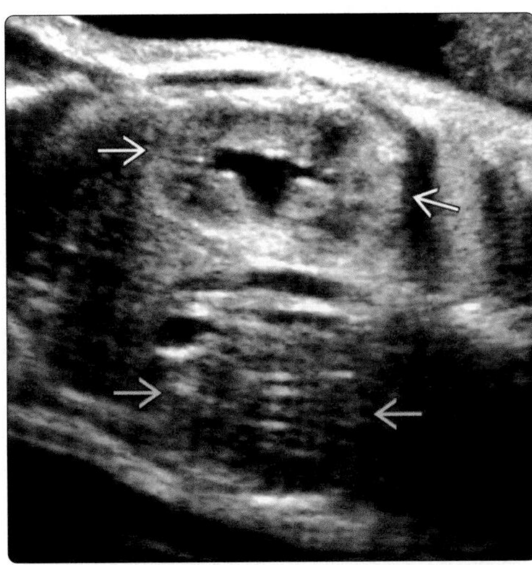

(Left) *Coronal US with Doppler in a fetus with unilateral renal agenesis in the setting of VACTERL shows a normal right renal artery ➡ but none on the left ➡.* **(Right)** *Coronal US shows a solitary left kidney ➡. The right renal fossa ➡ was empty. Before diagnosing unilateral renal agenesis, always look carefully for a pelvic kidney with high-resolution transducers and color Doppler to look for a renal artery in the pelvis.*

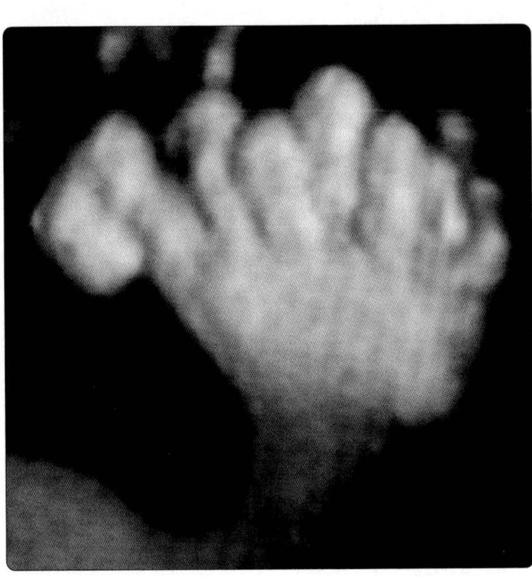

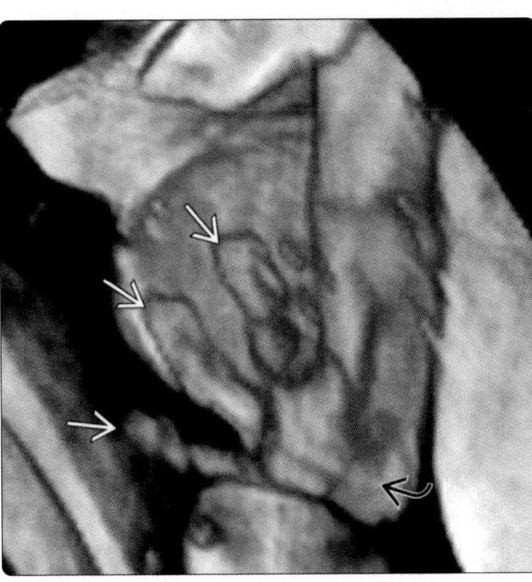

(Left) *3D US shows an abnormal foot with 8 toes in a fetus with additional findings of VACTERL, including esophageal atresia, absent anal dimple, short femur, hemivertebrae, and absent right upper extremity.* **(Right)** *3D US shows a radial ray defect. Notice the radially deviated wrist ➡ and oligodactyly. Only 3 digits ➡ are seen and the thumb is absent. A single bone was seen in the lower arm on 2D imaging. Radial ray defects are the most common limb abnormalities found in the VACTERL association.*

PART VI
SECTION 13
Infection

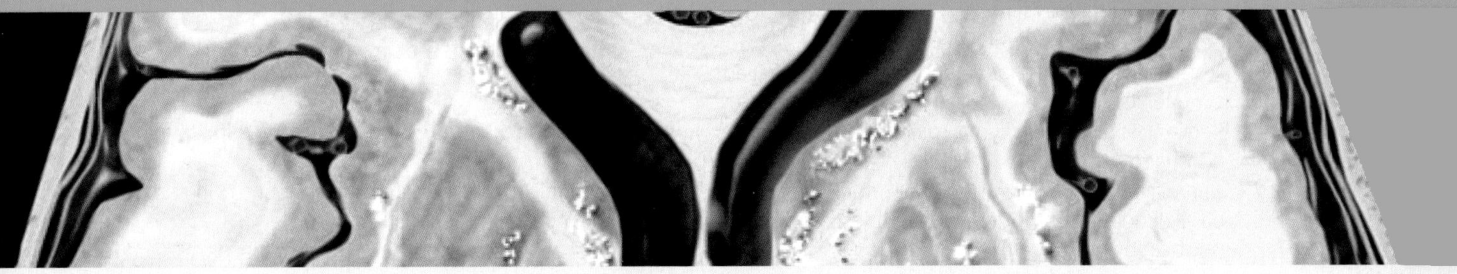

Cytomegalovirus

KEY FACTS

IMAGING

- Fetal growth restriction
- Brain findings
  - Microcephaly (up to 27%)
  - Ventriculomegaly (moderate to severe in 45%)
    - Intraventricular adhesions, abnormal periventricular echogenicity
    - Periventricular/parenchymal calcifications (often nonshadowing)
    - Uni-/bilateral curvilinear echogenic streaks within basal ganglia, thalami indicate lenticulostriate vessel calcification
  - Intraparenchymal cysts: Periventricular, anterior temporal, occipital, frontoparietal
  - Cortical dysplasia
  - Cerebellar/cisterna magna abnormalities (cerebellar volume loss in 67% of infants with congenital infection)
- Hepatosplenomegaly secondary to extramedullary hematopoiesis
- Echogenic bowel
- Cardiomyopathy ± hydrops

TOP DIFFERENTIAL DIAGNOSES

- Toxoplasmosis: Final diagnosis made on maternal serology as imaging findings are similar

SCANNING TIPS

- **Always check middle cerebral artery velocity in hydropic fetus**
  - Anemia maybe be cause: Alloimmune or due to bone marrow suppression in infection
- If cephalic presentation, use transvaginal ultrasound for highest resolution brain images
- **Do not overcall echogenic bowel**: Very technique-dependent observation
  - Use V4 transducer, turn off harmonics, turn down gain and see if bowel still visible as bone disappears
  - Bowel must be as bright as bone to call abnormal

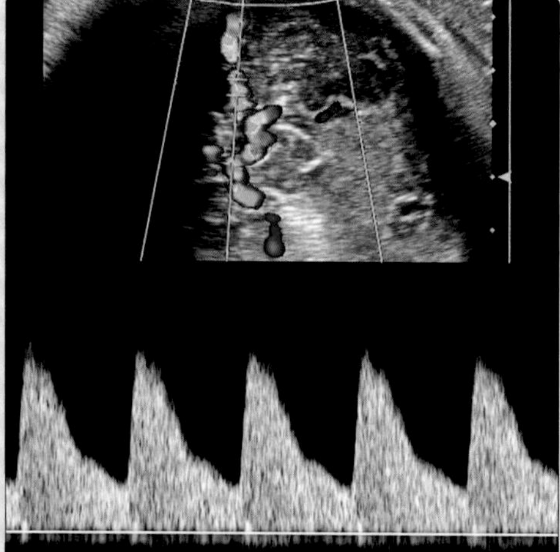
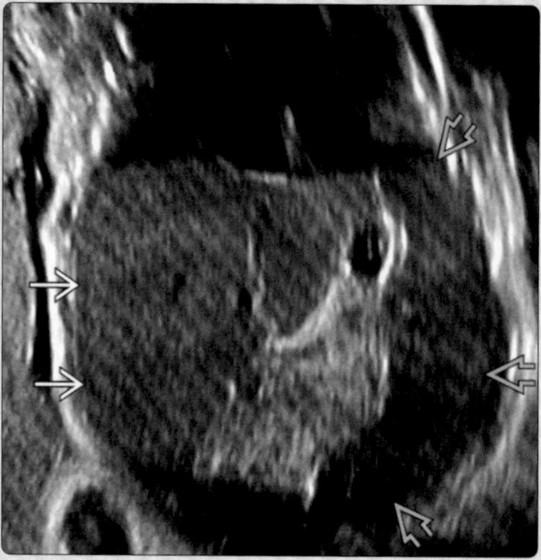

(Left) *Middle cerebral artery peak systolic velocity of 112 cm/sec in the 3rd trimester indicates anemia. The case was sent as alloimmune anemia, but marked hepatosplenomegaly was noted and work-up resulted in a diagnosis of cytomegalovirus infection (CMV).* **(Right)** *This fetus with hepatosplenomegaly from CMV infection shows a large liver ➡, but what is most striking is the dramatic enlargement of the spleen ⇨. The enlargement is caused by extramedullary hematopoiesis secondary to fetal anemia.*

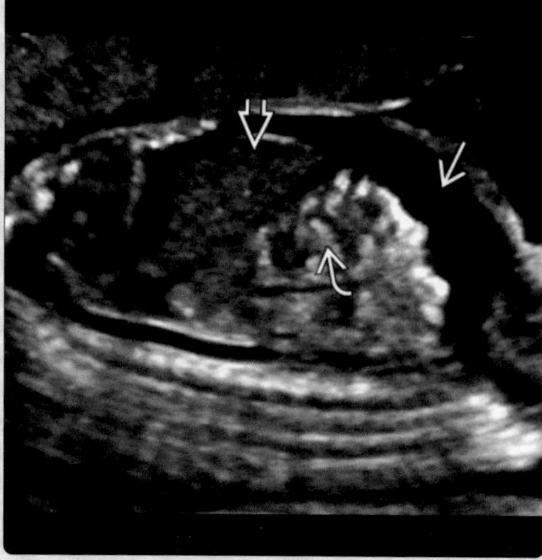
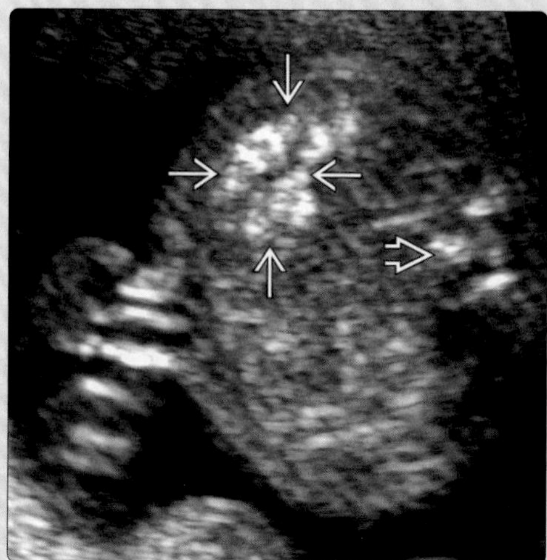

(Left) *Ultrasound at 27 weeks in a fetus with CMV infection shows new-onset ascites ➡ without other evidence of hydrops and mildly enlarged liver ➡. The bowel is also diffusely echogenic ➡. Intrauterine demise occurred shortly after the development of ascites.* **(Right)** *Axial ultrasound through the fetal abdomen shows focal echogenic bowel ➡, which is as bright as the bone in the adjacent spine ➡.*

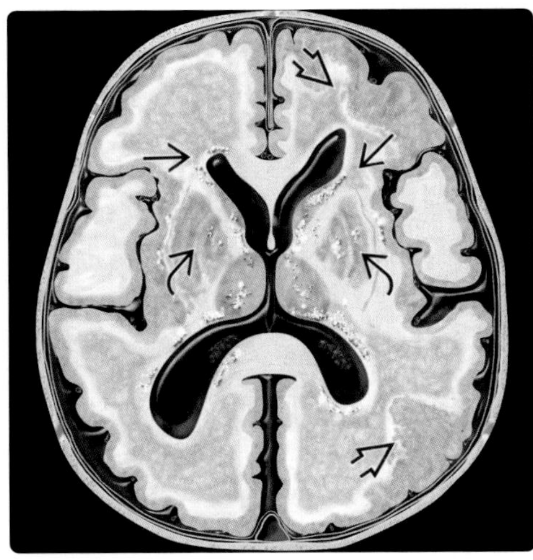

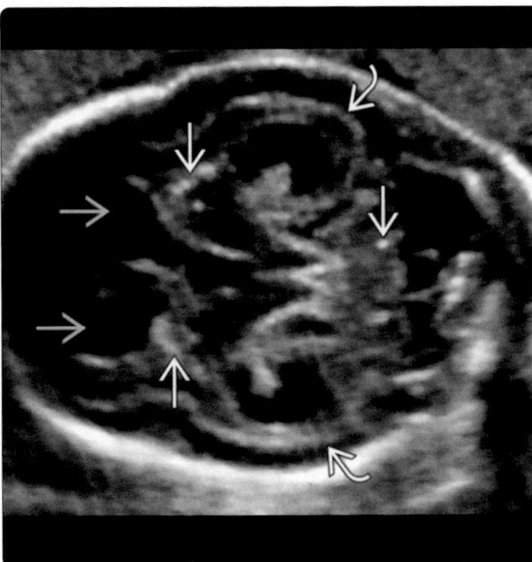

(Left) *Axial graphic shows periventricular ➔ and basal ganglia ➔ calcifications, regions of cortical dysplasia ➔ and ventricular dilation due to adjacent white matter volume loss. The yellowish white matter abnormalities reflect regions of edema, demyelination, &/or gliosis.* **(Right)** *Axial US at 25 weeks in a fetus with CMV infection shows ventriculomegaly ➔, cortical dysplasia ➔, and multiple periventricular and intraparenchymal calcifications ➔. Note that they do not cause acoustic shadowing.*

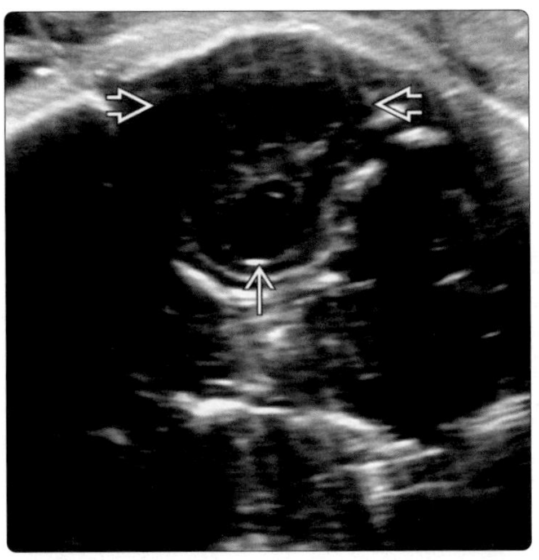

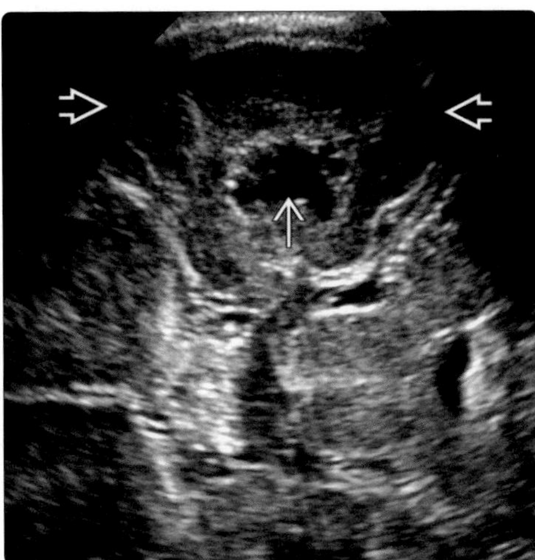

(Left) *Third trimester scan through the brain of a fetus with known CMV infection shows a new, irregularly shaped parenchymal cyst ➔ in the right temporal lobe ➔.* **(Right)** *Mastoid view neonatal head ultrasound in the same infant confirms the parenchymal cyst ➔ within the temporal lobe ➔. CMV infection causes inflammation and release of neurotoxic factors leading to focal parenchymal necrosis. The finding of anterior temporal cysts with associated white matter disease is particularly suggestive of CMV infection.*

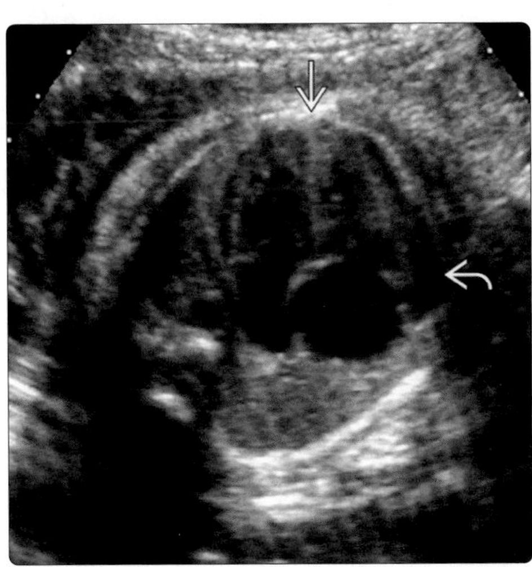

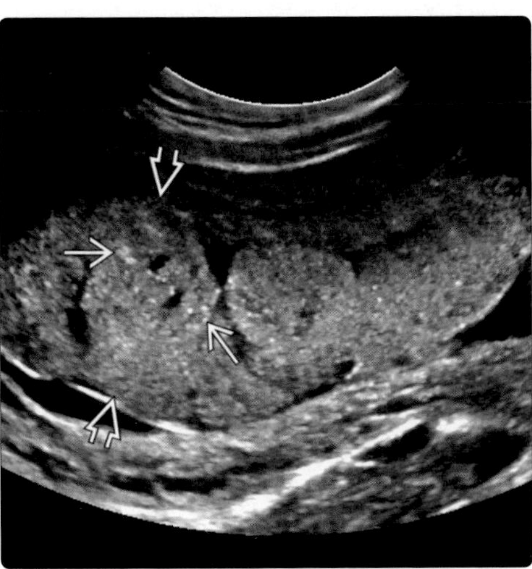

(Left) *Four-chamber view of the heart in a fetus with CMV shows cardiomegaly ➔ and a pericardial effusion ➔. Cardiomegaly may be due to viral cardiomyopathy or high-output failure from anemia, which is the result of bone marrow suppression.* **(Right)** *Ultrasound shows placentomegaly ➔ in the 2nd trimester. As a rule of thumb, normal placental thickness is ~ 1 mm per week of gestational age. Note also the irregular contour of the placenta and the punctate calcifications ➔ already at 22 weeks.*

PART VI
SECTION 14

Fluid, Growth, and Well-Being

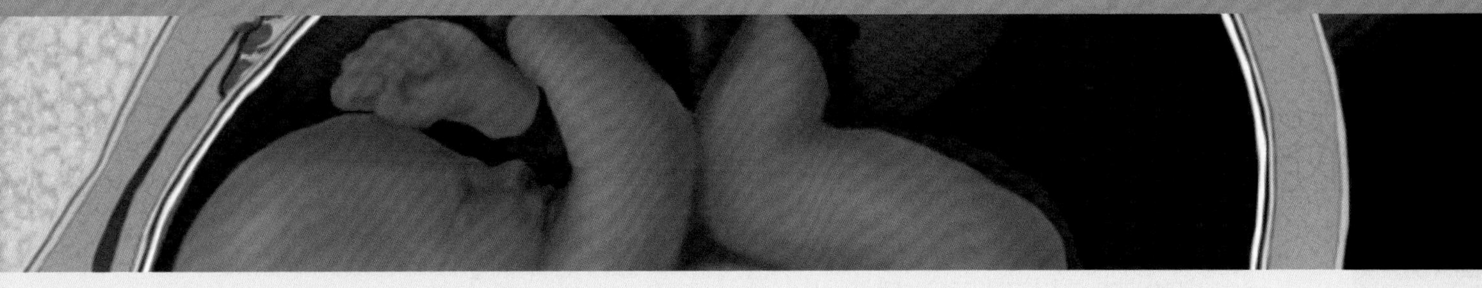

Parameters of Fetal Well-Being

KEY FACTS

IMAGING

- **Biophysical profile (BPP) score**: 0 or 2 points for 4 parameters in 30 min; numbers added for BPP score: 0, 2, 4, 6, 8 out of 8; can finish early if 8/8 scored < 30 min
  - Breathing (thoracic movement): 2 points if
    - ≥ 1 episode 30 seconds continuous breathing
    - Hiccups are acceptable
  - Gross body movement: 2 points if
    - ≥ 3 discrete movements (trunk roll, spine flexion/extension, gross limb movement)
  - Tone: 2 points if
    - ≥ 1 episode active extension then flexion of 1 limb
    - Hand opening and closing is acceptable
  - Amniotic fluid: 2 points if
    - ≥ 1 pocket measures ≥ 2 cm vertical and ≥ 1 cm width
- Doppler: Umbilical artery (UA), middle cerebral artery (MCA), ductus venosus (DV)
  - Normal UA and DV with ↑ diastolic flow
  - Abnormal UA and DV with ↓ or reversed diastolic flow
  - Normal MCA is high resistant (↓ diastolic flow)
  - Abnormal MCA has ↑ diastolic flow ("brain-sparing")
- Fetal growth assessment: Estimated fetal weight < 10th percentile considered growth restriction

CLINICAL ISSUES

- Well-being assessment goal: Identify fetuses at risk for in utero death (from hypoxia/asphyxia) → deliver early
- Conditions associated with fetal hypoxia: Hypertension, diabetes, collagen-vascular disease, postdates, infection
- BPP < 6/8 is abnormal (0 for fluid is most worrisome)
- Fetal monitoring non-stress test is additive

SCANNING TIPS

- Never give 1 point for partial credit in BPP
- Pregnancy can have oligohydramnios and score 2 for fluid
- Turn on color Doppler before measuring fluid pocket
- Do not let patient leave unit if BPP is < 6/8

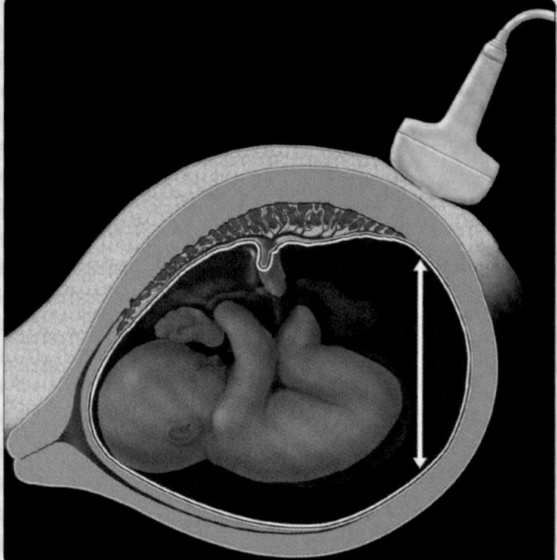

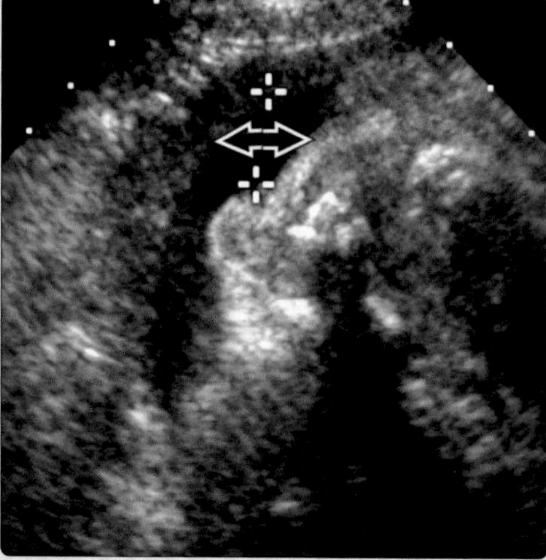

(Left) *For the purpose of amniotic fluid assessment in performing a BPP, the largest uterine fluid collection is found that is void of fetal parts and umbilical cord, and the maximum anterior-to-posterior distance is measured.* **(Right)** *The largest pocket of fluid in this pregnancy measured < 2 cm in depth (calipers) and < 1 cm in width ➡. This pocket does not meet criteria for a score of 2 for fluid in a BPP. A score of 0 for fluid in BPP is the most worrisome finding for fetal hypoxia/asphyxia.*

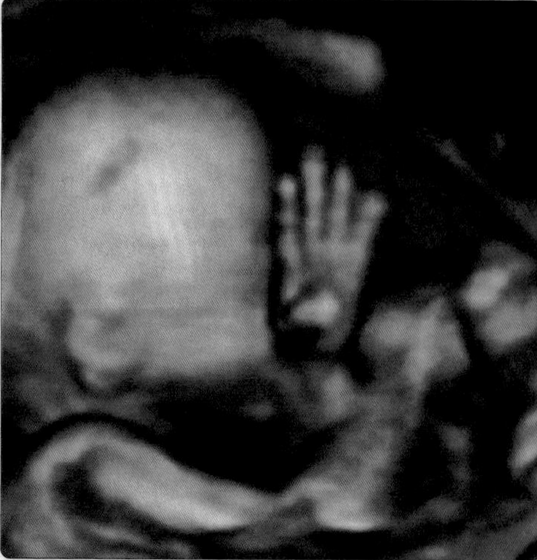

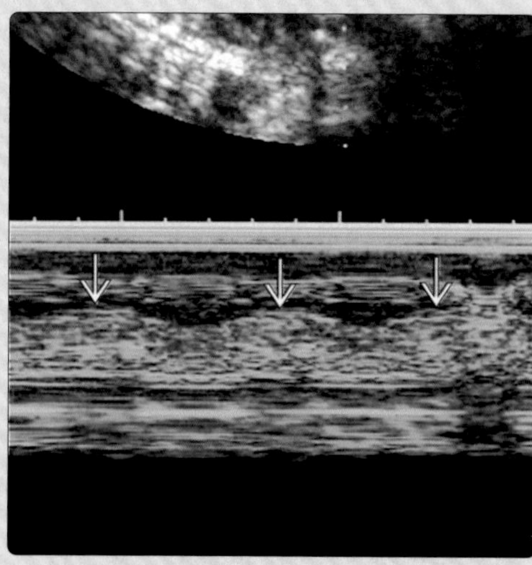

(Left) *3D ultrasound shows the fetal hand in an open position. To score a 2 for tone, the fetal extremity is seen to extend and return to flexion. Most sonographers report this finding without a need for documentation.* **(Right)** *M-mode ultrasound over the diaphragm can be used to document thoracic cage movement. Rhythmic continuous diaphragm motion ➡ is shown. Alternatively, a video clip of breathing can document breathing. Continuous breathing or hiccupping for 30 seconds is necessary for 2 points.*

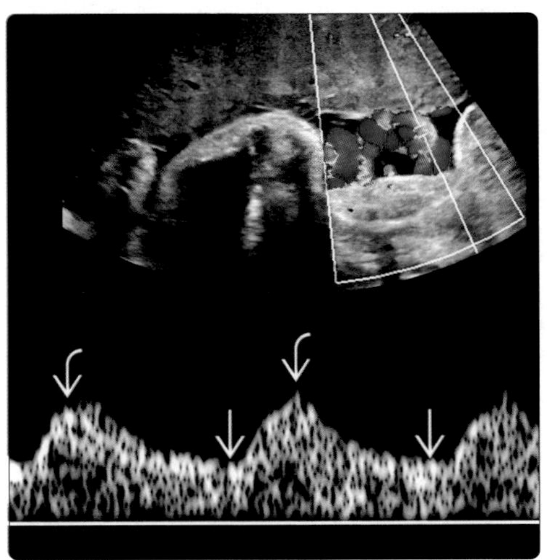

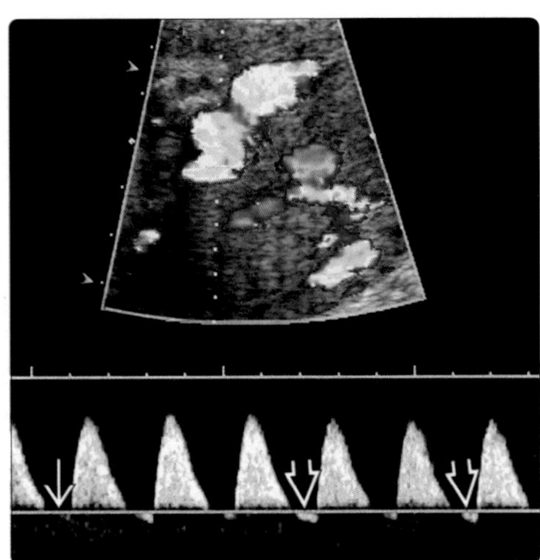

(Left) *The normal umbilical artery waveform has low resistive flow with continuous diastolic flow. The systolic/diastolic ratio is calculated by dividing the peak systolic velocity by the end-diastolic velocity.* **(Right)** *In this fetus with oligohydramnios and fetal growth restriction, the diastolic flow is occasionally absent and often reversed. This finding is associated with a higher risk for impending intrauterine fetal demise, and delivery should be considered.*

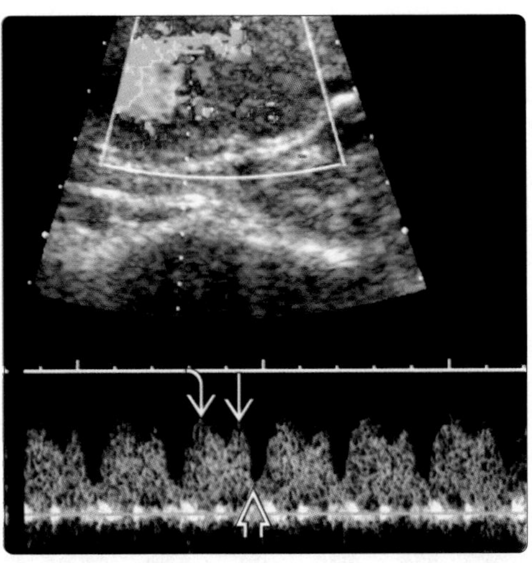

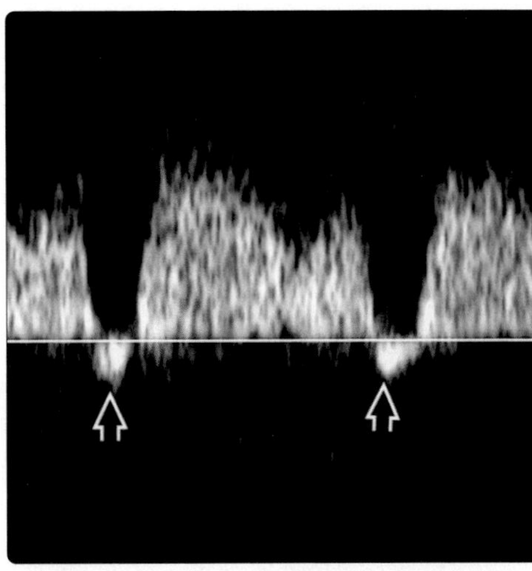

(Left) *Normal ductus venosus waveform in the liver demonstrates low-resistive systolic, diastolic, and atrial components with continuous flow toward the fetal heart throughout the cardiac cycle.* **(Right)** *Abnormal ductus venosus flow is seen in this case. The atrial contraction component (A-wave) shows reversal of flow, away from the heart. This finding is secondary to right heart stress, often from cardiac decompensation associated with fetal growth restriction.*

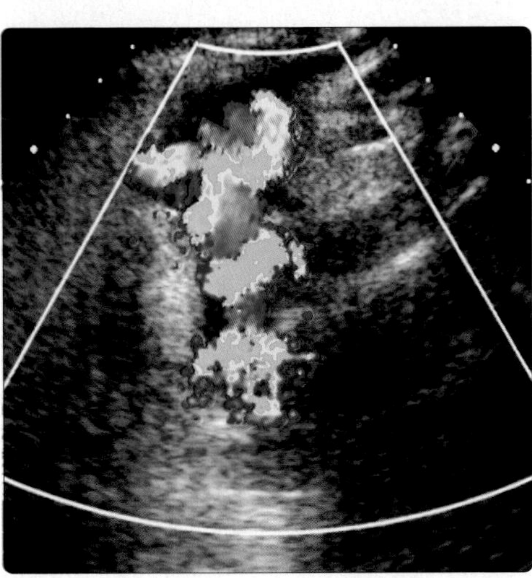

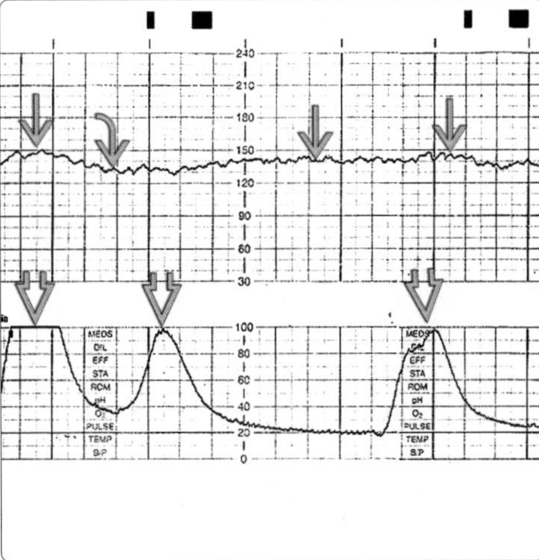

(Left) *Color Doppler shows umbilical cord filling a space that looked anechoic on grayscale images. Using color Doppler when measuring fluid pockets leads to more accurate assessment of amniotic fluid.* **(Right)** *Abnormal fetal monitoring non-stress test strip shows lack of cardiac acceleration and a mild deceleration during 3 uterine contractions in a nonlaboring patient. BPP is used in conjunction with fetal monitoring to decide when a fetus at risk for asphyxia should be delivered.*

Fetal Growth Restriction

KEY FACTS

TERMINOLOGY

- Fetus is pathologically small (growth restricted)
  - Fetal growth restriction (FGR)
  - Intrauterine growth restriction
- Small for gestational age
  - Fetus is small but healthy, not growth restricted

IMAGING

- Most common cause of FGR is placental insufficiency
  - Estimated fetal weight (EFW) < 5th-10th percentile
  - Abdominal circumference (AC) < 5-10 percentile
  - Abnormal umbilical artery (UA) Doppler values
    - Initial ↑ systolic:diastolic (S:D) ratio
    - Eventual absent end diastolic flow
    - Final reversed end diastolic flow
  - Oligohydramnios
- Other findings with FGR
  - Uterine artery postsystolic notch (early finding)
  - Ductus venosus shows reversed A-wave (late finding)
  - "Brain sparing" physiology (late finding)
    - Middle cerebral artery S:D ratio < UA S:D ratio
- FGR associations
  - Twin-twin transfusion
  - Triploidy, trisomy 18, trisomy 13
  - Anomalies (such as gastroschisis)

CLINICAL ISSUES

- Is pregnancy dated correctly
  - Cannot assess growth if dating is incorrect
- FGR fetuses have 4x higher rates of adverse outcome

SCANNING TIPS

- Good AC measurement necessary for accurate EFW
- Well-performed biophysical profile testing is key
  - Determines risk for fetal acidosis and drives delivery plan
- Perform UA Doppler at midcord level when fetus is at rest

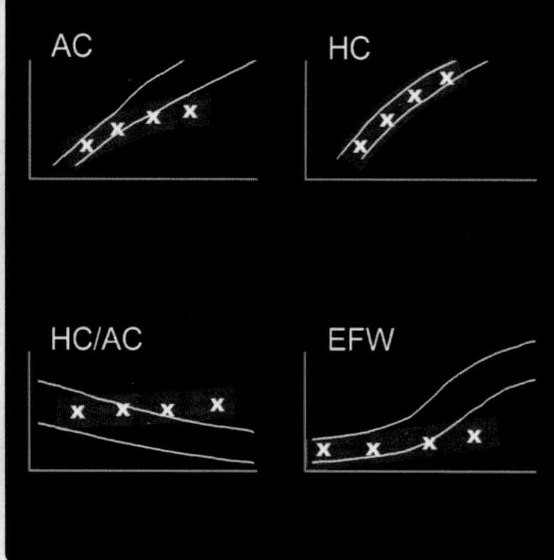

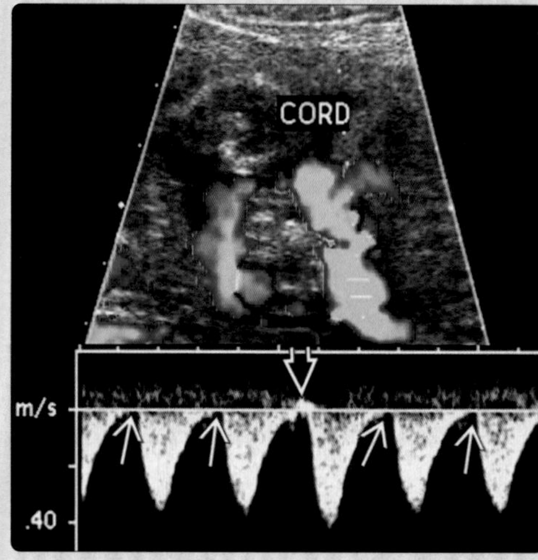

(Left) *Typical fetal biometric measurements of fetal growth restriction (FGR) from placental insufficiency shows estimated fetal weight < 5th percentile with most marked growth delay involving the AC.* **(Right)** *In this 28-week pregnancy with FGR and oligohydramnios, the UA demonstrates absent diastolic flow ➡ and occasional reversal of diastolic flow ⇨. High resistive flow in the UA is a hallmark finding with FGR from placental insufficiency. Reversal of flow is associated with a higher incidence of in utero fetal demise.*

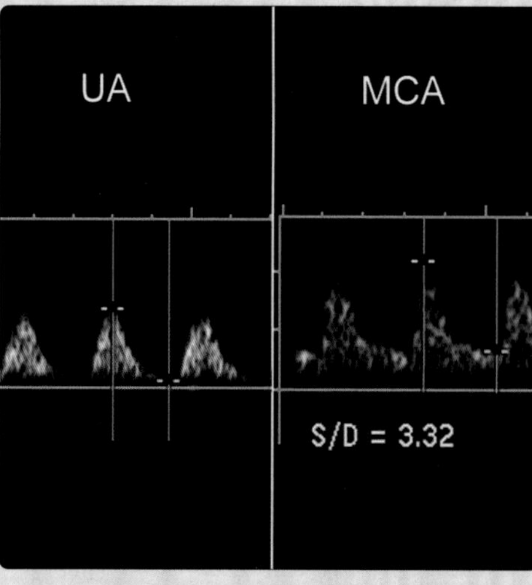

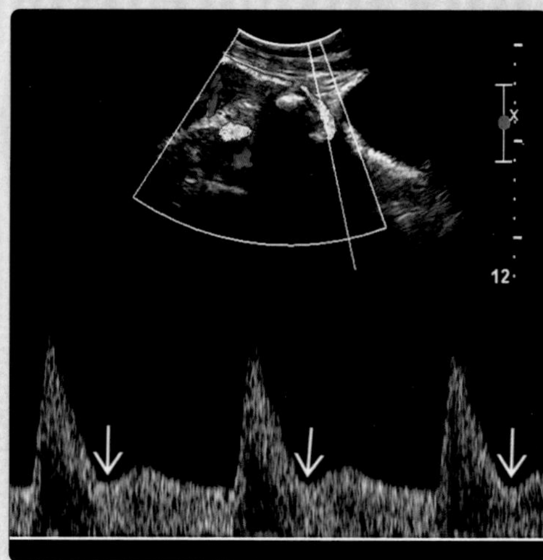

(Left) *"Brain-sparing" physiology of FGR is demonstrated in this fetus. Pulsed Doppler shows no diastolic flow in the UA (S:D ratio cannot be measured). Meanwhile, there is more diastolic flow in the MCA than expected. The MCA S:D ratio should always be > the UA S:D ratio.* **(Right)** *Abnormal uterine artery waveform is seen in a pregnancy complicated by early FDW. The presence of a postsystolic notch ➡ is not normal after the 1st trimester and suggests abnormal placentation as the cause of growth restriction.*

Macrosomia

KEY FACTS

TERMINOLOGY

- Newborn with birth weight > 4,000 or 4,500 g (10 lb)
- Fetus is considered at risk for macrosomia if estimated fetal weight (EFW) is > 90th percentile

IMAGING

- Large abdominal circumference (AC) is 1st clue
  - AC is heavily weighted in all EFW calculations
- Unfortunately, fetal weight prediction is not very accurate
  - High false-positive rates for macrosomia
    - Only 1/2 of newborns predicted to weigh > 4,500 g will actually weigh > 4,500 g
  - High negative predictive value of 97-99% is reassuring
    - EFW < 90th percentile is usually predictive that newborn will **not** be macrosomic
  - Growth graphs are useful visual tools
- Associated findings
  - Polyhydramnios
  - ↑ subcutaneous adipose tissue

TOP DIFFERENTIAL DIAGNOSES

- Beckwith-Wiedemann syndrome: Large tongue, liver, spleen, kidneys
- Hydrops: Skin edema, pleural effusion, ascites

CLINICAL ISSUES

- Associated with maternal diabetes
- Maternal complications: Prolonged, arrested labor
- Fetal complications: Shoulder dystocia, hypoglycemia, hypocalcemia
- Cesarean delivery recommended if EFW > 5,000 g and patient is not diabetic
- Cesarean delivery recommended if EFW > 4,500 g and patient is diabetic

SCANNING TIPS

- Perform several AC measurements and average good ones
- Macrosomia is critical finding, just like fetal growth restriction (need to alert referring clinician)

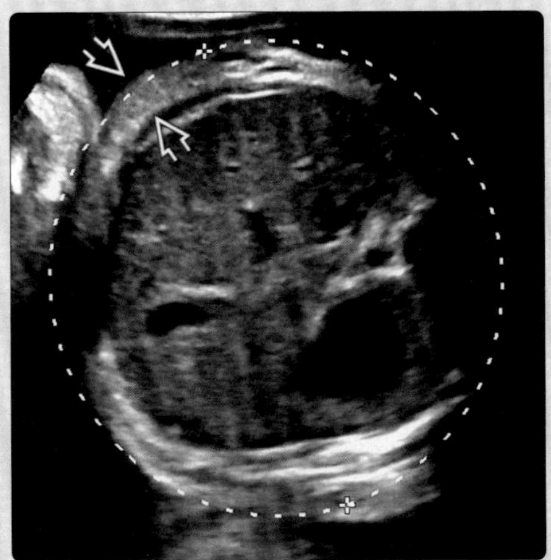

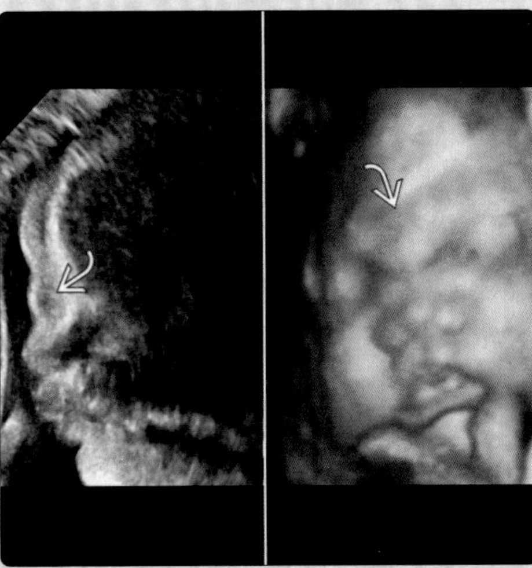

(Left) *The abdominal circumference (AC) in this fetus measured > 95th percentile, placing it at risk for macrosomia. Notice the abundant echogenic subcutaneous fat ➔.* **(Right)** *In this macrosomic fetus, there is abundant subcutaneous fat involving the head and face, particularly overlying the bridge of the nose and the forehead ➔. This finding should not be confused with skin edema, which tends to be more hypoechoic and is associated with hydrops.*

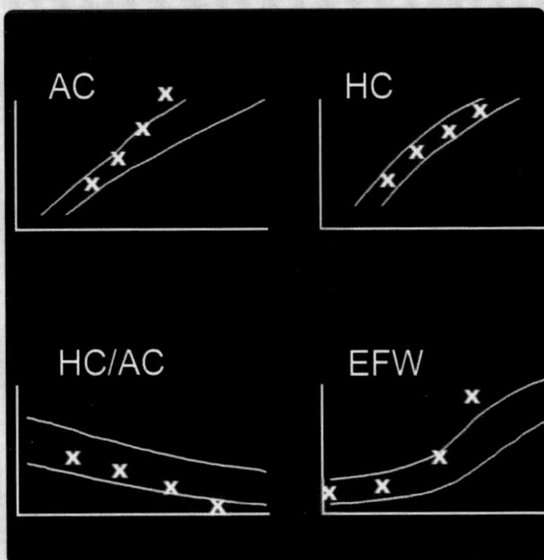

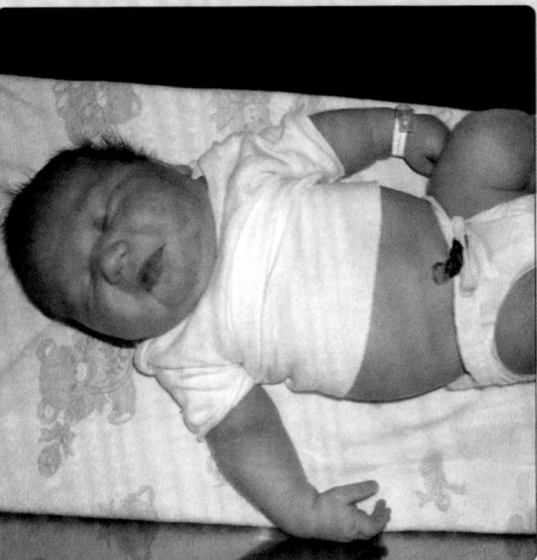

(Left) *Typical growth chart of a fetus with macrosomia shows excessive AC growth. Head circumference (HC) growth typically is normal, leading to ↓ HC:AC ratio. Estimated fetal weight is > 95th percentile in the 3rd trimester.* **(Right)** *At 12 lb 2 oz, this newborn is macrosomic. Note the protuberant abdomen and abundance of subcutaneous fat. Newborns with macrosomia are at risk for asphyxia (breathing difficulty), hypoglycemia (low blood sugar), and hypocalcemia (low calcium) and need extra monitoring.*

Fetal Anemia

KEY FACTS

IMAGING

- ↑ middle cerebral artery (MCA) peak systolic velocity (PSV) suggests diagnosis of fetal anemia
- High-output heart failure is late finding
  - Cardiomegaly, polyhydramnios
  - Hydrops
    - Pericardial &/or pleural effusion, ascites, anasarca

CLINICAL ISSUES

- Rhesus or other RBC antigen incompatibility
  - Antibodies cross placenta → fetal RBC lysis → anemia
  - Subsequent pregnancies with similar or more severe hemolysis
- Other causes of fetal anemia
  - Infection: Parvovirus most common
  - Fetal hemorrhage from any cause
  - Twin anemia-polycythemia sequence
    - From fetofetal transfusion in monochorionic twins
  - α-thalassemia

DIAGNOSTIC CHECKLIST

- Monitor anemia risk with serial MCA PSV measurements
  - Follow multiples of median (MoM) values
- Fetal intervention based on risk for significant anemia
  - ↑ risk of anemia if MCA PSV is ≥ 1.50 MoM
  - ↑ false-positive rates when > 35-week gestational age
- Ultrasound guidance used to access fetal circulation and give RBC transfusion
  - Cordocentesis: Umbilical vein (UV) blood sampled and sent to lab for fetal hematocrit value
  - Intrauterine transfusion: RBCs given to fetus via UV

SCANNING TIPS

- MCA waveform acquisition tips
  - Doppler gate placed near origin of MCA
  - Angle of insonation should be 0°
- Obtain several MCA PSV measurements
  - Choose best measurement with best technique, not average of MCA PSVs

(Left) *Axial color Doppler ultrasound of the fetal brain shows an intact circle of Willis. The optimal site of sampling the middle cerebral artery (MCA) is near its origin ➔ from the circle of Willis.* **(Right)** *The Doppler sample volume should be ~ 2 mm ➔ at the origin of the MCA, and no angle correction should be used to obtain the peak systolic velocity. Measurements are more accurate in the absence of fetal movement or breathing, which can cause variations in the peak velocity.*

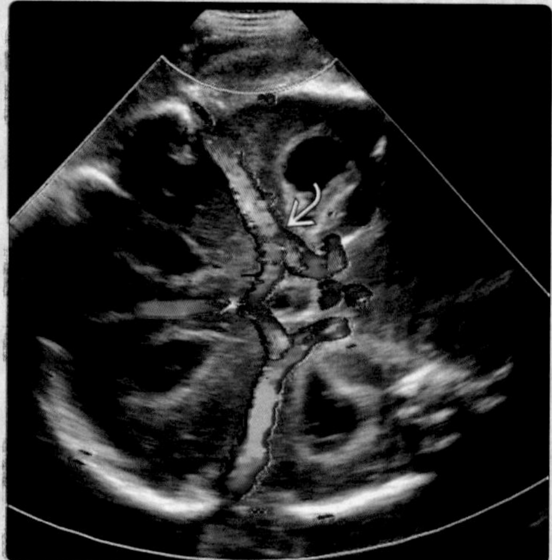

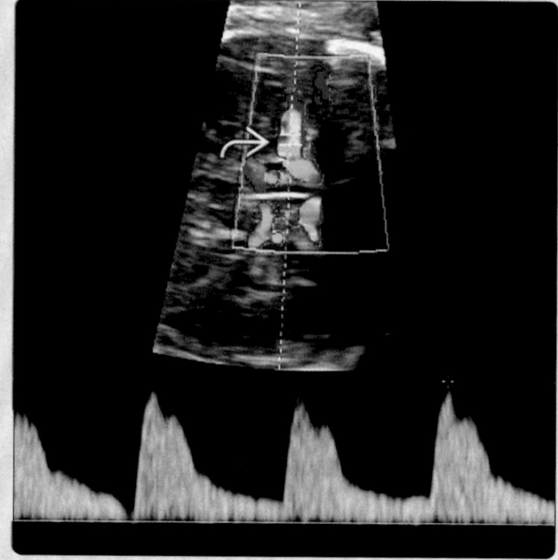

(Left) *Transabdominal ultrasound during cordocentesis and intrauterine transfusion shows the needle traversing the placenta ➔ into the base of the cord in a 28-week fetus. Transplacental needle placement can help stabilize the needle for transfusion.* **(Right)** *Chart shows the MCA velocities from a rhesus-sensitized fetus. Two intrauterine transfusions were required during gestation. The fetus was delivered at 35 weeks without complication.*

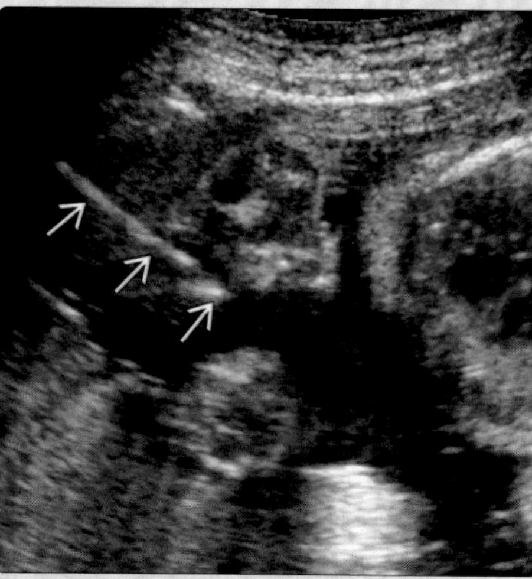

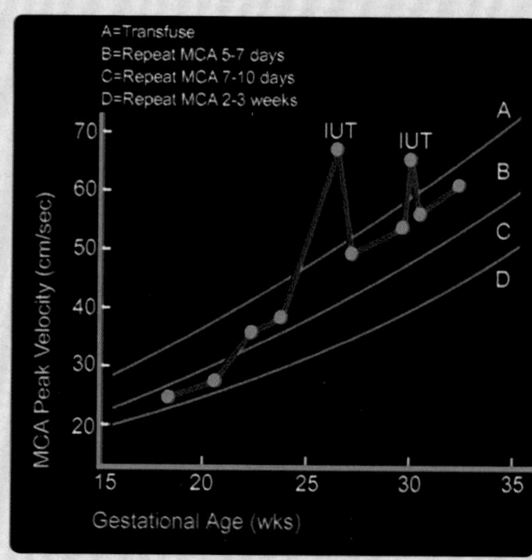

KEY FACTS

TERMINOLOGY

- Abnormal accumulation of fluid in 2 sites (pleural, pericardial, ascites, skin)

IMAGING

- Pleural effusion surrounds lung, which floats toward hilum: Angel wing sign
- Large pericardial effusion surrounds heart, displaces lungs to chest wall
- Polyhydramnios, placentomegaly may be seen but do not count toward areas of excess fluid accumulation

SCANNING TIPS

- Look for structural abnormalities: Hydrops may be due to chromosomal abnormality, infection, vascular malformation, skeletal dysplasia
- Do not confuse hypoechoic abdominal wall muscles with small volume of ascites
- Do not confuse hypoechoic, compacted peripheral myocardium with pericardial effusion
    - Myocardium ends at valves, effusion surround atria as well as ventricles
- Check cardiac rate and rhythm
    - Place M-mode cursor through 1 atrium/1 ventricle to assess atrioventricular conduction
    - Apparently isolated ascites may be sign of impending hydrops in fetus with tachycardia
- In any fetus with hydrops, measure middle cerebral artery (MCA) peak systolic velocity (PSV)
    - MCA PSV increases with fetal anemia
    - Anemia is treatable cause of hydrops
- Scan technique is critical for measurement of MCA PSV
    - Small sample volume placed within 2 mm of takeoff of MCA from circle of Willis
    - Angle of insonation must be 0, fetus at rest
    - Measure PSV and plot multiples of median for gestational age (> 1.5 indicates fetal anemia)

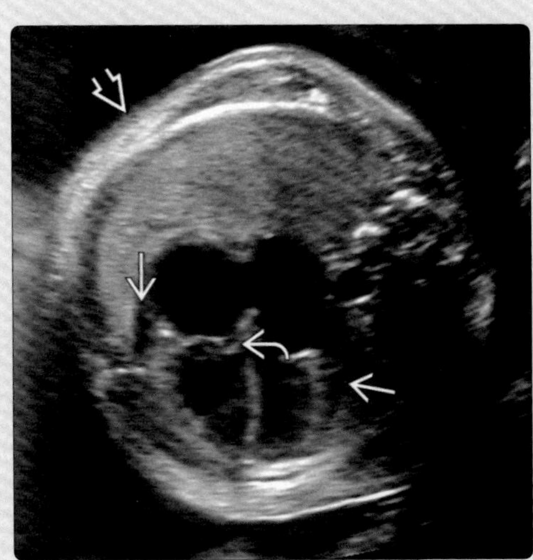

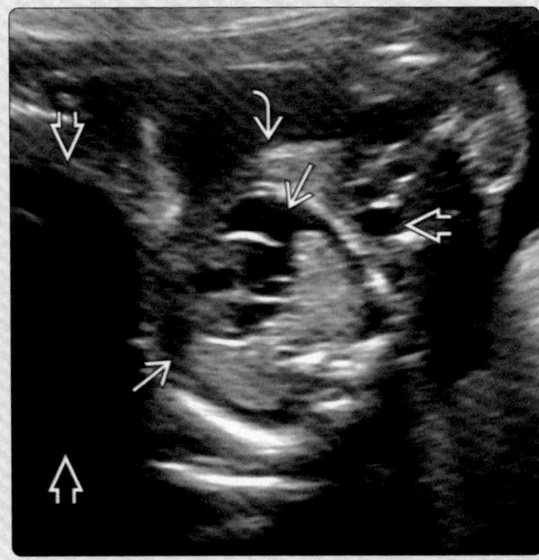

(Left) *Four-chamber US in an early case of developing hydrops shows cardiomegaly, subtle skin thickening ➡, and a small pericardial effusion ➡. Note that the hypoechoic fluid extends beyond the level of the valves ➡.* **(Right)** *Axial US through the chest of a hydropic fetus with Turner syndrome shows bilateral pleural effusions ➡ (note the angel wing appearance of the lungs) as well as skin thickening ➡ and incompletely visualized components of a massive cystic hygroma ➡.*

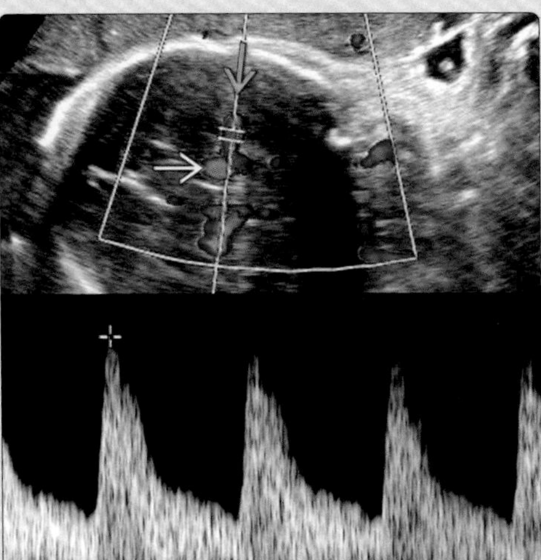

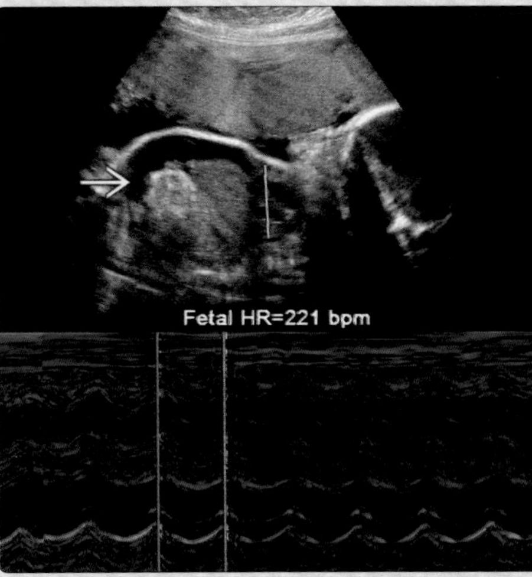

(Left) *Color Doppler US shows the correct technique for measurement of middle cerebral artery peak systolic velocity with zero angle of insonation ➡ and sample volume placement within 2 mm of takeoff from the circle of Willis ➡.* **(Right)** *M-mode US through the fetal heart shows supraventricular tachycardia with a rate of 221 BPM. Ascites ➡ is often the 1st sign of impending hydrops in fetuses with tachycardia. In this case, medical management was successful before onset of full-blown hydrops.*

PART VI
SECTION 15

Maternal Conditions in Pregnancy

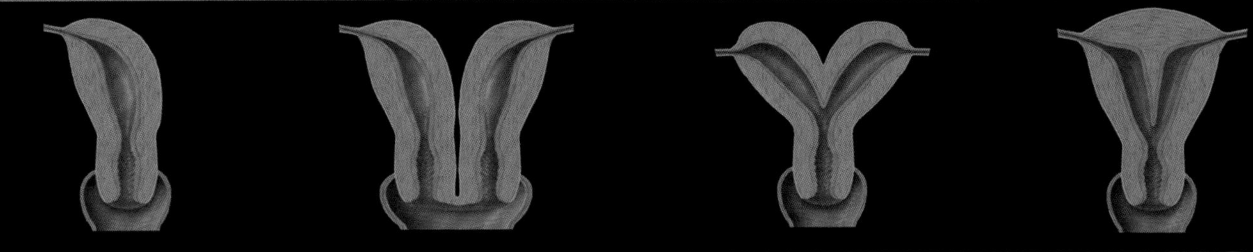

Myoma in Pregnancy

KEY FACTS

TERMINOLOGY

- Fibroid, leiomyoma
- Definition: Benign smooth muscle tumor of uterus

IMAGING

- Typically well-defined round or oval hypoechoic mass ± calcification
- Myomas can grow during first 1/2 of pregnancy
- Myomas can degenerate during pregnancy
  - Most common: Asymptomatic hyaline degeneration
    - Typically heterogeneous, septated, cystic myoma
  - Less common: Symptomatic hemorrhagic degeneration
    - Hyperechoic, heterogeneous, solid-appearing myoma
    - Can lead to preterm labor and pregnancy loss
- Placenta can implant upon myoma
- Color Doppler findings
  - Uterine vessels supply myoma
    - May see vascular pedicle to pedunculated myoma
  - Peripheral swirled pattern of flow is typical

CLINICAL ISSUES

- Complications related to size, number, and location
  - Lower uterine myoma with ↑ rates of malpresentation, cesarean delivery, and postpartum hemorrhage
  - Retroplacental myoma with ↑ rates of placental insufficiency, abruption, and preterm labor
  - Multiple myomas associated with fetal growth restriction and postpartum hemorrhage
- Acute pain, low-grade fever associated with hemorrhagic degeneration: MR best to show hemorrhage

SCANNING TIPS

- Note location, type, and size of myoma in every case
- Note relationship with placenta and cervix
- Adnexal and pedunculated myoma can mimic ovarian mass
  - Look for blood supply from uterus
  - Look for separate ovary
- If myoma is painful, consider hemorrhagic degeneration and alert provider

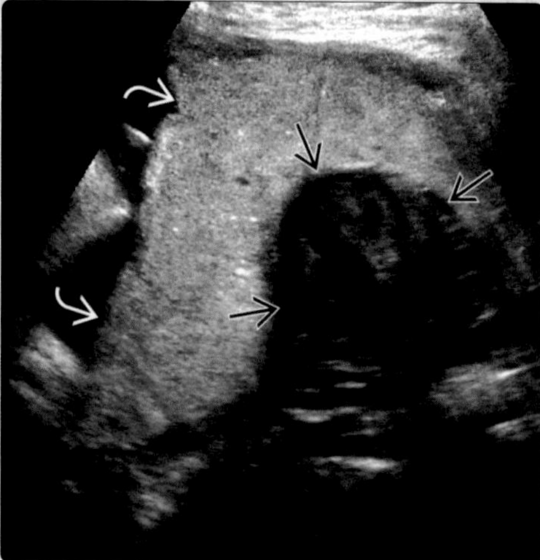

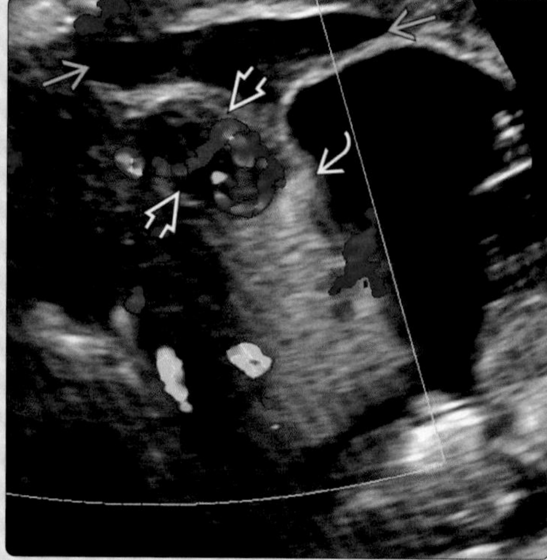

(Left) *In this asymptomatic pregnant patient, the placenta ➔ implants upon a submucosal myoma ➔. The myoma is homogeneous and hypoechoic. Placental implantation upon myoma is associated with abruption and fetal growth restriction.* **(Right)** *In this pregnancy complicated by early 2nd-trimester bleeding, the placental edge ➔ is implanted upon a myoma ➔, demonstrating typical swirled flow pattern on color Doppler. This is probably why a marginal abruption ➔ occurred in this pregnancy.*

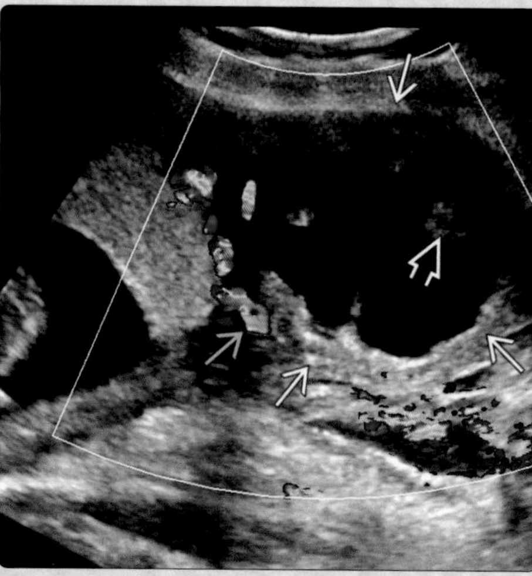

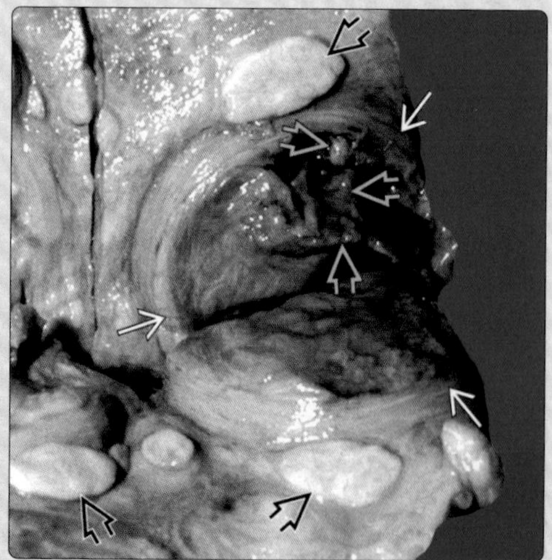

(Left) *In this pregnancy with cystic degeneration of a subserosal myoma ➔, the avascular central cystic region and wall nodularities ➔ mimic an ovarian neoplasm. However, the myoma blood supply is shown coming from the uterus ➔ and a separate normal ovary was documented (not shown).* **(Right)** *Gross pathology shows the inside of a cystic degenerated fibroid ➔. Note the internal septations and wall nodularity ➔. Smaller uncomplicated solid fibroids ➔ are also seen.*

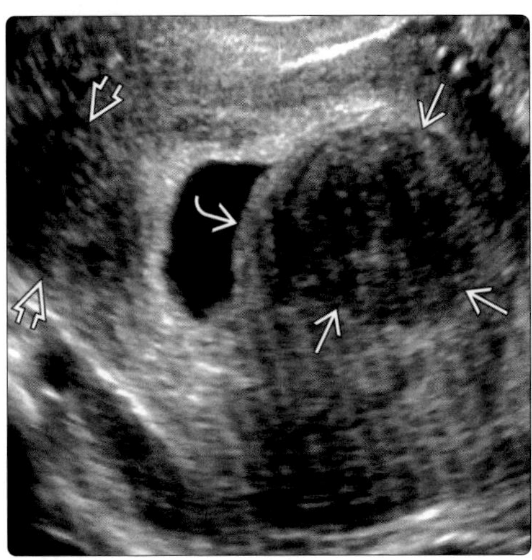

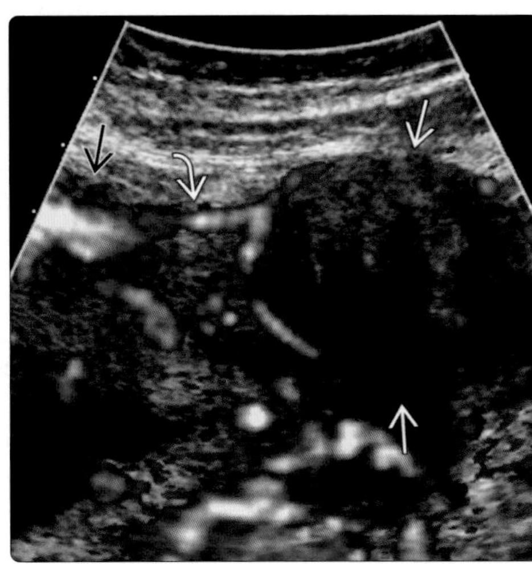

(Left) *Axial transvaginal US of a 1st-trimester case shows a submucosal myoma ➡. The fibroid indents the gestational sac ➡. A 2nd subtle mural myoma ➡ is also present. Submucosal myomas can cause recurrent pregnancy loss and infertility.* **(Right)** *Axial power Doppler US shows a pedunculated fibroid ➡ connected by a vascular stalk ➡ to the lateral edge of the uterus ➡. Pedunculated fibroids are at risk for torsion and can be confused with adnexal masses.*

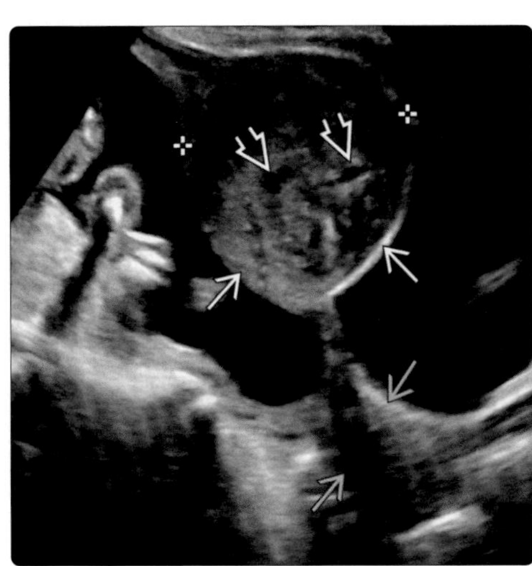

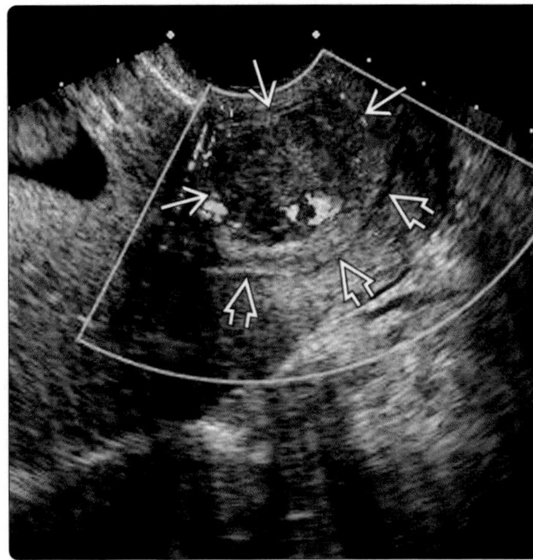

(Left) *Sagittal US of the lower uterine segment shows a large anterior myoma ➡ with a few scattered cystic areas ➡, most typical for hyaline degeneration. The proximity to the cervix ➡ should be noted.* **(Right)** *Sagittal transvaginal US shows a small anterior cervix myoma ➡. Note the mass effect upon the endocervical canal ➡ and the typical peripheral blood flow. Lower uterine segment and cervical myomas are associated with fetal malpresentation and cesarean delivery.*

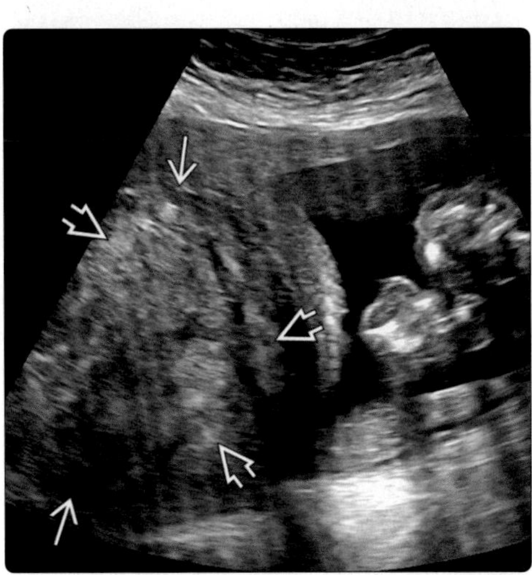

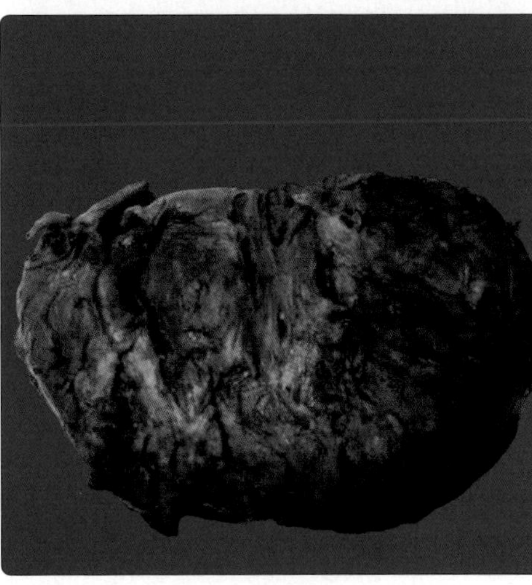

(Left) *Axial US in a 17-week pregnant patient presenting to the emergency department with RLQ and low-grade fever shows a heterogeneous myoma ➡ with focal echogenic areas ➡. On MR, the fibroid was hemorrhagic and the appendix was normal. The next day, the patient lost the pregnancy.* **(Right)** *In the same patient, the myoma was removed and was deemed to be the cause of the pregnancy loss. Hemorrhagic, red, carneous myoma degeneration is symptomatic and seen in 5% of cases with myoma degeneration.*

Müllerian Duct Anomalies in Pregnancy

KEY FACTS

TERMINOLOGY

- Spectrum of congenital uterine malformations
  - **20% unicornuate**: Single uterine horn ± rudimentary horns
  - **5% uterus didelphys**: 2 separate horns, 2 cervices
    - Often associated with vaginal septum (75%)
  - **10% bicornuate**: 2 horns with variable degree of fusion
    - Concave or heart-shaped external fundal contour
    - May have 1 cervix (bicornis unicollis) or 2 cervices (bicornis bicollis)
  - **55% septate**: Normal, convex external fundal contour
    - Septum length variable: When complete it extends to external os

SCANNING TIPS

- **Use 3D ultrasound**
  - Volume acquisition allows reconstruction of true coronal plane to show fundal contour
    - Septate uterus: Fundus mildly convex to mildly concave
    - Bicornuate: Concave or heart-shaped external fundal contour
- **Look for associated renal anomalies**
  - Occur in ~ 30% of patients with müllerian duct anomalies
  - Unilateral renal agenesis in majority but crossed-fused ectopia, pelvic kidney, horseshoe kidney, renal duplication, and cystic dysplasia all reported
- **Look for obstructed component if pelvic pain**
  - Hematometra: Blood-filled uterus (may involve single horn of duplicated system)
  - Hematometrocolpos: Blood-filled uterus and vagina
- Pregnancy failure increased especially with septate uterus
  - Use ultrasound guidance for dilatation and evacuation/curettage to ensure appropriate part of cavity is reached

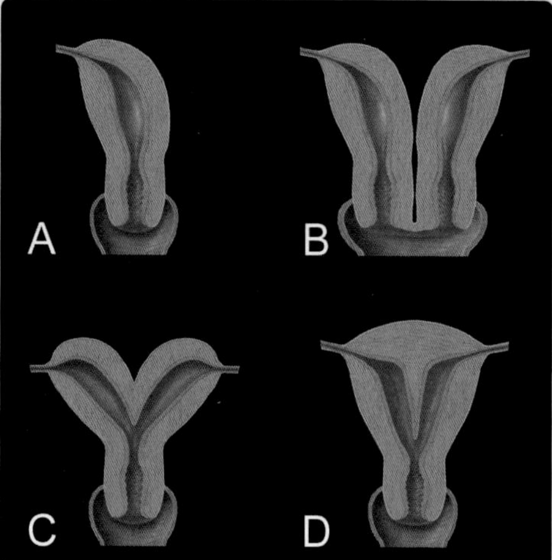

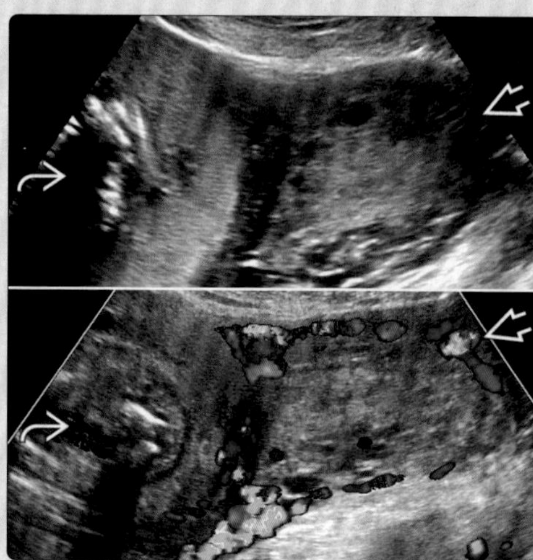

(Left) *Graphic of müllerian duct anomalies shows unicornuate (A) has 1 horn; didelphys (B) has 2 nonfused horns; bicornuate (C) has a concave external contour; septate (D) has a normal external contour. An accessory rudimentary horn may occur with A.* **(Right)** *Grayscale and color Doppler US show a rudimentary horn adjacent to the pregnancy, which is in a unicornuate uterus. Implantation in a rudimentary horn may result in rupture. Color Doppler shows bridging vessels between rudimentary horn & the unicornuate uterus.*

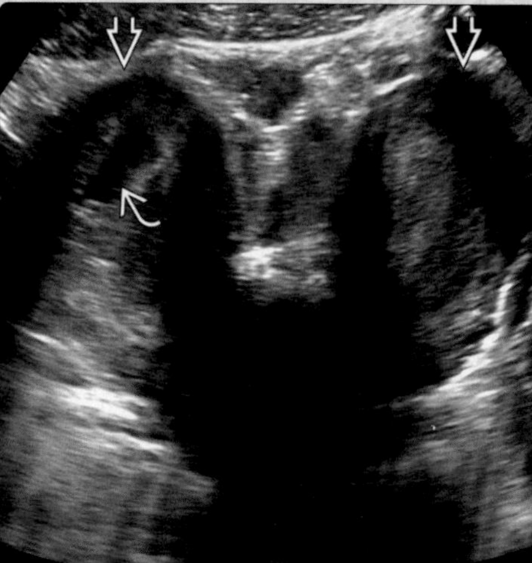

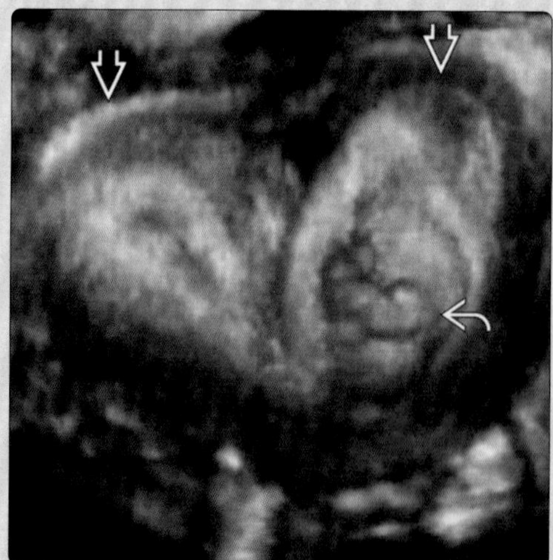

(Left) *Abdominal US shows the separate horns of a uterus didelphys. They are similar in size, excluding a unicornuate uterus with a rudimentary horn. The 2 horns never attach excluding a bicornuate uterus. The pregnancy is in the right horn.* **(Right)** *3D ultrasound in the same patient's next pregnancy shows the separate horns of the didelphys uterus with the pregnancy now in the left horn. The cervices are not visible in either image as they are out of the scan plane.*

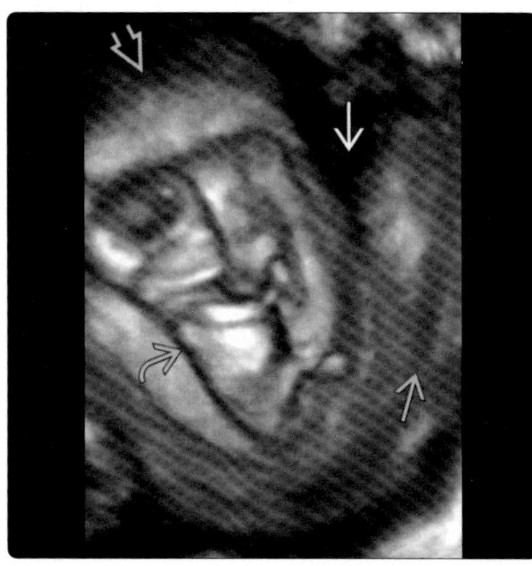

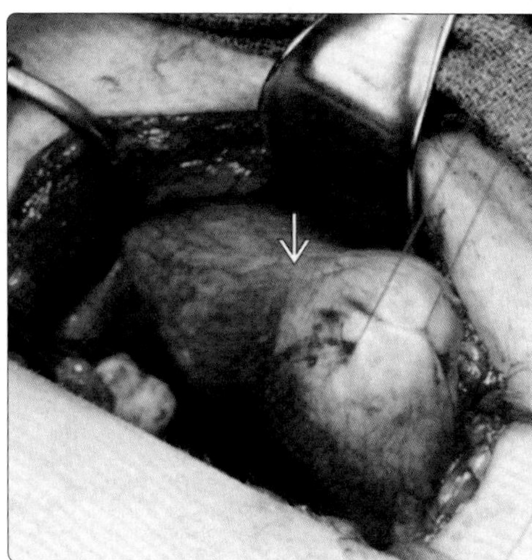

(Left) *3D ultrasound in the late 1st trimester shows the embryo ➢ in the right horn ➪ of a bicornuate uterus. The empty cavity ➪ of the left horn is visible at the edge of the picture. Note the cleft ➡ in the fundal contour, which proves that this is not a septate uterus.* **(Right)** *Intraoperative photograph in a different case shows the characteristic heart-shaped contour of a bicornuate uterus with the fundal cleft ➡ between the 2 horns. The fundal contour is either flat or convex outward in a septate uterus.*

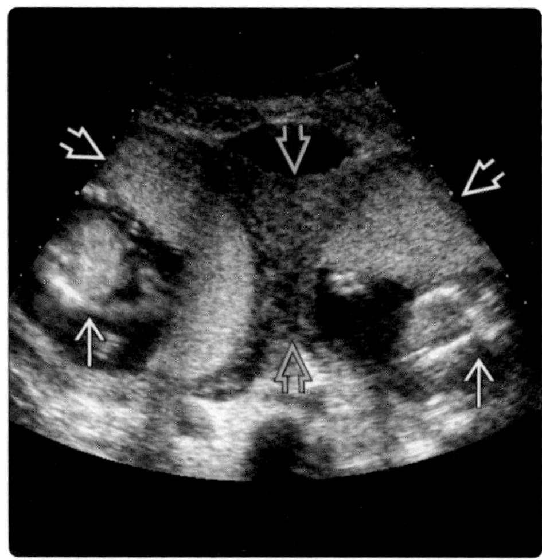

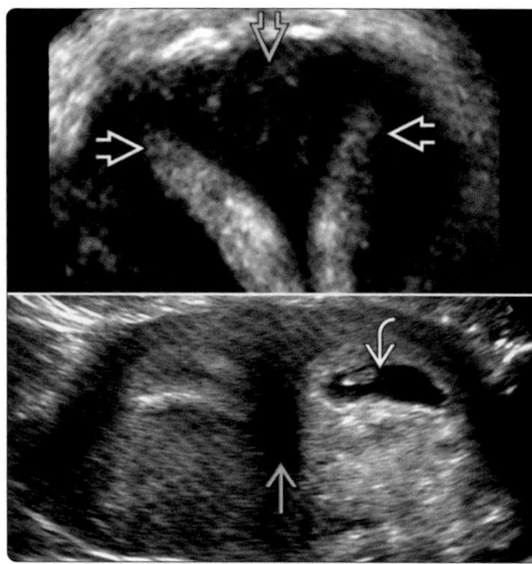

(Left) *Transverse US of a bicornuate uterus shows a twin pregnancy with a fetus ➡ and placenta ➡ in each uterine horn. Note the classic indentation of the external uterine contour ➪.* **(Right)** *Coronal 3D US performed for recurrent pregnancy loss shows normal fundal contour ➪ with a septum between the uterine cavities ➡. A transverse view through the pregnant uterus shows a gestational sac (embryo ➡) implanted to the left of the septum ➪. This patient had successful pregnancies after septal takedown.*

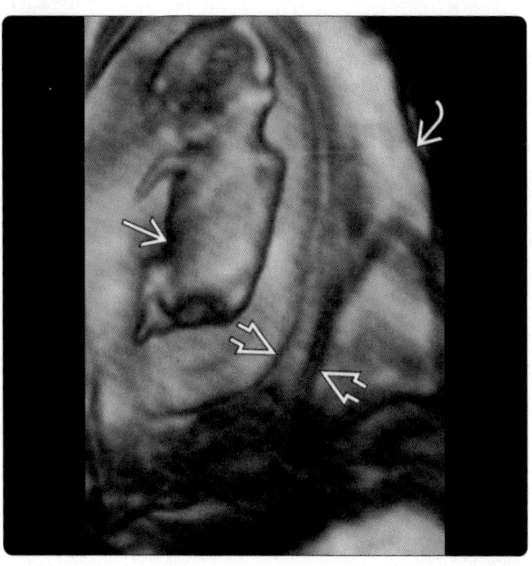

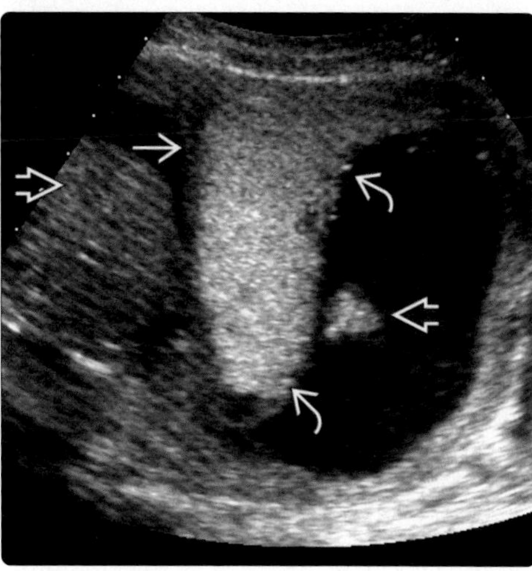

(Left) *Coronal 3D ultrasound in the 1st trimester shows a fetus ➡ on the right side of a septate uterus. Note the smooth uterine fundus ➡ and the long uterine septum ➡. The fundal contour differentiates this from a bicornuate uterus.* **(Right)** *Axial ultrasound shows a large portion of the placenta ➡ implanted on a uterine septum ➡. Because the septum is not as well vascularized as normal myometrium, these cases are at risk for fetal growth restriction. Fetal parts ➡ are seen on either side of the septum.*

Cervical Insufficiency/Short Cervix

KEY FACTS

TERMINOLOGY

- **Cervical insufficiency** is clinical diagnosis: Inability of cervix to retain pregnancy in absence of contractions or labor
- **Short cervix** is sonographic observation: Cervical length (CL) < 25 mm at < 24 weeks
- **Funneling**: Protrusion of amniotic membranes into cervical canal

SCANNING TIPS

- **Check CL at beginning of exam as cervix is dynamic**
- Length is shortest in patients who have recently been upright
- **Transvaginal US essential** in high-risk patients or if CL < 30 mm on transabdominal ultrasound
  - Observe for 3-5 minutes
    - Magnify image so cervix occupies 75% of screen
    - Avoid excessive vaginal transducer pressure
    - Measure from internal os to external os
    - Use fundal pressure to unveil short cervix
    - Look for amniotic fluid "sludge" (layering, inflammatory debris)
- Report single best, shortest cervical length; do not average measurements
  - Worse prognosis if short cervix + funneling
  - Funneling > 50% of CL is most significant (79% risk preterm birth)
- **Cerclage monitoring** is controversial
  - American College of Obstetrics and Gynecology bulletin says it is not required
  - Proponents argue that it helps counsel patients regarding prognosis if signs of stitch failure
  - If scan performed for cerclage follow-up
    - Measure functional CL (length of closed cervix regardless of sutures)
    - Document funneling to or beyond suture
    - Document presence of amniotic fluid sludge

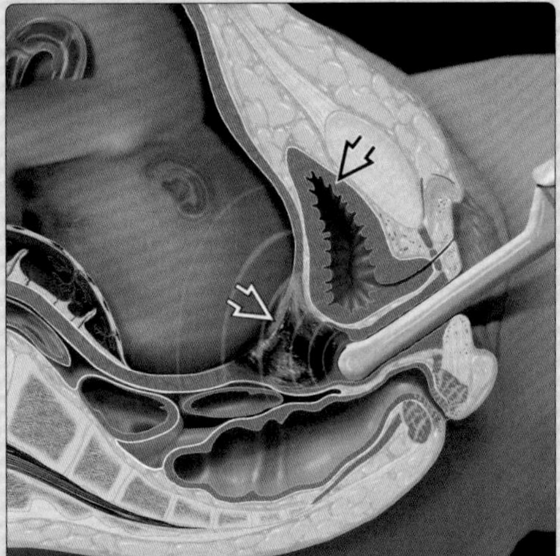

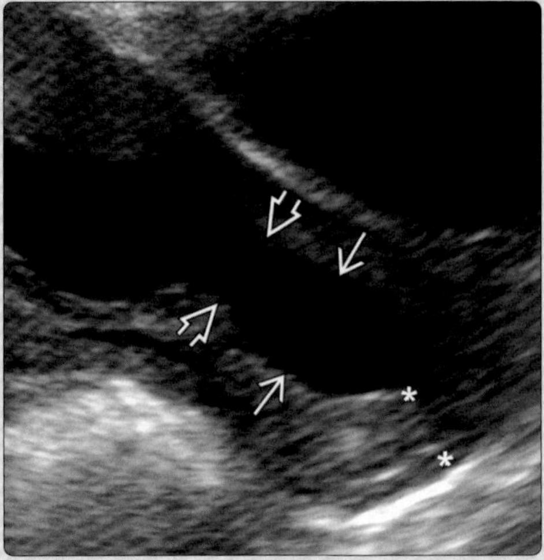

(Left) *Graphic illustrates cervical measurement. The transducer is positioned such that the cervix ⇨ is just in focus and not compressed. Compression may elongate the cervix and obscure dynamic changes. A full bladder ⇨ may also compress the lower uterine segment to mimic a long, closed cervix.* **(Right)** *Abdominal US shows a short cervix (calipers = 10 mm) with dilated internal os ⇨ and funneled membranes ➡. It is best to check cervical length at the start of the exam when the patient has been up and active.*

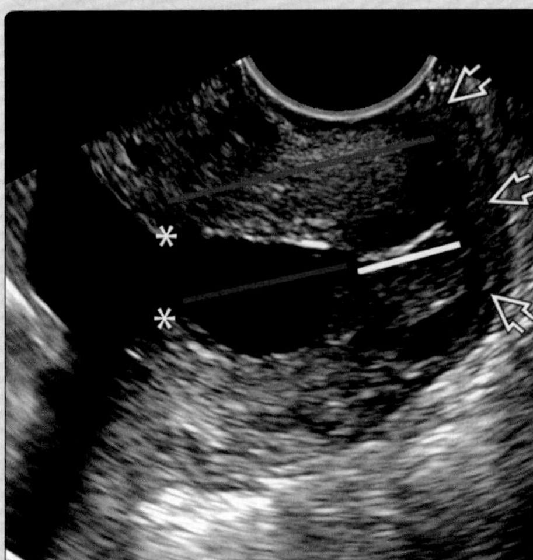

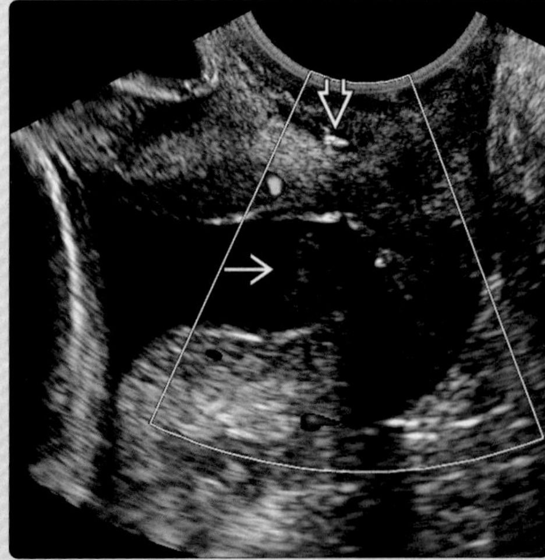

(Left) *Sagittal TVUS shows the length of the funnel (blue line), the functional cervical length (white line), and the total cervical length (red line). The funnel is > 50% of total cervical length. Visualization of the vaginal fornix ⇨ proves that the entire length of the cervix has been measured. The asterisks denote the internal os diameter.* **(Right)** *TVUS shows funneled membranes and amniotic fluid sludge ➡. The membranes are at the level of the cerclage stitch ⇨. This places the patient at further increased risk of preterm birth.*

Retained Products of Conception

KEY FACTS

TERMINOLOGY

- Incomplete uterine evacuation with retention of placental/trophoblastic tissue within endometrial cavity

IMAGING

- Solid, heterogeneous, echogenic mass
  - Early loss often has small cystic areas
  - Postpartum appears more like placenta
- Persistent, thickened endometrium
  - > 10 mm usually considered abnormal, but no consensus exists
- Perform color Doppler to look for flow
  - High-velocity, low-resistance flow
- Lack of increased flow does not rule out RPOC
  - 40% of cases may have no or minimal flow

TOP DIFFERENTIAL DIAGNOSES

- Normal postpartum uterus
  - Small echogenic foci and fluid common
  - Should decrease to < 8 mm with uterine involution
- Intrauterine blood/clot
  - Reported in up to 24% of postpartum patients
  - More hypoechoic than RPOC
  - No flow with Doppler

CLINICAL ISSUES

- Delayed postpartum bleeding
  - Most present within few days of delivery or abortion
- RPOC is risk factor for endometritis
  - Always consider RPOC in setting of postpartum fevers and pelvic pain

SCANNING TIPS

- Use transvaginal scanning with color and pulsed wave Doppler in all cases
- Carefully measure endometrial thickness
  - If no mass or fluid and endometrial thickness < 10 mm without increased flow, RPOC extremely unlikely

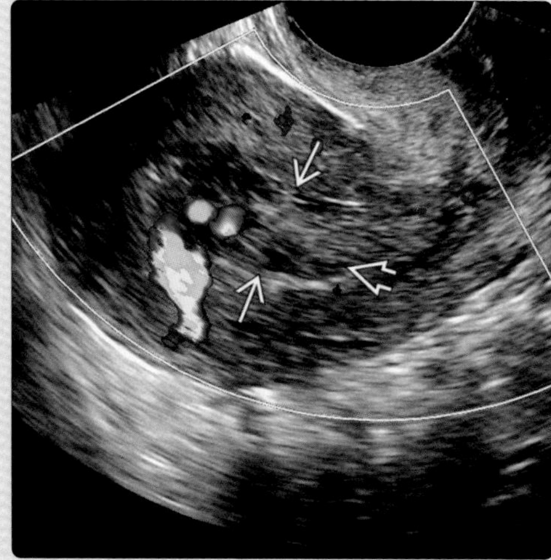

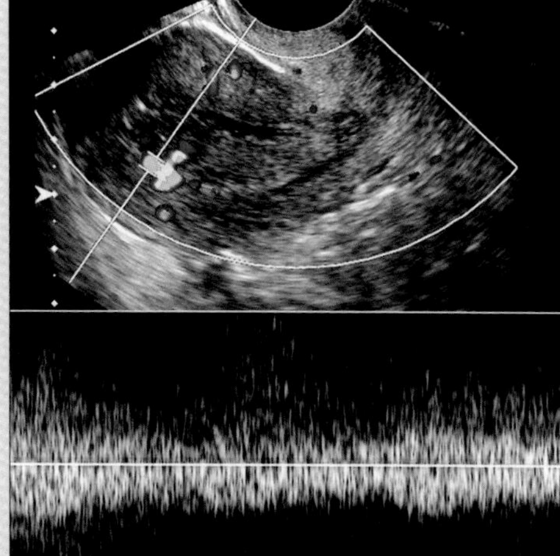

(Left) *Longitudinal transvaginal color Doppler ultrasound shows a complex, echogenic, vascular mass ➡ in the endometrial cavity of a woman with a 1st-trimester pregnancy loss. Note the small cystic areas ➡, which are common in RPOC after a spontaneous abortion.* **(Right)** *Pulsed wave Doppler ultrasound in the same case shows chaotic arterial and venous flow, which can be confused with an arteriovenous malformation. This flow will resolve after evacuation of the retained products.*

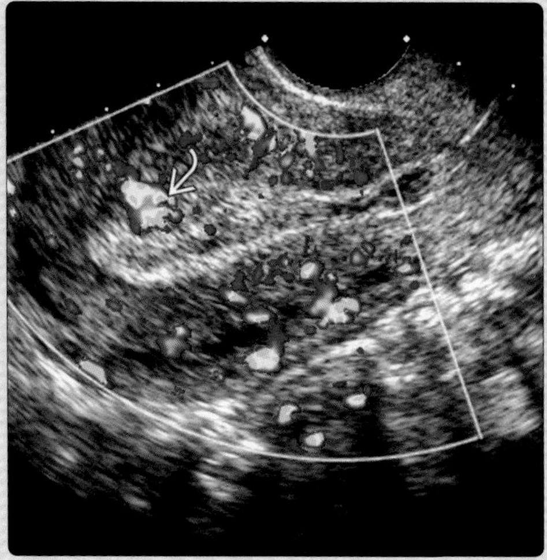

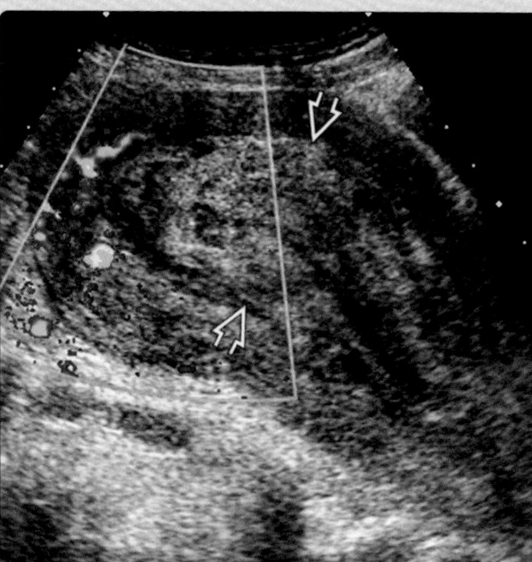

(Left) *In this case of RPOC, there is no endometrial mass, but there is diffuse endometrial thickening with an area of increased color flow ➡. Increased vascularity within a thickened postpartum endometrium is highly suggestive of RPOC.* **(Right)** *In this case, there is marked thickening of the endometrium ➡ but no flow on color Doppler. It is important to remember that in up to 40% of RPOC cases, there is little or no flow on Doppler imaging.*

PART VII
SECTION 1
Brain

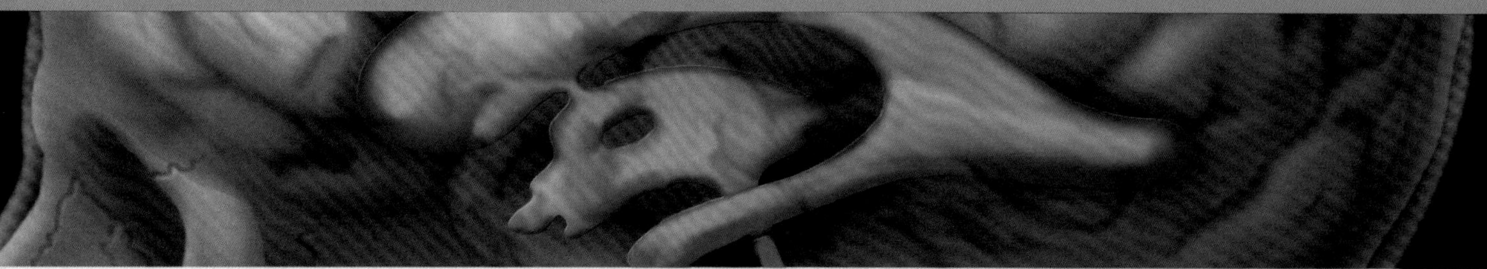

Anatomy and Approach

Brain Pathology

GROSS ANATOMY

Supratentorial Structures

- **Gyri**: Complex convolutions of brain cortex; hypoechoic on US
- **Sulci** (fissure): Cerebral spinal fluid (CSF)-filled grooves or clefts that separate gyri; echogenic on US
  - Sulci separate gyri, **fissures** separate hemispheres/lobes
- **Frontal lobe**
  - **Central sulcus separates frontal, parietal lobes**
  - Precentral gyrus contains primary motor cortex
- **Parietal lobe**
  - **Posterior to central sulcus**
  - Separated from occipital lobe by parietooccipital sulcus (medial surface)
  - Postcentral gyrus: Primary somatosensory cortex
- **Occipital lobe**
  - **Posterior to parietooccipital sulcus**
  - Primary visual cortex
- **Temporal lobe**
  - **Inferior to sylvian fissure**
  - Primary auditory cortex
  - Middle temporal gyrus: Connects with auditory, somatosensory, visual association pathways
- **Insula**
  - Lies deep in floor of sylvian fissure, overlapped by portions of frontal, temporal, & parietal lobes, called the opercula
- **Limbic system**
  - Includes amygdala, hippocampus, thalamus, hypothalamus, basal ganglia, & cingulate gyrus
    - **Cingulate gyrus** is directly above & parallels the corpus callosum
  - Important role in emotion, behavior, & long-term memory
- **Corpus callosum** is white matter tract, which links cerebral hemispheres
  - Genu is front-most portion; the body arches over the cavum septi pellucidi, ending at the splenium above vermis
    - Rostrum is short posterior extension from inferior portion of genu
- **Basal ganglia** are paired deep gray matter structures, including the **caudate nuclei**
- **Thalami** are paired, large nuclear complexes, which act as relay stations for most sensory pathways

Posterior Fossa (Infratentorial) Structures

- Protected space surrounded by calvarium
  - Bounded by tentorium cerebelli superiorly (an extension of the dura mater similar to falx) & foramen magnum inferiorly (where spinal cord exits skull)
- Posterior fossa contents
  - Brainstem (midbrain, pons, & medulla oblongata) anteriorly, cerebellum posteriorly
  - Cerebral aqueduct & 4th ventricle
  - CSF cisterns containing cranial nerves, vertebrobasilar arterial system, & veins
- **Cerebellum**
  - Integrates coordination & fine-tuning of movement & regulation of muscle tone
  - **2 hemispheres & midline vermis**
    - Vermis divided into lobes & lobules by multiple fissures
      - Appears highly echogenic on US
    - Hemispheres have thin, curved gyri called **folia**
  - Connected to brainstem by 3 paired peduncles
- **Brainstem**
  - **3 anatomic divisions**
    - **Midbrain (mesencephalon)**: Upper brainstem; connects pons & cerebellum with forebrain
    - **Pons**: Bulbous midportion of brainstem; relays information from brain to cerebellum
    - **Medulla**: Caudal (inferior) brainstem; relays information from spinal cord to brain

Ventricular System & Subarachnoid Space

- Cerebral ventricles consist of paired, lateral, midline 3rd & 4th ventricles
- Communicate with each other as well as central canal of spinal cord & subarachnoid space
- **Direction of CSF flow**
  - Lateral ventricles → foramen of Monro → 3rd ventricle → cerebral aqueduct (of Sylvius) → 4th ventricle → foramina of Luschka & Magendie → subarachnoid space
  - Bulk of CSF resorption through arachnoid granulations in superior sagittal sinus
- **Lateral ventricles**
  - Paired, C-shaped structures, which arch around/above thalami
  - Each has body, atrium, **3 horns (frontal, temporal, & occipital)**
    - Occipital horn typically largest
    - Asymmetry is common, often L > R
    - Sizes change with maturity, more prominent in preterm infants
  - **Atrium/trigone**: Confluence of horns
    - Contains glomus (thickened portion) of choroid plexus
  - Lateral ventricles communicate with each other & 3rd ventricle via Y-shaped foramen of Monro
- **3rd ventricle**
  - Thin, usually slit-like, between thalami
    - May not see fluid, just bright echogenic line on US
  - 80% have central adhesion between thalami (**massa intermedia**)
  - There are 4 small recesses: 2 projecting anteriorly (optic & infundibular recesses) & 2 projecting posteriorly (suprapineal & pineal)
  - Communicates with 4th ventricle via cerebral aqueduct (of Sylvius), passing through dorsal midbrain
- **4th ventricle**
  - Infratentorial, diamond-shaped cavity between brainstem & vermis
  - **Fastigial point**: Blind-ending, dorsally pointed midline outpouching from body of 4th ventricle
    - Important marker for true midline vermian plane on US
  - CSF exits 4th ventricle into subarachnoid space via foramina of Magendie (midline) & Luschka (lateral)
  - Inferiorly communicates with central canal of spinal cord
- **Choroid plexus**
  - Produces CSF

- **Glomus** (enlargement of choroid plexus in atrium) thickest area
- Tapers & extends anteriorly to foramen of Monro & roof of 3rd & 4th ventricles
- Tapers laterally into roof of temporal horns
- **Never extends into frontal or occipital horns**

- **Subarachnoid space/cisterns**
  - CSF-containing spaces around brain
  - Numerous trabeculae, septa, membranes cross subarachnoid space & create smaller compartments termed cisterns
    - **Cisterna magna** is large cistern in posterior fossa
  - All cisterns communicate with each other & with ventricular system
- Midline cystic structures (normal variants)
  - **Cavum septi pellucidi**
    - Anterior to foramen of Monro, between anterior horns of lateral ventricles
    - 85% closed by 3-6 months after birth, but some remain open into adulthood
      - Once closed called septum pellucidum
  - **Cavum vergae**
    - Posterior to foramen of Monro, interposed between bodies of lateral ventricles
    - Posterior extension of cavum septi pellucidi (**cavum septi pellucidi et vergae**)
    - Begins to close from posterior to anterior from 6-months gestation; 97% closed by full term
  - **Cavum velum interpositum**
    - Potential space, which may accumulate CSF, above choroid in roof of 3rd ventricle & below fornices
    - Typically seen in premature infants

ANATOMY IMAGING ISSUES

Imaging Approaches

- All scanning should be performed keeping the exposure as low as reasonably achievable, the **ALARA principle**
- Scans should be performed using a small footprint, high-frequency transducer, which allows sufficient penetration to see deep structures
  - Use linear high-frequency transducer for evaluating superficial structures, such as extraaxial fluid spaces (e.g., subdural hematoma) or superior sagittal sinus (e.g., thrombosis)
- Use Doppler (color, spectral, &/or power) as needed to evaluate vasculature structures
  - Always use to confirm an anechoic structure is truly a cyst & not a vascular malformation
- **Anterior fontanelle** most commonly used approach
- **Coronal scans**
  - Complete sweep from front to back documenting key landmarks
    - Begin anterior to frontal horns & extend to posterior to occipital horns, ensuring entire brain has been covered
      - May need to tilt transducer laterally to include superficial peripheral surfaces
    - Adjust transducer position as needed to keep image symmetric side to side
    - Adjust depth to include posterior fossa, including cerebellar hemispheres & cisterna magna
  - Symmetrical structures (from anterior to posterior) include frontal horns, bodies, trigones & occipital horns of lateral ventricles; caudate nuclei & thalami
    - Foramina of Monro seen extending inferomedially into 3rd ventricle creating a Y shape
      - Just posterior to this will be **3-dot sign**: Choroid plexus on floor of lateral ventricles & roof of 3rd ventricle
      - Choroid plexus does not extend anterior to this point; echogenic material anterior to this would represent hemorrhage
  - Midline structures include interhemispheric fissure, genu & body of corpus callosum, cavum septi pellucidi, 3rd ventricle, vermis, & 4th ventricle
- **Sagittal scans**
  - Midline scan: Best view for corpus callosum, cerebellar vermis, & 4th ventricle
  - Sweep side to side from this position documenting key areas
    - **Caudothalamic groove**: Site of germinal matrix (highly vascular area from which cells migrate during brain development)
      - Most common site of hemorrhage in premature infants
    - Size of lateral ventricle
    - Far lateral to assess degree of sulcal development
- **Posterior fontanelle**
  - Best view to evaluate occipital horns for intraventricular hemorrhage
    - Can misinterpret clot adherent to choroid plexus from anterior fontanelle approach alone
    - Use color Doppler to confirm flow in choroid plexus
- **Mastoid fontanelle**
  - Located at junction of squamosal, lambdoidal, occipital sutures
  - Transducer placed about 1 cm behind helix of ear & 1 cm above tragus
  - Allows assessment of brainstem & posterior fossa
  - Best view for 4th ventricle, posterior cerebellar vermis, cerebellar hemispheres, & cisterna magna
- **Transtemporal**
  - Temporal bone anterior to ear is thin, allowing imaging of brainstem even after sutural closure
  - Best view for cerebral peduncles & 3rd ventricle

Imaging Pitfalls

- Need to understand the normal development & changing appearance of the brain as it matures
- Must know not only age in days/weeks of infant but gestational age at birth
  - Normal gyral pattern in 26-week preterm infant would be abnormal in term infant
- Slit-like lateral ventricles common in infants, not to be mistaken for cerebral edema
- Glomus of choroid plexus can be bulbous & irregular, not to be mistaken for blood clot
  - Evaluate with color Doppler & posterior fontanelle view
- Echogenic material in frontal or occipital horns is clot; choroid does not extend into these horns

BRAIN

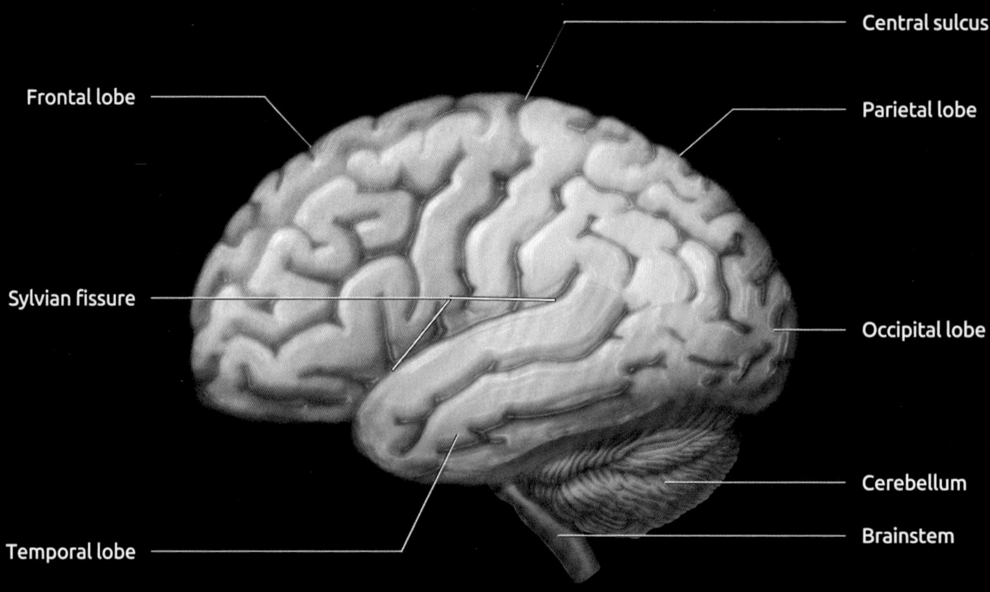

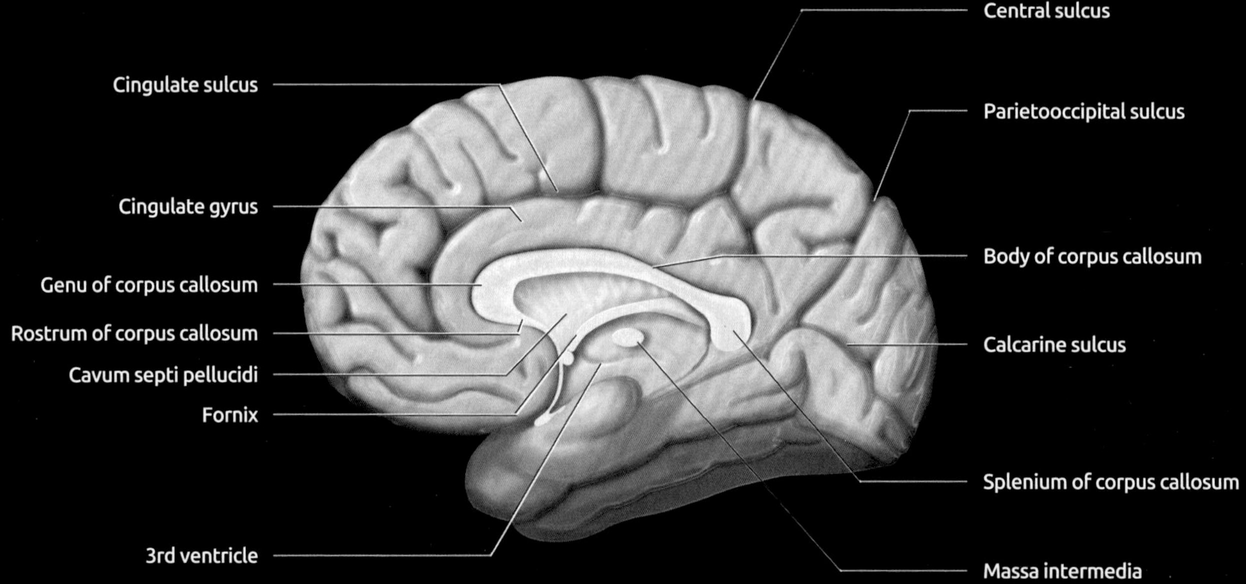

(Top) *Graphic of the brain viewed from the side shows the 4 lobes. The frontal lobe (pink) is separated from the parietal lobe (yellow) by the central sulcus. The occipital lobe (green) is the most posterior portion of the brain, and the temporal lobe (blue) lies below the sylvian fissure. The insula lies deep to the sylvian fissure and is covered by portions of the frontal, parietal, and temporal lobes, which are referred to as the opercula.* **(Bottom)** *Midline sagittal graphic shows the major structures, which should be seen on a midline US. The corpus callosum forms an arc over the cavum septi pellucidi. The cingulate gyrus has a similar arc-like configuration on top of the corpus callosum. In cases of agenesis of the corpus callosum, this configuration will be absent, and the gyri will fan out in a radial configuration, giving a sunray appearance. Several major sulci are shown, including the central, parietooccipital, calcarine, and cingulate sulci.*

VENTRICULAR SYSTEM

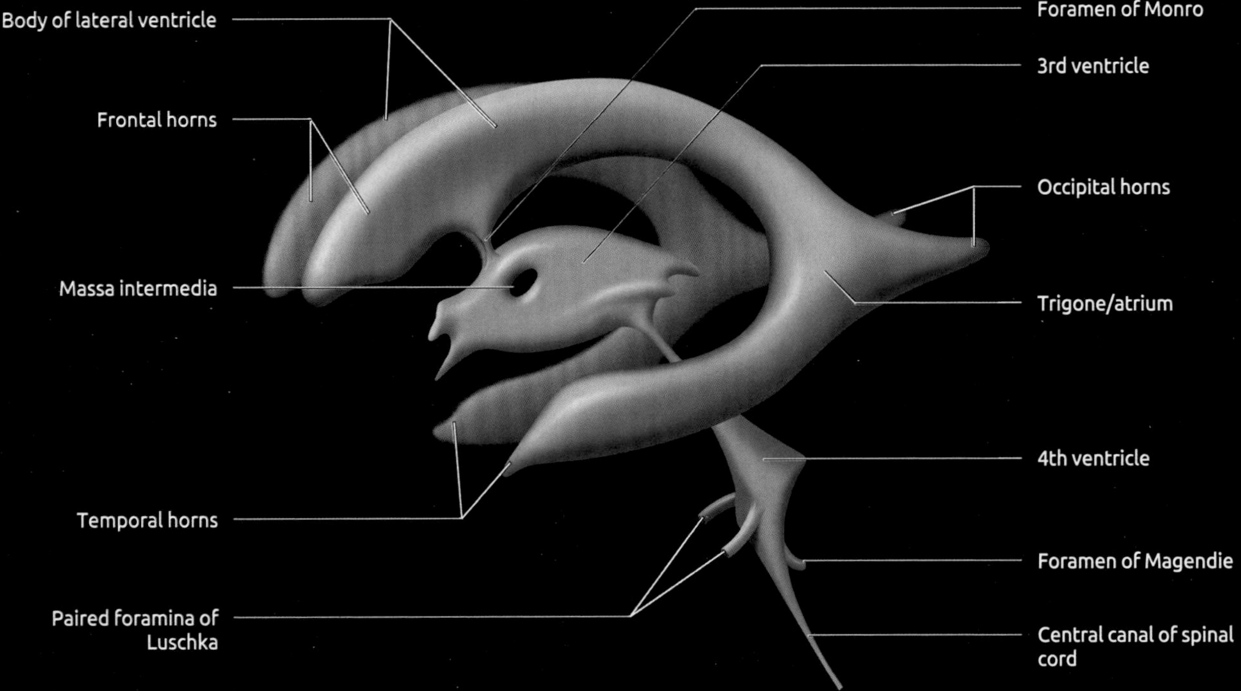

Schematic 3D representation of the ventricular system, viewed from the side, demonstrates the normal appearance and communicating pathways of the cerebral ventricles. Cerebral spinal fluid (CSF) flows from the lateral ventricles through the foramen of Monro into the 3rd ventricle and from there through the cerebral aqueduct into the 4th ventricle. CSF exits the 4th ventricle through the foramina of Luschka and Magendie to the subarachnoid space. There are 4 small recesses (2 anterior and 2 posterior) off the 3rd ventricle that are usually too small to be resolved on US.

STANDARD US PLANES VIA ANTERIOR FONTANELLE

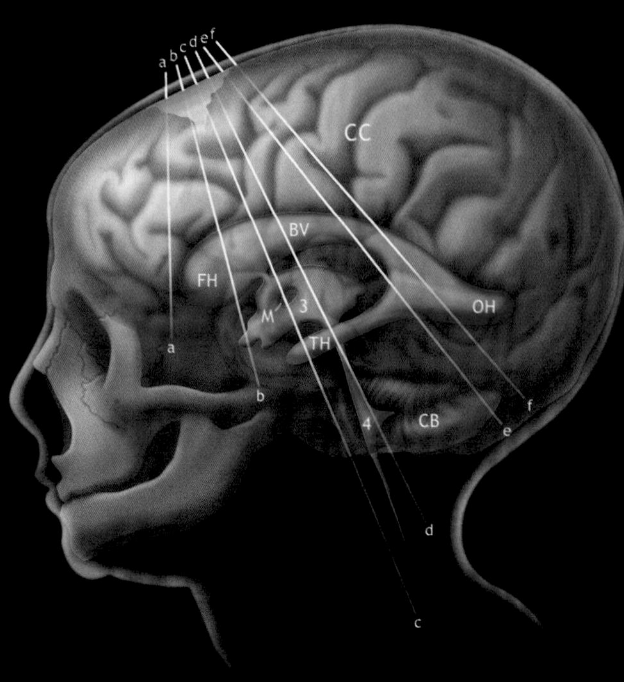

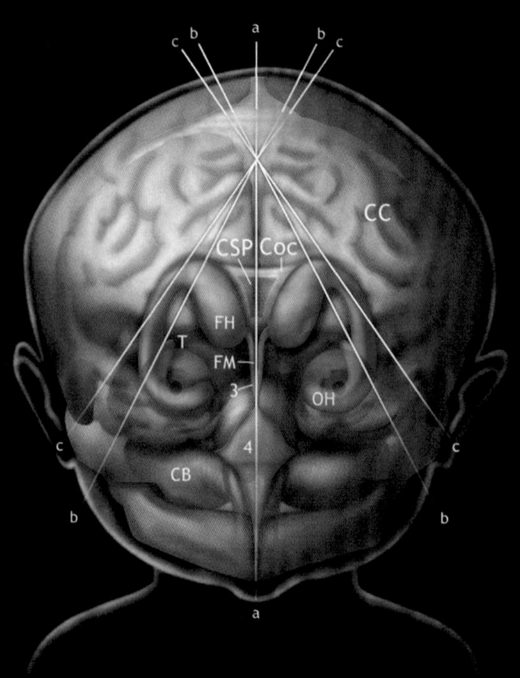

(Top) *Graphic shows the common coronal planes used in US brain scanning. The scan should include a complete sweep from front to back and side to side with still images as indicated [cerebral cortex (CC), body of lateral ventricle (BV), frontal horn (FH), occipital horn (OH), massa intermedia (M), 3rd ventricle (3), temporal horn (TH), 4th ventricle (4), cerebellum (CB)].* **(Bottom)** *Graphic shows the common sagittal planes used in US brain scanning: Planes A-C from midline to lateral [cerebellum (CB), cerebral cortex (CC), corpus callosum (Coc), cavum septi pellucidi (CSP), frontal horn (FH), foramen of Monro (FM), occipital horn (OH), temporal horn (T), 3rd ventricle (3), 4th ventricle (4)].*

CORONAL US VIA ANTERIOR FONTANELLE

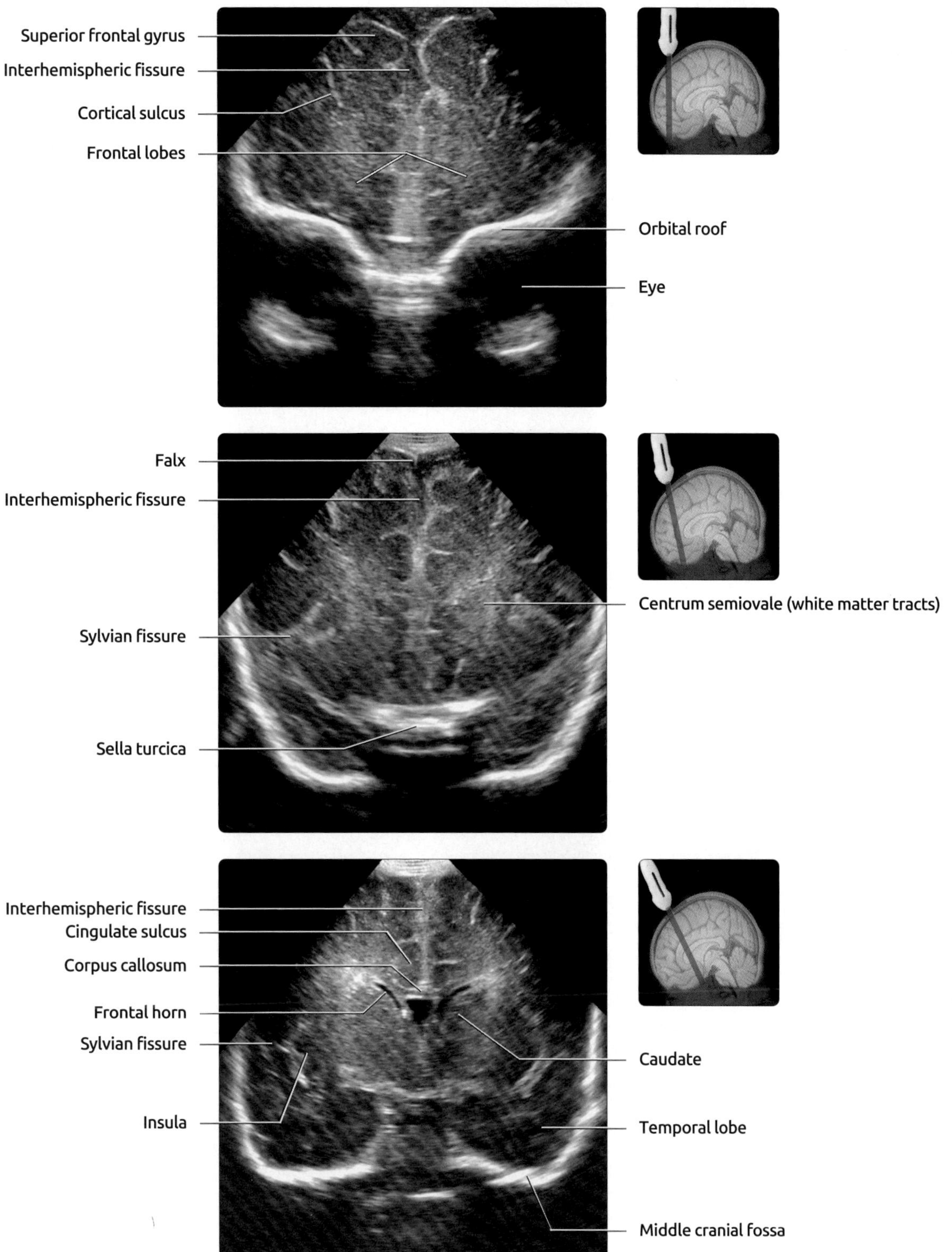

(Top) *The 1st of 9 coronal US of the brain through the anterior fontanelle in a term infant shows the frontal lobes lie in the anterior cranial fossa with orbital cavities deep to the floor of the skull base. The sulci are echogenic, and the gyri are hypoechoic. CSF is seen in the interhemispheric fissure.* **(Middle)** *US centered more posteriorly demonstrates a slightly more echogenic white matter region of the brain parenchyma known as the centrum semiovale. Parts of the skull base, including the sella turcica where the pituitary gland is located, can be seen.* **(Bottom)** *US acquired just anterior to the foramen of Monro is shown. The frontal horns of lateral ventricles are now seen. No choroid plexus should be present in the frontal horns. Any intraventricular echogenic material seen at this level should raise the suspicion of blood clot. The head of the caudate nucleus is inferior and lateral to the respective frontal horn.*

CORONAL US VIA ANTERIOR FONTANELLE

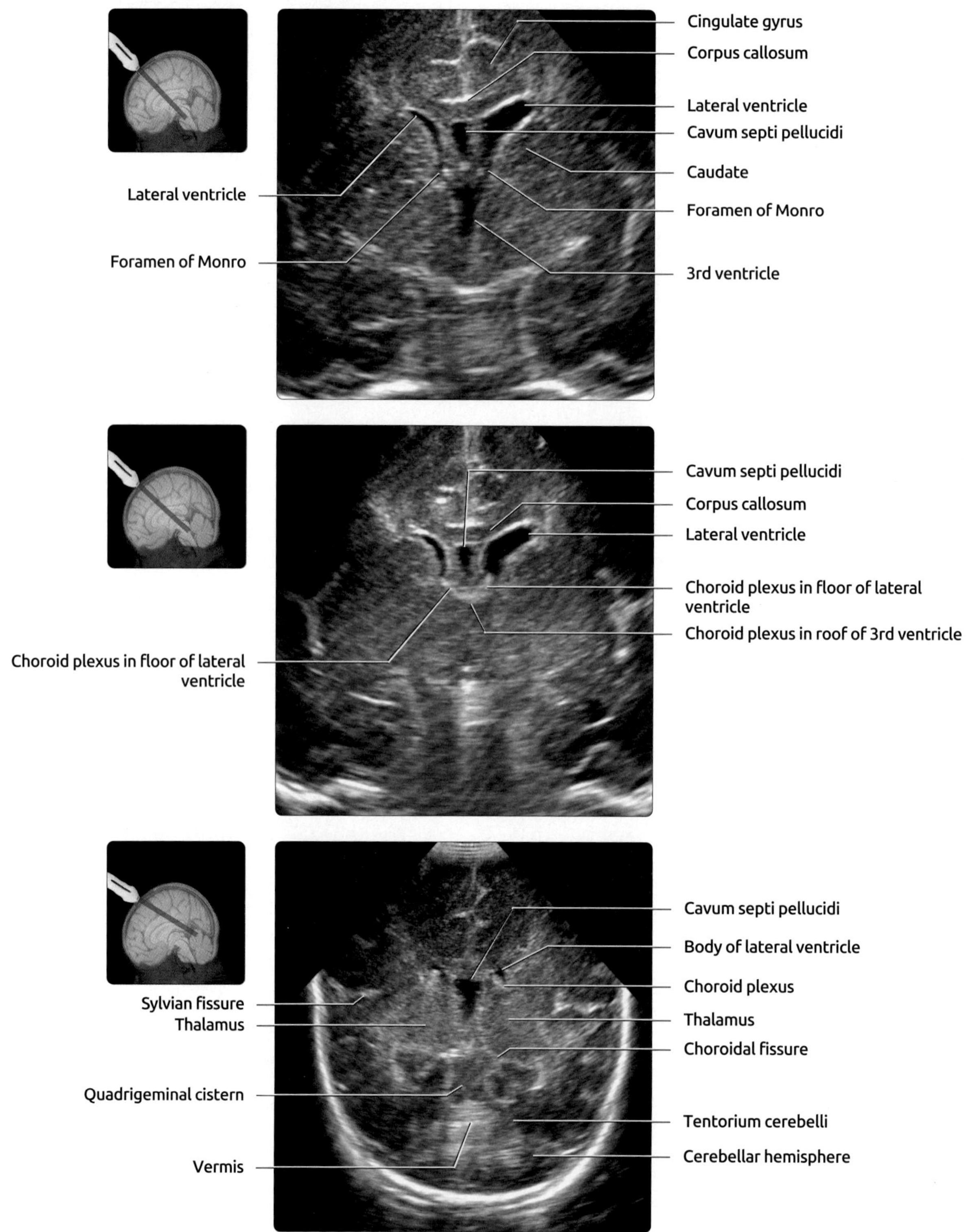

(Top) *US is taken at the level of the foramina of Monro, which connects the lateral ventricles to the 3rd ventricle, forming a Y shape. The caudate nucleus is slightly hypoechoic and located along the lateral inferior margin of the lateral ventricle. Some asymmetry, as seen here, is normal.* **(Middle)** *Just slightly more posterior, the choroid plexus is seen in the lateral and 3rd ventricles. They create 3 echogenic foci, 1 on the roof of the 3rd ventricle and 2 located bilaterally on the floor of the lateral ventricles, and are known as the 3-dot sign.* **(Bottom)** *A more posterior coronal US shows the thalami on either side of the midline. The quadrigeminal cistern forms a star-shaped CSF structure just above the vermis in this view.*

CORONAL US VIA ANTERIOR FONTANELLE

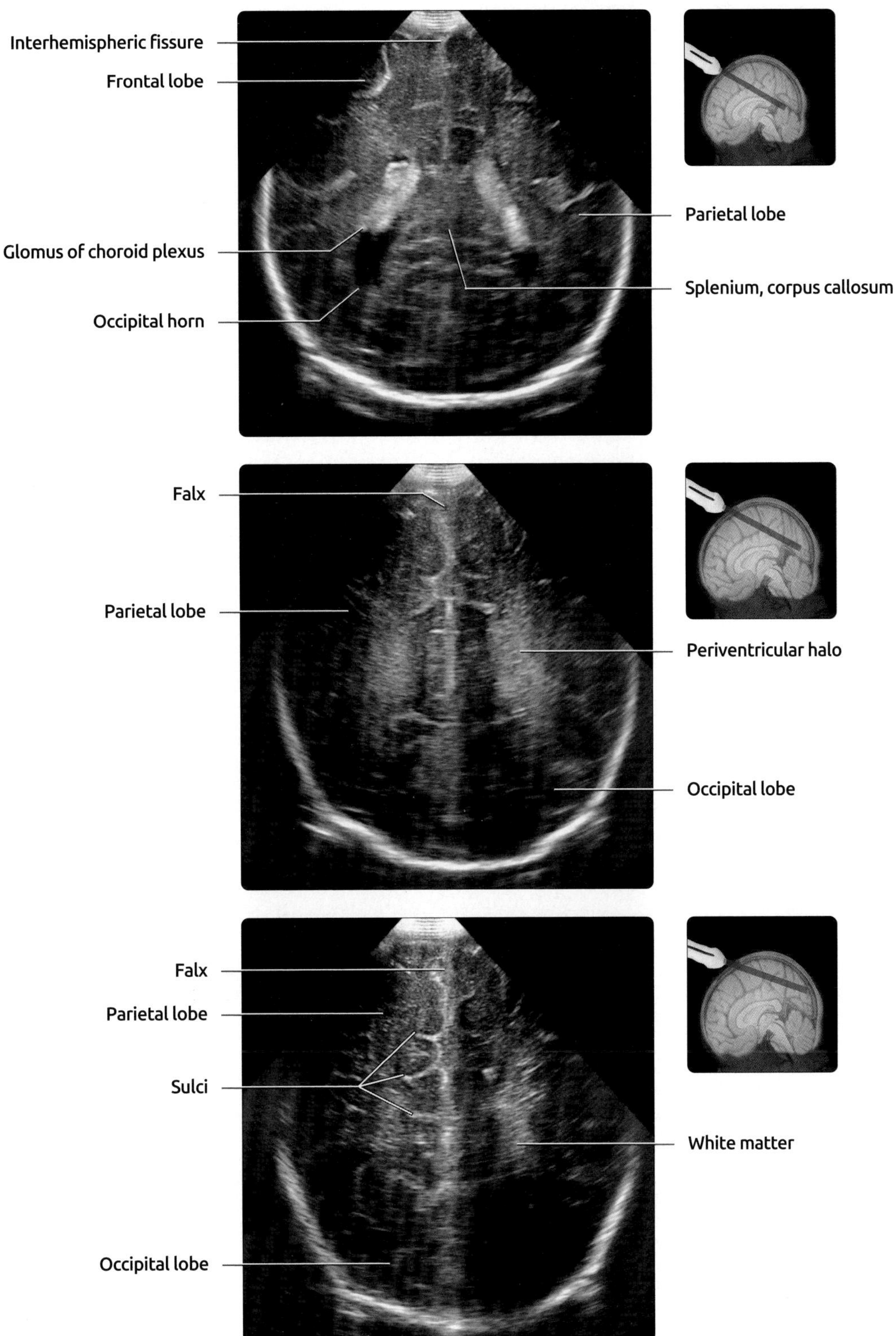

(Top) *US is taken at the trigone of the lateral ventricles. The glomus of the choroid plexus appears highly echogenic, nearly occupying the whole trigone. The splenium, the most posterior portion of the corpus callosum, is seen crossing the midline and connecting the 2 cerebral hemispheres.* **(Middle)** *US, slightly posterior to the trigone, shows mildly echogenic white matter regions lateral and parallel to both trigones of the lateral ventricles. These regions are known as the periventricular halo, a normal finding, present in almost all normal mature and premature neonates. The echogenicity of the halo should be less than that of the choroid plexus and symmetrical in appearance.* **(Bottom)** *The most posterior coronal US shows the cortex of the occipital lobe with multiple echogenic sulci extending medially from the lateral margin of the brain. The falx is in midline.*

SAGITTAL US VIA ANTERIOR FONTANELLE

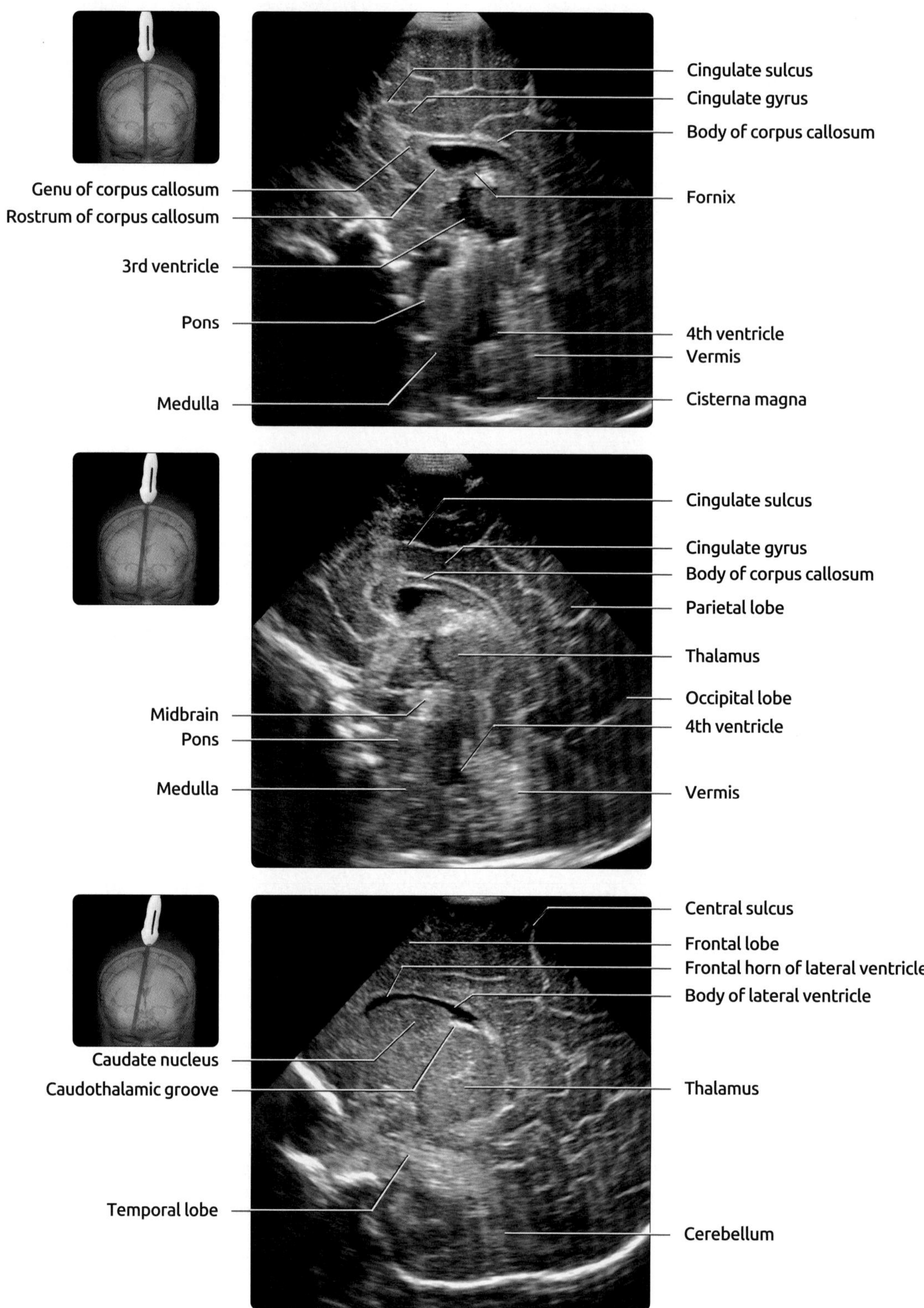

(Top) *The 1st of 6 sagittal US of the brain through the anterior fontanelle in a term infant is shown. This US, obtained in the midline, shows the corpus callosum as a hypoechoic, curving line. The cingulate gyrus is above and parallels the corpus callosum. The midline also allows evaluation of the posterior fossa structures, including the brainstem anteriorly and the vermis posteriorly. The 4th ventricle is well seen in this plane and appears as a triangular, CSF-filled structure at the level of the midvermis.* **(Middle)** *Slightly lateral to midline, the thalamus is more clearly seen.* **(Bottom)** *Parasagittal US obtained by angling more laterally shows the caudothalamic groove, the junction between the caudate nucleus and the thalamus. This is the area of the vascular germinal matrix, which is vulnerable to hemorrhage in preterm infants. This is a very important image to obtain when performing an exam.*

SAGITTAL US VIA ANTERIOR FONTANELLE

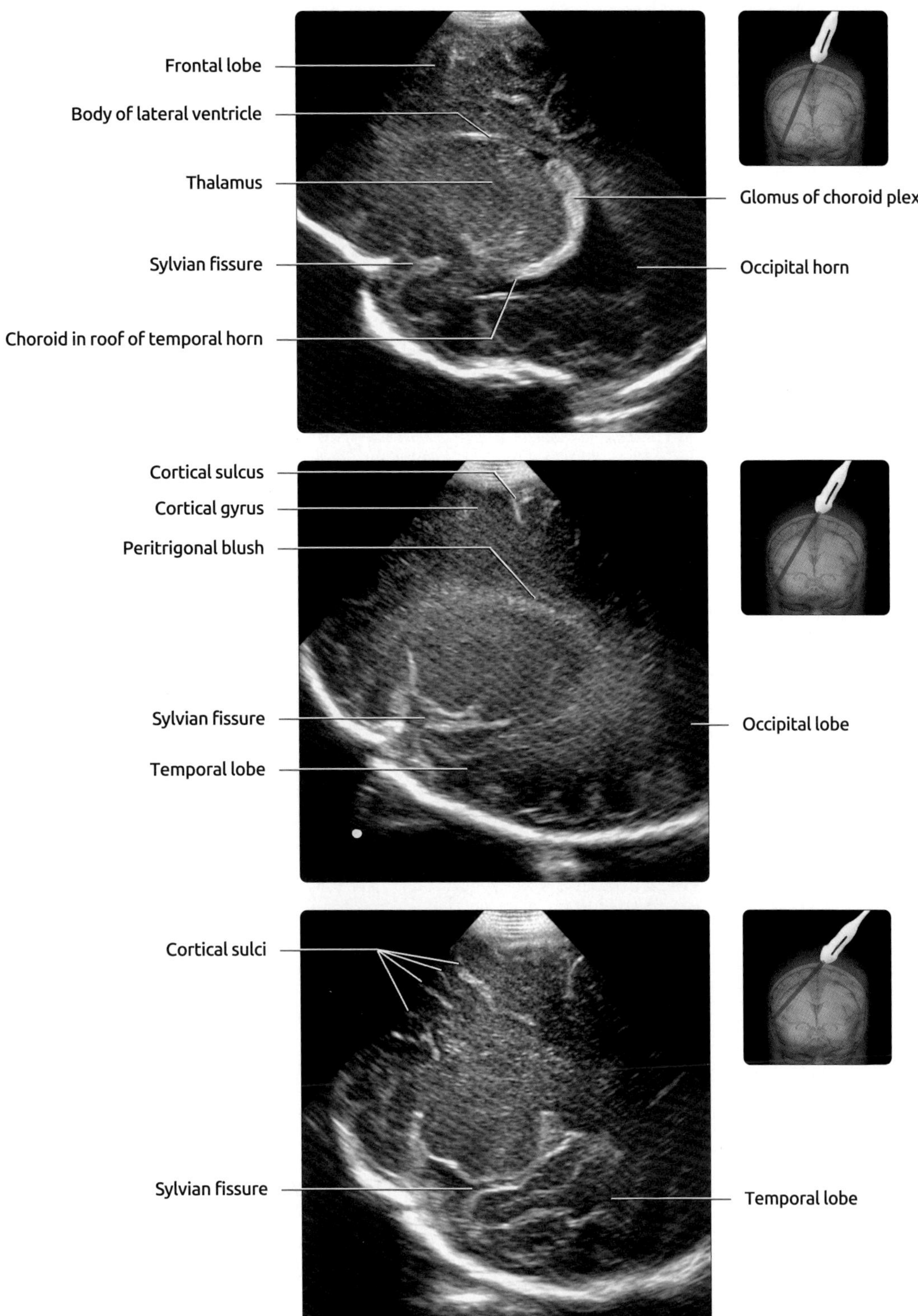

(Top) *Parasagittal US shows the glomus of the choroid plexus in the trigone. The glomus tapers anteriorly as it courses along the floor of the lateral ventricle to the foramen of Monro and continues along the roof of the 3rd ventricle. It also tapers posteriorly from the trigone into the roof of the temporal horn of each lateral ventricle. Glomus may appear bulbous and irregular at the trigone and should not be mistaken as a blood clot.* **(Middle)** *Parasagittal US is obtained just lateral to the lateral ventricle. The echogenic white matter of the brain just posterior and superior to the ventricular trigone is known as the peritrigonal blush or halo, representing radiating white fiber tracts (corona radiata). The peritrigonal blush is more prominent in premature than in term neonates.* **(Bottom)** *This is the last and most lateral sagittal US, showing the mature sulcal pattern with hyperechoic sulci and hypoechoic gyri.*

PREMATURE INFANT (23 WEEKS 6 DAYS)

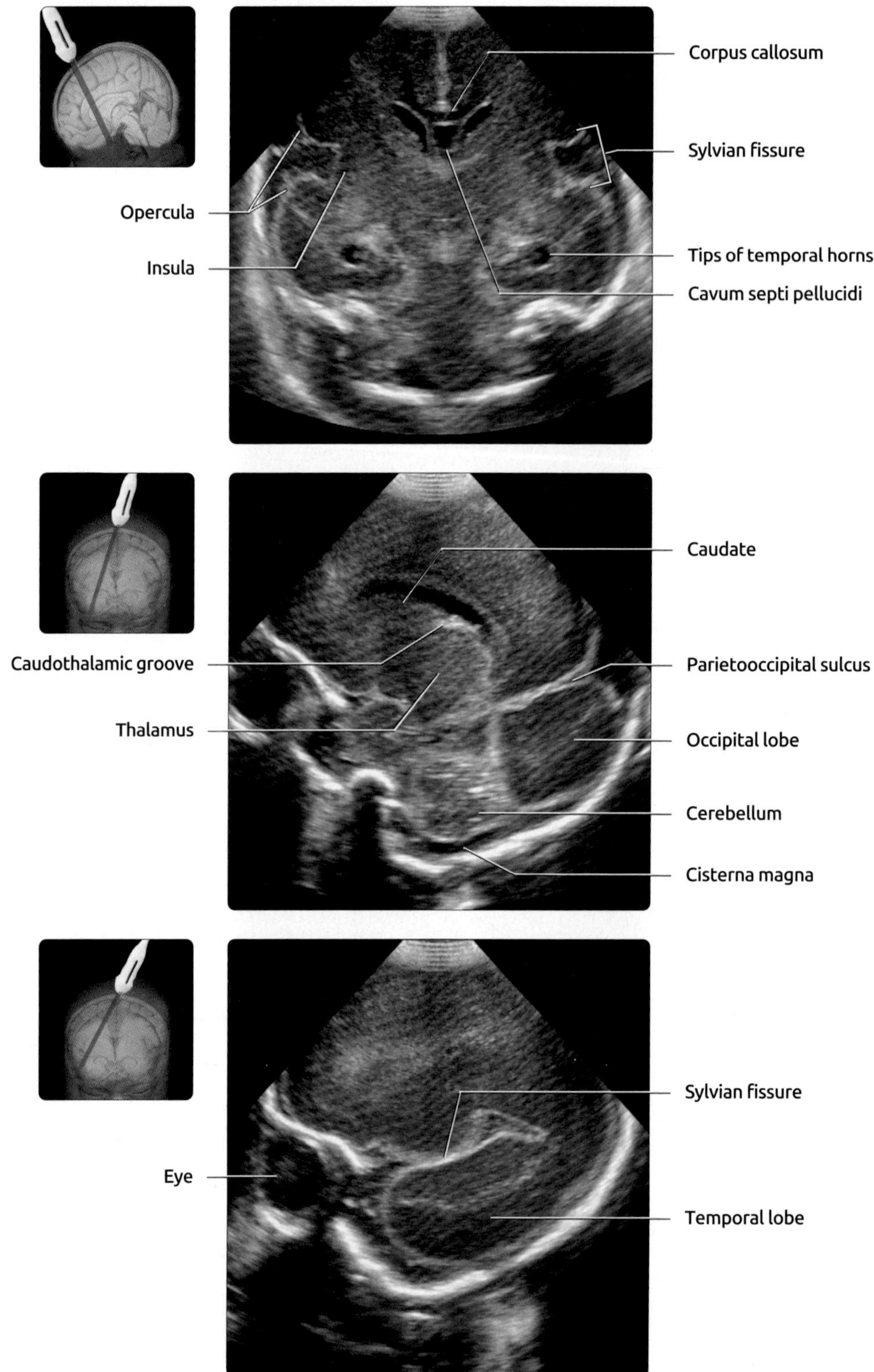

(Top) *Coronal US of a very premature infant, born at 23-weeks and 6-days gestational age, shows a very large, square, open sylvian fissure. The opercula of the frontal and temporal lobes have not yet grown to cover the insula.* **(Middle)** *Sagittal US through the caudothalamic groove in the same case shows the parietooccipital sulcus. The cortex otherwise appears "flat."* **(Bottom)** *Another sagittal US further lateral shows similar findings with no cortical gyri/sulci seen. This is normal for the gestational age at birth.*

SYLVIAN FISSURE AT DIFFERENT AGES

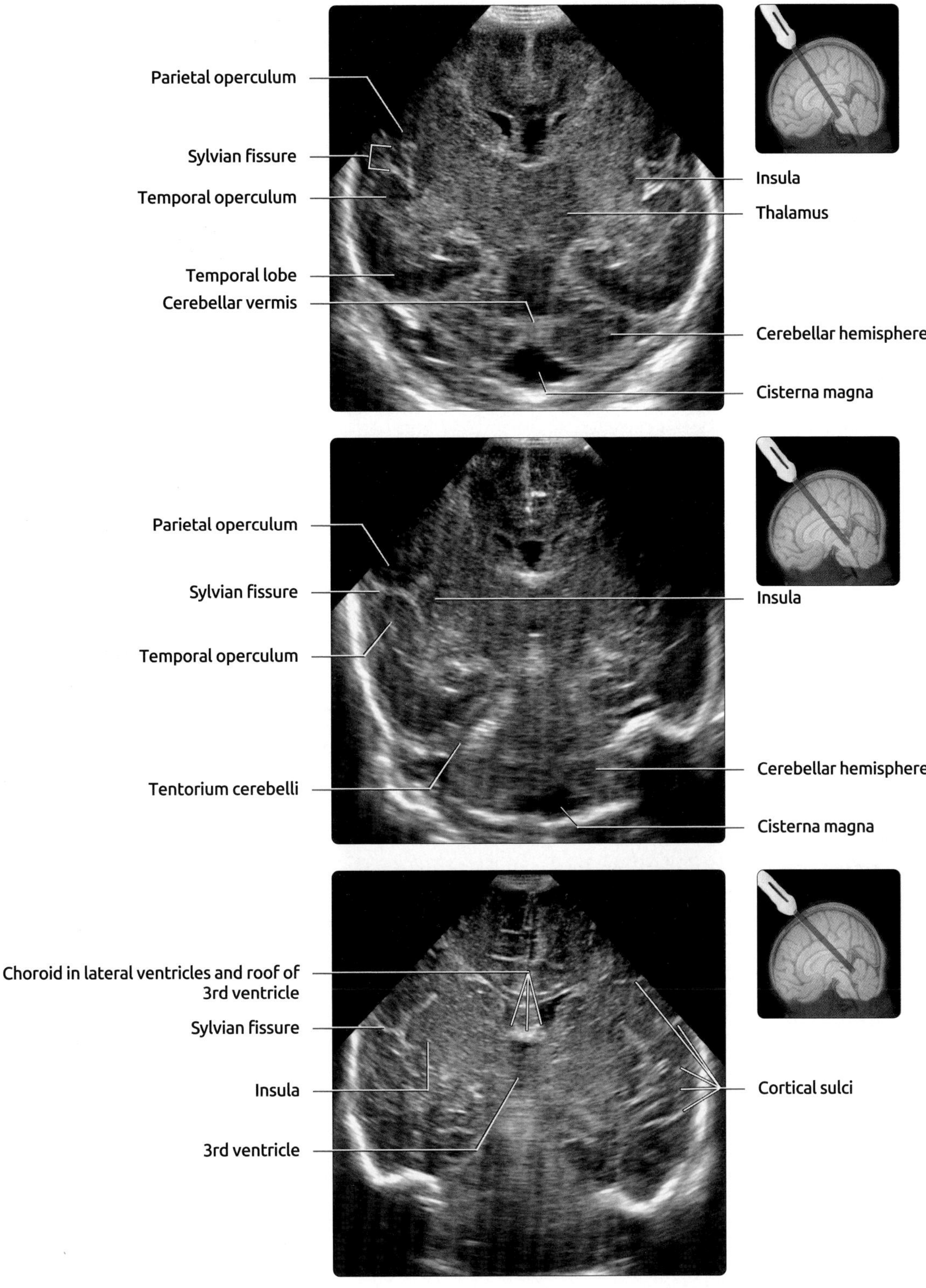

(Top) *An infant born at 29 weeks and 1 day shows more advanced development of the sylvian fissures. The frontal, temporal, and parietal lobes all have opercula, which are beginning to cover the insula.* **(Middle)** *At 31 weeks and 6 days, the opercula have grown to cover the insula, and the sylvian fissure appears closed.* **(Bottom)** *Another coronal US through the level of the sylvian fissure in a full-term infant shows multiple gyri and sulci over the convexities of the brain. It is important to understand the developmental anatomic changes; lack of cortical sulci may be normal for preterm infants, depending on the gestational age at delivery but is very abnormal at term.*

SAGITTAL US VIA POSTERIOR FONTANELLE

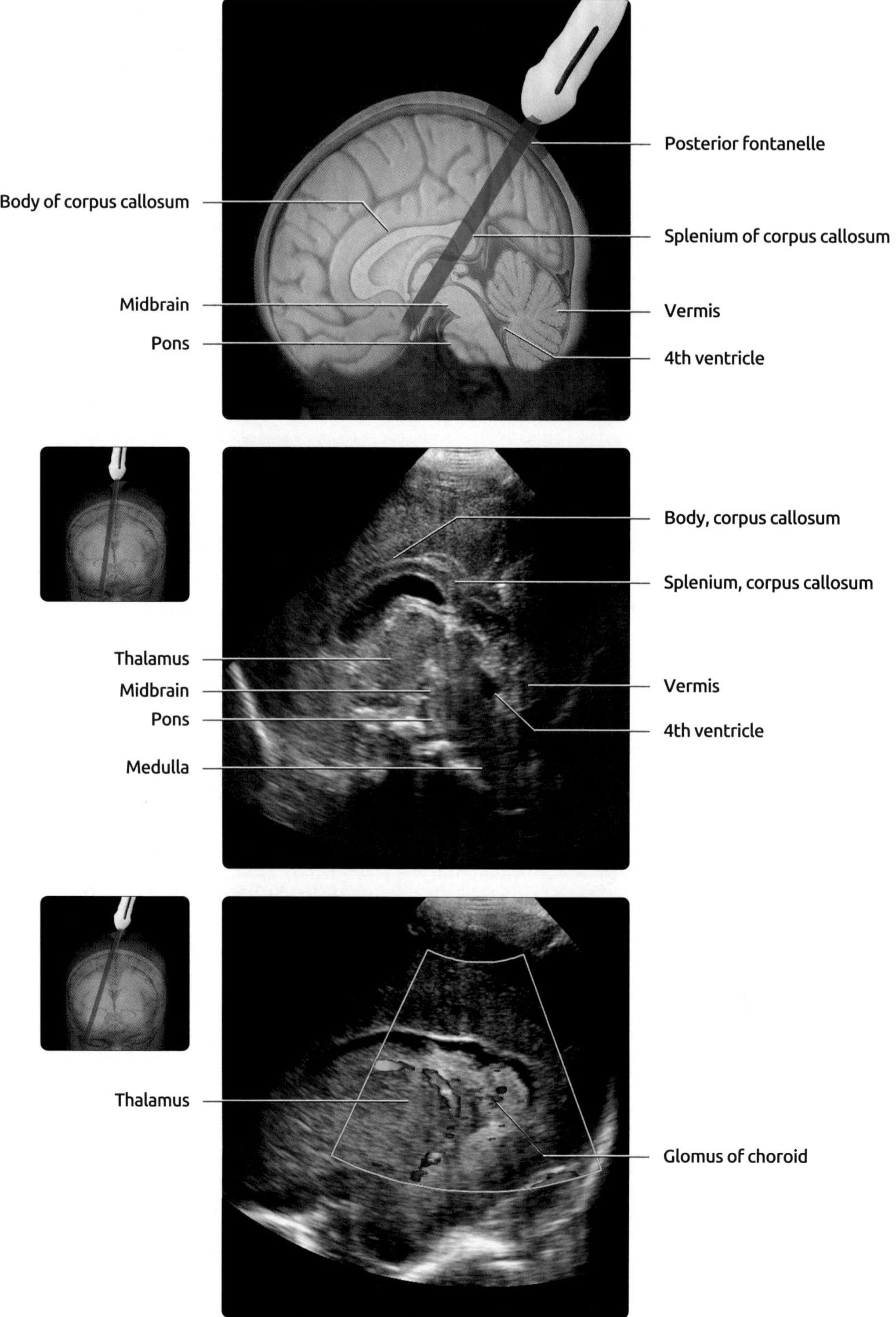

(Top) *Although routine scanning is performed via the anterior fontanelle, the posterior fontanelle is another alternative, particularly when it is difficult seeing more posterior structures in the brain.* **(Middle)** *Scan through the posterior fontanelle in a 26-week premature infant was performed to better evaluate the corpus callosum. The splenium is particularly well seen in this view.* **(Bottom)** *Color Doppler US shows flow within the choroid plexus at the glomus (thickening of choroid at in the trigone). The posterior fontanelle view can be helpful to differentiate bulky choroid from clot. The occipital horn does not contain choroid plexus, and any echogenic material in the occipital horn should raise the suspicion of intraventricular hemorrhage.*

AXIAL US THROUGH TEMPORAL BONE

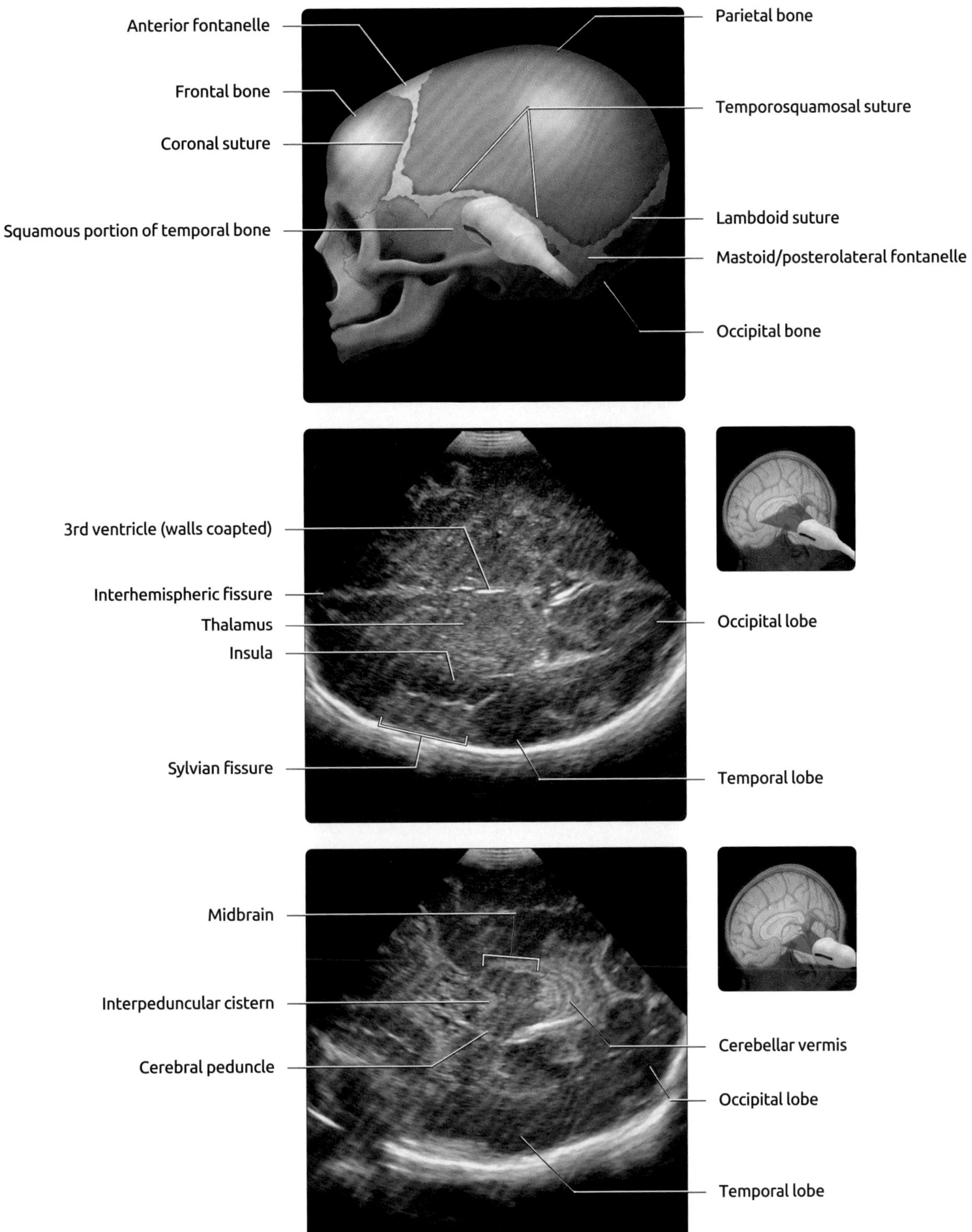

(Top) *Graphic of the transtemporal acoustic window is shown. The transducer is placed more anterior and superior than the mastoid fontanelle approach. The temporal bone anterior to the ear is thin enough to allow imaging of the brainstem even after closure of the temporosquamosal suture. This acoustic window allows the best assessment of cerebral peduncles and the 3rd ventricle.* **(Middle)** *Transtemporal axial scan in a 29-week premature infant shows intracranial anatomy in a plane similar to CT or MR.* **(Bottom)** *A plane slightly lower gives excellent axial views of the midbrain and upper vermis.*

CEREBELLUM AND POSTERIOR FOSSA

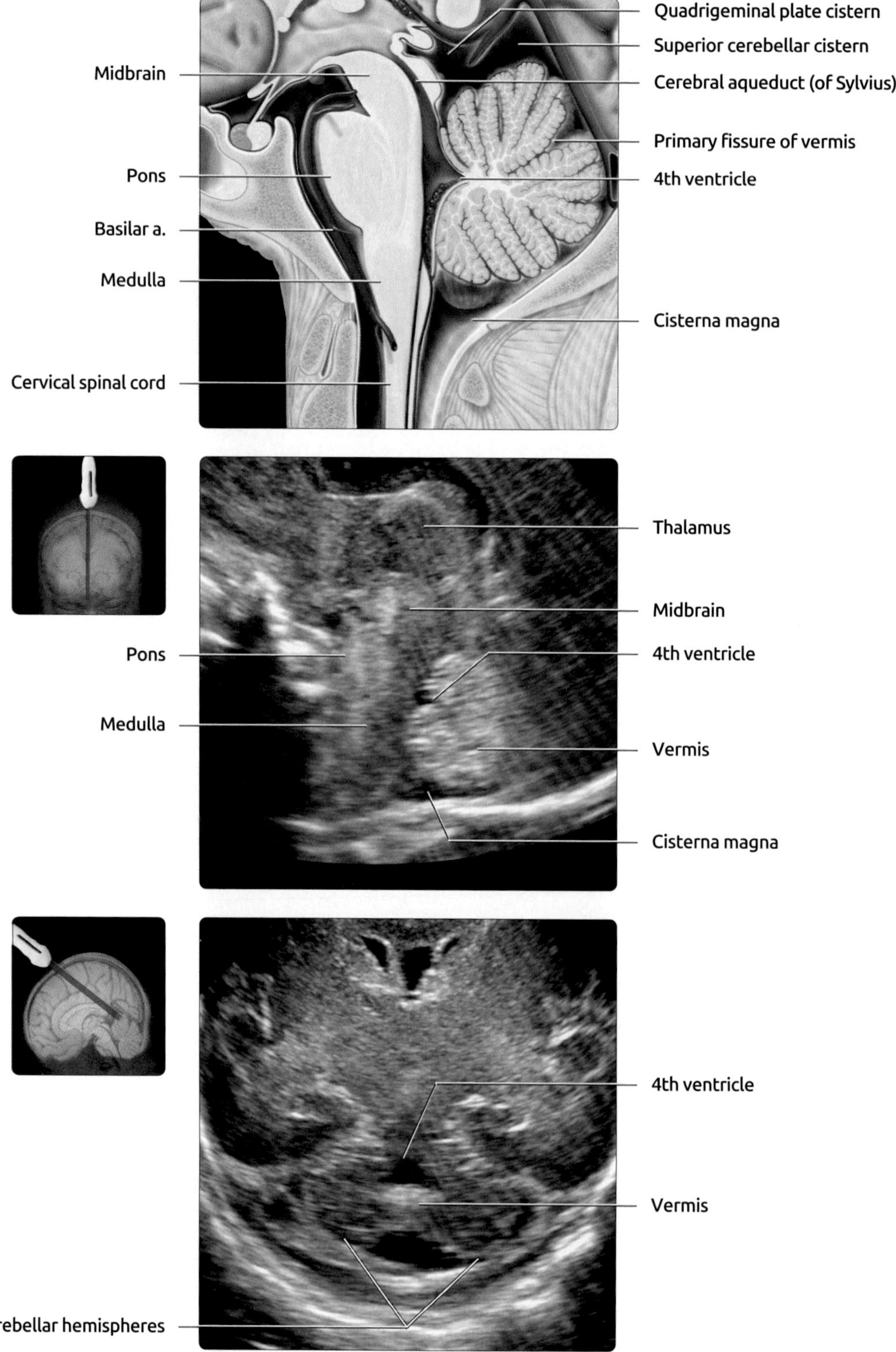

(Top) *Sagittal midline graphic of the posterior fossa shows the brainstem and vermis separated by the 4th ventricle. The brainstem consists of midbrain, pons, and medulla. The vermis has multiple fissures dividing it into lobules. CSF is seen above the vermis in the quadrigeminal plate and superior cerebellar cisterns and below in the cisterna magna.* **(Middle)** *This midline sagittal view of a premature infant, born at 29 weeks and 1 day, shows the brainstem. The pons is easily identified by its anterior bulge.* **(Bottom)** *Coronal US through the anterior fontanelle in the same infant shows symmetric cerebellar hemispheres. The vermis is midline, covers the 4th ventricle, and is more echogenic than the rest of the cerebellum.*

POSTERIOR FOSSA VIA MASTOID APPROACH

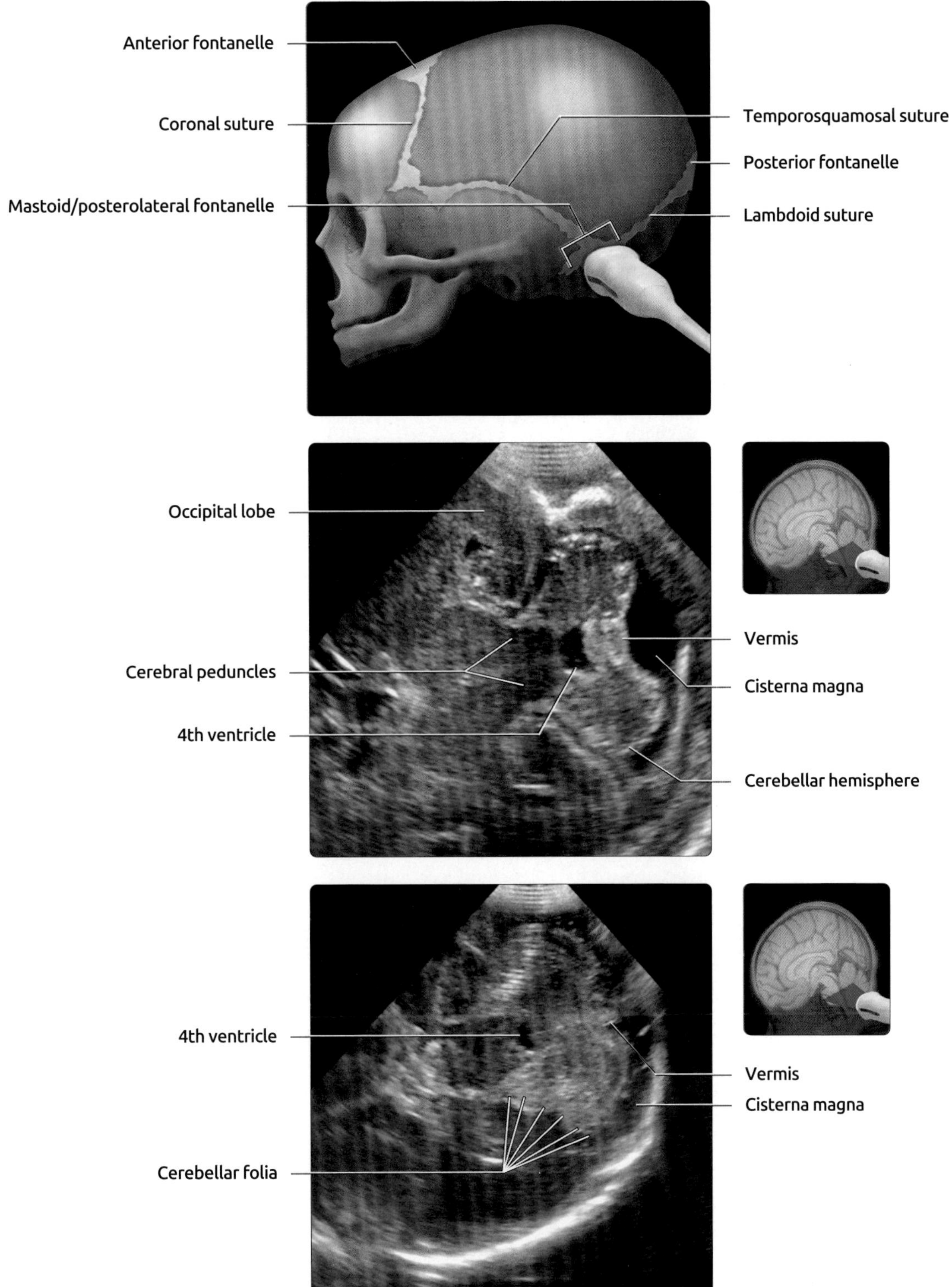

(Top) *The mastoid/posterolateral fontanelle is located at the junction of temporosquamosal and lambdoid sutures. It allows assessment of brainstem and posterior fossa structures, which are not well demonstrated in the standard planes through the anterior fontanelle. The transducer is placed ~ 1 cm behind the helix of ear and 1 cm above the tragus. This acoustic window allows the best visualization of the 4th ventricle, posterior cerebellar vermis, cerebellar hemispheres, and cisterna magna.* **(Middle)** *The mastoid approach allows for detailed evaluation of the posterior fossa structures. This is a premature infant (27 weeks and 5 days), which is evident by the lack of cortical gyri and cerebellar folia.* **(Bottom)** *Another mastoid view in an infant born at 37 weeks shows more advanced maturation with extensive folia on the surface of the cerebellum.*

CAVUM SEPTI PELLUCIDI ET VERGAE

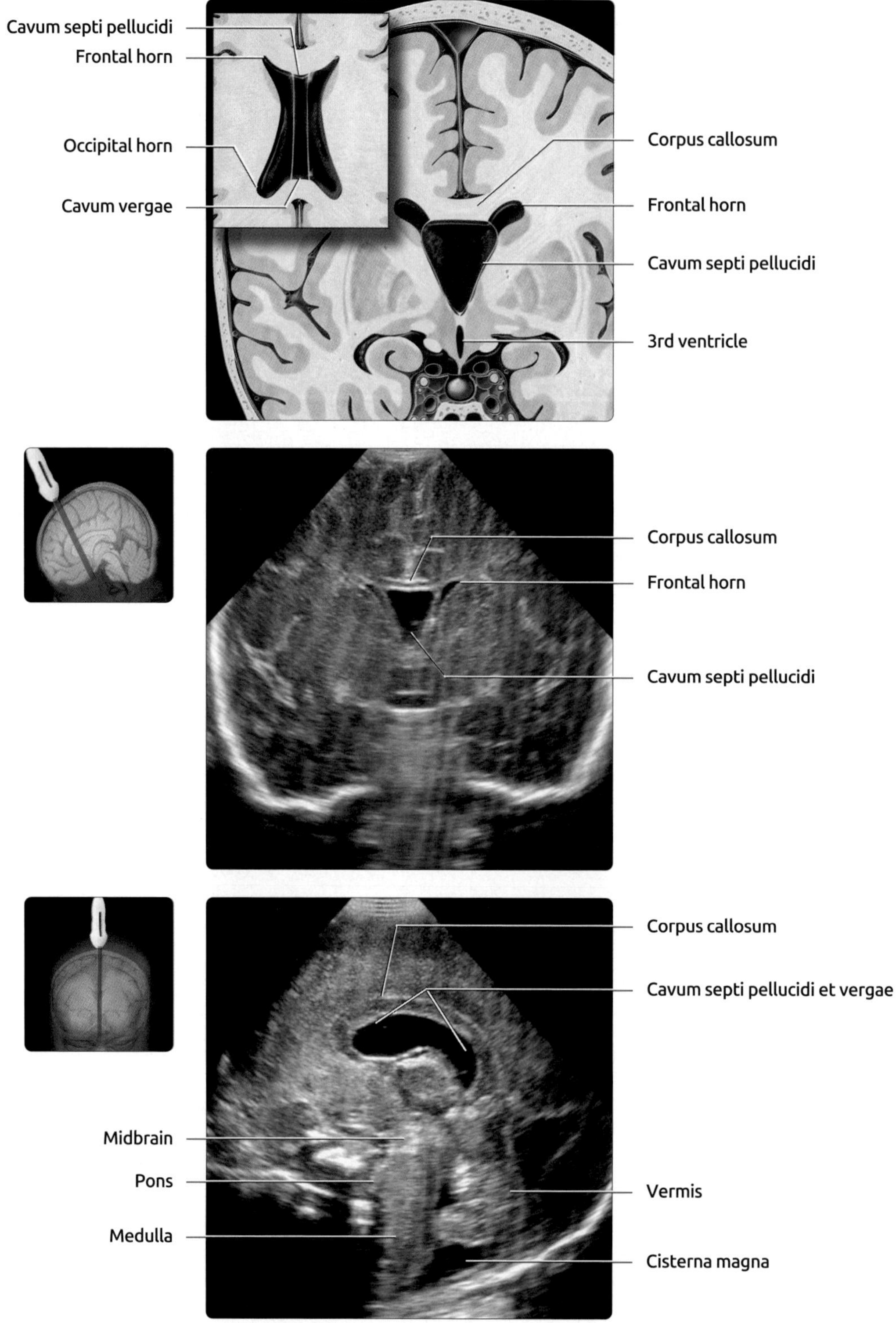

(Top) *Coronal graphic with an axial insert shows a classic cavum septi pellucidi with a posterior extension, the cavum vergae. It creates a finger-like CSF collection between the lateral ventricles.* **(Middle)** *The cavum septi pellucidi can be quite large, especially in premature infants, and should not be confused with an elevated 3rd ventricle or intracranial cyst.* **(Bottom)** *Midline sagittal US in this 27-week premature infant shows a cavum septi pellucidi continuing posteriorly into the cavum vergae. This is a common finding in premature infants. The cavum vergae is closed in 97% of full-term infants, and the cavum septi pellucidi is closed in 85% of infants by 3-6 months of age, becoming the septum pellucidum; however, it can remain open until adulthood.*

CAVUM VELUM INTERPOSITUM

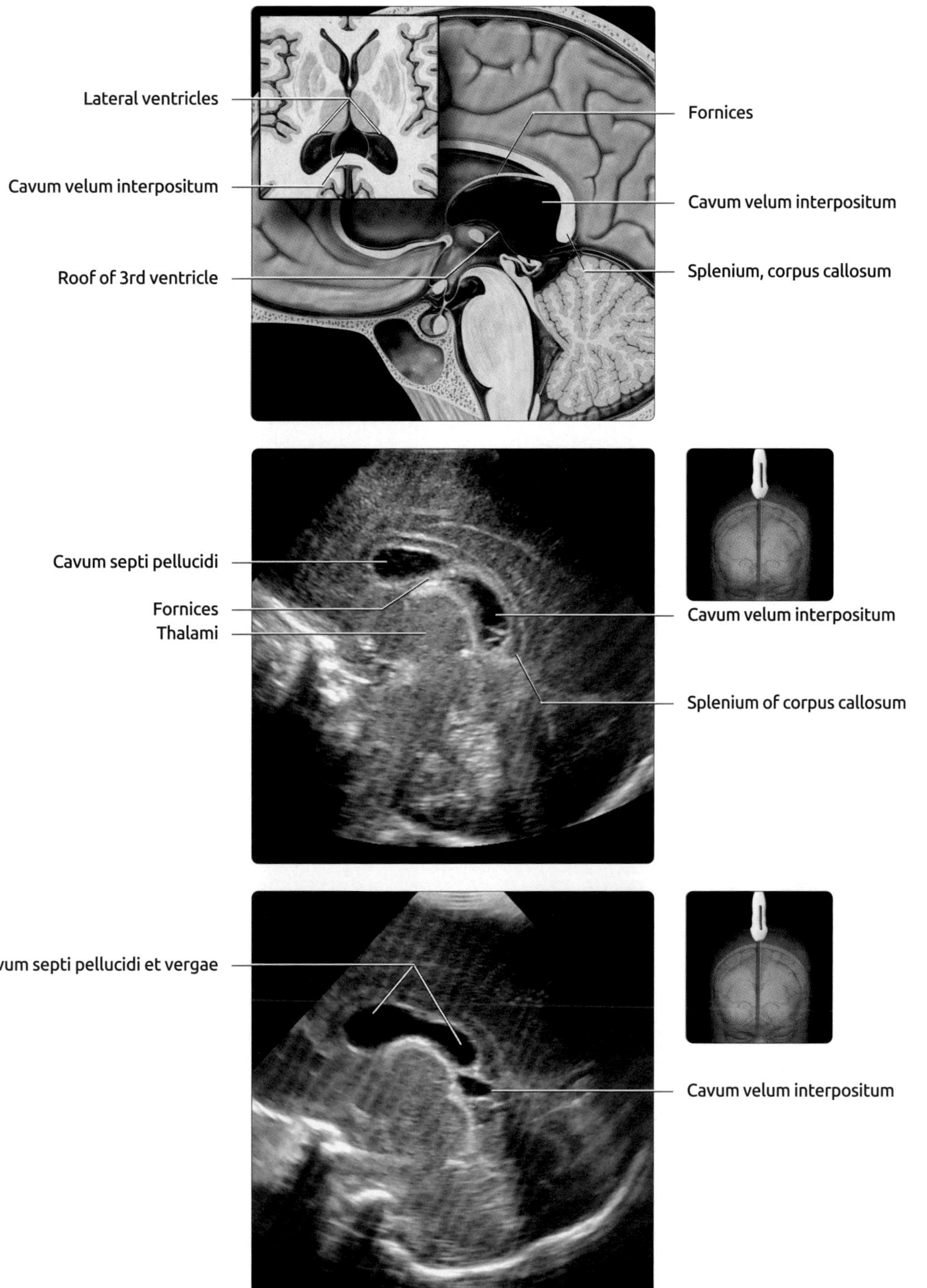

(Top) *Sagittal graphic with an axial insert shows a cavum velum interpositum. It is inferior to the fornices, superior to the 3rd ventricle, and anterior to the splenium of the corpus callosum. In the axial plane (insert), it appears as a cyst between the more posterior portion of the lateral ventricles.* **(Middle)** *Midline sagittal US shows a mildly complex cavum velum interpositum.* **(Bottom)** *This premature infant has a cavum septi pellucidi, vergae, and interpositum. Like a cavum septi pellucidi and vergae, a cavum velum interpositum is more common in premature infants.*

VASCULAR ANATOMY

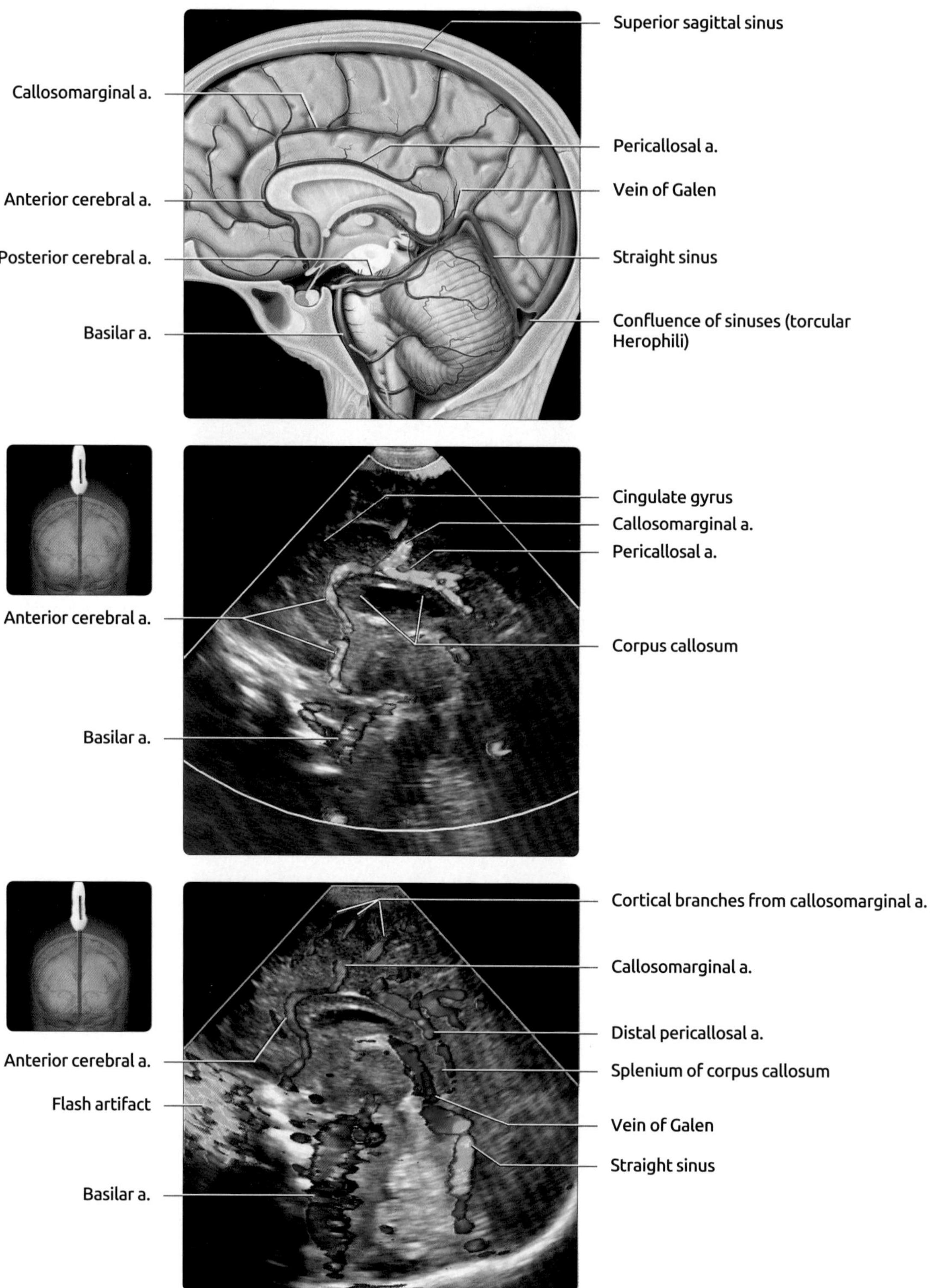

(Top) *Graphic shows the arteries, veins, and sinuses, many of which can be seen seen on a routine midline sagittal view. The anterior cerebral artery and its 2 main branches, the pericallosal and callosomarginal arteries, are easily seen on midline color Doppler US. The basilar artery is also easily identified, running anterior to the brainstem. The middle cerebral and posterior cerebral arteries are better evaluated in an axial plane using a transtemporal or mastoid approach.* **(Middle)** *Midline sagittal color Doppler US, obtained via the anterior fontanelle, shows the pericallosal artery running just above the corpus callosum. In a normal newborn, the pericallosal artery should be close to the surface of the corpus callosum. While in callosal agenesis, this artery takes an upward oblique direction.* **(Bottom)** *The vein of Galen can be seen beneath the splenium of the corpus callosum as it courses posteriorly to drain into the straight sinus.*

CIRCLE OF WILLIS

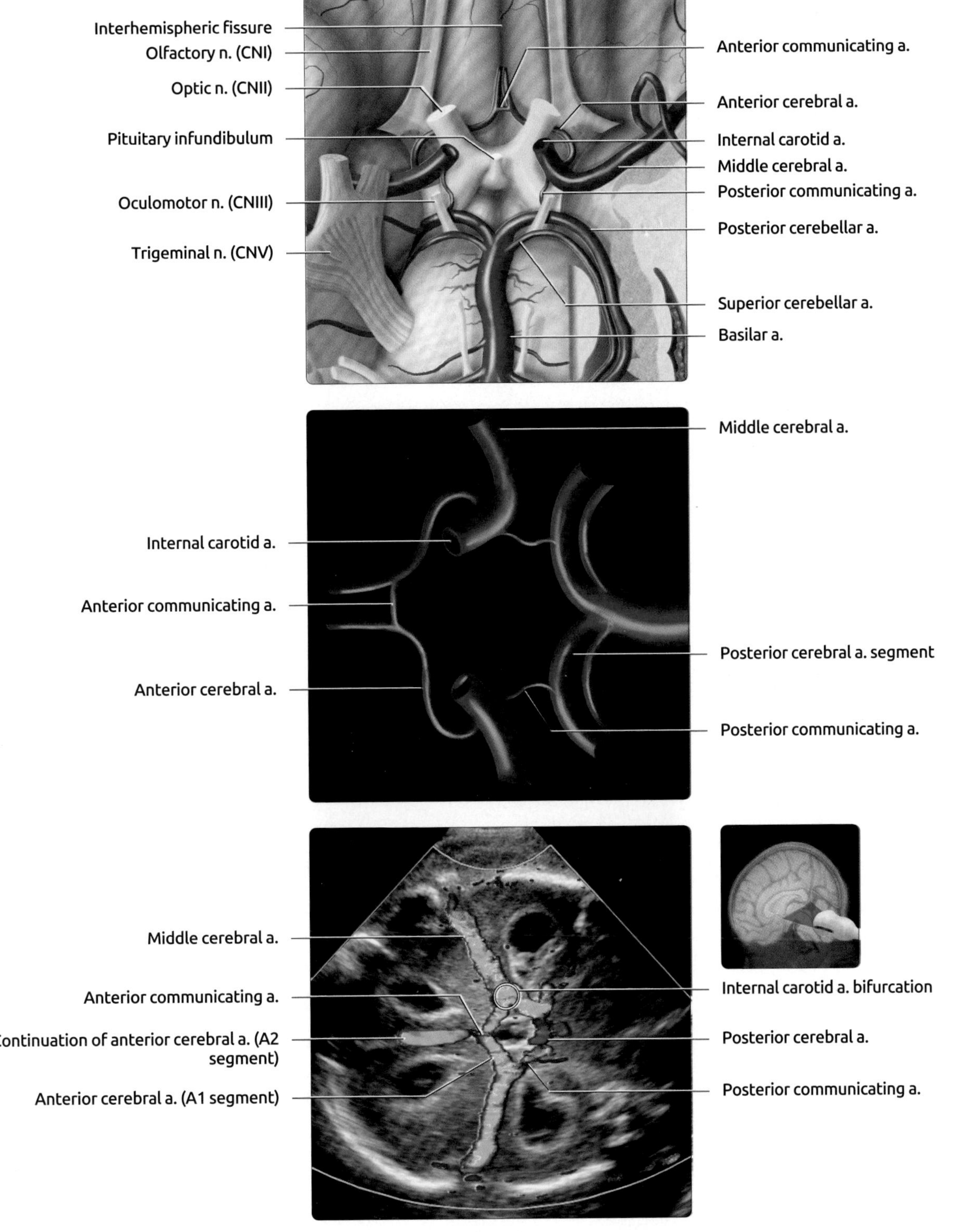

(Top) *The circle of Willis illustrated in situ shows its intricate relationship to adjacent structures. It is located in the suprasellar cistern; the pituitary infundibular stalk and optic chiasm lie in the middle of the circle, and it is surrounded by multiple cranial nerves.* **(Middle)** *The circle of Willis is shown in isolation and turned 90° counterclockwise to match the plane of the US.* **(Bottom)** *Transtemporal axial color Doppler US in a fetus with ventriculomegaly from an intracranial hemorrhage shows the circle of Willis. The anterior and middle cerebral arteries are the terminal branches of the internal carotid artery. The posterior cerebral artery is the terminal branch of the basilar artery. These 3 crucial arteries communicate via the anterior and posterior communicating arteries in a complete circle of Willis. The transtemporal approach provides the best window for evaluating the circle of Willis.*

CEREBRAL ARTERIES

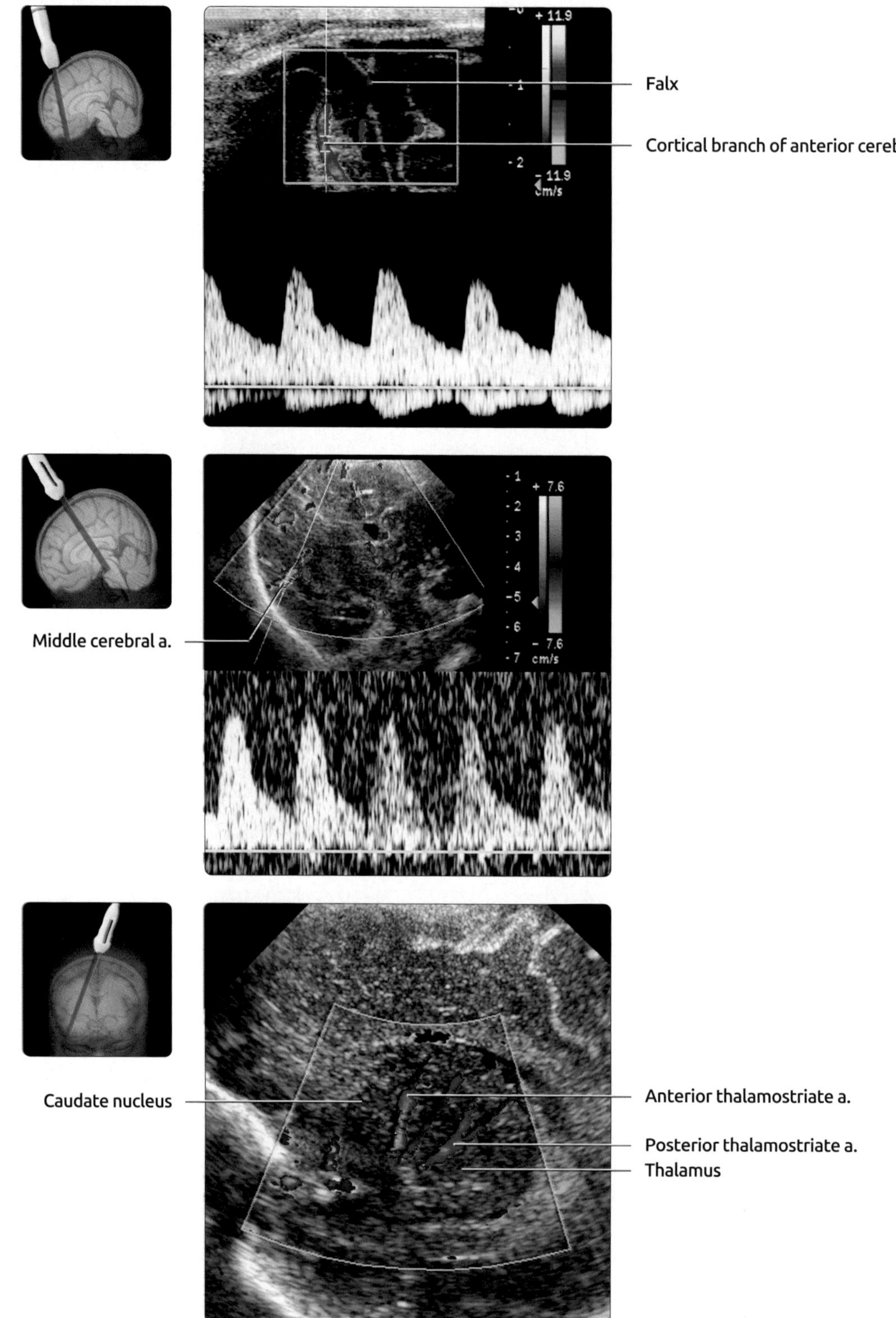

(Top) *Doppler waveform of a cortical branch of the anterior cerebral artery shows a low-resistance waveform with abundant diastolic flow.* **(Middle)** *Doppler waveform of the middle cerebral artery in the coronal plane is obtained by angling the beam laterally toward the sylvian fissure. A low-resistance arterial waveform is again noted.* **(Bottom)** *Color Doppler US obtained by a parasagittal scan through the anterior fontanelle shows the thalamostriate arteries. Anteriorly, the caudate nucleus is supplied by the anterior thalamostriate artery, while the thalamus posteriorly is supplied by the posterior thalamostriate artery. The thalamostriate arteries arise from the middle cerebral artery. Thalamostriate vasculopathy, also called lenticulostriate vasculopathy, can occur in infection (most commonly cytomegalovirus) and appear as hyperechoic linear or branching tubular structures.*

CEREBRAL VEINS AND SINUSES

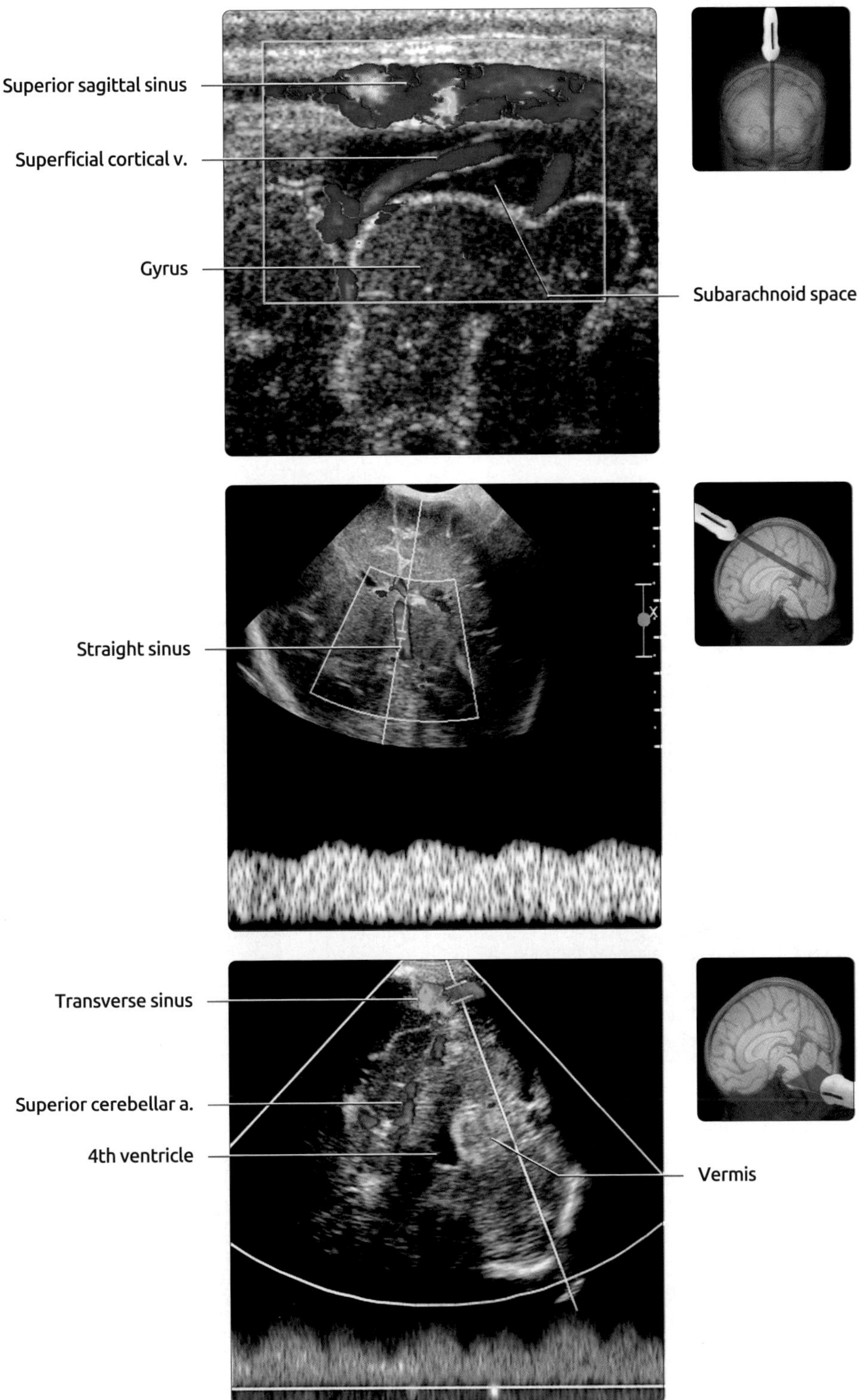

(Top) *Sagittal, high-frequency, linear, color Doppler US through the anterior fontanelle shows a superficial cortical vein traversing the subarachnoid space and draining into the superior sagittal sinus (SSS). The SSS appears as a curvilinear midline structure that hugs the inner cranial vault. It runs anterior to posterior between the falx and calvarium and drains the cortical veins. It joins with the straight and transverse sinuses at the confluence of sinus (torcular Herophili).* **(Middle)** *Doppler waveform of the straight sinus obtained by coronal scan through the anterior fontanelle is shown. The cerebral venous system is valveless, and pulsed Doppler waveforms typically show cardiac pulsations. There is wide fluctuation in venous flow velocity during forceful crying in infants.* **(Bottom)** *Other sinuses can be evaluated using different acoustic windows. The transverse sinus can be accessed via a mastoid fontanelle approach, as shown here.*

Germinal Matrix Hemorrhage

KEY FACTS

IMAGING

- Germinal matrix hemorrhage (GMH) most common at caudothalamic (CT) groove in vascular germinal matrix
- Grading system
  - **Grade 1**: GMH only with globular echogenic focus in CT groove
  - **Grade 2**: GMH + intraventricular hemorrhage (IVH), normal ventricle size
    - Look for fluid-debris levels in dependent occipital horns
  - **Grade 3**: GMH + IVH + ventricular expansion
    - Ventricular expansion some days after grade 2 IVH = secondary hydrocephalus
  - **Grade 4**: GMH + IVH + intraparenchymal hemorrhage
    - Venous compression leads to periventricular hemorrhagic venous infarction
    - Fan-shaped, echogenic, can liquefy, infarcted brain may be replaced by porencephalic cyst

TOP DIFFERENTIAL DIAGNOSES

- Hypoxic-ischemic encephalopathy: Ischemic injury due to perinatal insult
  - Abnormal echogenicity of affected deep gray &/or white matter
  - Heals as periventricular leukomalacia with Swiss cheese pattern in deep white matter

SCANNING TIPS

- Use small-footprint, high-frequency transducers with multiple focal zones
- Use multiple points of access (anterior/posterior fontanel, mastoid, temporal bone)
  - Look for fluid levels, blood in 3rd, 4th ventricles, cerebellar hemorrhage
  - Any grade of GMH has worse prognosis in setting of coexistent cerebellar hemorrhage
- Cine clips, color Doppler help differentiate avascular, variable-echogenicity clot from echogenic choroid

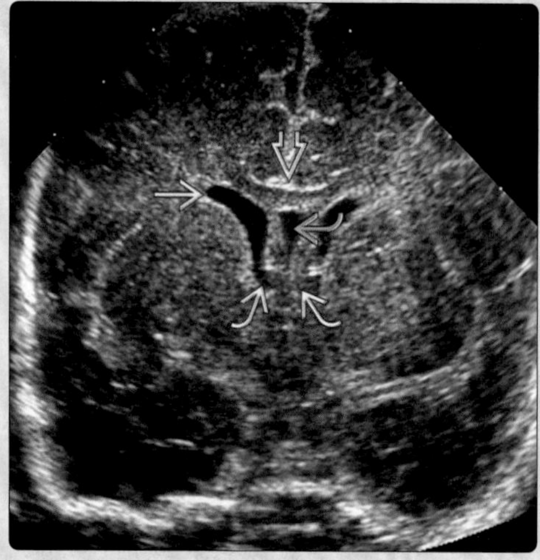

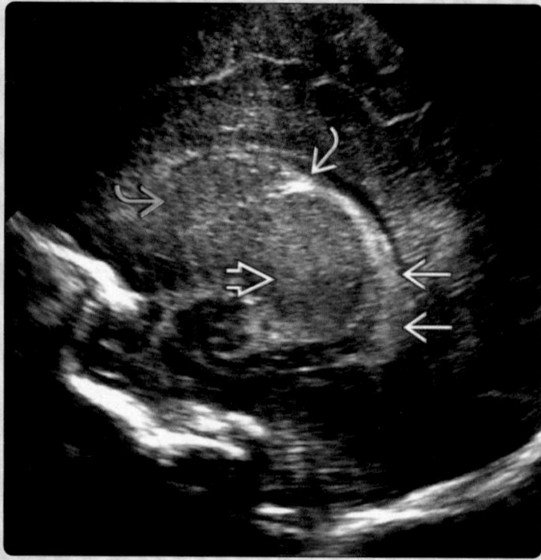

(Left) *Coronal US of a newborn delivered at 31-weeks gestation shows normal findings in the neonatal brain. The frontal horns ➔ are comma-shaped, on either side of the cavum septi pellucidi ⇨, and connected to the 3rd ventricle by the foramina of Monro ↪. The corpus callosum ⇩ is well seen.* **(Right)** *Corresponding sagittal view shows a normal caudothalamic groove ↪ (caudate ↪, thalamus ⇨). Normal, echogenic choroid ➔ never extends anterior to the caudothalamic groove or into the occipital horn.*

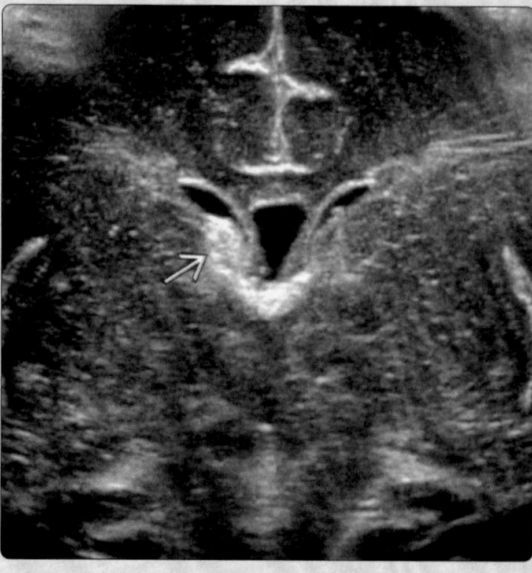

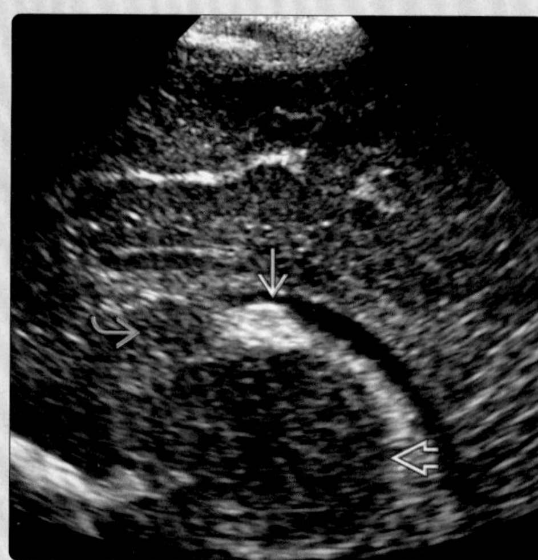

(Left) *Magnified view from a coronal head US in a 1-day-old infant born at 29-weeks gestation shows an asymmetric, globular, echogenic focus in the right caudothalamic groove ➔. This is a grade 1 germinal matrix hemorrhage (GMH).* **(Right)** *Magnified view of a sagittal US shows a rounded area of increased echogenicity in the caudothalamic groove ➔ (caudate ↪, thalamus ⇨), consistent with a grade 1 GMH. Note that there is no blood within the ventricles, which are not dilated.*

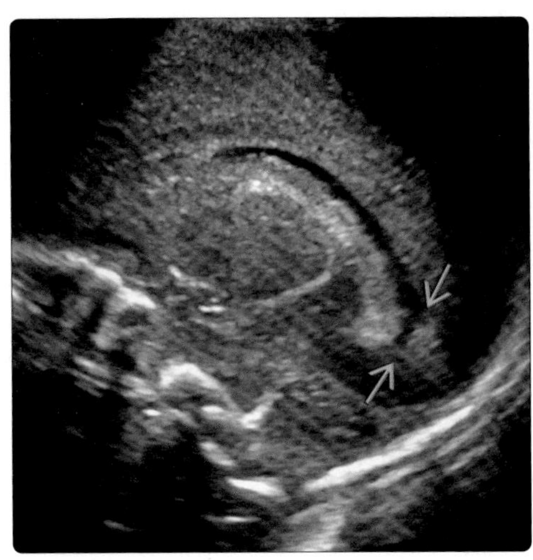

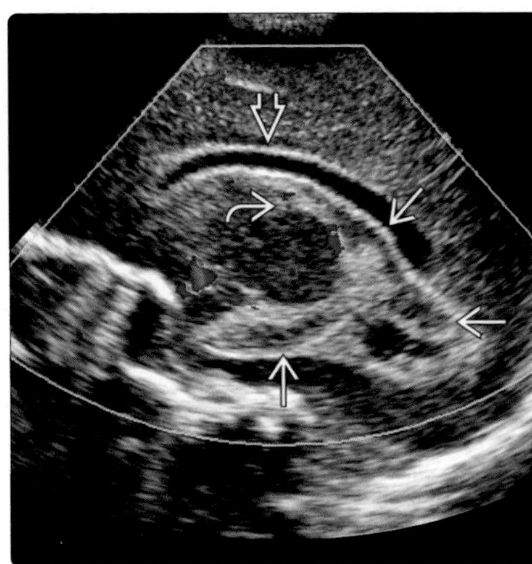

(Left) *Sagittal US in a 25-week twin at 4 days of life shows layering hemorrhage ➡ in the occipital horn of a nondilated lateral ventricle, consistent with grade 2 IVH. The posterior fontanel provides an excellent acoustic window to the occipital horn.* **(Right)** *Sagittal color Doppler US shows mixed echogenicity clot ➡ extending from the caudothalamic groove ➡ into the ventricle ➡, which is not dilated. Note the absence of color flow in the clot, which is useful in separating hemorrhage from choroid plexus.*

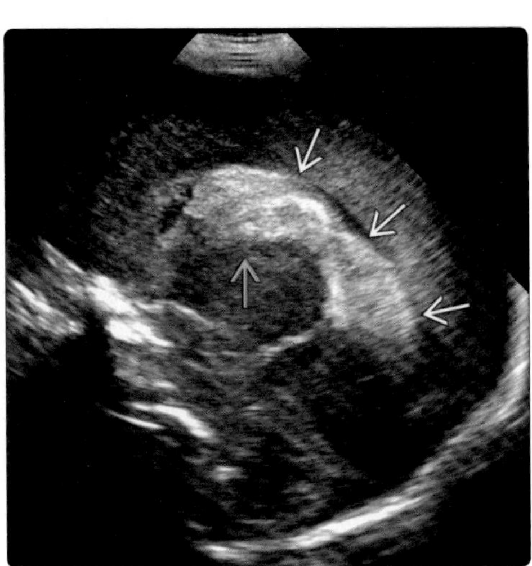

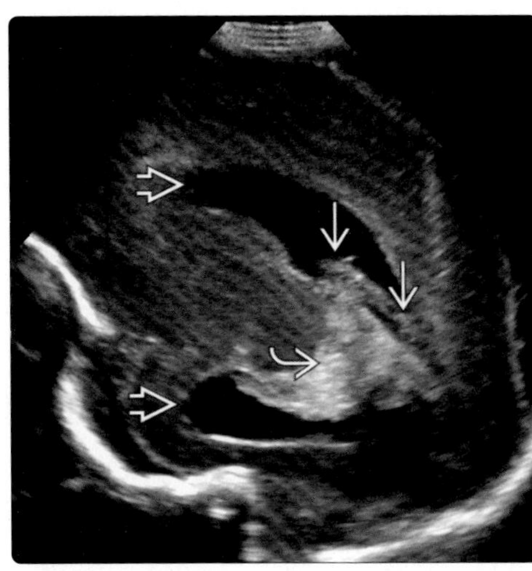

(Left) *Sagittal US in a 25-week gestation infant shows intraventricular hemorrhage (IVH) ➡ with clot filling and expanding almost the entire lateral ventricle. Note clot extends anterior to the caudothalamic groove ➡. This is a grade 3 GMH.* **(Right)** *Sagittal US in a 1-day-old, extremely premature infant shows mixed echogenicity clot ➡ adherent to the echogenic choroid ➡ as well as ventricular expansion ➡, indicating grade 3 GMH.*

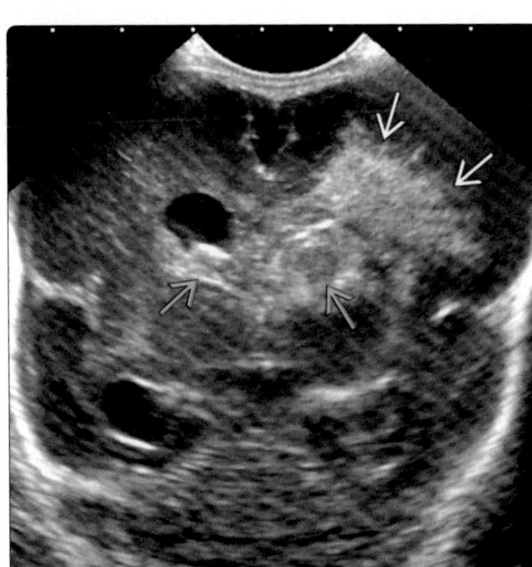

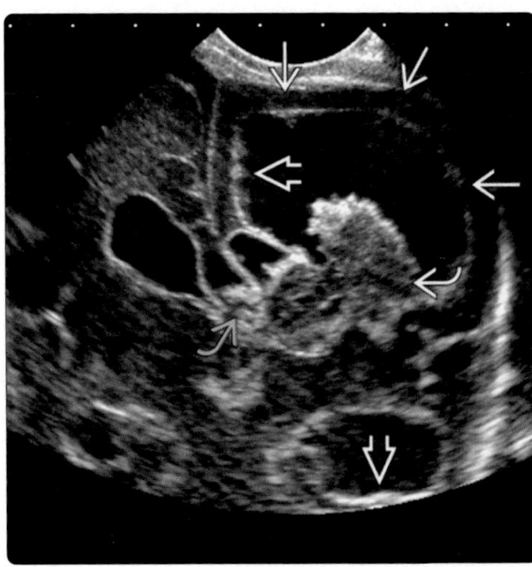

(Left) *Coronal US in a 28-week gestational age (GA) premature infant at 2 days of life shows bilateral GMH ➡ (left > right) and fan-shaped echogenic periventricular hemorrhagic infarction ➡ in the left deep white matter, consistent with grade 4 IVH.* **(Right)** *Coronal US in the same 28-week GA premature infant at 40 days of life shows that porencephaly ➡ has developed at the site of hemorrhagic infarction. Note the retracting clot ➡ and thick nodular ependyma ➡ as well as a clot in the 3rd ventricle ➡.*

PART VII
SECTION 2
Spine

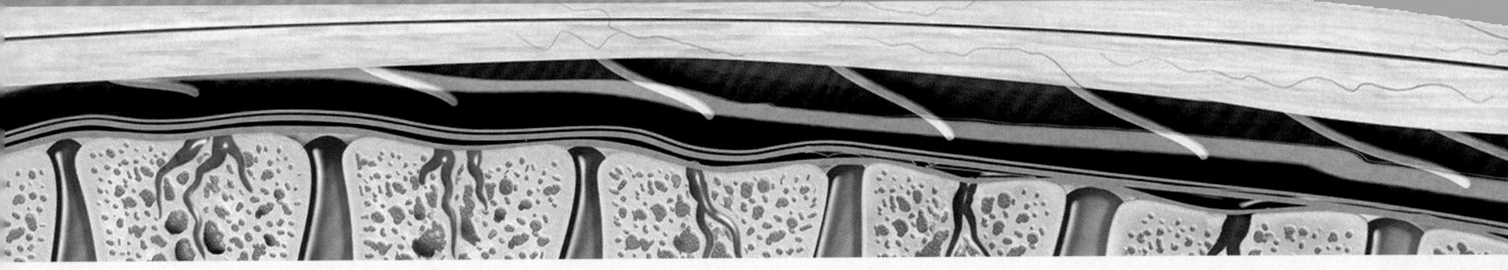

Anatomy and Approach

IMAGING ANATOMY

Vertebral Bodies

- Ossified vertebral body appears echogenic
  - Cartilaginous tip at spinous process appears hypoechoic
- **Cervical**: Upper 7 vertebrae
  - C1 (atlas): No body, spinous process; circular shape
  - C2 (axis): Body with bony peg (dens/odontoid process)
  - C3-C6 similar in size, shape; C7 marked by longest spinous process
- **Thoracic**: 12 vertebrae, which articulate with ribs
- **Lumbar**: 5 vertebrae
- **Sacrum**: Fusion of 5 segments
- **Coccyx**: Fusion of 3-5 segments
  - Cartilaginous coccyx is hypoechoic
  - Ossified coccygeal vertebral bodies have rounded central nucleus rather than square contour, as in sacrum

Spinal Cord

- **Hypoechoic with central echogenic complex**
  - Suspended within thecal sac, anchored to dura by denticulate ligaments, and surrounded by cerebral spinal fluid (CSF)
  - Central spinal canal: CSF-containing space throughout length of cord; contiguous with ventricular system
    - Typically do not see fluid in canal unless dilated (syrinx)
  - In contrast to brain, gray matter (which is roughly H-shaped) is on inside with white matter on periphery of cord
- **2 widened segments**: Cervical enlargement (C3-T2) and lumbar enlargement (T9-T12)
  - Cord tapers to diamond-shaped point (**conus medullaris**), normally ends between T12 to L2-L3 disc space, most common at T12-L1
- **Filum terminale**: Connective tissue extension of pia mater extending inferiorly from conus
  - Fuses distally into dura, attaches to dorsal coccyx
  - Should be < 2 mm in diameter
    - Hypoechoic center with more echogenic outer margin
    - Dorsal extension within thecal sac toward coccyx
- **Cauda equina**: "Horse's tail" of lumbar, sacral, coccygeal nerve roots below conus
  - Multiple, linear, diverging nerve roots drape dependently within thecal sac, undulate with each CSF pulsation
- **Thecal sac** usually ends at S2

ANATOMY IMAGING ISSUES

Imaging Recommendations

- Nonossified posterior elements provide ample acoustic window in newborns
- Spinal cord is best visualized by US within 1st month after birth for term infants
  - Transverse scan of cord possible in older infant as cartilaginous gap in vertebral ring allows penetration of US beam
- **Indications** include
  - Clinical suspicion of caudal regression syndrome or cord abnormality (e.g., tethered cord, diastematomyelia, syrinx)
  - Skin findings associated with spinal dysraphism and tethered cord, including midline discoloration or dimple, skin tags, hair tufts, hemangiomas
  - Looking for hematoma or other abnormality after unsuccessful lumbar puncture
- **Document level of conus medullaris termination in all cases**
- Real-time evaluation and cine loop documentation of **nerve root oscillation with CSF pulsations**

Imaging Approaches

- Infants are preferably scanned in prone position using high-frequency (9- to 12-MHz) linear transducer
  - Decubitus position is adopted to calm struggling baby by bottle or breast feeding
- Scan both longitudinally and transversely
  - Longitudinal images are ideally obtained in midline sagittal plane
  - In older infants with greater spine ossification, it may be necessary to obtain images in slightly off-midline parasagittal plane parallel to spinous processes
- Focus is generally on distal end of cord but prudent to scan from craniocervical junction to coccyx
- Ways to **determine vertebral level** where conus terminates
  - Count upward after defining lumbosacral junction
    - Lumbar vertebral bodies typically lie in horizontal plane in prone infant, while sacral vertebral bodies lie at angle
    - For more clear delineation of L5-S1, accentuate lumbar lordosis by elevation of shoulders
    - **Extended field of view** often facilitates identifying vertebral level and gives "big picture" of cord
  - Count downward from 12th rib
- Craniocervical junction can be assessed by scanning base of skull through foramen magnum

CLINICAL IMPLICATIONS

Clinical Importance

- **Tethered cord**
  - Conus terminates at or above inferior L2 vertebra in ≥ 98% of normal population
    - Conus at normal position by term to 2 months of age
  - **Conus terminating below L2-L3 disc is abnormal**
    - Significance questionable in absence of signs/symptoms particularly in preterm infants
      - □ Consider follow-up scan after infant attains corrected age of 40-weeks gestation
    - Important to evaluate appearance of nerve roots and filum terminale as well as conus level
  - Conus located over mid L3 or lower, or with lack of normal nerve-root pulsations, requires further evaluation with MR
  - Filum terminale thickened (> 2 mm at L5-S1 on axial/transverse images)
  - Cord may appear taut or directly apposed to dorsal thecal sac
    - Lack of conus/nerve root motion with CSF pulsations
    - Lack of dependent ventral shift of conus/nerve roots when prone
  - Look for associated **lipoma** (echogenic mass)

SPINAL CORD

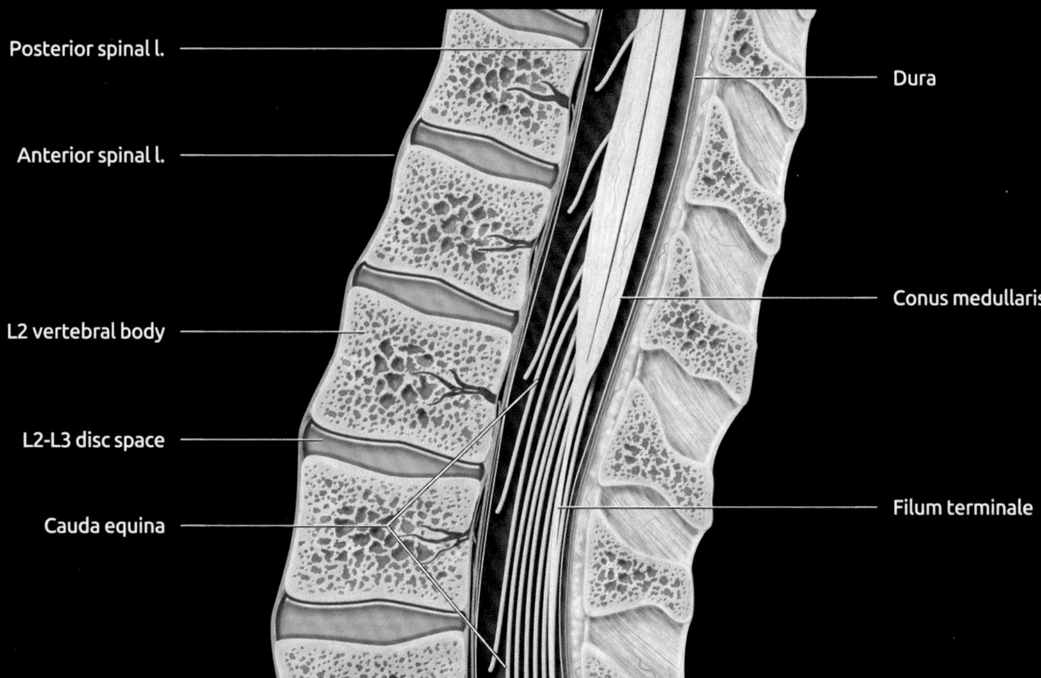

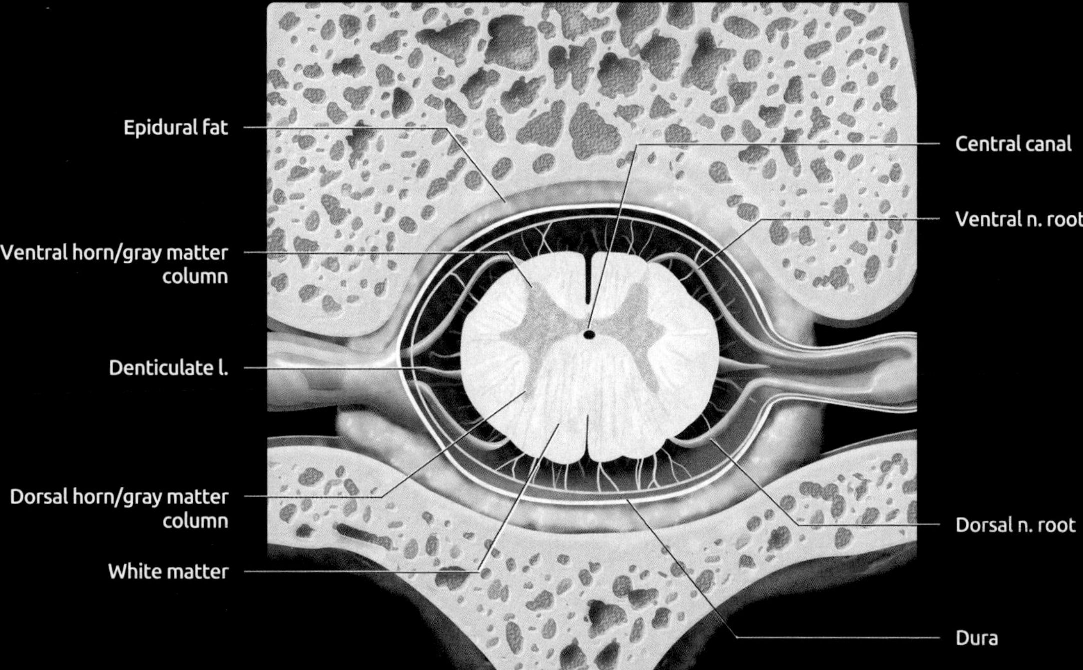

(Top) *Sagittal graphic of the thoracolumbar junction demonstrates a normal conus and cauda equina anatomy. The filum terminale lies amongst the cauda equina roots and affixes the conus dorsally to the terminal thecal sac. A normal conus should end above the inferior margin of L2. Extension below the L2-L3 disc space is concerning for possible tethered cord.* **(Bottom)** *Axial graphic shows the internal anatomy of the distal thoracic spinal cord. In contrast to the brain, the gray mater is on the inside, while the white matter is along the periphery. The gray matter forms columns that are roughly H-shaped in cross section. Nerve roots exit the cord on both the dorsal and ventral surfaces. The cord is surrounded by cerebral spinal fluid (CSF) and is attached to the dura by denticulate ligaments. Fluid is only seen in the central canal on US when it is abnormal (syrinx).*

CERVICAL SPINE

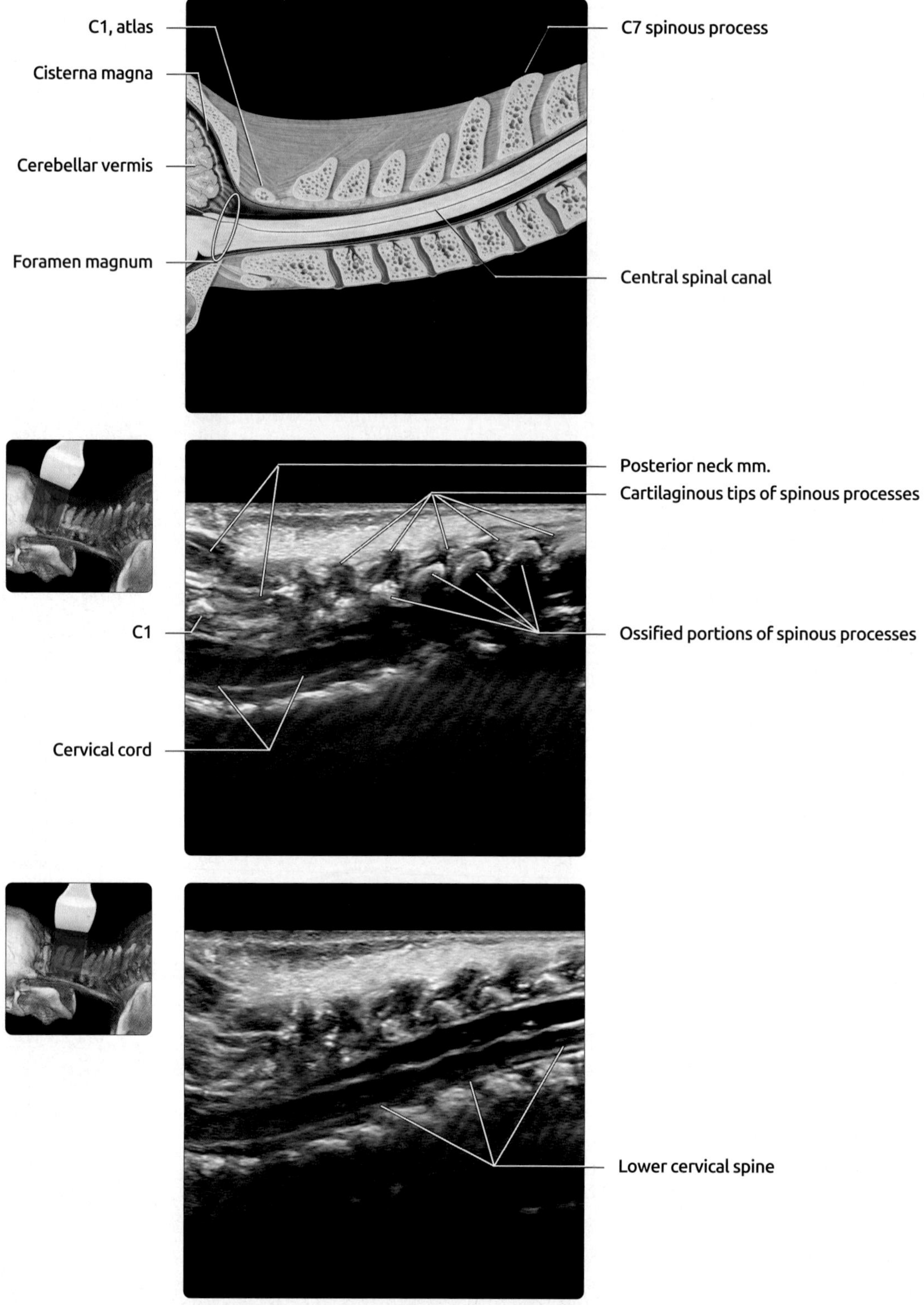

(Top) *Graphic shows the cervical portion of the spinal cord. The cervical spine has a gentle lordosis curving up toward the thoracic spine. The 1st cervical vertebral body (the atlas) has no spinous process. C7 has the longest spinous process and is usually identifiable on US.* **(Middle)** *The spinous processes of the cervical spine are longer and overlap more than in the lower spine making visualization of the cord more difficult, particularly in the transverse plane. Note the cartilaginous portion of the spinous processes appears hypoechoic, while the ossified portion of the vertebral body is echogenic and shadowing. The upper cervical cord is seen by scanning laterally through the neck and angling toward the spinal canal.* **(Bottom)** *Slightly lower and angled medially, the lower portion of the cervical cord can be seen.*

THORACIC SPINE

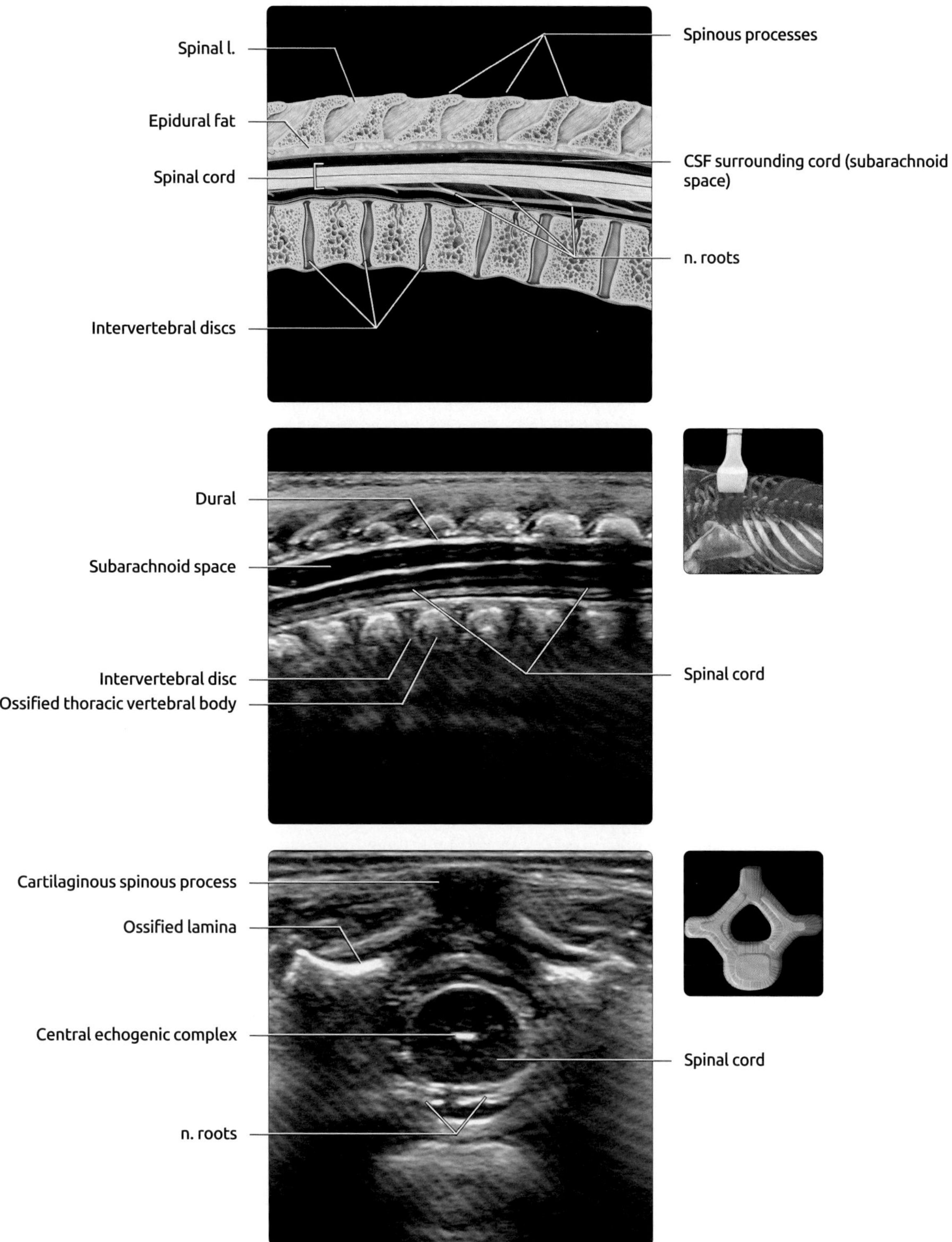

(Top) *The cord narrows in the thoracic portion. The thoracic spine has a gentle kyphosis.* **(Middle)** *Longitudinal US at the midthoracic level of the spinal cord shows the narrowest portion of the cord. The cord should lie dependently within the thecal sac with surrounding CSF in the subarachnoid space.* **(Bottom)** *Scout image shows the cartilaginous portion of the vertebral body in blue with the ossified portion in beige. The US in a transverse scan is taken at T12. At this point, the cord has started to widen again. The spinal cord is predominately hypoechoic with a central echogenic complex. Nerve roots are seen around the cord as it is approaching the conus medullaris.*

LONGITUDINAL US, CONUS MEDULLARIS AND CAUDA EQUINA

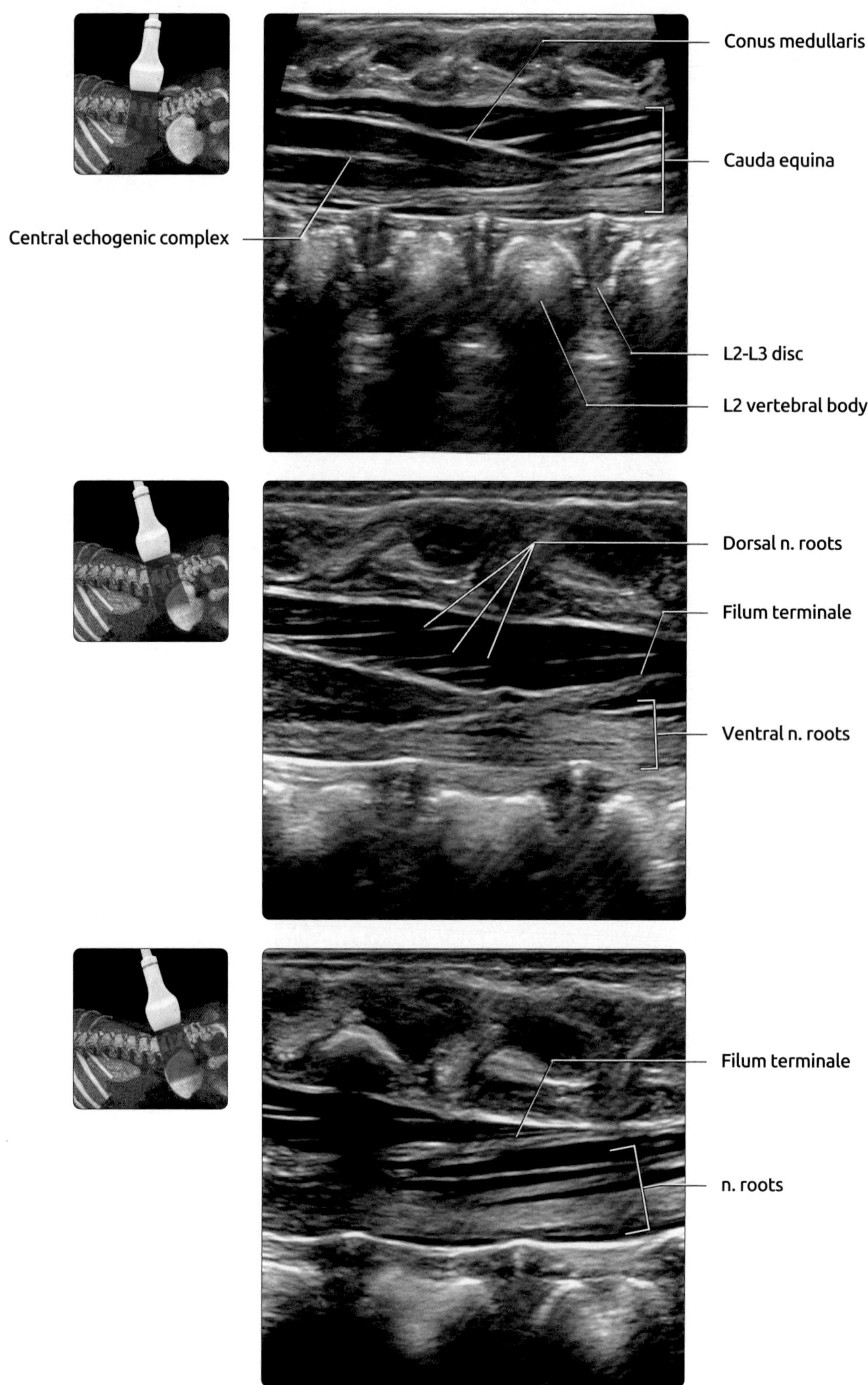

(Top) *The caudal portion of the cord tapers gradually, forming the conus medullaris. It should terminate above the L2-L3 disc space, as in this case. The nerve roots surrounding the conus tail form the cauda equina (horse's tail).* **(Middle)** *The filum terminale is a connective tissue continuation of the pia mater extending inferiorly from the conus. It extends dorsally through the thecal sac to insert on the dura of the dorsal coccyx. The nerve roots and filum should should move freely and undulate with CSF pulsations. The dorsal nerve roots are seen as they move to exit the canal, while the ventral nerve roots lie dependently within the thecal sac.* **(Bottom)** *More distally, the filum terminale is seen moving dorsally to insert on the dura at the level of the coccyx. Look for thickening or masses, such a lipoma, in cases of suspected tethered cord.*

AXIAL US, CONUS MEDULLARIS AND CAUDA EQUINA

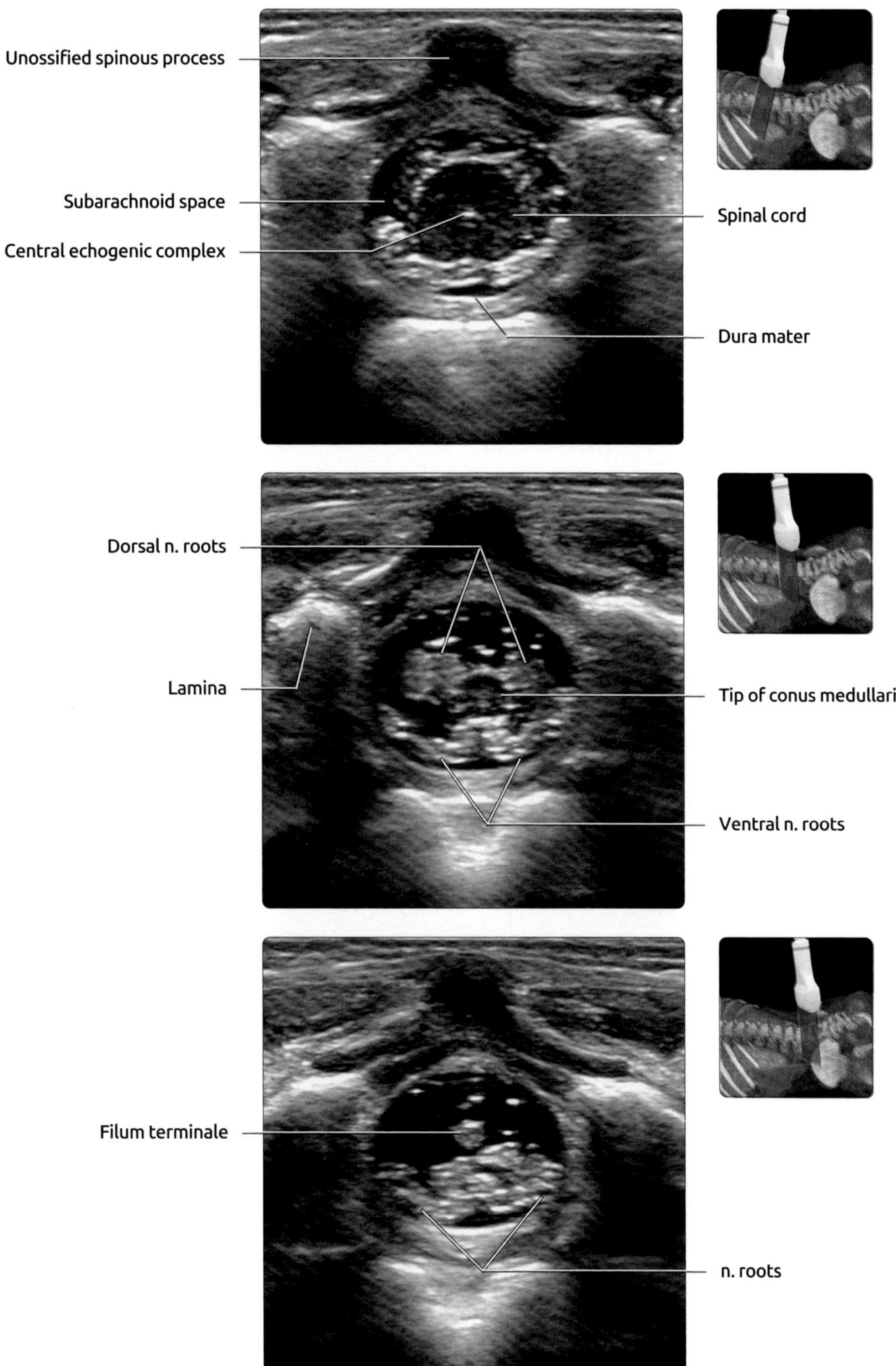

(Top) *Axial US in the upper lumbar spine at the level of the conus medullaris shows the normal hypoechoic cord with central echogenic complex. The spinal cord lies within the subarachnoid space, which is bound by the dura mater and filled with CSF. Echogenic nerve rootlets are seen draped around the cord.* **(Middle)** *Axial US scanning between L2 and L3 shows the tip of the conus. It is surrounded by free-floating nerve roots, collectively known as cauda equina. The conus should not extend below this level.* **(Bottom)** *Axial US at L4 level shows the filum terminale and nerve roots of cauda equina, all of which should float freely within the thecal sac. The filum terminale is the prolongation of the pia mater and attaches dorsally at the level of the coccyx. The filum terminale can be clearly distinguished from the nerve roots of the cauda equina and should be < 2 mm in diameter.*

SACRUM AND COCCYX

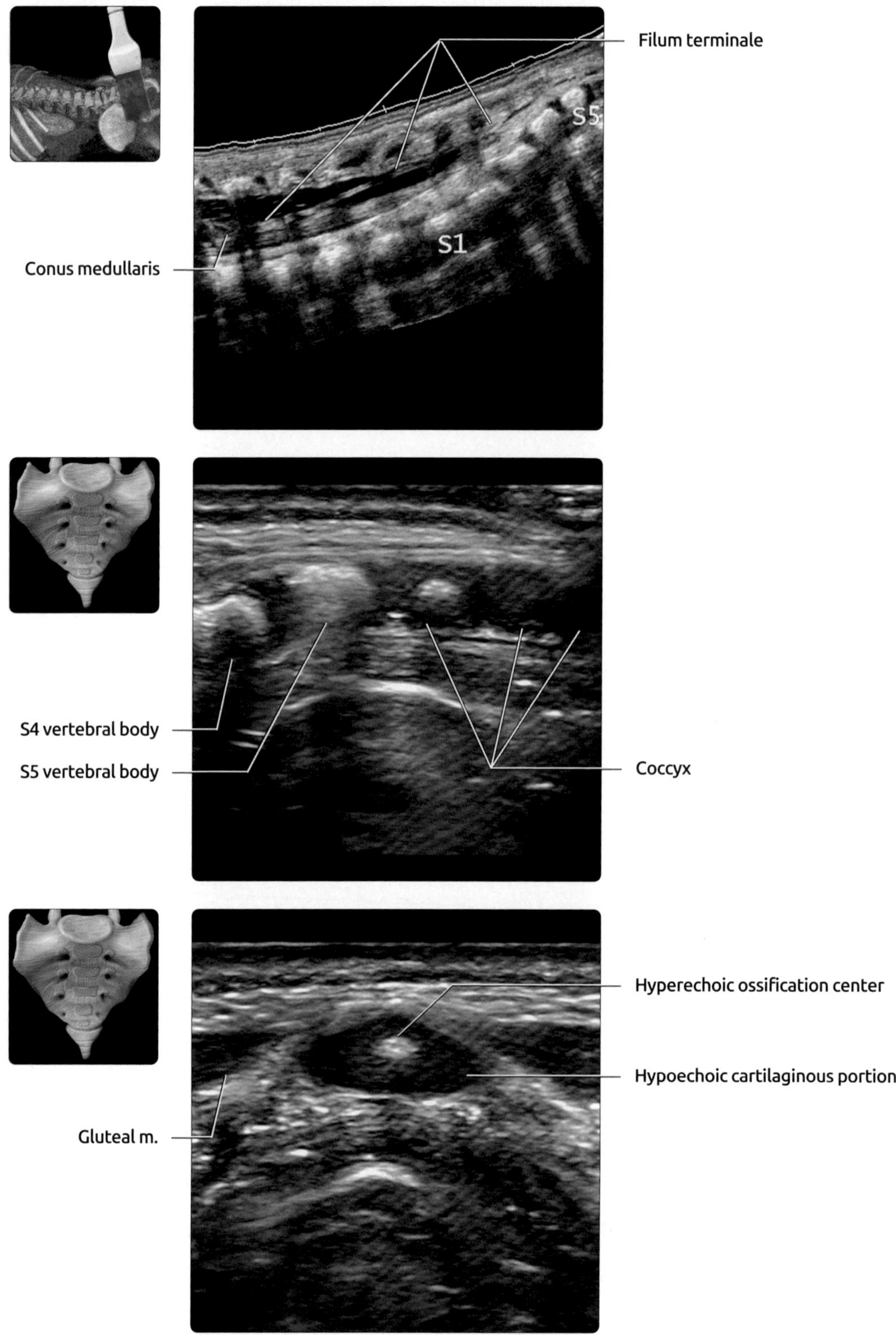

(Top) *Extended field of view shows the filum terminale extending dorsally within the thecal sac to insert on the dura at the level of the coccyx. One of the most difficult and crucial things in spinal sonography is accurately numbering the vertebral bodies. The angle at L5-S1 can be accentuated by raising up the shoulders; confirm your impression by counting down from the last rib. Only after confirming in both directions can you be confident in your determination of the conus level.* **(Middle)** *Scout image shows the cartilaginous portions of the sacrum and coccyx in blue with the ossified portions in beige. The coccygeal segments are the last vertebral bodies to ossify, so they often appear partially or completely hypoechoic by US.* **(Bottom)** *The ossification center of a coccygeal vertebral body is rounded, helping to distinguish it from a sacral vertebral body, which has a square ossification center.*

TETHERED CORD AND EPIDURAL HEMATOMA

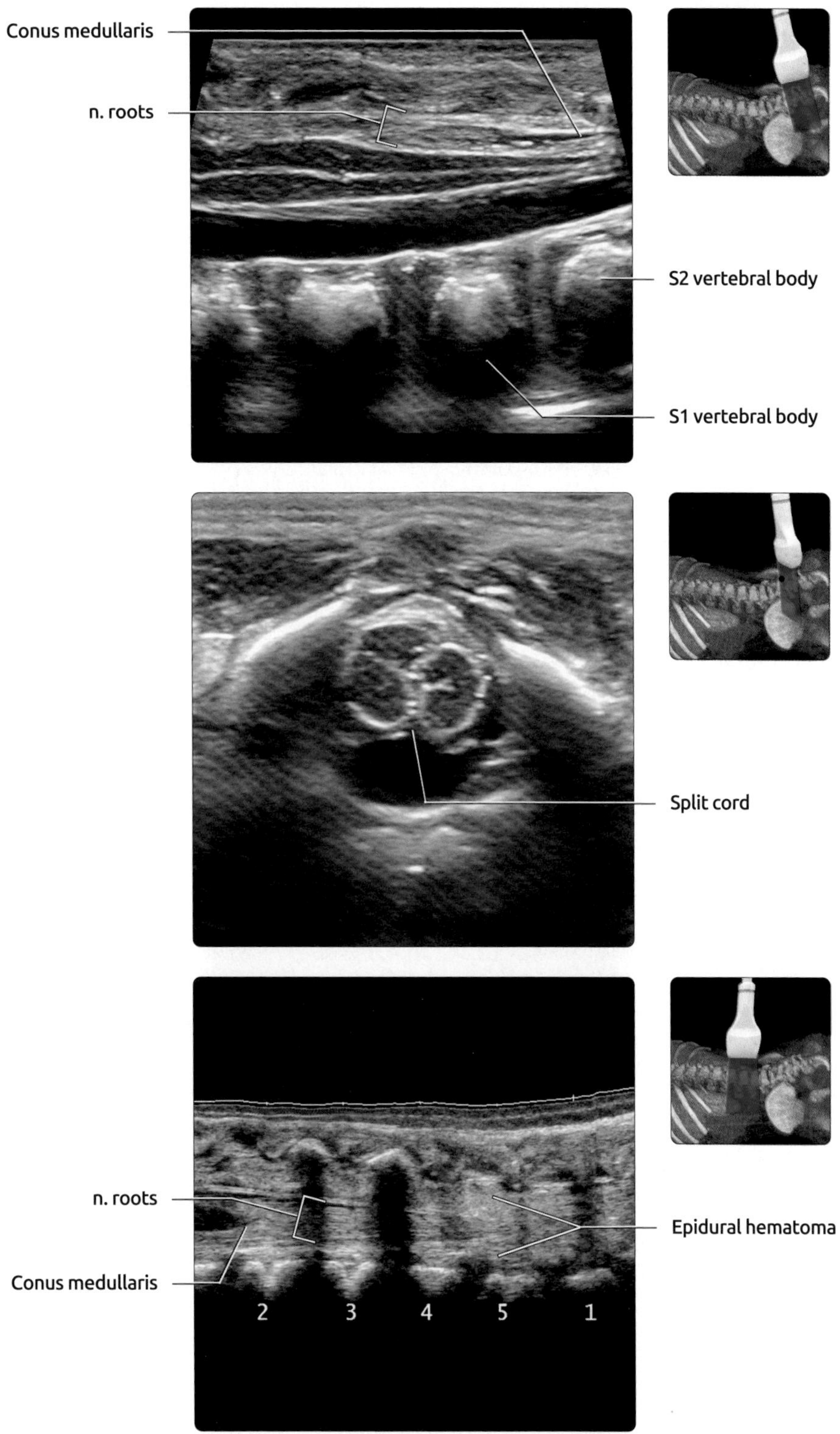

(Top) *In this case of tethered cord, the conus is ending very low at the level of S2. Also note the cord appears stuck to the dorsal surface of the sac and not lying dependently as would normally be seen. No free-floating nerve roots were seen during the real-time examination and are shown here in a conglomerate mass.* **(Middle)** *In the axial plane, not only is the position abnormal, but there is a cleft seen within the cord. A split cord was confirmed by MR.* **(Bottom)** *This scan was performed after a failed attempt at a lumbar puncture and shows the thecal sac is surrounded by a hyperechoic epidural hematoma. The nerve roots are compressed to the middle of the sac.*

INDEX

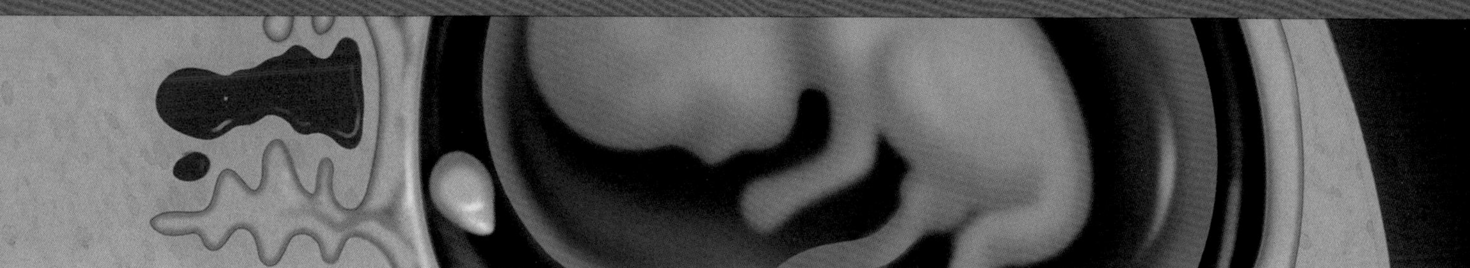

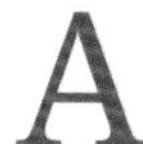

A

INDEX

INDEX

INDEX

B

INDEX

C

INDEX

INDEX

D

INDEX

E

F

G

H

INDEX

INDEX

I

INDEX

J

INDEX

K

L

M

INDEX

N

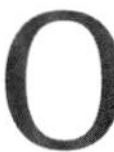

P

INDEX

Q

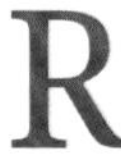

R

INDEX

S

INDEX

T

INDEX

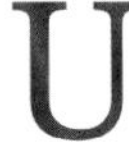

INDEX

V

W

X

Y